HISTOLOGY

FOURTH EDITION

HISTOLOGY

LEON WEISS
Professor of Cell Biology
Department of Animal Biology
University of Pennsylvania

ROY O. GREEP
Laboratory of Human Reproduction
and Reproductive Biology
Harvard University

McGRAW-HILL BOOK COMPANY
A Blakiston Publication

New York   St. Louis   San Francisco   Auckland   Bogotá
Düsseldorf   Johannesburg   London   Madrid   Mexico
Montreal   New Delhi   Panama   Paris
São Paulo   Singapore   Sydney   Tokyo   Toronto

HISTOLOGY

1 2 3 4 5 6 7 8 9 0   HDHD   7 8 3 2 1 0 9 8 7

This book was set in Souvenir Light by York Graphic Services, Inc.
The editors were Alice Macnow, J. Dereck Jeffers,
Peter R. Karsten, and Douglas J. Marshall;
the designer was Nicholas Krenitsky;
the production supervisor was Leroy A. Young.
The drawings were done by J & R Services, Inc.
Halliday Lithograph Corporation was printer and binder.

Library of Congress Cataloging in Publication Data

Main entry under title:

Histology.

    First-2d ed. edited by R. O. Greep; 3d ed. edited by R. O. Greep and L. Weiss.
Includes index.
    1. Histology. I. Weiss, Leon. II. Greep, Roy Orval, date– III. Greep, Roy Orval, date–   ed. Histology. [DNLM: 1. Histology.   QS504 H676]
QM551.G73   1977   599'.08'2   76-42251
ISBN 0-07-069091-X

Contents

List of Contributors

Leonard F. Bélanger, M.D.
Department of Anatomy
Faculty of Medicine
University of Ottawa
Ottawa, Ontario, Canada K1N 9A9

Richard J. Blandau, M.D., Ph.D.
Department of Biological Structure
University of Washington
School of Medicine
Seattle, Washington 98105

Ruth Ellen Bulger, Ph.D.
Department of Anatomy
University of Massachusetts
Medical School
Worcester, Massachusetts 01605

David G. Cogan, M.D.
Clinical Branch
National Eye Institute
National Institutes of Health
Bethesda, Maryland 20014

W. Maxwell Cowan, M.D., Ph.D.
Department of Anatomy and Neurobiology
Washington University
School of Medicine
St. Louis, Missouri 63110

Martin Dym, Ph.D.
Department of Anatomy
Harvard Medical School
Boston, Massachusetts 02114

Åke Flock, M.D., Ph.D.
Department of Physiology II
Karolinska Institutet
Stockholm, Sweden

Robert M. Frank, D.D.S., M.D.
Faculté de Chirurgie Dentaire
Université Louis Pasteur
Strasbourg, France

Geraldine F. Gauthier, Ph.D.
Laboratory of Electron Microscopy
Wellesley College
Wellesley, Massachusetts 02181

Burton D. Goldberg, M.D.
Department of Pathology
New York University
School of Medicine
New York, New York 10016

M. R. C. Greenwood, Ph.D.
Institute of Human Nutrition
College of Physicians and Surgeons
Columbia University
New York, New York 10032

Roy O. Greep, Ph.D.
Laboratory of Human Reproduction and
    Reproductive Biology
Harvard Medical School
Boston, Massachusetts 02115

Nicholas S. Halmi, M.D.
Department of Anatomy
University of Iowa
College of Medicine
Iowa City, Iowa 52242

Elizabeth D. Hay, M.D.
Department of Anatomy
Harvard Medical School
Boston, Massachusetts 02115

Susumu Ito, M.D.
Department of Anatomy
Harvard Medical School
Boston, Massachusetts 02115

Patricia R. Johnson, Ph.D.
Department of Biology
Vassar College
Poughkeepsie, New York 12601

Albert L. Jones, M.D.
Cell Biology Section
Veterans Administration Hospital
San Francisco, California 94121
Departments of Medicine and Anatomy
University of California
San Francisco, California 94122

Edward G. Jones, M.D., Ph.D.
Department of Anatomy and Neurobiology
Washington University
School of Medicine
St. Louis, Missouri 63110

Toichiro Kuwabara, M.D.
National Eye Institute
National Institutes of Health
Bethesda, Maryland 20014

John A. Long, Ph.D.
Department of Anatomy
University of California
School of Medicine
San Francisco, California 94122

A. Gedeon Matoltsy, M.D.
Department of Dermatology
Boston University Medical Center
Boston, Massachusetts 02118

Gwen C. Moriarty, Ph.D.
Department of Anatomy
Northwestern University
Medical School
Chicago, Illinois 60611

Helen A. Padykula, Ph.D.
Laboratory of Electron Microscopy
Wellesley College
Wellesley, Massachusetts 02181

Dorothy R. Pitelka, Ph.D.
Cancer Research Laboratory
University of California, Berkeley
Berkeley, California 94720

Wilbur B. Quay, Ph.D.
Department of Anatomy
University of Texas Medical Branch
Galveston, Texas 77550

Michel Rabinovitch, M.D.
Department of Cell Biology
New York University
School of Medicine
New York, New York 10016

Maia Simionescu, Ph.D.
Section of Cell Biology
Yale University
School of Medicine
New Haven, Connecticut 06510

Nicolae Simionescu, M.D.
Section of Cell Biology
Yale University
School of Medicine
New Haven, Connecticut 06510

Reidar F. Sognnaes, D.M.D., Ph.D.
School of Dentistry
The Center for the Health Sciences
University of California
Los Angeles, California 90024

Sergei P. Sorokin, M.D.
Department of Physiology
Harvard University
School of Public Health
Boston, Massachusetts 02115

Elinor Spring-Mills
Cell Biology Section
Veterans Administration Hospital
San Francisco, California 94121
Department of Anatomy
University of California
San Francisco, California 94122

John S. Strauss, M.D.
Department of Dermatology
Boston University Medical Center
Boston, Massachusetts 02118

Lois W. Tice, M.D.
Laboratory of Experimental Pathology
NIAMDD
National Institutes of Health
Bethesda, Maryland 20014

Leon Weiss, M.D.
Department of Animal Biology
School of Veterinary Medicine
University of Pennsylvania
Philadelphia, Pennsylvania 19174

Preface

Our major objective in this, the fourth edition of *Histology,* remains the same as in the third, viz., to present in depth, but not in undue detail, an up-to-date picture of the microscopic and submicroscopic structure of the mammalian body useful to students in the medical sciences, to graduate students, and to advanced undergraduates. This has been a thorough revision. A few chapters have been changed relatively little. Most have undergone considerable revision, and some have been entirely rewritten. The revision has affected the figures even more than the text. Many new transmission and scanning electron micrographs and freeze-fracture-etch preparations replace figures of the third edition or have been added. It is a delight to become scientifically current by so beautiful a means!

Drs. Bélanger, Blandau, Bulger, Flock, Frank, Gauthier, Halmi, Hay, Ito, A. Jones, Kuwabara, Long, Matoltsy, Padykula, Sognnaes, Sorokin, Spring-Mills, and Strauss remain with us from the third edition. We welcome, as new colleagues, Drs. Cowan, Dym, Goldberg, Greenwood, Johnson, E. Jones, Moriarty, Pitelka, Quay, Rabinovitch, Maia and Nicolae Simionescu, and Tice. We are most grateful to all these scholars for their contributions and their unfailing willingness to accept editorial suggestions. We hope we have retained the authority of a multiauthored text while achieving much more uniformity in depth and style of treatment.

We are indebted to Dr. James Lake for his revision of the section on ribosomes and to Dr. Helen Padykula, a contributor since the inception of *Histology,* for reviews of a number of the chapters in this edition. We have been fortunate in having the editorial and secretarial services of Ms. Nancie Brownley in setting up and concluding this revision and Ms. Gail Levy for the middle portion. This revision has been the opportunity to continue close relationships with Ms. Alice Macnow, Mr. J. Dereck Jeffers, and Mr. Peter R. Karsten, sponsoring editors; and Mr. Joseph J. Brehm, editor-in-chief, Blakiston Publications; and to begin work with Mr. Douglas Marshall, who has patiently and effectively supervised the making of a book from our manuscripts.

Few professional activities have been as satisfying for us as developing and editing this text. It has provided stimulating and enlightening relationships, international in scope, with many achieving and interesting scientists and teachers in histology and cell biology—with very little pain. It is a privilege for us to have had this opportunity to bring them together and edit their work. We hope this finished text makes a contribution to teaching worthy of them.

Leon Weiss

Roy O. Greep

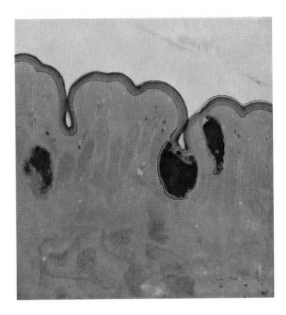

<FIGURE 2-12 Villus of small intestine stained by the periodic acid Schiff procedure, counterstained with fast green. Tissue fixed in OsO$_4$, embedded in methacrylate, and sectioned at 1 μm. The mucus in the goblet cells as well as that covering the striated border of the epithelial cells reacts intensely. ×1,700. (Micrograph courtesy of S. Ito.)

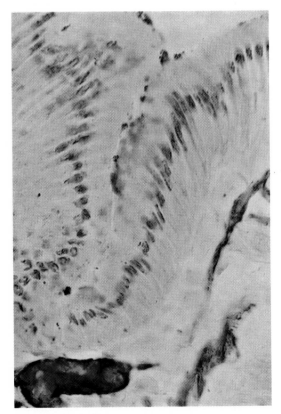

<FIGURE 2-17 Mucosa of stomach stained to demonstrate the activity of thiamine pyrophosphatase (nucleoside diphosphatase) by a modified Gomori metal-salt method. Note the color of the lead sulfide, the final reaction product. This enzyme is localized in the Golgi apparatus of the surface epithelial cells, as well as in capillary walls. ×800. (Courtesy of H. Ragins.)

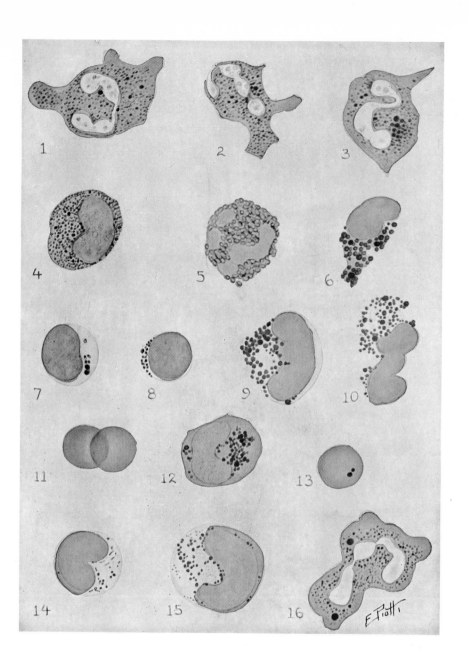

< **FIGURE 10-5** Human blood cells stained supravitally. All cells are from the same individual and are drawn the same scale. Cells 1-13 are stained with neutral red only (granules and phagocytic vacuoles). Cells 14-16 are stained with neutral red and Janus green (mitochondria). Legend on facing page. (Preparation Courtesy of E. Tompkins.)

1. Polymorphonuclear neutrophil stained for 20 min at 37°C. The small dots are the specific, refractive granules, which appear brown-red or gray, depending on focus. Unlike phagocytic vacuoles, these do not change with time. The pseudopodia are usually free of the streaming granules. The larger droplets represent the phagocytic vacuoles. There are few of these in a normal neutrophil within this period of time.

2. A neutrophil from the same field after the film has been at room temperature for 1 hr. Phagocytosis is slight at the lower temperature, and there is little change in the vacuoles.

3. The same cells as in 2 after the film has been at room temperature for 2 h. The number of lobes of the nucleus has changed somewhat as the result of ameboid movements. The cell has become toxically injured after long exposure and is phagocytosing abnormally.

4. Myelocyte film stained at 37°C for 1 h. There are no ameboid movements and little phagocytosis. The specific granules are more refractive and stain more on the acid side than the granules of polymorphonuclear neutrophils. This type of staining is considered an indication of youth when it occurs in the latter cells.

5. Polymorphonuclear eosinophil from the same film as 4. The granules are highly refractive, and the intensity of their color consequently varies with focus. They are large, rice-shaped, and fairly uniform in size. They are straw-colored when freshly stained but gradually take on an apricot tint with exposure. Eosinophils rarely contain phagocytic vacuoles.

6. Polymorphonuclear basophil. The granules are large, round, very uniform, and highly refractive; the intensity of staining therefore varies with focus. The granules stain a deeper crimson than phagocytic vacuoles or than the granules of any other cells of the blood. The nucleus rarely shows lobing, and the cells are practically never phagocytic.

7. Intermediate-sized lymphocyte from . same film as 4 after the film stood at room temperature for 1 h. The cytoplasm is very clear and contains few phagocytic vacuoles. These are much fewer than in monocytes and are arranged indiscriminately. Lymphocytes should rarely be confused with monocytes. Double staining with Janus green also serves to differentiate the two types (see 13 and 14).

8. Small lymphocyte from same film as 7 after the film has stood at room temperature for 2 h.

9. 10. Monocytes from the same film after it has stained for 5 min at 37°C, and 1 h and 2 h, respectively, at room temperature. Monocytes vary constantly in shape and degree of phagocytosis, depending upon ameboid movement. They have the greatest number of phagocytic vacuoles of all blood cells and no granules. The vacuoles vary in size and change position constantly. They increase in both size and number with time of exposure.

11. Two normal erythrocytes. They do not stain. Their color is due entirely to their content of hemoglobin.

12. Monocyte from same film as 9 and 10. The cell is somewhat younger than those, less ameboid, and tends to aggregate the phagocytic vacuoles into rosette formation.

13. Erythrocyte from same film as 12. The cell is younger than those in 11 and contains reticulum, which was stained with neutral red.

14. Lymphocyte stained with neutral red and Janus green (compare with 7). Janus green inhibits phagocytosis somewhat. The mitochondria stain blue-green, are definitely rod-shaped, and tend to cluster toward the nucleus. They are larger than the mitochondria of monocytes.

15. Monocyte stained with neutral red and Janus green. Phagocytosis has been inhibited somewhat. The mitochondria are smaller than those in lymphocytes and more scattered (compare with 14).

16. Polymorphonuclear neutrophil stained with neutral red and Janus green. The mitochondria are the size of those in monocytes but are less abundant. Janus green is soon toxic to cells, and this cell shows the toxic action in the form of unusual phagocytic vacuoles.

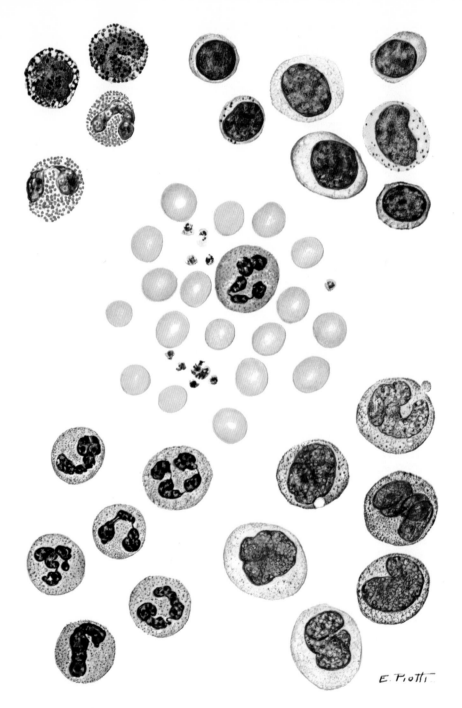

∧**FIGURE 10-7** Cells from a smear preparation of normal human blood. Wright's stain. In the center, adult red corpuscles, blood platelets, and a polymorphonuclear neutrophil. At left above, two polymorphonuclear basophils and two polymorphonuclear eosinophils. At right above, three large and four small lymphocytes. At left below, polymorphonuclear neutrophils. At right below, six monocytes.

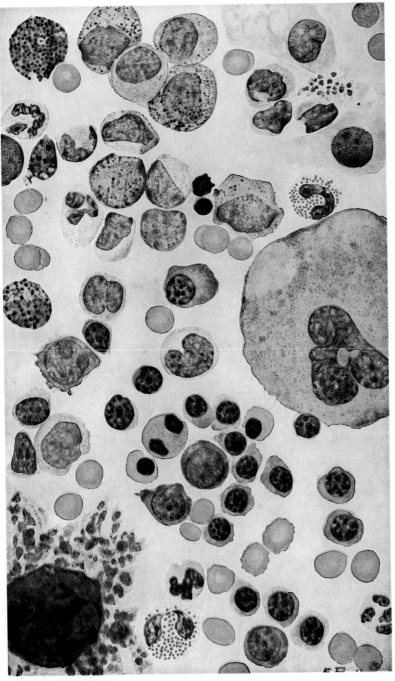

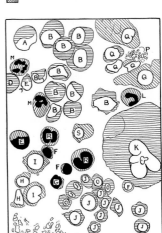

∧**FIGURE 11-7**   A and B. Composite plate of blood cells. A, eosinophilic myelocyte; B, myelocyte; D, blast form; E, basophilic leukocyte; F, small lymphocyte; G, medium-sized lymphocyte; H, large lymphocyte; I, blast form; J, basophilic erythroblast; K, megakaryocyte; L, eosinophilic leukocyte; M, neutrophilic leukocyte; O, polychromatophilic erythroblast; P, platelets; Q, reticulum cell; R, monocyte; S, plasma cell.

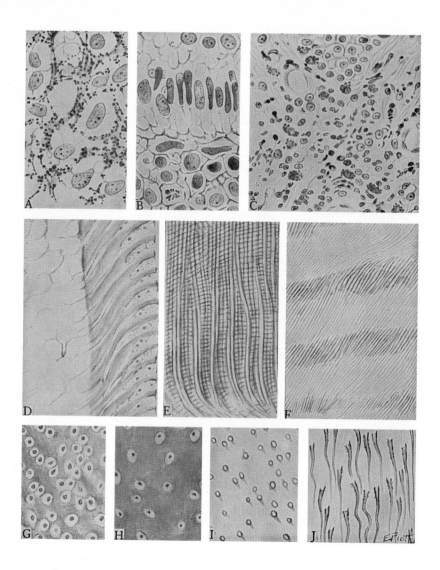

< **FIGURE 17-5** A. Stellate reticulum of enamel organ of human fetus (130-mm C-R length). Fixed in basic lead acetate and stained with 0.5% toluidine blue solution. The ground substance is intensely metachromatic. B. Odontoblasts and subjacent dental pulp of human fetus (130-mm C-R length). The small cells of the pulp are surrounded by metachromatic ground substance (toluidine blue). C. Gingiva of a young child, clinically normal, showing metachromasia of the ground substance and numerous mast cells. ×7 ocular; ×40 objective. D. Enamel from the growing portion of an incisor tooth of a 4-day-old rat, stained by the Prussian blue method for sulfhydryl and disulfide groups. The interprismatic areas stain brownish-red by the carmine counterstain. A well-defined greenish-blue reaction has taken place in the organic substance of the enamel prisms. ×7 ocular; ×90 objective. E. Enamel from the calcifying portion of an incisor tooth of a rat $1\frac{1}{2}$ months of age. Longitudinal ground section. Fixation in a 4% solution of basic lead acetate. Stained for $\frac{1}{2}$ h in 0.5% solution of toluidine blue. Note the metachromatic staining of the prism sheaths and the prism cross striations. ×10 ocular, ×40 objective. F. Enamel from an erupted human premolar tooth. Longitudinal ground section. Fixed in basic lead acetate and stained in toluidine blue. Note the metachromatic reaction of the alternating Hunter-Schreger's bands, which are relatively less calcified. ×10 ocular; ×20 objective. G. Dentin of an adult rhesus monkey's tooth, stained with Masson's connective tissue stain. Undecalcified section cut transversely. The dentinal matrix is stained green and the odontoblastic processes red by this mixture of acid dyes. The green staining of the matrix is due to collagen. H. Dentin of an adult human tooth. Fixed in Rossman's fluid and stained by McManus's periodic acid–Schiff technique. Undecalcified ground section. Observe that the dentinal matrix and odontoblastic processes are stained. I. Dentin of an adult rhesus monkey's tooth. Fixed in basic lead acetate and stained in methylene blue for 24 h at pH 2.9. Undecalcified ground section. The only objects stained at this pH are the areas located around the odontoblastic processes, indicating that these peritubular structures are strongly basophilic. J. Dentin of an adult human tooth. Fixed in basic lead acetate and stained with toluidine blue. Undecalcified ground section cut obliquely. The calcified dentinal matrix is unstained. Observe the metachromatic staining of the peritubular dentin. (Sections marked A, B, G, H, I, J courtesy of G. B. Wislocki, M. Singer, and C. M. Waldo, *Anat Rec.*, **101**:487, 1948; C, D, E, F, courtesy G. B. Wislocki and R. F. Sognnaes. *Am. J. Anat.*, **87**:239, 1950.)

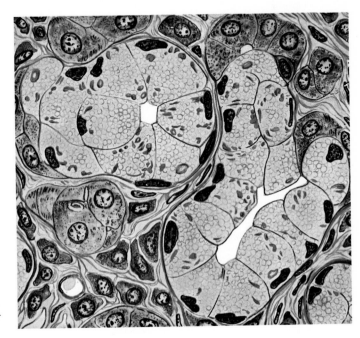

> **FIGURE 18-15** Section of the sublingual gland of a 30-year-old executed man. The mucus-secreting cells are stained blue; the serous cells are gray. Zenker fixation; iron-hematoxylin and Mallory's connective tissue stain. (Clara.)

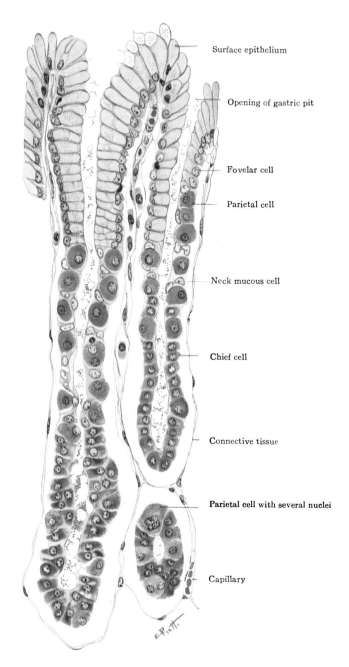

Surface epithelium

Opening of gastric pit

Fovelar cell

Parietal cell

Neck mucous cell

Chief cell

Connective tissue

Parietal cell with several nuclei

Capillary

∧**FIGURE 18-31** Drawing of two gastric glands of the adult human stomach. Four cell types are evident in the epithelium; the surface mucous cell (extending down into the pits), the neck mucous cell, the acidophilic parietal (or oxyntic) cell, and the basophilic chief (or zymogenic) cell. The epithelium has shrunk away from the underlying basement membrane and connective tissue. Zenker fixation; eosin and methylene blue.

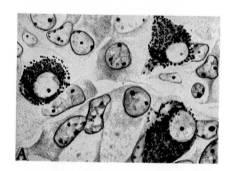

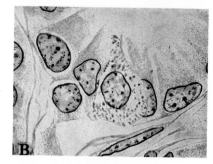

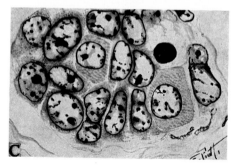

∧**FIGURE 18-38** Reactions of granules in argentaffin cells from the small intestine of a pig. A. Fixed in alcohol-formalin-acetic acid; stained by Bodian silver method. B. Fixed in acetone; stained by Gomori method for acid phosphatase. C. Fixed in Zenker-formalin; stained with eosin and methylene blue. ×1,200. (Courtesy of G. B. Wislocki and E. W. Dempsey.)

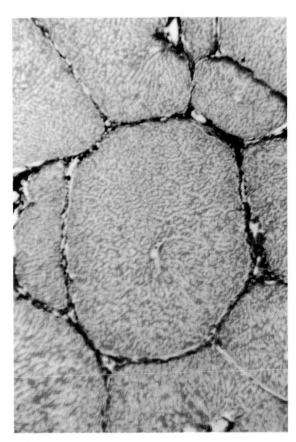

<FIGURE 19-7   Low-power photomicrograph of a section of pig liver, showing a classic lobule. Mallory-Azan.

∨ FIGURE 19-8   Low-power photomicrograph of a section of human liver, illustrating boundaries of a classic lobule. Mallory-Azan.

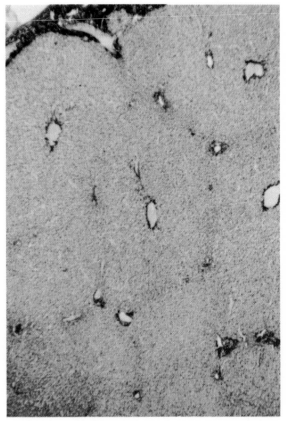

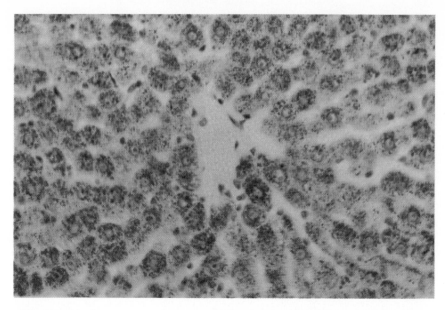

∧**FIGURE 19-12**   Glycogen deposits within the parenchymal cells are stained red by Best's carmine. The quantity of glycogen within the cells varies with the time interval after the last meal and the position of the cell in the lobule. Glycogen is not preserved in routine histologic preparations. Rat liver. Carnoy's fixative. Hematoxylin and Best's carmine.

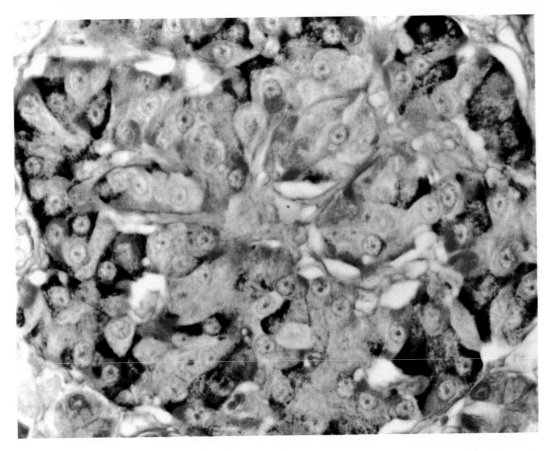

∧ **FIGURE 20-10** A photomicrograph of a human pancreatic islet stained with aldehyde fuchsin and light-green counterstain. The granular nature of the islet cell cytoplasm is evident at this magnification. The alpha cell granules are a deep purple, the beta cell granules are red, and connective tissue fibers are green. ×800. (Courtesy of A. Like.)

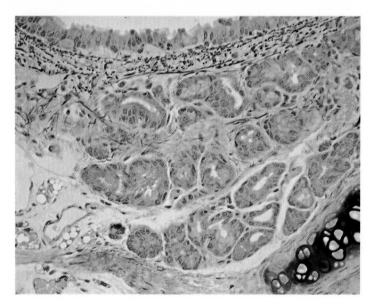

<FIGURE 21-12 Epithelium, fiber systems, and glands on the dorsal aspect of the trachea in a mouse. Resorcin-fuchsin, toluidine blue, and alcian green. ×175.

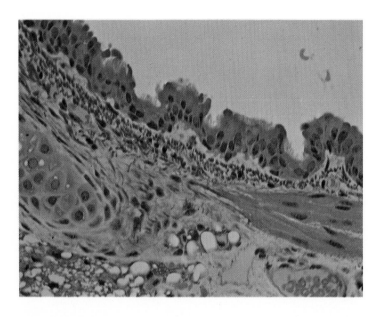

<FIGURE 21-13 Cross section of the upper trachea in a mouse showing connections between airway smooth muscle and the elastic fiber system. Tapering muscle cells are inserted on fibers just deep to the heavy longitudinal band separating lamina propria from submucosa. Resorcin-fuchsin, hematoxylin, and alcian green. ×300.

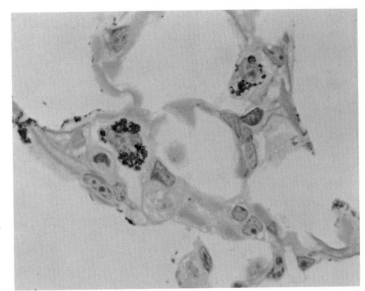

>**FIGURE 21-49** Alveolar macrophages ingesting inhaled iron oxide particles (blue) deposited in alveoli of a mouse's lung. Prussian blue reaction, resorcin-fuchsin, and basic fuchsin. ×1,100. (From S. Sorokin and J. Brain, *Anat. Rec.*, **181**:581, 1975.)

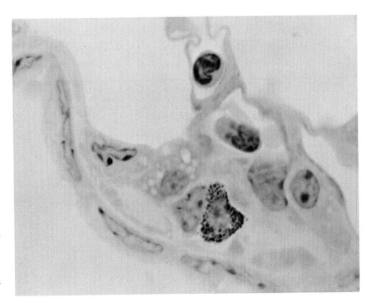

>**FIGURE 21-50** Mast cell beneath pleura in a guinea pig's lung. Leukocytes within blood vessels and a great alveolar cell (foamy cytoplasm) are adjacent, while the pleural mesothelium covers the outside. Toluidine blue. ×1500. (Work of J. Drazen and S. Sorokin.)

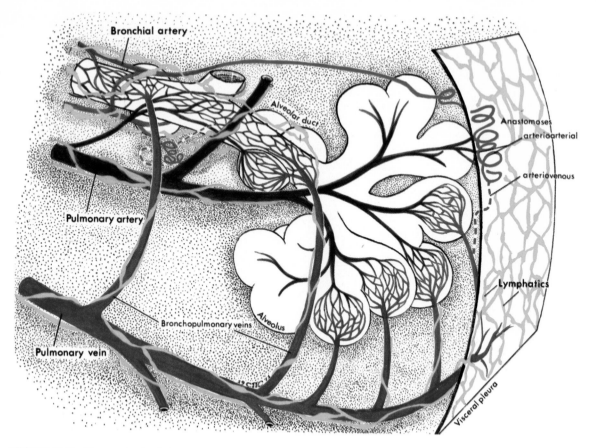

∧**FIGURE 21-58** Diagram showing the interrelationships among the airways, the vascular systems, and the lymphatic networks of the lung. (After diagrams of W. S. Miller and J. Lauweryns.)

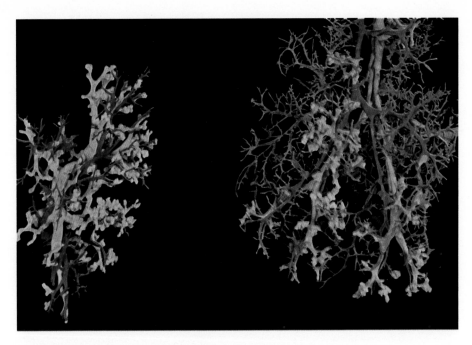

∧ **FIGURE 21-59**   The peripheral airway (greenish) with its accompanying pulmonary artery (red) on the left, and together with the pulmonary vein (blue) on the right, as they appear in casts. (From J. Lauweryns, "De Longvaten," pp. 1–302, Ed. Arscia, Brussels, 1962.)

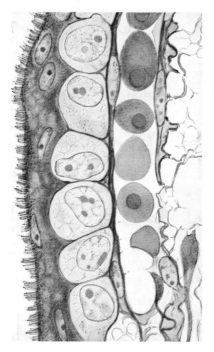

<FIGURE 25-17 Drawing illustrating the structure of the human placental villus at 3 months of gestation. The trophoblast consists of an internal layer of large, clear, chromophobic Langhans' cells and a superficial layer of darkly stained syncytial trophoblast. The free surface of the syncytium, bordering the intervillous space, possesses a brush or microvillous border. The Langhans' cells rest upon a basement membrane. Note the difference in the size of the nuclei of the cellular and syncytial trophoblast. A capillary, containing nucleated fetal erythrocytes and lined by endothelial cells, is closely applied to the trophoblast. The distance between the intervillous space and the lumen of the capillary constitutes the "placental barrier" through which transfer of substances between mother and fetus takes place. Mallory's connective tissue stain. ×1,520. (Courtesy of G. B. Wislocki and H. S. Bennett.)

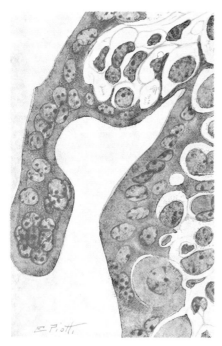

<FIGURE 25-19 Drawing of a section of a human placental villus at 13 weeks. On the left, a tag composed exclusively of syncytium protrudes from the surface of the villus. There is market cytoplasmic basophilia in the syncytium at the level of the nuclei, which indicates a high content of ribonucleoprotein, since this staining is eliminated by prior treatment with ribonuclease. In the cytoplasm of the Langhans' cells, there are only traces of basophilia. Methylene blue. ×1,140. (Courtesy of E. W. Dempsey and G. B. Wislocki.)

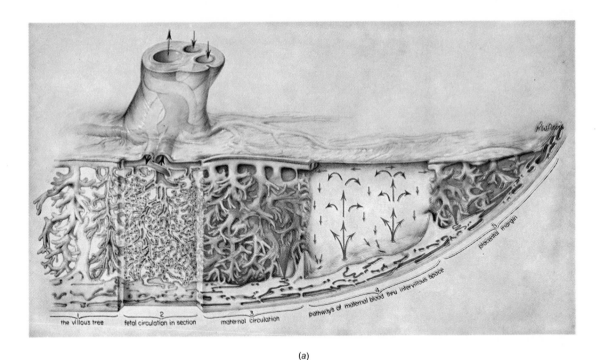

the villous tree   fetal circulation in section   maternal circulation   pathways of maternal blood thru intervillous space   placental margin

(a)

∧ **FIGURE 25-30** Structural organization and blood circulation in the human placenta. (a). Panel 1 illustrates the treelike form of a stem villus (fetal cotyledon), its origin at the chorionic plate, its branches in the intervillous space, and its anchorage to the basal plate. Panel 2 shows the CO_2-rich blood of the umbilical arteries entering the villous tree and being returned to the fetus in oxygenated form via the umbilical vein. In panels 3 and 4 maternal blood is shown entering the intervillous space through open-ended uteroplacental arteries. It enters in spurts and is driven toward the chorionic plate; then, as maternal pressure lessens, lateral dispersion occurs. Maternal blood drains into numerous venous openings along the basal plate. Panel 5 illustrates the peripheral portion of the intervillous space, which consists of a series of interrupted pools or lakes. (Harris and Ramsey, 1966.) [See next page for part (b).]

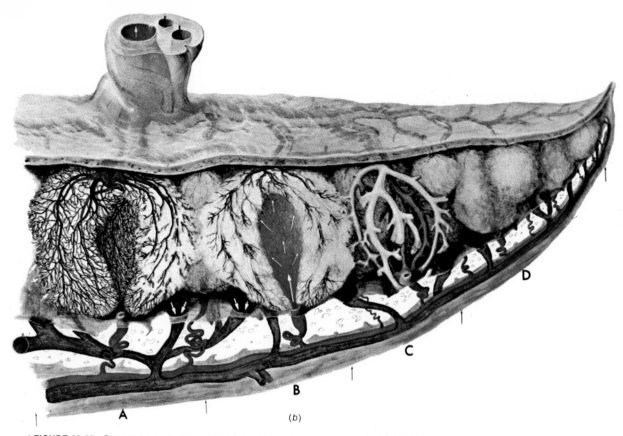

∧ FIGURE 25-30 Structural organization and blood circulation in the human placenta. (*b*). In this interpretation, the fetal cotyledon has a barrel-like configuration and the opening of a maternal uteroplacental (spiral) artery is aligned with the central cavity of the fetal cotyledon. See also Fig. 25-15. (From V. E. Freese, *Am. J. Obstet. Gynecol.*, **101:**8, 1968.) [See preceding page for part (*a*).]

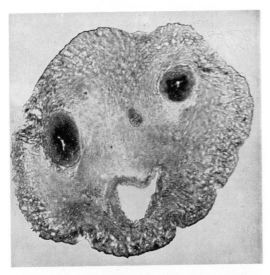

A

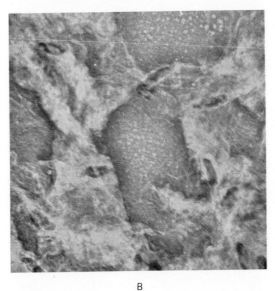

B

∧**FIGURE 25-34** Human umbilical cord at full term stained with
toluidine blue. A. The umbilical vein is the upper, single vessel with
a relatively thin wall and large lumen. The two lower vessels are the
umbilical arteries with their thick walls and constricted lumina. The
intense metochromasia of the ground substance of the mucous
connective tissue is evident. ×6. B. Higher-power view of A. Lakes
of metachromatic mucous ground substance fill the interstitial
spaces in the unstained collagenous framework. Only the nuclei of
the fibroblasts are evident; they are stained an orthochromatic blue.
×500. Frozen dried section fixed with formalin-ether vapor. (Courtesy E. H. Leduc and G. F. Odland.)

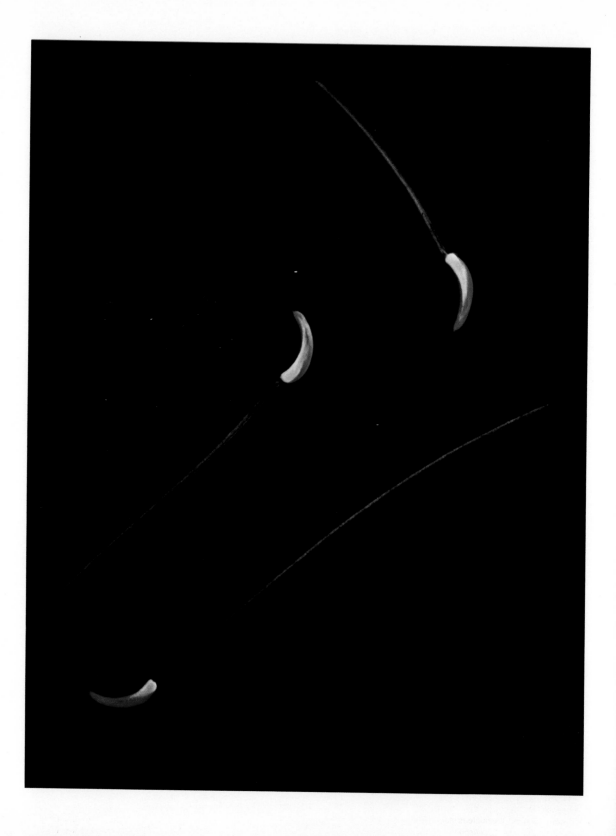

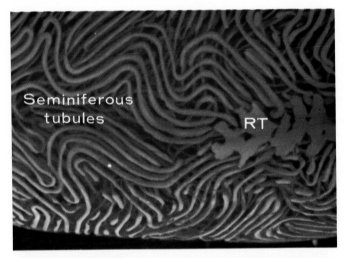

Seminiferous
tubules

RT

< **FIGURE 26-45** "Microfil," a compound used for microvascular injections, was introduced into the lumen of the rete testis of this rat's testis, using a 30-gauge needle. The lumina of the rete testis and the seminiferous tubules were filled with the compound. The rest of the tissue was cleared with methyl salicylate. Note the irregular outline of the superficial rete and the gentle undulating parallel pattern of the seminiferous tubules.

< **FIGURE 26-47** This preparation is similar to Fig. 26-45. The lumina of the ductuli efferentes contain the "microfil."

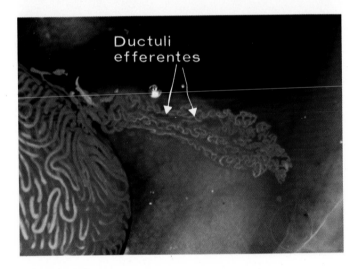

Ductuli
efferentes

<**FIGURE 26-18** These hamster sperm have been stained with a fluorescent aminoacridine dye. The lysosomal enzymes of the acrosome stain red, the nucleus stains yellow, and the tail stains blue. (*Courtesy of A. C. Allison.*)

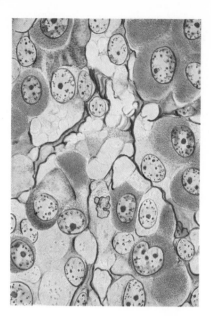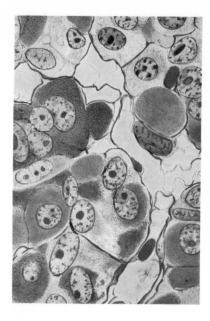

> **FIGURE 27-12** Anterior lobe of the cat hypophysis. A. Anestrous female. Orange acidophils, basophils (blue), and chromophobes (light blue) can be seen. B. Last week of pregnancy. Note presence of numerous red carmine cells. Modified azan stain. (Drawn from preparations of A. B. Dawson.)

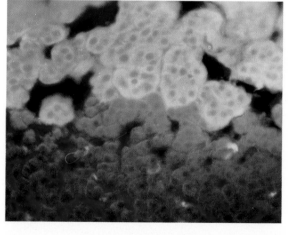

> **FIGURE 31-15** Fluorescence photomicrograph of a section of the adrenal medulla of the rat. Chromaffin cells have a characteristic yellow-green fluorescence, whereas cortical cells (bottom) are dark green. The capillaries are filled with a dye which appears red by this technique. ×100. (Courtesy of Dr. Donald McDonald.)

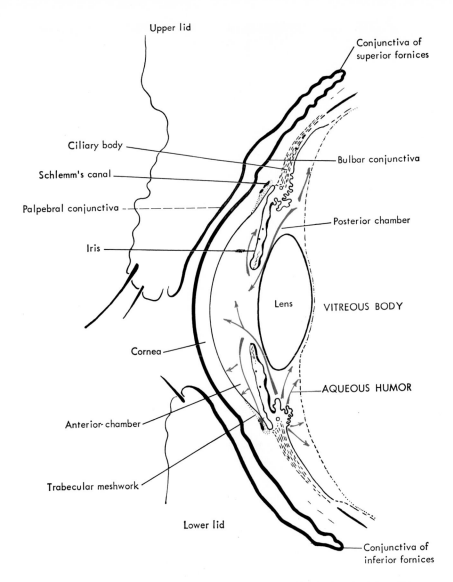

Upper lid

Conjunctiva of
superior fornices

Ciliary body

Bulbar conjunctiva

Schlemm's canal

Palpebral conjunctiva

Posterior chamber

Iris

Lens   VITREOUS BODY

Cornea

AQUEOUS HUMOR

Anterior chamber

Trabecular meshwork

Lower lid

Conjunctiva of
inferior fornices

∧**FIGURE 32-23**   Diagram of the anterior segment of the eye and lids, showing circulation within the eye. Aqueous humor is formed chiefly at the ciliary processes. From the posterior chamber it passes, for the most part, through the pupil into the anterior chamber and thence out of the eye by way of the trabecular meshwork and Schlemm's canal.

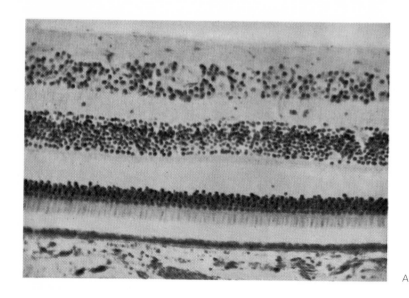

A

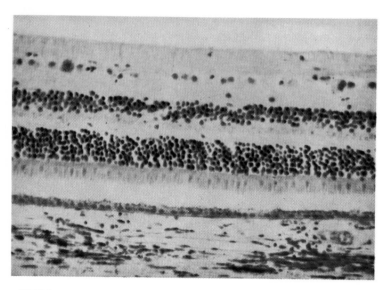

B

∧ **FIGURE 32-42** Cross section of the retina, showing thick ganglion cell layer. A. Near the macula. B. Some distance from the macula. (From Amer. J. Ophthal., **54**:347, 1962.)

The Cell

LEON WEISS

The cell is a physical entity that constitutes the unit of living structure. The tissues that form the body consist entirely of cells and of extracellular material elaborated by cells. The cell, moreover, can carry out an independent existence whereas none of its constituents can do so. Indeed, an entire phylum, the Protozoa, is unicellular, and isolated metazoan cells may be maintained in tissue culture. Furthermore, growth, reproduction, continued responsiveness to stimuli, and other attributes of life are characteristics of cells and not of their parts.

Most mammalian cells are microscopic, although in some instances they reach macroscopic visibility. The limits of cell size are exemplified by bacteria or bacterialike organisms, which may be less than 1 μm in largest dimension, and by avian egg cells, measured in centimeters (Fig. 1-1).

A cell is an intricate, complex, aqueous gel that consists chemically of protein, carbohydrate, fat, and nucleic acids as well as inorganic materials.

Protein is the major structural element of the cell. By itself or in combination with fat, as lipoprotein, or with carbohydrate, as glycoprotein or mucoprotein, it constitutes the substantive structural element both of the cell and of extracellular substances. Enzymes, large molecules which catalyze all essential metabolic reactions, are proteins. Products and secretions of cells may be proteins.

Carbohydrate is the major source of energy in mammalian cells. Among the principal carbohydrates are *glucose,* a monomeric utilizable form, and *glycogen,* a polymeric storage form. Carbohydrates built into complexes with protein may play a role linking cells or compounds together, are major components of extracellular tissues, have significant structural properties within cells, and may constitute enzymes. They may serve as distinctive receptors on the cell surface necessary for such phenomena as cell-homing.

Fat, too, may be a source of energy to the cell and may exist in a storage form. Fatty acids constitute the principal storage form of fat and are an efficient depot of energy. Lipids have major structural properties. Phospholipids and sphingolipids are major compounds in the structure of biological membranes, making them preferentially permeable to fats, and control the orientation and mobility of proteins intrinsic to the membranes.

Inorganic materials may be present in cells in a variety of combinations. They may be associated with enzymes and with other proteins or fats, or they may be free of combination with organic chemicals. They influence the adhesiveness and other physical properties of cells and extracellular materials. Thus calcium contributes to the rigidity of bone, to the adhesiveness of the constituents of the subcellular particles, the ribosomes, and to the capacity of cells to aggregate.

FIGURE 1-1 Equivalent measurements

10 angstroms (Å)	=	1 millimicrometer (mμm) or 1 nanometer (nm)
10,000 angstroms	=	1 micrometer (μm)
1,000 microns	=	1 millimeter (mm)
10 millimeters	=	1 centimeter (cm)
100 centimeters	=	1 meter (m)

It is one of the achievements of microscopic anatomy that selective chemical reactions revealing the presence and location of different chemical moieties may be carried out in tissue prepared for examination under the microscope. Chapter 2 is devoted to *histochemistry*, the term given to this division of histology.

There are two major classes of cells: *prokaryotes* and *eukaryotes*. Prokaryotes, exemplified by bacteria, contain aggregated nuclear material which lies free in the cell protoplasm. In eukaryotes, represented by fungi and higher forms, a true nucleus is present, bounded by a membrane and thereby separated from the cytoplasm. The nucleus is typically a prominent central spherical or ovoid structure. It contains the chromosomes, which harbor the genetic material, and typically one or more *nucleoli* which are concerned with the synthesis of protein. The cytoplasm surrounds the nucleus and typically contains many distinctive, highly ordered organelles, which are the structural

FIGURE 1-2 Hela cells, living in tissue culture; phase-contrast photomicrograph. Hela cells were derived by Dr. George Gey from a carcinoma of the uterine cervix explanted in tissue culture and are maintained as a cell strain in tissue culture and used in a variety of experimental procedures. The cell border is ruffled and in places retracted, resulting in spinelike processes. The nucleus is spherical, surrounded by refractile clear bodies. Mitochondria are evident as irregular linear structures. ×1200. (From the work of Dr. G. Gey.)

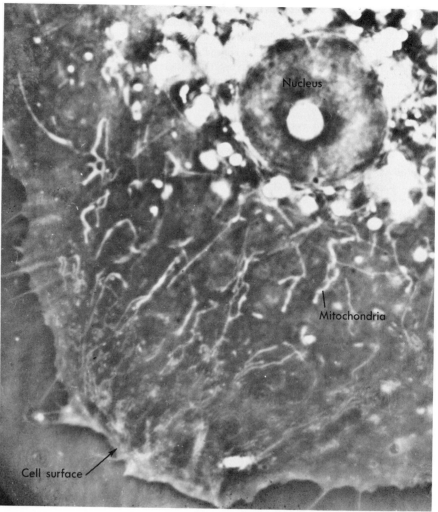

parts of the cytoplasm. These include *mitochondria, lysosomes, Golgi apparatus, endoplasmic reticulum, centrioles, microtubules, microfilaments, ribosomes, secretory granules,* and other structures which will be considered presently. The cytoplasm is limited by a membrane termed the *cell membrane, plasma membrane,* or *plasmalemma* (Figs. 1-2 to 1-4). In addition to these relatively large, organized vesicular, membranous, tubular, and fibrillar structures, both nucleus and cytoplasm contain an apparently amorphous ground or matrix, the *karyolymph* and *hyaloplasm,* respectively.

Metazoa consist of cells organized into tissues and organs, and the specializations developed in these cells are remarkable (Figs. 1-5 and 1-6). In humans, cells vary in shape and size from spherical blood cells 6 μm in diameter to branched nerve cells whose processes may reach a meter or more in length. Cells may display pronounced internal variation as well. Striated muscle cells are packed with cross-banded contractile filaments, adipose cells are distended with fat, and

secretory cells are filled with granules or other cell products. Osteoclasts may contain 25 or more nuclei, interstitial cells of the testis are packed with endoplasmic reticulum, parietal cells of the stomach have rich infoldings of plasma membrane, renal tubular cells and brown fat may contain extraordinarily large numbers of mitochondria, and immature blood cells may be unusually rich in ribosomes. Indeed, such variations in cell structure and function constitute a major theme of this book. So much has been learned of the functions of these cell constituents, moreover, that the function of a cell may be inferred from knowledge of its subcellular constituents. But despite pronounced and significant variations in cell structure, cells also have much in common. This chapter will explore some of these general features of cells. However, we first consider some of the techniques used by morphologists.

MICROSCOPY

To be suitable for most kinds of microscopic study, a tissue must be sufficiently thin to transmit light or electrons and its parts must have sufficient contrast or color difference for one part to be distinguishable from another. But beyond the simple identification of cell structures, there is considerable physical, chemical, and ultrastructural information to be obtained from cells. In quest of this information, refined methods of

tissue preparation have been worked out, and phase, fluorescent, dark-field, interference, polarizing, and electron microscopes have been developed.

TYPES OF MICROSCOPY

In most microscopy of biologic material, a thin piece of tissue modifies light passing through it. This is the

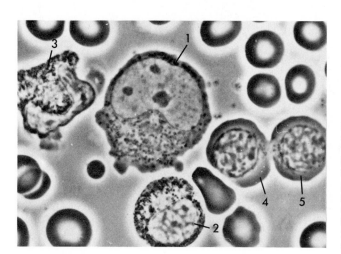

FIGURE 1-3 Human bone marrow cells, phase-contrast microscopy. This field shows immature white blood cells (myelocytes) which contain large indented nuclei and cytoplasmic granules. Erythrocytes are also present (see Chap. 12). Nucleated cells are numbered. Erythrocytes, lacking a nucleus, are not. ×1300. (From the work of G. A. Ackerman.)

FIGURE 1-4 Diagram of a cell, showing structures revealed by electron microscopy. The cell is enclosed by a membrane, the plasmalemma. The cell surface in this model is quite irregular. It is thrown up into microvilli (Mvl) and displays deep infoldings which ''pocket'' mitochondria (Mit). It is active in pinocytosis (Pin) and phagocytosis (Pha). The nucleus lies near the center of the cell and is indented by the cytocentrum which contains centrioles (Cen) and is contiguous to a Golgi complex (Gol). A spherical nucleolus is present. Chromatin is aggregated into heterochromatic masses (Chr). The nuclear membrane is a double membrane bearing nuclear pores (n.p.). The outer nuclear membrane is continuous with the endoplasmic reticulum in the cytoplasm. The endoplasmic reticulum may be entirely membranous or smooth (SER), or it may bear ribosomes on its outside surface (GER). Ribosomes are also present as clusters, polyribosomes (PRib), free in the cytoplasm unassociated with endoplasmic reticulum. The Golgi apparatus consists of stacks of membranes with the concave or distal face directed away from the nucleus and the convex or proximal face toward the nucleus. The edges of the sacs are expanded, and vesicles bud from the Golgi, increase in size, and lie free in the cytoplasm (LGr). These may be secretory granules or lysosomes. Pinocytotic (or phagocytic) vesicles may fuse with these Golgi-produced vesicles. Small packets of Golgi membranes and vesicles lie in the cytoplasm elsewhere than the centrosome. This diagram is representative of a free or unattached cell such as a macrophage. When cells lie next to one another in forming tissues, their contour is modified by contiguous cells and they may bear modifications of their cell surface, as discussed in Chap. 3.

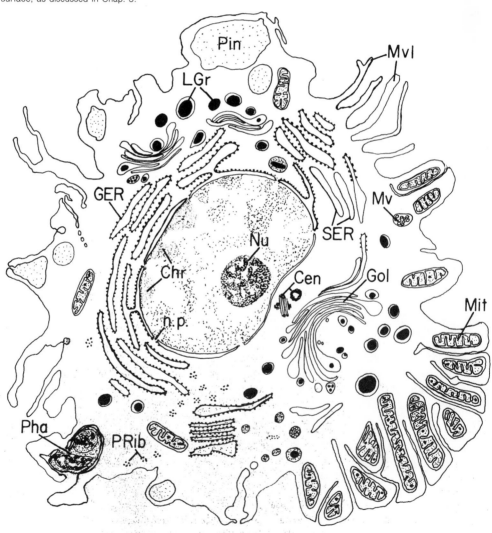

FIGURE 1-5 Variety of cells from the human body. a, Portion of a striated muscle fiber. b, Fibroblast from the umbilical cord. c, Osteocyte within a bone lacuna. d, Portion of the placental chorion, showing syncytial trophoblast and underlying cytotrophoblast cells. e, Squamous epithelial cell and bacteria from a vaginal smear. f, Three pigmented epithelial cells from the first layer of the retina. g, Macrophage in bone marrow, which has ingested masses of blood pigments. h, Two red blood cells; i, polymorphonuclear neutrophil; and j, small lymphocyte, all from a blood smear. k, Fat cell from loose connective tissue. l, Large motor neuron and adjacent small glial cell (process not revealed) from a hypoglossal nucleus in the medulla. m, Adjacent ciliated and secretory epithelial cells from the oviduct. n, Mature spermatozoon from semen. Cells a and d are multinucleate; g in binucleate; e has a pycnotic nucleus; c, f, j, and n have dense nuclei; the nucleus of l is extremely vesicular; i has a lobulated nucleus; the nuclei of a, g, and k are displaced by the cell contents. Some of the cells are rounded or polygonal, but a is extremely elongate, b and c have short processes, and the neuron in l has long processes (cut off here). The syncytium in d has a brush border; one cell in m has cilia; n, has a flagellum. Cells a and l display cytoplasmic fibrils; f, pigment granules; g, phagocytized masses; l, specific granules; k, a space left by dissolved fat; j and the neuron in l, conspicuous amounts of cytoplasmic basophilia. [The diameter of the red blood cells (approximately 7.5 μm) provides a useful measure of the other cells.] All ×700. (Prepared by H. W. Deane and E. Piotti.)

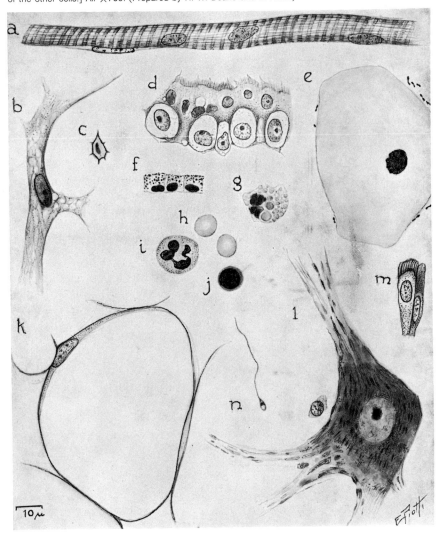

basis of transmission microscopy. This modified light contains information inherent in the specimen, and the function of the lens systems in any microscope is to amplify that information to a form discernible by eye.

The human eye is sensitive to the contrast of light and dark and to differences in color. A light train may be represented as electromagnetic sine waves, color being a function of wavelength and intensity a function of amplitude. In order to render visible the disturbance in the light train induced by a biologic preparation, the light must be modified in color or intensity. Thus some wave frequencies must be absorbed more than others so that the preparation will be seen to contain materials of different colors, or there must be a change in the amplitude of a wave so that the preparation will be seen to consist of darker and lighter parts. Because unstained tissue generally does not absorb light differentially and does not modify its amplitude to a useful degree, numerous staining techniques have been developed.

Bright-Field Microscopy

The *bright-field microscope* is a complex optical instrument consisting of three lens systems, a stage on which to place the preparation, and controls to permit focus, control of lens aperture, and centering of lenses and of light. The light, coming in parallel rays, is focused upon the preparation by the condenser lens. It passes through the specimen, where it is modified, and this modified beam enters the objective lens system. An image is formed in the focal plane of the objective. In that image lies whatever resolution the instrument is capable of providing. The bright-field microscope is theoretically capable of resolving points approximately 0.2 μm apart. The ocular or eyepiece then magnifies the image formed by the objective, presenting it to the eye as a visible magnified image.

The primary purpose in staining histologic preparations is to induce differential absorption of light so that various structures may be seen in distinguishing colors. Staining has expanded from this elementary function until it has become possible to stain many chemical compounds selectively and specifically (see Chap. 2).

Phase-Contrast Microscopy

Although unstained tissue does not absorb light, it does affect light by *retarding* some wave trains more than others. Thus the light may enter a specimen in phase, that is, with peaks and troughs of the component sine waves in register. But the components of the specimen, having different optical densities, retard the sine waves differentially, putting them out of phase with one another. These phase differences are not perceivable by the eye. The function of the *phase microscope* is to convert phase differences into ampli-

FIGURE 1-6 Various cytoplasmic organelles and cell inclusions. Because of their specific physical and chemical properties, these objects are not generally demonstrated by routine methods and are rarely revealed together. A. Cytocentrum in a cell of grasshopper testis, showing paired centrioles. B. Golgi material in a pancreas cell of guinea pig, as demonstrated with osmic acid fixation. [Redrawn from E. V. Cowdry (ed.), "Special Cytology," 2d ed., Paul B. Hoeber, Inc., New York, 1932.] C. Mitochondria in a hepatocyte of a dog, stained with hematoxylin. (Weatherford.) D. Crystal within the nucleus of a hepatocyte of a dog. (Weatherford.) E. Spaces in a young fat cell left by dissolved fat. F. Secretory granules in a human pancreas cell. Below and lateral to the nucleus lies ergastoplasm.

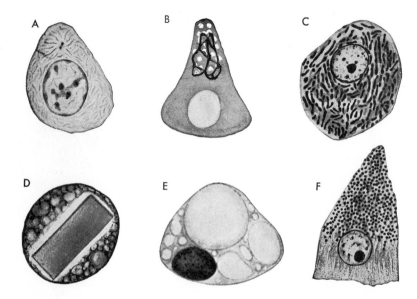

tude differences by matching the retarded waves with out-of-phase waves so as to cancel or diminish the amplitude of the retarded waves. The phase microscope thus permits one to observe considerable detail in unstained material and hence is suited to the study of living cells (Figs. 1-2 and 1-3).

Dark-Field Microscopy

The *dark-field microscope* is also able to provide contrast in unstained material. Its effectiveness depends upon excluding the central light train that comes into the objective from the condenser in the conventional bright-field microscope. Instead, the specimen is illuminated by light coming in from the side. Should there be objects of greater optical density than their surroundings in the field, such as bacteria moving in a fluid medium, they will deflect light into the microscopic objective and appear as light objects against a dark background. The effect is similar to motes visualized on a sunbeam in a darkened room (Tyndall effect) (Fig. 10-4). Little or no internal structure of the lighted particles is revealed. This technique, eminently suited to such examinations as the detection of bacteria in fluid, has been superseded by phase-contrast microscopy in many situations.

Interference Microscopy

The *interference microscope* provides not only contrast in unstained preparations but additional information on the physical properties and the submicroscopic organization of tissue. Like the phase microscope, the interference microscope depends upon phase differences induced in transmitted light by differences in optical densities in the parts of the biologic preparation. But this is a quantitative instrument in which the light trains subject to phase retardation are compared with a reference beam. Since the optical density and phase retardation are in proportion to specimen mass, the mass of different components of the cell may be calculated.

Fluorescence Microscopy

The *fluorescence microscope* depends upon exciting the emission of visible light in a specimen irradiated with ultraviolet light. Certain biologic substances, such as vitamin A, are autofluorescent; that is, they can absorb light of one frequency and emit light of another. In practice, light within one frequency range, usually in the ultraviolet spectrum, is focused upon the specimen, care being taken to protect the observer's eyes from this damaging radiation. This light is ab-

sorbed by certain structures within the specimen which then emit light within the visible range, the wavelength of the emitted light being dependent upon the chemical nature of the emitting substance. Although the autofluoresence of materials like vitamin A permits the use of this microscope with unstained material, the value of the technique is enormously enhanced by staining the tissue with fluorescent reagents. (See Fig. 1-7 and Chaps. 2, 14, and 15.)

Ultraviolet Microscopy

The *ultraviolet microscope,* like the fluorescence mi-

FIGURE 1-7 Fluorescence microscopy. A lymph node of a rabbit in the fourth day of a secondary antibody response to the antigen bovine serum albumin. The antibody, which has been tagged with a fluorescent tracer and is white in this photomicrograph, is present in the cytoplasm of plasma cells and lymphocytes. The nuclei are seldom stained and are present as negative (dark) images. See Chaps. 2 and 14. ×500. (From the work of A. H. Coons.)

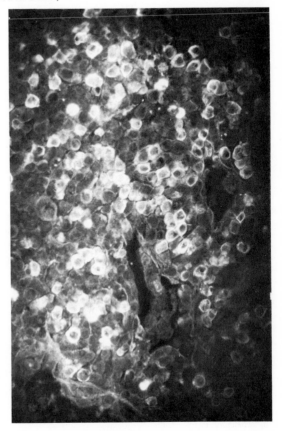

croscope, is built around the use of ultraviolet light instead of visible light. Its optical system is usually made of quartz which efficiently transmits ultraviolet light. The image-bearing ultraviolet light coming from the ocular of the ultraviolet microscope is recorded on a photographic film, since ultraviolet is both invisible and damaging to the eye. The value of the ultraviolet microscope lies in the fact that certain highly significant cellular structures, notably those containing nucleic acids, absorb ultraviolet light of specific wavelength and can therefore be demonstrated. Because the wavelength of ultraviolet is shorter than that of visible light, this microscope offers somewhat higher resolution than the bright-field microscope.

Polarizing Microscopy

The *polarizing microscope* permits one to determine whether biologic materials have different refractive indices along different optical axes. Such materials are *birefringent* or *anisotropic*. They have the capability of converting a beam of linear polarized light to elliptical polarized light, one axis of which can be transmitted by an analyzer and visualized. In the polarizing microscope, light is polarized below the stage of the microscope by a Nicol quartz prism or other suitable polarizer. This polarized light is passed through the specimen. An analyzer is placed at the ocular; like the polarizer, it is made of material capable of transmitting only polarized light in one plane or axis. By rotating the analyzer, the polarization of the light transmitted by the specimen may be determined and any change from the character of polarization of the source detected. Those substances incapable of affecting polarized light are termed *isotropic*. The capacity of biologic material to change linear to elliptical polarized light requires that submicroscopic particles which are asymmetric be present, and that these particles be oriented in an ordered nonrandom manner. *Thus, change of linear to elliptical polarized light by biologic material indicates that its submicroscopic structure consists of oriented asymmetric molecules.*

Filaments, fibers, and linear proteins are typically birefringent. Lipoprotein complexes, such as those composing membranes, may display complex polarizing properties. Typically the orientation of the lipid molecules, and hence their rotation of polarized light, is at right angles to that of the protein component. Polarization optics have been fruitfully applied to the study of muscle, connective tissue fibers, cell membranes, and the achromatic mitotic apparatus (Fig. 1-68).

Electron Microscopy

The *transmission electron microscope* (TEM), in contrast to light microscopes, uses a beam of electrons in place of a beam of visible light. Additional differences follow from the special properties of electrons. Electron beams are streams of negatively charged particles incapable of passing through or being refracted by glass. Hence the lenses of an electron microscope are electromagnetic coils which surround the beam at different levels, somewhat like a set of collars. The strength of these electromagnetic lenses may be changed by varying the current passing through their coils. By varying the strength of the projector lens (the counterpart of the ocular of the light microscope), the magnification of the image formed by the objective lens is changed.

Electrons are charged particles, and since collision with charged molecules of air will absorb and deflect electrons and distort the beam, the optical system of an electron microscope must be evacuated of air. A vacuum of 10^{-4}mm Hg is commonly required. The electron stream is produced by heating a tungsten filament. The electrons are directed and impelled by moderately high voltage, usually ranging from 40,000 to 100,000 V. The higher voltages produce electron streams with shorter wavelengths which are more penetrating and produce an image with less contrast but with higher resolution than lower voltages. Since electron beams are invisible to the eye, the images they form are revealed by causing them to strike a fluorescent screen, and they are then recorded on a photographic plate. Indeed, the eye and the whole body of the operator must be protected from the electron beam, not only because it can do damage but because it can produce x-rays, which are also damaging.

Stability of the specimen is always a major consideration, and efforts must be made to protect the structure of the specimen against sublimation, distortion, and other damage by the electron beam or the vacuum. Extreme thinness of the specimen is required so that the electrons, so easily absorbed, may pass through it and create an image on the fluorescent screen and photographic plate. Electron-microscopic sections are approximately $\frac{1}{40}$ μm (250 Å) thick. Obtaining sections of tissues this thin has required the development of new slicing machines, ultramicrotomes, and a new or highly modified technology of fixation and embedding of tissues. Because these thin sections have little intrinsic contrast, they must be stained with heavy electron-absorbing metals to provide the contrast necessary to reveal details of cell structure.

The value of the electron microscope lies in its great resolving power. *Resolution* of a microscope, measured as the distance between the closest two points it can resolve as two separate points, depends upon the wavelength of the radiation. An electron train has wave characteristics in addition to the characteristics of charge and mass. Its wavelength is small enough so that resolution of about 2 Å is possible and of about 30 Å is routine. This means that a useful magnification of more than 500,000 is possible. The bright-field microscope is capable of resolution of approximately 0.2 μm and useful magnification of 2,000. It has not proved practicable, so far, to examine living tissue by electron microscopy because of the vacuum and the damaging effects of electrons. However, the development of modified specimen chambers may permit this. New cytochemical techniques that make it possible to obtain histochemical information at electron-microscopic resolutions have made electron microscopy increasingly productive. Moreover, quantitative analytic methods are also being introduced.

Variations on the transmission electron microscope characterized above have been made. High-voltage electron microscopes capable of exceptionally high resolution exist. With accelerating voltages of a million electronvolts, they provide greater resolution and greater penetrating power of the electron beam and, therefore, the capacity to use thicker sections than is possible by conventional transmission electron microscopes (Fig. 1-9). Scanning electron microscopy, wherein a remarkably detailed three-dimensional view of the surface of a specimen is obtained, is increasingly useful (Fig. 1-8 and discussion below). New methods of preparing tissues, as discussed below, have considerably enhanced the versatility of electron microscopy.

Scanning Electron Microscopy

Scanning electron microscopy (SEM) provides a remarkably beautiful three-dimensional high-resolution image of cells and tissues (Figs. 1-8, 12-10, and 15-20). By relatively simple means, moreover, cytochemical data can be obtained and localized on the image. This technique has provided invaluable infor-

mation on the contours of cells and the organization of cells and extracellular elements into tissues.

In SEM the tissue is seldom sectioned, since it is the surface of the tissue which is studied. Whole mounts of tissue cultures or pieces of tissue are placed on the stage of the SEM. These tissues may be rather large, even a centimeter or more in one dimension. In the SEM, a slender electron beam or probe plays upon the surface, going back and forth in a regular way scanning the preparation. As the electron probe strikes the surface of the specimen, it generates several different kinds of signals. These include electrons (the so-called *secondary electrons*) and x-rays. The secondary electron may be collected and focused upon a cathode-ray tube or photographic film to form the striking three-dimensional image. X-rays are generated by the electron probe striking atoms having a mass greater than that of sodium. Each element is the source of x-rays of distinctive wavelength. The magnitude of the x-rays generated is a function of the concentration of the element. Analysis of the x-ray pattern of a tissue thus provides information on the concentration and distribution of elements.

Tissues prepared for SEM are fixed, often in glutaraldehyde and osmium tetroxide. They are then dehydrated. Drying at the critical point has become the preferred method. The tissue is introduced into a suitable fluid and that fluid brought to its *critical point,* which is the pressure and temperature at which the fluid and gaseous phase exist together without an interface or meniscus. Thus, there is no surface tension. The presence of surface tension during drying is disruptive to a tissue and causes visible shrinkage, distortions, and other types of damage. After drying, the surface of the tissue is commonly coated in a vacuum with an electrically conductive coat of gold, gold-palladium, or carbon. The preparation is now ready for study in the SEM. Too heavy a coat must be avoided or details of surface structure will be obscured. A number of methods which impregnate the tissue with heavy metals can make the coating unnecessary; and as the resolution of SEM improves, the detail-masking coating will likely be used less and less.

Resolution of the SEM is inversely proportional to the diameter of the electron probe. Accordingly, scanning microscopes are being developed which work with very narrow, very coherent electron beams. The beam must be broad enough, however, to have sufficient energy to generate a useful number of secondary electrons as it scans the preparation. Resolution of the scanning electron microscope in the images generated by secondary electrons may be from 25 to 75 Å at the present time.

BIOLOGIC MICROSCOPIC PREPARATIONS

Study of Living Cells

Living cells may be maintained in *tissue culture* for long periods and examined by microscopy while in culture through the use of suitable culture vessels. Tissue culture permits control over the environment of cells and isolation of single cells or of *clones,* which are colonies derived from proliferation of a single cell.

Maintenance of cells in tissue culture requires considerable attention, involving nutritive media, temperature control, and sterility. For short-term investigation, living cells such as leukocytes from a drop of blood may be placed on a clean slide, covered with a cover slip, sealed with petroleum jelly to prevent evapo-ration, placed on a warming stage, and studied under the microscope. This type of preparation is called *supravital* in distinction to more stable, longer-lasting preparations, such as whole animals or long-term tissue cultures, which are called *vital preparations.* Thus living cells may be observed with the conventional bright-field microscope or with the phase, interference, polarizing, or fluorescence microscopes. Living material may be studied unstained or it may be stained and remain alive, but such vital or supravital staining offers limited structural detail and damages the cells. Although it is of value in special situations, as in the staining of the reticulocytes of the blood (Chap. 10), it is no longer generally used.

The nucleus, cytoplasm, mitochondria, Golgi apparatus, and centriole may all be observed in the living state, as may such cell functions as motility of whole cells and the movement of structures within the cell.

FIGURE 1-8 Scanning electron microscopy of the surface of the yolk sac. Note the three-dimensional character of the scanning electron micrograph. The surface is thrown up into folds, and each of the folds is beset with many cobblestonelike protuberances. The surface drips down around these protuberances. The appearance of this surface by light microscopy and transmission electron microscopy is presented in Chap. 25. (From B. King, Jr., and A. C. Enders, *Am. J. Anat.,* **127:**397, 1970.)

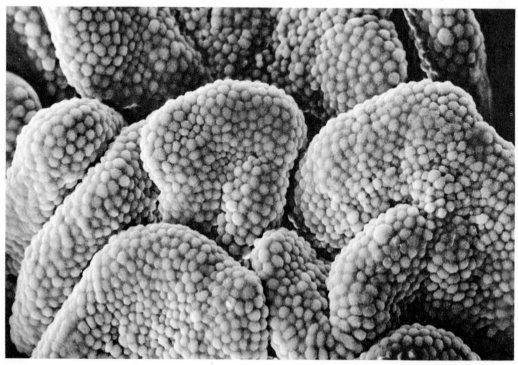

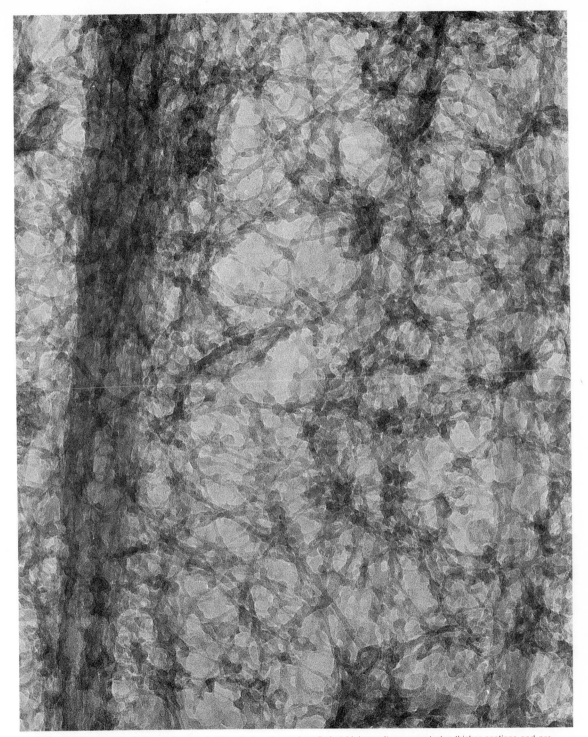

FIGURE 1-9 High-voltage electron micrograph. The electron beam, impelled at higher voltage, penetrates thicker sections and provides greater resolution than that in conventional transmission electron microscopes. This field includes the ground cytoplasm (hyaloplasm or cell sap). The ground substance of the cytoplasm contains a lattice of microtrabeculae. These form an irregular lattice which is continuous with the actin fibers (on the left) and support polysomes at their junction points. The microtrabeculae are about 30 to 50 Å in diameter and highly variable in length. The intertrabecular spaces provide for the rapid diffusion of water soluble metabolites. ×145,000. (Courtesy of John Wolosewick and Keith Porter.)

The behavior of the plasma membrane is rewardingly studied in living material. The membrane is in active movement and may be associated with such processes as pinocytosis and phagocytosis. The study of living material offers certain satisfactions. Any scientific study induces artefacts, or departures from the natural state of things. A question that a scientist must always consider is whether or not the artefacts induced in one's material are consistent, repeatable, and significant. Intuitively, one thinks that what is seen in the living cell is less apt to be an uncontrolled or misleading artefact and nearer to the undisturbed life of the unscrutinized cell than what can be inferred from killed, sectioned, and stained tissue.

In order to obtain greater resolution and more chemical and other information about the structure and function of cells, it is necessary to kill them by fixation, section them into thin slices, and stain them. The nature of these procedures will now be considered.

Fixation

Fixation is a step wherein a certain structure or function of interest in a cell or tissue is preserved. Fixation is usually accomplished by immersing the tissue in a solution of chemicals. It is important to realize that, although there are fixatives which may be of general use, fixation may be quite selective. Thus, to study the structure of fat droplets, the tissues must be fixed in formaldehyde or other materials which stabilize the fat and avoid the use of alcohol or other organic solvents which extract fats. Fixatives that fix or coagulate protein are widely used because they preserve the general structure of nucleus and cytoplasm. Greater resolution and less distortion of cellular structures are obtained with a fixative that produces a fine coagulum than with one that produces a coarse one. Thus glutaraldehyde and osmium tetroxide, which cause a very fine precipitation of protein, permit high resolution without appreciable distortion of structure. Indeed, so finely do they fix tissue that they are the most widely used fixatives for electron microscopy. Phosphotungstic acid is a coarse protein precipitant which causes the cell to be thrown into heavy strands. For general work, therefore, phosphotungstic acid is used little, but one consequence of its drastic action is that it may expose more reactive groups. Thus more sulfhydryl groups are free to react after the coarse

fixation with phosphotungstic acid than with fixatives that induce a finer coagulation of protein. For the special purpose of detecting sulfhydryl groups in tissue section this otherwise unsatisfactory chemical may be the fixative of choice.

It is important to emphasize that fixation induces chemical change in tissue. Thus fixatives containing heavy metals, such as Zenker's fluid which contains mercuric chloride, may react with the carboxyl groups of tissue proteins and influence their subsequent staining. Aldehyde-containing fixatives, as formaldehyde and gluteraldehyde, may react with amino groups in tissue and block them. Reagents as bromide in the fixative may saturate double bonds and influence the staining of lipids. Staining methods are available which detect enzyme activity. The fixative used for this purpose must be very gentle; most chemical fixatives tend to damage enzymes so much that they become inoperative and therefore undetectable.

Fixation is thus a procedure wherein a given cellular structure is preserved or stabilized, often at the expense of other structures, for subsequent viewing in microscopic preparations. Fixation may be achieved by immersing the tissue in a solution of chemicals, the form most commonly employed, or it may be physical, as heat denaturation, freezing, or air drying.

While fixation is commonly required as an early step in preparing tissue for study by light and electron microscopy, it must sometimes be avoided or its effects minimized because of unwanted chemical change or damage. Some living tissues, as a drop of blood or tissue cultures, lend themselves to direct study by light microscopy and need not be fixed. But the information so obtained, though valuable, is quite limited. The deleterious effects of fixation may be minimized by such maneuvers as freezing the tissue or using very dilute fixatives for very short times. Such alternatives to conventional fixation are discussed below. They may provide invaluable information of a specialized sort unattainable either by conventional fixation or from living tissue.

Embedding and Sectioning

After the tissue is fixed, it is usually necessary to section it into sufficiently thin slices so that the detail it contains can be inspected by microscopy. Only in exceptional cases, as in spreading out a drop of blood on a slide, can the required thinness of tissue be obtained without slicing. The slices must be thin enough to allow light or electrons, in the case of electron microscopy, to pass through them. Moreover, since the depth of focus of microscopic objectives is shallow, clarity of detail is favored by thin sections. For light microscopy, section thickness varies from less than 1 μm to about 100 μm. Most preparations are about 5 μm thick. Slices this thin are made with an instrument known as a *microtome,* which consists of a chuck that holds the tissue, a knife, and an advance mechanism. However, tissue after fixation is often pulpy or brittle and impossible to cut into thin slices. In order to cut tissue successfully for microscopy, it must be infiltrated with a material which is stiff and of a consistency that can be cut. Most of these infiltrating or embedding agents are fatty waxes, immiscible with the aqueous cytoplasm. Most fixing solutions, moreover, are aqueous. Therefore, to embed in the most commonly used embedding agents, which are paraffin or celloidin for light microscopy and the acrylic or epoxy resins for electron microscopy, the fixed tissues must be dehydrated. To this end the tissues are passed through a series of increasingly concentrated aqueous solutions of ethyl alcohol, acetone, or other dehydrating agent which is miscible with both water and fat. Thus the tissue may be passed through 50, 70, 80, 95 percent, and then into absolute ethanol. For here, either directly or through an intermediate organic solvent like toluene, the tissue is placed in the embedding agent in a liquid phase. The embedding agent replaces the solvent and thus thoroughly infiltrates the tissue.

Paraffin is made fluid by temperatures above the melting point, usually about 60°C, and the dehydrated tissue is allowed to steep in molten paraffin. The preparation is then cooled. Having infiltrated the interstices of the tissue, the paraffin becomes solid, forming a block that can be cut.

In plastic embedding for electron or light microscopy, the plastic is introduced in the fluid monomeric state. With sufficient steeping, it infiltrates the tissue. Then, by means of heat or ultraviolet light, the plastic is polymerized and becomes, like paraffin, a solid in which the tissue lies thoroughly infiltrated and embedded.

But a price must be paid to obtain such stable infiltrated blocks of tissue capable of being cut into microscopic sections. The alcohols employed to dehydrate tissues before infiltration extract fat, coagulate protein, and effect other chemical changes in a tissue. In order to infiltrate with paraffin, moreover, the tissue must be subjected to temperatures high enough to inactivate many enzymes. As plastic polymerizes, heat is given off and may damage the tissue undergoing

embedding. Moreover, paraffin and other embedding agents may shrink and thereby distort the structure of tissues. For these reasons, alternatives to these convenient types of embedding are often employed. Water-soluble embedding agents are available which circumvent the need for dehydration so that fatty materials may be preserved.

Some enzymatic activities, however, are so fugitive that they do not withstand infiltration with an embedding agent. In such circumstances the tissue may be frozen, and the frozen block of tissue has sufficient rigidity, elasticity, and other physical properties to permit sectioning. Freezing may speed up the processing of tissues, saving the time required for embedding. Tissues can be frozen and sections made, stained, and read in minutes, as is common practice in a surgical operating room. There a surgeon will expose a tumor, take a biopsy, and hand it to a pathologist, wait for the pathologist's interpretation of the tissue section, and then go ahead and do simple or radical surgery depending on whether the tumor, by microscopic examination, is benign or malignant.

More specialized methods of fixation and embedding have been developed

Freeze-drying is a significant refinement over fixation by freezing or chemical means because it allows minimal distortion and displacement of tissues, minimal chemical extraction, and maximal preservation of enzyme activity for light microscopy. A small block of tissue is quick-frozen or quenched by immersion in isopentane in liquid nitrogen at a temperature of -150 to $-160°C$. It is then placed in a vacuum and dried by sublimation of H_2O, thereby avoiding liquid H_2O which causes displacement and extraction of cellular components. The dried tissue, while still in vacuo, may be infiltrated with molten paraffin.

Tissues that have been quenched may have their sublimated water replaced by a chemical fixative in vapor form; this type of fixation is designated *free substitution.* It offers the results of freeze-drying coupled with chemical fixation. A new electron-microscopic technique, *freeze-fracture-etch,* has proved so valuable that it is described in some detail below.

Mounting and Staining

After the tissue is sectioned for light microscopy, it is usually mounted on a glass slide and stained, although, as with living cells, it is possible by the use of the phase-contrast or the interference microscope to study unstained tissue. The primary purpose of staining is to induce some parts of the cell to appear darker or of different color than others so that they can be recognized. Staining, however, is a chemical procedure, and it has been refined to a degree that it provides considerable information on the chemical constitution of the parts of cells in both light and electron microscopy (consult Chap. 2).

Freeze-Fracture-Etch

The technique of freeze-fracture-etch has become an invaluable method in cell biology necessary in the modern study of membranes (Figs. 1-10 and 1-25 to 1-27). The technique avoids embedding and sectioning of tissue and may even avoid fixation. It has been possible to recognize heterogeneity in biological membranes, to illuminate the nature of cell junctions and other specialized parts of the plasma membrane and of membranes within the cell. Its applications have not been restricted to study of membranes, however. Useful information has also been obtained on particles, filaments, ground substance within the cell, and extracellular substances. Much of the information obtained by freeze-fracture-etch depends upon the rather simple fact that when a tissue is frozen and fractured under certain circumstances, the fracture line tends to travel within membranes separating them into inner and outer leaflets thereby revealing structures heretofore hidden. So important is this technique and so frequently has it become the basis of the observations described in this text that it shall be described in steps.

1. The tissue is removed from the body and fixed in glutaraldehyde although fixation may be eliminated or other fixatives used.

2. After suitable rinses the tissue is transferred to glycerol. This infiltrates the tissue and protects against artefacts due to ice-crystal formation in the subsequent freezing.

3. The tissue is cut into small pieces approximately

2 mm^3 and placed on small metal (temperature conductive) discs.

4. The tissue is then plunged into a bath of isopentane, which is held in a temperature-conductive vessel partially immersed in liquid nitrogen. Temperature is low ($-160°C$) so that the tissue is almost immediately quenched or frozen below the eutectic point of water. This is most important because it permits freezing without ice-crystal formation in glycerated tissue. If ice crystals occur, they rotate as they are formed and literally cut and damage the tissue, causing artefacts visible by electron microscopy.

5. The frozen tissue is quickly transferred to the chamber of a freeze-fracture-etch machine. A number of operations can be carried out in the chamber. It can be cooled to low temperature. It contains a razor on an adjustable swinging arm which can intersect the tissue. It may be pumped out to achieve high vacuum (approximately 10^{-8} mm of mercury). It is set up with platinum electrodes, moreover, so that platinum may be evaporated to form a film over the specimen. Within the freeze-fracture-etch machine the tissue is maintained frozen and under vacuum through the production of a platinum replica (step 8).

6. The tissue, positioned on its disc, is now fractured by the razor blade on the swinging arm. The cutting edge of the blade strikes the tissue and starts a fracture rift. It is important to understand that the cut surface of the block is not caused by the razor slicing through the tissue but by the razor edge striking the edge of the tissue and inducing a fracture line which then travels across the tissue. The free piece of tissue above the fracture line flies off and is lost. The lower part of the tissue affixed to the disc now has an exposed fracture face. The face is relatively smooth with glasslike frozen water surrounding the tissue and filling in the spaces between membranes, particles, and other cellular and extracellular structures.

7. The freshly fractured face of tissue is permitted to remain under vacuum for a short time, usually a matter of minutes. This represents the etching phase of the process, since some of the frozen water at the fracture face sublimates into the vacuum. As a result membranes and granules, other cellular structures on the fractured surface, and the cell itself now stand out in relief, the level of the frozen water table being below them.

8. Current is passed through the platinum electrodes and

FIGURE 1-10 Guinea pig macrophage. A. A cell which has been fixed and sectioned and photographed in the electron microscope after staining with heavy metals. Nucleus (N), mitochondria (M), lysosomes (L), and the plasma membrane are visible by this standard technique. ×13,500. B. A freeze-fractured-etched macrophage, showing the nucleus (N), bearing nuclear pores, numerous globular profiles, two cisternae of the ER (ER), and an invagination (arrow) at the cell surface (CS). ×19,000. [From W. Th. Daems and P. Bredero, in R. van Furth (ed.), "Mononuclear Phagocytes," p. 29. F. A. Davis Company, Philadelphia, 1970.]

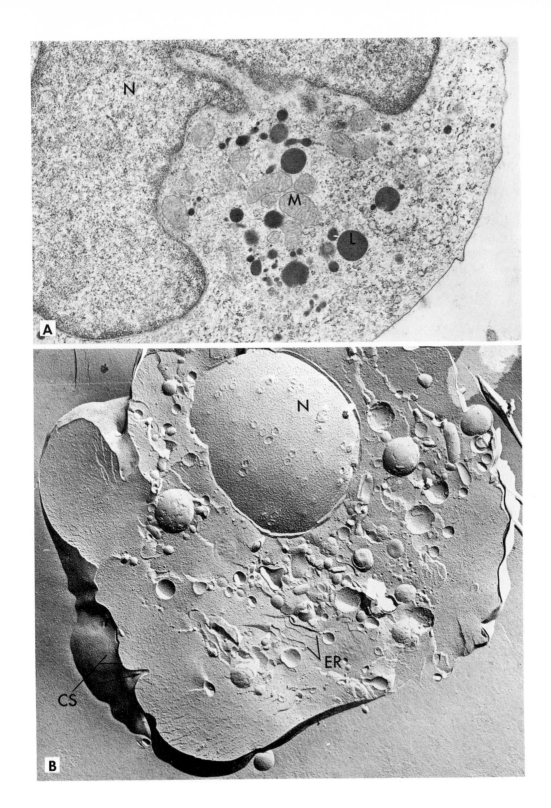

a layer of platinum is evaporated over the frozen-frac-tured-etched surface of the tissue. This platinum layer forms a tough membranous replica of the surface. It is important to note that the platinum is evaporated from a point source and reaches the tissue from a given point in a given direction. As the platinum comes over the tissue and lies on it, it covers the tissue very much as snow falling from a certain direction covers a landscape. It piles up on the near side of structures which rise from the surface and leaves a clear space or shadow on the far side.

9. The vacuum is broken, the chamber is opened, and the disc bearing the tissue covered with a platinum replica is removed from the machine.

10. The replica is freed from the tissue digesting the tissue away and is caught on a grid which fits into the specimen holder of a transmission electron microscope.

11. The replica is examined by electron microscopy. The grain of the platinum permits resolution to better than 30 Å.

ISOLATION OF WHOLE CELLS AND PARTS OF CELLS

The morphologic techniques outlined above have been extended by techniques whereby whole viable cells may be isolated from complex tissues and by other related techniques wherein cells are disrupted and their constituent parts isolated.

A single cell type may be purified in a viable state from a complex tissue containing many cell types. For example, *hepatocytes,* the distinctive parenchymal cell type of liver, can be isolated from blood vessels, lymphatics, nerves, fibroblasts, macrophages, extracellular substances, and other cells and extracellular materials of the liver. The first objective is to prepare a cell suspension of the tissue. In a few tissues, as blood, this is not necessary, since the cells already are in suspension in the liquid plasma. But in a solid tissue, such as the liver and kidney, the tissue is usually cut into small pieces and subjected to enzyme digestion while shaking or other mechanical agitation is applied. *Trypsin,* a proteolytic enzyme produced in large scale by the pancreas, will digest virtually any protein substrate and is widely used in cell-separation procedures. Judicious application will result in the destruction or depolymerization of extracellular substances and the loosening of intercellular junctional complexes without too much cell destruction. (A valuable related use of

trypsin is in the harvesting of cells in tissue culture adherent to the flask walls. Brief treatment loosens the cells. Overlong treatment digests and destroys them.) *Collagenase* rather selectively removes major components of the extracellular connective tissues and is therefore especially useful in freeing cells enmeshed in collagen and related proteins. *Neuriminidase* can remove a sticky extrinsic carbohydrate, that is, sialic acid, from the cell surface. (This highlights a refined use of enzymes in cell biology in which certain receptors or other molecules can be specifically removed from the cell surface, as fucose by fucase).

After enzymatic treatment and mechanical agitation a solid tissue is reduced to a suspension of diverse cell types and debris. A given cell type may be separated by one or more of a number of techniques. Cells will migrate differently in a countercurrent or in an electrophoretic system and a given cell type may thereby be removed. In certain instances cells may be selectively removed as destroying erythrocytes with hypotonic solutions or destroying other cells by anti-cell antibodies and complement. Cells may have different affinities for surfaces. If a suspension of macrophages and lymphocytes is poured through a column of glass wool, the macrophages will adhere to the glass fibers (from which they can later be removed) and the lymphocytes will go through. This technique may be refined by coating a surface with certain specific reactants which can hold certain cell types by interacting with specific cell surface receptors.

But the major methods for separating cells are centrifugal, whereby the cells are subjected to pulls greater than gravity. (The number of gravities, or *g,* is a function of the speed of rotation and the distance from the center of rotation to the material in the centrifuge tube.) The rate at which a structure reaches the bottom of the centrifuge tube depends upon its density and volume. Cells or other particles may thus be separated differentially by varying the time of centrifugation, with the denser and more voluminous structures coming down first. When centrifugation is complete, moreover, the larger denser structures are on the bottom of the tube and the smaller lighter ones lie on top of them. This is the technique of *differential centrifugation.* For example, the density of red cells is approximately 1077 and that of white cells, 1033. As a result, on differential centrifugation, the red cells and white cells are separated with the red cells below and the white cells above. (The sedimentation of red cells is enhanced by their tendency to aggregate into rouleaux, thereby increasing their effective unit volume.) But separation may be cleaner by interposing a density barrier. That is, a suspension of blood cells may be layered carefully over a solution of bovine albumin or sucrose of density intermediate between red cells and white cells. The red cells go through the density barrier and the white cells do not, and hence a better separation is achieved. This is the principle of *density-gradient separation*. The technique may be refined by using a number of layers of varying density, or going without steps from low to high density, resulting in *continuous, or linear, density-gradient centrifugation*. If the range of densities in such multiple or continuous density barriers encompasses the densities of the cells being centrifuged into them, the cells will come to rest in the layer whose density equals its own. This is *isopycnic* centrifugation.

In the separation and analysis of constituent parts of a cell, the main elements of the procedure are as follows. Fresh tissue is shred into small pieces or run through a grinder. Cells are then disrupted in a blender or in a mortar and pestle or ground by fine sand or in a mill by a closely fitting piston riding in a test tube. The tissue is thereby reduced to a pulpy heterogenous liquid which contains disrupted cells and their constituent parts, extracellular material, and debris. This homogenate is centrifuged and its different components are isolated, depending upon the force of the centrifugal field. The nucleus is a relatively large, heavy structure and is concentrated in fields of low gravity. Mitochondria, ribosomes, lysosomes, and other cellular elements may also be separated differentially. An isolated component may be studied by electron microscopy to confirm its nature and determine the damage, if any, done in its disruption and concentration, and the cleanness of separation. The pellet may also be studied chemically or by other means. Rich correlative chemical and morphologic data have been obtained by these procedures.

MICROCHEMISTRY AND HISTOCHEMISTRY

Microchemical methods have evolved from an extraordinary refinement of chemical methods. Thus it has been possible to take a section of a tissue and study it under the microscope and then take the section next to it and analyze it for inorganic salts, oxidative enzymes, or other components. It is possible, moreover, to dissect sections and carry out chemical analyses on small groups of similar cells or even upon single cells.

Histochemistry, the visualization of chemical reactions in microscopic preparations, is so valuable and well developed a field as to be accorded a full treatment in Chap. 2.

THE STRUCTURE OF THE CELL

THE NUCLEUS

The nucleus is the fundamental part of a cell that encodes the information from which the structure and function of the organism derive. The information is encoded in the genetic material, deoxyribonucleic acid (DNA), complexed to simple basic proteins, histones, to form deoxyribonucleoprotein (DNP). With some exceptions, notably mitochondria, DNA lies exclusively in the nucleus. DNA is capable of replicating itself, thereby providing precise copies of the genetic code that are passed on to daughter cells by cellular division.

The nucleus further plays a central role in synthesizing proteins and polypeptides from the genetic information it carries. All the nucleated cells of the body contain the same genes, yet cells differ in their structure, function, and products. The nucleus differentially controls the use of this information from cell to cell by repressing or derepressing the action of various genes. The nucleus, moreover, actually initiates the translation of its encoded information into the synthesis of proteins by means of ribonucleic acids (RNAs), a group of nucleic acids different in base composition and other critical respects from DNA. Some RNAs are complexed to proteins to form ribonucleoprotein (RNP). The RNAs are produced in or under the control of the nucleus and are released to the cytoplasm where they actually engage in protein synthesis. The "machine" which assembles proteins from amino acids is a complex of RNAs and protein, the *ribosome*, whose constituents are produced in a nuclear subdivi-

18

sion termed the nucleolus. Other RNAs are *messenger RNA* which links ribosomes into working units termed *polyribosomes* and *transfer RNA* which carries amino acids to the polyribosomes to initiate protein synthesis.

The nucleus, in summary, encodes genetic information, determines in any cell type which information is to be used in differentiation and maturity, and initiates and effects the utilization of this information in cellular synthesis. Moreover, it possesses mechanisms for replicating its DNA and passing it on to its progeny or utilizing it for augmented cellular activities.

A nucleus is present in virtually all differentiated metazoan cells, being absent only from mammalian erythrocytes and a few other end-stage cell types. Certain cell types have many nuclei or are polyploid (see below), thereby multiplying the number of genes and other elements in the protein-synthesizing apparatus of a cell, and permitting it to produce a greater volume of product. Hepatocytes, particularly with age, may develop two or more nuclei, and renal tubular cells may be binucleate. Giant cells with 100 or more nuclei exist as osteoclasts or foreign-body giant cells. A mechanism wherein nuclear function is increased without increasing nuclear number is *polyploidy,* an increase in the number of chromosomal pairs within a

FIGURE 1-11 Nucleus, isolated from an oocyte of *Xenopus laevis.* The nucleus was dissected from the oocyte, flooded with cresyl violet stain, and photographed. The deeply stained spots are those of the hundreds of nucleoli which are in the plane of focus. (From D. D. Brown and I. B. Dawid, *Science,* **160:**272, 1968.)

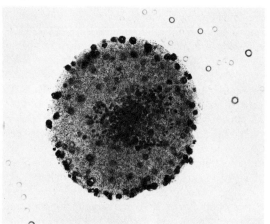

single nucleus. Most somatic cells are diploid (2n), having one pair of each chromosome characterizing its species, but cells may develop two pairs (4n) or more. Hepatocytes tend to increase in ploidy with age, in old rats often being 8n and 16n. Megakaryocytes, giant cells of the bone marrow containing a giant polymorphous nucleus, regularly become 32n or 64n. A more restricted mechanism for increasing nuclear components is that of increasing the number of nucleoli in certain oocytes, with a concomitant increase in ribosomal RNA production. The foregoing adaptations increase nuclear activities without increasing the number of cells in a tissue.

The nucleus may occur in a dividing (mitotic or meiotic) state, during which it reproduces itself, or in a nondividing or interphase state. The interphase nucleus is that most frequently encountered, since nuclear division takes only 1 h or more whereas, even in actively dividing cells, 6 h or more elapse between divisions.

The interphase nucleus is, in most cell types, a round or ovoid structure several micrometers in diameter (Figs. 1-11 to 1-16 and 1-18 to 1-22). In the leukocytes of blood and connective tissues, the nucleus is lobulated and hence termed *polymorphous* (see Chaps. 10 and 11). The nucleus is deformable and may therefore be pressed into a reniform or horseshoe shape. In contracted smooth muscle, it may be twisted like a corkscrew (Fig. 1-12), thereby adapting to the shortened space.

The interphase nucleus typically contains several distinctive structures. These include *chromatin, nuclear sap* or *karyolymph,* and one or more *nucleoli.* The protoplasm of the nucleus is termed *nucleoplasm* or *karyoplasm.*

Chromatin, by light microscopy, consists of irregular clumps or masses which, although not highly constant, tend to be characteristic in texture, quantity, and size in any given cell type. These clumps, sometimes termed *karyosomes,* have an affinity for basic dye because chromatin is a DNA-protein complex, DNP. DNA confers other distinctive staining reactions

FIGURE 1-12 Contracted muscle cell. The nucleus has been twisted into a corkscrew spiral. On relaxation, the nucleus will untwist and be cigar-shaped.

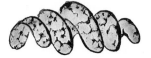

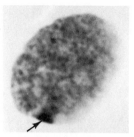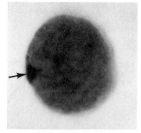

FIGURE 1-13 Sex chromatin of a human female. The chromatin lies against the nuclear membrane (arrows). This formation of sex chromatin appears to be due to the persistent coiling in interphase in one of the X chromosomes. Human buccal mucosa. ×4000. (From the work of B. R. Migeon.)

upon chromatin. In preparations stained with methyl green-pyronin, chromatin binds methyl green. In Romanovsky preparations which are stained with methylene blue and azures, chromatin masses are stained violet (Chap. 10). A highly significant staining reaction is the selective staining of DNA in the Feulgen method (Chap. 2). These distinctive DNA staining reactions are abolished by pretreatment of the specimen with the enzyme *deoxyribonuclease.*

Chromatin is the representation in the interphase nucleus of the DNP of the chromosomes. The chromosomes in the interphase nucleus are very slender, long, threadlike structures lying in a rather tangled mass. It is impossible to delineate individual chromosomes from this tangle. Indeed it was at one time thought that this mass was a continuous single thread instead of individual interlaced chromosomes, and the name *spireme* was applied to it.

In the early phases of mitosis, however, the chromosomes become highly coiled, so that in microscopic preparations they become shorter, broader, densely stained, and clearly visible (see later discussions of mitosis). Masses of chromatin visualized in the interphase nucleus by light microscopy represent the persistence of coiling along a segment of a chromosome. The dense chromatin is termed *heterochromatin* in contrast to the uncoiled or extended *euchromatin.* Thus, whereas DNA is present along the length of chromosomes, it is not visible by light microscopy in the extended chromosomes of interphase (euchromatin), being too finely dispersed. It is visible only where the coiling of a chromosome brings it to an aggregate size, above the limit of resolution of the light microscope, 0.2 μm (heterochromatin). Heterochromatin masses, moreover, may be an index to a cell's activity. Cells with large blocks of heterochromatin tend to be

relatively inactive in at least an early stage of protein synthesis, production of mRNA (see below). In the extended chromosome there is optimum exposure of its functional surface for transcription of mRNA. In cells of females a chracteristic mass of chromatin represents one of the female sex chromosomes which remains clumped through interphase. It may lie against the nuclear membrane or in other positions and is termed the *sex chromatin* or, after its discoverer, the *Barr body* (Fig. 1-13). It permits the determination of the genetic sex of an individual, a procedure of value in certain endocrinopathies or congenital disturbances in which the genetic sex may not be apparent. The Y (male) chromosome may be demonstrated in interphase nuclei by a special fluorescence staining method.

In addition to chromatin, nuclei may contain discrete RNA-rich bodies, nucleoli (see below). The clear space in the nucleoplasm between chromatin and nucleoli is the nuclear sap or karyolymph. The nucleus is bounded by a well-defined *nuclear membrane* (see below).

The elements of the interphase nucleus, namely chromatin, nucleoli, karyolymph, and nuclear membranes, are readily identified by electron microscopy (Figs. 1-14 to 1-26). But the correlation of electron-microscopic observations of interphase nuclei with what is inferred of the structure of chromosomes and other nuclear structures from genetic and other data is, at this time, rudimentary. It is known, for example, that an uncoiled chromosome may be of the order of 10,000 times the largest dimension of the nucleus. But it is difficult to gain any appreciation in sections of nuclei of the nature of the immense amount of folding and coiling which the chromosomes must undergo. Such inferences as electron microscopy affords come from preparations in which chromosomes are floated out of disrupted nuclei, dried down on supporting membranes, and examined whole. Here high degrees of coiling and folding are evident. Pure DNA may be prepared and examined as whole, unsectioned filaments by electron microscopy. These filaments are approximately 20 Å in diameter. DNA can be identified in sectioned interphase nuclei on the basis of selective staining. It is present in filaments of varying diameter, the slimmest being about 100 Å in diameter. The greater thickness of DNA in sections may be due to such factors as coiling, folding, or intertwining of

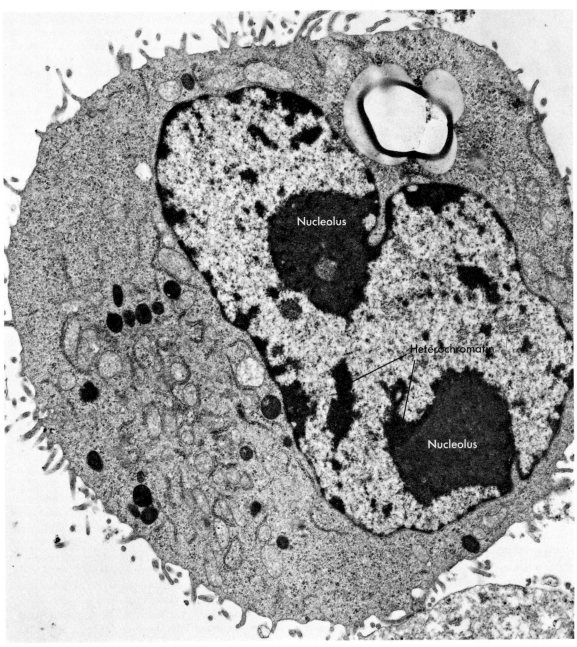

FIGURE 1-14 Tumor cell (Ehrlich's ascites tumor). The nucleus is somewhat irregular in shape and deeply indented at one point. Heterochromatin, densely stained, is present against the inner surface of the nuclear membrane and upon the nucleolus. Two nucleoli are present. They are darkly stained, but not as dense as the chromatin. The cell has been fixed in glutaraldehyde and osmium textroxide and stained with both lead and uranyl acetate. ×13,000. (From the work of A. Monneron.)

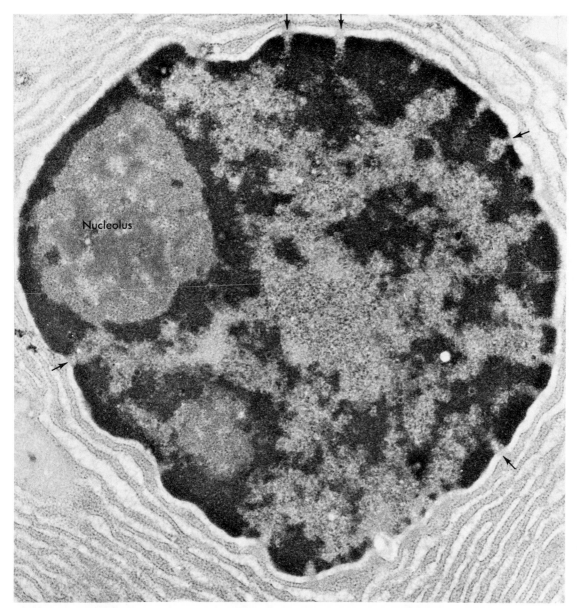

FIGURE 1-15 Pancreatic acinar cell. The nucleus of this cell, which secretes digestive enzymes, has been selectively treated to enhance the staining of DNA and to reduce the staining of the nucleoli and other RNA-containing structures. Chromatin is densely stained. Much of it is marginated on the inner surface of the nuclear membrane. Nuclear pores are prominent (arrow), their location marked by the lightly stained aisles between heterochromatin masses. The section was treated with picric acid, uranyl acetate, and lead. ×30,000. (From the work of A. Monneron.)

DNA filaments or complexing of DNA with histones or other substances.

NUCLEOLUS

A nucleolus is a discrete intranuclear structure consisting largely of protein and RNA whose function is the synthesis of the major components of ribosomes. The nucleolus is well developed in cells active in protein synthesis. Such cells may contain several nu-

cleoli. In cells inactive in protein synthesis, as spermatocytes and muscle cells, a nucleolus may not be evident. Nucleoli appear at certain specific sites in certain chromosomes, the *nucleolar organizing sites* (Fig. 1-17). These sites are secondary constrictions in the chromosomes. They represent the location on the chromosomes of the gene sequences (cistrons) which

FIGURE 1-16 Pancreatic acinar cell. The chromatin stands out sharply in this nucleus, having been stained with uranyl acetate and lead. The nucleolus and other RNA-containing structures are poorly stained because the section was treated with ribonuclease which digested away the RNA. The tissue was embedded in water-soluble methacrylate, an embedding medium which permits penetration of the ribonuclease. ×30,000 (From the work of A. Monneron.)

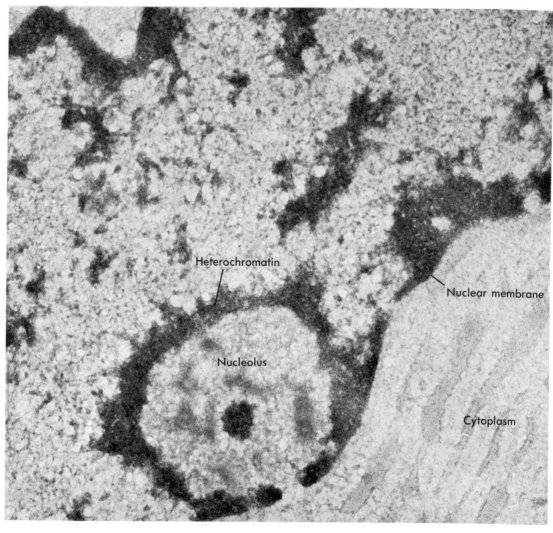

Wild
type

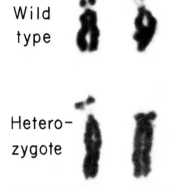

Hetero-
zygote

FIGURE 1-17 Chromosomes containing nucleolar organizing sites from the clawed toad *Xenopus laevis*. They are taken from the metaphase karyotype (see text). Each of the chromosomes in the wild type contains very slender zones, the nucleolar organizing sites. In the heterozygote, on the other hand, only one pair of chromosomes contains this site. The result in heterozygotes, as discussed in the text, is nucleolar-deficient mutants. (From the work of D. D. Brown.)

encode the genetic information for the synthesis of ribosomal RNA. Nucleoli remain attached to the chromosomes at nucleolar organizing sites.

Light Microscopy

Nucleoli by light microscopy are often dense, clearly outlined structures up to 1 μm or more in size (Figs. 1-18 and 1-19). They have a characteristic structure dependent upon cell type and activity. Often they are spherical, but they may be oval or even bow-tie-shaped. They are usually compact and sharply outlined, but they may be porous with fuzzy borders. Nucleoli may lie at random in the nucleus or against the inside of the nuclear membrane, an efficient location for the discharge of substances into the cytoplasm.

Nucleoli are demonstrated cytochemically by methods for RNA. Thus the nucleolus absorbs at about 2600 Å, in the ultraviolet. It is stained with pyronin in the methyl green-pyronin mixture and is blue in Romanovsky blood stains. RNA contains the characteristic nucleotide base uridine. DNA does not. Therefore, if radioactive uridine is given an animal, autoradiography of its cells shows positive nucleoli, because of the high concentration of RNA in nucleoli and the selective uptake of uridine (Fig. 1-20). Selective demonstration of nucleoli by staining or other means is not possible after pretreatment of the section with ribonuclease. A threadlike structure, the *nu-*

cleolonema, may be demonstrated in the nucleolus by silver or other selective stain. Although its composition is not yet known, and its significance is in doubt, it may be predominantly RNA.

Electron Microscopy

By electron microscopy, nucleoli contain two forms of RNA. One is granular, approximately 150 Å in diameter, similar but not identical to ribosomes. This form is typically the dominant nucleolar structure. The second form of RNA is fibrillar, 50 to 80 Å in thickness; the fibrils are probably precursor to the granules.

Nucleoli are not the only sites of RNP in the nucleus. Particles of different sizes and filaments of RNP lie against and between chromatin. It is likely that some of this widely dispersed nuclear RNA is mRNA (see below) produced on extended segments of DNA (euchromatin).

DNA is also present as a component of the nucleolus and has been designated *nucleolar chromatin.* It occurs in twisted or single filaments 200 to 300 Å in diameter.

Poorly defined granular material, probably protein, occurs throughout nucleoli. Rarefied vacuolar zones, not membrane-bounded, occur. Nucleoli are not confined by a membrane.

Functions

The nucleolus, a site of considerable molecular traffic, is a center for the synthesis of ribosomes. The size and number of nucleoli depend upon the level of ribosomal RNA synthesis. In actively synthesizing secretory cells (pancreatic acinar cells) the nucleoli are large and multiple, whereas in cells showing a low level of protein synthesis (muscle cells, certain small lymphocytes) nucleoli may be small or absent.

Ribosomes have several subunits (see section on Ribosomes). It appears, on the basis of isolation of nucleoli and sedimentation analysis, that they produce the subunits of ribosomes, and release them to the cytoplasm. It is likely that the release to the cytoplasm is facilitated by the nucleolus moving against the nuclear membrane and discharging through nuclear pores. Once in the cytoplasm, the nucleolar-produced ribosomal components may mature further, perhaps by adding protein, and combine to form ribosomes.

Support for the role of nucleoli in ribosomal synthesis comes from the work of Brown and his associates (1965) on amphibian mutants lacking nucleoli (Figs. 1-11 and 1-17). The embryo of the clawed toad, *Xenopus laevis,* synthesizes few ribosomes before the tail bud stage, the ribosomes from the oocyte serving until that time. A lethal anucleolate mutant of *Xenopus* may be bred from a spontaneously occurring heterozygote mutant with but one nucleolus per cell, instead of the normal two. Development of the anucleolate embryos is retarded after hatching. The embryos are microcephalic and edematous and die before feeding. The mutation which prevents the for-

mation of a normal nucleolus also prevents the synthesis of 28S and 18S ribosomal RNA, as well as high-molecular-weight ribosomal RNA precursor molecules.

The correlation between ribosome production and nucleoli is evident in multinucleolate amphibian oocytes where the DNA specifying the sequences for 28S and 18S ribosomal RNAs is selectively replicated. As many as 1000 nucleoli may occur per oocyte (Fig. 1-17)! Each of these nucleoli is analogous to the nucleoli of somatic cells and is an autonomous site for the synthesis of ribosomal RNA.

FIGURE 1-18 Rhesus kidney cell (strain MA 104) in culture. The nucleolus, stained with uranyl acetate and lead, is well developed. ×40,000. (From the work of A. Monneron.)

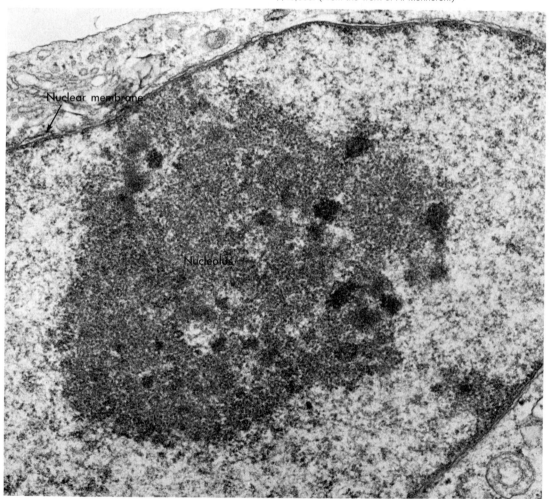

The nuclear membrane or envelope stands for a major evolutionary change, the development of eukaryotic organisms. In prokaryotic organisms such as bacteria,

nuclear material, although zonal, lies unseparated from the remainder of the protoplasm. In the higher fungi and on the eukaryotes, the nucleus becomes a discrete unit bounded by a complex discriminatory envelope.

The envelope consists of two concentric unit membranes. Each is approximately 70 Å in thickness, the inner one somewhat thinner. The space or cisterna

FIGURE 1-19 Hepatocyte. In this preparation RNP is preferentially stained and chromatin is bleached. The nucleolus stands out sharply. Stained granules, presumably containing RNA, lie outside the nucleolus in association with the chromatin. There are large (400 to 500 Å) perichromatin granules and small (200 Å) interchromatin granules. ×27,000. (From the work of A. Monneron; see also W. Bernhard, *J. Ultrastruct. Res.*, **27:**250, 1969.)

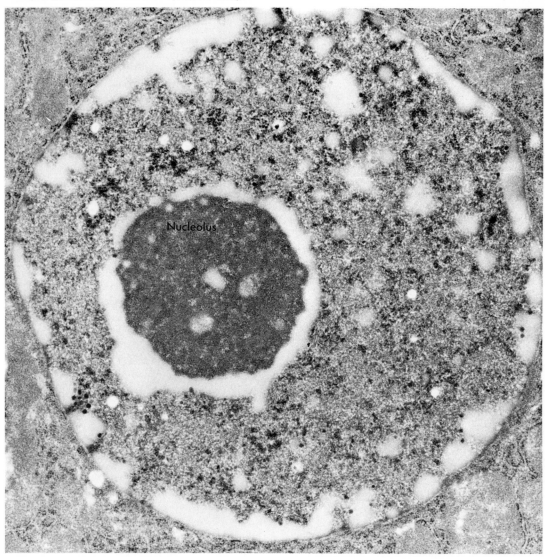

between inner and outer nuclear membranes varies in size and content. It is commonly about 150 Å wide and lucent. The outer nuclear membrane is continuous with the ER, both rough and smooth. The continuity of the outer nuclear membrane with the ER establishes the cytoplasmic character of these membranes. This character is underscored in the re-formation of nuclear membranes in the telophase. The nuclear membranes are clearly formed by segments of ER which line up around the reconstituted nuclear mass. In cells synthesizing protein the nuclear enve-

FIGURE 1-20 Monkey kidney cells (strain BSC). These cells, in tissue culture, were exposed to [³H] uridine (a precursor of RNA) for 30 min and then fixed and processed for EM autoradiography. The distribution of silver grains is only over the nucleus and mainly over the nucleolus. ×25,000. (From A. Monneron, J. Burglen, and W. Bernhard, *J. Ultrastruct. Res.,* **32:**370, 1970.)

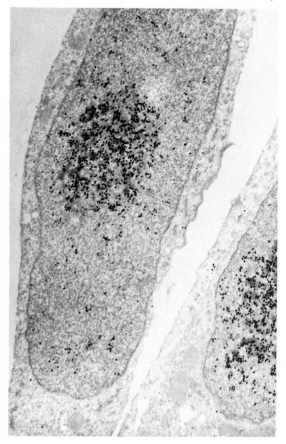

lope may, like the rough ER, contain the protein product. Thus, in antibody-producing cells the nuclear envelope may be distended with antibody and, indeed, is among the first places antibody accumulates. The chromosomes during the first meiotic prophase may be attached to the inner surface of the inner membrane and nucleoli may lie there (see above). Although the nuclear envelope cannot be resolved by light microscopy, its location is often revealed as a definite line representing the sum of the nuclear membranes, nuclear cisterna, and adherent material.

Nuclear pore complexes represent interruptions in the membranous structure of the nuclear membranes (Fig. 1-21). At a pore complex the inner and outer nuclear membranes appear to fuse and their margins thicken to form an *annulus* as great as 1000 Å in outside diameter and 600 Å inside. On surface view it is circular or octagonal in outline. By low-power electron microscopy the pore complex may appear as an aperture in the nuclear membranes with a thickened annulus, closed by a thin diaphragm which often contains a central granule. At high resolution the complex appears to be a granular and filamentous structure wherein eight regularly spaced granules, each about 100 Å in diameter, lie in the rim, perhaps in some matrical material. There is, moreover, a central granule or rod connected by filaments to the wall of the complex or to the annular granules. The granules, including the central one, may consist of particulate material or of condensed filaments.

There are very few cell types, such as the spermatozoa of bulls, which have few or even no nuclear pore complexes. In other cell types, 3 to 35 percent of the nuclear surface may be covered by complexes. They may be distributed over the whole nuclear surface or be clustered. They may lie irregularly or regularly, falling into square or hexagonal arrays.

Intuitively, nuclear pore complexes would seem to represent passageways, albeit encumbered ones, between nucleus and cytoplasm. There is, however, no experimental evidence for their functions.

ANNULATE LAMELLAE

In many cell types stacks of membranes which exactly resemble portions of nuclear membranes, pore complexes and all, may be found in the cytoplasm (Figs. 1-22 and 1-23). In certain germ cells they may be present in nucleoplasm. These membranes are termed *annulate lamellae* and are especially common in germ cells and in some tumor cells. They may be present in

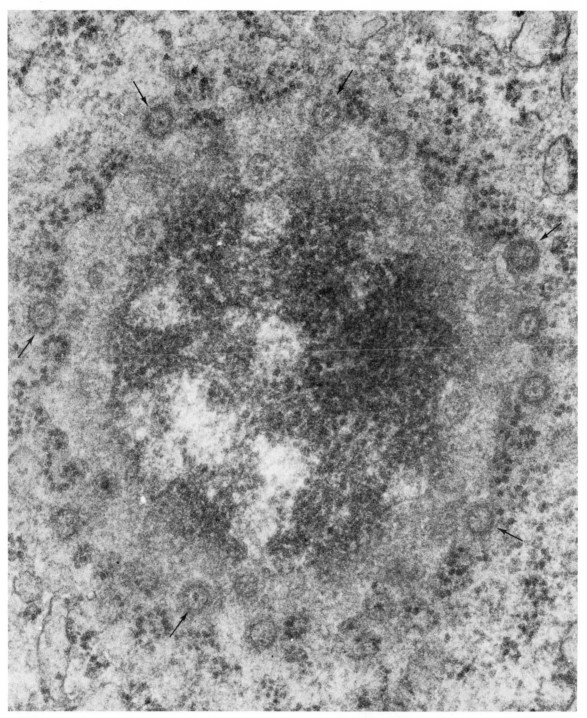

FIGURE 1-21 Rat hepatocyte. This is a tangential section of the nucleus, revealing nuclear pores all around (arrow), some with a dark central granule. Note that polyribosomes are in close association with the pores. This preparation is stained with uranyl acetate and lead. ×140,000. (From the work of A. Monneron.)

varying concentrations and in different parts of the cytoplasm and may be continuous with the endoplasmic reticulum (see below). Their significance is not known. It has been suggested that they may excise a type of nuclear control in parts of the cytoplasm distant from the nucleus.

THE CYTOPLASM

The cytoplasm surrounds the nucleus and is bounded

by the plasma membrane or plasmalemma. The cytoplasm is capable of energy formation and release, of protein synthesis, growth, motility, phagocytosis, and diverse other functions. It is dependent upon the nucleus for direction, renewal, and regeneration. Thus

FIGURE 1-22 Nuclear pores and annulate lamellae. The nucleus in the left upper corner is bounded by a double membrane, each component consisting of a unit membrane (see text). Within the nucleus, densely stained chromatin is arranged against the nuclear membrane, in which two nuclear pores (np) are present. Within the cytoplasm, occupying much of the field, are stacks of annulate lamellae. These appear identical in structure with the nuclear membrane and, like the nuclear membrane, have frequently spaced pore complexes. ×65,000. (From G. Maul, *J. Cell Biol.,* **46:**604, 1970.)

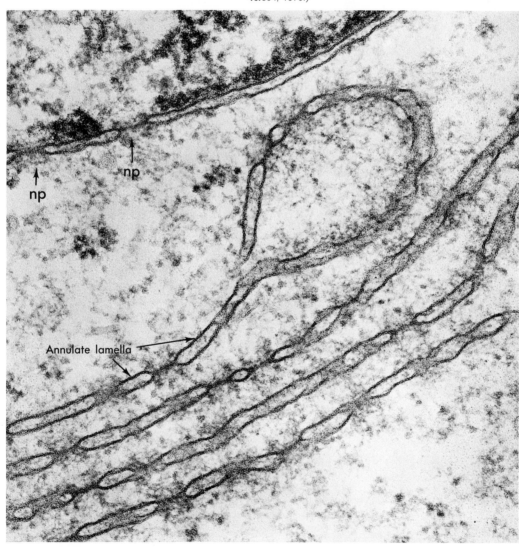

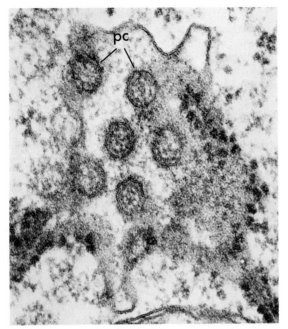

FIGURE 1-23 Annulate lamellae. In this face-on section, surface views of the pore complexes (pc) are presented. The pores appear limited by a unit membrane and have a complex, regular internal structure. ×65,000. (From G. Maul, *J. Cell Biol.,* **46:**604, 1970.)

Several zones may be recognized in cytoplasm. The cytoplasm in the center of the cell, next to the nucleus, may be gelated. It contains the centrioles and centrosphere but is usually clear of other organelles, and it is surrounded by the Golgi apparatus. Often it pushes the nucleus aside, deforming it into a U-shaped or reniform structure. This zone is designated the *cell center* or *cytocentrum*. Peripheral to this is a rather solvated part of the cell in which many vacuoles and granules, mitochondria, and elements of the endoplasmic reticulum are present. Active cytoplasmic streaming occurs here, carrying the cytoplasmic organelles in rapid movement. This zone is designated *endoplasm.* The peripheral cytoplasm in many cell types, particularly in free or motile cells, is gelated and free of organelles. This zone is the *ectoplasm.* The cytoplasm is capable of rapid sol-gel transformations. Areas of gelation of the ectoplasm may break down, particularly in motile cells or cells extending pseudopodial processes, and the solvated endoplasm bearing organelles then flows in.

BIOLOGICAL MEMBRANES

Membranes are essential to cells. They are broad, metabolically active sheets which enclose the cell as the *plasma membrane* and occur within the metazoan cell as *nuclear membranes, endoplasmic reticulum, Golgi membranes,* and such others as the membranes enclosing pinocytotic and phagocytic vacuoles. Membranes clearly bound or compartmentalize elements of the cell as the nucleus and indeed the cell itself. The organization and many of the functions of the cell depend upon its membranes. These functions include the secretion of protein, the synthesis of fat, the detoxification of certain drugs, the control of phagocytosis, the respiratory functions of mitochondria, and active transport.

The plasma membrane is the outer limit of the living cell and its face to the environment. It possesses distinctive and vital functions. It rigorously controls the readiness or difficulty by which substances enter the cell, providing *selective permeability* for the cell. The plasma membrane contains many and diverse receptor molecules in its surface which form linkages with outside substances. Some receptors occur in virtually *every* cell type; others vary with the cell type. The degree of selectivity and affinity of the receptor vary.

isolated units of cytoplasm, exemplified by blood platelets and mature erythrocytes, are capable of protein synthesis and of such specific functions as respiration and the retraction of blood clots. But the cytoplasmic structures, as membranes and microfilaments, which are the basis of such cytoplasmic functions, were synthesized and accumulated in the cytoplasm from ribosomes and other materials derived from a viable nucleus present at an early phase in the life cycle of these anucleated structures. The volume of cytoplasm in proportion to the nucleus, the *nuclear-cytoplasmic ratio,* varies considerably from cell type to cell type. In some cells, such as the spermatozoa, the cytoplasm is scant and, structurally, highly specialized, whereas in others, such as the lymphocytes, it is scant and apparently unspecialized. In most cells the cytoplasm is relatively abundant, exceeding the nuclear volume by a factor of 3 to 5 or more. The cytoplasm possesses several distinctive organelles with specialized functions of protein synthesis, energy production, etc. They lie in the ground substance or hyaloplasm. The volume of cytoplasm and its functions are determined by the number and nature of its organelles.

In the case of antibody molecules which function as receptors on the cell surface of lymphocytes, for example, selectivity for such outside substances, namely antigens, may be quite specific. These receptors are the key to essential cell functions, such as, in the above example, antibody production. Metabolic control of cells, the actions of hormones and of toxins, and such phenomena as cellular differentiation depend upon the mediation of receptors in the plasma membrane. The capacity of cells to interact with one another to form tissue and to "home" to distinctive sites is controlled by the plasma membrane. Again with respect to lymphocytes, these circulating cells move through blood and lymphatic vessels in definite pathways. Within lymphatic tissue, moreover, they lie in specific sites and associate with certain cell types. The capacities for cellular association and for controlled migration depend upon the carbohydrate *sialic acid,* which is linked to protein in the lymphocyte plasma membrane. If this carbohydrate is removed as it may be by the action of the enzyme neuriminidase, lymphocytes will lose their distinctive capacity for homing and aggregating. The phenomenon of *contact inhibition* is related to properties of the cell surface. Normal cells, as can be shown in tissue culture, cease to grow or move away on establishing contact with other cells; they show contact inhibition. Malignant cells, on the other hand, are not inhibited but continue to move over other cells. This phenomenon appears to be mediated by substances in the plasma membrane. The plasma membrane is thus necessary for cells to specialize and to interact with other cells in the formation of multicellular organisms.

Plasma membranes, as other membranes, are complex and diverse. Their composition and functions have been studied by a number of techniques. They can be isolated by cell disruption followed by differential centrifugation. The techniques of x-ray diffraction, freeze-fracture-etch, and microchemistry are among those which are applied to membranes. The erythrocyte plasma membrane has been one of the most extensively studied because large amounts can be easily prepared. As is the case with most membranes, it is preponderantly protein (50 to 60 percent of dry weight). This reflects high metabolic activity and structural stability. A notable exception is the lipid-rich membrane of myelinated nerves, whose high concentration of myelin appears to serve as an insulator. The

majority of proteins, associated with cell membranes, are regarded as intrinsic to the membrane since they can be removed only by drastic procedures of extraction, digestion, or denaturation. The remainder of the protein is easily removed and thus considered extrinsic. Intrinsic or extrinsic proteins include structural proteins, enzymes, and receptor substances. Many of these proteins, notably the intrinsic ones, appear to be *amphipathic,* that is, asymmetric or polarized with hydrophilic groups at one pole and hydrophobic groups at the other. The implications of amphipathety are discussed below.

Lipids are a second major component of membranes, representing 20 to 30 percent of the dry weight of membranes of erythrocytes. Lipid accounts for certain permeability characteristics of plasma membrane. Thus, fat-soluble compounds may readily enter cells, whereas fat-insoluble compounds enter with difficulty. The dominant lipid in the cell membrane is phospholipid, which is amphipathic, since the glycerol end is water-soluble, carrying as it does phosphate and other ionized groups, whereas the fatty acid end is not, being lipid-soluble and hydrophobic. Other lipids include cholesterol and a minor component linked to protein or carbohydrate as lipoprotein or liposaccharides. Carbohydrate accounts for less than 10 percent of the weight of plasma membranes in most cells studied. It may be free as oligosaccharide or linked to protein or fat. Carbohydrate moieties may function as receptor molecules and in such phenomena as homing and cell degradation.

The structure and organization of plasma membranes and of other cell membranes are subjects of intensive study in cell biology (Figs. 1-24 to 1-32). By conventional transmission electron microscopy the plasma membrane is approximately 75 Å in thickness with a range of about 60 to 90 Å. As with most intracellular membranes, it is seen as a trilaminar structure, termed the *unit membrane,* with outer darker lines approximately 20 Å in width (Fig. 1-24). With very high resolutions, suggestions of bridges across the lucent central zone or of granular structures within the membrane may be present, but usually little or no specialization is evident in the unit membrane as seen in sectioned material. By negative staining there are membranes which do display distinctive structures such as the mitochondrial membranes (see below); but plasma membranes do not. Perhaps the most valuable morphologic technique in revealing membrane structure is freeze-fracture-etch (see above). By this method membranes are typically split into outer and inner leaflets, the split tending to occur in the central lucent zone (Fig. 1-25). A major finding in such material is that membranes are heterogeneous. Large numbers of particles may be seen on the split surface of the plasma membrane and other membranes. The number, size, and pattern of these particles differ from place to place in a given membrane and from membrane to membrane. By the use of labeled antibodies or other cytochemical procedures, it is evident that at least certain of these particles are protein. ATPase and adenylate cyclase are membrane proteins.

A number of models for the organization of the plasma membrane have evolved. That of Singer and Nicholson has received wide support (Fig. 1-25). As is the case with many other models, it postulates a lipid bilayer consisting primarily of phospholipid molecules oriented with their hydrophilic ends directed out to the outside and to the inside surfaces. Being hydrophilic, the surfaces of the membrane thus interact with watery environments. Within the membrane, on the other hand, lie the long-chain nonpolar hydrocarbon por-

tions of the fatty acid constituents of the phospholipid bilayer. The internum of the membrane is, therefore, fatty and hydrophobic. The phospholipid constituents of the outside and inside surfaces of the membrane, moreover, are somewhat different. Cholesterol molecules are dispersed through the membrane. Lying in the phospholipid bilayer like "icebergs in a lipid sea" are the proteins. These proteins are likely amphipathic, as discussed above, with their hydrophobic ends lying within the membrane among the hydrophobic fatty acids and the hydrophilic pole protruding from the outside or inside hydrophilic surface of the membrane. Certain intrinsic proteins are longer than the width of the membrane and, therefore, cross it protruding from both inside and outside surfaces. These proteins are presumably hydrophilic at the ends and hydrophobic in the center. There are places in some membranes as the *synaptosome* of nerve and

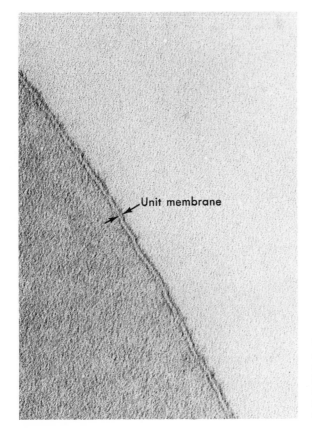

FIGURE 1-24 Erythrocyte, peripheral cytoplasm. Note the trilaminar character of the plasmalemma, there being two dark laminae separated by a light one. This membrane is a unit membrane. ×280,000. (From the work of J. D. Robertson.)

junctional complexes, where there are many proteins which may be closely linked to one another and the membrane is unusually rich in protein. In most instances, however, the proteins appear rather isolated from one another. Moreover, they appear to move about in the plane of the membrane. A notable experiment disclosing such movement involved the staining of certain receptor substances in the plasma membrane of the cells of the mouse with a fluorescent marker of one color and of cells of man with a fluorescent marker of another color. The plasma membranes, and thereby the cells, were then fused by the action of sendai virus. At first the labeled receptor substances remained apart, but within 40 min they appeared completely intermixed. The mixing was temperature-dependent, moreover, occurring at physiological temperature but inhibited at 4°C. This suggests simple diffusion as the basis of mixing. The antibody molecules in the surface of B lymphocytes which serve as receptors also move about in the plane of the membrane, as can be shown by their moving to one pole of the cell, *capping,* when cross-linked by antigen or other reagents (see Chap. 10). Other receptors are capable of being capped and are, therefore, mobile.

In addition to proteins which are intrinsic to the membrane, there are proteins, the extrinsic proteins, which are linked to the membrane. The actin-containing contractile protein, *spectrin,* appears attached to the inside surface of erythrocyte membranes. Certain proteins as cytochromes may be attached loosely to the outside surface of membranes. Carbohydrates are often present, attached to the outside surface of the plasma membrane. These include sialic acid and other glyco- or mucoproteins. The carbohydrate-rich extrinsic coat may be so heavy as to be visible as a fuzzy layer and can be selectively stained by ruthenium red or lanthanum (Fig. 1-28). If sufficiently thick, it can be visible by light microscopy stained by the periodic acid Schiff procedure. The carbohydrate-rich cover to cells has been designated *glycocalyx.* The sarcolemma of muscle and basal laminae in general may be regarded as sites of massive accumulation of glycoprotein extrinsic to the plasma membrane.

ENDOPLASMIC RETICULUM

The endoplasmic reticulum (ER) is a cytoplasmic system of tubules, vesicles, and sacs or cisternae fash-

FIGURE 1-25 Fluid mosaic model of cell membrane. The bulk of the phospholipids (solid circles represent polar head groups and wavy lines their fatty acid chains) are organized in a discontinuous lipid bilayer. Intrinsic or integral proteins are embedded in the bilayer but can protrude from the membrane. Extrinsic or peripheral proteins may bind to phospholipid polar head groups or to the membrane via protein-protein interactions. The arrow shows the position of the natural cleavage plane within the center of a lipid bilayer in freeze-fracture-etch techniques. (From R. S. Weinstein, ''The Red Blood Cell,'' p. 239, Academic Press, Inc., New York, 1974.)

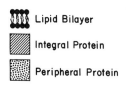

▓▓ Lipid Bilayer

▨ Integral Protein

▨ Peripheral Protein

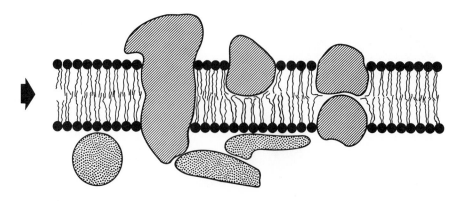

ioned of unit membranes. The ER is subject to characteristic variations in complexity and extent, depending upon cell type and cell function. It is continuous with the outer membrane of the nuclear envelope (Fig. 1-29).

The ER has been defined by electron microscopy, although it has been observed by light microscopy in some cells, notably as the *sarcoplasmic reticulum,* the specialized ER of striated muscle. The ER was first described in electron micrographs of fibroblasts in tissue culture examined as whole mounts without sectioning. Ordinarily whole cells are too thick for electron-microscopic study, but cells in culture may put out cytoplasmic processes thin enough to pass an electron beam. In such preparations a cytoplasmic network, the endoplasmic reticulum, may be seen (Fig. 1-30).

The ER is subject to specialization. Perhaps the most important is the differentiation of *rough* or *granular* ER (Fig. 1-31), with ribosomes on its outside surface, and *smooth* ER, whose surface is free of ribosomes. Ribosomes synthesize protein (see below) and need not be associated with ER. The association of ER and ribosomes occurs in cells which either secrete the protein they synthesize, or isolate it within membrane-bounded sacs. Thus in *polychromatophilic erythroblasts* which synthesize the pigmented respiratory protein *hemoglobin* that remains free in the cytoplasm, ribosomes are plentiful but little ER is present. In plasma cells, on the other hand, which synthesize large volumes of antibody protein, confine it by membranes, and then *secrete* it, rough ER is abundant. Peptide chains are synthesized in the ribosomes and sent across the ER membrane into the lumen of the

ER (see below). The ER thereby isolates synthesized material from the rest of the cytoplasm, permits further assembly of peptides into larger molecules, and channels the material into the Golgi where further synthesis, aggregation, complexing, condensation, and packaging occur. Although rough ER is well developed in secretory cells, it is also abundant in certain phases in the life cycle of cells which synthesize a protein product and hold it membrane-bounded within their cytoplasm, as in blood leukocytes and in macrophages. These cells contain enzyme-rich membrane-bounded granules. The formation of these granules parallels the formation of a secretory vacuole, except that the granules tend to be retained rather than released (secreted).

In nerve cells rough ER exists as large, flattened sacs lying upon one another in lamellated fashion to form masses, *Nissl bodies,* identifiable by light microscopy. Hepatic parenchymal cells contain smaller blocks of rough ER. In plasma cells the rough ER is rather uniformly distributed through the cytoplasm, except for the region of the cytocentrum. It may be tubular, vesicular, or flattened, depending upon the phase of antibody secretion. Rough ER occupies the base of the pancreatic acinar cell, its development varying with the secretory cycle. This rough ER, recognizable in light microscopy as basophilic material (because of the affinity of ribosomes for cationic dye), is termed *ergastoplasm.*

Smooth ER, free of ribosomes, occurs in a number of cell types and may have diverse functions. It

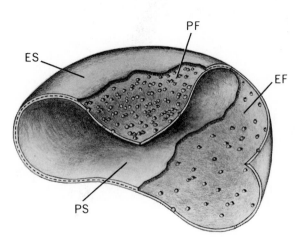

FIGURE 1-26 Diagrammatic representation of the four membrane "faces" that can be studied with the freeze-fracture-etch technique as shown on an erythrocyte. Note the terms used to designate the four surfaces: ES, the true outside surface of the plasma membrane; PS, the true inside surface of the plasma membrane; PF, the split surface of the plasma membrane which faces away from the cytoplasm; EF, the split surface of the plasma membrane which faces toward the cytoplasm. Particles, representing protein molecules, are shown only on faces PF and EF. (From R. S. Weinstein, "The Red Blood Cell," p. 247, Academic Press, Inc., New York, 1974.)

34

may well have a role in the production of steroid hormones since it is abundant in such cells as the Leydig cells of the testis which produce the steroid testosterone. There is evidence that smooth ER synthesizes complex lipids from fatty acids. It may be active in the detoxification of certain drugs, becoming very prominent in hepatocytes during the inactivation of phenobarbital by the liver, for example. In striated

FIGURE 1-27 Replicas of freeze-fractured human red cell membranes. (A) Freeze-fracture face PF originating from within the interior of the membrane shows more or less randomly distributed membrane-associated particles (MAP) which may represent sites of integral membrane proteins. ×120,000; (B) Face-EF has fewer MAP than face-PF. ×140,000; (C) Freeze-etching has exposed the true exterior surface of the red cell membrane (*) which appears barren and smooth. The fracture has entered the membrane (arrows) and exposed a PF-face for replication. ×100,000; (D) Small fibrils (arrows) apparently extend from the cytoplasm of intact cells into the interior of the cell membrane. ×90,000. (From R. S. Weinstein, "The Red Blood Cell," Academic Press, Inc., New York, 1974.)

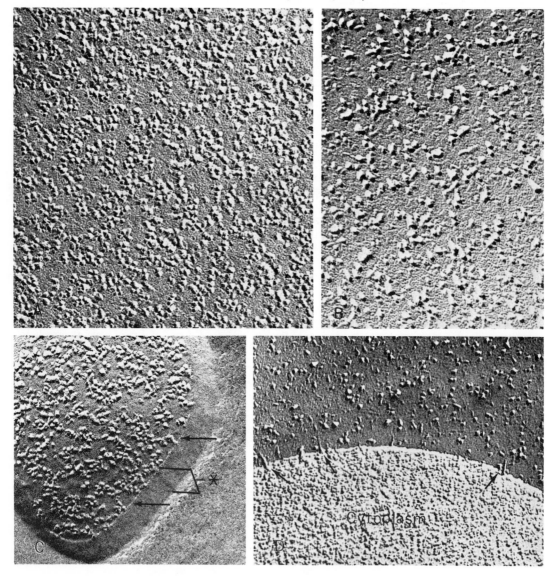

muscle, smooth ER is distinctively organized as the *sarcoplasmic reticulum* whose functions include the delivery of high concentrations of Ca^{2+} and other ions to critical places in the sarcomere for muscular contraction and relaxation. Smooth ER in megakaryocytes delimits platelet zones in the cytoplasm and, by fusing, frees platelets from the megakaryocyte. Carbohydrate synthesis is associated with smooth ER and the Golgi apparatus. The re-formation of the nuclear membrane in telophase is accomplished by smooth ER.

The smooth ER may be continuous with rough ER. Possibly the rough ER synthesizes the smooth. It is likely that ER is a dynamic system whose tubules may extend or retract and which may dilate into cisternae or separate into vesicles or vacuoles that lose continu-

ity with the main body. Indeed, the membranes of the ER appear to possess a self-healing capacity when disrupted. When ultracentrifugation fractions rich in ER are recovered from disrupted cells, the ER is found as small spheroid vesicles (*microsomes*) (Fig. 1-32). Evidently the tubular system is fragmented, but the membranes reunite or "heal" to form small vesicles. After fixation with osmium tetroxide, the tubular T system of sarcoplasmic reticulum is revealed as a system of vesicles—another example of the readiness with which the tubules of ER may be broken up and re-formed as small vesicles. See Chap. 7.

GOLGI APPARATUS

The Golgi apparatus or complex is a system of membranes and vesicles, usually located in the region of the cytocentrum. It is active in processing proteins

FIGURE 1-28 Cell surface, human buccal epithelium; electron micrograph. The free surface of an epithelial cell having large and small villi (v) is shown. A surface coat has been stained selectively with the dye ruthenium red. The coat, where it lies upon the plasmalemma, is relatively dense. On its free surface, on the other hand, the surface coat has a flocculent or filamentous character. ×40,000. (From John Luft, *Anat. Rec.*, **171**:347, 1971.)

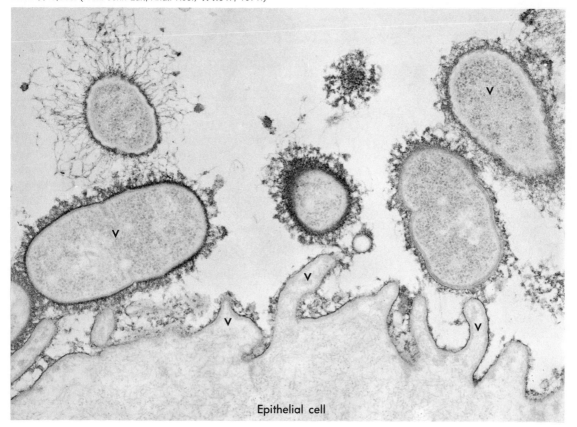

Epithelial cell

which are secreted or which remain membrane-bounded within a cell, in distinction to those proteins, such as hemoglobin and keratin, which lie free in the

FIGURE 1-29 Connective tissue cell from human embryo spleen. Here the continuity of the outer nuclear membrane and the smooth ER is evident. Thus the perinuclear space and the lumen of the ER are continuous. ×12,000.

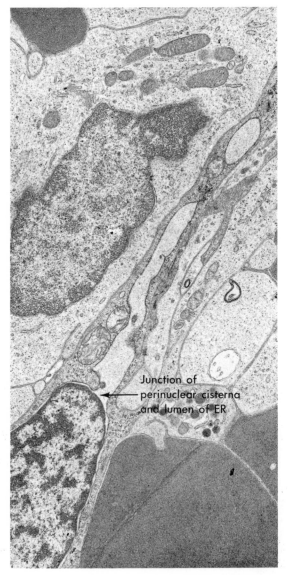

Junction of perinuclear cisterna and lumen of ER

cytoplasm. It is associated with the synthesis of lipoprotein and of glycoprotein.

Light Microscopy

The Golgi complex has a characteristic appearance by light microscopy. It may be a small compact structure; it may be a cluster of small structures (termed *dicytosomes* in earlier literature); or it may be a large netlike structure, the *internal reticular apparatus* as initially defined by C. Golgi in nerve cells. The Golgi is often juxtanuclear and, in the intestinal epithelium, for example, lies toward the apical surface. It may partially enclose the centrioles. Its size fluctuates with cell type and cell activity. It is well developed in secretory cells, especially in the mucus-producing intestinal epithelial cells which elaborate a product rich in carbohydrate. It is subject to waxing and waning during the secretory cycle. The Golgi has the capacity to reduce metal salts, such as salts of osmium and of silver (Figs. 1-6 and 1-33), and may, therefore, be stained with these compounds. In such polarized secretory cells as the mucus-producing intestinal epithelial cells where one major product is produced and follows a distinct secretory pathway within the cell toward its apical surface, the Golgi is present as a large reticular apparatus. On the other hand, in secretory cells, such as hepatocytes, elaborating diverse products released or stored in different places in the cell, there may be a number of Golgi complexes.

Electron Microscopy

By electron microscopy the Golgi is fabricated of unit membranes about 60 Å thick, thinner than the plasmalemma and even the ER (Figs. 1-34 to 1-37). The proximal membranes (those facing the nucleus) are thinner than the distal (those facing out toward the bulk of the cytoplasm), which are more like those of plasmalemma and ER. The Golgi apparatus contains large flat sacs or cisternae lamellated on one another. They are relatively compressed at their centers and somewhat dilated peripherally. The sacs tend to be bowed, presenting a convex proximal face and concave distal face. These cisternae thus form bowl-shaped structures. The Golgi apparatus therefore looks like a stack of shallow bowls with the concavity directed away from the nucleus. The cisternae communicate with one another by slender channels at places along their contiguous surfaces. At the edge of the lamellated sacs, near their expanded peripheries, vesicles 400 to 800 Å in diameter are typically present. Some contain dense lipoidal material. Similar vesicles may also be abundant at the distal face. These vesicles may be attached to the most superficial sac. The vesicles vary in size and probably fuse to form larger vesicles. They, like the lateral vesicles, may contain a dense material. The proximal face (toward the nucleus) is relatively free of vesicles and has been termed the *forming face*, but in certain cell types, notably leukocytes, this face is active in a distinct type of membrane-bounded granule formation. The distal

face (away from the nucleus), which is typically engaged in granule and vacuole formation, has been termed the *maturation face*.

Peptides destined to be secreted or enclosed by membrane into vesicles or granules are synthesized by ribosomes lying on the outside surface of ER. The peptides are collected within the luman of the rough ER, linked by peptide bonds into polypeptides, and move into contiguous ER free of ribosomes (Figs. 1-34 and 1-35). This smooth ER has been termed *transitional* ER since it has been considered contiguous with

FIGURE 1-30 Fibroblast, tissue culture. The preparation in this electron micrograph has not been sectioned. It is a whole mount of the cell, and only the peripheral region is sufficiently thin to permit passage of the electron beam. (From the work of K. R. Porter.)

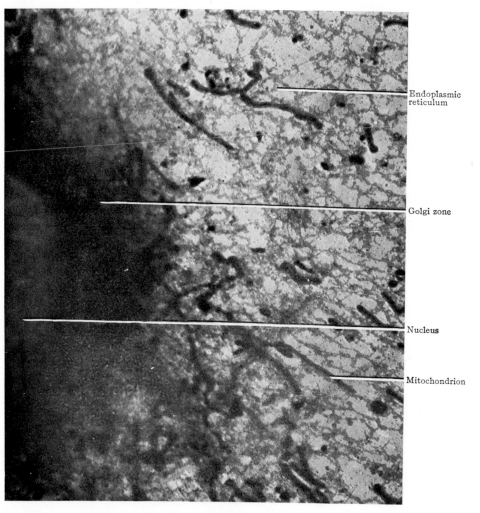

Endoplasmic reticulum

Golgi zone

Nucleus

Mitochondrion

the rough ER on the one side and the Golgi complex on the other and may convey the polypeptides synthesized by the rough ER to the Golgi. In fact, it may be that the transitional ER breaks up into vesicles, the *transport vesicles,* which carry the polypeptides to the Golgi. The Golgi saccules are rich in intrinsic enzymes and are active metabolically. They may process the polypeptides they receive from the transport vesicles in several ways, depending upon the cell type and the phase of the synthetic cycle. The Golgi complex may assemble polypeptide chains into proteins by disulfide bonds or other linkages. Many protein products of cells, moreover, are complexed to carbohydrate and become glycoproteins. Such is the case with immunoglobulins, the antibody proteins, and many pancreatic enzymes. The carbohydrate moiety is synthesized and affixed to the protein in the Golgi complex. The high concentration of the intrinsic enzyme *glycosyl transferase* on the inside surface of Golgi membranes reflects this function. Aliquots of this protein product are now enclosed by membrane at the forming face of the Golgi, resulting in *primary storage granules.* These move out from the Golgi. In epithelial cells they move toward the apical pole from which they will be secreted. The proteins in the primary storage granules become concentrated by as many as 25 times, and the granules may now be recgonized as *condensing vacuoles* or *granules.* Depending upon the cell type, the granules may remain within the cell, as the granules of

FIGURE 1-31 Hepatocyte of a rat. In this portion of the cytoplasm most of the cisternae of the rough ER were cut transversely (top), and others tangentially. In the latter (arrow) the membrane of the ER and the attached polysomes are seen *en face.* A section of a mitochondrion (mit) is present. ×64,000. (From the work of G. E. Palade.)

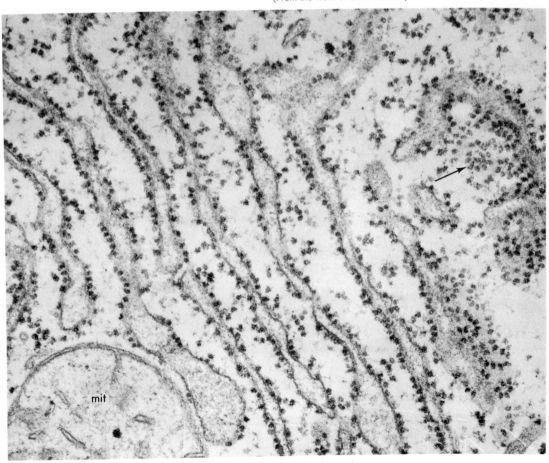

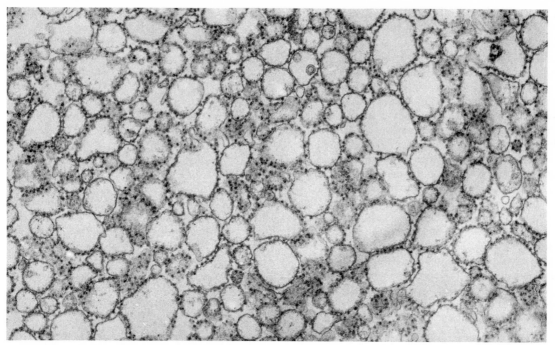

FIGURE 1-32 Microsomes of rat liver. The liver was disrupted and various fractions recovered by ultracentrifugation. This is the microsome fraction. It consists almost entirely of rough ER which had been disrupted and ''healed'' as vesicles. Ribosomes remain attached to the outer surface. ×40,000. (From the work of D. Sabatini and M. Adelman.)

leukocytes or as primary lysosomes, or they may become *secretory granules.* On secretion a granule moves toward the plasma membrane and its membrane fuses with the plasma membrane. At the site of fusion the membranes break down and the contents of the secretory granule are released from the cell. There are several patterns of secretion. In the case of the plasma cell, secretion is continuous and is characterized by small secretory granules, perhaps 50 nm in diameter. In the case of the pancreatic acinar cells, on the other hand, secretion is intermittent, dependent upon physiological stimuli associated with food ingestion. Here the secretory granules accumulate in the cell and may reach rather large size, up to 1500 nm in diameter.

The Golgi complex functions in lipoprotein synthesis. Lipids enter the Golgi cisternae from smooth ER where they are synthesized from fatty acids. In the Golgi they are complexed to protein produced in rough ER. Membrane-bounded lipoprotein granules

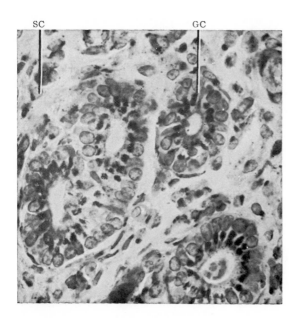

FIGURE 1-33 Golgi material in cells of guinea pig uterus. The Golgi material was blackened with silver by the method of Da Fano. Large quantities of it lie above the nuclei of the glandular cells (GC); smaller amounts lie next to the nuclei of the stromal cells (SC). ×500.

are then released from the Golgi (Figs. 1-34 and 1-35).

The major technique by which the sequences just given has been delineated is *pulse-chase electron-microscopic autoradiography*. Here a radioactive metabolite, such as an amino acid or sugar which will be incorporated into the product undergoing synthesis, is injected in a single rapidly administered dose into an experimental animal. This radioactively labeled compound now enters the metabolic pool. After a short time it is followed, or "chased," by the identical but nonradioactive compound which dilutes out the radioactive compound. As a result, a short, sharply delineated "pulse" of radioactively labeled metabolite enters the synthetic process and is carried through it. By sampling tissue at appropriate times and carrying out autoradiography, the radioactive complex is used to mark the sequence of intracellular sites associated in synthesis. By carrying out correlative microchemistry on such labeled cells, moreover, the level of synthesis can be ascertained.

The Golgi has been isolated by differential centrifugation and characterized cytochemically. It consists of approximately equal parts of lipid and protein and tends to be unusually rich in *nucleoside diphosphatases*. Histochemical demonstration of these phosphatases may serve as a marker for Golgi membranes.

RIBOSOMES[1]

Light Microscopy

A single ribosome is below the limit of resolution of the light microscope, but in aggregate, the presence of

---

[1]The section on ribosomes was revised by Dr. James A. Lake.

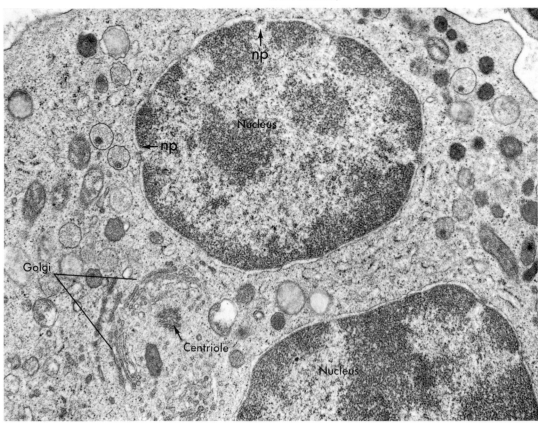

FIGURE 1-34 Human myelocyte. In this developing blood cell (see Chap. 11) the nucleus is lobed. Nuclear pores (np) are present. The cytoplasm contains granules, vesicles, rough and smooth ER, mitochondria, and free ribosomes. A Golgi apparatus is present, partially surrounding a centriole. ×26,000. (From the work of G. A. Ackerman.)

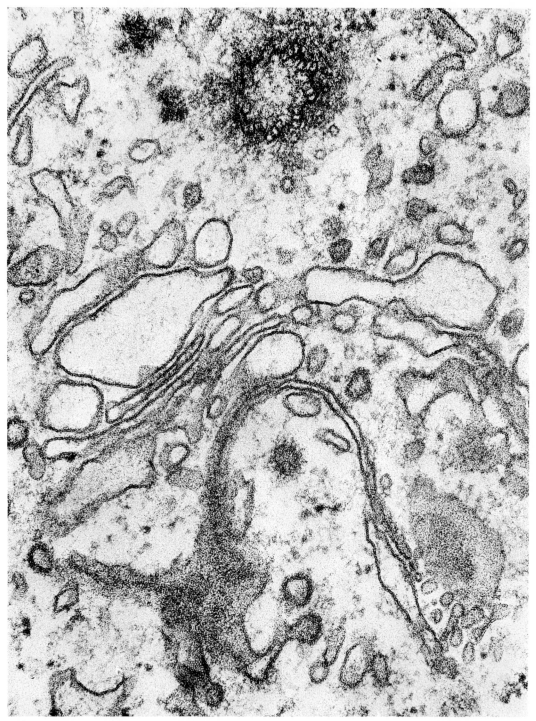

FIGURE 1-35 Golgi complex. It is evident, in this field, that the Golgi membranes and vesicles are made of the trilaminar unit membrane. A centriole is also present. (From the work of E. D. Hay and J. P. Revel.)

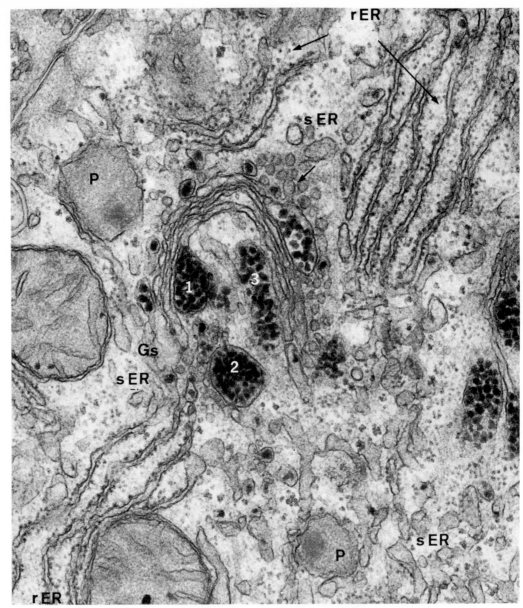

FIGURE 1-36 Golgi complex from a rat hepatocyte. The complex lies near the center of this field. The forming face of the Golgi, where the development of secretory product is initiated, is at the convex side of the apparatus, with extensions from the smooth ER network (sER) piling up from below and above, along the curved structure. This smooth ER is probably produced by the rough ER (rER) which surrounds the Golgi. The smooth ER may be continuous with the Golgi saccules or may break up into transport vesicles which move to the Golgi and fuse with it. A cluster of small vesicles, on top of the Golgi structure and next to a concentrating or secretory vesicle, is interpreted as representing cross sections of tubular, smooth ER extensions, with one of them (arrow) connecting with the concentrating vesicle. At the concave or maturing face of the Golgi three concentrating or secretory vesicles (1 to 3) are present. Each contains many small granules. At P, there are two peroxisomes (see text). Compare this process of lipoprotein granule formation with that of the formation of granules within leukocytes, described in Chap. 11. ×56,500. (From A. Claude, *J. Cell Biol.,* **47:**745, 1970.)

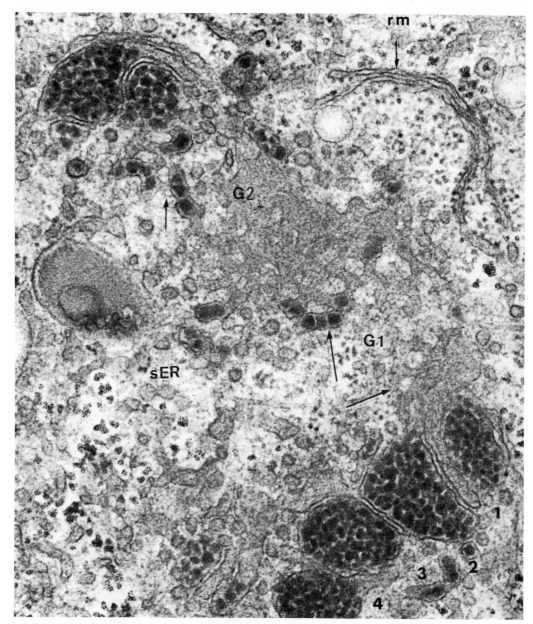

FIGURE 1-37 Golgi complex from a rat hepatocyte. Smooth-surfaced membranes (rm) similar to those in Fig. 1-36 are cut in cross section. As they are traced to the right they are continuous with rough ER. At G2 Golgi membranes at the forming surface are cut in a plane parallel to their surface. These membranes are fenestrated and, in all probability, are formed by coalescence of smooth ER (sER) tubules (arrows) carrying rows of dense lipoprotein granules. Four large concentrating or secretory vesicles are present (numbered 1 to 4). These would develop from the maturing face of the Golgi, corresponding to the concave portion in Fig. 1-36. ×67,800. (From A. Claude, *J. Cell Biol.,* **47:**745, 1970.)

ribosomes can be recognized. Owing, in all likelihood, to their PO_4^{3-} groups, they have a pronounced affinity for cationic or basic dyes such as methylene blue$^+$. As a result, cells rich in ribosomes are basophilic; this basophilia may be abolished by pretreament of the tissue with ribonuclease. The intensity and disposition of the basophilia are highly characteristic of cell type. The material by light microscopy has been designated *chromidial substance* or *ergastoplasm*. Consult the description of the *pancreatic acinar cells, lymphocytes,* and *erythroblasts* for a description of the patterns of chromidial substance.

Electron Microscopy

Ribosomes are flattened, spheroidal, complex cytoplasmic particles measuring approximately 150 × 250 Å which synthesize protein (Figs. 1-38 to 1-44). They consist of RNA and protein. Their RNA is classed as *ribosomal RNA,* which accounts for 85 percent of the RNA of the cell. In addition to this form of RNA, there is *messenger RNA* (mRNA) and *transfer RNA* (tRNA). The instruction for protein synthesis is encoded in DNA. This information is transcribed to messenger RNA, which is about 300 to 600 nm long, depending upon the protein. Messenger RNA is produced in the nucleus, on a template of uncoiled DNA. It moves to the cytoplasm where it associates itself with

ribosomes that lie along the mRNA like beads on a necklace. Ribosomes occurring singly in the cytoplasm are not active; only when they are linked by mRNA to form *polyribosomes* do they play a part in protein synthesis. The ribosomes are the small machines which receive the amino acid constituents of protein, assemble them into peptide chains, and release these chains into the cytoplasm or into the lumen of the ER where they continue to aggregate to form protein. The amino acids are brought to the ribosomes by tRNA, a low-molecular-weight nucleic acid (see below) that may be produced in the nucleolar region of the nucleus (as is ribosomal RNA) and passes out of the nucleus into the cytoplasm. There is a different tRNA for each of the amino acids. In protein synthesis, a ribosome moves along mRNA and reads the genetic message which has been transcribed from DNA. As the ribosome translates the message it binds on its surface the proper activated amino acyl-tRNA specified by the codon being read and synthesizes the peptide linkage of this amino acid to the earlier ones.

FIGURE 1-38 Ribosomes, hepatocyte, of a guinea pig. Ribosomes at high magnification show a larger and smaller component. When associated with the ER, the larger component lies upon the membrane. In this field a single cisterna (c) of the ER is present. The arrows indicate the position and orientation of the partitions separating the large from the small subunits of the ribosomes. Note that these partitions lie generally parallel to the surface of the membranes (m). This specimen was fixed in osmium tetroxide, embedded, sectioned, and stained with uranyl acetate. ×270,000. (From the work of D. Sabatini, Y. Toshiro, and G. E. Palade.)

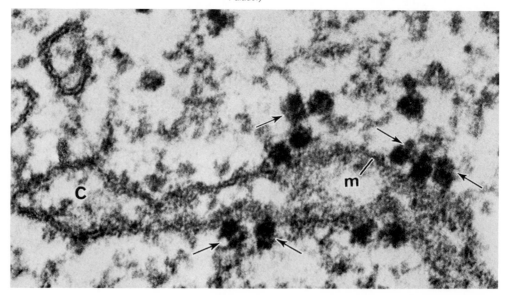

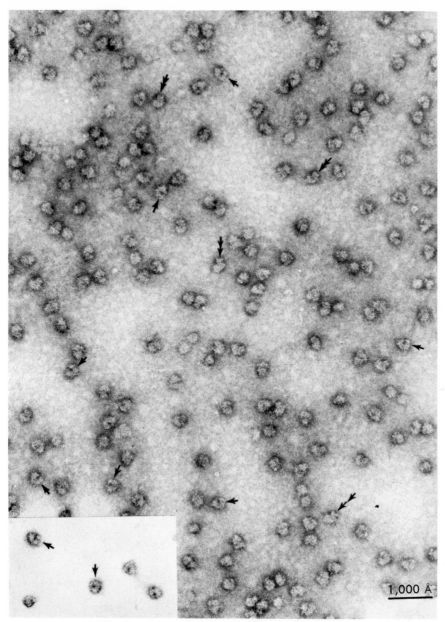

FIGURE 1-39 Ribosomes of a guinea pig. General view of a field of native monomeric ribosomes. Several image types are predominant. Frontal images (arrows) have an elongated small subunit profile and a dense spot toward the side of the separation between subunits. All frontal images in the field have this spot to the left of the observer if the particle image is oriented with the elongated small subunit horizontally and toward the top. In lateral images (double arrows) the small subunit produces a small rounded or rectangular profile toward one side of the large subunit profile. The insert shows images of monomeric ribosomes, reconstituted in vitro from the isolated large and small subunits. This preparation was made from ribosomes isolated by differential centrifugation of disrupted cells. The ribosomes were then floated on a membrane-covered electron-microscopic grid, dried, and negatively stained with phosphotungstic acid. ×125,000. (From the work of D. Sabatini, Y. Nonomura, and G. Blobel.)

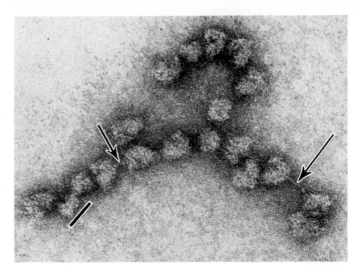

FIGURE 1-40 Ribosomes of a guinea pig. Here a strand of messenger RNA (arrows) links ribosomes into a polyribosomal unit. The mRNA runs between the small and large subunits. ×240,000. (From the work of D. Sabatini, Y. Nonomura, and G. Blobel.)

The peptide chain grows larger as the ribosome moves along the mRNA, and as the ribosome slides off the mRNA, it releases the peptide chain. As one ribosome slides off one end of the mRNA, another slides onto the other end and several ribosomes "read" or translate the mRNA at any time. The ribosomes lie on the mRNA approximately 340 Å apart (Fig. 1-40). For a polypeptide chain of hemoglobin 150 amino acids long, 1 to $1\frac{1}{2}$ min is required for the ribosome to run the length of mRNA.

The ribosome is composed of two unequal sub-

units, a large and a small subunit. Both are highly organized macromolecular assemblies consisting of one or more RNA molecules and numerous different proteins. In humans, as in most eukaryotes, the

FIGURE 1-41 An electron micrograph of *E. coli* small ribosomal subunits reacted with antibodies directed against ribosomal protein S14. The antibodies attach at only a single region in the upper one-third of the subunit, and are indicated by arrows. The centrally located pairs of subunits are connected by single IgG molecules, while the pair of subunits on the left is connected by two different IgG molecules, both attached to the same region of the subunit surface. (From the work of J. Lake, M. Pendergast, L. Kahan, and M. Nomura.)

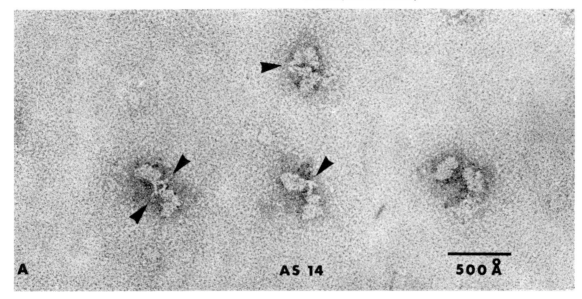

A   AS 14   500 Å

smaller subunit has a molecular weight of 1.5×10^6 daltons and is composed of a single molecule of RNA with a sedimentation constant of 18S and approximately 30 different, rather small (10,000 to 40,000 daltons) proteins. The small subunit functions in binding the messenger RNA to the ribosome and forms part of the tRNA binding site as the codon is being read by the anticodon of the tRNA. The larger subunit with a molecular weight of 3.0×10^6 daltons has a sedimentation constant of 60S and contains two RNA molecules (5S and 28S) and probably a third (5.8S). The approximately 40 different proteins contained in the large subunit are on the average slightly larger than those in the small subunit. The large subunit functions in protein synthesis by forming part of the tRNA binding sites, catalyzing peptidyl transfer, and holding the growing polypeptide chain. Ribosomes bound to the rough endoplasmic reticulum are attached through the large subunit (see Fig. 1-38). In bacteria, and prokary-

otes in general, ribosomes (70S) and their subunits (30S and 50S) are somewhat smaller. Bacterial ribosomes differ from eukaryotic ribosomes in their responses to antibiotics affecting protein synthesis. Some antibiotics, such as *puromycin,* inhibit protein synthesis on both prokaryotic and eukaryotic ribosomes; others, such as *streptomycin,* affect only prokaryotic ribosomes; and others, such as *cycloheximide,* affect only eukaryotic ribosomes. [The ribosomes found in the mitochondria of eukaryotes differ from others in their cytoplasm, since mitochondrial ribosomes resemble bacterial ribosomes in their responses to antibiotics. (see the discussion of mitochondria below.)] Eukaryotic and prokaryotic ribosomes have important similarities in spite of their differences. The sequence of events that occur during the protein synthesis cycle is the same in both eukaryotic and prokaryotic ribosomes, and although there are differences in size, ribosomes from both greatly resemble each other in gross morphology as observed in the electron microscope.

The structure of the ribosome is being studied intensively by electron microscopy, and the three-dimensional locations of specific ribosomal proteins are being mapped using antibodies directed against individual ribosomal proteins. In the electron micrograph of Fig. 1-41, small subunits of *E. coli* ribosomes have been reacted with antibodies against a protein (S14) thought to function in tRNA binding. Pairs of small subunits can be seen to be linked by either one

FIGURE 1-42 A diagrammatic representation of three views of the *E. coli* smaller ribosomal subunit illustrating the locations of some of the ribosomal proteins. The views from left to right represent rotations of the subunit about its long axis of 0°, 50°, and 110°, respectively. The cleft formed between the vertically oriented platform and the upper one-third of the subunit is best seen in the +50° view. The platform itself is attached to the lower two-thirds of the subunit. The vertical axis of the subunit is approximately 250 Å long. Many of the proteins are located at only a single region of the subunit but some, such as S4 and S19, are elongated and extend through the subunit. Three different regions of S4 are exposed and indicate that this protein must be at least 170 Å long. Protein S4 is required for the proper self–assembly of subunits and its extended nature may be related to its role in subunit assembly. (From the work of J. Lake, M. Nomura, and L. Kahan.)

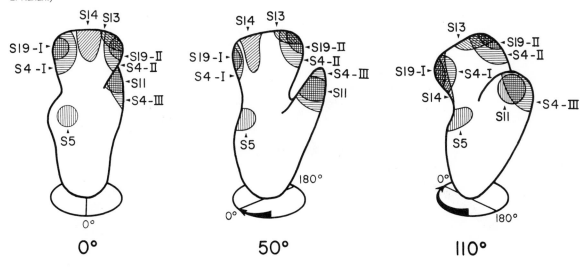

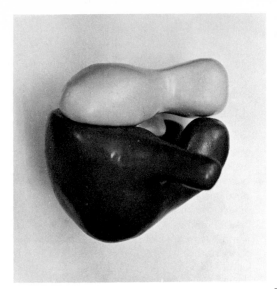 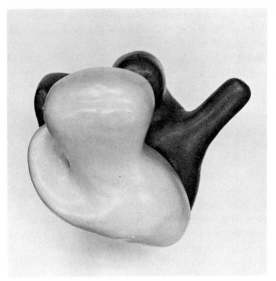

FIGURE 1-43 Model of the *E. coli* ribosome showing the relationship of the large and the small subunits. The view on the left shows the interface between the small subunit (light color) and the large subunit (dark color). This interface is an important region where the tRNAs, the mRNA, and factors involved in protein synthesis are located. In the view at the right showing the ribosome viewed from above, a prominent feature of the large subunit is the elongated projection extending from the subunit. At present, the function of this feature of the large subunit is not well understood. (From the work of J. Lake.)

FIGURE 1-44 Model of the relationship between ribosomes and ER membrane. Attachment by the large subunits and orientation of the partition separating the two ribosomal subunits are strongly suggested by the evidence presented. The central channel in the large subunit and the discontinuity in the subjacent ER membrane are tentative features of the model, included only to indicate a possible pathway for the release of the newly synthesized protein in the cisternal space. (From the work of D. Sabatini and G. Blobel.)

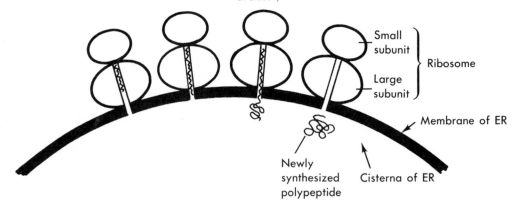

or two IgG antibodies, indicated by arrows, that are attached to a single region of the subunit. By observing the site of specific antibody attachment in different views or orientations of a subunit, it is possible to map the locations of proteins in three dimensions. The distributions of some of the small subunit proteins that have been localized are indicated in Fig. 1-42. Their locations have suggested functionally important regions of the ribosome. For example, the cleft, best seen in the +50° view in Fig. 1-41, that is formed between the winglike structure, called the platform, and the remainder of the subunit is likely to be the region where the condon-anticodon interaction occurs. In the monomeric ribosome, the small subunit is oriented with the platform and the cleft on the side of the small subunit adjacent to the large subunit (Fig. 1-42) so that the anticodon-codon interaction occurs near the interface between both subunits. The strand of messenger RNA traverses this region and can be seen (Fig. 1-40) to approach this region of the ribosome in electron micrographs of polyribosomes. Ribosome structure is being determined at a rapid pace and it is now possible that a detailed structural model of the molecular events occurring during protein synthesis will be available in the near future.

Polyribosomes may lie free in the cytoplasm, releasing their peptide chains into the cytoplasm for further combination and complexing. This is the means by which hemoglobin is synthesized. Where the ribosomes attach to the outer surface of ER, it is the larger unit which maintains attachment. The mRNA and the ER membranes are parallel. Further, there may be a canal which runs through the larger ribosomal component at right angles to the mRNA and the ER. This canal has been postulated to run through the membranous wall of the ER, with the result that the amino acids, in peptide linkage, are "spun out" by the ribosomes directly into the lumen of the ER (Fig. 1-44).

Ribosomes probably have a short life-span. With cessation of protein synthesis they are quickly metabolized and disappear.

MITOCHONDRIA

Mitochondria are membranous cytoplasmic organelles capable of releasing, by oxidation, chemical energy present in compounds obtained from food and of fixing that energy in a form readily utilizable by the cell. They are present, in suitably prepared light-microscopic sections, as punctate or linear structures

just within the resolving power of the microscope (Figs. 1-6 and 1-45). By electron microscopy they are tubular structures bounded by one membrane and containing an internal folded membrane (Figs. 1-46 to 1-49).

A cell obtains energy from substrates derived from food. Thus amino acids derived from protein, fatty acids from fat, and glucose from carbohydrate may be sources of energy, but the major source is glucose. Glucose is broken down in the cell by *glycolytic* enzymes to form pyruvic acid, which is then oxidized to *acetyl coenzyme A*. This compound then proceeds to a cycle of further oxidations, the *Krebs tricarboxylic acid cycle,* which has as its end products carbon dioxide and water. Approximately 690,000 calories of energy per mole lie in the chemical bonds of glucose. Its oxidation to pyruvate yields approximately 40,000 calories per mole, but its complete oxidation to carbon dioxide and water through the Krebs cycle yields approximately another 650,000 calories per mole. The energy-capturing mechanism of cells is at best only about 50 percent efficient, however, losing half the energy as heat, so that the total caloric content of glucose is never available. Only about 350,000 calories per mole are useful to the cell. The glycolytic breakdown of glucose to lactic acid is anaerobic—that is, it does not utilize oxygen—in contrast to the mechanism of the Krebs cycle which does require oxygen, and is, therefore, respiratory in nature. The oxidation through the Krebs cycle is clearly of great importance, as indicated by its caloric yield; indeed, it is necessary to life. Blocking this system, as can be done with fluoroacetate, causes death. *The Krebs cycle enzymes are present in mitochondria.*

The oxidation of pyruvate to carbon dioxide and water by itself, however, would yield only heat. Another enzyme system is coupled into the Krebs cycle. This is an *electron-transfer system* of cytochromes which accepts the energy liberated in each of the steps of the Krebs cycle and incorporates it into so-called *high-energy phosphate compounds,* notably *adenosine triphosphate,* or ATP. This is accomplished by the conversion of adenosine diphosphate (ADP) to ATP. The additional phosphate bond so formed represents approximately 7300 calories of stored energy. *The cytochrome electron-transfer system capable of fixing the energy obtained from the oxidations of the Krebs cycle into ATP lies in mitochondria.* The ATP appears to diffuse from mitochondria into surrounding cytoplasm. Its energy is released by ATPase which lie at different locations in a cell. One depot rich in ATPase is the cell membrane. Here the energy obtained from the conversion of ATP to ADP is used in the active transport of compounds across the cell membrane.

Mitochondria may be observed in living cells by phase-contrast microscopy (Fig. 1-2). They are quite pliant and appear to be carried passively in cytoplasmic streams, twisted, bent, and changing shape. On occasion they appear contractile or motile. They are subject to swelling in certain physiologic states.

Mitochondria may be vitally stained with Janus green B, pinacyanole, or other vital dyes which exist in a colored oxidized form and colorless reduced form. Because of their oxidative enzymes, mitochondria are capable of maintaining the dye in its oxidized form (a

green or blue in the case of Janus green B), whereas the remainder of the cytoplasm is, in most instances, unable to do so.

In fixed and stained light-microscopic preparations, mitochondria are usually demonstrated by virtue of the phospholipid contained in their membranous walls. For this reason, solvents which extract phospholipid must be avoided in making these preparations or the subsequent staining will be markedly reduced or absent. The reason for using iron hematoxylin, an excellent stain for mitochondria utilized in the Regaud, Baker, and other methods, is the

FIGURE 1-45 Light micrograph of a portion of the stomach lining. The preparation has been stained for NAD$^+$-dependent isocitric dehydrogenase activity (consult Chap. 2). This constitutes a selective stain for mitochondria. Nuclei are present in negative image. Two cell types are present. One, the parietal cell, is rich in granular mitochondria and carries out active transport. The second, the chief cell, has relatively few filamentous mitochondria and is concerned with the synthesis of protein. These cell types are discussed in Chap. 18. ×1500. (From the work of D. G. Walker.)

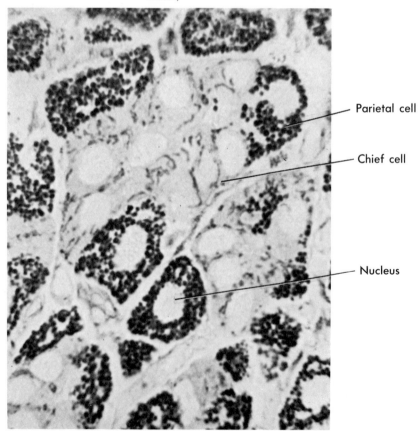

Parietal cell

Chief cell

Nucleus

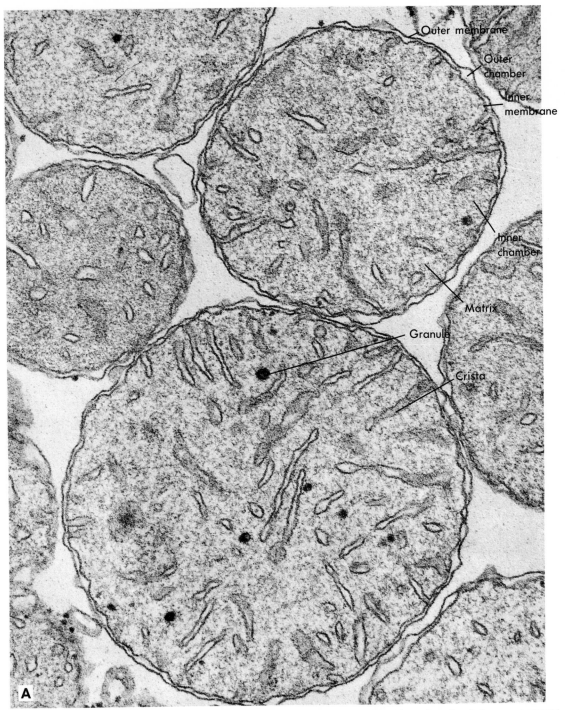

Outer membrane

Outer chamber

Inner membrane

Inner chamber

Matrix

Granule

Crista

FIGURE 1-46 Mitochondria of a rat hepatocyte. Mitochondria undergo reversible ultrastructural transformations between a condensed and an orthodox conformation in relationship to the level of oxidative phosphorylation (see text). These changes may be observed in isolated mitochondria and in tissue section. Mitochondria are isolated from disrupted hepatocytes and sectioned.

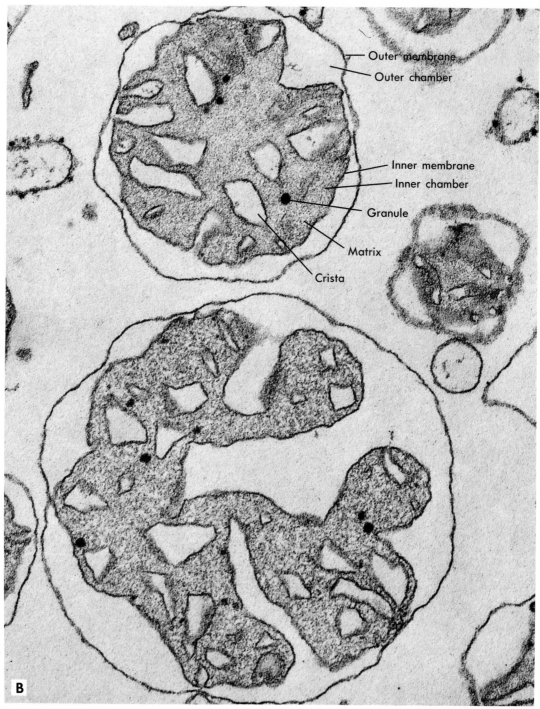

Outer membrane

Outer chamber

Inner membrane

Inner chamber

Granule

Matrix

Crista

B

A. The conventional conformation, the outer membrane, outer chamber, inner membrane with cristae, and inner chamber containing matrix and granules may be seen. B. The condensed state; the outer chamber is considerably enlarged and the inner membrane and matrix thereby condensed. Each ×110,000. (From C. R. Hackenbrock, *J. Cell Biol.*, **37**:345, 1968.)

staining of phospholipid. Sudan black B or other dyes which dissolve in lipid stain mitochondria faintly.

Mitochondria may also be demonstrated with light microscopy by histochemical staining of the activity of their enzymes (Fig. 1-45). Thus stains for succinic dehydrogenase, malic dehydrogenase, isocitrate dehydrogenase, fumaric dehydrogenase, and other oxidative enzymes are effective. The cells must be carefully fixed to limit diffusion of enzymes and to achieve good morphology; even slightly prolonged fixation destroys enzyme activity and renders the methods valueless. These methods also provide valuable physi-

ologic information. For example, mitochondria may appear identical by methods dependent upon phospholipid staining, by supravital staining, or by phase microscopy. Yet in such mitochondria, Krebs cycle enzymes may have different activities; and by staining for a variety of these enzymes, different functional classes of mitochondria may be recognized on the basis of different intensities of staining.

By electron microscopy, mitochondria may be recognized as distinctive tubular structures made of inner and outer unit membranes (Figs. 1-45 to 1-49). The outer limiting membrane is unfolded. The inner membrane is typically corrugated or folded to form cristae which extend into the center of the mitochondrion. In most mammalian cells the cristae are plates or shelves which extend partway across the internal cavity of the mitochondrion. Some variation in cristal

FIGURE 1-47 Mitochondria of an ascites tumor cell. A. Mitochondria are present in the orthodox conformation. A mitochondrion is enclosed in an outer membrane. The inner membrane is folded into cristae which extend into the matrix of the inner chamber. ×26,800. B. The condensed form, wherein the outer chamber is expanded, is evident. The cytoplasm also contains polyribosomes and rough ER. ×26,800. (From C. R. Hackenbrock, T. G. Rehn, E. C. Weinbach, and J. J. Lemasters, *J. Cell Biol.*, **51**:123, 1971.)

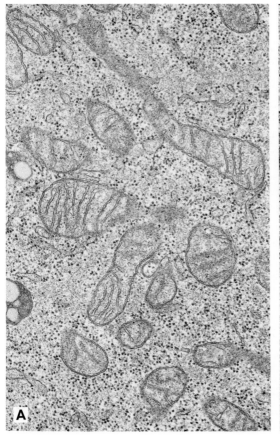
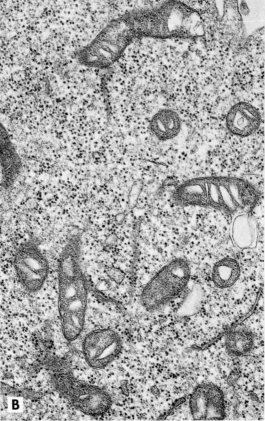

pattern is evident. In cardiac muscle there may be many cristae which reach across the mitochondrion, whereas in macrophages there are usually few cristae, and these are short. In kidney tubular cells the cristal pattern is quite regular, and the cristae reach almost all the way across the interior of the mitochondrion. In cells secreting steroid hormones, the cristae may be tubular rather than shelflike.

The unit membrane is modified in the cristae of mitochondria. The membrane surface which is exposed to the inner chamber of the mitochondrion possesses knoblike repeating units attached to a basal membrane by slender stalks (Fig. 1-49). These units, designated *elementary particles*, are revealed at high magnification with negative staining after osmotic shock. Their significance has not been established, although they may contain the enzymes associated

with the electron-transfer system. It is possible, moreover, that these particles, under normal conditions, are embedded in the membrane rather than projecting from it.

The inner chamber (the space enclosed by the inner membrane) of the mitochondrion contains finely granular material called *matrix*. It may contain dense granules.

Mitochondria are, however, subject to conformational change (Figs. 1-46 and 1-47). The *orthodox form* just described is typical of mitochondria in tissue section when the level of ADP is low and the mitochondria inactive in oxidative phosphorylation. If oxi-

FIGURE 1-48 Mitochondria of a rat hepatocyte. Freeze-fracture-etch of isolated mitochondria. The fracture line exposed the inner surface of the outer membrane and the inner surface of the inner membrane. Note the rather regularly arranged system of granules on the inner surface of the outer membrane. The granules are the size of certain enzymes and may represent membrane-associated enzymes. ×110,000. (From the work of C. R. Hackenbrock.)

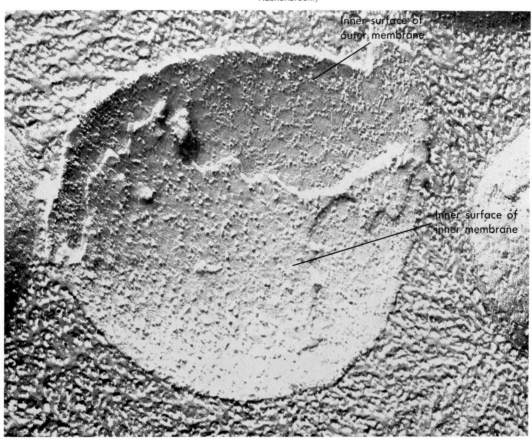

dative phosporylation is induced in isolated mitochondria by the addition of ADP to a mitochondrial
pellet, or if suitable measures are taken to preserve
mitochondria in the process of oxidative phosphorylation in tissue sections, a condensed conformation is
revealed. Here the crests of the inner membrane are
not present. Instead, the outer chamber (the space
between the inner and outer membranes) is increased
to approximately 50 percent of the volume of the
organelle.

Methods for demonstrating oxidative enzymes by
electron microscopy have been developed. With them,
cytochrome oxidase activity and the activity of related
enzymes have been demonstrated within mitochondria.

Mitochondria may be isolated with relative ease
from cells by a technique which requires disruption of
cells and then centrifugation of the fragments. In density-gradient centrifugation, the mitochondria form a
tan-colored stratum lying between the nuclei below
and the lysosomes and ribosomes above.

Mitochondria isolated under these circumstances
exhibit the various reactions delineated above. In addition, they may be studied by standard chemical and
microchemical methods. They may be dissociated by
application of deoxycholate and other surface-active
agents, and by this method it has been ascertained that
the electron-transfer system of cytochromes appears
firmly bound to membranes whereas the enzymes of
the Krebs tricarboxylic acid cycle are not.

Freeze-fracture-etch methods have been used
to reveal particles on mitochondrial membranes (Fig.
1-48). Both orthodox and condensed forms may be
seen. Particles are seen within both inner and outer

FIGURE 1-49 Mitochondrion from beef heart; negatively stained
electron micrograph. A. The cristae of the mitochondrion are outlined at a magnification of 62,000. Note that small bodies (arrow)
appear on the outer cristal membrane facing the interior of the
mitochondrion. B. Under 420,000 magnification these small bodies, the elementary particles (EP), are seen attached to the cristal
membrane by a slender stalk. (From H. Fernández-Morán.
T. Oda, P. V. Blair, and D. E. Green, *J. Cell Biol.*, **22:**63, 1964.)

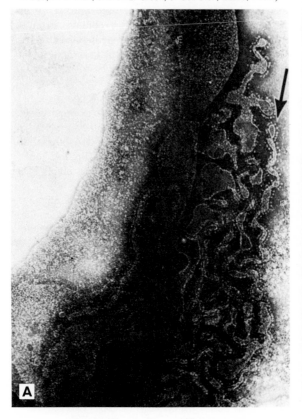

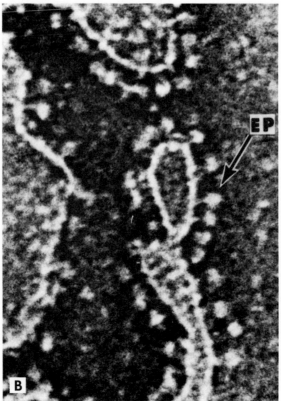

membranes. Those on the inner membrane are numerous and may constitute the enzymes of the electron-transfer chain.

In ameboid-free cells, mitochondria have no special distribution aside from being excluded, as a rule, from the cell center and the gelated cytoplasm of the ectoplasmic zones. In cells which maintain a marked polarity, as the renal tubular cells which present an apical surface to the lumen of a tubule and a basal surface to blood vessels, the mitochondria may have a characteristic location. In these cells the mitochondria are concentrated in the basal portion of the cell, lying at right angles to the basal surface between folds of the invaginated cell membrane.

The number of mitochondria is subject to variation. Hepatocytes may each contain around 1000 to 1500 mitochondria. At the other extreme, mature erythrocytes, totally dependent for energy on glycolysis, contain none.

Mitochondria may bear characteristic relationships to other organelles and cell structures. This relationship is often of great functional significance, as the mitochondrion is the primary source of energy in a cell. Thus in cells synthesizing protein, mitochondria may occur close to ribosomes. In cells engaged in large-scale active transport of materials across a cell membrane, as in the parietal cell of the stomach (which pumps protons across a membrane in the production of hydrochloric acid) or the salt gland parenchymal cell of marine birds (which pumps sodium ions), the plasma membrane dips into the cell in many folds and mitochondria are closely held in these folds. In striated muscle cells, which contain myofilaments responsible for contraction, the mitochondria are present in characteristic relation to the contractile elements. In the development of fat cells, the minute fat droplets which form and then coalesce are intimately associated with mitochondria.

As has been discussed, mitochondria possess a primary respiratory function. They may display other activities as well, notably the concentration of cations. The dense granules of the mitochondrial matrix in the inner chamber may represent concentrations of Ca^{2+}.

Mitochondria may constitute an extraordinary symbiotic event. On first discovery by Altmann, mitochondria were believed to be intracellular parasites termed *bioblasts*, a conception considered unacceptable at that time. However, mitochondria have now been found to contain DNA and RNA, of types typical of prokaryotes. (See discussion of ribosomes above.) Moreover, although the method of mitochondrial biogenesis has not been definitively resolved, there is evidence that existing mitochondria may produce new mitochondria. It thus must be considered possible that in the evolution of eukaryotes, ancestral prokaryote structures established a felicitous symbiotic relationship and permitted the considerable eukaryotic evolution which has occurred. A similar but far less fully documented case can be made for centrioles.

LYSOSOMES, PEROXISOMES, AND MULTIVESICULAR BODIES

Lysosomes are a class of cytoplasmic particles 50 to 80 Å in diameter, bounded by a unit membrane and containing hydrolytic enzymes active at acid pH. Lysosomes may be isolated by differential centrifugation of disrupted cells. They lie in the fraction centripetal to mitochondria. In electron micrographs they are oval or round membrane-bounded bodies containing variably dense granular material (Figs. 1-50 and 1-51). They may be identified cytochemically by reactions for acid phosphatase, a commonly used marker, or by reactions for other enzymes they contain. In such cytochemical preparations they may be visualized as punctate structures by light microscopy. Only under the electron microscope can their detailed structure be resolved.

The lysosomes of liver cells have been isolated and extensively studied. They contain a dozen or more hydrolytic enzymes. It is evident that even within a given tissue, as the liver, subclasses of lysosomes may be isolated, each somewhat different in enzymatic constitution. A hepatocyte may contain about 200 lysosomes.

Lysosomes occur in a number of states, accounting for heterogeneity of appearance. The *primary lysosome* or *storage body* is produced at the Golgi complex. Its genesis involves production of its enzymes in the rough ER, their movement into the Golgi, where a carbohydrate may be added, and their release

TABLE 1-1 ENZYMES PRESENT IN RAT LIVER LYSOSOMES*

Acid ribonuclease	α-Glucosidase
Acid deoxyribonuclease	β-N-Acetylglucosaminidase
Acid phosphatase	β-Glucuronidase
Phosphoprotein phosphatase	β-Galactosidase
Cathepsin	α-Mannosidase
Collagenase	Aryl-sulfatase

*From C. de Duve, "The Lysosome Concept," Ciba Foundation Symposium, Little, Brown and Company, Boston, 1963.

as enzyme-rich membrane-bounded particles. Lysosomes, with their complement of hydrolytic enzymes, are digestive organelles, and their heterogeneity must be understood in relationship to the incorporation of outside substances into the cell. A cell may engulf particulate matter (*phagocytosis*) or imbibe fluid (*pinocytosis*). Pinocytosis may be of a macrotype visible by light microscopy or of a microtype seen only in the electron microscope. In any case, the invaginated plasmalemma forms a membrane-bounded cytoplasmic vacuole, termed a *phagosome* or *pinosome*. On moving into the cytoplasm, phagosomes or pinosomes may meet primary lysosomes and fuse by coalescence of their membranes to form a *secondary lysosome, heterolysosome, heterophagosome,* or *definitive lysosome*. These structures may be stable structures, as in macrophages. They may later fuse with new phagosomes. Following fusion of a primary lysosome

with a pinosome or phagosome the hydrolytic enzymes of the lysosome may digest the contents of the pinosome or phagosome. Indeed, following fusion of the primary lysosome to form a heterolysosome, new substances and heightened hydrolytic enzyme activity may become apparent. Many of the substances brought into lysosomes may be digested and their products released to the cytoplasm, and the lysosome, with the selective addition of certain materials and with augmented enzyme activity, may constitute a relatively long-lived, active cellular component. At the end of their development, secondary lysosomes become *residual bodies*. These are membrane-bounded structures containing pigment, myelin bodies, lipid, and variegated materials: the residues of incompletely digested materials. These bodies may be expelled from the cell, as in macrophages and many invertebrate cells. On the other hand, they may accumulate as indices of "wear and tear" or aging.

Another group of secondary lysosomes is *auto-*

FIGURE 1-50 Lysosomes of the epithelioid cell of chicken. In this cell, derived from a macrophage, the cytoplasm is filled with lysosomes. They crowd out the centrosome. From the centriole, rays of gelated cytoplasm free of organelles radiate. At one place a small pocket of Golgi membranes is present. (From J. Sutton and L. Weiss, *J. Cell Biol.,* **28:**303, 1966.)

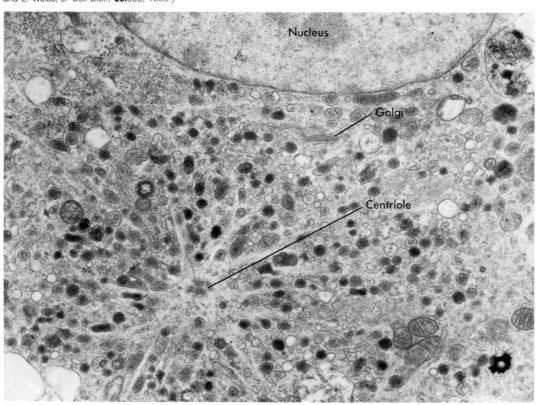

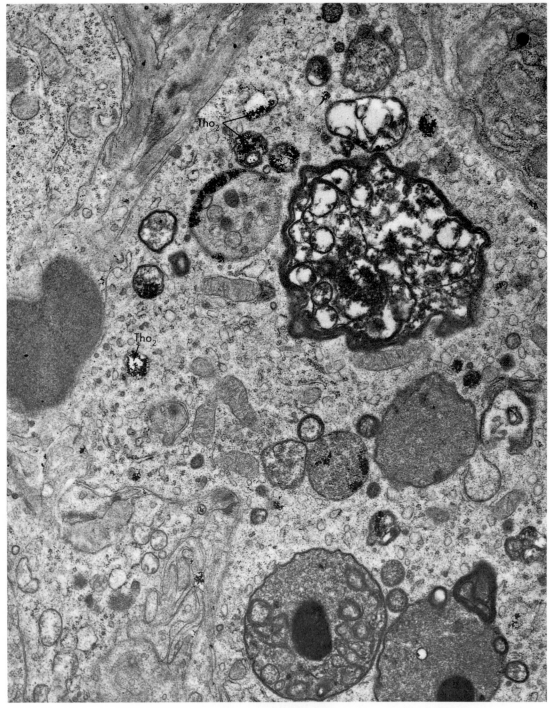

FIGURE 1-51 Lysosomes of a macrophage from a rabbit. This animal was given thorium dioxide (ThO$_2$) and electron-dense salt of the heavy metal shortly before this cell was fixed. Heterolysosomes, considerably different in appearance, are present. Many contain some ThO$_2$ ×40,000. (From L. Weiss, *Bull. Hopkins Hosp.*, **115:**99, 1964.)

phagocytic vacuoles or cytolysosomes. These are membrane-bounded structures containing some of the cells' own mitochondria, ribosomes, etc. They may originate from segments of smooth ER which curve about some cytoplasm and fuse to enclose it in a vacuole. These vacuoles may then fuse with primary lysosomes just as phagosomes do. Another mechanism may be the incorporation of some cytoplasm directly into a lysosome. The formation of autophagosomes may well be a mechanism of "internal policing" of a cell, removing damaged or senescent cell substance. Autophagocytic vacuoles increase in starvation, aging, and after tissue injury. They may well be the basis of permitting the turnover of cell organelles by destroying the aged ones. Thus, mitochondria have a half-life of only 10 days in rat hepatocytes and autophagocytic vacuoles may remove and digest the replaced mitochondria.

Lysosomes have many metabolic functions in normal cells. They may play a role in the degradation of glycogen, since in a type of *glycogen storage disease,* an illness of children characterized by a marked increase in liver size (*hepatomegaly*) due to the accumulation of glycogen, lysosomes are the site of glycogen accumulation and are deficient in α-glucosidase, the enzyme responsible for glycogen breakdown. Lysosomes function in hormone production and destruction. The thyroid hormone *thyroxin* is produced as a conjugate of globulin. Its separation or hydrolysis from globulin would appear to depend on incorporation of the thyroglobulin into lysosomes and its hydrolysis by the hydrolytic enzymes in lysosomes. The destruction of excess hormones, or structures containing hormones, is a function related to autophagocytosis, and can be seen by the autophagy of granules containing *mammotrophic hormone* by lysosomes of the secretory cells of the pars distalis of the pituitary gland.

Lysosomes constitute a product similar in many ways to secretory granules. However, lysosomes are typically not released but remain within the cytoplasm. It is likely, however, that macrophages in such loci as the red pulp of the spleen do selectively release lysosomes.

The membrane limiting the lysosome must protect the cell against the lytic effect of lysosomal enzymes. The lysosome represents an adaptation whereby a cell may concentrate powerful digestive enzymes without undergoing autodigestion (except in the controlled way associated with the development of autophagosomes). Cell death and postmortem autolysis may result from lysosomal disruption. That

point at which the membrane of a lysosome is either maintained or disrupted is clearly a critical matter. A number of diseases have been identified in which lysosomes play a part. The lysosomal membrane in leukocytes in Chediak-Higashi disease and chronic granulomatous disease of childhood is abnormally resistant to breakdown. Phagocytized bacteria are not exposed to the lysosome's lytic enzymes. As a result, control of bacteria is impaired and affected individuals die of infection. Gout appears to be a lysosome-dependent disease. As a result of genetically induced high uric acid levels in the body fluids, urate crystals form in the synovial cavities and other connective tissue spaces. Leukocytes engulf these crystals. As the crystals become incorporated into secondary lysosomes they disrupt the lysosomes, loosing the hydrolytic enzymes. The leukocytes are destroyed and the enzymes, released to the tissue, induce inflammation characteristic of gouty arthritis.

Peroxisomes or *microbodies* are membrane-bounded particles somewhat larger than lysosomes, distinctive in containing peroxidase and catalase, D-amino acid oxidase, and urate oxidase. They have a variegated granular internum which may be condensed or crystalline (Fig. 1-36). They are present in high concentration in liver, kidney, macrophages, and a number of other cell types. Peroxisomes reduce H_2O_2 into O_2 and H_2O. H_2O_2 is necessary to a number of cell functions including the killing of microorganisms (see Chap. 10). But only low concentrations of H_2O_2 can be tolerated by cells. Peroxisomes appear to have the important oxidative function of regulating H_2O_2 metabolism, providing necessary but not excessive concentrations. Peroxisomes are associated with α-keto acid formation, moreover, and thereby play a role in the formation of glucose from lipids and other noncarbohydrate precursors, a process termed *gluconeogenesis.*

Multivesicular bodies are found in liver and relatively few other cell types. They are somewhat larger than lysosomes and consist of a number of small clear vesicles lying within a larger vesicle. Their relationship to lysosomes and peroxisomes is not known.

MICROFILAMENTS

There appear to be two groups of fine filamentous strands in nonmuscle cells. One is approximately 50 Å in diameter (Fig. 1-52). Evidence has steadily accu-

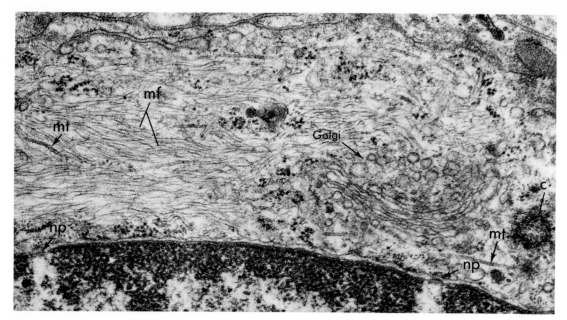

FIGURE 1-52 Microfilaments of human spleen, endothelium or lining cells of arterial capillary. The cytoplasm is filled with microfilaments (mf) 50Å in width. Although the identity of these filaments has not been established in these vessels, it is likely they are made of actin and are contractile. They would thereby control blood flow through the control of the caliber of the vessel by contractility of the endothelium. Some microtubules (mt), nuclear pores (np), a Golgi complex, and centriole (c) are also present. ×60,000. (From L. T. Chen and L. Weiss, *Am. J. Anat.*, **134:**425, 1972.)

mulated on the basis of studies with heavy meromyosin (see below) that these are actin in composition. They are present in virtually every cell type and are believed to underlie the locomotion of cells, ruffling and invagination of cell membranes, contraction, and other aspects of motility. This class of filaments form the terminal web of epithelial cells and enter microvilli. They form the contractile ring in dividing cells (Fig. 1-53). These filaments are termed *microfilaments*. The second group of fine intracellular filaments is stouter, approximately 90 to 120 Å in diameter. They appear to represent a more diverse population of filaments than the microfilaments. Groups of such filaments run in many cell types without evident relationship to motility. They may attach to the cytoplasmic surface of desmosomes. In epidermal cells they may fill the cell and be constituted of keratin. In endothelial cells they may run along the base of the cell. In general they would appear to have a supporting or stiffening function. They have been termed *tonofibrils* or *tonofilaments* and *intermediate-sized* filaments.

Microfilaments are part of the actomyosin system and very likely achieve their contractile functions by sliding over myosin in a manner similar to that in muscle cells. In nonmuscle cells, microfilaments are visible by electron microscopy while myosin is not. Yet myosin is also present, as shown in a number of cell types, by histochemical stains for myosin, that is, fluorescent staining following treatment of cells with a cytochemical reagent consisting of antimyosin antibody linked to a fluorescent dye. Thus, in the mitotic contractile ring in which actin microfilaments have been demonstrated by electron microscopy, the presence of myosin has been shown by fluorescence histochemistry. It is likely that myosin is not visible in electron micrographs because it occurs in short nondescript segments representing oligomers which do not aggregate into filaments. Actin can be detected by an excellent cytochemical test—its specific reaction with heavy meromyosin (HMM) (Fig. 1-53). The tissue is first extracted with glycerol to increase permeability and permit the penetrance of HMM. After irrigation with HMM, the result is that microfilaments are "decorated" with HMM, which gives them a characteristic fuzzy appearance and they may appear as arrowheads. Microfilaments, moreover, are disaggregated and rendered functionless by the antibiotic *cytochalasin B*. While the specificity of this reagent is uncertain, it has provided information about these microfilaments.

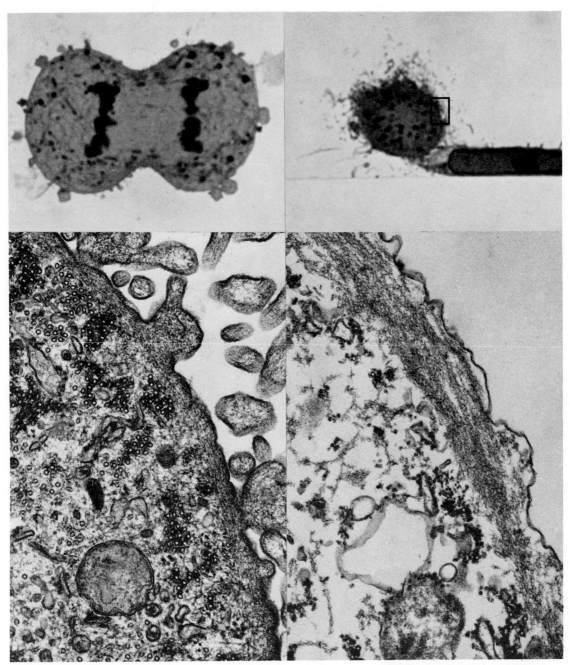

FIGURE 1-53 Cytoplasmic microfilaments in many cells are composed of actin. These micrographs illustrate this point for the contractile ring in dividing HeLa cells. The upper figures are light micrographs ($\times$2000) of 1 μm Epon sections of cells midway through cleavage: at the left parallel to the plane of the monolayer and at the right perpendicular to it at the level of the furrow constriction, hence the cell's circular profile. Electron micrographs below ($\times$50,000) illustrate portions of perpendicular sections, as indicated by the black rectangle. In standard preparations (lower left) the contractile ring appears as a layer of thin microfilament encircling the cell just beneath its membrane. After extraction in glycerol and irrigation with heavy meromyosin these same microfilaments appear "fuzzy" (lower right) in a way which is characteristic of actin filaments. Small circles in the electron micrographs are transverse profiles of microtubules of the mitotic apparatus. (From T. E. Shroeder, *Proc. Natl. Acad. Sci. U.S.A.*, **70:**1688, 1973.)

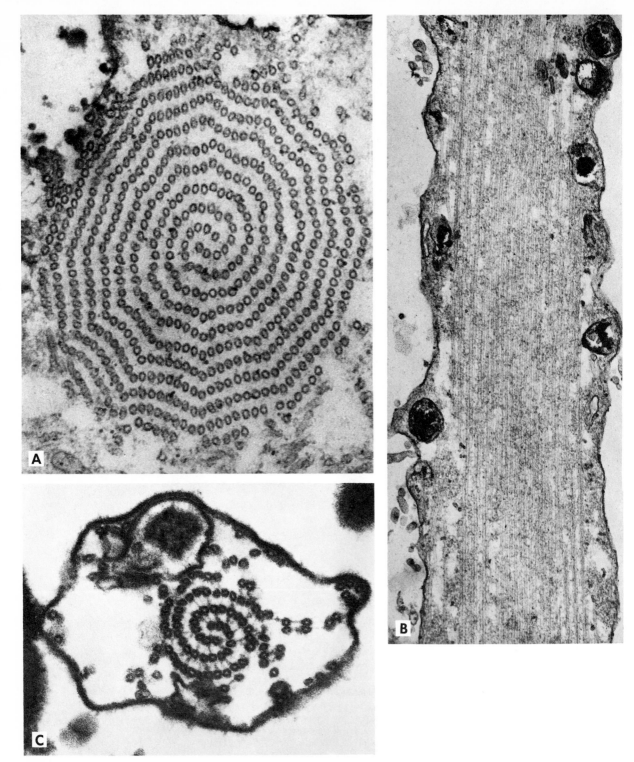

FIGURE 1-54 Microtubules in axoplasm of *Echinoshaerium*. Much correlative morphologic work in chemistry, physiology, and morphology has been done on invertebrates. A. Transverse section of an axoneme at the base of an axopodium. There are 12 sections of microtubules in cross section. ×70.000. B. Longitudinal section of an axoneme. Peripheral to the parallel array of microtubules constituting the axoneme are dense granules which undergo saltations. ×40,000. C. Transverse section of an axoneme heavily stained with MnO$_4$ to emphasize the bridges which connect the microtubules. ×110,000. (From L. G. Tilney and K. R. Porter, *Protoplasma,* **60:**317, 1965.)

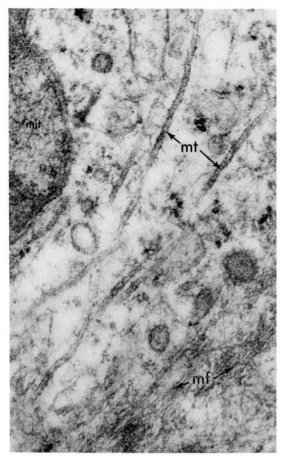

FIGURE 1-55 Microtubules of a human splenic reticular cell. This field is from the peripheral cytoplasm and contains sections of microtubules (mt), microfilaments (mf), and a mitochondrion (mit). ×90,000. (From L. T. Chen and L. Weiss, *Am. J. Anat.,* **134:**425, 1972.)

MICROTUBULES

Microtubules are major structures in prokaryotic and eukaryotic cells. They play a part, as a cytoskeleton, and operate in creating cell shape. They are responsible for asymmetry in the shape of cells. This is necessary for cell movement and for cellular differentiation. For example, the development of axons appears to depend on alignment of great numbers of microtubules in the axonal processes. Dispersal of the microtubules prevents axon formation. Microtubules appear to be important in intracellular transport. A fluid interface between the microtubular surface and the surrounding cytoplasm may facilitate the directed and rapid movement of large molecules. The movement of particles and organelles, such as mitochondria, often in a saltatory or jumplike fashion, appears directed along microtubules.

Microtubules appear as hollow, nonbranching cylinders 210 to 240 Å in diameter and many micrometers long (Figs. 1-54 and 1-55; see also succeeding figures on centrioles and mitosis). Their dense wall appears to be fabricated of globular subunits 40 Å in diameter, arranged in a helix with 13 subunits per turn. The center zone is lucent in most microtubules, giving the structures the appearance of hollow cylinders. Microtubules often appear in groups of 30 or 40 or more and may be connected by slender bridges.

Microtubules are the basis of such complex and well-defined structures as centrioles and cilia. In addition, there are bands of microtubules in the axons of nerve cells (neurotubules), beneath the plasma membrane of many cylindrical or asymmetric cells, within the endoplasm of such cells as macrophages, and constituting the achromatic mitotic apparatus. Microtubules may originate from nucleating or initiating sites in the cell. The centriole is a nucleating site for microtubular structures such as the cilia and achromatic apparatus. Most groups of microtubules are less stable than those in cilia and centrioles. They disappear on fixation in the cold and after fixation with many fixatives such as osmium tetroxide. Microtubules are relatively easily dispersed by the action of colchicine, vinblastine, or high hydrostatic pressure. With the removal of such dispersing factors, the subunits quickly reassociate to re-form microtubules.

CENTRIOLES

Centrioles are minute cylinders, 0.25 to 2 μm in length and 0.1 to 0.2 μm in diameter, whose walls are composed primarily of microtubules. Centrioles lie in the cytocentrum or centrosome, and may be surrounded by microtubules which can radiate out into the cytoplasm. Diploid metazoan cells contain two centrioles. Multinucleate cells may contain many centrioles: In osteoclasts and foreign-body giant cells, which may have 50 or more nuclei, the central regions of the cells are comprised of fused cytocentra strewn with centrioles. Higher plants are exceptional in lacking centrioles.

Centrioles are active in mitosis, in the genesis of

cilia, and in the production of new centrioles. Such activities may depend on a role in the production and orientation of microtubules. Unlike other cytoplasmic structures, centrioles are duplicated synchronously and precisely with division of the nucleus.

Light Microscopy

By light microscopy, centrioles are resolved as minute rods. They are well stained with a number of dyes, of which iron hematoxylin is the most commonly used (Fig. 1-6).

Electron Microscopy

The centriolar wall is made up of nine vanes or blades, each consisting of three fused microtubules (Figs. 1-56 to 1-58). The nine blades are set next to one another, their long axes parallel; the edge of one is slightly shingled beneath the edge of its neighbor, curving about to form the cylinder which is the outer wall of the centriole. In cross section, this array of the vanes resembles a pinwheel.

The fused microtubules, making up each of the blades, extend the length of the centriole and lie almost in a plane, with the result that the long blades they form are slightly curved from side to side. In addition, each of the blades, as one follows along its length, is subject to a slight twist about its long axis. Each of the microtubules is approximately 250 Å in diameter. Its wall is 45 Å in thickness. The lumen of the tubule, about 160 Å in diameter, is clear.

The principal structure within the lumen of the centriole is a 75-Å filament wound into a helix curving against the inside surface of the wall, apparently held in place by small spurs. The lumen of the centriole may also contain a large clear vesicle. An end of the centriolar cylinder may show spokes, radiating from a hub out to the wall.

Satellites, amorphous masses about 750 Å in diameter, may be observed close to the surface of centrioles, near the end, and may be material from which new centrioles are assembled.

Duplication

A new centriole is assembled at an end of each extant centriole a few hours before DNA replication. It is oriented at right angles to the parent centriole and requires several hours to complete.

In its development a centriole is preceded by a

FIGURE 1-56 Centrioles of a Chinese hamster fibroblast. A. The centriole is cut in cross section (from an interphase cell). B. The centriole is cut in longitudinal section (from a metaphase cell). ×100,000. (From the work of B. R. Brinkley.)

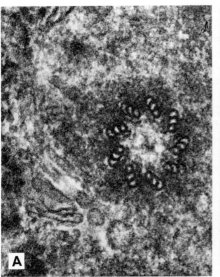
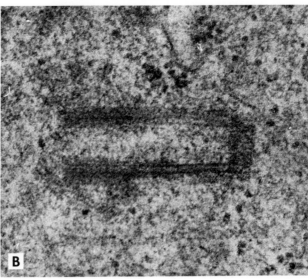

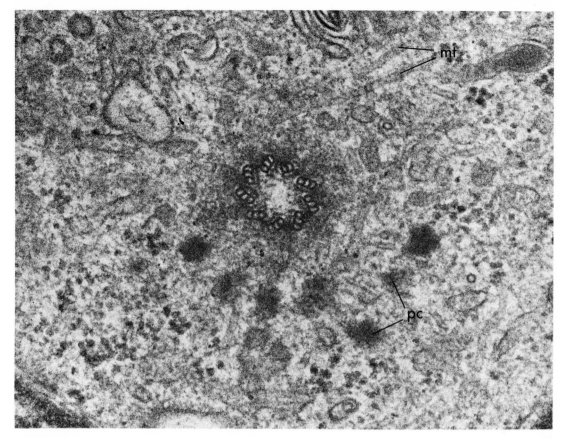

FIGURE 1-57 Centriole of a Chinese hamster fibroblast. The centriole is cut in cross section. Paracentriolar material (pc) is evident around the lower half of the centriole. Microtubules (mt) are also present, particularly in the upper half of the field. ×92,000. [From B. R. Brinkley and E. Stubblefield, in D. M. Prescott, L. Goldstein, and E. McConkey (eds.), "Advances in Cell Biology," vol. 1, Appleton-Century Crofts, New York, 1970.]

procentriole, a cylinder 150 nm in diameter with nine single microtubules in its wall. These singlets probably develop into the triplets of the centriole. The procentrioles are themselves preceded by small, dense procentriolar precursor bodies which are apparently transformed into procentrioles by the stimulation of "procentriole organizers," dense amorphous surrounding masses.

Functions

Centrioles are associated with cell division. They separate, move to opposite poles, and become focuses for the arrangement of the mitotic apparatus. Centrioles move beneath the cell surface and, as basal bodies, initiate the formation of cilia. Flagella are similarly related to centrioles. Basal bodies are structurally different from centrioles, primarily in possessing a basal plate which closes the end directed toward the cell membrane. The other end, directed toward the nucleus, is open and may contain spokes. In spermatocytes, a given centriole may be involved in both the mitotic apparatus and the flagellum. Microtubular formations other than the mitotic apparatus, cilia, and flagella may send bundles of microtubules into the cytocentrum in characteristic alignment with centrioles.

The role of the centriole in microtubular formation is not known, but it is likely that centrioles induce and direct the formation of microtubules.

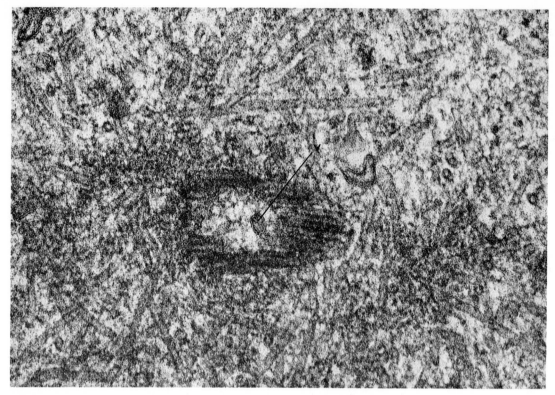

FIGURE 1-58 Centriole of a melanoma cell. The centriole is cut in oblique section. It contains a small vesicle (v). The field surrounding the vesicle abounds in microtubules. ×120,000. (From the work of G. G. Maul.)

THE LIFE CYCLE OF CELLS

Two major types of cell may be recognized: *somatic cells,* which are the diverse cells making up the somatic structure of the body, fated to die with or before the individual they constitute; and *germ cells,* which are the gametes capable of uniting sexually with those of another individual to form a new individual.

A somatic cell begins its life-span as one of the daughter cells of a mitotic division. Directly after this division the cell may undergo a period of intense protein synthesis, as a result of which emerge those granules, filaments, or other specific structures which mark the cell as mature and specialized. As the cell matures and morphologic signs of specialization occur, the cell is differentiating from an unspecialized, perhaps multipotential, cell into a highly specialized unit of limited cellular potency. But although a cell may appear undifferentiated, its direction of matura-

tion may be fixed and limited genetically, only time being required to disclose the nature of the differentiation by the appearance of morphologic specializations. In short, a cell which appears morphologically undifferentiated may, in fact, be highly differentiated.

The frequency of mitotic division varies with the cell type and tissue. Tissues may be classified as showing no mitotic division, resulting in no renewal (nervous tissue); little division, resulting in slow renewal (liver, skin, thyroid); and active division, resulting in fast renewal (gastrointestinal tract, hematopoietic tissue). Some slowly renewed tissues may be termed "conditional renewal" systems because their renewal rate can be considerably increased under certain circumstances. After partial hepatectomy, for example, the remaining hepatocytes divide very actively, providing fast renewal. Even some cells showing no mitotic division may, with appropriate stimulation, proliferate and differentiate. Certain small lymphocytes (T cells) may circulate and recirculate for many years in humans without dividing, but when stimulated by the appropriate antigen, or with certain mitogens, such as phytohemaglutinin or poke weed, they may divide rapidly, producing clones of immunologically competent cells. In neurons, mitosis occurs only prenatally and neonatally until the full number of neurons is reached. Thereafter, no replacement occurs; a cell lost diminishes the total number and its absence may cause functional impairment. The cells in tissues undergoing slow renewal tend to be long-lived. The relatively low levels of mitotic division provide new cells to replace those dying off or to permit the growth and increased functional capacity of the tissue. The increase in genetic material in certain tissues by increased nuclear number and polyploidy has been discussed earlier. Rapidly renewing tissues are characterized by short-lived cells replaced by active cell division, so that a rather stable number of cells results. In the replacement of intestinal epithelial cells, new cells formed in the depths of the intestinal glands appear to move up the wall of the gland with unremitting pressure, toppling the apparently still viable topmost cells into the detritus of the gut lumen. As a result, the entire intestinal epithelium is renewed in a span of days. The

The duration of G_1 varies greatly with cell types and mitotic turnover. In rapidly dividing cells it may be a matter of several hours. In nonrenewing tissues it may last the life of the organism. Such prolonged G_1 periods may be designated G_0. S is demonstrated by autoradiography. Indeed, it is the ability to delineate the S period by this means that makes possible the determination of the whole of the generation time. In a rapidly renewing tissue S is approximately 7 h. It is a matter of great interest that the DNA in a given chromosome does not all replicate at the same time. Instead, different segments of the chromosome replicate at different times in the S, and in a characteristic sequence. G_2 is very short—in time, about an hour—in rapidly renewing tissues. In cells destined to be polyploid, G_2 may last indefinitely. The whole of the cycle in such rapidly dividing rodent tissues as germinal centers or thymus may be about 12 h. In the epithelium of the gastrointestinal tract in humans G_2 is 1 to 7 hr, the S phase 10 to 20 hr, G_1 10 to 20 hr, and the whole of the cycle 1 to 2 days. In rodents this cycle may take but a third of this time.

The sequences in the generation cycle may be illustrated as follows*:

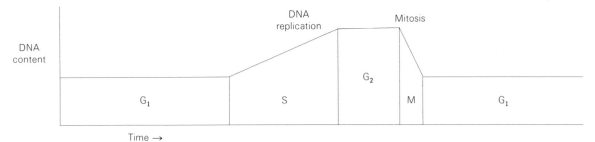

kinetics of hematopoietic tissues, particularly of the granular leukocytes, also exemplifies this pattern.

It is possible to define a *generation time* for a population of similar cells, relating the interphase state, the period of DNA replication, and the process of mitotic division. A series of four periods follows mitosis: G_1, S, G_2, and M. G_1 is an interval or gap which follows cell division; S is the period of DNA replication; G_2 is the gap between replication of DNA and the start of mitosis; and M is mitosis.

After functioning as a mature cell for varying lengths of time, a cell dies, its death often presaged by a period of senescence. Perhaps the best-studied case history of this sort is that of the erythrocyte, whose life-span in the circulation of humans is approximately 120 days. Near the end of its life-span, the activity of glucose-6-phosphatase and certain other enzymes declines, and the cell becomes mechanically more fragile. There are no morphologic concomitants of these senile changes.

* After L. F. Lamerton, in R. J. M. Fry, M. L. Griem, and W. H. Kirsten (eds.): "Normal and Malignant Cell Growth," Springer-Verlag, New York, 1969.

In other cell types, however, morphologic changes may signify senescence and coming cell death. These include, in muscle cells, attenuation, decrease in specific functional elements such as contractile filaments, and accumulation of pigment. Other changes include diminution in mitochondria, accumulation of fat, and vacuolization of cytoplasm and nucleus. Dead cells may disappear by lysis, by phagocytosis, or by displacement from the tissue, as exemplified by desquamated skin cells, respiratory cells, and intestinal cells.

CELL DIVISION

The division of one cell into two virtually identical cells is the basis of the continuity of life and underlies the complexity of metazoan organisms. The life-span of an individual protozoon is limited, but by cell division the line of Protozoa goes on. In Metazoa, division provides the cells constituting these organisms and the replacement of lost cells, underlies the phenomena of cellular differentiation and specialization, and permits the continuity of the species despite the death of individuals. Several types of cell division exist. We shall consider *mitosis, amitosis,* and *meiosis.* Cell division may be separated into two events: *karyokinesis,* or nuclear division, and *cytokinesis,* or cytoplasmic division. As indicated above, karyokinesis may occur without cytokinesis, resulting in binucleate or multinucleate cells.

Mitosis

DNA is capable of precise replication, ensuring constancy of genetic information from generation to generation and, thereby, maintenance of the characteristics of the species. (Occasionally, however, the replication of DNA is inexact and a change or *mutation* in a cell line results.) Mitosis is a complex, highly ordered process wherein the original and replicated molecules of DNA are separated from one another and distributed to two nuclei. Cytokinesis typically follows karyokinesis and two cells result. The DNA with associated protein is organized as chromosomes, whose number is highly characteristic for a species. These chromosomes are typically matched in pairs or homologues.

The human nucleus contains 46 chromosomes, paired as 23 homologues. The partners in 22 of these pairs, the *autosomes,* are morphologically alike. The remaining two chromosomes in the female are also matched and alike; they are the X chromosomes. In the male, however, these two chromosomes are morphologically different from one another; they are the X and Y, or sex, chromosomes. Chromosomes in the interphase nucleus are so long and thin that it is not possible to recognize 46 of them.

The first phase of mitosis is *prophase* (Figs. 1-59, 1-60, 1-63, and 1-64). Here the extended chromo-

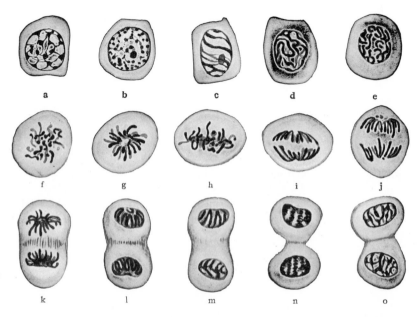

FIGURE 1-59 Mitosis. Epidermal cells of a mouse. These drawings are arranged in sequence from early prophase into telophase. a to f. Prophase. g and h. Metaphase. i and j. Anaphase. k to o. Telophase. Bouin fixation: iron hematoxylin. (From the work of Ortiz-Picón.)

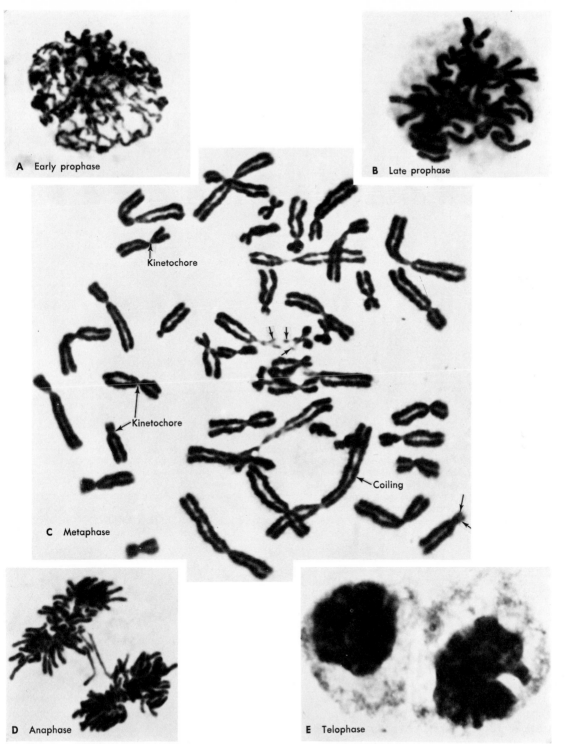

FIGURE 1-60 Mitosis. Human leukocytes. Only the chromosomes are stained. Each chromosome is seen to consist of two chromatids joined at the kinetochore. Note the secondary constrictions in several of the chromosomes and the presence of satellites (arrows). Note, too, the coiling evident in several of the chromatids. In anaphase, two chromosomes lie near the equatorial plane, lagging behind the others in joining the two diverging masses of chromosomes. This happens frequently. Note the sharp separation furrow in telophase. Aceto-orcein stain. ×4000. (From the work of B. R. Migeon.)

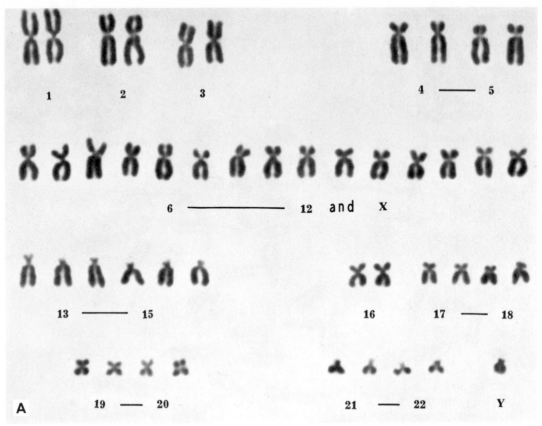

FIGURE 1-61 A. Human karyotype. Metaphase chromosomes have been arranged into morphologically similar groups of paired chromosomes and numbered. Pairs 1, 2, 3, and 16 can be identified as different from other chromosomes. It is impossible to separate 4 from 5, but 4 and 5 may be separated from the remainder. Similarly it is impossible to separate 6, 7, 8, 9, 10, 11, 12, and the X chromosome as different from one another, but this large group may be recognized as different from the other chromosomes. Chromosomes 13, 14, and 15; 17 and 18; 19 and 20 form similar groups. This individual is male, having an X and Y chromosome. B. The metaphase from which the karyotype was prepared. An interphase nucleus is present for comparison of size. Aceto-orcein stain. ×2400. (From the work of B. R. Migeon.)

somes characteristic of the interphase become progressively thicker and more and more tightly coiled. The coils may undergo secondary coiling. As perceived by light microscopy, the individual chromosomes emerge from the nuclear substance as strands which appear progressively shorter, thicker, and more intensely stained. Moreover, as prophase goes on, one can see that each of the chromosomes is split longitudinally into precisely equal halves, or *chromatids*. This longitudinal splitting of the chromosome actually occurs in the S and G_2 phases just preceding mitosis, but it becomes apparent only in late phophase. Through most of prophase the individually emerging chromosomes remain confined within the nuclear envelope and are too bunched together to be clearly characterized as to size and shape. Near the end of prophase,

when the chromosomes are maximally contracted, the nuclear membrane disappears and so do the nucleoli.

In prophase the centriole divides, if it had not divided preceding mitosis, and the two centrioles diverge from one another and move to opposite poles of the cell. From the polar centrioles, radiating toward the center of the cell, into and around the mass of chromosomes, is a system of poorly stained fibers, the *spindle*. Some of these, the discontinuous fibers, attach to chromosomes. Others, the continuous fibers, pass around the chromosomes, going from one centriole to the other. In addition, a set of fibers radiates about each centriole, forming an *aster*. The fibers of the spindle and of the asters are actually microtubules, as may be observed in electron micrographs. They are designated the *achromatic apparatus* because of their

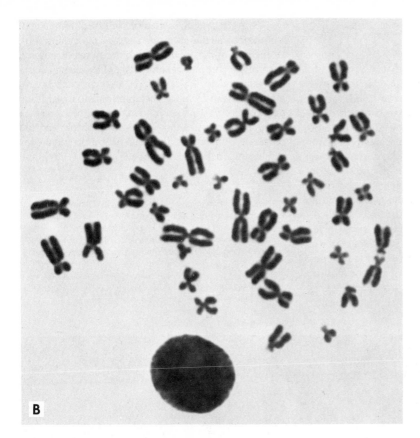

B

lack of affinity for dyes and are thus distinguished from the deeply stained ensemble of chromosomes, termed the *chromatic apparatus* (Figs. 1-59 to 1-68).

In the next phase of mitosis, *metaphase,* the chromosomes arrange themselves in an equatorial plane, forming an *equatorial plate* (Figs. 1-59, 1-60, 1-65 to 1-68). Viewed from the side, this plate appears as a somewhat irregular, dense line transecting the cell. Viewed from one of the poles, the chromosomes form a circlet. It is in polar view that the morphology of the chromosomes may best be studied in histologic preparations. Metaphase chromosomes are linear, densely stained structures. Each chromosome is constricted at one place along its length. An unstained zone, the *centromere* or *kinetochore,* lies at this place. The two chromatids of the chromosomes are free of one another except at the centromere, and the spindle fibers also attach there. Chromosomes may be divided into three groups, depending upon the location of the centromere. If the centromere divides the chromosomes into segments of equal length, the chromosome is *metacentric.* Those chromosomes separated into larger and smaller limbs by the centromere are *sub-*

median. Those in which the centromere is almost at the end of the chromosomes, so that there is virtually only one limb, are *telocentric.*

The chromatic material of the chromosome may have another *secondary constriction* in one of the limbs. This constriction may have some length, and so it isolates the chromatic material at the end of the chromosome into a *satellite.* Typically, nucleoli develop in certain zones of constriction in satellited chromosomes on reconstitution of daughter nuclei.

The chromosomes of each species may be classified on the basis of the location of the centromere, the size and shape of the limbs, and the presence of secondary constrictions and satellites. These characteristics make up the *karyotype,* or the morphology of the metaphase chromosomes singly and in aggregate. The karyotype of the human male is presented in Fig. 1-61A. The metaphase plate from which the karyotype was prepared is shown in Fig. 1-61B. The karyotype is prepared by cutting out the chromosome pairs from a photograph of a squash preparation of a metaphase cell selectively stained with a dye such as aceto-orcein. The cutout chromosomes are then arranged in clusters of similar chromosomes. It is not possible to differentiate chromosomes occurring within a cluster by the standard aceto-orcein procedure. Thus, in the human male karyotype one cannot separate chromosomes 6, 7, 8, 9, 10, 11, 12, and the X chromosome from one another. Certain fluorochromes produce a banded staining pattern in each of the chromosomes (Fig. 1-62). The banding pattern can also be shown in a more stable preparation by staining a squash preparation of a metaphase cell with dilute giemsa stain at pH 6.8. By this means it has proved possible to identify chromosomes not differentiable otherwise. Correlations of genetic diseases such as Down's syndrome (mongolism) and leukemia with abnormal karyotypes are being made in increasing number. The fluorochrome and giemsa methods are providing impetus for such correlation with individual chromosomes.

At the beginning of metaphase, the chromatids of a chromosome are connected only at the centromere. At the end of metaphase the centromeres divide and each of the chromatids, now a daughter chromosome and attached to the spindle by its own centromere, moves outward from the metaphase plate toward one pole of the cell. Thus, in human somatic cells, one set of 46 chromosomes moves to one centriole and the other set to the other. This divergent movement constitutes the *anaphase* of mitosis (Figs. 1-59, 1-60, and

FIGURE 1-62 Karyotype of normal male (XY) cultured human leukocyte, showing quinacrine fluorescence patterns. Note the bandings present in each of the chromosomes. Although the significance of this banding is not understood, it has proved useful in differentiating chromosomes which are morphologically alike. Compare with the conventional karyotype in Fig. 1-61A and B. ×2500. (From the work of W. R. Breg.) Very recently it has proved possible to obtain a similar banding pattern by staining a chromosomal preparation with a giemsa stain at a pH of about 6.8. The latter is a relatively easy procedure and may become more widely used than fluorescence staining.

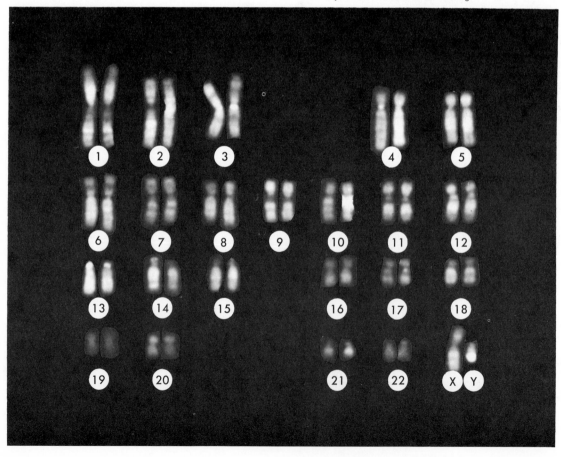

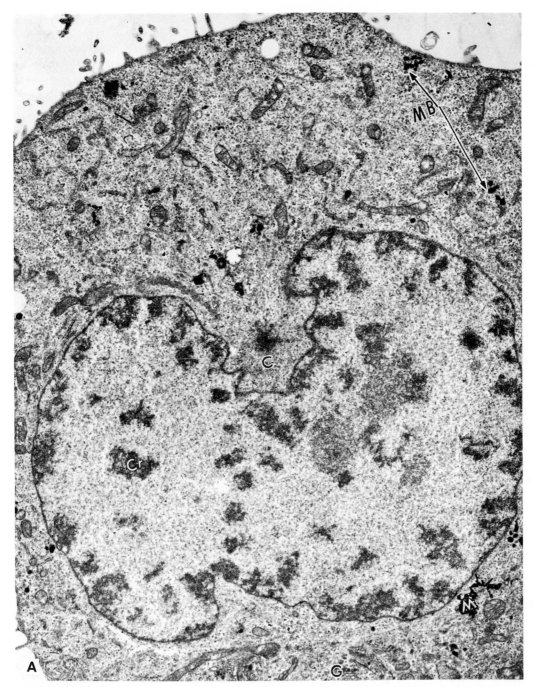

FIGURE 1-63 Electron micrograph of mitosis in a human Hela cell in tissue culture. These cells, originally derived from a carcinoma of the uterine cervix, form a strain of cells maintained in tissue culture. A. In early prophase, the chromatin becomes clumped because of the condensation of chromosomes (Cr). The nuclear membrane is still intact, and the centriole (C) and multivesicular bodies (MB) are prominent. Approximately ×3850. (From E. Robbins and N. K. Gonatas, *J. Cell Biol.,* **21:**429, 1964.)

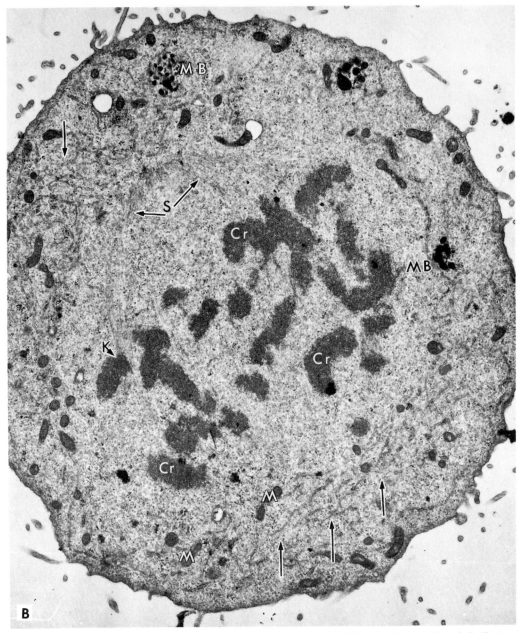

FIGURE 1-63 (continued) B. In later prophase the chromosomes are close to the equatorial plate and metaphase. The spindle fibers (S) are seen radiating from the centriole and attached to a chromosome at the kinetochore (K). Approximately ×5640. (From E. Robbins and N. K. Gonatas, *J. Cell Biol.*, **21:**429, 1964.)

C. In late anaphase, the two chromosomal masses have moved apart. They are already surrounded by a double nuclear membrane. At the lower pole, a portion of a centriole and spindle fibers may be seen. Note how the spindle fibers are present, together with some mitochondria, in the constriction between what will be the two daughter cells. Note, too, the blebs of cytoplasm (BL) about the periphery of these cells, indicating the frothing that occurs in this phase. Approximately ×5225. (From E. Robbins and N. K. Gonatas, *J. Cell Biol.*, **21:**429, 1964.)

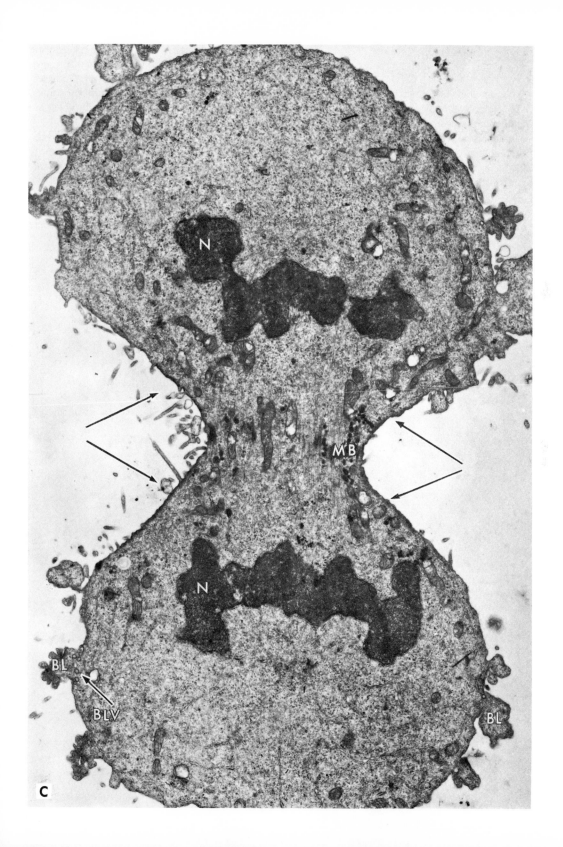

C

1-63C). The spindle fibers attached to the centromeres are responsible, to a considerable degree, for the characteristic orderly diverging movement of the chromosomes in anaphase. The drug colchicine interferes with the spindle by breaking up microtubules, leaving dividing cells suspended in metaphase and unable to complete the cell division.

Anaphase is concluded when the two chromosomal masses have moved to opposite poles of the cell. There now begins the final stage of nuclear division, *telophase* (Figs. 1-59, 1-60, and 1-63), during which two daughter nuclei are formed. Nuclear membranes form about each of the chromosomal masses, nucleoli appear at the satellite-bearing chromosomes, and segments of the chromosomes uncoil to become euchromatin.

Although primary attention must be accorded the nucleus in mitosis, characteristic changes occur in the cytoplasm. The division of the centrioles and the formation of the achromatic apparatus in prophase have already been discussed. In anaphase, frothing or bubbling of the cytoplasm occurs as the putative daughter nuclei separate. This is an index of the considerable

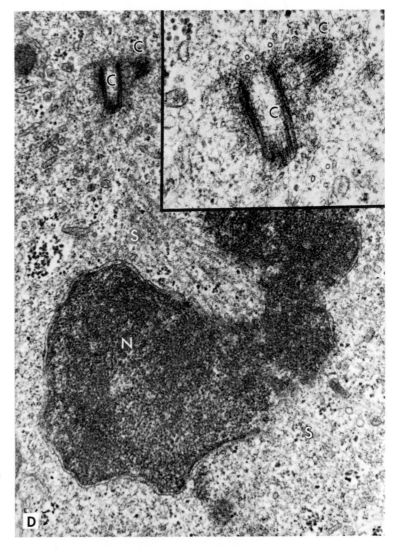

FIGURE 1-63 (continued)   D. Telophase. Note the presence of a double nuclear membrane about a daughter nucleus. The centriole (at higher magnification in the insert) has already been duplicated. Approximately ×13,750 (insert ×30,800). (From E. Robbins and N. K. Gonatas, *J. Cell Biol.*, **21**:429, 1964.)

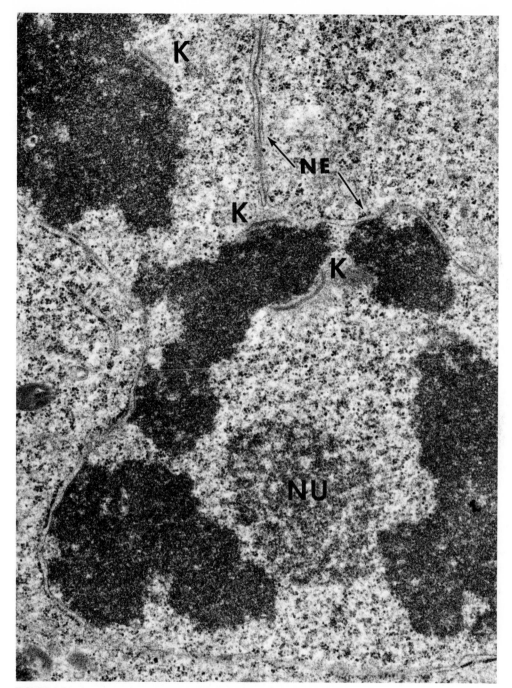

FIGURE 1-64 Late prophase. Chinese hamster fibroblast. Fully formed kinetochores (K) and a nucleus (NU) are present. The nuclear envelope (NE) is almost completely intact. [From B. R. Brinkley and E. Stubblefield, in D. M. Prescott, L. Goldstein, and E. McConkey (eds.), "Advances in Cell Biology," vol. 1, Appleton Century Crofts, New York, 1970.]

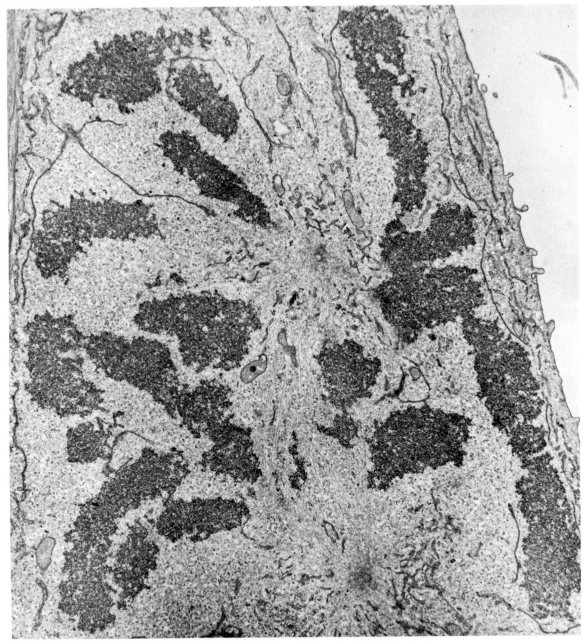

FIGURE 1-65 Prometaphase, rat kangaroo fibroblast. Here each of the chromosomes is tightly coiled and, although not evident, split into two chromatids. The chromosomes are moving to take positions on the metaphase plate. A centriole and microtubules are present in the cytoplasm. ×14,000. (From the work of B. R. Brinkley.)

change in solvation and gelation that attends mitosis. During this bubbling phase, the cell surfaces are covered with microvilli and other process. Indeed, microvilli occur throughout mitosis, being most prominent in anaphase. They also occur during G, but are usually absent or scanty in the rest of the cell cycle (Fig. 1-69). In mitosis, there are major changes in cell surface receptors: those binding lectins, for example, become reactive. With the separation of the nuclear masses in

anaphase, a partition of cytoplasmic constituents occurs. Mitochondria, lysosomes, ribosomes, and cytoplasmic membranes become distributed in approximately equal amounts about the two newly formed nuclei. As the nuclear membrane is reconstituted, the cytoplasm becomes deeply constricted between the two masses of chromosomes; as the nuclei form, the cytoplasm divides, forming two equal daughter cells. For a short time, the spindle may persist as a transient bridge between daughter cells. In the latter part of telophase, a cytocentrum and Golgi elements are formed.

FIGURE 1-66 Metaphase, rat kangaroo fibroblast. The metaphase plate is present in edge-on view. On the left, two centrioles (C) may be observed; on the right, one centriole. The microtubules of the spindle radiate from the centrioles. Both chromosomal (attached to kinetochore) and continuous (pole to pole) microtubules are present. ×10,350. (From B. R. Brinkley and J. Cartwright Jr., *J. Cell Biol.,* **50:**416, 1971.)

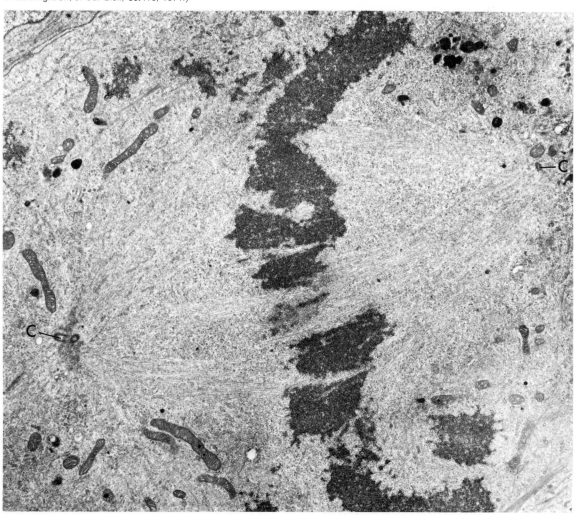

The electron microscope has elucidated several aspects of mitosis despite its disappointingly scanty information on chromosomal structure. The tubular nature of the spindle fibers and structural details of the centromere and attachment of the spindle are among these findings. An observation of particular interest relates to the formation of the nuclear membranes in telophase. Here the masses of chromosomes, before they are aggregated into a single mass, are surrounded

FIGURE 1-67 Metaphase, rat kangaroo fibroblast. Chromosomal microtubules are inserted into kinetochores (K). Note the double nature of the kinetochore. Continuous microtubules pass between the chromosomes running from pole to pole without insertion into kinetochores. ×30,800. (From B. R. Brinkley and J. W. Cartwright, *J. Cell Biol.,* **50:**416, 1971.)

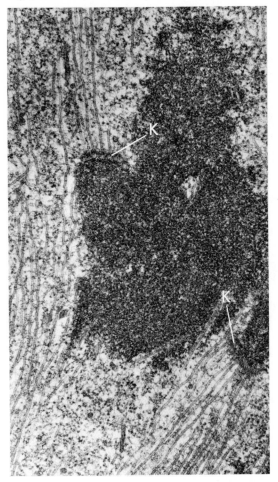

by membranes similar to the nuclear membranes, derived from the ER. Later, when the chromosomes unite into a single zone to become the nucleus, the membranes formed about each of the dispersed chromosomal groups coalesce to form a definitive nuclear membrane. The cell surface of cells in tissue culture shows interesting changes during mitosis, as shown by SEM. These are illustrated in Fig. 1-69.

Amitosis

Occasionally forms of somatic nuclear division besides mitosis occur; these are grouped under the term *amitosis* (Fig. 1-70). Amitosis may occur in terminal or highly transient cell types such as certain cells of the placenta or of the blood. It may also occur in some multinucleated cells, as the giant cells of the connective tissue. In amitosis the nuclear membrane appears to constrict deeply and a single nucleus becomes pinched into two. Although equal-sized daughter nuclei may sometimes result, it is clearly impossible that a precise separation of chromosomal material can thus be achieved.

Polyteny and Poliploidy

DNA replication may occur without nuclear division. It is characteristic of certain cell types, as the salivary gland cells of diptera, that DNA replication occurs without subsequent chromosomal division, resulting in *polytene* chromosomes. These are chromosomes which replicate themselves many times over. But the replicates remain together rather than move apart into separate chromosomes and thereby form giant chromosomes. Polytenic chromosomes readily show a type of banding which requires fluorochromes or special giemsa staining (Fig. 1-62) to demonstrate in other chromosomes. DNA replication may occur with subsequent chromosomal duplication but without karyokinesis, resulting in polyploid nuclei. Polyploid nuclei thus contain more than a diploid number of chromosomes, and may become larger than diploid nuclei as in some hepatocytes and megakaryocytes.

Meiosis

Meiosis is a type of nuclear division, restricted to gametes, that is, spermatocytes and oocytes, wherein the number of chromosomes characteristic of somatic cells, the *diploid* number (2n), is halved to the *haploid* number (1n). For this reason meiosis is termed *reduction division.* The haploid nuclei of the gametes unite and the diploid number of chromosomes is restored in the process of fertilization. The fertilized ovum, and all

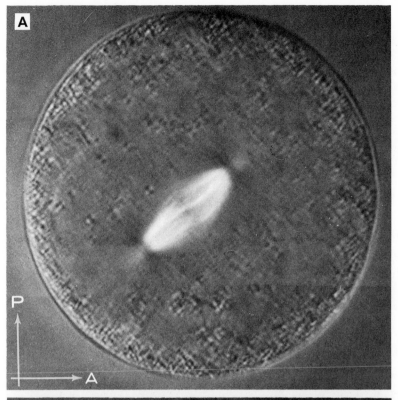

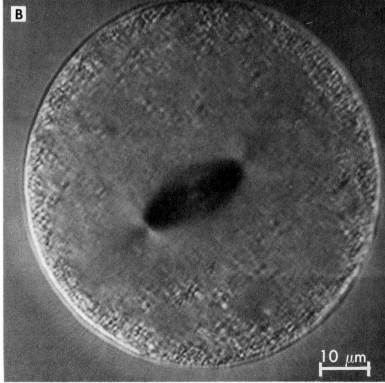

FIGURE 1-68 Metaphase spindle. Oocyte of *Pectinaria goulde.* The birefringence of the spindle is evident in these fields photographed by polarization microscopy. P represents the axis of polarized light and A corresponds to the direction of the analyzer. A. The optical axes of the polarizing plates (analyzer and polarizer) are crossed. B. Optical axes are parallel. See text under Polarizing Microscopy. (From H. Sato and S. Inoué, *J. Gen. Physiol.,* **50:**259, 1967.)

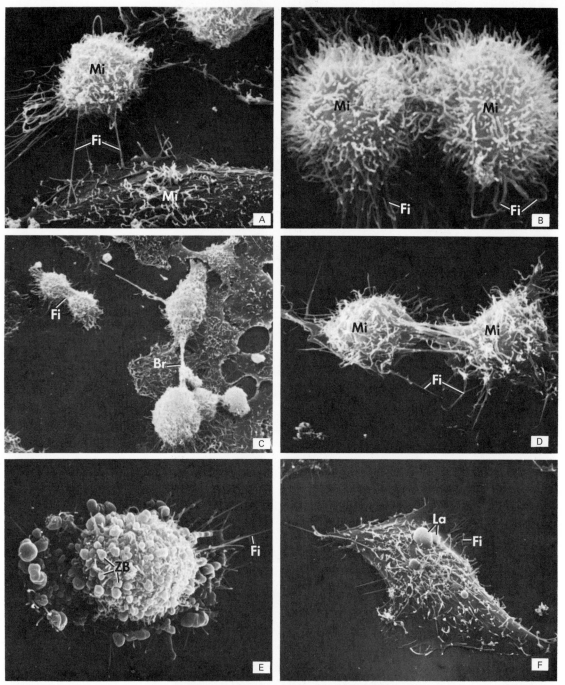

FIGURE 1-69 Scanning electron microscopy of cultured HeLa (A, C, and F) and KB cells (B, D, and E) in mitosis. Late stages in cell division are illustrated in B to D; interphase cells are illustrated in C, E, and F. Note the long bridge (Br) connecting the daughter cells in C. Other surface specializations identified are microvilli (Mi), filopodia (Fi), lamellapodia (La), and blebs (ZB). A, ×1664; B, ×3600; C, ×684; D, ×2040; E, ×1889; F, ×1680. (From H. W. Beams and R. G. Kessel, *Am. Sci.,* **64:**279, 1976.)

its descendants except the gametes, divide by mitotic division, and the diploid number is thereby maintained in somatic cells. But meiosis has the second major function of providing genetic variation by the exchange of segments of homologous chromosomes and the random selection of one of the two homologues during the reduction division.

Meiosis involves two successive nuclear divisions with only one division of chromosomes (Figs. 1-71 and 1-72). The first meiotic division is characterized by a prolonged prophase. In this prophase the homologous chromosomes come to lie together, closely and exactly paired in a point-for-point correspondence along their entire length (*synapsis*). During the process the chromosomes shorten by coiling, but not as much as in the prophase of mitosis. Moreover, each of the chromosomes is observed to be longitudinally split into two chromatids. The homologous paired chromosomes, termed a *bivalent,* therefore consist of four chromatids. A spindle forms and the bivalents arrange themselves on a metaphase plate. The divergent movement of anaphase begins as the homologues, consisting of two chromatids each, move apart to opposite poles and are then separated into daughter cells at telophase. Thenceforth, after the first meiotic division, each of the daughter cells contains one of the homologous chromosomes. It is of great significance that in the first meiotic division the kinetochore does not divide, as it does in mitosis, and so the chromatids remain together. A second meiotic division ensues in which the chromosomes become arranged in a metaphase plate and the kinetochores divide. The chromatids which make up each of the chromosomes are now free of one another and diverge from the metaphase

plate in an anaphase movement. Later in telophase they form daughter nuclei and then daughter cells. The two meiotic divisions have thus sorted the four homologous chromatids present in prophase of the first meiotic division into four separate gametes, each of which has the haploid number of chromosomes. In a male, four functional spermatozoa will result from the two meiotic divisions. Curiously, the completion of cytokinesis in the spermatozoa may be delayed so that four otherwise mature spermatozoa may remain linked in Siamese-quadruplet style. In a female four ova are produced as well, but the cytoplasmic division leaves virtually all the cytoplasm with one nucleus. The remaining nuclei, surrounded by minimal cytoplasm, cannot survive. They are called *polar bodies.* This unequal cytoplasmic division provides one nucleus with sufficient cytoplasm to support fertilization and embryogenesis. Each of the gamete nuclei contains 23 chromosomes. In female gametes one of these is an X chromosome, whereas in male gametes one is either an X or a Y. During fetal life in a human female, oocytes migrate into the ovary, proliferate a short time, and then enter prophase of the first meiotic division, and remain in that state until shortly before ovulation. Since a woman may ovulate until about 45 years of age, oocytes may remain in meiosis for more than 45 years. It may well be that the first meiotic prophase constitutes a particularly stable state for DNA.

The second major function of meiosis is to provide genetic variation. It will be recalled that in diploid

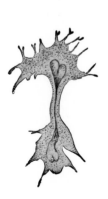
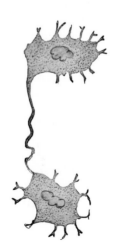
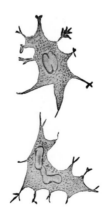

FIGURE 1-70 Amitosis in a histiocyte of a frog. The drawing is prepared from a cell in tissue culture. (From the work of Arnold.)

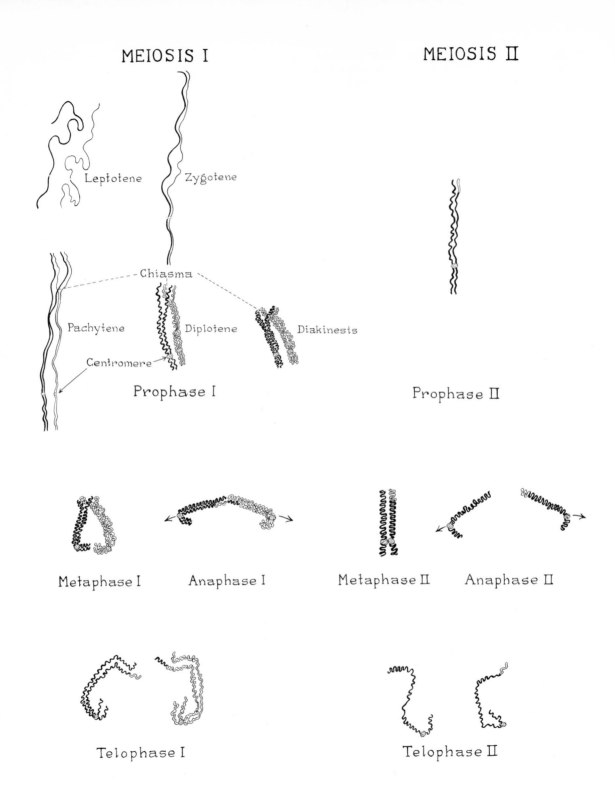

MEIOSIS I

MEIOSIS II

Leptotene

Zygotene

Chiasma

Pachytene   Diplotene   Diakinesis

Centromere

Prophase I

Prophase II

Metaphase I   Anaphase I   Metaphase II   Anaphase II

Telophase I   Telophase II

FIGURE 1-71 The stages of meiosis I and II shown schematically. A pair of homologous chromosomes, one dark and the other light, is followed through meiosis I. Then chromatids of a daughter cell are traced through meiosis II. The events are as follows:

Prophase I. Leptotene: The chromosomes become apparent as thin linear structures. Zygotene: Homologous chromosomes line up and pair with one another point to point (synapsis). Pachytene: With pairing completed, the chromosomes become shorter and thicker, and each longitudinally splits into chromatids, the centromere remaining single. The four chromatids of the two chromosomes constitute a bivalent. Chromatids from each of the homologous chromosomes may cross over one another, forming a chiasma. Diplotene: The chromosomes further shorten and broaden; they also coil. Homologous chromosomes begin to move apart but are held together at the chiasma. Diakinesis: The chromosomes become broader, thicker, more tightly coiled; they move further apart.

Metaphase I. The chromosomes are on the equatorial plate.

Anaphase I. The chromosomes diverge, exchanging chromosomal segments at the site of the chiasma.

Telophase I. Each chromatid pair, joined by a single centromere, lies in a daughter cell. The chromatids uncoil and lengthen to some extent.

Chromatids in the left-hand daughter cell pass through the following stages in meiosis II:

Prophase II. This stage is transient and possibly absent, since the chromatids may move directly to metaphase II.

Metaphase II. Chromatids become shorter, broader, and coiled. The centromere divides.

Anaphase II. Chromatids separate and move to opposite poles.

Telophase II. Each of the chromatids is now a daughter cell.

Thus in the course of these two divisions the four chromatids forming the bivalent of prophase I are separated, first into two daughter cells of telophase I, each containing two chromatids ($4n \rightarrow 2n$), and then into two daughter cells again in telophase II, each containing one chromatid ($2n \rightarrow 1n$). A total of four daughter cells is produced, each having the haploid ($1n$) number of chromosomes. In a male individual four sperms are produced; in a female, one ovum and three polar bodies. On fertilization the diploid ($2n$) number is restored.

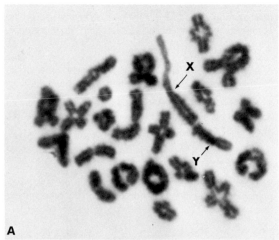

A

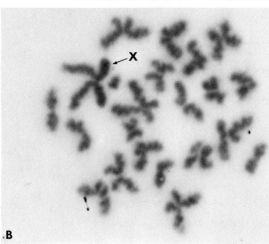

.B

FIGURE 1-72 Meiosis in the golden hamster *Mesocricetus auratus*. A. Primary spermatocyte showing the 22 bivalents at the first meiotic metaphase. The X and Y chromosomes are associated terminally, the X being distinguished by its length. The autosomal bivalents demonstrate chiasmata in various stages. Note the coiling of the chromatids. B. Secondary spermatocyte at the second meiotic metaphase, containing the haploid number of 22 chromosomes. This cell has received the Y chromosome. At this stage, the chromosomes show "relic" spirals, which are probably remnants of coiling from the first meiotic division. Aceto-orcein stain. ×2200. (From the work of M. Ferguson-Smith.)

cells one chromosome in a homologous pair is contributed by the spermatozoon and the other by the oocyte. When the homologous chromosomes are arranged upon the first meiotic metaphase plate, it is a matter of chance whether the homologue contributed by the sperm or the homologue contributed by the ovum faces a given pole. As a result, in each cell produced in the first meiotic division, the number of chromosomes derived from the sperm and the number derived from the egg are a matter of chance. This random separation is one mechanism of genetic mixture. A second mechanism is the exchange, by homologous chromosomes, of corresponding segments. This exchange occurs when the homologues are in synapsis during the early phases of meiotic prophase I. The extent of the exchange becomes apparent as the homologues pull away from their synaptic union. It is then seen that they frequently remain attached in one or more places. This persistent link between diverging chromosomes is termed a *chiasma.* The exchange of segments is termed *crossing over.*

The stages in meiosis are as follows:

1. The first prophase, prophase I, is long and may be divided into five stages. In *leptotene* the chromosomes are long and thin. In *zygotene* the homologous chromosomes move toward one another and pair, lying in close touch with one another in a point-for-point correspondence along their length (synapsis). In *pachytene* the chromosomes coil considerably, appearing shorter and thicker. At about this time it becomes apparent that each of the chromosomes of the bivalent contains four chromatids. The centromere does not split. In *diplotene* the chromosomes begin to separate from one another, but the separation is incomplete, with chiasmata forming. The separation continues into the *diakinesis,* a stage which shows the chiasmata and the thickened, coiled, partially separated chromosomes to good advantage. The nuclear membrane disappears.

2. In metaphase I the bivalent chromosomes are arranged upon an equatorial plate. There are two centromeres, one for each of the chromosomes, and these are attached to spindle fibers.

3. In anaphase I the chromosomes, each of which consists of two chromatids, move to opposite poles.

4. Telophase I follows, but the chromosomes may remain in a shortened form.

In the first meiotic division, therefore, the diploid number of chromosomes has been reduced to the haploid number; an exchange of genetic information may have occurred between the chromosomes; the distribution of chromosomes of a given bivalent to each pole has been a matter of chance, further increasing genetic variation; and each of the chromosomes is longitudinally split to form two chromatids.

5. Interphase, or *interkinesis,* is brief.

6. In prophase II a spindle forms, the nuclear membrane breaks down, and the chromosomes move equatorially.

7. In metaphase II the chromatids are arranged upon an equatorial plate and their centromeres divide and become attached to spindle fibers.

8. In anaphase II the chromatids, now daughter chromosomes, move to opposite poles.

9. Telophase II finds the appearance of a nuclear membrane, uncoiling of the chromosomes, and the development of daughter cells.

References

General

BAKER, J. R.: "Principles of Biological Microtechnique: A Study of Fixation and Dyeing." John Wiley & Sons, Inc., New York, 1958.

BRACHET, J., and A. E. MIRSKY (eds.): "The Cell." I. Biochemistry, Physiology, Morphology; II. Cells and Their Component Parts; III. Mitosis and Meiosis; IV. Specialized Cells, pt. 1; V. Specialized Cells, pt. 2, Academic Press, Inc., New York, 1961.

BROWN, W. V., and E. M. BERTKE: "Textbook of Cytology," The C. V. Mosby Company, Saint Louis, 1969.

BULGER. R. E. and J. M. STRUM: "The Functioning Cytoplasm" Plenum Press, Plenum Publishing Corporation, New York, 1974.

COWDRY, E. V. (ed.): "Special Cytology," 2d ed., vols. 1 to 3. Paul B. Hoeber, Inc., New York, 1932.

DE ROBERTIS, E. D. P., F. A. SAEZ, and E. M. F. DE ROBERTIS, JR.: "Cell Biology," 6th ed., W. B. Saunders Company, Philadelphia, 1975.

DOWBEN, R. M.: "Cell Biology," Harper & Row, Publishers Incorporated, New York, 1971.

GOMORI, G.: "Microscopic Histochemistry," The University of Chicago Press, Chicago, 1952.

LOEWY, A. G., and P. SIEKEVITZ: "Cell Structure and Function," Holt, Rinehart and Winston, Inc., New York, 1963.

PORTER, K. R., and M. A. BONNEVILLE: "An Introduction to the Fine Structure of Cells and Tissues," 2d ed., Lea & Febiger, Philadelphia, 1964.

Specific Aspects of Cytology

ACKERMAN, G. A.: Histochemistry of the Centrioles and Centrosomes of the Leukemic Cells from Human Myeloblastic Leukemia, *J. Biophys. Biochem. Cytol.,* **11:**717 (1961).

ADELMAN, M. R., G. G. BRISY, M. L. SHELANSKI, R. C. WEISENBERG, and E. W. TAYLOR: Cytoplasmic Filaments and Tubules, *Fed. Proc.,* **27:**1186 (1968).

BAKER, J. R.: The Cell-theory: A Restatement, History, and Critique, *Q. J. Microbiol. Sci.,* **89:**103 (1948); **90:**87 (1949); **93:**157 (1952).

BARR, M. L.: Sex Chromatin and Phenotype in Man, *Science,* **130:**679 (1959).

BEAMS, H. W. and R. G. KESSEL: Cytokinesis: A Comparative Study of Cytoplasmic Division in Animal Cells. *Am. Sci.* **64:**279 (1976).

BENEDETTI, E. L.: Cell Membrane Organization, *First Int. Symps. Cell Biol. Cytopharmacol.,* Venice, July 1969.

BENSLEY, R. R., and I. GERSH: Studies on Cell Structure by the Freezing-Drying Method. I. Introduction; II. The Nature of the Mitochondria in the Hepatic Cell of Amblystoma; III. The Distribution in Cells of the Basophil Substances, in Particular the Nissl Substance of the Nerve Cell, *Anat. Rec.,* **57:**205, 217, 369 (1933).

BENSLEY, R. R., and N. L. HOERR: Studies on Cell Structure by the Freezing-Drying Method. VI. The Preparation and Properties of Mitochondria, *Anat. Rec.,* **60:**449 (1935).

BRANDT, P. W., and G. D. PAPPAS: An Electron Microscopic Study of Pinocytosis in Ameba. I. The Surface Attachment Phase, *J. Biophys. Biochem. Cytol.,* **8:**675 (1960).

BRANTON, D.: Freeze-etching Studies of Membrane Structure, *Philos. Trans. R. Soc. Lond.* [*Biol.*], **261:**133, 1971.

BRINKLEY, B. R.: The Fine Structure of the Nucleolus in Mitotic Divisions of Chinese Hamster Cells In Vitro, *J. Cell Biol.,* **27:**411 (1965).

BRINKLEY, B. R., and E. STUBBLEFIELD: Ultrastructure and Interaction of the Kinetochore and Centriole in Mitosis and Meiosis, in D. M. Prescott, L. Goldstein, and E. McConkey (eds.), "Advances in Cell Biology," vol. 1, Appleton Century Crofts, New York, 1970.

BROWN, D. D., and J. B. GURDON: Absence of Ribosomal RNA Synthesis in the Anucleate Mutant of *Xenopus laevis,* in E. Bell (ed.), "Molecular and Cellular Aspects of Development," Harper & Row, Publishers, Incorporated, New York, 1965.

BUSCH, H., and K. SMETANA: "The Nucleolus," Academic Press, Inc., New York, 1970.

CATLEY, C. W.: "The Scanning Electron Microscope," Cambridge University Press, New York, 1972.

DALTON, A. J., and M. D. FELIX: A Comparative Study of the Golgi Complex, *J. Biophys. Biochem. Cytol.,* **2:**79 (1956).

DE DUVE, C.: Lysosomes and Phagosomes, *Protoplasma,* **63:**95 (1967).

DE DUVE, C.: Lysosomes, a New Group of Cytoplasmic Particles, in T. Hayashi (ed.), "Subcellular Particles," The Ronald Press Company, New York, 1958.

DE DUVE, C., and P. BAUDHUIN: Peroxisomes (Microbodies and Related Particles), *Physiol. Rev.,* **46:**323 (1966).

ESSNER, E., A. B. NOVIKOFF, and B. MASEK: Adenosine Triphosphatase and 5-Nucleotidease Activities in the Plasma Membrane of Liver Cells as Revealed by Electron Microscopy, *J. Biophys. Biochem. Cytol.*, **4:**711 (1958).

FAWCETT, D. W.: Cilia and Flagella, in J. Brachet and A. E. Mirsky (eds.), "The Cell," vol. 2, Academic Press, Inc., New York, 1961.

FELDHERR, C. M.: The Nuclear Annuli as Pathways for Nucleocytoplasmic Exchanges, *J. Cell Biol.,* **14:**65 (1962).

FERNANDEZ-MORAN, H., T. ODA, P. V. BLAIR, and D. E. GREEN: A Macromolecular Repeating Unit of Mitochondrial Structure and Function Correlated Electron Microscopic and Biochemical Studies of Isolated Mitochondria and Submitochondrial Particles of Beef Heart Muscle, *J. Cell Biol.,* **22:**71 (1964).

FRANKE, W. W.: Structure, Biochemistry and Functions of the Nuclear Envelope, *Int. Rev. Cytol* (Suppl) **4:**72 (1974).

FREEMAN, J. A., and B. O. SPURLOCK: A New Epoxy Embedment for Electron Microscopy, *J. Cell Biol.,* **13:**437 (1962).

GHOSH, S.: The Nucleolar Structure, *Int. Rev. Cytol.,* **44:**1 (1976).

GOSS, R. T.: Turnover in Cells and Tissues, in D. M. Prescott, L. Goldstein, and E. McConkey (eds.), "Advances in Cell Biology," vol. 1, Appleton Century Crofts, New York, 1970.

GRISHAM, J. W.: Cellular Proliferation in the Liver, in R. J. M. Fry, M. L. Griem, and W. H. Kirsten (eds.), "Normal and Malignant Cell Growth," Springer-Verlag New York Inc., New York, 1969.

HARRIS, E. J.: Transport through Biological Membranes, *Am. Rev. Physiol.,* **19:**13 (1957).

HOLTER, H.: Pinocytosis, *Int. Rev. Cytol.,* **8:**481 (1960).

HUGHES, A.: "The Mitotic Cycle," Academic Press, Inc., New York, 1952.

INOUÉ, S.: On the Physical Properties of the Mitotic Spindle, *Ann. NY Acad. Sci.,* **90:**529 (1960).

ITO, S.: The Endoplasmic Reticulum of Gastric Parietal Cells, *J. Biophys. Biochem. Cytol.,* **11:**333 (1961).

JAMIESON, J. D.: Role of the Golgi Complex in the Intracellular Transport of Secretory Proteins, in F. Clementi and B. Ceccarelli, Raven Books, Abelard-Schuman, Limited (eds.), "Advances in Cytopharmacology," vol. 1, p. 83, New York, 1971.

KARNOVSKY, M. J.: Simple Methods for "Staining with Lead" at High pH in Electron Microscopy, *J. Biophys, Biochem. Cytol.,* **11:**729 (1961).

LAJTHA, L.: Proliferative Capacity of Hemopoietic Stem Cells, in R. J. M. Fry, M. G. Griem, and W. H. Kirsten (eds.), "Normal and Malignant Cell Growth," Springer-Verlag New York Inc., New York, 1969.

LAMERTON, L.: General Introduction, in R. J. M. Fry, M. L. Griem, and W. H. Kirsten (eds.), "Normal and Malignant Cell Growth," Springer-Verlag New York Inc., New York, 1969.

LEBLOND, C. P., and Y. CLERMONT: The Cell Web, a Fibrillar Structure Found in a Variety of Cells in Animal Tissues, *Anat. Rec.,* **136:**230 (1960).

LEBLOND, C. P., and B. E. WALKER: Renewal of Cell Populations, *Physiol. Rev.,* **36:**255 (1956).

LESHER, S., and J. BAUMAN: Cell Proliferation in the Intestinal Epithelium," in R. J. M. Fry, M. L. Griem, and W. H. Kirsten (eds.), "Normal and Malignant Cell Growth," Springer-Verlag New York Inc., New York, 1969.

LIMA-DE-FARIA, A. (ed.): "Handbook of Molecular Cytology," North-Holland Publishing Company, Amsterdam, 1969.

MAUL, G. G.: On the Relationship between the Golgi Apparatus and Annucleate Lamellae, *J. Ultrastruct. Res.,* **30:**368 (1970).

MAZIA, D.: Mitosis and the Physiology of Cell Division, in J. Brachet and A. E. Mirsky (eds.), "The Cell," vol. 3, Academic Press, Inc., New York, 1961.

MC QUILLAN, K.: Ribosomes and Synthesis of Proteins, *Prog. Biophys. Biochem.,* **12:**69 (1962).

MIRSKY, A. E., and S. OSAWA: The Interphase Nucleus, in A. E. Mirsky and J. Brachet (eds.), "The Cell," vol. 2, Academic Press, Inc., New York, 1961.

MITCHELL, J. S. (ed.): "The Cell Nucleus," Academic Press, Inc., New York, 1960.

NEUTRA, M., and C. P. LEBLOND: The Golgi Apparatus, *Sci. Am.,* **220:**100 (1969).

NOVIKOFF, A. B.: Mitochondria (Chondriosomes), in J. Brachet and A. E. Mirsky (eds.), "The Cell," vol. 2, Academic Press, Inc., New York, 1961.

NOVIKOFF, A. B.: Lysosomes and Related Particles, in J. Brachet and A. E. Mirsky (eds.), "The Cell," vol. 2, Academic Press, Inc., New York, 1961.

PALADE, G. E.: Functional Interrelations of Cytoplasmic Organelles: Current Concepts and Outlook, *First Int. Symp. Cell Biol. Cytopharmacol.,* Venice, July, 1969.

PALADE, G. E.: A Small Particulate Component of the Cytoplasm, *J. Biophys. Biochem. Cytol.,* **1:**59 (1955).

PALADE, G. E.: A Study of Fixation for Electron Microscopy, *J. Exp. Med.,* **95:**285 (1952).

PALADE, G. E., P. SIEKEVITZ, and L. G. CARO: Structure, Chemistry and Function of the Pancreatic Exocrine Cell," in A. V. S. de Reuck and M. P. Cameron (eds.), "The Exocrine Pancreas," Ciba Foundation Symposium, Little, Brown and Company, Boston, 1962.

PELC, S. R.: Labelling of DNA and Cell Division in So-called Non-dividing Tissues, *J. Cell Biol.,* **22:**21 (1964).

POLLARD, T. D.: Functional Implications of the Biochemical and Structural Properties of Cytoplasmic Contractile Proteins, in S. Inove and R. E. Stephens (eds.), "Molecules and Cell Movement," Raven Books, Abelard-Schuman, Limited, New York, 1975.

PORTER, K. R., and G. E. PALADE: Studies on the Endoplasmic Reticulum. V. Its Form and Differentiation in Striated Muscle Cells, *J. Biophys. Biochem. Cytol.,* **3:**269 (1957).

PORTER, K. R., and E. YAMADA: Studies on the Endoplasmic Reticulum. V. Its Form and Differentiation in Pigment Epithelial Cells of the Frog Retina, *J. Biophys. Biochem. Cytol.,* **8:**181 (1960).

PRESCOTT, D. M.: Structure and Replication of Eukaryotic Chromosomes, in D. M. Prescott, L. Goldstein, and E. McConkey (eds.), "Advances in Cell Biology," vol. 1, Appleton Century Crofts, New York, 1970.

PRETLOW, T. G., II., E. E. WEIR, and J. G. ZETTERGREN: Problems Connected with the Separation of Different Kinds of Cells, *Int. Rev. Exp. Pathol.,* **14:**91, 1975.

RAFF. M. C. and S. DE PETRIS: Movement of Lymphocyte Surface Antigens and Receptors: The Fluid Nature of the Lymphocyte Plasma Membrane and Its Immunological Significance, *Fed. Proc.,* **32:**48 (1973).

RHOADES, M. M.: Meiosis, in J. Brachet and A. E. Mirsky (eds.), "The Cell," vol. 3, Academic Press, Inc., New York, 1961.

RICH, A., J. R. WARNER, and H. M. GOODMAN: The Structure and Function of Polyribosomes, *Cold Spring Harbor Symp. Quant. Biol.,* **28:**269 (1963).

ROBBINS, E., and N. K. GONATAS: The Ultrastructures of a Mammalian Cell during the Mitotic Cycle, *J. Cell Biol.,* **21:**429 (1964).

ROBERTSON, J. D.: The Unit Membrane, in J. D. Boyd, F. R. Johnson, and J. D. Lever (eds.), "Electron Microscopy in Anatomy," The Williams & Wilkins Company, Baltimore, 1961.

SCHROEDER, T. E.: Actin in Dividing Cells: Contractile Ring Filaments Bind Heavy Meromyosin, *Proc. Natl. Acad. Sci. U.S.A.,* **70:**1688, 1973.

SCHROEDER, T. E.: Dynamics of the Contractile Ring, S. Inove and R. E. Stephens (eds.), in "Molecules and Cell Movement," Raven Books, Abelard-Schuman, Limited, New York, 1975.

SIEGEL, B. M. (ed.): "Modern Developments in Electron Microscopy: The Physics of the Electron Microscope; Techniques: Applications," Academic Press, Inc., New York, 1964.

SINGER, S. J. and G. L. NICOLSON: The Fluid Mosaic Model of the Structure of Cell Membranes, *Science,* **175:**720 (1972).

SJÖSTRAND, F. S.: The Structure of Cellular Membranes, *Protoplasma,* **63:**248 (1967).

STERN, H.: Function and Reproduction of Chromosomes, *Physiol. Rev.,* **42:**271 (1962).

STRAUS, W.: Occurrence of Phagosomes and Phagolysosomes in Different Segments of the Nephron in Relation to the Reabsorption, Transport, Digestion, and Extrusion of Intravenously Injected Horseradish Peroxidase, *J. Cell Biol.,* **21:**295 (1964).

TAYLOR, J. H.: The Duplication of Chromosomes, in P. von Sette (ed.), "Probleme der biologischen Reduplikation," Springer-Verlag OHG, Berlin, 1966.

TAYLOR, J. H.: The Time and Mode of Duplication of Chromosomes, *Am. Naturalist,* **91:**209 (1957).

VALENCIA, J. I., and R. F. GRELL (eds.): Genes and Chromosomes, Structure and Function, *Natl. Cancer Inst. Monogr.* 18, 1965.

WATSON, M. L.: Staining of Tissue Sections for Electron Microscopy with Heavy Metals, *J. Biophys. Biochem. Cytol.,* **4:**475 (1958).

WEINSTEIN, R. S.: The Morphology of Adult Red Cells, in D. Moe and N. Surgenor (eds.), "The Red Blood Cell," 2d ed., vol. 1, p. 213, Academic Press, New York, 1974.

WEISS, J. M.: The Ergastoplasm; Its Fine Structure and Relation to Protein Synthesis as Studied with the Electron Microscope in the Pancreas of the Swiss Albino Mouse, *J. Exp. Med.,* **98:**607 (1953).

WHITE, M. J. D.: "The Chromosomes," 5th ed., Methuen & Co., Ltd., London, 1961.

WILBRANDT, W., and T. ROSENBERG: The Concept of Carrier Transport and Its Corollaries in Pharmacology, *Pharmacol Rev.,* **13:**109 (1961).

WOLSTENHOLME, G. E. W., and M. O'CONNOR (eds.): "Principles of Biomolecular Organization," Ciba Foundation Symposium, J. & A. Churchill, London, 1966.

Histochemistry and Cytochemistry

HELEN A. PADYKULA

Histochemistry-cytochemistry is a biological approach which permits a precise interpretation of the chemistry of cells and tissues in relation to structural organization. A student of histology quickly becomes aware of the intrinsic heterogeneity in the structure of multicellular organisms. Biochemical analysis alone is inadequate because homogenization of an organ obscures the structural heterogeneity, which extends to the molecular level. In histochemistry-cytochemistry, by using tissue sections, morphologic relationships are maintained. In its current stage of development, it is primarily a qualitative science, although significant advances in quantitation in situ have been made. The principal question asked by the cytochemist is the following: Where, within the organized framework of the cell, is a particular chemical component located? To identify and localize the component, a specific procedure derived from well-established reactions in inorganic or organic chemistry is used to yield a reaction product visible with microscopes. The result offers qualitative and spatial precision; for example, it has been established that glucose-6-phosphatase is localized in the rough and smooth endoplasmic reticulum as well as in the nuclear envelope of the hepatocyte and that galactose is incorporated into mucoprotein in the Golgi complex of the intestinal goblet cell. Such information is essential to an understanding of cell physiology.

Another major approach to the chemical characterization of cells and tissues is the isolation of cellular and tissue components by ultracentrifugation. Current procedures of ultracentrifugation and electron microscopy are so refined that ultrastructural entities (for example, the outer mitochondrial membrane or the Golgi complex) can be isolated, recognized, and characterized quantitatively. A limitation of this powerful methodology is that cell and tissue organization is dismantled with consequent loss of the interrelationship of component parts. Thus, the two major approaches to chemical characterization of cells are complementary in terms of the kinds of information yielded.

The potential for study of biological organization unleashed by the electron microscope's resolving power of 2 Å offers an exciting challenge to cytochemistry. Already many significant chemical localizations have been made at the ultrastructural level. The new impetus provided by electron microscopy is extending most of histochemistry (intratissue localizations) to cytochemistry (intracellular localizations). Much current effort centers heavily on immunocytochemistry, which has also advanced to the ultrastructural level. This powerful methodology uses the high precision of the antigen-antibody reaction to identify the location of an individual exogenous or endogenous protein.

Many significant biological concepts have emerged from the application of histochemistry and cytochemistry, only a few examples of which are cited here. Concepts of the mechanism of cellular defense have been shaped in part from information gained through the cytochemical study of phagocytosis (via identification of lysosomal derivatives by localization of acid phosphatase) and through identification of antibody-producing cells by fluorescent and other labels. Interpretations related to cell differentiation, migration, and replacement have been heavily dependent on information gained through radioautography, which permits visualization of the location of an incorporated radioactive label. The characterization of chemical differences along the nephron is accomplished mainly through histochemistry, since the complex histologic organization of the kidney makes biochemical analysis exceedingly difficult. Modern exploration of the heterogeneity of vertebrate skeletal muscle fibers received its direction from histochemical observations; zonation of the hepatic lobule is largely a histochemical concept. In all problems involving multicellular systems, some information can be derived through histochemistry. It is necessary, however, for an observer to have an adequate background in microscopic anatomy as well as in chemistry.

GENERAL PRINCIPLES OF HISTOCHEMISTRY

1. *The essential first step is the preservation and immobilization of the chemical substance by appropriate fixation and processing.* Cellular structure and selected chemical features must survive the procedures required to prepare a suitable tissue section for transmission microscopy. Special fixation is usually required to ensure retention of the chemical entity with its characteristic reactivity. In fixation for morphologic purposes, only the macromolecular protein framework (for example, nucleoproteins, lipoproteins, glycoproteins) is retained, since the proteins are denatured and new cross-linkages are established which render them insoluble. Thus, the cytochemistry of macromolecules is more readily approached than that of small molecules, such as simple sugars, amino acids, and electrolytes, which are usually washed out of tissue sections. To preserve triglycerides and other lipids, organic solvents such as acetone, chloroform, and xylol must be avoided. The fact that glycogen is soluble in water but insoluble in concentrated ethanol should be considered in selecting an appropriate fixative. Most enzymes are inactivated to some degree by fixation, and some enzymes, in addition, are soluble. Thus, fixation preceding a cytochemical demonstration of enzymatic activity usually represents a compromise between the quality of morphologic preservation and the degree of activity.

2. *A specific chemical-identifying reaction is needed which will yield an insoluble product* composed of particles small enough to be localized among the tissue and cell components and large enough to be resolved by light and electron microscopes. In addition, the reaction product should be visible by virtue of its color (ordinary light microscope), fluorescence (ultraviolet microscope), or high electron opacity (electron microscope).

3. *The specificity of the histochemical test must be defined by the appropriate use of control preparations.* The importance of this principle cannot be overemphasized, since the tissue section is a heterogeneous system with highly varied chemical reactivity. Common control preparations are ones in which a significant reagent has been omitted from the reaction or ones in which the reactive substance has been removed or masked.

4. *The accuracy of the localization of the reaction product must be evaluated* to eliminate the possibility that one of the reagents may have been bound nonspecifically to a tissue component or that the reaction product may migrate or be soluble in adjacent cell inclusions, such as lipid droplets.

5. *The sensitivity of the histochemical test must be considered when evaluating results.* A negative histochemical reaction may or may not indicate the absence of a substance. Negative results may mean that the material is not present or is in insufficient amount for detection, that an interfering reaction is present, that the substance has been chemically altered, or that the substance has been lost from the tissue during preparation.

To introduce the rationale of the histochemical-cytochemical approach, these principles are illustrated in a few commonly employed procedures. For more information about these and other procedures, the books by Barka and Anderson, Pearse, Gomori, and Burstone should be consulted.

ACIDOPHILIA AND BASOPHILIA

Staining with a cationic (basic) dye and an anionic (acid) dye is the principal way of creating the color contrasts necessary for morphologic study (see Chap. 1). A cellular or tissue component that binds a basic dye is described as being *basophilic;* conversely, a component that binds an acid dye is *acidophilic.* The designations *acidophilia* and *basophilia* are primary distinctions drawn to characterize cellular and tissue components. Understanding of the meaning of these terms is therefore of fundamental importance.

Here we shall consider how these cationic and anionic dyes may be used as histochemical reagents to characterize the cell. Figure 2-1 illustrates the chemical structure of a representative anionic (so-called acidic) dye, orange G, and a representative cationic (basic) dye, methylene blue.

Acidic and *basic* dyes are inherited designations that unfortunately do not conform to current chemical definitions for an acid and a base (that is, an acid is a substance capable of donating protons and a base is capable of accepting protons). However, through long-standing usage in biological and medical sciences, an acidic dye is one capable of forming a salt linkage with a positively charged tissue group; therefore, the dye molecule is negatively charged (anionic). A basic dye is positively charged (cationic) and hence forms a salt with a negatively charged tissue group. This usage is analogous to the naming of the nucleic acids.

Commonly used basic dyes are methylene blue, toluidine blue, basic fuchsin, carmine, and hematoxylin. (Note below the special usage of mordants with hematoxylin.) Common acid dyes are eosin, orange G, phloxine, anilin blue, and light green. For further information on dyes, consult texts in organic chemistry and Conn's book (1965).

Many substances in the protein scaffolding of the tissue section—simple proteins, nucleoproteins, glycoproteins, and lipoproteins, as well as many lipids, glycolipids, and glycosaminoglycans—have ionizable radicals that allow formation of electrostatic (salt) linkages with these dyes. This staining capacity is more easily appreciated in relation to the chemical structure of proteins. A protein is a polymer of a variety of amino acids; it is amphoteric because of the side groups of these acids, since some residues contain additional anionic functions (for example, phenolic hydroxyl or carboxyl groups) and others have addi-

tional cationic functions (for example, amino, imidazole, or guanidine) (Fig. 2-2). The basis of the amphoteric property is illustrated in Fig. 2-3, which indicates that the charge of an amino acid depends on the pH of the medium. Thus, the protein as a whole may act either as an anion or cation, depending on the algebraic sum of its positive and negative charges at the pH of its environment. The pH at which the protein approaches electrical neutrality is known as the *isoelectric point.*

The fixed proteins of a tissue section retain their amphoteric properties but are modified by denaturation. Actually fixation causes increased affinity for stains, since secondary groups are ruptured and become available for combination with the dye molecules. Certain fixatives (for example, those containing osmium or mercury) combine with various reactive groups in the tissue and can influence subsequent stainability considerably.

Evidence that the binding of acid (anionic) and basic (cationic) dyes by proteins is principally an electrostatic phenomenon can be obtained by experiments involving the dye-binding of a single pure protein, fibrin, at various pH levels (Fig. 2-4). The intensity of staining at each pH—that is, the amount of light absorbed—can be measured with a photometer; and

FIGURE 2-1 Formulas of a typical anionic (acid) dye, orange G, and a typical cationic (basic) dye, methylene blue. The formula for methylene blue depicts it as a resonance hybrid of three main structures; it was taken from Bergeron and Singer (1958).

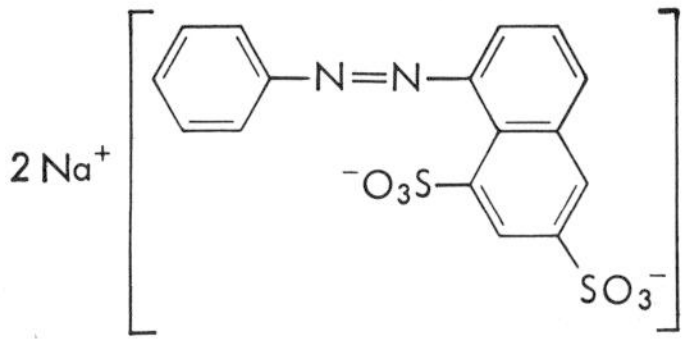

Disodium orange G

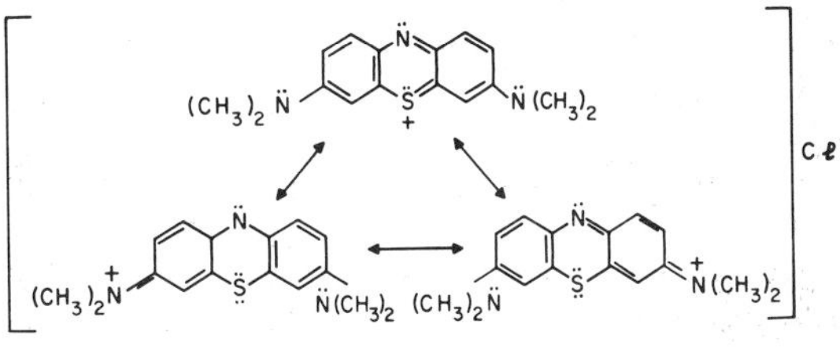

METHYLENE BLUE

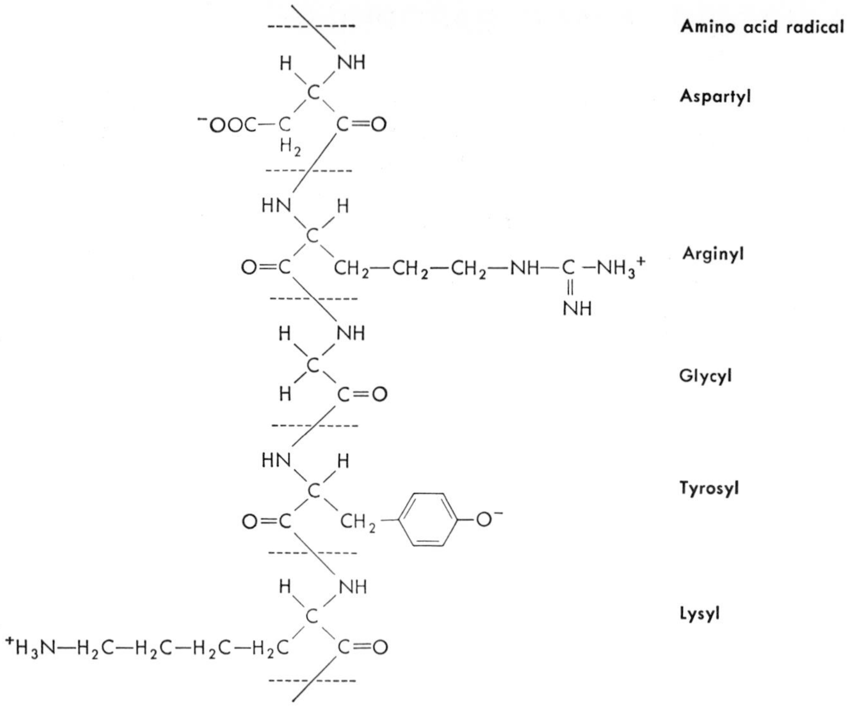

FIGURE 2-2 Structural formula of a portion of a hypothetical protein chain, showing the presence of ionizable radicals.

when plotted against pH, curves representing the acidophilia and basophilia of the protein can be drawn. Study of Fig. 2-4 shows that the least binding of cationic and anionic dyes occurs near pH 6.0, which is near the isoelectric point of fibrin. Below its isoelectric pH, the fibrin is acidophilic (that is, it binds the anionic orange G) by virtue of its overall positive charge, as $-NH_2$ ionizes to $-NH_3^+$. Above the isoelectric point, the fibrin is basophilic (that is, it binds the cationic methylene blue) because of its overall negative charge as $-COOH$ ionizes to $-COO^-$.

A tissue section, however, contains a myriad of proteins that differ in their amino acid composition and thereby have different isoelectric points, so at a pH that creates good color contrast for morphologic study, certain tissue components will show a relative acidophilia (for example, mitochondria, collagen, hemoglobin of red blood cells) while others display a relative basophilia (for example, chromatin, nucleoli, and ergastoplasm). However, the dye-binding of pro-

teins is not only related to their amino acid content but is also profoundly affected by the presence of associated groups, such as the phosphoric acid of the nucleoproteins (Fig. 2-5). Much of the cellular basophilia commonly observed in the chromatin, nucleoli, and endoplasmic reticulum (Fig. 2-6) is based on the dissociation of the phosphate groups of DNA and RNA to form negative radicals, even at relatively low pH (Fig. 2-7). Other highly basophilic structures (granules of mast cells and blood basophils, cartilage matrix, mucus of goblet cells) contain sulfated mucopolysaccharides; the high electronegativity of the sulfate group causes a basophilia that persists even at pH 2 (Fig. 2-7).

To identify basophilia originating from nucleoproteins, other information is required which can be derived from control preparations. For example, if the cytoplasm exhibits marked basophilia, a control section may be exposed to the action of the enzyme ribonuclease before staining. RNase will hydrolyze and

FIGURE 2-3 The amino acid zwitterion: the net charge is zero at the isoelectric point. The substance is anionic above the isoelectric point and cationic below it.

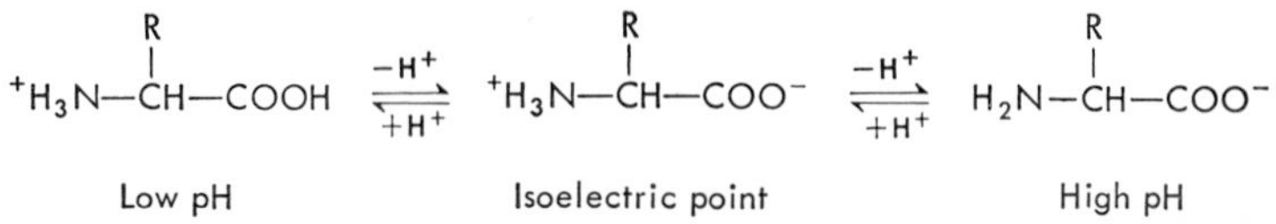

$$\overset{R}{\underset{|}{^+H_3N-CH-COOH}} \underset{+H^+}{\overset{-H^+}{\rightleftharpoons}} \overset{R}{\underset{|}{^+H_3N-CH-COO^-}} \underset{+H^+}{\overset{-H^+}{\rightleftharpoons}} \overset{R}{\underset{|}{H_2N-CH-COO^-}}$$

Low pH   Isoelectric point   High pH

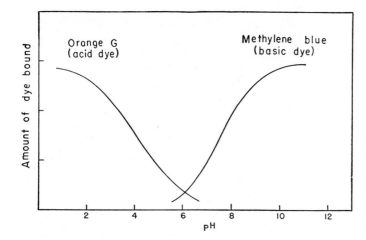

thus remove RNA present in the control, so areas in the section whose dye affinity is due to RNA will not be basophilic after such treatment. Similarly, DNase can be used to remove DNA from control preparations. Also, useful information concerning the relative basophilia of various radicals on protein molecules can be uncovered rather simply by staining at different pH levels, as shown in Fig. 2-7. The basophilia caused by the carboxyl groups of muscle proteins will be extinguished at a higher pH than that originating from the

FIGURE 2-5 Structure of a portion of DNA. The component responsible for the basophilia of chromatin is its content of phosphate radicals that can dissociate to form anions at the OH group. The arrow indicates the point between the purine and deoxyribose residues where acid hydrolysis occurs, an essential step in the Feulgen nucleal reaction.

Adenine   Deoxyribose   Phosphate

Thymine

phosphate groups of ribonucleoprotein. Basophilia persisting at pH 2 is usually indicative of the presence of the sulfate group, as in the heparin (Fig. 2-8) of mast cells or chondroitin sulfate of cartilage matrix. There are, of course, other procedures for distinguishing among basophilic substances.

Intense acidophilia over a wide pH range may reflect the presence of certain proteins. For example, red blood cells are strongly acidophilic because they are rich in hemoglobin, which contains an abundance of the amino acid lysine. The eosinophilic leukocytes obtain their name from the presence of strongly acidophilic (eosinophilic) cytoplasmic granules that contain arginine. It should be added, however, that there are also substances, such as elastic fibers, which are relatively chromophobic and which therefore show little reactivity toward these aqueous dyes.

Since the dyes hematoxylin and eosin are commonly used in routine study, it should be noted that the color-bearing moiety of the hematoxylin is actually an anionic substance called hematein that is bound (or chelated) to tissue components by a multivalent metallic cation, such as aluminum or iron, which is known as a mordant. The hematein-mordant *complex* (referred to as a *lake*) carries a positive charge. Although it behaves generally as a cationic dye, certain hematoxylin mixtures will stain mitochondria and other structures which are not basophilic under the conditions previously described. For critical distinction between acidophilic and basophilic structures, the use of methylene blue and eosin at controlled pH levels yields more evident color distinctions than a hematoxylin and eosin preparation.

Some special staining mixtures (Mallory's trichrome, Heidenhain's azan, Masson's trichrome, that is, the so-called connective tissue stains) employ a

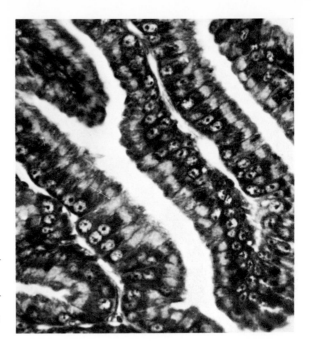

FIGURE 2-6 Epithelium, prostate, rat. Stained with methylene blue (basic or cationic dye) and eosin (acid or animic dye). Dark areas represent basophilia. In the nuclei, the basophilia of the nucleoli is evident. Most of the cytoplasm is strongly basophilic, except for a supranuclear acidophilic region, which is occupied by the Golgi complex.

combination of acid dyes, and the mechanism of their differential staining of tissue structures is still largely unanalyzed. In each mixture, however, one dye (light green, aniline blue) shows a particular affinity for collagen after the preparation has been pretreated with a tanning agent such as phosphotungstic or phospho-molybdic acid. This produces selective staining although not specific staining.

The semithin (or "thick") plastic section (1 or 2 μm), a by-product from electron microscopy, is a valuable recent addition to light microscopy. It offers the excellent preservation derived from the double

FIGURE 2-7 Staining characteristics, or "signatures," of several basophilic constituents of tissues. Methylene blue staining was employed under constant conditions of salt and dye concentration. The chemical constituents responsible for the basophilia of these cells and tissue components are the sulfate groups of chondromucoprotein in cartilage, heparin (see Fig. 2-8) of mast cell granules, the phosphate groups of ribonucleoprotein in the Nissl bodies of neurons, and the carboxyl groups of muscle proteins. In routine preparations, most cell and tissue basophilia originates from the strongly anionic phosphate group of DNA and RNA and from the sulfate groups of certain polysaccharides. (Courtesy of Dr. Marcus Singer.)

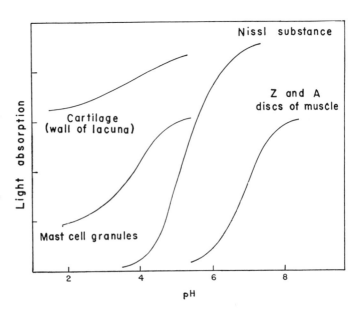

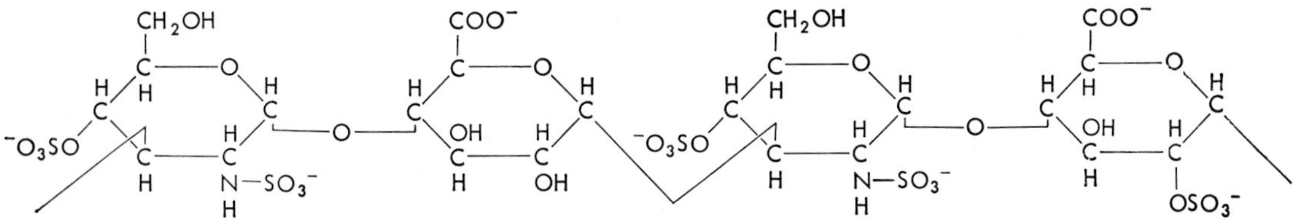

FIGURE 2-8 Tetrasaccharide unit of one type of heparin, showing the presence of sulfated radicals, which account for the marked basophilia and the metachromatic staining, and also of an unsubstituted uronic acid residue, which apparently accounts for the moderate PAS-reactivity of this substance.

fixation of electron microscopy (glutaraldehyde followed by osmium tetroxide) as well as thinness that facilitates intracellular distinctions. Such sections are most commonly stained with a single basic dye—methylene blue or toluidine blue, which are thiazine dyes that exhibit metachromasia (see below). Thus,

tissue components are usually stained blue (orthochromatic) or pink-rose (metachromatic). Osmium tetroxide blocks most of the reactive groups of macromolecules, and binding of these cationic dyes can be achieved only by staining at highly alkaline pH. As a result, the terms basophilia and acidophilia are not strictly applicable. In this system, mitochondria (usually nonbasophilic structures) will bind these cationic dyes, along with the usual basophilic cellular components.

METACHROMASIA

In a tissue section, *metachromasia* signals the change in the absorption spectrum of certain basic dyes when they are bound to polyanionic polymers, such as heparin (Fig. 2-8), chondromucoprotein, and nucleoprotein. Thiazine dyes (such as toluidine blue, thionine, and to a lesser extent, methylene blue) are *orthochromatic* blue when seen in a dilute solution where they exist in a monomeric state; however, when they are concentrated in a solution, they aggregate as

dimers and polymers which absorb at a lower wavelength and thus appear *metachromatic* red. Thus, different colors may be obtained from a single thiazine dye, depending on the state of aggregation of the molecules, and this state may be altered by the tissue components themselves.

For a histochemical demonstration of metachromasia, a tissue section is exposed to a dilute solution of toluidine blue. This cationic dye will bind

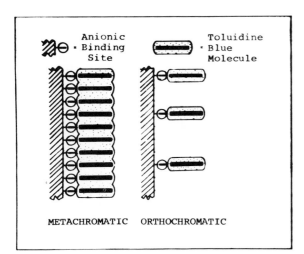

FIGURE 2-9A Hypothesis concerning the basis of metachromasia in tissue sections. The polyanionic polymer on the left possesses a series of closely, uniformly spaced negative sites which react electrostatically with cationic molecules of toluidine blue. This alignment allows interaction of dye molecules that results in a metachromatic shift (red). On the right, the anionic sites are more widely and irregularly spaced; this results in an orthochromatic effect (blue). (Modified from Bradley and Wolf, *Proc. Natl. Acad. Sci.*, **45**:944, 1959.)

electrostatically with anionic sites. Wherever the anionic sites are close enough, as in polyanionic polymers, the dye molecules will be aggregated by certain constituents of the tissue (Fig. 2-9A). Their interaction on the surface of the polyanion will result in a shift in absorption that creates the metachromatic effect. It is postulated that the distance between dye molecules should be about 5 to 7 Å for such interaction and that the presence of water is essential (Fig. 2-9B). Metachromasia is illustrated in Fig. 25-34; here the nuclei stain an orthochromatic blue, but the ground substance of the connective tissue is metachromatic red. Under certain conditions, nucleoproteins will also stain metachromatically but less obviously than the sulfated mucopolysaccharides. For the expression of metachromasia, the chemical nature of the binding site does not seem so important as the distribution and

frequency of the negative charges (Fig. 2-9A). For a stimulating analysis of metachromasia, see Bergeron and Singer (1958).

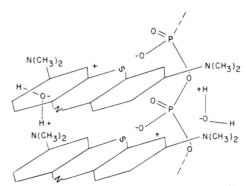

FIGURE 2-9B Hypothetical representation to illustrate the alignment of two methylene blue cations with adjacent anionic groups of a phosphate polymer such as RNA or DNA. Methylene blue cations are separated by 7 Å and dipolar water molecules intervene (from Bergeron and Singer, 1958).

REACTIONS OF THE SCHIFF REAGENT WITH ALDEHYDE GROUPS

THE PERIODIC ACID SCHIFF (PAS) REACTION

The histochemistry of carbohydrates centers around the periodic acid Schiff reaction, a procedure used routinely in most histology and pathology laboratories. It permits the localization of carbohydrate-rich macromolecules such as glycogen, mucoproteins, and glycoproteins. Glycogen is the principal storage form of carbohydrate in animals, and its identification and localization is often important.

The specificity of the PAS reaction is derived from the sequential use of two selective reagents, periodic acid (HIO_4) and the Schiff reagent. Periodic acid oxidizes the free hydroxyl groups on two adjacent carbon atoms, such as the 1,2-glycol linkage in hexoses or the adjacent hydroxyl and amino groups in hexosamine (Fig. 2-10). The hydroxyl groups are converted to aldehydes, the carbon-to-carbon bond is cleaved, and under the conditions of the PAS procedure, the oxidation does not proceed further. The resulting aldehydes react readily with the Schiff reagent to produce a stable-colored complex. The usual Schiff reagent is leukofuchsin, or fuchsin-sulfurous

acid, a chromogenic bisulfite compound which, when it forms an additional product with aldehydes, produces a stable red product (Fig. 2-11).

Numerous substances, especially in the epithelia and connective tissues, are reactive in the PAS method. Common reactive tissue components are glycogen, epithelial mucins, the Golgi apparatus, cell coats (see Fig. 2-12, color insert, and Fig. 7-47), basement membranes, and polysaccharide-protein complexes occurring in the ground substance of the various connective tissues (proteoglycans). To establish that the PAS-reactive material is glycogen, a control preparation is used which has been pre-

FIGURE 2-10 Oxidation of hexosamine residue of a polysaccharide or glycoprotein by periodic acid to form dialdehydes. The point of attack is shown by the arrow.

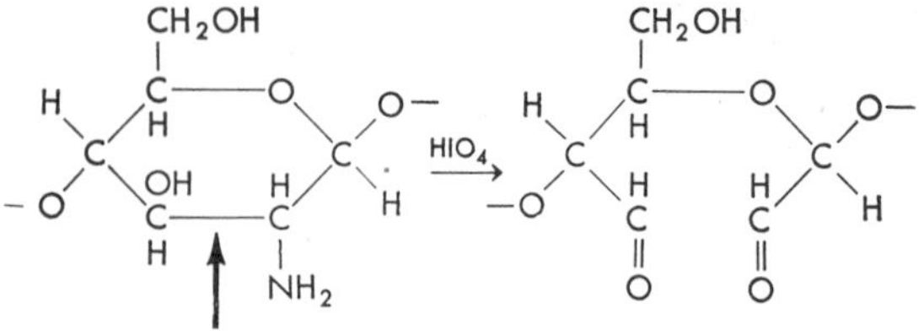

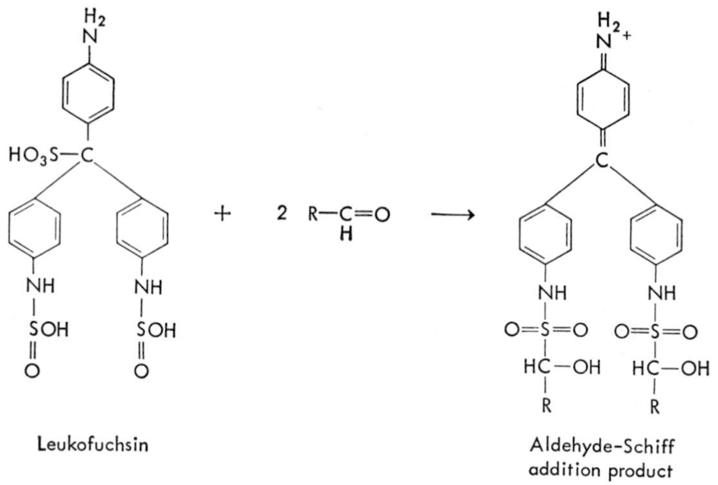

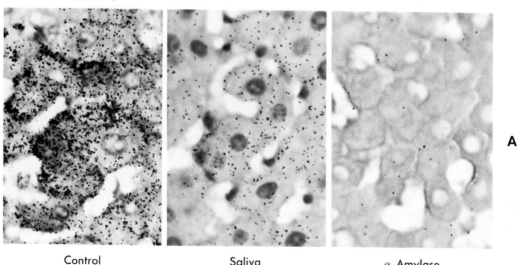

Leukofuchsin + 2 R—C=O (H) ⟶ **Aldehyde–Schiff addition product**

FIGURE 2-11 Reaction of colorless leukofuchsin with a dialdehyde to form a magenta-colored complex (see Fig. 2-12, color insert).

digested with α-amylase, an enzyme that hydrolyzes glycogen specifically (Fig. 2-13). At the ultrastructural level, glycogen particles are recognizable as aggregates called α particles (Fig. 2-14) and single β particles as in muscle fibers (Figs. 7-29 and 7-31). The sorting out

FIGURE 2-13 Glycogen synthesis in liver slices. Radioautographs of sections stained with PAS and hematoxylin. These three sections were taken from a single liver slice (obtained from a rat fasted for 24 h) that had been incubated in a medium containing [³H] glucose for 15 min. In the control, silver grains overlay PAS-positive material, especially at the periphery of the hepatocytes. That this reactive material is glycogen is demonstrated by its complete removal by α amylase. The amylase of saliva removes the glycogen only partially. ×680. (From Coimbra and Leblond, *J. Cell Biol.*, **30:**151, 1966.)

of the PAS-reactive substances not digested by amylase is a more difficult task, since there is considerable chemical variation among the carbohydrate polymers. Moreover, many of the carbohydrate-rich substances that have been localized histochemically have not yet been characterized biochemically (see Spicer et al., 1967). However, it must be appreciated that some carbohydrate units built into cellular and extracellular materials fail to stain by the PAS procedure, including several of the hyaluronic acids and most chondroitin sulfates.

An important application of the PAS reaction will be encountered in Chap. 27; the identification of the

| Control | Saliva | α Amylase |

A

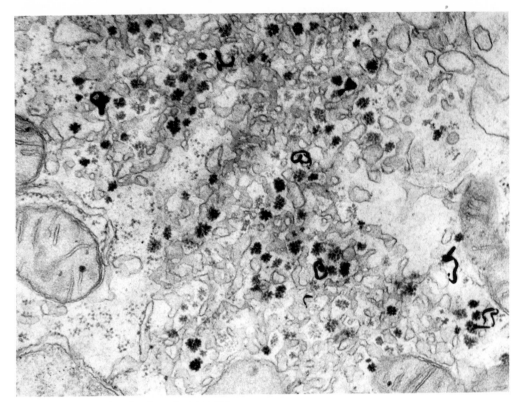

B

FIGURE 2-14 Electron-microscopic radioautograph of a portion of the cytoplasm of a hepatocyte (from liver of a fasted rat 1 h after administration of glucose-^{3}H). Most of the field is occupied by a glycogen area composed of profiles of smooth endoplasmic reticulum and dense alpha particles of glycogen in the cytoplasmic matrix. Note that the curled silver grains occur primarily in the glycogen area and not over mitochondria. ×63,000. (From Coimbra and Leblond, *J. Cell Biol.,* **30:**151, 1966.)

cells producing the glycoprotein hormones FSH, LH, and TSH is facilitated by this histochemical reaction. At the ultrastructural level carbohydrate macromolecules may be detected by oxidation with periodic acid followed by silver methenamine as a substitute for the Schiff reagent, which yields a final reaction product of sufficient electron opacity.

Further characterization of a carbohydrate-rich substance that can be made easily is the determination of its degree of basophilia, such as the strong basophilia caused by the heparin (Fig. 2-7) of mast cell granules. The presence of sulfate groups or sialic acid in polysaccharides (glycans) confers a distinct basophilia in appropriately fixed material. Glycans with polyanionic groups can also be identified by staining with Alcian blue. Sialoglycans can be removed from the tissue section by digestion with neuraminidase.

THE FEULGEN REACTION FOR DNA

A highly specific reaction for the cytochemical localization of DNA was devised by Feulgen and Rossenbeck in 1924. This widely used technique permits the localization of high-polymer DNA, and this can be followed by quantitative estimation using microspectrophotometry. The specificity is derived from the presence in DNA of a unique sugar, deoxyribose.

The procedure involves the hydrolytic removal of the purine groups by *mild* acid hydrolysis (Fig. 2-5). The furanose ring of deoxyribose thus opens and forms an aldehyde group which can react with Schiff reagent. A magenta-colored product marks the locus of DNA. One control for this test involves predigestion of the section with deoxyribonuclease; this control preparation is then stained in parallel with a standard preparation. A comparison of the two preparations allows identification of the DNA.

In most normal cells, the material reactive in the Feulgen test is limited to nuclear chromatin. Although mitochondria contain DNA, the amount is too low for the sensitivity of this procedure. Usually the same material is basophilic, but in some instances the high

isoelectric point of the protein (a protoamine) associated with the DNA competes with the cationic dye and prevents expression of basophilia.

SUDANOPHILIA OF LIPIDS

The most common cellular lipids are triglycerides and phospholipids. Triglycerides are metabolic reserves that occur in droplet form in cells, and their fluctuations within a tissue can be followed cytochemically. Phospholipids are structural components of membranes and are more difficult to localize visually. Lipids are usually preserved by formalin fixation, and frozen sections are then prepared to avoid the extraction of lipids that occurs in the routine paraffin technique.

A widely used procedure for localizing lipids is based on the properties of the Sudan dyes. These lipid "stains" are weakly ionizable and hence can be dissolved only in nonaqueous media (Fig. 2-15). The carrier for the Sudan dye is an organic solvent in which lipids are relatively insoluble, such as 70% ethanol or propylene glycol. The dye should also be only moderately soluble in this carrier but more soluble in lipids, so "staining" occurs with substances in which the dye is partitioned, as in a separatory funnel. The stained sections are then mounted in glycerol or some other water-soluble medium to avoid extraction of either the dye or the lipid. Sudanophilia therefore depends on solubility rather than salt formation or the reactivity of certain end groups. The Sudan dyes will dissolve in droplets containing triglycerides and color them intensely.

Sudan black is widely used because of its color and its ability to demonstrate lipoprotein structures such as mitochondria and myelin. Structures containing polymerized lipids, such as lipofuscin granules, can also be stained with Sudan dyes, but crystallized lipids cannot be colored. One type of control preparation consists of extraction prior to staining with an organic solvent such as acetone or chloroform plus methanol. Such extraction will remove triglycerides and cholesterol but not the phospholipids. Another important control is based on the extraction of the Sudan dye from the stained tissue section by excess solvent; this helps identify any chemical binding that might occur.

Special techniques are available for localizing cholesterol and other lipids. For a critical discussion of the cytochemistry of lipids, see the review by Deane (1958).

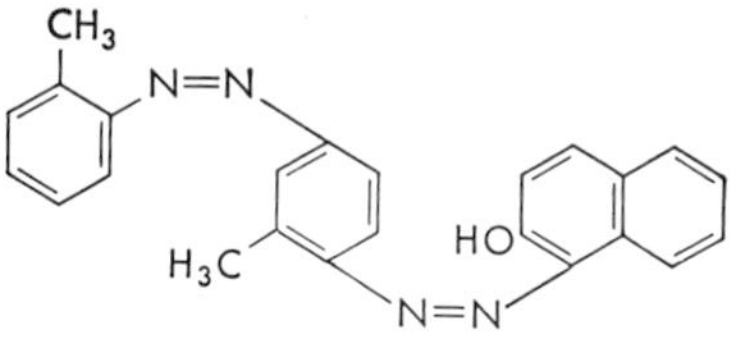

FIGURE 2-15 Sudan IV; representative oil-soluble dye.

SPECIFIC PROTEINS: ENZYMES, ANTIGENS, AND ANTIBODIES

The inherent specificity of an enzyme for its substrate or of an antibody for its antigen constitutes the basis for precise cytochemical localizations, some of which can be performed at the ultrastructural level. A colored reaction product is needed for a light microscopic localization, whereas visualization with the electron microscope requires an electron-opaque product, such as one containing a heavy metal. Furthermore, the great resolving power of the electron microscope demands that reaction products be composed of exceedingly fine particles, ideally as close as possible to the limit of resolution.

ENZYMATIC ACTIVITY

In cytochemical localizations, *the enzyme itself is not directly visualized, but as a result of its catalytic activity, a visible reaction product is formed that marks its site.* A typical cytochemical reaction for hydrolases and oxidoreductases can be formulated, in simple fashion, as follows: *AB* is the *substrate,* which undergoes an enzyme-catalyzed reaction to *A* + *B.* In the presence of *R,* a reagent capable of precipitating one of the products of the enzymatic reaction (in this case *A*), an insoluble complex *AR* is formed:

$$AB \xrightarrow[R]{\text{enzyme}} AR\downarrow + B$$

The initial insoluble complex *AR* may itself be colored or electron-opaque and hence readily visualized; more frequently, it is insoluble but not colored and must usually be converted secondarily to a colored precipitate for visualization with the light microscope. During incubation, conditions favorable for enzymatic activity—proper pH, ionic composition, and temperature—are maintained as closely as is compatible with the requirements for visualizing the product.

The choice of fixative is critical, since most fixatives inhibit enzymatic activity to some degree. Enzymes vary in their sensitivity to fixation as well as in their solubility; these properties present problems to the cytochemist. To avoid denaturation and other inhibition, frozen sections of fresh tissue are prepared, usually in a cryostat (a refrigerated chamber held usually at -15 to $-20°C$ and containing a microtome). The frozen sections are incubated in an appropriate medium for demonstrating enzymatic activity. Usually the activity of fixed and unfixed sections is compared. Fixation is generally necessary, particularly at the ultrastructural level, to preserve the macromolecular structure during the subsequent cytochemical processing. Aldehydic fixatives such as formalin or glutaraldehyde are most frequently used, the latter

being especially effective for dual preservation of cellular structure and protein reactivity.

As representatives of this principle of histochemistry, two examples will be cited: the Gomori procedure for phosphatases and a method for a pyridine nucleotide–dependent dehydrogenase.

PHOSPHATASES

A valuable cytochemical approach was introduced by Gomori in 1939 for localizing phosphatase activity, and it possesses a versatility that is still being explored. Phosphatases hydrolyze the ester linkages of natural organic phosphates such as ATP, glucose-6-phosphate, or glycerophosphate, and liberate phosphate ions as one of the reaction products (Fig. 2-16). The released phosphate ions are then trapped, ideally at the site of the enzyme, by either lead or calcium ions, to form a relatively insoluble primary reaction product, lead or calcium phosphate, which lacks color. Therefore, for light microscopy, lead phosphate is customarily converted to lead sulfide, which is black (Fig. 2-17, see color insert).

However, the interference and the phase-contrast microscopes can be used to detect the primary project; also for electron microscopy, the second step is unnecessary, since the lead phosphate itself is electron-opaque (Fig. 2-18A and B). Calcium phosphate is converted in a two-step reaction to cobalt sulfide, a brown-black precipitate for light-microscopic study. The Gomori principle is thus termed metal-salt visualization.

This rationale permits localization of phosphatases over a wide range of pH. Below pH 8, lead is the trapping ion. Though lead is useful for both light and electron microscopy, it tends to combine with hydroxyl ions about pH 8 and precipitates from the medium, so calcium is used as the capture agent above pH 8. To localize acid phosphatase, which has a pH optimum near 5, the incubating medium would contain the substrate (for example, glycerophosphate), buffer (for example, tris maleate), and lead ion as the capture reagent (Fig. 2-16). The morphologic identi-

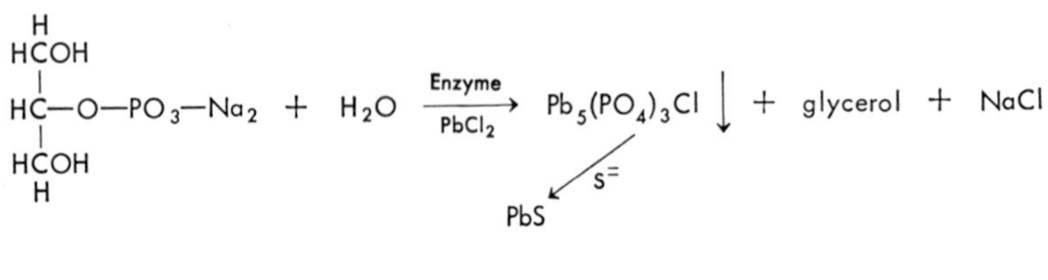

FIGURE 2-16 The Gomori acid-phosphatase reaction, pH 5.0, performed in two steps, the first yielding lead phosphate, the second, lead sulfide, both of which are insoluble reaction products.

$$\begin{array}{c} \text{H} \\ \text{HCOH} \\ | \\ \text{HC}-\text{O}-\text{PO}_3-\text{Na}_2 \\ | \\ \text{HCOH} \\ \text{H} \end{array} + \text{H}_2\text{O} \xrightarrow[\text{PbCl}_2]{\text{Enzyme}} \text{Pb}_5(\text{PO}_4)_3\text{Cl} \downarrow + \text{glycerol} + \text{NaCl}$$

$$\xrightarrow{\text{S}^=} \text{PbS}$$

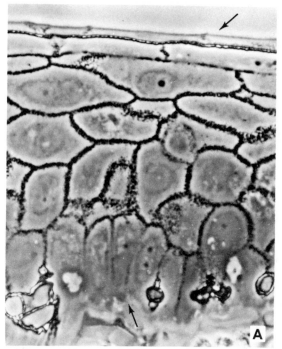

FIGURE 2-18A ATPase activity of the frog epidermis. In this photomicrograph, the shapes of the cells making up the stratified squamous epithelium are evident because the lead sulfide reaction product, which reflects ATPase activity, is located at most of the cell boundaries. It is absent, however, from the free and basal surfaces of the epithelium (see arrows). Dendritic portions of pigment cells are also reactive in the deeper layers of the epidermis. Glutaraldehyde-fixed tissue, incubation in a Gomori-type medium for ATPase activity at pH 7.2, postfixation in OsO_4, araldite section 1 μm treated with $(NH_4)S$ to produce PbS ×900. (From Farquhar and Palade, *J. Cell Biol.*, **30**:359, 1966).

preservation than that needed for cytochemistry at the light-microscopic level. It became apparent in early attempts at ultrastructural cytochemistry that osmium tetroxide, although an excellent preserver of ultrastructure and a creator of contrasting densities, is a potent inhibitor of enzymes. To circumvent this problem, two different kinds of fixation are employed. Initial fixation by glutaraldehyde preserves ultrastructure while retaining the reactive groups of many enzymes, antibodies, and other proteins (Sabatini et al., 1963). Then a cytochemical demonstration, such as that of the Gomori procedure, may be performed, preferably on tissue slices. Such aldehyde-fixed tissues tend, however, to be too low in contrast for morphologic examination, and a second fixation (or postfixation) with osmium tetroxide is performed to create the usual density contrasts associated with the ultrastructural image (Fig. 2-18B).

Various controls are required to ensure that the reaction product is a result of enzymatic activity and that its location accurately reflects the site of the enzyme. The most common control preparation is one in which the substrate has been omitted; a positive reaction here would signify the presence in vivo of metallic precipitates such as calcium or iron salts or nonspecific binding of the capture reagent. Diffusion of a reaction product to another locus is also a possibility that must be considered. In addition, special problems sometimes arise; for example, lead ion at certain concentrations can hydrolyze ATP and thus contribute a nonenzymatic component to the reaction product (Rosenthal et al., 1969). Generally the specificity of enzymatic localization and identification is greatest for enzymes that are tightly bound to cellular organelles and that also have a high substrate specificity or are selectively inhibited or activated by certain compounds.

It should be pointed out that hydrolases can also be demonstrated through the so-called azo-dye procedures which depend on a different principle. For example, phosphatase can be demonstrated by using an artificial substrate, such as naphthyl phosphate. The primary reaction products are naphthol and phosphate, but in this system, the naphthol instead of the phosphate is visualized by precipitation with a chromogenic diazonium compound. An azo dye is thereby formed as the final reaction product. This principle is illustrated in Fig. 2-19.

fication of lysosomal derivatives rests heavily on this ultrastructural cytochemical demonstration of the presence of acid phosphatase. In contrast, the muscle protein myosin has ATPase activity with an alkaline pH optimum; thus, frozen sections are incubated with ATP, barbital buffer (pH 9), and calcium ion as the capture agent. Phosphatases with a pH optimum near 7, such as glucose-6-phosphatase or mitochondrial ATPase, can be demonstrated by suitable adjustment of buffer and substrate. In addition, known activators can be incorporated to enhance catalysis and specificity.

Because it yields an electron-opaque, lead-containing reaction product, the Gomori procedure has had widespread use in ultrastructural localizations. The great resolving power of the electron microscope carries a more stringent requirement for morphologic

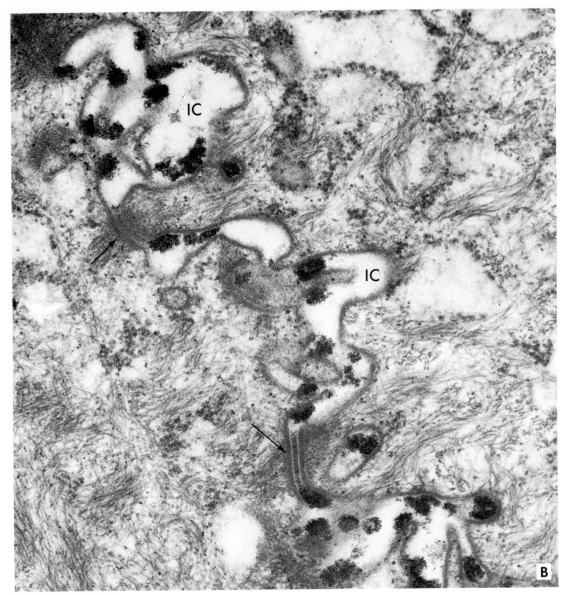

FIGURE 2-18B Electron micrograph of the junction of two cells of the stratum corneum. Lead phosphate deposits occur as aggregates of small particles (approximately 50 Å) which are located irregularly along the apposed cellular surfaces as well as in the intercellular spaces (IC). No reaction product occurs at the site of the desmosome (arrows). Fixation in glutaraldehyde, incubation in a Gomori-type medium for ATPase activity at pH 7.2, postfixation in OsO$_4$, and embedding in araldite. ×72,000. (From Farquhar and Palade, *J. Cell Biol.*, **30**:359, 1966.)

The azo-dye principle was originally introduced in 1944 by Menten, Junge, and Green for the demonstration of alkaline phosphatase activity. The coupling of the primary reaction product α-naphthol with the diazonium salt, which thus allows localization of many enzymes, can be performed over a wide pH range. The versatility of this approach was rapidly recognized by several laboratories (Seligman; Gomori; Burstone; Pearse). It was applied to demonstrate phosphatase, esterase, sulfatase, aminopeptidase, and β-glucuroni-

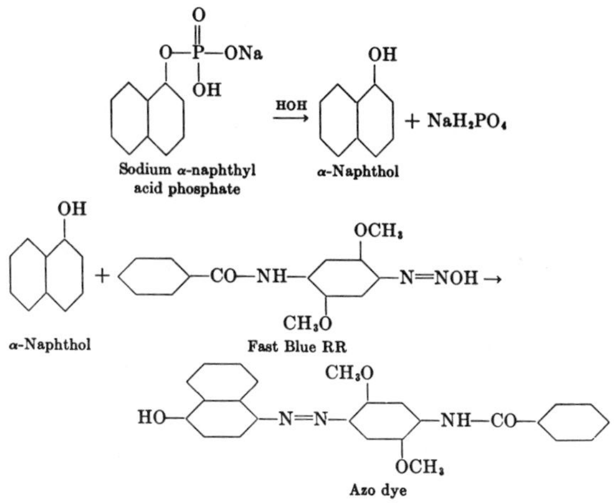

Sodium α-naphthyl acid phosphate

α-Naphthol

$+ NaH_2PO_4$

α-Naphthol

Fast Blue RR

Azo dye

FIGURE 2-19 Azo-dye procedure for localizing alkaline phosphatase activity. The enzyme hydrolyzes the substrate, naphthyl phosphate, to yield α-naphthol and phosphate ion. The diazonium salt, fast blue RR, couples with the α-naphthol to yield a bright-colored insoluble azo-dye pigment. (From Barka and Anderson, 1963.).

dase activities as well as the —SH, —NH$_2$, and —COOH groups of proteins. These variations could be achieved by synthesis of an appropriate napthyl substrate that would be hydrolyzed rapidly and specifically by the enzyme. Diazonium salts exist in considerable variety and are selected in relation to the pH of the reaction and the desired color of the final azo-dye pigment. For additional information, consult Barka and Anderson (1963), and Burstone (1962), Pearse (1968) texts and the publications of Seligman and his associates.

REPRESENTATIVE OXIDOREDUCTASE REACTIONS

This class of enzymes catalyzes the transfer of hydrogen and electrons. Many biologic oxidations take place with loss of hydrogen and electrons and without the addition of oxygen; the enzymes catalyzing such oxidations are called *dehydrogenases*. The majority of the available histochemical methods employ a reagent known as a *tetrazolium salt*. Such compounds are nearly colorless, water-soluble substances that become insoluble and colored formazans upon reduction (Figs. 2-20 and 2-21).

Chemically, the reduction of tetrazoles requires quite vigorous reducing agents acting at high pH and temperature, but in the presence of specific enzymes and substrates, the reaction will proceed at biologic

temperature and pH. Normally, when substrates are oxidized, hydrogen ions and electrons are transferred through a pyridine nucleotide coenzyme (NAD or NADP) to cytochrome *c* and thence through the electron-transport chain to oxygen. The tetrazolium can substitute for the cytochrome *c*. The enzyme capable of transferring hydrogen ions to the tetrazolium from the reduced pyridine nucleotide is called a diaphorase, or more specifically in the histochemical reaction, a tetrazolium reductase.

A representative reaction, using lactate as the initial hydrogen donor, a pyridine nucleotide coenzyme (NAD) as the initial hydrogen acceptor, and a tetrazolium salt as the final acceptor, involves a minimum of two linked enzymes, lactate-NAD oxidoreductase (lactase dehydrogenase) and NADH$_2$-tetrazolium reductase (diaphorase) (Fig. 2-21). Thus, histochemically, one is demonstrating the activity of the second, not the primary, enzyme, although the primary one is necessary for obtaining reduced coenzyme.

The reaction in which NADH$_2$ itself is supplied as substrate may be used to demonstrate the locations of the NADH$_2$-cytochrome *c* reductases. The insoluble dehydrogenases, those capable of reliable visualization, reside in mitochondria and, in some cell types, also in the endoplasmic reticulum.

Control procedures to confirm the enzymatic nature of the reaction and to establish that the provided substrate is the source of the hydrogen ions include (1) inactivation by pretreatment with heat or an —SH reagent such as *p*-chloromercuribenzoate (since like most dehydrogenases, lactate dehydrogenase is —SH-dependent) and (2) omission of the primary substrate or of the coenzyme from the incubation medium. Control preparations to confirm the location of the enzyme are more complex, especially in this

FIGURE 2-20 Reduction of a soluble tetrazolium salt to its formazan, which is insoluble in aqueous solution and is colored. R is a substituted phenolic radical.

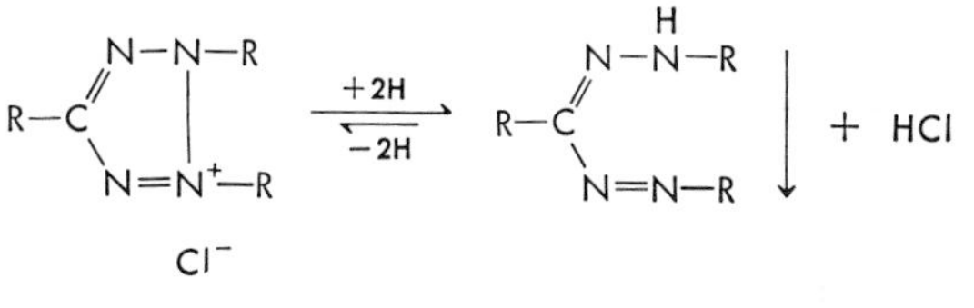

$$R-C \overset{N-N-R}{\underset{N=N^+-R}{|}} \quad Cl^- \quad \underset{-2H}{\overset{+2H}{\rightleftharpoons}} \quad R-C \overset{\overset{H}{N}-N-R}{\underset{N=N-R}{|}} \quad + HCl \downarrow$$

Tetrazolium salt   Formazan

example, where one is, at best, localizing the second of two enzymes.

A major problem in the use of tetrazoles in histochemistry has been the frequency of false localization of the formazans owing to their solubility in lipids. This difficulty has now been largely overcome by the substitution of additional water-soluble radicals on tetrazolium salts, rendering their formazans virtually insoluble in lipids. Illustrations in this book have used nitro-blue tetrazolium (nitro-BT) and tetranitro-blue tetrazolium, both of which yield highly insoluble formazans. With the tetrazoles that yield highly insoluble formazans composed of fine particles, attempts have been made to localize enzymatic activity with the electron microscope.

The diaphorase reaction is of key importance for many biologic processes, since oxidative metabolism of nutrients provides energy. Many of the oxidative enzymes are located within mitochondria, presumably in a spatial organization that permits ordered activity.

Other methods utilizing tetrazoles as hydrogen-ion acceptors from oxidative enzymes are those for the succinate oxidase system (Fig. 2-22) and monoamine oxidase. These reactions do not require pyridine nucleotides as coenzymes. In addition, at high pH, tetrazoles can accept hydrogen ions from —SH and ketol groups.

THE VISUALIZATION OF ENZYMATIC AND NONENZYMATIC HEMOPROTEINS

An important research tool in cell physiology was introduced originally by Werner Straus (1957) when

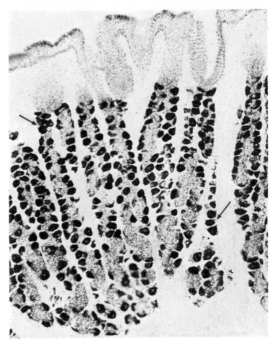

FIGURE 2-22 Succinic dehydrogenase activity, gastric glands of the cat. This cryostat section was incubated with succinate and neotetrazolium at pH 7.5 for 10 min. The diformazan deposits reveal various levels of succinic dehydrogenase activity in the cells of the gastric epithelium. The most reactive cells are the parietal cells (arrows), which have numerous mitochondria. The mucous cells of the gastric surface and pits are considerably less reactive. ×150.

he intravenously administered an exogenous enzyme, horseradish peroxidase (an oxygen transferase that is a hemoprotein), to trace the pathway of protein absorption in the kidney. The location of the tracer was identified by demonstrating its enzymic activity at the light microscopic level by incubating tissue sections with the substrate hydrogen peroxide H_2O_2 and the reagent benzidine which upon oxidation yields a blue color. Graham and Karnovsky (1966) provided ultrastructural visibility by substituting benzidine with 3,3'-diaminobenzidine (DAB) (Fig. 2-23), which upon oxidation yields an insoluble, highly colored polymeric indamine or phenazine polymers that are osmiophilic (Fig. 2-23). In the horseradish peroxidase reaction the DAB serves as the donor of two electrons to hydrogen peroxide. Subsequent osmication of the polymers yields a distinct electron-opaque reaction product called osmium black. Variations and limitations of the procedure are described by Essner (1974) and Hanker (1976).

This procedure involving oxidative polymerization

FIGURE 2-21 Production of a formazan deposit as the end result of the oxidation of sodium L-lactate, with nicotinamide-adenine dinucleotide (NAD) serving as the coenzyme.

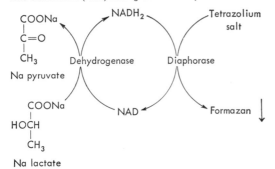

of diaminobenzidine has been used effectively to achieve ultrastructural identifications of the pathway of protein transport in a variety of cellular systems. Moreover, this principle can be used to localize endogenous hemoproteins, both enzymic and nonenzymic (catalase of peroxisomes, mitochondrial cytochrome *c* and cytochrome oxidase, hemoglobin, and myoglobin). Most hemoproteins contain the iron porphyrin prosthetic group which has peroxidatic activity, as illustrated for cytochrome *c* in Fig. 2-24.

The significance of the DAB procedure is enhanced by its effectiveness in immunocytochemical identifications of exogenous or endogenous proteins (see Fig. 2-25 and the next section). Current effort centers also on adaptation of this principle of osmiophilic polymer generation to localize a wide variety of

oxidoreductases and hydrolases with the electron microscope (see Hanker, 1976).

IMMUNOCYTOCHEMISTRY: ANTIGENS AND ANTIBODIES

Our understanding of the immune response in lymphatic organs and elsewhere in the body has been significantly advanced by the techniques of immunocytochemistry. The high specificity that resides in the mutual recognition of an antigen and its antibody makes these cytochemical identifications potentially the most precise. This powerful approach was introduced in 1941 by Albert H. Coons who, in essence, adapted immunologic procedures for use with tissue sections. *The technique is based on the use of a specific antibody that carries a label capable of being visualized.* In his highly original investigations, Coons conjugated a fluorescent dye in vitro with an antibody and thus labeled it without destroying its ability to form a complex with its antigen. The corresponding antigen could then be identified in tissue sections by "stain-

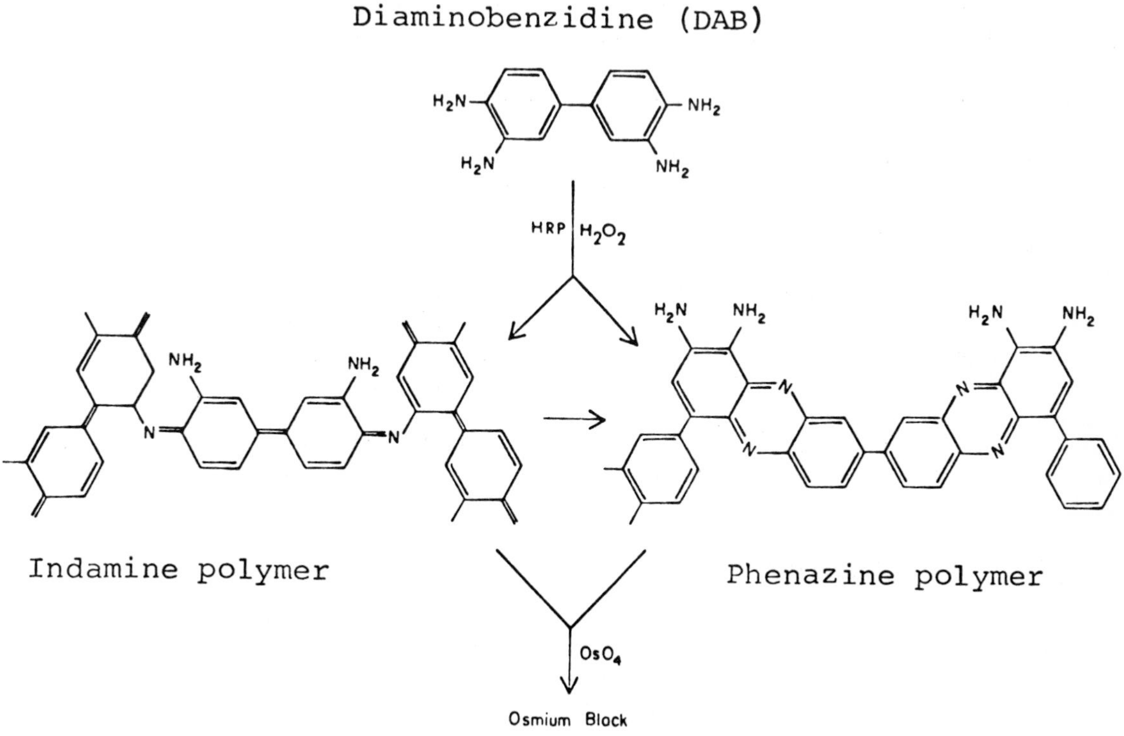

FIGURE 2-23 The DAB procedure for demonstrating peroxidase activity. Hypothetical reaction for the peroxidative or oxidative polymerization of 3,3'-diaminobenzidine (DAB) as a consequence of the catalytic action of the hemoprotein enzyme horseradish peroxidase (HRP). The oxidation of DAB results in the formation of insoluble, colored indamine or phenazine polymers at the site of peroxidase activity. The indamine polymer may also cyclize to form the phenazine polymer. Visibility of these polymers with the electron microscope is dependent on their osmiophilia. Osmication results in the formation of discrete, electron-opaque osmium blacks. (Courtesy of Dr. Jacob S. Hanker.)

Diaminobenzidine (DAB)

Indamine polymer

Phenazine polymer

Osmium Block

ing" with the fluorescein-labeled antibody and then studying the preparation with an ultraviolet microscope to localize the characteristic fluorescence of the dye-immune complex. Fewer molecules of a fluorescent dye are required for detection than of a visible dye, giving this method great sensitivity. A modification of this procedure allows recognition of the cells that produce antibody to a given antigen. Antibody is usually localized by an indirect approach which involves exposing the antibody-containing tissue section first to the corresponding antigen and then allowing the attached antigen to be "stained" with a fluorescein-labeled antibody. The specificity of the reaction is only as good as the purity of the antigen used for immunizing the animal that supplies the antibody. The importance of adequate control preparations in immunocytochemical localizations cannot be emphasized too much.

The significance of immunocytochemistry extends beyond study of the immune response because theoretically one can localize any *endogenous* protein that can be isolated and is highly purified so that specific antibody can be prepared to it. Applications of immunocytochemistry to the identification and localization of endogenous proteins have already been made in relation to the origin and location of myosin in developing muscle (Pepe, 1966) and to the cellular origin of the various protein hormones of the anterior pituitary (Nakane, 1967; see also Chap. 27). Much current effort is directed toward immunocytochemical mapping of the surfaces of cells (for example, lymphocytes.

Ultrastructural localizations have also been effected by using antigens that can be seen with the electron microscope. The protein ferritin is identifiable ultrastructurally and has been used as an antigenic stimulus to identify antibody-producing cells (de Petris et al., 1963). The ferritin molecule (MW 650,000) contains ferric hydroxide micelles arranged in a tetrahedral lattice, so it is opaque to electrons and has a characteristic ultrastructure. When ferritin is introduced as an antigenic stimulus into the footpad of a

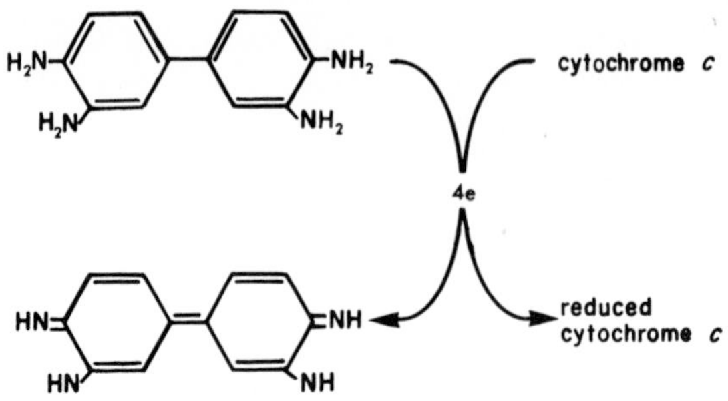

FIGURE 2-24 Diagram representing the reduction of a nonenzymic hemoprotein, cytochrome *c*, by 3,3'-diaminobenzidine (DAB) (top left). Oxidized polymeric products of DAB (lower left) after osmication (see Fig. 2-23) have been localized along the inner mitochondrial membrane through electron microscopy. Reduced cytochrome *c* is oxidized by O_2 through the action of cytochrome oxidase. (From Hanker, 1976.)

rabbit, antibody to ferritin is produced by plasma cells in the popliteal lymph node; then exposure of tissue sections of lymph node to ferritin reveals the presence of antiferritin antibody in the cisternae of the rough endoplasmic reticulum, including the nuclear envelope, of the plasma cell. Ferritin has also been used as an ultrastructural tag for antibodies, in a manner comparable to the use of fluorescent dyes as labels in light microscopy.

Immunocytochemistry has recently received considerable impetus from the use of horseradish peroxidase (MW 44,000) as an antigenic stimulus and also as a label for antibody. The use of an enzymatic label on an antibody increases the sensitivity of the identification since relatively few enzyme molecules can generate considerable reaction product (see Avrameas, 1975).

Antibodies labeled with horseradish peroxidase and other enzymes have been used as sensitive identifiers of cellular antigens (Nakane, 1970); and of the enzyme-labeled antibodies, they are currently receiving wide application to biomedical problems.

The use of horseradish peroxidase as an antigen to study the immune response is illustrated in Fig. 2-25.

Ludwig Sternberger's (1974) monograph on immunocytochemistry should be consulted for an authoritative review of current knowledge.

RADIOAUTOGRAPHY

Radioautography is a cytochemical procedure for localizing sites of radioactivity within biologic specimens, usually by using tissue sections. An animal is injected with a biologically important molecule that is labeled with a radioactive isotope, usually tritium (^3H), an isotope of hydrogen that emits particles of low energy and thus short range. For example, thymidine-^3H is injected to label DNA for a study of cellular origin and

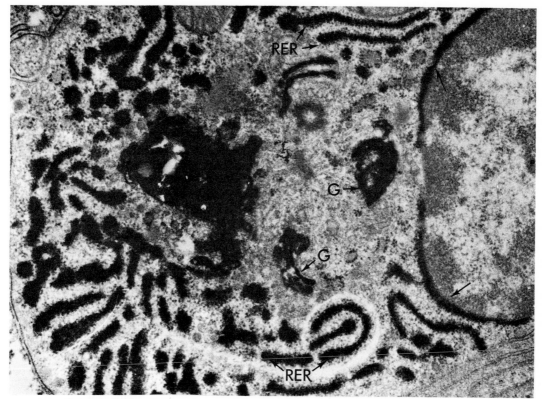

FIGURE 2-25 Ultrastructural localization of an antienzyme antibody produced in response to the injection of horseradish peroxidase, which binds specifically to its antibody. The DAB procedure of Graham and Karnovsky was used to visualize the enzymic activity of the antibody-attached horseradish peroxidase; the reaction product was then rendered electron-opaque by OsO_4, as shown in Fig. 2-23. In this immature plasma cell, antibody is located within the cisternae of the rough endoplasmic reticulum (RER) [including the perinuclear cisterna (see arrow)], and also within the cisternae of the Golgi complex (G). ×23,000. (From E. H. Leduc and S. Avrameas, Triangle, *Sandoz J. Med. Sci.,* **9:**220, 1970.)

turnover; to investigate protein synthesis, a tritiated amino acid is used; or for a study of glycogen synthesis. [^{3}H]-glucose serves as the precursor for this carbohydrate macromolecule (Figs. 2-13 and 2-14). After appropriate time intervals, the animal is sacrificed and tissue sections are prepared for light and electron microscopy. Such radioactive precursors are rapidly incorporated into macromolecules that can be readily preserved in tissue sections. Then in a darkroom, a very thin layer of photographic emulsion (suspension of silver halide crystals in gelatin) is placed on top of the tissue section (Fig. 2-26). During the subsequent period of exposure, β particles are emitted from the sites of radioactivity, and some of them pass through

the photographic emulsion and hit some of the silver halide crystals to produce a latent image (that is, small sites within a crystal where ionic silver is converted to metallic silver). After an appropriate interval of exposure, chemical development is used to convert the entire silver halide crystal that has been hit by β particles into metallic silver (a true image). Finally, the unexposed crystals are dissolved out as silver thiosulfate complexes by the photographic fixer.

The reaction product is a pattern of metallic silver grains (Figs. 2-13 and 2-14) that localizes the position of the isotope. A resolution of 0.1 μm can be achieved under good conditions, and this is certainly adequate for light microscopy. In the ultrastructural image, however, precise localization may require statistical analysis, since 0.1 μm can include a variety of structures. Resolution is influenced by geometric factors such as section and emulsion thickness, and also by the size of the silver halide crystal and the resulting developed grain.

Dynamic aspects of cellular and tissue morphology can be followed through radioautography, and many important concepts have been derived from such studies, only a few of which are noted here.

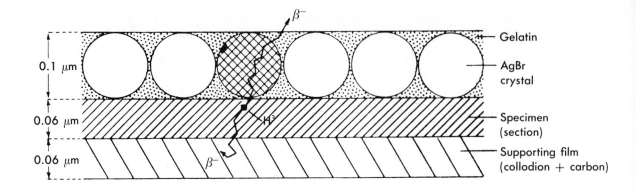

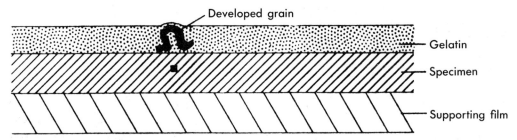

FIGURE 2-26 Diagram of a radioautographic preparation for electron microscopy. Top. A β particle emanating from a tritium source within a tissue section hits a silver halide crystal in the overlying gelatin photographic emulsion. This exposure creates a latent image in that crystal. Bottom. After photographic processing, the exposed crystal has been converted to a true image of metallic silver (developed grain) whereas the unexposed crystals have been dissolved out by the hypo solution. (Caro).

Concepts of epithelial replacement, as in the gastrointestinal tract, have evolved from labeling dividing cell populations and following their subsequent migration and differentiation. The first clue that galactosyl trans- ferase might be an enzyme of the Golgi complex was obtained from the radioautographic observation that galactose-³H is incorporated in the Golgi region of intestinal goblet cells (Neutra and Leblond). The site of macromolecular synthesis and the subsequent path of migration can be traced by ultrastructural radioautography, for example, the synthesis, storage, and secretion of digestive enzymes by the pancreatic acinar cell (Caro and Palade, 1964).

REFERENCES

AVRAMEAS, S.: Studies on Antibody Formation with Enzyme Markers, in W. Hijmans and M. Schaeffer (eds.), 5th Int. Conf. Immunofluorescence and Related Staining Technique, *Ann. NY Acad. Sci.,* **254:**175 (1975).

BARKA, T., and P. J. ANDERSON: ''Histochemistry-Theory, Practice and Bibliography.'' Paul B. Hoeber, Inc., New York, 1963.

BERGERON, J. A. and M. SINGER: Metachromasy: An Experimental and Theoretical Reevaluation, *J. Biophys. Biochem. Cytol.,* **4:**433 (1958).

BURSTONE, M. S.: ''Enzyme Histochemistry and Its Application in the Study of Neoplasms,'' Academic Press, Inc., New York, 1962.

CARO, L. G.: High Resolution Autoradiography, in David M. Prescott (ed.), "Methods in Cell Physiology," vol. 1, chap. 16, Academic Press, Inc., New York, 1964.

CARO, L. G., and G. E. PALADE: Protein Synthesis, Storage, and Discharge in the Pancreatic Exocrine Cell. A Radioautographic Study, *J. Cell Biol.,* **20:**473 (1964).

CONN, H. J.: "Biological Stains," 7th ed., Biotechnical Publications, Geneva, N.Y., 1965.

COONS, A. H.: Some Reactions of Lymphoid Tissues to Stimulation by Antigens, *Harvey Lectures,* Series L111, p. 113, 1959.

DEANE, H. W.: Intracellular Lipides: Their Detection and Significance, in S. L. Palay (ed.) "Frontiers in Cytology," Yale University Press, New Haven, 1958.

DEPETRIS, S., G. KARLSBAD, and B. PERNIS: Localization of Antibodies in Plasma Cells by Electron Microscopy, *J. Exp. Med.,* **117:**849 (1963).

ESSNER, E.: Hemoproteins, in M. A. Hayat (ed.), "Electron Microscopy of Enzymes: Principles and Methods," vol. 2, chap. 1, D. Van Nostrand Company, Inc., Princeton, N.J., 1974.

GOMORI, G.: "Microscopic Histochemistry," University of Chicago Press, Chicago, 1952.

GRAHAM, R. C., and M. J. KARNOVSKY: The Early Stages of Absorption of Injected Horseradish Peroxidase in the Proximal Tubules of Mouse Kidney: Ultrastructural Cytochemistry by a New Technique, *J. Histochem. Cytochem.,* **14:**291 (1966).

HANKER, J. S.: Catalytic Osmiophilic Polymer Generation in the Demonstration of Membrane-Bound Enzymes and Ultrastructural Tracers in Cytochemistry, in R. J. Barrnett (ed.), "Symposium in Electron Cytochemistry: Electron Microscopy Society of America, 32nd Annual Meeting," John Wiley & Sons, Inc., New York, 1976.

KARNOVSKY, M. J.: The Ultrastructural Basis of Capillary Permeability Studied with Peroxidase as a Tracer, *J. Cell Biol.,* **35:**213 (1967).

KASTEN, F. H.: The Chemistry of the Schiff's Reagent, *Int. Rev. Cytol.,* **10:**1 (1960).

LEDUC, E. H., S. AVRAMEAS, and M. BOUTEILLE: Localization of Antibody in Plasma Cells by Electron Microscopy, *J. Exp. Med.,* **127:**109 (1968).

NAKANE, P. K., and G. B. PIERCE, JR.: Enzyme-labeled Antibodies for the Light and Electron Microscopic Localization of Tissue Antigens, *J. Cell Biol.,* **33:**307 (1967).

NAKANE, P. K.: Classifications of Anterior Pituitary Cell Types with Immunoenzyme Histochemistry, *J. Histochem. Cytochem.,* **18:**9 (1970).

NEUTRA, M., and C. P. LEBLOND: Synthesis of the Carbohydrate of Mucus in the Golgi Complex, as Shown by Electron Microscopic Radioautography of Goblet Cells from Rats Injected with Glucose-H^3, *J. Cell Biol.,* **30:**119 (1966).

PEARSE, A. G. E.: "Histochemistry—Theoretical and Applied," 3d ed., vols. 1 and 2, Little, Brown and Company, Boston, 1968.

PEPE, F. A.: Some Aspects of the Structural Organization of the Myofibril as Revealed by Antibody-Staining Methods. *J. Cell Biol.,* **28:**505, 1966.

ROSENTHAL, A. S., H. L. MOSES, C. E. GUNOTE, and L. TICE: The Participation of Nucleotide in the Formation of Phosphatase Reaction Product: A Chemical and Electron Microscope Autoradiographic Study. *J. Histochem. Cytochem.* **17:**839 (1969).

SABATINI, D. D., K. BENSCH, and R. J. BARRNETT: Cytochemistry and Electron Microscopy. The Preservation of Cellular Ultrastructure and Enzymatic Activity by Aldehyde Fixation, *J. Cell Biol.,* **17:**19 (1963).

SALPETER, M. M., L. BACHMANN, and E. E. SALPETER: Resolution in Electron Microscope Radioautography, *J. Cell Biol.,* **41:**1 (1969).

SINGER, M.: Factors Which Control the Staining of Tissue Sections with Acid and Basic Dyes, *Int. Rev. Cytol.,* **1:**211 (1951).

SPICER, S. S., T. J. LEPPI, and P. J. STOWARD: Suggestions for a Histochemical Terminology of Carbohydrate-rich Tissue Components, *J. Histochem. Cytochem.,* **13:**599 (1965).

SPICER, S. S., R. G. HORN, and T. J. LEPPI: Histochemistry of Connective Tissue Mucopolysaccharides, in "The Connective Tissue," Internat. Acad. Pathol. 7, chap. 17, The Williams & Wilkins Company, Baltimore, 1967.

STERNBERGER, L. A.: "Immunocytochemistry," Prentice-Hall, Inc., Englewood Cliffs, New Jersey, 1974.

STRAUS, W.: Segregation of an Intravenously Injected Protein by "Droplets" of the Cells of Rat Kidney, *J. Biophys. Biochem. Cytol.,* **3:**1037, 1957.

SWIFT, H.: Cytochemical Techniques for Nucleic Acids, in E. Chargaff and J. N. Davidson (eds.), "The Nucleic Acids," vol. 2, Academic Press, Inc., New York, 1955.

Epithelium

ELIZABETH D. HAY

A *tissue* is defined by the histologist as a group of similar cells that work together to perform a role in the structuring and functioning of the body. For example, the tissue called muscle provides locomotion; nervous tissue integrates body activities; and connective tissue furnishes support and a source of mobile cells. *Epithelium is the tissue that covers the free surfaces of the body,* from the exposed external surface to the smallest free facets within the internal organs. The term, which was introduced in the eighteenth century by the Dutch anatomist Ruysch, probably refers to the fact that the tissue grows (G. *theleo*) upon (G. *epi*) another tissue. The cells are contiguous and rest upon a supporting extracellular layer, the *basement membrane.* There is very little intercellular material in the tissue. The free surface of the outer cells may exhibit small immobile cytoplasmic projections, called *microvilli,* and other structural specializations such as *cilia.* The total free surface of the tissue itself is frequently increased by means of folds, tubules, and, in the intestine, large multicellular projections called *villi.* The various epithelia of the adult originate from all three of the primary embryonic germ layers (ectoderm, mesoderm, endoderm).[1]

The functions of the epithelia are related to the fact that the *tissue lines free surfaces. Protection* of underlying tissues is the main role of the epithelium covering the external surfaces and body orifices. *Surface transport* of mucus and other substances is performed by the ciliated epithelium found in the respiratory and genital ducts. The epithelium of the intestine, kidney, and certain other organs is concerned primarily with *absorption* and *secretion* of products into and from a lumen. The exocrine glands are devoted exclusively to the job of providing secretory materials that will reach a free surface. Most of the endocrine glands derive from epithelium, and in some cases the fundamental relation of the tissue to a free surface is retained (follicles of thyroid gland).

By virtue of their exposed position on free surfaces, epithelial cells are also natural candidates for a role in *sensory reception,* as in the case of the taste buds and olfactory mucosa. Highly modified epithelia nourish and sustain the *reproductive cells* of the ovary and testis, but these very specialized epithelia will not be taken up in any detail in this chapter.

---

[1] *Ectoderm* gives rise to epidermis, epidermal appendages, lining of body orifices, ameloblasts, sensory epithelium, and the lens; *mesoderm* gives rise to mesothelium, endothelium, epithelium of the upper part of the urinary system, adrenal cortex, Mullerian ducts, and synovial membranes; *endoderm* gives rise to the epithelium of the respiratory and gastrointestinal tracts excepting the orifices, lining of the bladder, urethra and upper part of vagina, lining of middle ear, parenchyma of thyroid and thymus glands.

CLASSIFICATION OF EPITHELIA

An epithelium that consists of one cell layer is said to be *simple*. A simple epithelium is usually found where transfer of materials must take place across the tissue, by secretion, absorption, or diffusion. On the other hand, the protective epithelia on exposed surfaces of the body are usually *stratified;* that is, they consist of two or more layers of cells. Simple epithelium is sometimes erroneously identified as stratified in oblique sections which pass through two or more adjacent cells. One should survey large areas of an epithelium before deciding that it is really stratified.

The simple and stratified epithelia are classified as *squamous, cuboidal,* or *columnar* according to the shape of the cells on the free surface of the tissue. The cell form is actually more irregular than these terms imply, for the lateral cell surface usually has a dozen or more facets, and cell processes from adjacent cells often interdigitate to form numerous intercellular clefts. In the stratified epithelium of the urinary tract, the shape of the cells varies continually as mechanical tension changes. Nevertheless, the general differences in stratification and cell form make it convenient to subdivide the epithelia proper—that is, the sheets of contiguous cells lining free surfaces—into the following eight categories:

Simple epithelium
  Simple squamous epithelium
  Simple cuboidal epithelium
  Simple columnar epithelium
  Pseudostratified columnar epithelium

Stratified epithelium
  Stratified squamous epithelium
  Stratified cuboidal epithelium
  Stratified columnar epithelium
  Transitional epithelium

GENERAL STRUCTURE AND DISTRIBUTION OF EPITHELIA

SIMPLE SQUAMOUS EPITHELIUM

The cell in a simple squamous epithelium (Fig. 3-1) is shaped like a flat plate or "scale" (L. *squama*). Interdigitations of adjacent cell surfaces (Fig. 3-2) and specialized attachment plates along the cell facets keep the tissue intact as a sheet. The *mesothelium* lining the

FIGURE 3-1 Section showing simple squamous epithelium (below) and simple cuboidal epithelium (above) from adherent allantois and amnion of a pig embryo measuring 60 mm. At the surface of the allantois, terminal bars are evident. Zenker fixation; H & E.

FIGURE 3-2 Surface view of mesothelial cells of cat mesentery. The cell outlines are demonstrated by silver nitrate impregnation. The serrated facets of the cells interdigitate extensively.

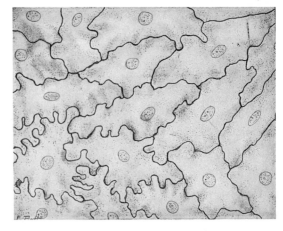

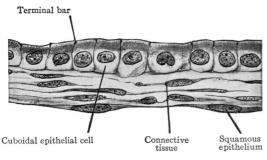

Terminal bar

Cuboidal epithelial cell   Connective tissue   Squamous epithelium

body cavities and the *endothelium* of the blood and lymphatic vessels are simple squamous sheets of attenuated cells whose nuclei bulge into the lumen. Good examples of simple squamous epithelium are also found in the air sacs of the lung, in the glomerulus and thin segment of the loop of Henle in the kidney, in the rete testis, and in certain small ducts of glands.

SIMPLE CUBOIDAL EPITHELIUM

A single-layered epithelium is said to be cuboidal if the height of each component cell is approximately equivalent to its width. The increased height permits a more extensive development and more polarized arrangement of the cytoplasmic organelles. Thus, it is not surprising to find that cuboidal cells often take a more active role in secretion and absorption than do the attenuated cells of the squamous epithelia. The best examples of simple cuboidal epithelium in the adult occur in the kidney, ciliary body, and choroid plexus. Many of the organs of the embryo are lined with a cuboidal type of epithelium (Figs. 3-1 and 3-3).

SIMPLE COLUMNAR EPITHELIUM

The cells comprising a simple columnar epithelium are usually tall and prismatic in shape. The height exceeds the width of the cell. The absorptive epithelia of the intestine and the ciliated epithelia lining the uterine tubes and small bronchi of the lung are typical examples of simple columnar epithelium (Fig. 3-4).

FIGURE 3-3 Surface view of allantois of a pig embryo. The cell outlines are more regular than those of the mesothelial cells in Fig. 3-2. The cell has on the average six lateral facets, and at each corner three cells meet.

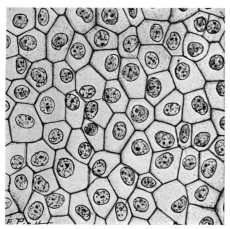

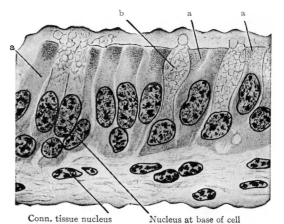

Conn. tissue nucleus   Nucleus at base of cell

FIGURE 3-4 Section of simple columnar epithelium from intestinal mucosa of Necturus. The epithelial cells are of two types: (a) cells that absorb foodstuffs, (b) goblet-shaped cells that secrete mucus.

There are, of course, cells whose shape is intermediate between that of the typical columnar and that of the typical cuboidal cell. The secretory cells of the exocrine glands are mostly low columnar or pyramidal in shape. In the thyroid gland and seminal vesicles, the epithelial cells vary in height from low cuboidal to columnar, depending on the degree of hormonal stimulation. In general, the taller the gland cell, the more polarized the arrangement of its organelles and the greater its secretory activity.

PSEUDOSTRATIFIED COLUMNAR EPITHELIUM

When a simple columnar epithelium lines a large tube, an additional layer of less differentiated cells is often added to the basal region (Fig. 3-5). The tissue usually does not become truly stratified. A careful dissection would reveal that the differentiated surface cells have retained their attachment to the basement membrane, even though their nuclei lie at different levels in the tissue. Such an epithelium is regarded as pseudostratified and is much more common than the truly multilayered columnar type. Pseudostratified columnar epithelium with cilia lines the large ducts of the respiratory tract, including the trachea, large bronchi, and much of the pharynx. Pseudostratified columnar epithelium also occurs in the vas deferens and epididymis, the male urethra, and large ducts of glands.

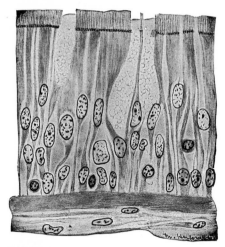

FIGURE 3-5 Pseudostratified columnar epithelium from the human trachea. All the cells rest upon the basement membrane, but not all reach the surface. The lateral cell membranes are difficult to distinguish. Three goblet cells are present, and three lymphocytes are seen migrating between the ciliated epithelial cells.

STRATIFIED SQUAMOUS EPITHELIUM

True stratification of an epithelium provides a complete basal layer of proliferating cells. The cells that will replace the superficial layer differentiate in the intermediate regions of the epithelium. The disadvantage is that the outer cells are displaced away from the vascular system in the underlying connective tissue. A ciliated or secretory cell on an epithelial surface might not function well if it were removed so far from its source of nutrition. It is not surprising, then, to find that most of the truly multilayered epithelia in the adult are stratified squamous epithelia (Fig. 3-6) whose growing basal cells are cuboidal or even columnar in form, but whose *outer cells* are flattened and relatively inert metabolically.

In regions exposed to air, the outer cells lose their nuclei and transform into keratinized plates (skin). In regions covered with fluid (cornea, esophagus, mouth, vagina), the superficial cells generally do not lose their nuclei. Such epithelium is spoken of as *nonkeratinized* to distinguish it from the *keratinized* epithelium of the skin. The difference, however, is merely one of degree, since keratin occurs in both types of stratified squamous epithelia.

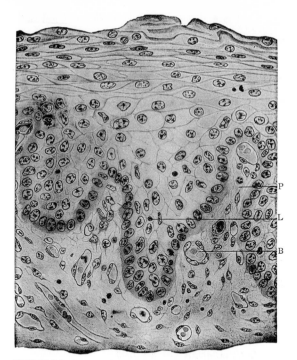

FIGURE 3-6 Section of stratified squamous epithelium from human esophagus. The cells are flattened at the surface, large and polygonal in the intermediate regions, and small and cuboidal at the base of the epithelium. The connective tissue under the epithelium forms projections (such as P) which are called papillae (L., nipple). Blood vessels are prominent in the connective tissue (such as B), but they do not extend into the epithelium. Cell L is a small lymphocyte that is migrating through the epithelium.

STRATIFIED CUBOIDAL AND STRATIFIED COLUMNAR EPITHELIUM

The two-layered epithelium of the sweat gland ducts and the epithelium in intermediate zones of the anal canal, conjunctiva, and female urethra are sometimes classified as stratified cuboidal, because the superficial cells are shaped more like cubes than squames.

Stratified columnar epithelium occurs in the intermediate zones between pseudostratified columnar epithelium and stratified squamous epithelium in the larynx, pharynx, and ducts of large glands (mammary, parotid). It is distinguished with difficulty from the more common pseudostratified columnar epithelium; if the plane of sectioning is perpendicular to the long axis of the cells, the regular appearance of the outer row of cells can be used as an identifying characteristic of the stratified epithelium. Both stratified cuboidal

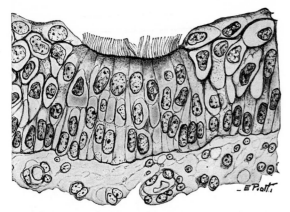

FIGURE 3-7 A section of stratified epithelium from the esophagus of a 4-month-old human fetus. In the central portion the superficial cells are ciliated and columnar, whereas laterally the epithelium is stratified cuboidal.

and stratified columnar epithelia occur more extensively in the embryo (Fig. 3-7) than in the adult.

TRANSITIONAL EPITHELIUM

The arrangement of the cells in transitional epithelium is a truly remarkable adaptation for the special tensions that may develop in the bladder, ureters, and upper part of the urethra. When the bladder is relaxed, the multilayered epithelium resembles a nonkeratinized stratified squamous or cuboidal type. The large surface cells are round and bulge into the lumen; the basal cells are small and they interdigitate with the overlying cells. It was once believed that the cells slide past each other to become a flattened, seemingly simple layer when the wall is stretched. It now seems more likely that the cells do not move over one another during distension of the organ but only become more flattened, with less interdigitation of cell processes.

The interdigitations of cell processes and folding of the luminal surface that occur in transitional epithelium are best appreciated in electron micrographs (Fig. 3-8). The cells rest on a connective tissue substratum which is not organized into rigid layers, for it also must be adapted to stretching. A rather unusual feature of the cytoplasm of bladder epithelium is the presence of numerous membrane-bounded oblong vacuoles (inset, Fig. 3-8). These may serve as reservoirs of membranous material for expansion of the cell surface. Both the surface plasmalemma and the vacuolar membrane have a unique anatomy (see Chap. 22).

CYTOLOGICAL FEATURES OF EPITHELIA

The most fundamental property of epithelial cells is their tendency to cover surfaces and maintain closely knit sheets. Structural specializations of the cytoplasm and the *lateral and basal surfaces* of the cells help to maintain cell contiguity and to give strength to the epithelial sheets. Such specializations are particularly well developed in epithelia that have a protective role, as in the skin and oral mucosa. The keratin of the epidermis protects the body surface from desiccation and abrasion. The dense tonofibrils and terminal webs of the superficial cells in the stratified squamous and transitional epithelia also protect against abrasion. Simple epithelia subject to wear and tear likewise have a tough superficial *cytoskeleton*, as in the gastrointestinal tract. Secretory and absorptive cells and ciliated cells usually have a highly specialized *free surface* and are more strikingly *polarized*. The lateral surface may also be greatly modified by extensive interdigitations.

In the discussion below, the various cytological features of the epithelial cells and their immediate environment will be considered in the following order:

1. Specializations of the lateral surface
2. The cytoskeleton
3. Specializations of the basal surface
4. Specializations of the free surface
5. Polarity of the cells

SPECIALIZATIONS OF THE LATERAL SURFACE

Intercellular Junctions

Epithelial cells are linked on their lateral surfaces by several kinds of intercellular junctions. Two of these contribute greatly to the strength of the adhesion be-

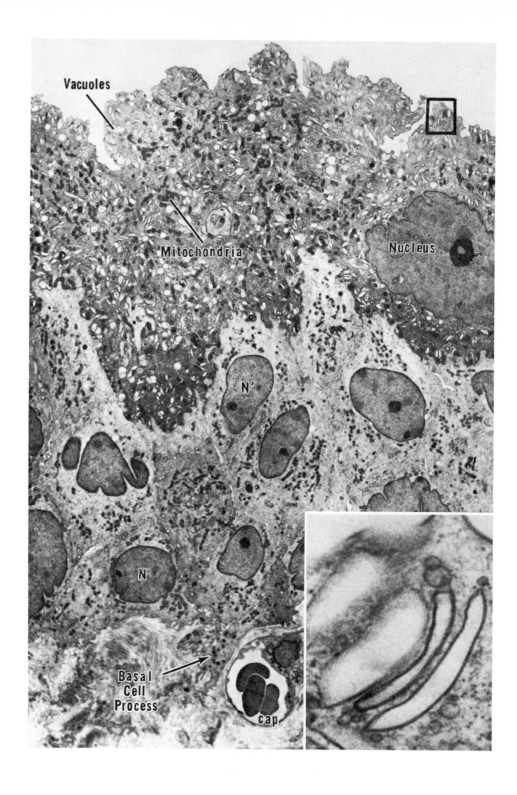

Vacuoles

Mitochondria

Nucleus

N'

N

Basal
Cell
Process

cap

tween the cells and are called adhering junctions: (1) the *macula adhaerens* or *desmosome*, which is plate-shaped and is widely distributed along the intercellular facets; and (2) the *zonula adhaerens*, which is belt-shaped and occurs around the juxtaluminal border of certain epithelia where it is the principal component of the *terminal bar.* A third type of junction, the *zonula occludens*, seals the intercellular space from contact with the lumen; and a fourth, the *gap junction* or *nexus*, seems to play a role in intercellular communication.

Maculae adhaerentes (desmosomes) are particularly well developed in the epidermis, where they occur on intercellular bridges between the cells (D, Fig. 3-9). There was considerable debate among light microscopists about whether or not the cytoplasm of adjacent cells was continuous through the bridges containing the desmosomes. Microdissection studies by Chambers and Rényi showed the desmosome to be a point of very strong attachment at the very least. Electron-microscopic studies have now demonstrated that the intercellular bridge is not a region of actual cytoplasmic continuity between cells (Fig. 3-10). The intercellular space, however, is narrow (about 200 Å) between the two halves of the desmosomes and is filled by extracellular material of low density, often bisected by an electron-opaque central or intermediate line (arrow, Figs. 3-11 and 3-12). Both the extracellular intermediate line and the amorphous material are believed to contain sialic acid, acid mucopolysaccharide (glycosaminoglycan), and protein which together presumably act as a glue. The most characteristic intracellular morphologic feature of the desmosome is the dense *attachment plaque* in the cytoplasm next to each apposed plasma membrane (DP, Figs. 3-11 and 3-12). Tonofilaments (see Cytoskeleton) are inserted into the attachment plaque. Within the plaque, each filament makes a hairpin loop and then passes back into the cytoplasm. Desmosomes fall into two main categories: those associated with stratified squamous and glandular epithelia, which are sensitive to trypsin;

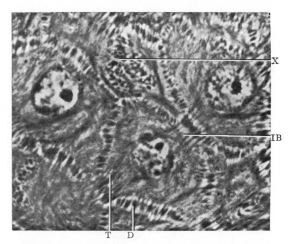

FIGURE 3-9 Light micrograph showing desmosomes (D) and tonofibrils (T) in stratified squamous epithelium. Tonofibrils course through the cells and into the intercellular ''bridges'' (IB). The midpoint of each bridge is marked by a dense body known as a desmosome. At X, the desmosomes are cut in cross section. Buccal epithelium. Zenker Formalin fixation, photographed unstained under a phase-contrast microscope. × 1,500. (Courtesy of P. H. Ralph.)

and those associated with simple columnar epithelia, which are sensitive to ethylenediaminetetraacetic acid (EDTA). Certain desmosomes can be disrupted only by detergent (desoxycholate). The bipartite structure of desmosomes is demonstrated by their mode of development. In the embryonic corneal epithelium, hemidesmosomes have been described as forming first between the cells; the halves are subsequently joined to make whole desmosomes.

The *zonula adhaerens* surrounding the lateral surface of epithelial cells near the junction of their luminal borders is similar in some respects to the desmosome (Fig. 3-12). The apposed cell membranes are separated by a very regular extracellular space,

FIGURE 3-8 Low-magnification electron micrograph of transitional epithelium from empty bladder of a mouse. The superficial cells in transitional epithelium are large and vary from cuboidal to squamous in shape, depending on the degree to which the bladder is distended. The surface cells of the mouse bladder (above) have large nuclei and are probably polyploid. Superficial cells are characterized by the presence of numerous mitochondria and oblong vacuoles. Several of these vacuoles are shown at high magnification in the inset. The square on the larger picture indicates approximately the area that appears in the inset. The nuclei of the cells in the intermediate layer (N′) and basal layer (N) are diploid and are smaller than nuclei in the superficial layer. A basal cell process extends into the connective tissue near a capillary (cap). Osmium fixation; lead tartrate stain. × 1,600; inset, × 50,000. (Courtesy of J. Rhodin.)

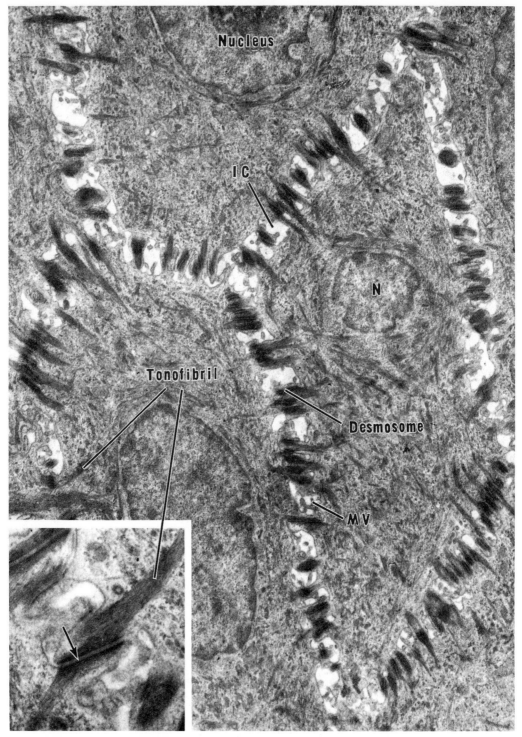

FIGURE 3-10 Electron micrograph of tonofibrils and desmosomes in stratified squamous epithelium of human oral mucosa. The desmosome is resolved as consisting of two dense attachment plates into which the tonofibrils of adjacent cells insert. The tonofibrils do not pass from cell to cell; the intercellular space, however, is very narrow between the two ''halves'' of the desmosome. One of the opposed plasmalemmas is labeled here (arrow, inset). The lateral surface of the epithelial cells have a few microvilli (MV) which project into the interfacial canals (IC). Osmium fixation. ×10,000; inset, ×30,000. (Courtesy of M. A. Listgarten.)

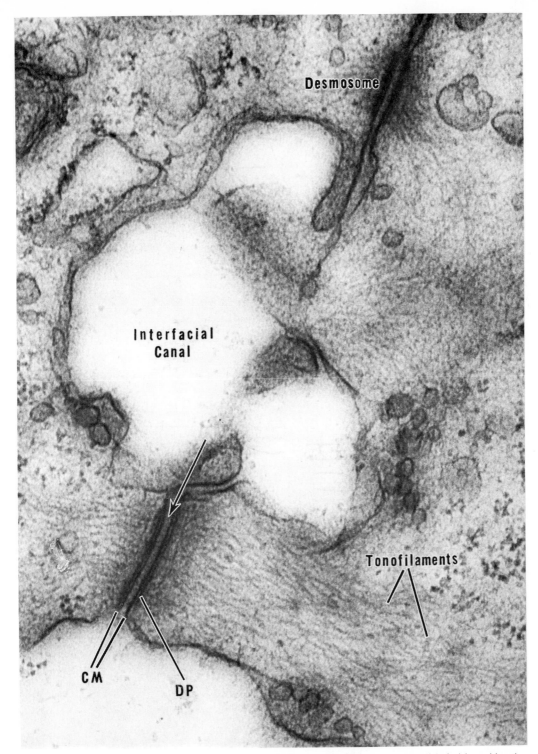

FIGURE 3-11 Electron micrograph at higher magnification showing two desmosomes and a large interfacial canal in salamander epidermis. A plaque of dense intracellular material (DP) is seen subjacent to the cell membrane (CM) on each side of the desmosome. The rather vague electron-opaque "line" (arrow) in the intercellular space may represent condensed ground substance. The component filaments of the tonofibril (tonofilaments) are resolved clearly at this magnification. They appear to be firmly anchored in the cytoplasm adjacent to the dense plaques of the desmosomes. Osmium fixation; lead hydroxide stain. × 75,000.

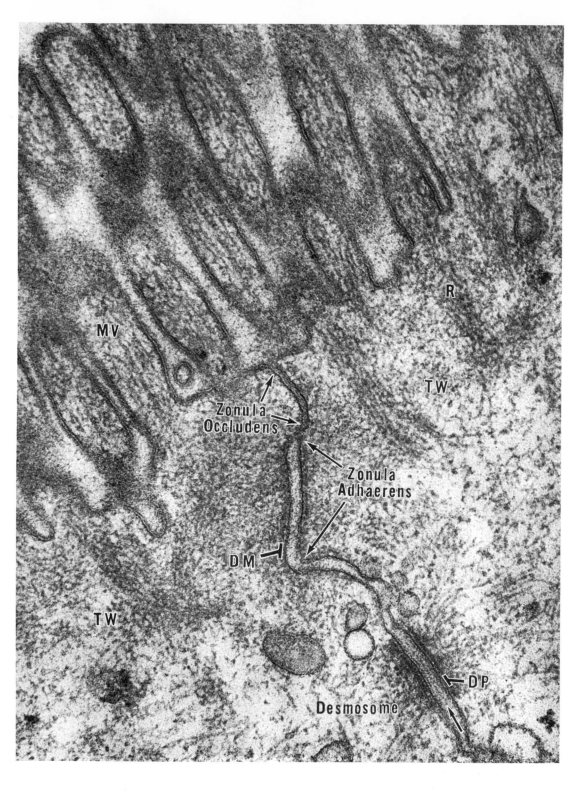

200 Å wide, in the contact zone. The dense extracellular intermediate line of the macula adhaerens is not found in the zonula adhaerens. A well-developed attachment plaque does not occur, but a moderately dense material associated with filaments of the *terminal web* is usually present in the cytoplasm next to the plasmalemma of the adjacent cells (DM, Fig. 3-12). This cytoplasmic component of the zonula adhaerens probably contributes to the darkly staining, or chromophilic, component of the terminal bar that can be visualized with the light microscope around the luminal borders of epithelial cells (Fig. 3-1).

The outermost component of the terminal bar—called the *zonula occludens*—can be appreciated only with the electron microscope. At low magnification, the zonula occludens may appear to be an area where the outer leaflets of the plasma membranes of the apposed cells are broadly fused (Fig. 3-12). Higher-magnification micrographs of thin sections show that membranes are in contact only at points within the zonula occludens (arrows, inset, Fig. 3-13). These close contacts have been called tight junctions because outer leaflets of the two apposed membranes appear as a single line and the total distance between inner leaflets is less than the sum of the width of two membranes, suggesting that the membranes really do fuse at these points. Freeze-cleave preparations reveal the three-dimensional disposition of the seemingly punctate contacts. Each contact point in fact represents a tiny ridge that, together with other ridges, forms an anastomosing network (Figs. 3-13 and 3-14). The zonula occludens network extends completely around the apical border of the cell to seal the underlying intercellular clefts from contact with the outside environment. Electron-dense tracers placed in the tissue space do not reach the free surface of the tissue (Fig. 3-15C). Interestingly, such a tracer may pass into the zonula occludens between incomplete ridges, but it is invariably stopped by the final ridge in the assembly

before it reaches the cell surface. Alternatively, one can place an electron-dense tracer in the lumen and show that the material cannot penetrate directly into the extracellular space within the epithelium.

The term *junctional complex* is used to refer to the assortment of cell junctions along the lateral interfaces next to the lumen of an epithelium. In simple columnar epithelia subjected to wear and tear, such as the intestinal epithelium, the junctional complex is especially well developed and includes, in addition to the beltlike zonula adhaerens and the zonula occludens, a band of desmosomes (Figs. 3-12 and 3-17). In other epithelia, the zonula occludens may be the only component of the junctional complex present at the luminal border (Figs. 3-13 and 3-14). In some epithelia, even the zonula occludens seems to be poorly developed or absent; the rather permeable endothelium lining capillaries is an example of this kind. Sometimes the terms *terminal bar* and *junctional complex* are used synonymously, but this is not quite correct because the terminal bar is the beltlike zone around the lateral surface of epithelial cells which can be visualized in the light microscope after appropriate staining. It probably corresponds principally to the zonula adhaerens and zonula occludens (Fig. 3-17), whereas the junctional complex is any combination of one or more juxtaluminal contacts. Since the zonula occludens and zonula adhaerens are specializations of the juxtaluminal surface of epithelia, they obviously do not occur as such in tissues lacking a lumen. However, the intercalated disc of cardiac muscle is so similar to an epithelial-adhering junction that it has been called a *fascia adhaerentes*. Moreover, punctate tight junctions have been described in sections of connective tissue cells and incompletely developed desmosomes occur in fibroblasts, cardiac muscle, and possibly other cell types.

FIGURE 3-12 Electron micrograph of the junctional complex between two epithelial cells of the rat intestine. The tight junction (zonula occludens) and the intermediate junction (zonula adhaerens) form an attachment belt which extends around the luminal surfaces of the cells. A row of desmosomes disposed under the zonula adhaerens may be present as a third component of the junctional complex. The terminal bar visualized by the light microscope corresponds to the zonula occludens and zonula adhaerens together. A dense material (DM) is usually associated with the cell membranes in attachment belts. It is similar to but not so well developed as the dense plaque (DP) of the desmosome. Intercellular material (arrow) is also more prominent in the desmosome. The terminal web (TW) is a filamentous meshwork in the apical cytoplasm of columnar and cuboidal cells. Actin filaments (R) extend into the web from the cores of the microvilli (MV) of intestinal cells. Osmium fixation; stained with lead hydroxide. × 100,000. (Courtesy of M. G. Farquhar and G. E. Palade.)

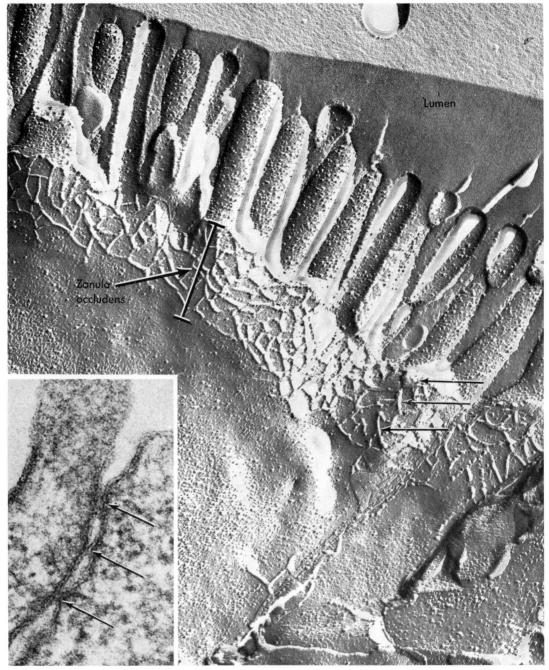

FIGURE 3-13 The zonula occludens on the luminal border of two intestinal cells is shown here in a freeze-cleave preparation viewed in the electron microscope. Numerous microvilli broken in different planes can be seen across the top of the cells. It is believed that the cell membrane cleaves through the middle, thus exposing the two inside surfaces of the plasmalemma. The surface viewed in this electron micrograph is studded with many small particles and is therefore probably the outside surface (face A) of the inner lamella (LM 1) of the plasma membrane (Fig. 3-14). The ridges (arrows, main picture) correspond to what in thin section appear to be points of tight contact (arrows, inset). An electron-dense marker, such as lanthanum entering from below, can penetrate partly into the zonula occludens by passing between incomplete ridges, but it is eventually stopped before it reaches the lumen (Fig. 3-15C). Were the other cleaved surface of the plasmalemma visible (face B), it would be seen generally to be smooth except for a few particles and, in area of zonula occludens, rows of indentations (Fig. 3-14). × 75,000 (Courtesy J. P. Revel); inset × 200,000 (Courtesy R. L. Trelstad, E. D. Hay, J. P. Revel.)

Still another kind of junction has now been demonstrated in epithelium and in all other tissues that exhibit electrotonic coupling between component cells. Termed a *gap junction,* or *nexus,* this contact specialization is a platelike junction of variable size which occurs on the deep lateral surfaces of epithelial cells. It has been widely misnamed a tight junction because the minute gap (20 Å wide) between apposed cell membranes is obscured by the lead stains routinely used in electron microscopy, thus giving the false impression that the outer regions of the membranes are fused in

the area. However, the distance between the inner leaflets of the apposed membranes is greater than the width of two fused membranes. In thin sections stained with uranyl acetate and viewed at high magnifications, the so-called gap can be seen (arrows, Fig. 3-15A). The fact that the outer leaflets of the plasma membranes are not fused in this widely distributed junction has now been conclusively demonstrated with electron-dense tracers. Tracers such as lanthanum can and do penetrate into the gap (Fig. 3-15B). The presence of such a tracer, interestingly, reveals the existence of an unexpected subunit, within the gap, which accounts for its highly uniform width. In preparations treated with lanthanum, the minute subunit is revealed in areas where the plane of section passes tangential to the plasma membrane (Fig. 3-15B). The term *gap junction* initially used to describe these contacts is thus incorrect in the sense that the term implies that a blank space separates the membranes. Each subunit of the gap junction has been called a *connexon* by Goodenough and a protein, *connexin,* has been isolated from the junction. Lipids also occur; their removal with polar organic solvents disrupts the lattice of connexons, thereby obliterating the 20-Å gap. In the lattice, each connexon is arranged hexagonally around the others and each contains a central density (arrow, Fig. 3-15B). The distance from the center of

FIGURE 3-14 This diagram depicts the junctional specializations adjacent to the bile canaliculus (BC) of a liver cell. The bile canaliculus is an example of an intercellular canaliculus (Fig. 3-27); it represents an extension of the free surface between two cells for the purpose of collecting secretory products. As for any free surface, a zonula occludens seals the adjacent lateral cleft. In routine sections, the zonula occludens is seen as a series of tiny membrane contacts immediately adjacent to the free surface. In three dimensions (inner surface, above), it is represented by a weblike array of ridges. The gap junction, or nexus, is seen in routine sections as an area of close membrane apposition where the outer leaflets of the apposed cell membranes are separated by a very regular 20-Å gap. The so-called gap is traversed by a polygonal array of subunits that extend across each apposed plasma membrane. The artist has taken some freedom in depicting the inner surface of the cell below. Freeze-cleave preparations view the outer side (face p) of the inner leaflet (LM 1) or inner face (face e) of the outer leaflet (LM 2) of the plasmalemma, so the real inner cell surface is rarely seen. The p (protoplasmic) face is also called the A face and the e (extracellular) face is sometimes called the B face. (Diagram based on unpublished illustrations by D. A. Goodenough.)

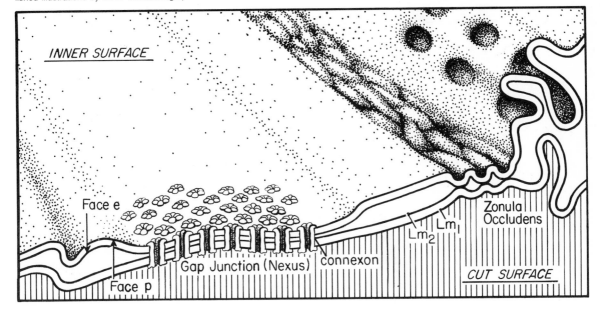

INNER SURFACE

Face e

Face p

Gap Junction (Nexus) connexon

Lm₂ Lm₁

Zonula Occludens

CUT SURFACE

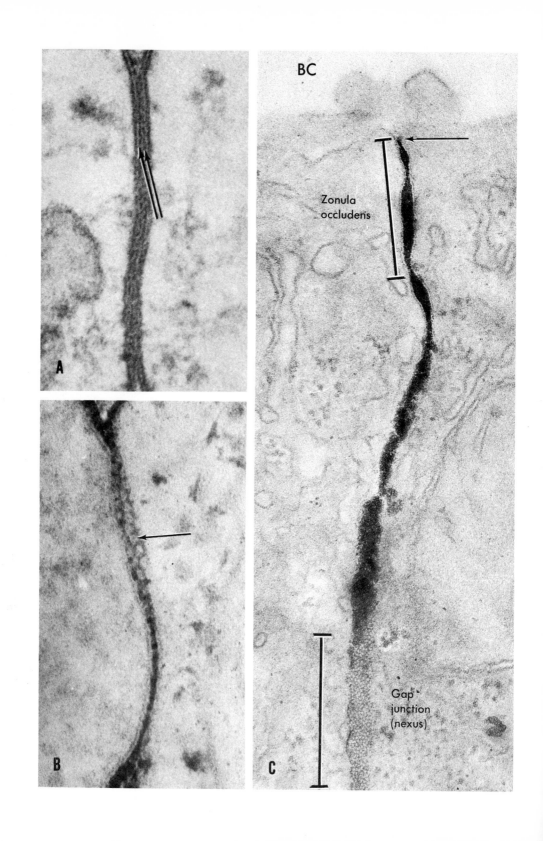

one subunit to the next is 90 Å. The freeze-cleave technique demonstrates that the polygonal lattice of connexons penetrates both junctional membranes to form a continuous connection between the cytoplasms of each apposing cell (Figs. 3-14 and 3-16).

The gap junction, or nexus, has received particular attention recently because of the possibility that it is the principal or even the only junction which mediates electric (electrotonic) coupling between cells. Furshpan and Potter (1968) and Loewenstein (1967) have shown that most normal epithelial cells are electrically coupled by placing a stimulating electrode in one cell and a recording electrode in an adjacent cell. Current passed through the first electrode meets less resistance going from cell to cell than it would if it had gone via the surrounding extracellular space. Electric coupling between cells does not imply that currents normally are passing from one cell to the other, but it shows that regions exist for preferential exchange of small ions between cells. Moreover there is now evidence that small biological molecules (up to MW 2,000) can pass preferentially from one cell to the other, presumably through gap junctions. It has been speculated that the small hole in the middle of the subunit (arrow, Fig. 3-15B) is the pore through which molecules flow. The gap junction seems to mediate impulse transmission in electrical synapses within the nervous system and may have a similar function in smooth and cardiac muscle. The myocardium beats and electrotonic coupling between heart cells persists as long as gap junctions are intact, even though desmosomes and intercalated discs are disrupted by calcium removal. When cells tear away from each other, the gap junctions do not split in half but go with one cell or the other, and coupling is lost. Loewenstein

(1967) has stressed the correlation between loss of intercellular communication of this kind and neoplasia, and he has also presented evidence that electrical coupling accompanies contact inhibition of movement when migrating cells meet during wound repair.

The Lateral Extracellular Compartment

The lateral extracellular compartment in many epithelia is narrow (200 to 300 Å), even in regions lacking junctions, suggesting that there are invisible bonds holding the cells together along their entire opposed surfaces. Such bonds may be contributed by the mucopolysaccharides demonstrated by Leblond to coat all the surfaces of the cells, and they may even be the same bonds that bring disaggregated epithelial cells together so specifically. In some epithelia, the lateral extracellular compartment may be quite large in its dimension. In stratified squamous epithelia, for example, the intercellular spaces are so dilated that they are referred to as *interfacial canals* (Figs. 3-10 and 3-11). It is likely that nutrients are circulated to the middle of the thickened epithelium through these canals between the cell facets. It is a characteristic of true epithelia that neither blood nor lymphatic vessels are present between the cells. White blood cells and macrophages can be found migrating through the intercellular spaces of epithelia on exposed surfaces of the body, particularly in the oral mucosa. Processes of unmyelinated sensory nerves extend into the interfacial canals of the epithelium of the cornea and the lip.

Interdigitation of lateral cell processes occurs to some extent in all epithelia and probably contributes to

FIGURE 3-15 Fine structure of the gap junction as seen in thin sections. A. Two trilaminar unit membranes are closely apposed along most of their length in this view. A 20-Å-wide gap can be made out between the outer leaflets of the two apposed membranes (arrows). B. A section at the same magnification showing tissue which had been soaked in lanthanum while fixing. The electron-dense marker has filled the extracellular space and penetrated the gap junction. The junction is cut tangential to the cell membrane along part of its length, and this plane of section reveals the hexagonally arrayed subunits that occupy the gap. The electron-dense dye has penetrated around the subunits, making them easy to see. The significance of the dot in the center of each 90-Å subunit (arrow) is unknown; it could mark the location of a tiny canal linking the cells. C. A lower-magnification view of a section of a piece of liver that had been soaked in lanthanum while fixing. The bile canaliculus at the top of the figure is an extension of free surface between two cells. The electron-dense marker, which entered from below, has passed around the gap junction cut tangentially near the bottom of the figure. It penetrated the zonula occludens, presumably through incomplete ridges in the zonula meshwork, but it was finally stopped by the outermost tight contact (arrow). A and B, ×300,000; (Courtesy of A. J. Hudspeth and J. P. Revel.) C, ×170,000; (Courtesy of D. A. Goodenough and J. P. Revel.)

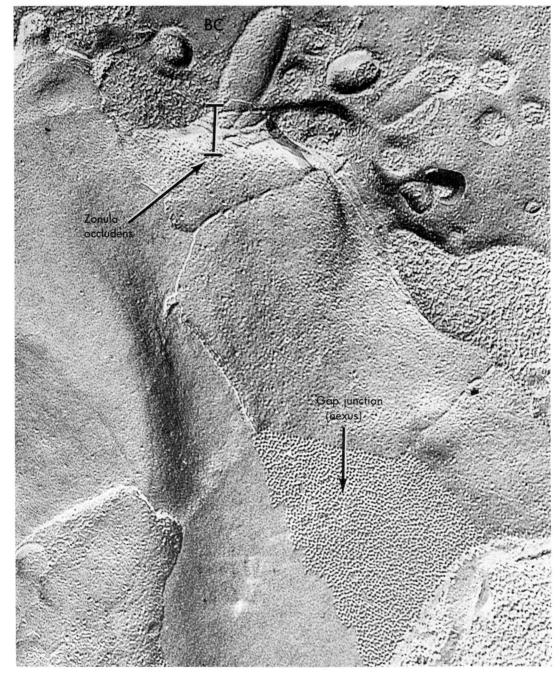

FIGURE 3-16 This electron micrograph shows, in a freeze-cleave preparation of liver, a portion of cell similar to that depicted in Fig. 3-15C. The bile canaliculus (BC) at the top of the picture is flanked by microvilli cleaved longitudinally and obliquely. The small part of the zonula occludens included in the plane of cleavage can be seen to have a typical weblike structure. Several microns below the luminal surface, a gap junction (nexus) can be seen. The surface of the membrane visualized above is the outer side (face A) of the inner leaflet (LM 1); it contains numerous closely packed particles that are more evident when the micrograph is viewed in the proper orientation, which is upside down from the way it is mounted here (carbon was sprayed onto the cleaved surface from above). The particles in the membranes of the nexus are spaced approximately 90 Å apart, as are the subunits visible in the extracellular space, or so-called gap (Figs. 3-15B and C). It is likely that each particle within the plasmalemma is situated next to one of the subunits within the extracellular space. ×90,000. (Courtesy of J. P. Revel.)

contiguity. In stratified squamous epithelia subjected to abrasion, the desmosomes are dispersed along interlocking lateral cell processes (Fig. 3-10), an arrangement which may help to space the plasmalemma from shearing forces. In the kidney, particularly in the distal renal tubule, the epithelial cells interdigitate so extensively with one another that it is difficult to tell

where one cell ends and the next begins. The interdigitations of renal tubule cells enormously increase the lateral surface membrane, which presumably plays a role in water and salt transfer across the cells. Salt-secreting cells in birds have the same highly elaborate interdigitating cell processes, and so do the cells of the secretory ducts of salivary glands and sweat glands and the lining epithelium of the ciliary body, gall bladder, and choroid plexus. Diamond (1964) has postulated a standing osmotic gradient between such epi-

FIGURE 3-17 Diagram illustrating the principal surface specializations that would be found on a simple columnar epithelial cell. The junctional complex at the luminal surface consists of a zonula occludens and zonula adhaerens (together they form a terminal bar) and a row of desmosomes. Under the row of desmosomes, gap junctions occur. Other desmosomes and gap junctions are located deeper in the tissue. The intercellular canaliculi are bound off from the rest of the lateral cell compartment by zonulae occludentes. Canaliculi are, in fact, extensions of the free surface and communicate with it. Microvilli therein and on the free surface are covered with a glycoprotein ''fuzzy'' coat. The basal surface of the cell rests on another glycoprotein layer called the basement or basal lamina, which is the main component of the basement membrane.

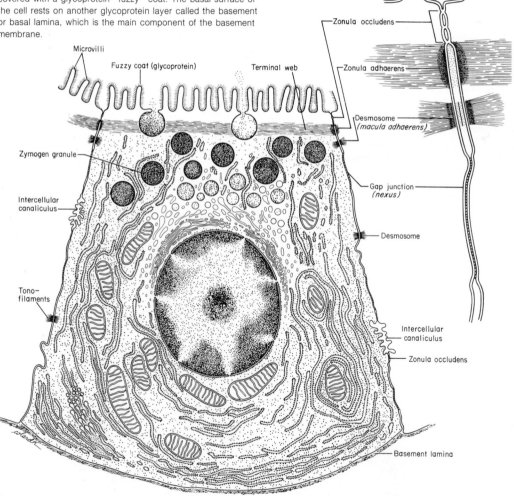

thelial cells caused by active pumping of sodium by the cells from the lumen into the intercellular space. He suggests that osmotic pressure causes water to flow passively across the cells into the same space. Transport of water out of the epithelium into underlying capillaries is thought to result from hydrostatic pressure caused by swelling of the water-filled extracellular compartment. Kaye et al. (1966) have shown by electron microscopy that the extracellular clefts become enormously dilated during water transport by the gall bladder epithelium.

Intercellular canaliculi often connect the lateral facets of secretory epithelial cells to the free surface (Figs. 3-17 and 3-27). They are bounded by a zonula occludens which seals the rest of the lateral extracellular compartment from contact with their contents. Within such a canaliculus (BC, Fig. 3-14), microvilli project as on a typical free surface. Thus the intercellular canaliculus is really an extension of the free surface into the tissue.

CYTOSKELETON

It is tempting to think that mechanical tension developing at the desmosome or terminal bar is not borne by the cell membrane alone but is transmitted to the tough fibrous elements of the cytoplasm. Cytoplasmic

filaments approximately 100 Å in diameter form thick bundles called *tonofibrils* in stratified squamous epithelia (Fig. 3-10). The filaments are developed to some extent in most epithelial cells, and they usually insert into the dense placodes of the desmosomes (Fig. 3-11). The *terminal web* in the apical cytoplasm of the intestinal absorptive cell is composed of a meshwork of small myosinlike filaments, which seem to be attached to the zonula adhaerens (TW, Fig. 3-12). The *tonofilaments* constituting tonofibrils are responsible for the birefringence of epidermal cells and are probably composed of the fibrous protein keratin in its less highly cross-linked form. This precursor protein is rich in sulfhydryl, whereas the true keratin of the outer cornified layers of the epidermis contains disulfide bonds (see Chap. 16). On the other hand, the small filaments in the intestinal microvilli are composed of actin. The tonofilaments of the epidermis, the small filaments of the terminal web, and other cytoplasmic filaments 50 Å or more in diameter may be considered together as *filaments*, but they obviously constitute a heterogeneous class with respect to

FIGURE 3-18 Basement membranes taken from different sites in adult monkey tissue and viewed with the light microscope. × 300. A. Palmar skin, showing thick basement membrane (BM) underlying epidermis: stained by the PAS procedure for carbohydrate-containing complexes. B. Kidney, showing relatively thin membranes around renal corpuscles (RC) and various tubules (T): stained by Pap's ammoniacal-silver nitrate method, illustrating the argyrophilia of reticular fibers in basement membranes. (Courtesy of H. W. Deane.)

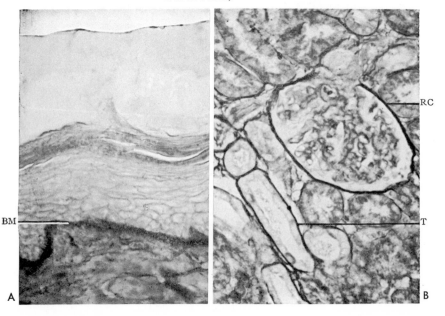

protein composition and possible function. In addition to filaments, *microtubules* help maintain the shape of some epithelial cells and thus can also be classified as part of the cytoskeleton (Chap. 1).

SPECIALIZATIONS OF THE BASAL SURFACE

The *basement membrane* is an extracellular condensation of glycoprotein, mucopolysaccharide and pro-

FIGURE 3-19 Electron micrograph of the basal surface of corneal epithelium of the albino rabbit. Basal attachment plates called half desmosomes help to anchor the epithelial cells to the basement lamina. The basement lamina is a glycoprotein layer about 0.1 μm thick, composed of fine filaments, and is seen to be intimately related to the epithelium and to the underlying collagen fibrils. The collagen fibrils (Cf) are embedded in ground substance and are arranged in a condensed network, the reticular lamina. The reticular lamina and the basement lamina together correspond to the basement membrane (BM) usually visualized in the light microscope. It is known that the corneal epithelium makes the basement membrane shown here. Stained with phosphotungstic acid in block after osmium fixation. × 15,000. (Courtesy of M. Jakus, relabeled according to the nomenclature suggested by Fawcett.)

teins that occurs under the basal surface of all epithelia (Fig. 3-18). It reaches its greatest width under epithelia that are subject to abrasion, such as the epidermis. In addition to providing support, the basement membrane undoubtedly serves as a semipermeable filter under the epithelium. Its most consistent component is a dense filamentous sheet 500 to 1,000 Å thick, called the *basement lamina* (*basal lamina*). This layer seems attached to the plasmalemma of the basal epithelial cell and to the underlying reticular tissue (Fig. 3-19). The underlying tissue, or *reticular lamina*, of the basement membrane is composed of condensed ground substance and small irregular bundles of collagen fibrils termed *reticular fibers* (Fig. 3-19). In the trachea, elastic fibers are also present in the reticular lamina of the basement membrane. In certain epithelia, the basement membrane is so poorly developed that it seems to consist only of basement lamina (Fig. 3-20). Some electron microscopists refer to the basement lamina alone as the basement membrane, even

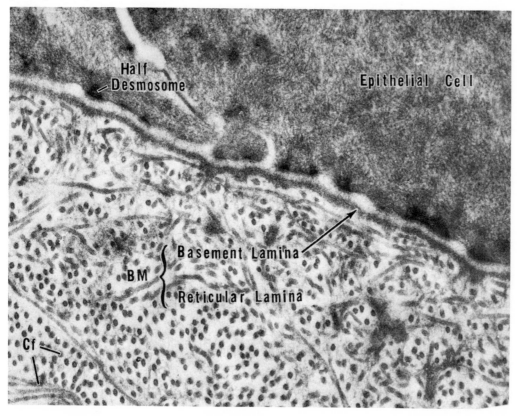

132

when describing tissue such as the epidermis. This practice leads to confusion because it ignores the reticular lamina.

The capsule of the vertebrate lens is a very thick basement lamina which can be readily separated from surrounding tissues and analyzed biochemically. Kefalides (1973) has shown that this basement lamina is composed of a large and a small molecular weight glycoprotein, both unnamed, and a third glycoprotein that is a collagen of the type IV class. The collagen molecule is richer in hydroxylysine and sugar (glucosylgalactose) than most interstitial collagens and contains only α1 units. It also seems to retain a telopeptide (extension peptide) rich in half-cystine which is not present on the final version of the interstitial (type I or II) collagen molecule. Thus, instead of polymerizing into fibrils, these collagen molecules seem to link to each other by disulfide and covalent bonds and to interact by hydrogen bonds with noncollagenous glycoproteins, giving the final rather

amorphous "membrane," in which component glycoprotein filaments can barely be distinguished by electron microscopy (arrow, Fig. 3-20). Dische (1970) reported that acid mucopolysaccharide (glycosaminoglycan) could also be detected in the lens basement lamina; and recently Trelstad et al. (1974) published a histochemical study illustrating a regular pattern of chondroitin sulfate aggregates within embryonic corneal basement lamina. The corneal reticular lamina (Fig. 3-19) also contains chondroitin sulfate, but the component collagen fibrils are of the interstitial type. It is possible that the mucopolysaccharide and perhaps even the collagenous component of both layers vary somewhat in type from tissue to tissue. The intense

FIGURE 3-20 High-power electron micrographs of the junction between renal epithelium and capillary endothelium in rat glomerulus. Foot processes of the renal epithelium (Epi) rest on the basement membrane (arrow). The basement membrane in this case represents the combined basement laminas of the capillary endothelium (End) and the renal epithelium. There is no reticular lamina throughout most of the glomerulus, for the narrow adepithelial layer is the effective filter between the blood and nephron cavities. The inset shows basement membrane under higher magnification. Osmium fixation; stained with lead citrate and uranyl acetate. ×75,000; inset, ×150,000. (Courtesy of E. Reynolds.)

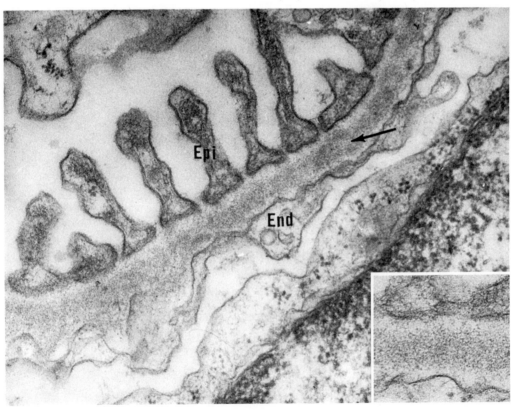

periodic acid Schiff (PAS) reaction of most basement membranes as viewed in the light microscope (Fig. 3-18) is probably a result of the large amount of sugar in basement lamina collagen and in the associated reticular fibers (when present).

There is considerable evidence in the recent and past literature to support the idea that the epithelium makes its own basement lamina (reviewed by Hay and Revel, 1969). It is clear that the lens epithelium produces the lens capsule discussed above. Dodson and Hay (1971) have shown, moreover, that isolated corneal epithelium can produce striated collagen fibrils of the interstitial type, as well as basal lamina, in vitro. Whether or not underlying fibroblasts also contribute collagen to the reticular lamina in vivo is not clear.

Basal cell processes that extend into the underlying connective tissue increase the attachment surface of the basal epithelial cells, particularly in stratified squamous and transitional epithelia (Fig. 3-8). Adhesion plates that occur on the basal plasmalemma in certain stratified epithelia are called *hemidesmosomes* because there is no matching counterpart in the underlying connective tissue (Fig. 3-19).

SPECIALIZATIONS OF THE FREE SURFACE

Microvilli are narrow (0.1 μm) cylindrical cytoplasmic processes that project from the free surface of the cell. They constitute the *brush border* of the absorptive cells of the proximal renal tubule, the choroid plexus, and the placental epithelium. The so-called striated border of the intestinal epithelium (Fig. 3-21A) has essentially the same structure as a brush border. The free surface of one absorptive cell may contain as many as 2000 of the minute cytoplasmic projections which give the border a refractile, brushlike, or striated appearance as viewed in the light microscope. The plasmalemma of the microvillus is an extension of the cell membrane. The moderately dense cytoplasm within the microvillus contains actin filaments which connect with the underlying terminal web (Fig. 3-12).

The increased free surface provided by microvilli undoubtedly contributes to the absorptive function of cells. The brush border of the intestine contains enzymes which hydrolyze sugar phosphate esters and disaccharides to monosaccharides. Active transport mechanisms exist in or near the microvilli (see Chap. 18). In the kidney, the microvilli are quite long and may fill the entire lumen of the proximal tubule. The urine must filter through the cytoplasmic processes of these epithelial cells. Large molecules such as hemo-

globin, which sometimes traverse the glomerulus to reach the lumen of the proximal tubule, are taken up through membrane-bounded invaginations at the base of the microvilli. The same kind of process occurs between the microvilli of intestinal cells during lipid absorption (see Chaps. 1 and 18).

Stereocilia are very long microvilli which are quite numerous on the surface of the epithelial cells lining the epididymis and vas deferens (Fig. 3-22). This epithelium regulates the specialized environment in

FIGURE 3-21 Specialization of free surface of epithelial cells as viewed with light microscope. A. Striated border (SB) of cells covering duodenal villus of monkey. The dense line (L) corresponds to the outer portion of the terminal web. H & E. B. Brush border (Br) of cells lining proximal convoluted tubule of mouse. The border is stained by the PAS method for demonstrating glycoprotein. C. Cilia (C) emerging from a cell lining human oviduct. The basal bodies (BB) can be seen. Iron alum hemtoxylin. All × 1,600. (Courtesy of H. W. Deane.)

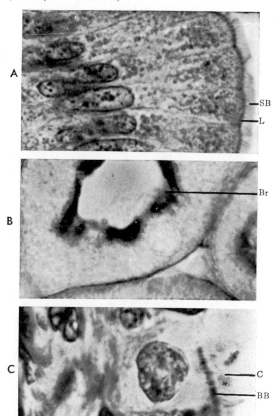

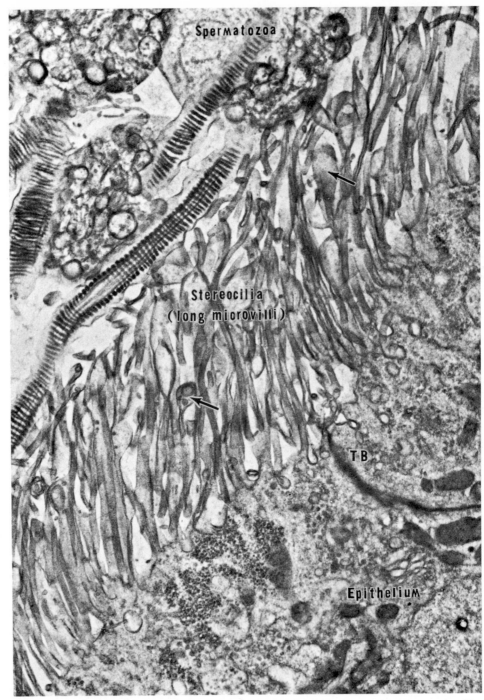

FIGURE 3-22 Electron micrograph of the free border of the epithelium of the epididymis of bat. Stereocilia are unusually long microvilli that extend from the free surface of the epithelium into the lumen. The microvilli are often dilated (arrows) and may contain secretory products. A terminal bar between two epithelial cells is obliquely sectioned at TB. Osmium fixation; no counterstain. × 12,000. (Courtesy of A. Mitchell.)

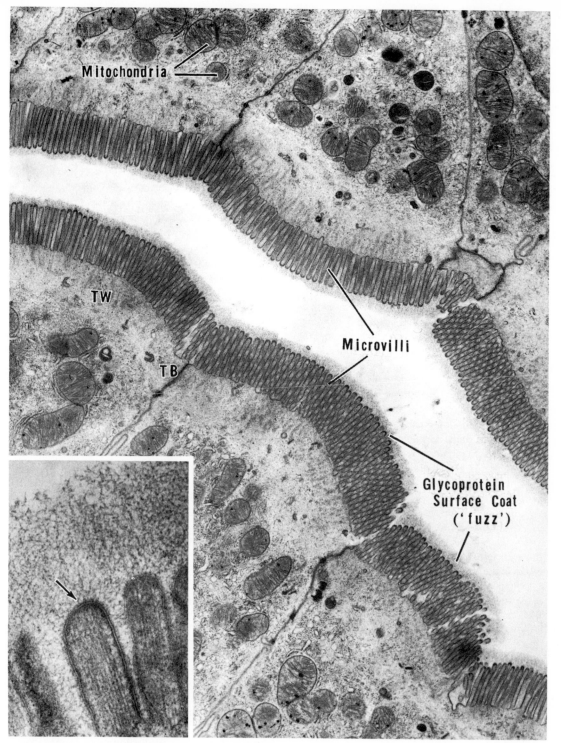

FIGURE 3-23 Electron micrographs of intestinal epithelium, showing the filamentous glycoprotein surface coat which covers the surface of the microvilli. Glycoprotein surface coats are particularly well developed in the bat intestine (large micrograph), cat intestine (inset), and human intestine (not illustrated). They account for the positive staining of the striated border with Schiff's reagent after periodic acid oxidation (Fig. 2-21B). The filaments of ''fuzz'' (arrow, inset) are closely related to the cell membrane. In the large micrograph the terminal bar (TB) and terminal web (TW) in the apical cytoplasm are shown to good advantage. Osmium fixation; stained with uranyl acetate and lead citrate. ×8,000; inset, ×100,000. (Courtesy of S. Ito.)

which the spermatozoa mature, and perhaps the stereocilia play a role in secretion as well as absorption of the surrounding medium. The secretory cells of exocrine glands possess a few microvilli on their free surface.

Glycoprotein surface coats cover the luminal surface of the microvilli in the proximal renal tubule (Fig. 3-21B) and can be demonstrated in the intestine (inset, Fig. 3-23). When present, they give the brush and striated borders a positive PAS reaction and probably contribute to the gel-like rigidity of the regular array of microvilli on such surfaces. The surface glycoprotein coat has been called *fuzz* by Ito (1965) and *fluffy coat* by Farquhar and Palade (1963) because it is filamentous in its fine structure (Fig. 3-23).

Cilia and *flagella*[2] are motile cell processes with a complex inner structure adapted for rapid bending (Fig. 3-21C). They are not to be confused with microvilli. Viewed in cross section in the electron microscope, each cilium is seen to contain two central fibrils and nine peripheral fibrils enclosed in the plasmalemma (Fig. 3-24). Each peripheral fibril is actually composed of two smaller fibrils (microtubules). The fibrils run from the tip of the cilium to the basal body, where the central fibrils terminate (Fig. 3-25). The nine outer fibrils originate next to nine longitudinal fibrils in the peripheral wall of the basal body. Fibrous rootlets, which may be striated, extend from the basal body into the apical cytoplasm (Fig. 3-25). The basal body is a modified centriole and often an additional centriole is oriented more or less perpendicular to it (Fig. 3-25). During development of the multiciliated cell, the centrioles, which give rise to the cilia, are duplicated a hundred or more times. In other cell types, a single centriole lying close to the plasmalemma may give rise to an isolated cilium of no apparent function. In developing cells, newly forming fibrils within the cilium can be disrupted by colchicine and thus resemble ordinary microtubules (Chap. 1). In fully formed cilia, the fibrils are considered to be modified microtubules because they are sensitive to colchicine treatment.

The cilium is within the resolution of the light microscope in diameter (0.2 μm) and is 5 to 10 μm in length, much longer than the usual microvillus (1 to 2 μm). Thus, the living cilia of the cells of the respiratory and genital epithelia can be resolved fairly readily with the light microscope and ciliary action observed directly. During the forward or *effective stroke,* the cilium is rigid and curved slightly forward. The return or *recovery stroke* is slower, and to effect it the cilium curves backward and then progressively stiffens from base to tip. It has been suggested that the impulse causing the movement first spreads from the basal body to the forward-placed peripheral fibrils. These fibrils may then slide along adjacent fibrils via the so-called arms of the fibrils, much as actin filaments slide past myosin filaments in muscle. Gibbons has called the class of protein constituting the arms of the fibrils *dynein.* Dyneins have molecular weights (MW 600,000) similar to myosins (MW 500,000) and both proteins are mechanicochemically coupled ATPase enzymes.

The proteins (α- and β-tubulin) which constitute the microtubules exist as dimers in solution and they polymerize into tubular form by a poorly understood mechanism. Tubulin resembles actin in that it binds nucleotides and interacts with an ATPase, but it has a higher molecular weight (54,000 as against 40,000 for actin), different amino acids, and a different morphologic assembly (microtubules instead of filaments). Nevertheless, a similar sliding mechanism of motility exists in cilia, flagella, and muscle. Glycerin-extracted cilia and flagella will beat if supplied with ATP and ciliary fibrils (microtubules) remain the same length during the beat cycle (forward and backward stroke). Gibbons (1975) has removed the plasmalemma, added ATP, and photographed the peripheral fibrils sliding past each other. The role of the central fibrils is unknown, but they may determine the plane of the stroke.

The cilia of the columnar epithelia of the respiratory tract, oviduct, and uterus do not beat syncronously; rather, they exhibit a *metachronal rhythm,* which results in forward-spreading ciliary waves that effectively move mucus or other materials over the free surface of the organ. Acetylcholine and acetylcholinesterase occur in ciliated cells, and it has been speculated that the coordinated metachronal rhythm is caused by a propagated impulse passing from cilium to cilium and cell to cell. Gap junctions that could transport small molecules exist between the cells. Al-

---

[2] *Flagella* are motile cell processes similar to cilia in their fine structure, but they are much longer and occur only once per cell when they are present. The term flagellum should probably be reserved for the long motile processes that were observed by light microscopy in certain nephrons and ducts, and not be applied to the individual, often poorly developed cilia that electron micrographs have revealed on the surface of so many supposedly nonciliated epithelial cells. A true flagellum is a specialized form of the cilium, such as is exemplified by the tail of the spermatozoon (Chap. 26).

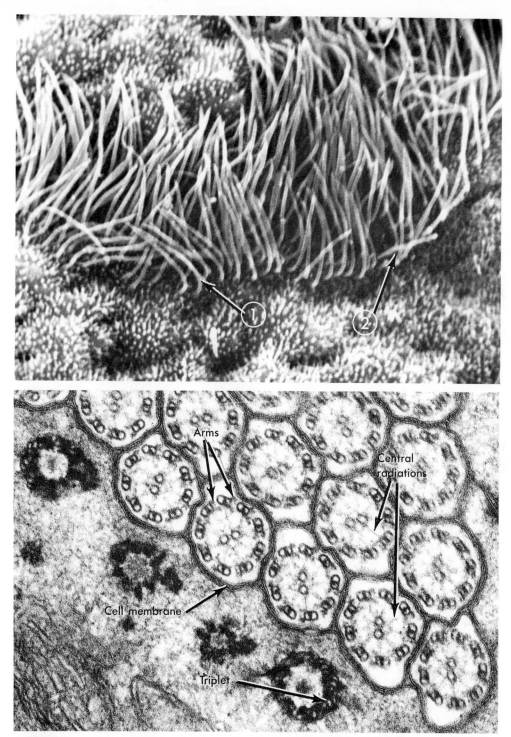

FIGURE 3-24 A (top). Low-power scanning electron micrograph reveals the three-dimensional configuration of a group of cilia on the outer surface of a planarian. Some cilia seem to have been caught by the fixative while in their forward stroke, as at 1, others while in their back stroke, as at 2. The smaller protrusions are microvilli. B (bottom). Higher-magnification transmission electron micrograph reveals a group of closely apposed cilia in cross section. Each cilium has two central fibrils or microtubules from which fine condensations (central radiations) pass toward the peripheral fibrils. Each of the nine peripheral fibrils is a pair of microtubules. The arms on the fibrils contain ATPase and are thought to cause sliding of the fibrils during ciliary bending. Several centrioles in an adjacent cell appear on the left. Unlike the cilium, the centriole has no central fibrils. Each of its nine peripheral fibrils is a triplet of microtubules. A, ×4,000; B, ×90,000. (Courtesy of S. J. Coward and R. O. Vitale-Calpe.)

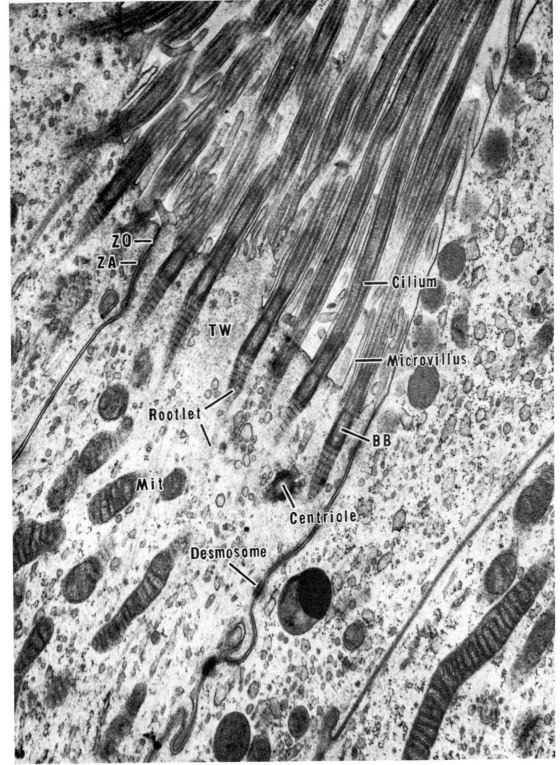

FIGURE 3-25 Electron micrograph of a longitudinal section through the apex of a ciliated cell in human fallopian tube. Cilia and micro-villi are shown to good advantage. The centriole adjacent to the basal body (BB) of one cilium appears but is obliquely sectioned. Note the moderately well-developed terminal web (TW). Also shown are the zonula occludens (ZO) and zonula adhaerens (ZA) of a terminal bar, Mit, mitochondrion. Osmium fixation; stained with lead hydroxide. ×25,000. (Courtesy of N. Bjorkman and B. Fredricsson.)

ternatively, cilia may trigger subsequent bending of their neighbors by means of a physical interaction (for example by touching them or by changing the intercentriolar tension).

POLARITY OF THE EPITHELIAL CELLS

An epithelial cell whose apex differs from its base is said to be *polarized*. The most striking examples of polarity occur in the columnar epithelia. In the absorptive epithelial cells of the intestine (Fig. 3-26A), digested lipid enters the apical cytoplasm, where it is processed by the Golgi complex and then transported to the intercellular space. Mitochondria tend to be preferentially located in the apical cytoplasm of intestinal epithelial cells (Fig. 3-26B) and ciliated columnar cells (Fig. 3-25). Mitochondria also show striking polarity in the simple cuboidal and columnar epithelium associated with water and electrolyte transport. In the

secretory ducts of the salivary gland (Fig. 18-24) and convoluted tubules of the kidney (Figs. 24-13 and 24-18), they are concentrated in the basal cytoplasm. Their striking orientation parallel to the long axis of the cell gives the basal cytoplasm its characteristic striated appearance as viewed in the light microscope. The highly interdigitated lateral cell membranes of these cells are intimately related to the mitochondria.

In exocrine gland cells, the well-developed endoplasmic reticulum is located primarily in the basal cytoplasm. The Golgi apparatus, or "packaging" center, occurs in the apical juxtanuclear cytoplasm (Fig. 3-17). Mitochondria tend to be disposed to the base of the cell, particularly when secretory product has accumulated in the apical cytoplasm (Fig. 3-30).

REGENERATION OF EPITHELIA

Epithelia on exposed surfaces of the body and the epithelia of the intestinal tract, holocrine glands, and

FIGURE 3-26 Intestinal cells viewed in the light microscope. A. The supranuclear Golgi net, (G) small intestine of guinea pig. Da Fano's silver nitrate method. B. Mitochondria in rat intestine. M, mitochondria; G. negative image of Golgi apparatus; T, terminal bar. Compare with electron micrograph shown in Fig. 3-20. Iron alum-hematoxylin stain. Both ×1,600. (Courtesy of H. W. Deane.)

female genital tract exhibit a remarkable degree of physiologic regeneration. In most of the stratified squamous epithelia, the relatively undifferentiated cuboidal cells of the basal layer proliferate to supply new cells which move to the outer surface. The cells differentiate along the way, a process called *cytomorphosis*. The continuing growth of hairs and nails involves a similar proliferation of basal epithelial cells which sub-

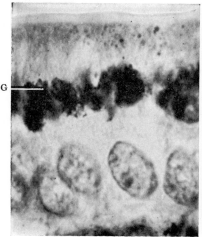
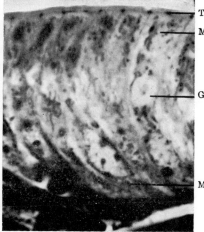

A   B

sequently are converted to hard keratin plaques. In *holocrine glands,* such as the sebaceous gland, the cells are secreted as part of the product and so must be renewed constantly. In the alimentary tract, relatively undifferentiated cells in the intestinal crypts and necks of the gastric glands serve as a reservoir of new cells to replace surface epithelia. The epithelium of small intestinal villi is entirely replaced every 2 to 4 days.

In addition to its capacity for physiologic regeneration, epithelium in general shows considerable ability to proliferate after a traumatic wound. If a lesion occurs in the epidermis, for example, the basal cells

adjacent to the wound migrate over the underlying connective tissue as a single sheet of contiguous cells which gradually increases in thickness as more cells move in. Interestingly enough, the migrating cells do not usually divide. The synthesis of new DNA and mitosis occur in the epithelium at the margin of the wound. It seems likely that in exocrine glands, regeneration is accomplished by proliferation of the relatively undifferentiated cells of the ducts. In the bladder, the less differentiated basal cells seem to have the greatest proliferative capacity. Nevertheless, the relation between degree of differentiation and ability to divide is not an absolute one. Some highly differentiated epithelial cells do retain the capacity to proliferate after injury, as, for example, in the liver.

CLASSIFICATION OF GLANDS

The glands of the body fall into two major groups: the exocrine glands, which secrete products that reach a free surface, and the endocrine glands, which produce hormones that enter the bloodstream.

The *endocrine glands* usually arise as invaginations of the surface epithelium but later lose their connection with the surface and thus are ductless. In some cases, typical epithelial characteristics are retained by the secretory cells (thyroid gland). In most cases the epithelial origin of the tissue is difficult to recognize. The cells may be arranged in anastomosing sheets or as irregular cords. Such cells are often said to be *epithelioid* because they resemble epithelium in

that they are contiguous; however, other epithelial characteristics, such as a free surface, are not present. Certain endocrine cells are more like fibroblasts (the interstitial tissue of testis, the theca interna of ovarian follicles). The cytology of endocrine cells will be considered in subsequent chapters.

Exocrine glands are usually classified according to the branching of the ducts and shape of the secretory units. In some cases, the gland cells are dispersed throughout a lining epithelium as single units, called *unicellular* glands. More commonly, the secretory cells are arranged in *tubules* or saclike endpieces called *alveoli (acini),* which connect to a duct (Fig. 3-27). If the duct goes directly to the surface without branching, the gland is considered to be a *simple tubular* or *simple alveolar* gland (Fig. 3-28). If the duct branches, connecting more than one secretory unit to the surface, the gland is a *compound tubular* or *compound*

FIGURE 3-27 Diagrams of glands. A. Duct ending in alveolus and tubule with wide lumina, as in a mixed serous and mucous gland. B. Duct ending in alveolus with narrow lumen, as in a purely serous gland. Intercellular canaliculi are shown.

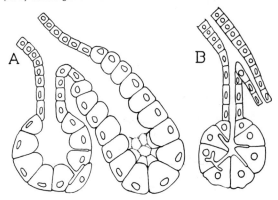

FIGURE 3-28 Diagrams of simple and compound forms of tubular and alveolar glands, including a compound tubuloalveolar gland.

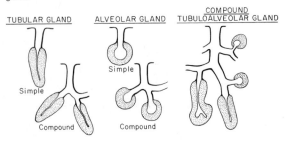

alveolar gland. Both tubular and alveolar secretory units are present in a *compound tubuloalveolar* gland.

An exocrine gland is said to be <u>holocrine</u> if whole cells are secreted (sebaceous gland); <u>apocrine</u> if protrusions of apical cytoplasm are lost; and <u>merocrine</u> if no actual cytoplasm is lost. Most secretory cells are merocrine. The "part" (G., *meros*) that is secreted is a protein synthesized in the endoplasmic reticulum and combined with oligosaccharide or polysaccharide as it passes through the Golgi zone (see Chap. 1).

The secretory cells of merocrine glands are usually classified as serous or mucous. <u>Serous cells</u> are common in glands of the alimentary tract. <u>Mucous cells</u> occur as unicellular glands throughout the gastrointestinal and respiratory tracts and are a prominent component of many of the salivary glands. In some of

the salivary glands, serous and mucous cells occupy the same endpieces. The serous cells are pushed away from the lumen to form a crescent, or *demilune,* at the periphery of the alveolus or tubule (Fig. 3-29).

Serous cells produce a secretion which is watery but high in enzyme content. The protein precursor accumulates in the apical cytoplasm in the form of small zymogen, or "preenzyme," granules. Nuclei are round and located near the base of the cell (Fig. 3-29). The abundant endoplasmic reticulum gives the basal cytoplasm a strong affinity for basic dyes. Cell borders are indistinct as viewed with the light microscope, and the lumen of a typical serous acinus or alveolus is usually quite narrow (Fig. 3-29). The serous secretion is rich in protein and contains some mucopolysaccharide.

Mucous cells produce a protein secretion richer in sugar and more viscous than the serous secretion. It forms large masses in the apical cytoplasm of the mucous cell and compresses the flattened nucleus to the basal surface (Fig. 3-30). Secretion extruded from the cells often dilates the lumen of the secretory

FIGURE 3-29 Light micrograph showing typical serous and mucous alveoli in human submandibular gland. The irregular, branching mucous endpieces are often so elongate that they are called tubules instead of alveoli, and the gland is said to be tubuloalveolar. Serous cells may form caps (demilunes) on the ends of mucous tubules. Isolated serous cells also occur in mucous tubules in a mixed salivary gland such as the submandibular. The plasma cells located in the connective tissue adjacent to the glandular alveoli (upper part of picture) are commonly seen in organs associated with the gastrointestinal tract. Bouin's fixation; H & E. × 850.

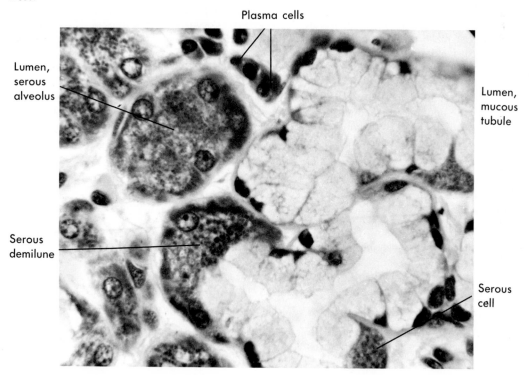

Plasma cells

Lumen, serous alveolus

Lumen, mucous tubule

Serous demilune

Serous cell

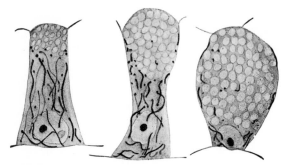

FIGURE 3-30 Mucous cells from the sublingual gland of a dog in various phases of secretion. The mitochondria appear as blackened filaments; the mucous droplets have been dissolved out and are represented by empty vacuoles. Potassium dichromate and formaldehyde fixation; mitochondria stained by acid fuchsin. (Hoven.)

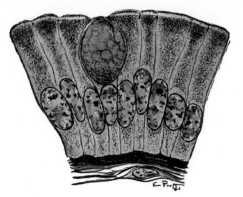

FIGURE 3-31 Columnar epithelium of a bile duct of a rhesus monkey. Goblet cell appears in the center of the field. Susa fixation; azan stain.

alveolus. In the unicellular mucous gland, the *goblet cell* (Fig. 3-31), the accumulated mucus in the apical cytoplasm gives the appearance of the "globe" of a goblet; the narrow, compressed basal cytoplasm is the "stem." Mucus usually stains poorly in routine histologic preparations, so the cells often appear empty with well-defined borders (Fig. 3-29). Endoplasmic reticulum is present in the basal cytoplasm when the cells are making the protein component of mucus. Examples of cells that make products intermediate between typical mucous and serous secretions can be found (Brunner's glands of the duodenum, mucous neck cells of the stomach).

It will become apparent in subsequent chapters that secretion of protein and mucoid products is not an exclusive property of the typical exocrine gland cells discussed above. *Connective tissue cells* secrete mucopolysaccharide and protein to form the extracellular matrix that surrounds these cells, and certain *neurons* produce neurosecretory materials which are rich in polypeptides and polysaccharides. The connective tissue cells that form the bone matrix, the osteoblasts, are often arranged in sheets and are said to be epithelioid, so closely do they resemble true epithelial cells. It might be pointed out, too, that even *muscle* can take on so-called epithelial characteristics where contiguity is essential to function; true desmosomes and modified adhering zonules called *intercalated disks* occur in cardiac muscle. The distinction between the epithelia and other tissues of the body is, in last measure, an arbitrary one, a matter of the degree to which the cells express the criteria that we assign to a particular tissue category. The principal distinguishing feature of a true epithelium is that the contiguous cells comprising it actually line a lumen or external surface and thus possess a free border.

REFERENCES

Specializations of the Lateral Surface

BORYSENKO, J. Z., and J. P. REVEL: Experimental Manipulation of Desmosome Structure, *Am. J. Anat.,* **137:**403 (1973).

CHAMBERS, R., and G. S. RÉNYI: The Structure of the Cells in Tissues as Revealed by Microdissection. I. The Physical Relationships of the Cells in Epithelia, *Am. J. Anat.,* **35:**385 (1925).

DIAMOND, J. M.: The Mechanism of Isotonic Water Transport, *J. Gen. Physiol.,* **48:**15 (1964).

DOUGLAS, W. H. J., R. C. RIPLEY, and R. A. ELLIS: Enzymatic Digestion of Desmosomes and Hemidesmosome Plaques Performed on Ultrathin Sections, *J. Cell Biol.,* **44:**211 (1970).

FARQUHAR, M. G., and G. E. PALADE: Junctional Complexes in Various Epithelia, *J. Cell Biol.*, **17:**375 (1963).

FURSHPAN, E. J., and D. D. POTTER: Low Resistance Junctions between Cells in Embryos and Tissue Culture, in "Current Topics in Developmental Biology," vol. 3, Academic Press, Inc., New York, 1968.

GOODENOUGH, D. A.: Methods for the Isolation and Structural Characterization of Hepatocyte Gap Junctions, in E. D. Korn (ed.), "Methods in Membrane Biology," vol. 3, Plenum Publishing Corporation, New York, 1975.

GOODENOUGH, D. A., and J. P. REVEL: A Fine Structural Analysis of Intercellular Junctions in the Mouse Liver., *J. Cell Biol.*, **45:**272 (1970).

HAY, E. D., and J. P. REVEL: "Fine Structure of the Developing Avian Cornea," vol. 1, "Monographs in Developmental Biology," A. Wolsky and P. S. Chen (eds.), S. Karger, Basel, 1969.

KAYE, G. I., H. O. WHEELER, R. T. WHITLOCK, and N. LANE: Fluid Transport in the Rabbit Gall Bladder. A Combined Physiological and Electron Microscopic Study, *J. Cell Biol.*, **30:**237 (1966).

LOEWENSTEIN, W. R.: On the Genesis of Cellular Communication, *Dev. Biol.*, **15:**503 (1967).

MATOLTSY, A. G.: Desmosomes, Filaments, and Keratohyaline Granules: Their Role in the Stabilization and Keratinization of the Epidermis, *J. Invest. Dermatol.*, **65:**127 (1975).

MCNUTT, N. S., and R. S. WEINSTEIN: The Ultrastructure of the Nexus. A Correlated Thin-section and Freeze-cleave Study, *J. Cell Biol.*, **47:**666 (1970).

MUIR, A. R.: The Effect of Divalent Cations on the Ultrastructure of the Perfused Rat Heart, *J. Anat.*, **101:**239 (1967).

RASH, J. E., J. W. SHAY, and J. J. BIESELE: Urea Extractions of Z-bands, Intercalated Discs, and Desmosomes, *J. Ultrastruct. Res.*, **24:**181 (1968).

Specializations of the Basal Surface

DISCHE, Z.: Collagen of Embryonic Type in the Vertebrate Eye and Its Relation to Carbohydrates and Subunit of Tropocollagen, *Dev. Biol.*, suppl., **4:**164 (1970).

DODSON, J. W., and E. D. HAY: Secretion of Collagenous Stroma by Isolated Epithelium Grown in Vitro, *Exp. Cell Res.*, **65:**215 (1971).

KEFALIDES, N. A.: Structure and Biosynthesis of Basement Membranes, *Int. Rev. Connect. Tissue Res.*, **6:**63 (1973).

TRELSTAD, R. L., K. HAYASHI, and B. P. TOOLE: Epithelial Collagens and Glycosaminoglycans in the Embryonic Cornea. Macromolecular Order and Morphogenesis in the Basement Membrane, *J. Cell Biol.*, **62:**815 (1974).

Specializations of the Free Surface

CRANE, P. K.: Structure and Functional Organization of an Epithelial Cell Brush Border, in K. B. Warren (ed.), "Intracellular Transport," p. 71, Academic Press, Inc., New York, 1966.

GIBBONS, I. R.: The Structure and Composition of Cilia, in K. B. Warren (ed.), "Formation and Fate of Cell Organelles," p. 99, Academic Press, Inc., New York, 1967.

GIBBONS, I. R.: The Molecular Basis of Flagellar Motility in Sea Urchin Spermatozoon, in S. Inoué and R. E. Stephens (eds.), "Molecules and Cell Movement," p. 207, Raven Books, Abelard-Schuman, Limited, New York, 1975.

ITO, S.: The Enteric Surface Coating of Cat Intestinal Microvilli, *J. Cell Biol.*, **27:**475 (1965).

MOOSEKER, M. S., and L. G. TILNEY: Organization of an Actin Filament-Membrane Complex. Filament Polarity and Membrane Attachment in the Microvilli of Intestinal Epithelial Cells, *J. Cell Biol.*, **67:**725 (1975).

SATIR, P.: Studies on Cilia. II. Examination of the Distal Region of the Ciliary Shaft and the Role of the Filaments in Motility, *J. Cell Biol.*, **26:**805 (1965).

SLEIGH, M. A.: Metachronism and Frequency of Beat in the Perisomial Cilia of *Stentor, J. Exp. Biol.*, **33:**15 (1956).

STEPHENS, R. C.: On the Apparent Homology of Actin and Tubulin, *Science*, **168:**845 (1970).

General

BENNETT, G., and C. P. LEBLOND: Formation of Cell Coat Materials for the Whole Surface of Columnar Cells in the Rat Small Intestine, as Visualized by Radioautography with L-Fucose-^{3}H, *J. Cell Biol.*, **46:**409 (1970).

MESSIER, B., and C. P. LEBLOND: Cell Proliferation and Migration as Revealed by Radioautography after Injection of Thymidine-H^3 into Male Rats and Mice, *Am. J. Anat.*, **106:**247 (1960).

Connective Tissue

BURTON GOLDBERG AND MICHEL RABINOVITCH

Connective tissues provide the supporting matrix for almost every organ in the body. They consist of an indigenous population of cells surrounded by *fibers* and amorphous *ground* substance. The fibers are mainly assembled from the proteins *collagen* and *elastin,* and the ground substance consists mostly of *proteoglycans.*[1]

The fibroblast, chondroblast, osteoblast, odontoblast, and reticular cells are mesenchymally derived connective tissue cells which are differentiated for the synthesis and secretion of the fibrous proteins and proteoglycans. The connective tissues can also contain lipid-laden adipose cells, phagocytic macrophages, and pharmacologically reactive mast cells. We classify all these types as *resident cells* because they are constantly present in relatively fixed numbers and patterns in certain types of adult connective tissue. The resident cells contrast with *immigrant cells,* which usually appear transitorially in connective tissues as part of the inflammatory reaction to cell injury. Under these conditions, neutrophils, eosinophils, basophils, cells of lymphocytic lineage, and monocytes can be observed to pass in large numbers from blood vessels into the surrounding connective tissues. These hematogenous cells tend to disappear from the tissues as the inflammatory reaction subsides. In certain connective tissues one may observe small numbers of lymphoid cells, neutrophils, and eosinophils in the absence of documented injury.

When connective tissues from different organ systems are compared, considerable morphologic diversity may be observed. The proportion of cells to fibers and ground substance, and the amounts, kinds, and organization of the extracellular materials may vary greatly from tissue to tissue. Table 4-1 provides a general classification of connective tissues and indicates their range of morphologic diversity. Mesenchyme is an embryonic connective tissue containing stellate-shaped cells in an abundant ground substance. It originates from the middle embryonic layer (mesoderm) and from the neural crest. Mesenchymal cells are capable of rapid division and are dispersed throughout the embryo to become the progenitors for most of the resident cells of the connective tissues. Because resident cells in adult tissues may expand their numbers greatly under certain circumstances, it has been postulated that these expanding cell populations are derived from primordial mesenchymal cells which have persisted in adult tissues. However, since differentiated cell types such as the fibroblast can undergo serial replication in vivo and in vitro, there is no need to postulate the existence of a primordial progenitor cell for this cell type.

---

[1] *Proteoglycans* (proteinpolysaccharides) are molecules in which polymers of disaccharide units are covalently linked to protein, and in which the sugar components account for most of the molecular weight. Mucopolysaccharide, glycosaminoglycan, and glycosaminoglucuronoglycan are all terms for the polysaccharide components of proteoglycans. *Glycoproteins* are molecules in which the protein component rather than the sugars accounts for most of the weight. In contrast to proteoglycans, the sugar moieties of glycoproteins are not generally formed from repeating disaccharide units.

TABLE 4-1 CLASSIFICATION OF CONNECTIVE TISSUES

Embryonic: mesenchyme
Adult
  Connective tissues proper
    General
      Loose
        Subcutaneous, mesentery, omentum, lamina propria of
        tubular epithelial organs
      Dense
        Irregular (periosteum, dermis, organ capsules)
        Regular (tendons, ligaments, cornea)
    Special
      Adipose
      Reticular
  Cartilage
  Bone

Loose (areolar) connective tissue is abundantly distributed in the body and is characterized by a relative excess of cells over fibrous elements. Adipose cells, macrophages, and mast cells are relatively abundant in areolar connective tissues. Collagen fibers predominate in dense connective tissue; they show little preferential orientation in dense irregular tissue (for example, the dermis) but are strikingly oriented in the regular variety (for example, in tendons and ligaments). In adipose tissues, fat-laden cells predominate. These will be described in Chap. 5. Reticular tissues consist of a network of very thin collagen fibrils and matrix supporting hemopoietic, epithelial, and endothelial cells.

Cartilage and bone are traditionally placed in separate categories because of their special architecture; they are characterized by a predominance of extracellular materials over cells (see Chap. 6).

The cells and extracellular materials of connective tissues can be thought of as a functional complex subserving structural and mechanical roles in tissues and organs throughout the body. Additionally, the fibers and ground substance influence the extracellular transport of molecules. The cells in the connective tissues also play important roles in storage of metabolites, in immune and inflammatory responses, and in healing of wounds. In this chapter we will discuss the structure and functions of the macrophage, the mast cell, and the fibroblast. The fibrous proteins and the proteoglycans will then be described in sufficient detail to afford some understanding of how these molecules are generally organized into functional units in tissues.

MACROPHAGES

The importance of phagocytic cells in antibacterial defense was first delineated in 1882 by Elie Metchnikoff. Starting with observations of transparent starfish larvae, Metchnikoff examined phagocytosis in the various animal phyla. He found that vertebrates characteristically possessed two types of cells able to fight invading microorganisms. The cell types were the *microphages* (small eaters), now known as polymorphonuclear leukocytes (PMN), and the *macrophages* (big eaters). The latter included the monocytes of the blood and phagocytic cells found in many tissues and organs. Early in the twentieth century, other investigators showed that acid disazo dyes (trypan blue, isamine blue, or pyrrhol blue, for example) injected into animals accumulated in cells present in different tissues and organs. This collection of cells was named by Aschoff the "reticuloendothelial system" (RES), a term which is still used in the current literature. Aschoff proposed that the RES was not only involved in defense but had other functions such as hematopoiesis, blood destruction, and metabolism of iron, bilirubin, and fat. Several of the cells listed under the RES (see Table 4-2) belong to the original macrophage population described by Metchnikoff. It is now clear that the disazo dyes are bound to plasma albumin and then taken into cells by pinocytosis. Indeed, the dyes administered in vivo are also captured by

TABLE 4-2 COMPONENTS OF THE RETICULOENDOTHELIAL SYSTEM (RES)

Sinus lining macrophages
  Lymph sinuses
  Blood sinuses
    Liver (Kupffer cells)
    Spleen
    Bone marrow
    Adrenal cortex
    Anterior pituitary
Microglia (central nervous system)
Reticular cells of lymphatic tissues
Tissue macrophages (histiocytes)
Blood macrophages (monocytes)

Source: Lord Florey, "General Pathology," 4th ed., p. 156, Lloyd-Luke (Medical Books) Ltd., London, 1970.

other cells such as renal tubular epithelia, so dye uptake alone cannot be used to define the macrophage system. Several cells included in the RES, such as those lining the sinusoids of the spleen or the reticular cells of hematopoietic tissues are only weakly phagocytic and differ from monocytes and macrophages in their recognition of particulate matter.

In recent years the RES has been reexamined and a new concept, named the *mononuclear phagocyte system* (MPS), has been proposed in its stead. As shown in Table 4-3, the MPS excludes some of the cells of the RES and adds others. The criteria for inclusion of cell types in the MPS are (1) derivation from bone marrow precursors cells; (2) characteristic cell morphology; and (3) high level of phagocytic activity mediated by immunoglobulin and components of the serum complement system. Other cell types, such as fibroblasts, thyroid epithelium, or pigmented retinal cells can ingest certain particles, but such uptake is not increased by immunoglobulins and complement. PMNs are arbitrarily excluded from the MPS classification even though they possess many of the properties of the cells of the MPS.

STRUCTURE OF MACROPHAGES

Macrophages can best be studied and identified by means of electron microscopy. The cell surface is

TABLE 4-3 THE MONONUCLEAR PHAGOCYTE SYSTEM

CELLS	LOCALIZATION
Stem cell (committed) ↓	Bone marrow
Monoblasts ↓	Bone marrow
Promonocytes ↓	Bone marrow
Monocytes ↓	Bone marrow Peripheral blood

Macrophages	Tissues
	   Connective tissue (histiocytes)
	   Liver (Kupffer cells)
	   Lung (alveolar macrophages)
	   Lymph nodes (free and fixed macrophages)
	   Spleen (free and fixed macrophages)
	   Bone marrow (macrophages)
	   Serous cavities (pleural and peritoneal
	     macrophages)
	   Bone tissue [osteoclasts(?)]
	   Nervous system (microglial cells)

Source: R. van Furth, "Mononuclear Phagocytes in Immunity, Infection and Pathology, Blackwell Scientific Publications, Ltd., Oxford, 1975. (Reproduced by permission of the author and publisher.)

thrown into numerous folds, or fingerlike processes (Figs. 4-1 and 4-2). The surface processes participate in spreading, phagocytosis, and cell movement. The cell nucleus is often indented and the cytoplasm characteristically contains abundant endocytic vacuoles, lysosomes, and phagolysosomes (Fig. 4-3). Mitochondria and bundles of microtubules and microfilaments are also present. The cytoskeletal constituents are often arranged under the plasma membrane. They not only may be involved in adhesion, endocytosis, and movement but may also control the fusion of lysosomes and phagosomes with the plasma membrane. There is a relatively large Golgi region which participates in the maturation of the lysosomes. Smooth and rough endoplasmic reticulum are prominent and the latter compartment is the site of synthesis of lysosomal hydrolases. Mature and functionally activated macrophages have more complex and abundant surface folds, increased numbers of vacuoles, lysosomes, phagosomes, and endoplasmic reticular elements.

With the light microscope and the usual hematoxylin-eosin-stained tissue sections, it is difficult to identify quiescent macrophages with certainty. An

FIGURE 4-1 Scanning electron micrograph of freshly explanted mouse macrophage in the process of ingesting aldehyde-treated erythrocytes. Small fingerlike processes decorate the surface of the phagocyte. The macrophage periphery extends as a collar over the erythrocytes. × 4600. (J. P. Revel, M. Rabinovitch, and M. J. DeStefano).

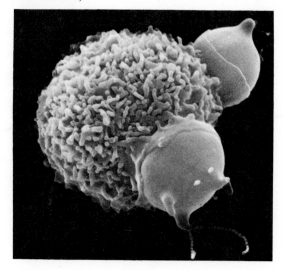

irregularly shaped nucleus and abundant and eosino-philic cytoplasm may help in the identification, but fibroblasts, lymphoid cells, or pericytes may have sim-ilar morphology. In tissue sections or imprints, mac-rophages may be better identified by cytochemical methods for lysosomal enzymes such as acid phos-phatase, aryl-sulfatase, or fluoride-resistant esterases. Monocytes and macrophages are well stained by these techniques.

BIOLOGICAL PROPERTIES OF MACROPHAGES

ENDOCYTOSIS

Macrophages are very active in pinocytosis and pha-gocytosis, processes collectively known as *endocy-tosis*. In pinocytosis, droplets of fluid are interiorized together with dissolved solute and macromolecules, or small particles (Figs. 4-1 and 4-3). The efficiency and selectivity of this form of uptake is often increased by

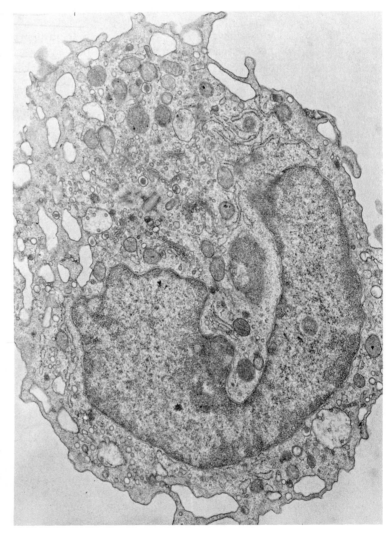

FIGURE 4-2 Transmission electron micrograph of normal mouse macro-phage. Notice the pinocytic vacuoles, lysosomes, and abundance of Golgi elements. ×16,000. (From R. van Furth, J. G. Hirsch, and M. Fedorko, *J. Exp. Med.*, **132:**794, 1970.)

binding of the material to the cell surface. Pinocytic vacuoles can be seen with the light microscope (macropinocytosis), but often they can be resolved only with the electron microscope (micropinocytosis).

FIGURE 4-3 Normal macrophage incubated with horseradish peroxidase for 1 h, washed, and left in peroxidase-free medium prior to fixation and staining with the diaminobenzidine method for peroxidatic activity. Intensely stained lysosomes indicate uptake and accumulation of peroxidase by pinocytosis. ×20,000. (R. M. Steinman.)

The vacuoles (pinosomes) are formed by invagination at the plasma membrane and thus they contain solutes and fluid from the extracellular space. The vacuoles pinch off from the membrane and are translocated toward the Golgi region. Their movement is probably dependent on the microtubular cytoskeleton. Pino-

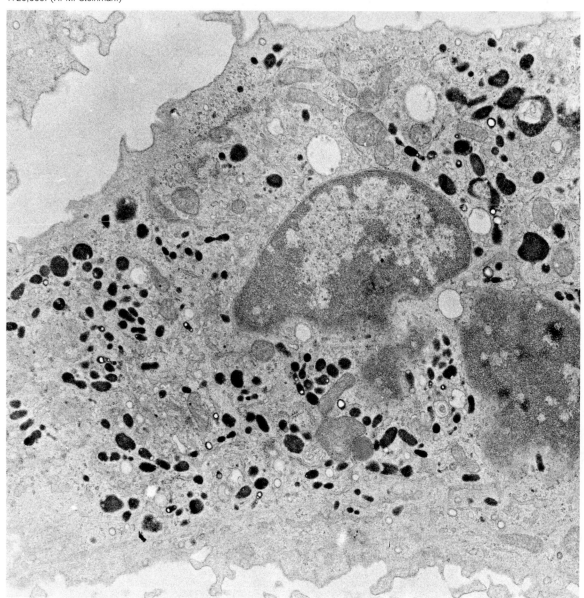

somes fuse with primary lysosomes to form secondary lysosomes, in which ingested material can be stored and enzymatically degraded.

In contrast to pinocytosis, phagocytosis generally allows the uptake of particles larger than 0.5 μm in diameter; but the distinction between pinocytic and phagocytic uptake is not always clear. Phagocytosis requires the attachment of the particle to the surface of the macrophage before interiorization occurs (Fig. 4-4). Herein may lie a difference between pinocytosis and phagocytosis: only the latter requires the interaction of the material with the plasma membrane. For this reason, pinocytic uptake may be of lower specificity than phagocytic uptake. Some particles as well as cells (lymphocytes are an example) can attach to the macrophage surface with only a slow rate of interiorization. Because binding is not necessarily followed by the ingestion step, the latter is the hallmark of phagocytosis.

Particle attachment is not an energy-dependent step, but particle ingestion is blocked by low temperatures or by metabolic inhibitors. Ingestion is accomplished by progressive spreading of the phagocyte plasma membrane and underlying cell cortex over the surface of the attached particle (Figs. 4-1 and 4-4). The membrane motility required for particle ingestion possibly utilizes forces generated by submembranous actin-rich microfilaments. The formation of a phagocytic vacuole requires resealing of the plasma membrane and of the membrane which envelops the particle. Similar to the pinosome, the phagocytic vacuole is transported toward the cell center. In this engulfment only a small amount of medium is trapped in the phagocytic vacuole (phagosome).

PHAGOCYTIC RECOGNITION

The process by which the phagocytes select the particles to be taken up is called *phagocytic recognition*. Some inert materials as well as certain bacteria, may be ingested in the absence of specific recognition factors from the serum. The interaction of such particles with phagocytes is apparently due to relatively nonspecific electrostatic or hydrophobic interactions between the particles and the macrophage surface. This nonimmunological phagocytosis is particularly relevant to the function of lung (alveolar) macro-

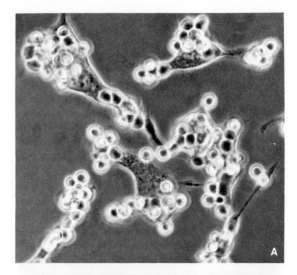

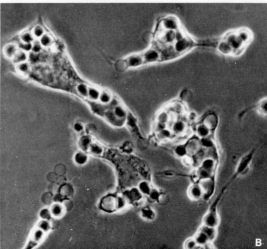

FIGURE 4-4 Cultivated macrophages, phase contrast. Macrophages were incubated with erythrocytes coated with immunoglobulin G antibody. The cells were rinsed to remove free erythrocytes, photographed (A), incubated in medium of lower osmolarity, fixed, and photographed again (B). In A, refractile erythrocytes are attached to the macrophages. These erythrocytes are lysed by the low osmolarity medium and thus ingested red cells (which escape lysis) are clearly seen in B. Some erythrocyte ghosts remained attached to the macrophages. $\times 500$.

phages, which have the task of clearing the airways of such materials as carbon, silica, berylium, asbestos, cellulose, cotton fibers, and other industrial pollutants.

The ingestion of many pathogenic microorganisms and intact cells requires that they first be coated with certain serum proteins (opsonins). The main recognition factors in serum are certain immunoglobulins (IgG, IgM) and the third component of complement. Complement is a system of proteins in serum which interact with each other and antibody to kill cells or bacteria by lysis. Antibody and complement provide a finer degree of selectivity than the nonimmunologic, nonspecific form of phagocytosis. In essence, the phagocytes recognize not the particle proper but the antibody or complement fractions bound to the particle. The particle-bound recognition factors interact with specific receptors present on the phagocytic surface to trigger particle attachment and ingestion. Because macrophages interact with a certain portion of the heavy chains of the IgG molecules (the Fc domain), the macrophage receptors for IgG are often called the *Fc receptors*. Similarly, complement receptors are present; they are designated *C3 receptors*. Phagocytosis is most efficient when both IgG and C3 are present on the particle. C3 potentiates the ingestion by ensuring the approximation of particle and phagocyte. It is also of interest that certain bacteria possess capsules with antiphagocytic properties. An example is the M protein of *Streptococci*, which inhibits uptake of the bacteria by the phagocytes.

It is the presence of phagocytic receptors for IgG and complement on the surface of macrophages that distinguishes these cells ("professional" phagocytes) from other phagocytic cells (epithelial cells and fibroblasts, for example). The latter, "nonprofessional" phagocytes, will not specifically ingest particles coated with immunoglobulin or complement. Damaged cells or extracellular materials are also avidly phagocytized by macrophages, but the mechanisms involved are unknown. This recognition of damage is important under normal and pathological conditions. For example, macrophages phagocytize cells and extracellular materials which become altered in the course of normal morphogenesis and inflammation.

POSTENGULFMENT EVENTS

Pinocytic and phagocytic vacuoles fuse with lysosomes, membrane-bounded vesicles that contain a battery of hydrolytic enzymes. The outcome of this fusion is the formation of phagolysosomes or secondary lysosomes. The pH within these organelles is around 4, which is close to the optimum pH of the lysosomal hydrolases. The hydrolases digest macromolecules, and digestion intermediates of molecular

weights below 300 daltons may diffuse out of the lysosomes. Materials that cannot be digested may be stored in lysosomes for long periods of time. It is of interest that genetically determined defects of lysosomal hydrolases can lead to a variety of "storage diseases" in which undigested materials accumulate within macrophages and other cells.

Many kinds of bacteria are killed within phagosomes of the macrophages, but the mechanisms involved are not well understood. It was pointed out that the pH inside the phagosomes is rather low, and this factor by itself may reduce the viability of microorganisms. Lung macrophages contain the polysaccharidase lysozyme, active on many bacteria. A peroxidase involved in bactericidal activity is detectable in monocytes but probably absent in most tissue macrophages.

Certain organisms thrive and multiply within macrophages. Examples are the leprosy and tubercle bacilli and the protozoa, *Toxoplasma* and *Trypanosoma cruzi*. Recent experiments have shown that phagocytic vacuoles containing *Toxoplasma* or tubercle bacilli do not fuse efficiently with primary lysosomes, which thus explains the survival of these organisms within the macrophages.

EXOCYTOSIS

When macrophages bind to particles or to immune complexes under conditions where ingestion is inhibited, or the phagocytes interact with certain complement fragments (C5a), lysosomal enzymes are released to the extracellular space. This occurs by fusion of lysosomes with the phagocytic pouch or with the plasma membrane. The enzymes released can increase tissue damage in several forms of inflammation. Experimentally, partial release of lysosomal enzymes can be obtained by incubation of cells with particles (for example, yeast cell walls) in the presence of the fungal product cytochalasin B, which inhibits membrane motility by interfering with the function of actin-rich microfilaments. Alternatively, lysosomal enzyme release can be obtained by plating of phagocytes over substrate-bound immune complexes. Macrophages spread over the immobilized complexes, and the situation can be likened to a frustrated attempt at phagocytosis of a particle of large diameter.

Exocytosis in toto of undigestible materials, as

found in amoebae, has not been demonstrated in macrophages, but release of small amounts of processed or semidigested macromolecules such as hemocyanin previously fed to the phagocytes has been reported.

CHEMOTAXIS

Monocytes and macrophages are attracted toward certain substances named chemotactic factors, that is, they move directionally up concentration gradients of these factors. Chemotactic factors include C5a, a split product of the fifth component of complement, certain bacterial products, and many denatured proteins. Chemotaxis is often assayed by placing cells on top of a filter which has pores of sufficient diameter to admit the cells (about 5 μm). Solutions of chemotactic factors are placed in the bottom chamber (with an appropriate control medium in the upper compartment) and thus a concentration gradient of chemotactic factors is established across the membrane. Chemotactic activity is measured by counting cells that migrate into or through the membrane over time intervals. The relevance of the chemotactic assays in vitro to the situation in vivo needs additional evaluation.

MACROPHAGES AS SECRETORY CELLS

Macrophages produce and secrete molecules other than lysosomal hydrolases, and in some instances this secretion is unrelated to phagocytosis. Among biologically important substances thus released are certain proteins of the complement system (C2 and C4), a pyrogen (fever-inducing protein), certain interferons (antiviral agents), the enzymes lysozyme, elastase, collagenase, plasminogen activator, and colony-stimulating factors that increase the number of hematopoietic colonies in bone marrow. The list of materials secreted by macrophages can be expected to grow in the future, which highlights the importance of these cells in events other than phagocytosis.

MACROPHAGE ACTIVATION

In vitro and in vivo experiments demonstrate that macrophages subjected to appropriate stimuli undergo morphological, biochemical, and functional changes consistent with increased activity. Examples of such stimuli are the injection of certain irritant materials into a serous cavity (for example, thioglycollate broth), parenteral administration of bacterial lipopolysaccharides, or systemic infection with obligatory or facultative intracellular microorganisms, such as the agents of leprosy, tuberculosis, listeriosis, toxoplasmosis, leishmaniasis, etc. Among the parameters that characterize activated macrophages are increases in size, adhesiveness, glucose oxidation, lysosomal hydrolase content, production of enzymes such as collagenase or plasminogen activator, and endocytic and bactericidal activities. These cellular changes are most often correlated with increased numbers of macrophages either by recruitment from monocytes or proliferation of fixed macrophages.

Of particular interest is macrophage activation during infection of the host with microorganisms. There is good evidence that this activation requires the triggering of sensitized thymus-derived (T) lymphocytes by the microbial antigens. The T cells release soluble products (lymphokines) which activate the macrophages. The activation is nonspecific in the sense that macrophages activated during the course of infection by one organism are also better able to kill other bacteria. The importance of this area of investigation is highlighted by the recent findings that activated, or "irate," macrophages are selectively cytotoxic toward tumor cells in vitro but spare normal cells. Inhibition of the growth of certain tumors can be induced by local or systemic administration of bacterial products to animals and humans, but it remains to be shown that this form of immunotherapy is primarily mediated by macrophage activation.

ORIGIN, FATE, AND LIFESPAN OF MACROPHAGES

It has been demonstrated in rodents that macrophages of inflammatory exudates are derived from circulating monocytes. It was later shown that macrophages in the peritoneal cavity, or in the parenchyma of liver or lung, are also similarly derived. The present concept of the origin of macrophages is the following (Fig. 4-5). A stem cell for the monocyte is presumably derived from a pluripotential marrow cell. Maturation occurs in the bone marrow and mature monocytes are released into the circulation. Release must occur steadily and rapidly inasmuch as there does not appear to be an appreciable pool of monocytes in the marrow. Monocytes remain in circulation for about 40 h, enter the connective tissues, and increase in size, lysosomal enzyme content, and endocytic activity, and are thus operationally recognized as macrophages. Under normal conditions, but particularly under certain experimental or pathological situations, macrophages can show replicative activity. The lifespan of macrophages varies in different tissues but may be as long as 2 or 3 months. This agrees with the extended longevity of macrophages maintained in culture. There is in vivo evidence of macrophage translocation within the body: for example, labeled macrophages transferred to the peritoneal cavity can be found at later times in the liver, spleen, and thymus.

In response to foreign bodies and to certain bacterial infections (for example, tuberculosis, leprosy), macrophages fuse to form giant cells that can have 20 or more nuclei. Alternatively, in chronic granulomas, macrophages may establish tight junctions, become less phagocytic, and show fewer lysosomes; they are then called epithelioid cells. Epithelioid cells seem to wall off the inflammatory sites.

QUANTITATION OF THE IN VIVO FUNCTION OF MONONUCLEAR PHAGOCYTES

The rate of clearance of colloids (carbon, colloidal gold, aggregated albumin, radioiodinated lipid emul-

sions) from the blood has been used in experimental animals and human beings as a measure of the activity of the MPS. After a single intravenous injection, these materials are taken up predominantly by phagocytes in the liver and spleen. Therefore, the clearance studies evaluate only a fraction of the MPS. Rates of clearance depend not only on the endocytotic activity of individual cells but also on the numbers of phagocytes present in the liver. These numbers may vary in pathological or experimental conditions.

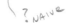

PARTICIPATION IN THE IMMUNE RESPONSE

There is no doubt that macrophages ingest and degrade many particulate antigens and may thus prevent inhibition of the immune response by antigen overload. In addition, it has been proposed that certain antigens may be retained on the macrophage surface long enough to be able to stimulate lymphocytes and lead to antibody production. Macrophage-associated antigen is more immunogenic in vivo and in vitro than an equivalent amount of free antigen. There is also evidence of a minor release of semiprocessed antigen molecules from macrophages, but the generality and importance of this mechanism remains to be evaluated.

FIGURE 4-5 Cell lineage of mononuclear phagocytes. (From R. van Furth, "Mononuclear Phagocytes in Immunity, Infection and Pathology," p. 162, Blackwell Scientific Publications, Ltd., Oxford, 1975.)

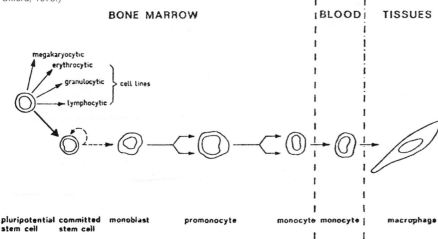

BONE MARROW　　　　**｜BLOOD｜　TISSUES**

megakaryocytic
erythrocytic
granulocytic 〉 cell lines
lymphocytic

pluripotential　committed　monoblast　　　promonocyte　　　monocyte　monocyte｜　macrophage
stem cell　　stem cell

MAST CELLS

While a medical student, Paul Ehrlich demonstrated (1877) that certain cells in connective tissues contained granules which stained characteristically with basic aniline dyes. He presumed that the granules represented stored nutrients and he named the cells "mast cells" (a reference to "feeding" in German). The granules were also metachromatic, that is, the color of the stained granules differed from that of the original dye. It is now known that mast cells stain with basic and metachromatic dyes such as toluidine blue or thionine because the cells contain a high concentration of heparin, a sulfated proteoglycan (see below).

Rat mast cell granules are easily demonstrated with conventional fixation and staining, but staining of mast cell granules in humans and other species requires that ethanol and lead ions be present in the fixative. For this reason, whereas mast cells are widely distributed, they are not usually observed in normal or pathological human tissues prepared by routine methods of fixation and staining. Rat mast cells found in the mesentery or in the peritoneal fluid have been a favorite subject for experimental studies, but there are morphological, compositional, and pharmacological differences between the human and the rodent cells.

Mast cells are quite common in connective tissues and are most often observed adjacent to blood vessels (Figs. 4-6 and 4-7). Granules similar in composition and function to those of mast cells are also present in blood basophils, a type of marrow-derived granulocyte.

Under the light microscope, in appropriately prepared total mounts or sections, mast cells are relatively large (20 to 30 μm) and filled with characteristic

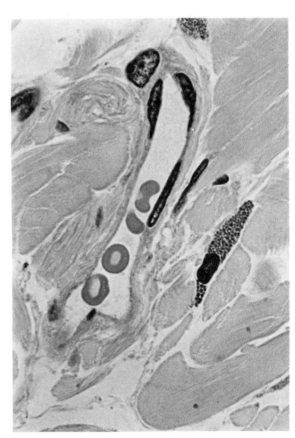

FIGURE 4-6 Human mast cell between collagen bundles in thin section of skin. A venule is also shown. × 800. (E. S. Robbins.)

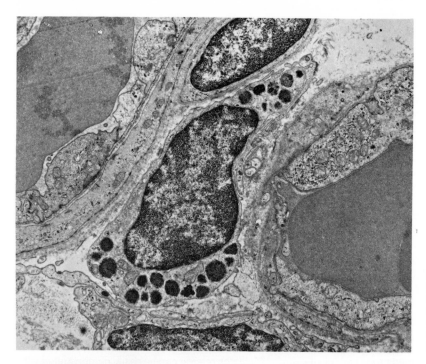

FIGURE 4-7 Electron micrograph of human mast cell from a biopsy of the rectal submucosa. The mast cell is situated between two small blood vessels. ×7500. (From D. Lagunoff, *J. Invest. Dermatol.,* **58:**296, 1972.)

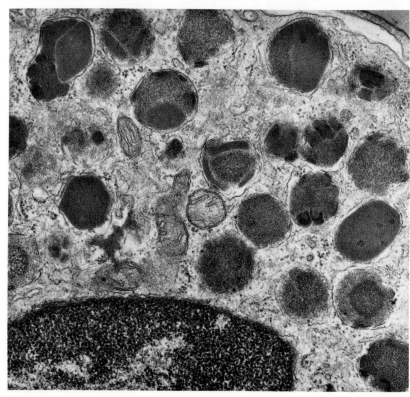

FIGURE 4-8 Portion of human mast cell showing granules with denser cores or with lamellar or paracrystalline arrays. ×25,800. (From D. Lagunoff, *J. Invest. Dermatol.,* **58:**296, 1972.)

basophilic granules which often obscure the cell nucleus. Under the electron microscope mast cell granules are bounded by a unit membrane. Human granules are heterogeneous, containing lamellar bodies, whorls, or paracrystalline structures (Fig. 4-8), whereas the granules are more homogenous in the rat (Fig. 4-9). Besides the specific granules, mast cells contain the usual cytoplasmic organelles such as mitochrondria, Golgi, endoplasmic reticulum, microtubules, and microfilaments.

Mast cells are rather long-lived. They may originate from mesenchymally derived cells in tissues; there is no evidence for their origin from the bone marrow. It is now possible to clone mast cells from suspensions of mouse thymus. Further information on the origin and differentiation of these cells may be available in the near future.

Mast cells and basophils, like macrophages, polymorphonuclear neutrophils, and platelets store pharmacologically potent mediators that are secreted after appropriate stimulation. These mediators can elicit such phenomena as edema, pain, shock, hypercoagulation, and fever. In humans, mast cells are mainly involved in immunologically mediated "immediate hypersensitivity" reactions, which occur within a short period after a sensitized individual is challenged with the homologous antigen. Thus, mast cells participate in conditions such as asthma, hay fever, urticaria, sensitization to drugs, or anaphylactic shock.

The mediators produced by human mast cells and basophils are histamine (beta imidazole ethylamine), the proteoglycan heparin, the slow-reacting substance of anaphylaxis (SRS-A), and the eosinophil chemotactic factor of anaphylaxis (ECF-A). In the human being, the main mechanism that triggers the release of mediators from mast cells and basophils involves a class of immunoglobulins known as IgE. These immunoglobulins are synthesized preferentially after exposure to certain antigens such as those present in ragweed pollen. IgE is present in serum in very low concentrations, but its Fc domain has a very high avidity for specific surface receptors on mast cells and basophils. Consequently, most of the IgE in the body is fixed to the surface of these cells. When the sensitized host is reexposed to minute amounts of the antigen (e.g., micromicrograms of ragweed antigen), the antigen may interact with mast-cell-bound IgE antibody and this in turn causes the release of histamine, SRS-A, and ECF-A. In human beings heparin may not be released by this mechanism.

Mediator release can be easily demonstrated with suspensions of mast cells or basophils, or with slices of tissues, such as lung, which are rich in mast cells. These preparations have furnished important information about the mechanisms of release of mediators, and they have helped in the development of drugs which inhibit or facilitate the release reaction.

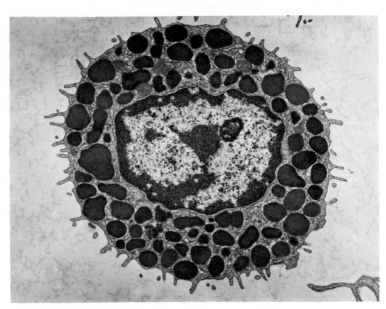

FIGURE 4-9 Electron micrograph of the peritoneal mast cell from a rat. Note relative uniformity in granule densities. × 6200. (From *J. Invest. Dermatol.*, **58**:296, 1972).

Ultrastructural studies of the release reaction (Figs. 4-9 and 4-10) show that the peripheral granules fuse with the plasma membrane to discharge their contents. The membranes of granules toward the center of the cell may fuse with each other, creating channels which connect with the cell surface (Fig. 4-10). The process of mediator release or secretion is energy-dependent, requires Ca^{2+}, and seems to involve microfilaments.

Some relevant properties of mast cell mediators are as follows. Histamine induces increased permeability of small venules, presumably because gaps form between adjacent endothelial cells. Leakage of plasma protein and fluid accounts for edema (swelling), one of the features of inflammation. Not all the histamine in the body, however, is present in mast cells and basophils. SRS-A is an ethanol-soluble substance of about 400 daltons, which causes smooth muscle cells to contract slowly and which increases vascular permeability. SRS-A may not exist preformed in mast cells, but its synthesis seems to be induced soon after anaphylactic challenge, that is, when an antigen gains access to the surface of sensitized mast cells. ECF-A in contrast is preformed. ECF-A, which is a chemotactic factor for eosinophils, is an acidic peptide of about

500 daltons. Accumulation of eosinophils at sites of allergic reactions, such as the nasal mucosa in hay fever, the bronchial mucosa in asthma, and the gut submucosa in parasitic infestations, is ascribed to the release of ECF-A.

IgE-dependent mediator release is inhibited by agents which increase the cyclic AMP (cAMP) concentration in mast cells. Drugs such as isoproterenol act on beta-adrenergic receptors of mast cells and increase the synthesis of cAMP. Other drugs, such as theophylline (a methylxanthine), increase cAMP levels by reducing the degradation of the nucleotide by a diesterase. On the other hand, agents that lower the cAMP content of mast cells (or increase cyclic GMP) increase mediator release. These responses are relevant to the pathogenesis and the treatment of allergic conditions. There is a rare disease called diffuse urticaria pigmentosa associated with increased numbers of mast cells. The mast cells in such patients are abnormally fragile, and simple stroking of the skin results in mediator release with the formation of wheals (*dermographism*).

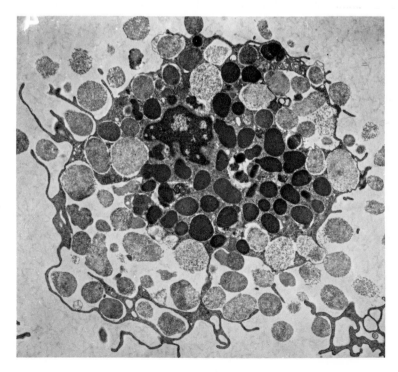

FIGURE 4-10 Rat mast cell degranulated by exposure to polymyxin B sulfate (0.5 μg/ml). The peripheral granules are swollen and exhibit decreased density and frayed margins; channels are present within the cytoplasm. ×6200. (From D. Lagunoff, *J. Invest. Dermatol.* **58:**296, 1972.)

THE FIBROBLAST

In connective tissue the fibroblast is identified as a spindle-shaped cell with tapering eosinophilic cytoplasmic extensions (Fig. 4-11). Its nucleus generally has a regular elliptical contour, contains two to four nucleoli, and has sparse and scattered chromatin. In very dense connective tissue, fibroblasts appear to be compressed between the thick bundles of collagen, for their nuclei are more elongated and darkly stained, and their cell borders usually cannot be resolved in routine preparations. Fibroblasts are motile, and they change their shape as they move over surfaces. When inoculated at low cell density into culture plates, fibroblasts flatten onto the surface, send out long cytoplasmic projections, and move about, assuming stellate, rectangular, and elliptical shapes (Fig. 4-12). The fibroblast is capable of serial replication in vivo and in vitro; and when the cell enters the mitotic phase, it loosens its attachment to a surface and becomes spherical. After telophase, the daughter cells flatten onto available surfaces and once again assume extended forms.

The ultrastructural organization of the differentiated fibroblast reflects that cell type's commitment to the synthesis of molecules destined for secretion into the extracellular space. Accordingly, the typical fibroblast has a well-developed granular endoplasmic reticulum on which the precursor polypeptides of collagen, elastin, and the proteoglycans are synthesized (Fig. 4-13). The cisternae of that compartment contain finely granular or filamentous material, which presumably represents the soluble precursor molecules that have been artefactually precipitated in the course of fixation and staining. The molecules in the cisternae are transported to a well-defined Golgi zone by transitional vesicular elements. Although the molecules are chemically modified in the Golgi, they do not generally appear to be subject to concentration and storage in condensing vacuoles. Accordingly, smooth-surfaced secretory vesicles which move from the Golgi zone to the plasma membrane do not usually appear to contain greater concentrations of material than the cisternae of the granular endoplasmic reticulum. The secretory vesicles fuse with the plasma

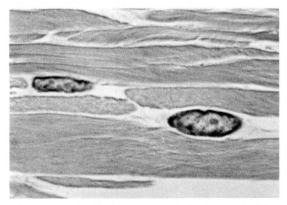

FIGURE 4-11 General appearance of fibroblasts in moderately dense connective tissue. The nuclei are regularly elliptical and the cytoplasmic borders are not well resolved from the adjacent collagen fibers. × 1500.

membrane to release their soluble contents into the extracellular space (Fig. 4-14). Further biochemical modifications of the soluble-secreted molecules may follow, and deposition of insoluble collagen and elastic fibers occurs in the extracellular space, usually in close proximity to the cell surface.

The fibroblast contains the usual complement of cytoplasmic organelles and inclusions. The mitochondria tend to be long and slender, and fat droplets and primary and secondary lysosomes are occasionally prominent. Microtubules are present and appear to be required for the translocation of secretory vesicular elements. Additionally, bundles of microfilaments thought to represent actin are identified and are implicated in both secretion and general cellular motility. Fibroblasts in healing wounds frequently have large bundles of microfilaments and other morphologic features which make them resemble smooth muscle cells. Such "myofibroblasts" are thought to play a role in the contraction of wounds.

For discussions of the functional morphology of the osteoblast, chondroblast, and smooth muscle cell, the reader is referred to the chapters on bone, cartilage, and muscle.

FIGURE 4-12 Cultured human-skin fibroblasts. Photomicrographs illustrate the variety of shapes fibroblasts may take when their movement is not restricted by adjacent cells or fibrous elements. ×500.

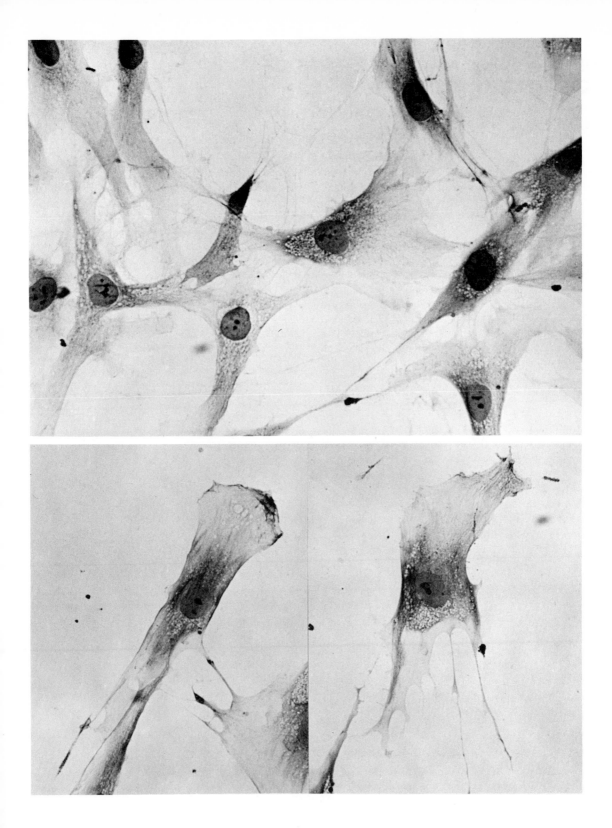

EXTRACELLULAR COMPONENTS OF CONNECTIVE TISSUE

COLLAGEN

Collagen is a protein which forms extracellular fibers or basement membrane networks in practically every tissue of the body. Depending upon the structural and functional requirements of a particular tissue, the collagenous elements may be abundant (dense connective tissue) or sparse (loose connective tissue) and may be arranged in distinctive patterns. For example, in tendons and ligaments, the collagen fibers are thick and long and grouped into large parallel bundles to provide the required tensile strength. By contrast, collagen fibers tend to be wrapped helically around the long axes of tubular expansile structures such as blood vessels, intestine, and glandular ducts. In cartilage and bone, calcium phosphate crystals are deposited on collagen fibers, so the latter help to determine the mechanical properties of the skeleton. In the cornea the collagen fibers form alternating orthogonal lamel-

lae, which by their spacing and angular orientation permit the cornea to function as a refractive element of the eye. The cornea is continuous with the sclera, but in the latter coat the orthogonal arrangement of collagen fibers is not present. In the transparent vitreous humor, the collagen fibrils are thin, sparse, randomly oriented, and embedded in a gel of hyaluronic acid.

For most of the examples cited, the collagenous units are in the form of fibers, and such fibers most

FIGURE 4-13 Electron micrograph of cytoplasm of a fibroblast shows a tangential section through the granular endoplasmic reticulum (E_g). The polysomes are seen as curved chains; the cisterna contains granular material. Arrows indicate profiles of agranular ergastoplasm in continuity with granular reticulum. Smooth vesicles could represent transitional vesicles moving to the Golgi zone. $\times 74,000$. (From B. Goldberg and H. Green, *J. Cell Biol.*, **22**:227, 1964.)

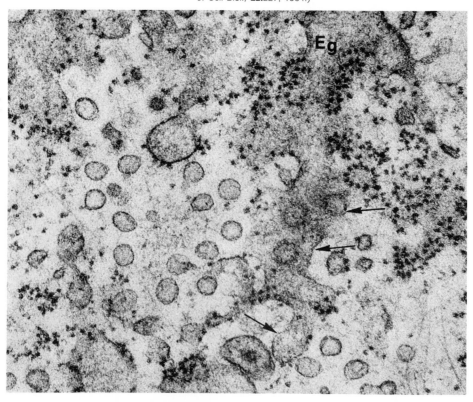

usually display a characteristic "native" pattern of transverse bands when examined by means of the electron microscope (Fig. 4-15). Collagen molecules are also a major component of the basal lamina, the extracellular supporting layer which is characteristically interposed between epithelial surfaces and the underlying connective tissue. In the electron microscope the basal lamina (basement lamina) is seen as a meshwork of fine fibrils lacking any banding pattern (Fig. 4-16). The endothelium of capillaries is also supported by a basal lamina; and in the case of the capillaries of the renal glomerulus, this layer achieves a thickness of about 1500 Å (0.15 μm). The capsule of the lens of the eye is an example of an epithelial basal lamina with a thickness of about 15 μm. As will be discussed, the collagen molecules of the basal laminae differ somewhat from the collagen molecules which form the native cross-banded fibers.

Collagen thus serves a wide variety of structural and mechanical functions, and as a component of basal laminae it plays an important role in the control of vascular and epithelial permeability. Histologic stains for light microscopy aid in identifying the various fibrous and fibrillar forms of collagen in different tissues, but they are not specific for the protein. Collagen fibers or fibrils can be uniquely identified only by their banding pattern in the electron microscope, by their wide angle x-ray diffraction pattern, or by their amino acid composition.

MOLECULAR STRUCTURE

It is of value to study the general structure of the collagen molecule, for such study provides a basis for understanding the biosynthesis of the protein and the manner in which the molecules aggregate to form the characteristic fibers in the extracellular space. Cold neutral salt or weakly acidic solutions will extract the collagen molecule (tropocollagen) from the connec-

FIGURE 4-14 Electron micrograph shows surfaces of two fibroblasts. Smooth vesicles (V_s) appear to be fusing with the plasma membranes and discharging their contents into the extracellular space (ECS). A banded collagen fiber (C) is present between the cells. × 74,000. (From B. Goldberg and H. Green, *J. Cell Biol.,* **22:**227, 1964.)

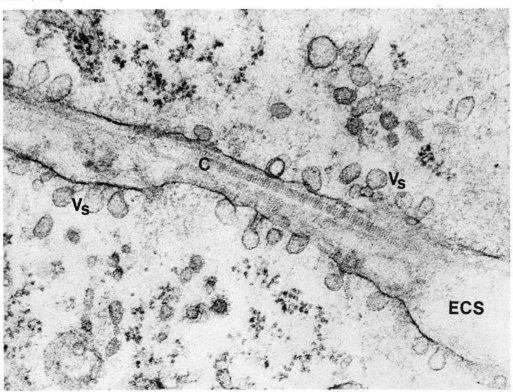

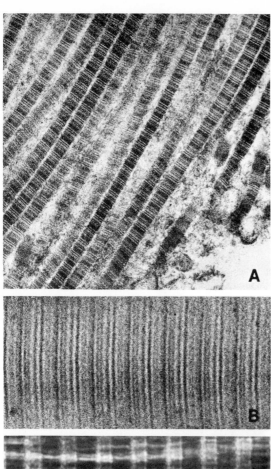

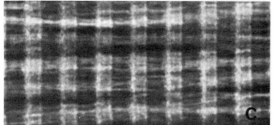

FIGURE 4-15 Electron micrographs of native collagen fibers. A. Positively stained collagen fibers with characteristic cross-striations and periodicity. ×59,000. (Courtesy of Dr. E. Robbins, New York University.) B. Positively stained rat tail tendon. Higher magnification emphasizes regularity of bands across the fiber and the repeat period of 670 Å. ×149,000. C. Negatively stained collagen fiber formed by warming a neutral salt solution of human collagen to 37°C. The repeat period is 670 Å, but only two major intraperiod bands are present. ×149,000.

FIGURE 4-17 Schematic of the triple helical collagen (tropocollagen) molecule. The three chains are helical except for the short terminal segments (the telopeptides) of 16 to 25 residues. The amino termini of all three chains are at the same end of the molecule. The dotted line indicates that one chain may differ in primary structure from the other two chains, as is the case for type I collagen (see Table 4-4).

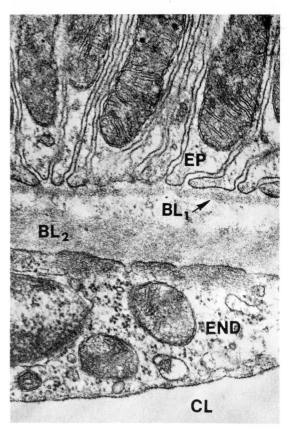

FIGURE 4-16 Electron micrograph of basal laminae of proximal convoluted tubule of kidney (BL₁) and capillary (BL₂). Note lack of banding in the laminae. EP, epithelium of renal tubule; END, endothelial cell of capillary; CL, capillary lumen. Molecules exchanged between the renal tubule and the capillary must traverse the collagenous basal laminae. ×41,000. (Courtesy of Dr. E. Robbins, New York University.)

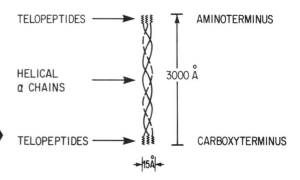

tive tissues of growing animals. Analysis has shown tropocollagen (Fig. 4-17) to consist of three polypeptide chains (α chains) of equal length, each with a molecular weight of approximately 95,000. The amino termini of the three chains are at the same end of the molecule. The individual chains form a left-handed helix, but the three chains are coiled around the central axis to form a right-handed major helix. The molecule overall has the shape of a rod, about 3000 Å long and 15 Å in diameter. The molecular structure is determined by its unique amino acid composition: in particular, every third residue in the helical chains is glycine, and the imino acids proline and 4-hydroxyproline together account for about another 20 percent of the residues. The imino acids direct the helical conformation by virtue of their rotational restrictions, and hydroxyproline also helps to stabilize the triple helix by contributing to interchain hydrogen bonds. The other amino acids of the chains are not critical for the general helical structure, but their polar and nonpolar side chains are directed out from the central axis and thus are available for interactions with other collagen molecules or noncollagenous components of the connective tissues. Such interactions play a role in the assembly of collagen molecules into fibers.

Hydroxyproline is a convenient analytical marker for collagen inasmuch as it occurs only in one other animal protein (elastin) and then in much lesser amounts. 5-Hydroxylysine is another amino acid that is unique for collagen, but it is much less abundant than hydroxyproline. Galactose, or the disaccharide galactose-glucose, is covalently linked to the hydroxyl group of some of the hydroxylysine residues. The function of these sugars is unknown. At both the amino and carboxy termini of each α chain are 16 to 25 residues which are nonhelical because of their low glycine and low imino acid content. These abbreviated nonhelical regions are called telopeptides. They are represented by the pleated lines in Fig. 4-17. Lysine and hydroxylysine residues in the telopeptides participate in covalent cross-linking of collagen molecules after the molecules aggregate to form fibers.

It is now known that at least four molecular types of collagen may be extracted from tissues. These genetically distinct molecules do not differ greatly with respect to glycine and imino acid content, so they all possess the general molecular form depicted in Fig. 4-17. However, there are minor but distinctive differences among the four molecular types with respect to amino acid composition and sequence. The nomenclature, chain composition, and tissue distributions of the four collagen types are given in Table 4-4.

TABLE 4-4

MOLECULAR TYPE	CHAIN COMPOSITION*	PREDOMINANT DISTRIBUTION
I	$[\alpha 1(I)]_2\alpha 2$	Dermis, bone, tendons, ligaments, dentine
II	$[\alpha 1(II)]_3$	Hyaline cartilage
III	$[\alpha 1(III)]_3$	Dermis, cardiovascular system, uterus, intestine
IV	$[\alpha 1(IV)]_3$	Basal laminae

* $\alpha 2$ notation signifies that type I collagen contains two chain classes. Roman numerals signify that the $\alpha 1$ chains of each collagen type have a unique primary structure.

Type I is the most abundant of the collagens and it is this molecule that was first extensively analyzed and considered to be prototypic. Only two of the three chains of type I collagen are identical; but in each of the other molecular types, only one chain class is present. Type II collagen has been found only in cartilage, and one of its characteristics is a higher content of glycosylated hydroxylysine relative to type I collagen. Type III collagen was first isolated from fetal skin. It is distinguished by the presence of half-cystine residues at the carboxy termini. Type IV collagen has been extracted exclusively from basal laminae. Relative to the other types, type IV α chains generally have a higher molecular weight (10 to 20 percent) and more half-cystine and glycosylated hydroxylysine residues, and they contain significant amounts of 3-hydroxyproline in addition to 4-hydroxyproline. Type IV molecules are also unique because they are covalently linked to glycoproteins. The various types of epithelial and endothelial basal laminae may differ in chemical composition. Either the constituent collagen chains or the glycoproteins could be the source of these compositional differences.

The genetic heterogeneity of collagen molecules presumably reflects an evolutionary selection for different functions in particular tissues. It remains a task for future research to relate the unique primary structure of each molecular type to its function in a morphologic unit of a given tissue.

COLLAGEN SYNTHESIS BY DIFFERENTIATED CELL TYPES

Most of the collagen of the body is synthesized by cells derived from the mesenchyme. The fibroblast is responsible for synthesizing the bulk of type I collagen, but its counterpart, the osteoblast, synthesizes the type I collagen of bone. Cartilage collagen (II) is synthesized by the chondroblast. Type III collagen of skin is synthesized by the fibroblast. It appears that a skin fibroblast may simultaneously synthesize both type I and type III collagens. The type III collagen found in the muscularis of arteries, intestine, and uterus is probably synthesized by smooth muscle cells. Smooth muscle cells may also synthesize type I collagen.

Basement membrane collagen (IV) is synthesized by endothelial cells of vessels and by surface epithelia of various types. Epithelia are not derived from mesenchyme; and correspondingly, a variety of nonfibroblastic cell types of ectodermal, neuroectodermal, and endodermal origin have been shown to synthesize small amounts of collagen in culture.

Most of what we know about collagen biosynthesis has been learned from studying fibroblastic systems synthesizing type I collagen, but the mechanisms to be described are probably generally valid for the other cell types synthesizing the other molecular forms of collagen. The biosynthetic steps are schematized in Figs. 4-18 and 4-19.

Like other proteins destined for secretion from the cell, collagen is synthesized on polysomes attached to the endoplasmic reticulum with the nascent chains vectorially oriented into the cisternae. Incorporation of the amino acids into the nascent chains via transfer RNAs proceeds by the usual mechanisms with the exceptions of hydroxyproline and hydroxylysine. These residues of collagen arise from the enzymatic hydroxylation of specific prolyl and lysyl residues in peptide linkage in the growing nascent chains. The two hydroxylating enzymes (prolyl and lysyl hydroxylase)

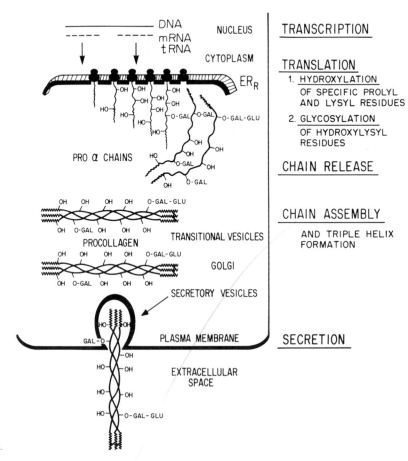

FIGURE 4-18 Collagen biosynthesis: intracellular events and secretion.

are contained within the granular endoplasmic reticulul, and atmospheric O_2, α-ketoglutarate, ferrous ions, and ascorbate are utilized as substrates or cofactors in both the hydroxylations.

Galactosyl and glucosyl transferases catalyze the sequential addition of the sugars to specific hydroxylysyl residues in the nascent chains. Chains released from the polysomes pass into the cisternae of the rough endoplasmic reticulum where some of the hydroxylations and glycosylations might be completed. The released chains are larger precursor forms (pro α chains) of collagen chains, for they have nonhelical polypeptide extensions at both the amino and carboxytermini which are larger than the telopeptides of tropocollagen. These nonhelical extensions ("propeptides," "registration peptides") aid in the correct and rapid assembly of the chains, and they keep the assembled triple helical molecule (procollagen) in solution. Assembly of procollagen probably begins in the cisternae, and the molecule is then transported to the Golgi complex via transitional elements of the rough endoplasmic reticulum. The nonhelical propeptides also have covalently attached sugar residues, and perhaps the Golgi complex is the site where these additional enzymatic glycosylations occur. Procollagen is transported from the Golgi complex to the cell surface via secretory vesicles which then fuse with the plasma membrane to discharge the soluble precursor molecule. The transcellular movement and secretion of procollagen requires energy, and the microtubular system is required for the translocations of the vacuolar elements. Once secreted from the cell, procollagen is enzymatically converted to collagen (Fig. 4-19). The fibroblast secretes one or more enzymes ("procollagen

peptidase") which excise most of the nonhelical peptides from the ends of the precursor, generating tropocollagen, the triple helical molecule which retains only the abbreviated telopeptides. Once generated, tropocollagen tends to come out of solution and aggregate in a specific manner to form collagen fibers.

Some elements of the general biosynthetic scheme presented in Figs. 4-18 and 4-19 should be considered as provisional. For example, some of the registration peptides of procollagen may be enzymatically excised just before secretion occurs. This may be the explanation for the fibrous aggregates observed in secretory vesicles of the odontoblast. Another possibility is that the final excision of propeptides may occur after the molecules have aggregated as fibers in the extracellular space.

The biosynthesis of collagen is evidently complex, for it involves the balanced synthesis of pro α chain classes, hydroxylation and glycosylation of specific residues, and extracellular modifications of the precursor so that the final molecule can be incorporated into a type of fiber appropriate to the tissue. If a cell synthesizes two molecular forms of collagen simultaneously, the complexities are increased. Controls must clearly operate at the level of genomic transcription so that the proper kinds and amounts of messenger RNA are released to the cytoplasm. Translational controls may further modulate the balanced synthesis of different chain classes. One presumes that the hydroxylations, glycosylations, assembly, and extracellular processing of the precursors are critically de-

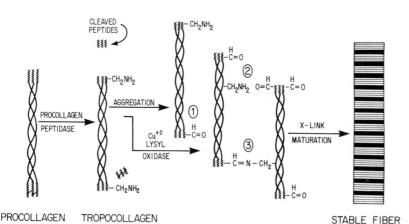

PROCOLLAGEN   TROPOCOLLAGEN   STABLE FIBER

FIGURE 4-19 Collagen biosynthesis: extracellular events. The propeptides are enzymatically cleaved from the ends of the procollagen molecule, leaving the abbreviated telopeptides of tropocollagen. Tropocollagen molecules aggregate to form fibers. Enzymatic oxidative deamination (1) of lysyl or hydroxylysyl residues in the telopeptides introduces reactive aldehydic groups. The latter groups react with the ε-amino groups of lysine or hydroxylysine in adjacent molecules (2) to form Schiff bases (3).

termined by the primary structure of the pro α chains, but controls affecting the activities of the various enzymes could also be superimposed. The biosyntheses of types II and IV collagens illustrate some of the possible variations which may be imposed on the general scheme. In chondroblasts, type II pro α chains are released into the cisternae of the rough-surfaced endoplasmic reticulum, but their assembly into a three-chain molecule in this compartment proceeds more slowly than it does for type I pro α chains. Assembly of type II pro α chains may not be completed until the chains are transported to smooth-surfaced compartments, and this delay may allow for the more extensive glycosylation of the hydroxylysine residues in this type of collagen. In the case of type IV procollagen, it has been suggested that the propeptides of the secreted molecule may not be subject to extensive excision by a peptidase, and the relatively intact procollagen molecule may be incorporated into the structure of basal laminae.

FIBRILLOGENESIS

The bulk of collagen in the body is in the form of fibers which display a characteristic "native" pattern of cross-banding when positively or negatively stained with heavy metal ions and examined by electron microscopy (Fig. 4-15). The native pattern is characterized by a major axial repeat period of 670 Å within which 12 dark bands may be resolved under optimal conditions of positive staining. Negatively stained native fibers show the same repeat period, but within it are only two major bands: a dark zone where the stain penetrates, and a light zone produced by exclusion of the stain.

Native fibrils will form in vitro if neutral salt solutions of collagen are warmed to 37°C. This result suggests that fibrillogenesis in vivo might be determined only by the primary structure and the limited solubility of the tropocollagen molecule. However, we must still explain how the collagen molecules are packed to give the ultrastructure of the native fibril. The discovery of another aggregated form of tropocollagen has provided an explanation. If ATP is added to acidic solutions of collagen, the precipitates which form are not fibrils but aggregates with lengths of only 3000 Å (Fig. 4-20). These segment long spacing

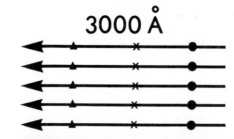

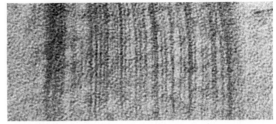

FIGURE 4-20 Electron micrograph of segment long spacing (SLS) aggregate of human collagen. Arrows represent tropocollagen molecules, and indicate that aggregate is formed by parallel packing of molecules with amino termini and all other residues in register. Vertical lines are formed by binding of stain to charged residues. × 187,000.

(SLS) forms result from tropocollagen molecules aggregating in parallel with all their amino termini in register. Consequently, all the amino acid residues are in register across the SLS aggregate, the polar residues bind the heavy metal stains, and the resultant cross-striations represent a map or fingerprint of the distribution of polar side chains along the length of the molecule. Fibrils are formed when molecules are aligned end to end, or when they are overlapped along their long axes. Accordingly, it was found that when SLS forms were overlapped by approximately one-quarter of their length, the band pattern of the native fibril could be reconstructed. A quarter-stagger model of molecular packing for the native fibril was therefore proposed, a current modification of which is reproduced in Fig. 4-21. The essential elements of the model are as follows. (1) The tropocollagen molecule has a length of $4.4D$; D equals 670 Å. (2) The molecules in the fibril are polarized. (3) Axial displacement of adjacent molecules by a distance D produces fibrils with a repeat period of D. (4) Mass per unit length alternates within the period, corresponding to an overlap zone of $0.4D$ and a hole zone of $0.6D$. The model accounts for the banding pattern of positively and negatively stained native fibrils. In the latter case,

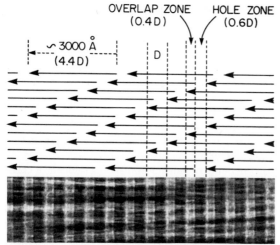

OVERLAP ZONE   HOLE ZONE
(0.4D)   (0.6D)

~3000 Å
(4.4D)   D

FIGURE 4-21 Two-dimensional model for packing of tropocollagen molecules (arrows) in the native-type fibril. Arrowheads indicate amino terminal ends. Adjacent molecules are longitudinally displaced by a distance D (approximately 670 Å) to form a fibril of repeating period D. The electron micrograph of a negatively stained fibril (below) shows that each period consists of a light overlap zone $(0.4D)$ from which the stain is mostly excluded, and a dark hole zone $(0.6D)$ into which the stain penetrates. [Adapted from the model of A. J. Hodge, J. A. Petruska, and A. J. Bailey, "Structure and Function of Connective and Skeletal Tissue," p. 31, Butterworths & Co. (Publishers), Ltd., London 1965.]

molecules prevent native fibrillar packing. Although lacking periodicity, the fibrillar networks of basal laminae have a structural order which determines their capacity to function as molecular sieves.

When loose connective tissues are stained with alkaline solutions of silver salts, a delicate network of very thin silver-stained fibers can be seen by light microscopy. These reticular fibers (reticulin) often underlie basal laminae of various types and contribute to the supporting stroma of epithelial and hematopoietic tissues. Thick collagenous fibers do not stain intensely with the silver stain; accordingly, reticulin and collagen were once assumed to be different fibrous proteins. However, we now believe that most reticulin is collagen, because electron microscopy shows that argyrophilic reticular fibers may have the characteristic periodicity of collagen. The current view is that the argyrophilia of reticulin is best ascribed to a coating of proteoglycans and glycoproteins on these thin collagen fibrils. In some tissues reticulin may fail to show collagen periodicity (see Chaps. 14 and 15). In these instances, the collagen may have aggregated randomly or be of the basal laminar type, or the observed fibrils might be composed almost entirely of proteoglycans and glycoproteins.

The proteoglycans are polyanions (see below), so they can interact with positively charged side chains of tropocollagen. Such interactions might favor one form of molecular packing over another, alter the rate of packing, or control the size of the fibril generated. However, we are far from understanding in detail how connective tissue components interact to control the size and orientation of collagen fibers in particular tissues.

the stain penetrates maximally into the hole zone to produce the dark band. Additionally, the model is in accord with currently available biochemical sequence data for various residues in the chains.

The native fibril and the SLS form are only two of many possible periodic structures which can result from electrostatic and hydrophobic interactions between collagen molecules. Moreover, if collagen molecules precipitate without statistical symmetry, nonperiodic aggregates will be generated. Fundamentally, the specificity for all the possible forms of aggregation resides in the primary structure of tropocollagen, but pH, temperature, ionic strength, and noncovalent interactions with noncollagenous molecules can favor one form of collagen packing over another. The essential point is that the chemical environment in vivo is controlled so that collagen types I, II, and III generally pack as native fibrils. Type IV collagen represents an exception, for basement laminae are characterized by a feltwork of nonperiodic fibrils. It has been suggested that the disaccharide or bulky heteropolysaccharide groups which are covalently linked to type IV collagen

CROSS-LINKING OF COLLAGEN FIBERS

Noncovalent interactions between collagen molecules are responsible for the assembly of the collagen fiber, but once formed, the fiber becomes stabilized by covalent intermolecular cross-links. The latter bonds are initiated when a specific copper-dependent amine oxidase (lysyl oxidase) secreted by the fibroblast causes the oxidative deamination of the side chains of the lysyl and hydroxylysyl residues in the telopeptide regions of tropocollagen. After deamination, these side chains terminate in an aldehyde group which can then condense spontaneously with the epsilon-amino groups of lysyl and hydroxylysyl residues in adjacent molecules. Collagen molecules are thus linked through a reducible aldimine bond (a Schiff base) which is later transformed to a more thermally stable, nonreducible cross-link by an unknown mechanism. These events are schematized in Fig. 4-19, but it should be emphasized that our understanding of the structure and locations of all the cross-links of collagen is still incomplete.

The cross-linking process is an extracellular event, and it is suspected that oxidative deamination of the lysyl and hydroxylysyl residues occurs after procollagen peptidase has removed the propeptides from procollagen. Noncovalent associations bring the molecules into the staggered array of the native fibril; and where aldehydic and epsilon-amino groups are approximated, the cross-links form nonenzymatically.

Introduction of covalent cross-links into the fiber increases its tensile strength by preventing slippage between molecules, renders the fiber less soluble, and decreases the fiber's susceptibility to proteolytic turnover. The cross-linking process is finely controlled, because collagen fibers from particular tissues have characteristic kinds and amounts of certain cross-links which determine in large part the mechanical properties of the fibers. When normal cross-linking is inhibited, as may occur in certain inherited and acquired diseases, the consequences are dramatic. For example, the skin may become hyperextensible and easily torn, wounds may heal poorly, bones may be deformed, and blood vessels may dilate and rupture. Excessive and abnormal cross-linking of collagen has also been invoked as a possible cause of some of the changes occurring in various tissues in the course of aging.

Collagen fibers are resorbed during growth, remodeling, involution, and inflammation and repair of tissues. The resorption is initiated by specific collagenases which can digest the tropocollagen molecules of the fiber under conditions of physiologic pH and temperature. These collagenases cleave all three α chains of tropocollagen at a specific site 750 Å from their carboxy termini, thus generating two triple helical fragments which represent, respectively, 75 and 25 percent of the original molecule. Occasionally a collagenase may make secondary clips through the three chains of the larger fragment. If the fragments are not bound by intermolecular cross-links to other molecules of the fiber, they go into solution and diffuse away. The triple helical fragments have lower melting points than the parent molecule and so are denatured to random coils at body temperature. Once denatured, they are susceptible to further digestion by the collagenases or by other neutral proteases present in the extracellular space. Additionally, the molecular fragments, or partially digested fibrils, may be phagocytosed by macrophages and degraded within secondary lysosomes by proteases with acid pH optima.

Several different cell types can synthesize and release collagenases in normal and injured tissues. Among these are fibroblasts, polymorphonuclear leucocytes, macrophages, squamous epithelium of skin, and synovial epithelium. For the normal remodeling of connective tissues during growth, or following injury and repair, there must be a proper balance between the formation and the resorption of collagen fibers. How this balance is achieved is not known in detail, but there is some evidence about how collagenase activity might be regulated. Some collagenases are synthesized as inactive precursors (zymogens) which must react with other proteins (presumably activator proteases) before they can digest collagen. Additionally, potent inhibitors (usually proteins) of collagenase activity have been demonstrated in extracellular fluids.

ELASTIC FIBERS

Elastic fibers have rubberlike properties, that is, they stretch easily and return to their original length when the deforming force is removed. Elastic fibers are found in tissues which are normally subject to stretching and expansile forces, for example, arteries, the vocal cords, the pleura, the trachea, bronchi, pulmonary alveolar septums, certain ligaments (ligamenta flava of humans, ligamentum nuchae of ruminants), auricular cartilage, Scarpa's fascia of the anterior abdominal wall, and the skin. Special stains (Verhoeff's

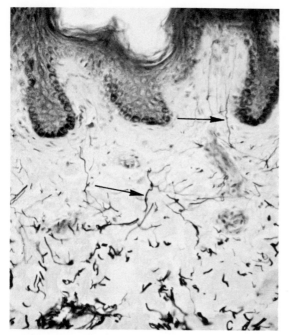

FIGURE 4-22 Elastic fibers in dermis of skin (arrows) are stained black with Verhoeff's stain. × 600.

stain, Weigert's resorcin-fuchsin) are usually required for the identification of elastic fibers in histologic preparations for light microscopy (Fig. 4-22). The thickness, length, and disposition of the fibers are different for different tissues. In arteries, elastic fibers form two thick concentric lamellae, the elastica interna and externa, and elastic fibers are also dispersed through the media of the artery as a concentric highly fenestrated network. In mesentery, fasciae, and skin, the thin and scattered fibers form networks between bundles of collagen. In the peripheral portions of the respiratory tree, very thin elastic fibers follow the course of the bronchioles, alveolar ducts, and sacs.

When examined with the electron microscope most of an elastic fiber appears to be composed of material which has neither fibrillar nor periodic structure and which has little affinity for the standard staining reagents (Fig. 4-23). However, at the periphery of the amorphous component the stains define microfibrils which are about 110 Å in diameter. When elastic fibers are being formed, the microfibrillar component appears first and then the amorphous component accumulates to form the bulk of the fiber.

The chemical compositions of the amorphous and microfibrillar components of the fiber are quite

different. *Elastin,* the insoluble protein which remains after connective tissues are digested with dilute alkali, is derived from the amorphous component of the elastic fiber. Like collagen, about one-third of the residues of elastin are glycine and about 11 percent are proline. Unlike collagen, elastin is composed mostly of nonpolar hydrophobic amino acids, and it has little hydroxyproline and no hydroxylysine. Also, elastin uniquely contains desmosine and isodesmosine (Fig. 4-24), which function as covalent cross-links in and between the polypeptide chains. Elastin stains poorly with ionic dyes because it contains relatively few charged amino acids, and the preponderance of hydrophobic residues and the presence of cross-links account for elastin's insolubility.

The microfibrillar protein is composed mainly of hydrophilic amino acids. It contains much less glycine than elastin, and has no hydroxyproline, desmosine, or isodesmosine. It contains a relatively large number of half-cystine residues which are absent from elastin. Accordingly, when elastic fibers are treated with chemical agents which break disulfide bonds, the microfibrils are solubilized and the elastin is left as an insoluble residue. Neutral sugars represent about 5 percent of the weight of the microfibrillar protein.

Fibroblasts and smooth muscle cells synthesize the molecules which form the elastic fiber. Given the

FIGURE 4-23 Electron micrograph of elastic fibers. The fibers are composed of amorphous elastin (E) and a fibrillar protein. × 84,400. (Courtesy of Dr. R. Ross.)

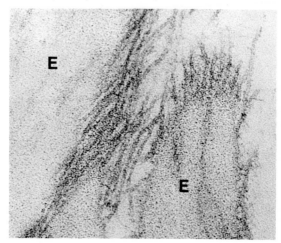

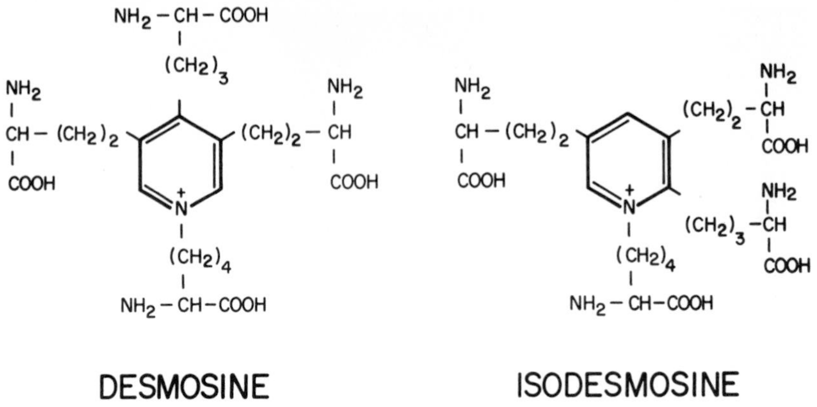

FIGURE 4-24 The structure of desmosine and isodesmosine. These isomers function as cross-links in elastin.

DESMOSINE   ISODESMOSINE

example of collagen, we suspect that elastin is synthesized and secreted as a precursor molecule (proelastin), which remains soluble by virtue of having additional hydrophilic amino acids on its polypeptide chains. Insoluble elastic fibers would be formed in the extracellular space by the assembly of modified proelastin molecules. It is possible that the microfibrillar protein of the elastic fiber might originate from the extra hydrophilic sequences of proelastin.

The desmosine and isodesmosine cross-links of elastin are initiated by an enzymatic reaction equiva-lent to that described for the cross-linking of collagen. A copper-dependent lysyl oxidase catalyzes the oxidative deamination of the ε-amino groups of specific lysyl residues in the polypeptide chains of elastin. Three aldelydic residues ("allysyl" residues) formed by this reaction condense with a fourth intact lysyl residue to give the carbon and nitrogen ring structure of the desmosines (Fig. 4-25). Thus, the desmosines have the potential of cross-linking four separate elastin chains. The formation of the cross-links could be the nucleation step for the aggregation of elastic fibers,

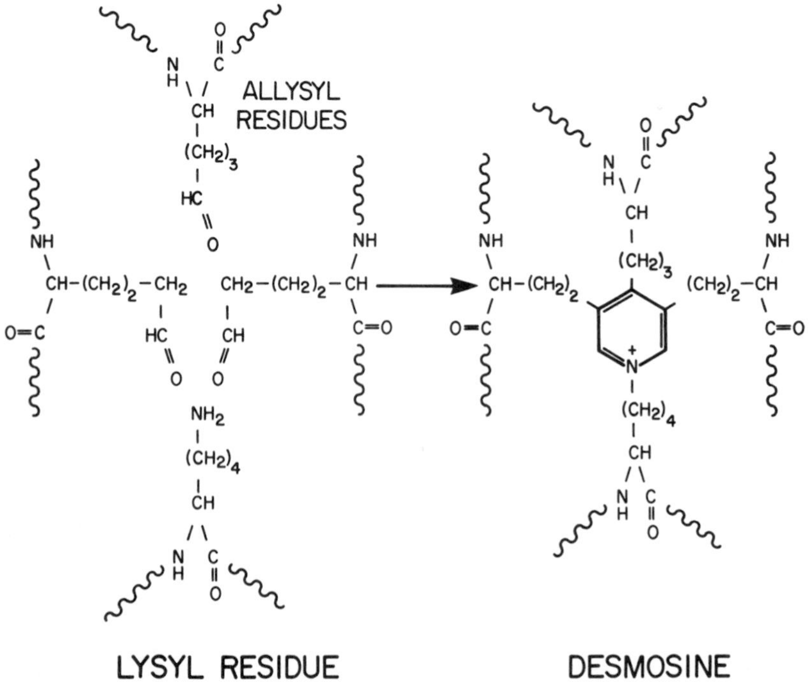

FIGURE 4-25 Schematic showing how four lysine residues form the desmosines and how the latter may potentially link four elastin chains.

LYSYL RESIDUE   DESMOSINE

could be utilized to add soluble proelastin chains to an insoluble fiber matrix, or could occur with time in a completely formed fiber.

The available data have suggested various structural models for elastin. One model, derived from the known structure of rubber, consists of a three-dimensional network of randomly coiled chains joined by covalent cross-links. The noncovalent interchain forces are considered to be weak and the covalent cross-links to be widely spaced. Thus, minimal unidirectional forces would produce extensive slippage of

the chains (stretching) before the cross-links restricted their movement. Because the thermodynamics of stretching of elastin do not fit those of rubber, other models have been proposed which depict elastin as a syncytium of easily deformable globular or fibrillar corpuscles which behave as an array of interconnected springs.

THE GROUND SUBSTANCE

The cellular and fibrous (collagen and elastin) components of connective tissue are surrounded by ground substance. Proteoglycans of various types are the major components of ground substance. The proteoglycans are polyanions (see below) and hence, when present in sufficient concentrations (for example, in cartilage), they stain with conventional basophilic dyes such as hematoxylin. When present in lower concentrations, they may be detected with special cationic dyes (for example, colloidal iron, alcian blue) which have a high affinity for the anionic groups of these macromolecules. Toluidine blue and crystal violet are cationic dyes which undergo characteristic spectral shifts (metachromasia) when reacting with the anionic groups of the proteoglycans. Whether viewed in the fresh or stained state, the ground substance lacks a fibrous organization and so it is described as being amorphous.

THE STRUCTURE OF PROTEOGLYCANS

These molecules consist of multiple polysaccharide chains covalently linked to protein. The polysaccharide chains are polymers of repeating disaccharide units, one of which is always a hexosamine. The five major classes of proteoglycans described below are defined by the chemical structure of their polysaccharide components.

Hyaluronic Acid

The repeating disaccharide unit is N-acetylglucosamine and D-glucuronic acid, and it is estimated that about 2500 such units form the chains (molecular weight about 10^6 daltons). Hyaluronic acid has been found in cartilage, blood vessels, skin, and the umbilical cord, and it is a major component of synovial fluid and vitreous humor.

Chondroitin Sulfate

The repeating unit is N-acetylgalactosamine and D-glucuronic acid, and the hexosamine is variously sulfated at carbons 4 or 6. About 60 repeating units contribute to an estimated molecular weight of about 30,000. This molecule predominates in cartilage, bone, and blood vessels, but it has also been identified in skin, cornea, and other connective tissues.

Dermatan Sulfate

The repeating unit is N-acetylgalactosamine-4-sulfate and L-iduronic acid. This is a stereoisomer of chondroitin 4-sulfate in which L-iduronic acid has generally replaced D-glucuronic acid, although a few of the latter groups may still occur in each polysaccharide chain. Its molecular weight is comparable to that of chondroitin sulfate. Dermatan sulfate is found mostly in the skin, but it has also been demonstrated in blood vessels, heart valves, tendons, and the connective tissues of the lung.

Keratan Sulfate

The repeating unit is N-acetylglucosamine-6-sulfate and galactose. The structure is unusual inasmuch as galactose replaces the uronic acid moiety in the repeating unit. Considerable variation exists in the structure with respect to the degree of sulfation of the hexosamine group. Moreover, the galactose groups may be sulfated in position 6 and galactosamine may also be present. Keratan sulfate probably has the lowest average molecular weight of the tissue polysaccharides. It has been extracted from the cornea, cartilage, and nucleus pulposus.

Heparan Sulfate

The repeating unit is *N*-acetylglucosamine and D-glucuronic acid, but it also contains *N*-sulfate glucosamine and L-iduronic acid. Its molecular weight has been estimated to be 15,000 daltons. Heparan sulfate has been identified in aorta, liver, and lung.

Heparin, the anticoagulant and antilipemic agent, has a structure similar to that of heparan sulfate, but the disaccharide repeating unit of heparin is more heavily sulfated. Heparin is synthesized and stored in mast cells.

Relatively less is known of the chemistry of the protein moieties of the proteoglycans. It is currently believed that the polysaccharide chains extend laterally from the protein core. More than one class of polysaccharide chain may be attached to a single core protein. Compositional and structural analyses of the proteoglycans are made difficult by the heterogeneity of these molecules. For example, there may be tissue-specific variations in both the protein and polysaccharide moieties of a given proteoglycan.

The complex organization of the proteoglycans is illustrated by the model recently proposed for the proteoglycans of articular cartilage (Fig. 4-26). The fundamental structural unit is called the *proteoglycan subunit;* it appears to consist of a core protein of variable length, to which are covalently linked chondroitin sulfate and keratan sulfate chains. The length of the core protein appears to determine the number of polysaccharide chains attached. The proteoglycan subunits in turn form a *proteoglycan aggregate* by noncovalent attachments to a hyaluronic acid backbone. Subunits are associated with hyaluronic acid through an invariant region of the core protein and an additional link protein.

BIOSYNTHESIS AND TURNOVER

The proteoglycans are generally synthesized and secreted by cells derived from the primitive mesen-

PROTEOGLYCAN   SUBUNIT

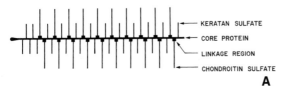

KERATAN SULFATE
CORE PROTEIN
LINKAGE REGION
CHONDROITIN SULFATE

A

FIGURE 4-26 Model for molecular organization of articular cartilage. A. Chondroitin sulfate and keratan sulfate are covalently attached to a core protein to form the proteoglycan subunit. B. The subunits are noncovalently associated with hyaluronic acid to form the macro-molecular proteoglycan aggregate. (From L. Rosenberg, in M. Burleigh and R. Poole (eds.), "Dynamics of Connective Tissue Macro-Molecules," p. 105, North-Holland Publishing Company, Amsterdam, 1975.)

PROTEOGLYCAN   AGGREGATE

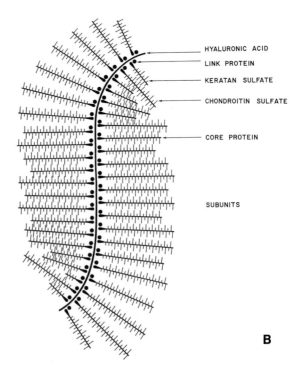

HYALURONIC ACID
LINK PROTEIN
KERATAN SULFATE
CHONDROITIN SULFATE
CORE PROTEIN
SUBUNITS

B

chyme, for example, fibroblasts, chondroblasts, osteoblasts, synovial cells, smooth muscle cells, mast cells, etc. Relatively little detailed information is available about the precise intracellular sites where polysaccharide synthesis is initiated and about where and how the covalent attachment to the protein moiety is effected. However, much is known about the biochemical mechanisms whereby polysaccharides are assembled by stepwise transfers from sugar nucleotides and about how individual sugar groups are sulfated, epimerized, oxidized, and reduced. By analogy with other secretory proteins, the translation of the protein moiety of these molecules is probably restricted to the rough-surfaced endoplasmic reticulum, and the sugar components are most likely synthesized in greatest part in the Golgi complex or other smooth-surfaced membrane compartments. Secretion of the molecules occurs by transport to the plasma membrane via smooth-surfaced vesicles. Perhaps, like collagen, proteoglycans may undergo additional biochemical modifications after secretion into the extracellular space.

The proteoglycans turn over more rapidly than collagen, both in growing and in adult individuals. The catabolic turnover of these molecules requires several enzymes which cleave specific linkages in the polysaccharide chains; these enzymes are generally contained within lysosomes of the cellular elements of the connective tissues. Much of our knowledge of the degradative pathways has come from studying patients with hereditary deficiencies in these enzymes. In these diseases (the mucopolysaccharidoses) partially digested proteoglycans accumulate in the tissues, thereby causing characteristic clinical and biochemical disturbances.

STRUCTURE AND FUNCTION

The polysaccharide chains of these molecules are thought to be generally unbranched. The sulfate and carboxyl groups in the repeating disaccharide units of

the chains provide a high density of anionic charges which promote an elongated chain configuration. The protein moieties of the molecules may also impose configurational restraints. The proteoglycans thus extend through a larger volume of solution ("domain") than do uncharged, highly folded molecules with similar molecular weights. The elongated proteoglycans tend to become entangled and form three-dimensional nets with themselves and other polymeric molecules in the connective tissue spaces.

Most of the functions of the proteoglycans can be related to the chemical and physical properties mentioned above. We have noted the affinity of cationic dyes for the anionic groups of the polysaccharide chains. In vivo, the proteoglycans presumably interact electrostatically with a variety of cationic molecules, and through such binding play a significant role in the transport of electrolytes and water. We have already mentioned that proteoglycans may interact with positively charged tropocollagen molecules to affect the kinetics of collagen fiber formation. The permeability, transport, and osmotic functions of interstitial fluid can also be modified by the entangled proteoglycans acting as molecular sieves to exclude or entrap molecules of different sizes. Such networks increase the viscosity of interstitial fluids and can thus contribute to their lubricative and mechanical functions. Because of its high molecular weight, hyaluronic acid makes an important contribution to the viscosity of interstitial fluids. The viscous or gel-like nature of tissue fluids may also play a role in limiting the spread of bacteria. Additionally, special antilipemic and anticoagulant functions are recognized for heparin and dermatan sulfate.

In summary, the proteoglycans help to maintain the proper homeostatic environment for cells and fibrous elements. Their diversity and heterogeneity no doubt reflect their adaptation for different functions in different types of tissue.

CONNECTIVE TISSUES AND DISEASE

Injury or destruction of tissues by chemical, physical, or infectious agents induces a local protective response called inflammation. The inflammatory reaction is initiated, in part, by the release of substances from mast cells which alter the tone and permeability of capillaries and venules. The vascular response is accompanied by the migration of leukocytes from the blood vessels, and these cells and macrophages serve

174

to neutralize infectious agents and to phagocytose and digest tissue debris. Fibroblasts proliferate at the site of injury, collagen and proteoglycans are secreted, and any tissue defects are eventually bridged by collagen fibers. Thus, the cellular and extracellular components of connective tissue play a critical role in the general response to tissue injury.

Certain diseases are caused by primary disturbances in the synthesis or catabolism of collagen. For example, scurvy, a disease due to a lack of vitamin C (ascorbic acid), is characterized by an inability to form collagen fibers. Consequently, bone growth and dentition are abnormal, wounds and fractures do not heal, and small blood vessels are prone to rupture. The disease complex can be related to the role of vitamin C as a cofactor in the enzymatic hydroxylation of the prolyl and lysyl residues of collagen. A procollagen molecule lacking hydroxyproline has an unstable triple helix and is prone to denaturation and proteolytic turnover. Moreover, such molecules are secreted at a very slow rate from the fibroblast; and if a few fibers do form extracellularly, they may not be adequately cross-linked because of their lack of hydroxylsine residues.

Inherited disorders of collagen, elastin, and proteoglycan metabolism are well documented. For example, patients with a genetic deficiency in the enzyme lysyl hydroxylase have poorly cross-linked collagen as manifested by deformities of bone, dislocation of joints, hyperextensibility of skin, and fragility of the globe of the eye. We have already mentioned that patients having inherited defects in enzymes required for the catabolic cleavage of the proteoglycans suffer from excessive storage of these molecules in their tissues.

The morbidity of many diseases of unknown etiology can be related to disturbances in the normal structure of connective tissue elements. Among these diseases we may list arthritis, degenerative vascular disease as it occurs in diabetes mellitus and in the course of aging, and several autoimmune disorders. Future studies of the normal and abnormal structure and function of connective tissues will no doubt provide the bases for prevention and rational treatment of these diseases.

REFERENCES

MACROPHAGES

Books

BELANTI, J. A., and D. H. DAYTON (eds.): "The Phagocytic Cell and Host Resistance," Raven Books, Abeland-Schuman, New York, 1975.

CARR, I: "The Macrophage: A Review of Ultrastructure and Function," Academic Press, Inc., New York, 1973.

METCHNIKOFF, E: "Immunity in Infective Diseases," Trans. F. G. Binnie, Johnson Reprint Corporation, New York, 1968.

NELSON, D. S.: "Macrophages and Immunity," North-Holland Publishing Company, Amsterdam, 1969.

NELSON, D. S. (ed.): "Immunobiology of the Macrophage," Academic Press, New York, 1976.

PEARSALL, N. N., and R. S. WEISER: "The Macrophage," Lea & Febiger, Philadelphia, 1970.

STUART, A. E.: "The Reticulo-endothelial System," E. & S. Livingstone, Edinburgh, 1970.

VAN FURTH, R. (ed.): "Mononuclear Phagocytes," Blackwell Scientific Publications, Ltd., Oxford, 1970.

VAN FURTH, R. (ed.): "Mononuclear Phagocytes in Immunity, Infection and Pathology," Blackwell Scientific Publications, Ltd., Oxford, 1975.

VERNON-ROBERTS, B.: "The Macrophage," Cambridge University Press, New York, 1972.

Articles and Reviews

BIANCO, C., F. M. GRIFFIN, JR., and S. C. SILVERSTEIN: Studies of the Macrophage Complement Receptor. Alteration of Receptor Function upon Macrophage Activation, *J. Exp. Med.,* **141:**1278–1290 (1975).

COHN, Z. A.: The Structure and Function of Monocytes and Macrophages, *Adv. Immunol.,* **9:**163–214 (1968).

GORDON, S., and Z. A. COHN: The Macrophage, *Int. Rev. Cytol.,* **36:**171–214 (1973).

GORDON, S., J. C. UNKELESS, and Z. A. COHN: Induction of Macrophage Plasminogen Activator by Endotoxin Stimulation and Phagocytosis, *J. Exp. Med.,* **140:**995–1010 (1974).

GOUD, T. J., C. SCHOTTE and R. VAN FURTH: Identification and Characterization of the Monoblast in Mononuclear Phagocyte Colonies Grown in Vitro, *J. Exp. Med.,* **142:**1180–1199 (1975).

JAFFE, R. H.: The Reticuloendothelial System, in H. Downey (ed.), "Handbook of Hematology," vol. 2, pp. 973–1271, Paul B. Hoeber, Inc., New York, 1938.

LEVY, M. H., and E. F. WHEELOCK: The Role of Macrophages in Defense against Neoplastic Disease, *Adv. Cancer Res.,* **20:**131–163 (1974).

NELSON, D. S.: Macrophages as Effectors in Cell-mediated Immunity, *CRC Crit. Rev. Microbiol.,* **1:**353–384 (1972).

NORTH, R. J.: T-Cell Dependent Macrophage Activation in Cell-mediated Anti-Listeria Immunity, in W. H. Wagner and H. Hahn (eds.), "Activation of Macrophages," pp. 210–220, Excerpta Medica, Amsterdam, 1974.

RABINOVITCH, M. Phagocytic Recognition, in R. van Furth (ed.), "Mononuclear Phagocytes," pp. 299–313, Blackwell Scientific Publications, Ltd., Oxford, 1970.

RABINOVITCH, M.: Macrophage Spreading In Vitro, in R. van Furth (ed.), "Mononuclear Phagocytes in Immunity, Infection and Pathology, pp. 369–383, Blackwell Scientific Publications, Oxford, 1975.

RABINOVITCH, M., and M. J. DESTEFANO: Macrophage Spreading In Vitro. III. The Effect of Metabolic Inhibitors, Anesthetics and Other Drugs on Spreading Induced by Subtilisin, *Exp. Cell Res.,* **88:**153 (1974).

RABINOVITCH, M., R. E. MANEJIAS, and V. NUSSENZWEIG: Selective Phagocytic Paralysis Induced by Immobilized Immune Complexes, *J. Exp. Med.,* **142:**827–838 (1975).

REAVEN, E. P., and S. G. AXLINE: Subplasmalemmal Microfilaments and Microtubules in Resting and Phagocytizing Cultivated Macrophages, *J. Cell Biol.,* **59:**12–27 (1973).

STOSSEL, T. P. Phagocytosis: Recognition and Ingestion, *Semin. Hematol.,* **12:**83–116 (1975).

VAN FURTH, R., Z. A. COHN, J. G. HIRSCH, J. H. HUMPHREY, W. G. SPECTOR, and H. L. LANGEVOORT: The Mononuclear Phagocyte System: A New Classification of Macrophages, Monocytes, and Their Precursor Cells, *Bull. WHO,* **46:**845–852 (1972).

MAST CELLS

AUSTEN, K. F.: Reaction Mechanisms in the Release of Mediators of Immediate Hypersensitivity from Human Lung Tissue, *Fed. Proc.,* **33:**2256–2262 (1974).

BECKER, E. L., and P. M. HENSON: In Vitro Studies of Immunologically Induced Secretion of Mediators from Cells and Related Phenomena, *Adv. Immunol.,* **17:**93–193 (1973).

CHI, E. Y., D. LAGUNOFF, and J. K. KOEHLER: Electron Microscopy of Freeze-fractured Rat Peritoneal Mast Cells, *J. Ultrastruc. Res.,* **51:**46–54 (1975).

ISHIZAKA, T., H. OKUDAIRA, L. E. MAUSER, and K. ISHIZAKA: Development of Rat Mast Cells *in vitro.* I. Differentiation of Mast Cells from Thymus Cells. *J. Immunol.,* **116:**747 (1976).

LAGUNOFF, D.: Contributions of Electron Microscopy to the Study of Mast Cells, *J. Invest. Dermatol.,* **58:**296–311 (1972).

MICHELS, N. A.: The Mast Cells, in H. Downey (ed.), "Handbook of Hematology," vol. 1 pp. 231–372, Paul B. Hoeber, Inc., New York, 1938.

ORR, T. S. C.: Mast Cells and Allergic Asthma, *Br. J. Dis. Chest,* **67:**87–106 (1973).

SELYE, H.: "The Mast Cells," Butterworths, Washington, 1965.

WHIPPLE, H. E. (ed.): Mast Cells and Basophils, *Ann. N.Y. Acad. Sci.,* **103:**1–492 (1963).

THE FIBROBLAST

GABBIANI, G., G. MAJNO, and G. B. RYAN: The Fibroblast as a Contractile Cell: The Myofibroblast, in E. Kulonen and J. Pikkarainen (eds.), "Biology of the Fibroblast," p. 139, Academic Press, Inc., New York, 1973.

GOLDBERG, B., and H. GREEN: An Analysis of Collagen Secretion by Established Mouse Fibroblast Lines, *J. Cell Biol.,* **22:**227 (1964).

MOVAT, H. Z., and N. V. P. FERNANDO: The Fine Structure of Connective Tissue. I. The Fibroblast, *Exp. Mol. Path.,* **1:**509 (1962).

REVEL, J. P., and E. D. HAY: An Autoradiographic and Electron Microscopic Study of Collagen Synthesis in Differentiating Cartilage, *Z. Zellforsch. Mikrosk. Anat.,* **61:**110 (1963).

WEINSTOCK, M., and C. P. LEBLOND: Formation of Collagen, *Fed. Proc.,* **33:**1205 (1974).

COLLAGEN

General References

BAILEY, A. J.: The Nature of Collagen, in M. Florkin and E. H. Stotz (eds.), "Comprehensive Biochemistry," vol. 26B, p. 297, Elsevier Publishing Company, Amsterdam, 1968.

GALLOP, P. M., and M. A. PAZ: Posttranslational Protein Modifications, with Special Attention to Collagen and Elastin, *Physiol. Rev.,* **55:**418 (1975).

GROSS, J.: Collagen Biology: Structure, Degradation, and Disease, *Harvey Lect.,* **68:**351 (1974).

KUHN, K.: The Structure of Collagen, in P. N. Campbell and G. D. Greville (eds.), "Essays in Biochemistry," vol. 5, p. 59, Academic Press, Inc., New York, 1969.

PÉREZ-TAMAYO, R., and M. ROJKIND (eds.): "Molecular Pathology of Connective Tissues," Marcel Dekker, Inc., New York, 1973.

RAMACHANDRAN, G. N. (ed.): "Treatise on Collagen," vol. 1, "Chemistry of Collagen," Academic Press, Inc., New York 1967.

Structure, Biosynthesis, Fibrillogenesis, Cross-Linking, Degradation

BAILEY, A. J., and S. P. ROBINS: Development and Maturation of the Crosslinks in the Collagen Fibres of Skin, in L. Robert and B. Robert (eds.), "Frontiers Matrix Biology," vol. 1, p. 130, Karger, Basel, 1973.

BORNSTEIN, P.: The Biosynthesis of Collagen, *Ann. Rev. Biochem.,* **143:**567 (1974).

BORNSTEIN, P., H. P. EHRLICH, and A. W. WYKE: Procollagen: Conversion of Precursor to Collagen by a Neutral Protease, *Science,* **175:**544 (1972).

BRUNO, R. R., and J. GROSS: High Resolution Analysis of the Modified Quarter-Stagger Model of the Collagen Fibril, *Biopolymers,* **13:**931 (1974).

DOYLE, B. B., D. W. L. HUKINS, D. J. S. HULMES, A. MILLER, and J. WOODHEAD-GALLOWAY: Collagen Polymorphism: Its Origins in the Amino Acid Sequence, *J. Mol. Biol.,* **91:**79 (1975).

GOLDBERG, B., and C. J. SHERR: Secretion and Extracellular Processing of Procollagen by Cultured Human Fibroblasts, *Proc. Natl. Acad. Sci. USA,* **70:**361 (1973).

GOLDBERG, B., M. B. TAUBMAN, and A. RADIN: Procollagen Peptidase: Its Mode of Action on the Native Substrate, *Cell,* **4:**45 (1975).

GREEN, H., B. GOLDBERG, and G. J. TODARO: Differentiated Cell Types and the Regulation of Collagen Synthesis. *Nature,* **212:**631 (1966).

GROSS, J.; The Behavior of Collagen Units as a Model in Morphogenesis. *J. Biophys. Biochem. Cytol.* **2** (suppl.): 261 (1956).

GROSS, J., J. H. HIGHBERGER, and F. O. SCHMITT: Collagen Structures Considered as States of Aggregation of a Kinetic Unit: The Tropocollagen Particle, *Proc. Natl. Acad. Sci. USA,* **40:**679 (1954).

HARRIS, E. D., JR., and S. M. KRANE: Collagenases, *N. Engl. J. Med.,* **291:**557, 605, 652 (1974).

HARWOOD, R., A. K. BHALLA, M. E. GRANT, and D. S. JACKSON: The Synthesis and Secretion of Cartilage Procollagen, *Biochem. J.,* **148:**129 (1975).

HENNING, B-H., C. M. COBB, R. E. TAYLOR, and H. M. FULLMER: Synthesis and Release of Procollagenase by Cultured Fibroblasts, *J. Biol. Chem.,* **251:**3162 (1976).

HODGE, A. J., J. A. PETRUSKA, and A. J. BAILEY: The Subunit Structure of the Tropocollagen Macromolecule and its Relation to Various Ordered Aggregation States, in "Structure and Function of Connective and Skeletal Tissue," p. 31, London Butterworths Ltd. 1965.

KEFALIDES, N. A.: Comparative Biochemistry of Mammalian Basement Membranes, in E. A. Balazs (ed.), "Chemistry and Molecular Biology of the Intercellular Matrix," p. 535. Academic Press, Inc., New York, 1970.

LAPIÈRE, C. M., A. LENAERS, and L. D. KOHN: Procollagen Peptidase: An Enzyme Excising the Coordination Peptides of Procollagen, *Proc. Natl. Acad. Sci. USA* **68:**3054 (1971).

MARTIN, G. R., P. H. BYERS, and K. A. PIEZ: Procollagen, *Adv. Enzymol.,* **42:**167 (1975).

MILLER, E. J., and V. J. MATUKAS: Biosynthesis of Collagen: The Biochemist's View, *Fed. Proc.,* **33:**1197 (1974).

MINOR, R. R., C. C. CLARK, E. L. STRAUSE, T. R. KOSZALKA, R. L. BRENT, and N. A. KEFALIDES: Basement Membrane Procollagen is Not Converted to Collagen in Organ Cultures of Parietal Yolk Sac Endoderm, *J. Biol. Chem.,* **251:**1789 (1976).

ROSS, R.: Connective Tissue Cells, Cell Proliferation and Synthesis of Extracellular Matrix—A Review, *Philos. Trans. R. Soc. Lond. [Biol. Sci.],* **271:**247 (1975).

TANZER, M.: Cross-Linking of Collagen, *Science,* **180:**561 (1973).

VEIS, A., and A. G. BROWNELL: Collagen Biosynthesis, *Crit. Rev. Biochem.,* **2:**417 (1975).

ELASTIC FIBERS

FRANZBLAU, C.: Elastin, in M. Florkin and E. H. Stotz (eds.), "Comprehensive Biochemistry," vol. 26C, p. 659, Elsevier Publishing Company, Amsterdam, 1971.

ROSS, R., and P. BORNSTEIN: The Elastic Fiber, *J. Cell Biol.,* **40:**366 (1969).

ROSS, R., and P. BORNSTEIN: Studies of the Components of the Elastic Fiber, in E. A. Balazs (ed.), "Chemistry and Molecular Biology of the Intercellular Matrix," vol. 1, p. 641, Academic Press, Inc., New York, 1970.

ROSS, R., and P. BORNSTEIN: Elastic Fibers in the Body, *Sci. Am.,* **224:**44 (1971).

GROUND SUBSTANCE

General References

BALAZS, E. A. (ed.): "Chemistry and Molecular Biology of the Intercellular Matrix," vol. 2, "Glycosaminoglycans and Proteoglycans," vol. 3, "Structural Organization and Function of the Matrix," Academic Press, Inc., New York, 1970.

SCHUBERT, M., and D. HAMERMAN: "A Primer on Connective Tissue Biochemistry," Lea & Febiger, Philadelphia, 1968.

Macromolecular Structure

HARDINGHAM, T. E., and H. MUIR: The Specific Interaction of Hyaluronic Acid with Cartilage Proteoglycans, *Biochim. Biophys. Acta,* **279:**401 (1972).

HASCALL, V. C., and D. HEINEGÅRD: Aggregation of Cartilage Proteoglycans. I. The Role of Hyaluronic Acid, *J. Biol. Chem.,* **249:**4232 (1974).

HEINEGÅRD, D., and V. C. HASCALL: Aggregation of Cartilage Proteoglycans. III. Characteristics of the Proteins Isolated from Trypsin Digests of Aggregates, *J. Biol. Chem.,* **249:**4250 (1974).

ROSENBERG, L.: Structure of Cartilage Proteoglycans, in M. Burleigh and R. Poole (eds.), "Dynamics of Connective Tissue Macromolecules," p. 105, North-Holland Publishing Company, Amsterdam, 1975.

ROSENBERG, L., W. HELLMANN, and A. K. KLEINSCHMIDT: Electron Microscopic Studies of Proteoglycan Aggregates from Bovine Articular Cartilage, *J. Biol. Chem.,* **250:**1877 (1975).

DISEASES OF CONNECTIVE TISSUES

BORNSTEIN, P.: Disorders of Connective Tissues, in P. K. Bondy and L. E. Rosenberg (eds.), "Duncan's Diseases of Metabolism: Genetics and Metabolism," p. 881, W. B. Saunders Company, Philadelphia, 1974.

MCKUSICK, V. A.: "Heritable Disorders of Connective Tissue," C. V. Mosby Company, St. Louis, 1972.

ADDITIONAL REFERENCES

GRIFFIN, F. M., J. A. GRIFFIN, and S. C. SILVERSTEIN: Studies on the Mechanism of Phagocytosis. II. The Interaction of Macrophages with Anti-Immunoglobulin IgG-coated Bone Marrow derived Lymphocytes. *J. Exp. Med.,* **144:**788–809 (1976).

STEINMAN, R. M., and Z. A. COHN: The Metabolism and Physiology of the Mononuclear Phagocytes, in B. W. Zweifach, L. Grant, and R. T. McCluskey (eds.), "The Immunoflammagory Process, Vol. I", pp. 449–510, Academic Press, New York, 1974.

UNANUE, E. R.: Secretory Function of Mononuclear Phagocytes. A Review. *Am. J. Pathol.,* **83:**396–417 (1976).

The Adipose Tissue

M. R. C. GREENWOOD AND PATRICIA R. JOHNSON

ADIPOSE TISSUE MORPHOLOGY

INTRODUCTION

Adipose tissue occurs in virtually every mammalian organism; it is commonly referred to as fat. It has long been considered a type of connective tissue and can be described as a loose association of lipid filled cells known as adipocytes, with associated stromal-vascular cells, held in a matrix of collagen fibers. Adipocytes occur in two major forms: *unilocular,* with a single large inclusion of lipid, and *multilocular* with many smaller lipid inclusions. The unilocular adipocyte is the characteristic cell type of white adipose tissue, which constitutes the primary energy-storage compartment of the mammal. The multilocular adipocyte is characteristic of brown adipose tissue which functions as a heat-production organ in the mammal.

In humans, roughly 15 percent of the body weight in a normal adult male is white adipose tissue and approximately 22 percent of body weight is found as fat in females. The capacity of adipose tissue to change its size is remarkable and distinctly different from any other mammalian tissue. Although in the normal organism it would appear that the percent of body weight which remains as fat is fairly constant throughout the adult life-span, in pathological conditions such as obesity or anorexia nervosa, this tissue displays the amazing property of being able to increase its total weight upwards of 100 percent or to decrease its weight to 3 percent of normal.

This unique property of the tissue reflects the function of the unilocular white adipocyte itself. Although adipose tissue of the adult mammal contains many cell types in addition to the adipocyte, most of the physiological functions of the tissue are thought to result from changes in lipid storage and mobilization by the adipocyte. The other cell types that exist in the tissue and may account for as much as 80 percent of tissue DNA consist of cells in the vascular bed, fibroblastic connective tissue cells, leukocytes, and macrophages. Although these cells are obviously necessary for tissue integrity, support, and nutrition, they have no known specialized role in adipose tissue function per se.

DISTRIBUTION OF ADIPOSE TISSUE

In mammals the two types of adipose tissue—white adipose tissue and brown adipose tissue—serve different functions, occur in different amounts, and are distributed differently in the body.

179

White adipose tissue is characterized by a white or yellow color and is less well vascularized and innervated than brown adipose tissue, and the fat cells are unilocular. In the rat, major deposits of white adipose tissue occur (1) subcutaneously, as a sheath around the scapular, axillary, and cervical regions and in the inguinal area with minor amounts around the buttocks; (2) intraabdominally in retroperitoneal, mesenteric, and omental regions; and (3) in association with the gonads—the intraabdominal parametrial pad in the female and the well-known epididymal pad which lines the epididymis and testis of the male and normally lies at least partially in the scrotal sac. In the human, there is a more or less continuous subcutaneous layer that shows sexual dimorphism, being more well developed, particularly in abdominal and buttocks regions, in the female than in the male. This difference in the subcutaneous adipose depot between male and female accounts, in large measure, for the difference in total body fat seen in the two sexes. Unlike the rat, the human male has no epididymal fat pad. The retroperitoneal, mesenteric, and omental depots are well developed in both sexes.

Brown adipose tissue, the only known function of which is heat production, has been found in newborn mammals of nearly all species that have been examined (Fig. 5-1). In nonhibernators, the relative weight of the tissue declines during the course of maturation. However, in rats it may increase again during prolonged exposure to cold.

In the adult rat, brown adipose tissue occurs mainly in the interscapular region and the axillae. Some minor deposits exist adjacent to the thymus and in the dorsal midline region of the thorax and abdomen. In the adult human, brown adipose tissue deposits are essentially absent, but tissue closely resembling the brown adipose tissue of rodents does occur

in human fetuses and newborns. According to Merklin, the major brown fat deposits in the human fetus are located in the posterior cervical, axillary, suprailiac, and perirenal regions (Fig. 5-1). Lesser deposits exist in the interscapular, anterior mediastinal, intercostal, anterior abdominal, and retropubic areas. As the individual ages, a gradual and selective replacement of these brown fat deposits by white adipose tissue takes place.

MORPHOLOGY

White Adipose Tissue

LIGHT MICROSCOPY The cells of white adipose tissue are characterized by one large lipid inclusion giving the cell a signet-ring shape that results from distension of the cytoplasm and apposition of the nucleus to the plasmalemma. In tissue sections these cells are typically polygonal and range in size from 25 to 200 μm. At the light microscopic level, the cytoplasm is a thin rim surrounding the bulk lipid droplet. Cytoplasmic organelles are difficult to decipher, but mitochondria may be demonstrated by the use of vital dyes such as Janus green. Mitochondria are generally noted in the thicker part of the cytoplasmic rim near the nucleus. The nucleus is flattened against the plasma membrane because of the presence of the large central lipid inclusion.

Between 60 and 85 percent of the weight of white adipose tissue is lipid, 5 to 30 percent water and 2 to 3 percent protein. The lipid is 90 to 99 percent triglyceride. Thin-layer chromatographic analysis has demonstrated that small amounts of free fatty acid, diglyceride, cholesterol, and phospholipid and trace quantities of cholesterol ester and monoglyceride are present. The fatty acid composition of the triglyceride component is a complex array which reflects the influence of dietary fat as well as patterns of synthesis from carbohydrate. Six fatty acids contribute more than 90

FIGURE 5-1 1. Anterior view of the fetus illustrating the position of brown fat bodies and fat cell composition. 2. Posterior view of the fetus illustrating the position of brown fat bodies and fat cell composition. (1) posterior cervical, (2) axillary, (3) intercostal, (4) anterior mediastinal, (5) anterior abdominal, (6) perirenal, (7) urachal, (8) inferior epigastric, (9) retropubic, (10) suprailiac, (11) interscapular, (12) deltoid, (13) lateral trapezial.

Predominantly multilocular fat cells (dense dot pattern)

Mixed multilocular and unilocular fat cells (light dot pattern)

3. Suprailiac brown fat body of a 7-month fetus. Multilocular cells predominate. H&E ×250. 4. Axillary brown fat body of a 7-month fetus. There is a mixture of unilocular and multilocular fat cells. H&E ×250. (From Robert J. Merklin, *Anat. Rec.* **178:**637, 1973.)

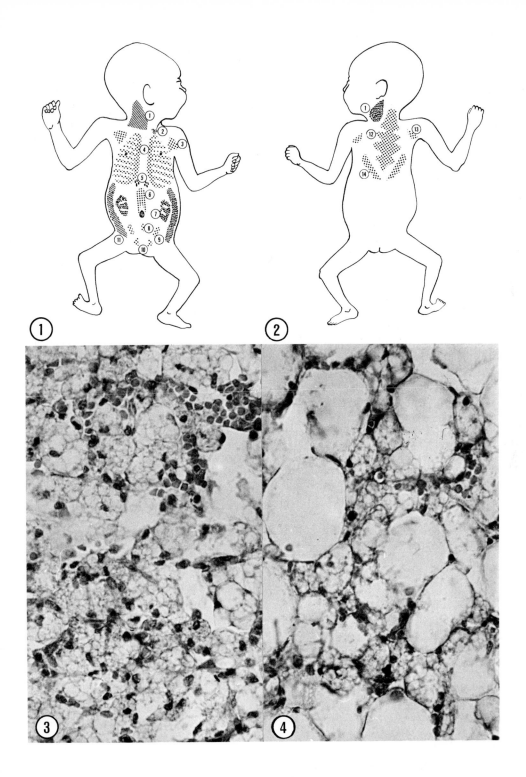

percent of the total mixture: myristic, palmitic, palmit-oleic, stearic, oleic, and linoleic.

ELECTRON MICROSCOPY The electron microscope has not been used extensively in studies of adipose tissue until recently. This is probably a result of preparation difficulties encountered when dealing with the large amounts of lipid present in adipose cells. The early investigations of Chase showed that adipose cells had a peculiarly filamentous structure, either closely applied to the plasmalemma or as an intergral part of the cell membrane. Wasserman (1960) noted that rather than having such a closely applied extracellular collagenous structure, the fat cell was enveloped by a structure similar to, and probably identical to, the basement membrane complex described by Robertson. However, Chase's suggestion that a filamentous collagenous structure is in immediate contact with the adipocyte plasmalemma has been recently confirmed by scanning electron microscopic studies of adipocytes from rat bone marrow (Fig. 5-2). More recent studies, which meet current standards for well-fixed material, have all demonstrated that properly fixed adipose cells show normal cell membranes: Golgi, endoplasmic reticulum, a basement membrane complex, and pleomorphic mitochondria (Figs. 5-3 and 5-4). These intracellular structures are present in adipocytes from chick bone marrow tissue and adipocyte cell culture and in isolated adipocyte preparations, as well as in mammalian whole-tissue preparations. All the intracellular organelles are present in the cytoplasmic rim of the adipocyte (Fig. 5-3). The predominant morphological characteristic of the adipocyte is, of course, the large lipid inclusion. The lipid inclusion itself seems devoid of any inclusions or intracellular organelles. It is not entirely clear how the lipid inclusion enlarges. However, time-lapse photography demonstrated that viable cells in culture show coalescence of lipid droplets after a few days. Pinocytotic vesicles were observed in cells from both in vivo and in vitro studies. Cushman reported that mature adipocytes would pinocytose and remove serum albumin from media. It has been suggested that the pinocytotic vesicles deliver their contents directly to the large lipid inclusion (Fig. 5-4).

Although there has been no suggestion that the multilocular droplets in fat cells are membrane-bound, a question still exists about whether or not the central lipid inclusion of the unilocular adipocyte is membrane-bound. Some investigators have reported an electron-dense region at the edge of the lipid droplet, whereas others have found fine filaments (80 to 100 Å in diameter) arranged in an orderly array and proximate to the lipid droplet. It seems reasonable to conclude that some specialized structures may be associated with the large lipid droplet but that a true membrane boundary does not exist.

INNERVATION AND VASCULARIZATION OF WHITE ADIPOSE TISSUE

According to Ballantyne and Rafferty, the sole innervation of rat epididymal adipose tissue is postganglionic sympathetic and noradrenergic and is arranged as periarteriolar plexuses. Adipocytes are not directly in contact with nerve terminals (Fig. 5-5). Innervation of white adipose tissue appears to be vasoconstrictor in nature, since neural stimulation causes reduction in the volume of the tissue. However, stimulation also causes an increase in lipolysis, the breakdown of triglyceride in the central droplet, and the release of free fatty acids and glycerol from adipose tissue. The explanation for this finding, in view of the lack of direct innervation to the adipocyte, is that adrenergic-stimulated lipolysis is the result of noradrenaline (NA) release from the perivascular plexuses and its transport through the plasma to adipocyte membrane receptors. Since the adipocyte itself is not innervated, studies of the effects of autonomic agonists or antagonists on the release of nonesterified fatty acids (NEFA) from white adipose tissue should be reexamined. Studies showing that NA increases the rate of release of NEFA and that adrenergic antagonists inhibit catecholamine-stimulated lipolysis have led to the proposition that lipolysis is, in part, under direct sympathetic regulation. The more likely interpretation based upon morphological grounds is that a direct interaction between drugs and receptors at the adipocyte plasma membrane is responsible for these effects. The fact that catecholamines act in vitro to stimulate lipolysis is in accord with this interpretation.

Although white adipose tissue has been considered to be a poorly vascularized tissue, each adipocyte is actually in contact with at least a single capillary. The blood supply is adequate to support the very active metabolism of the thin rim of cytoplasm which surrounds the large lipid inclusion. Moreover, adipose

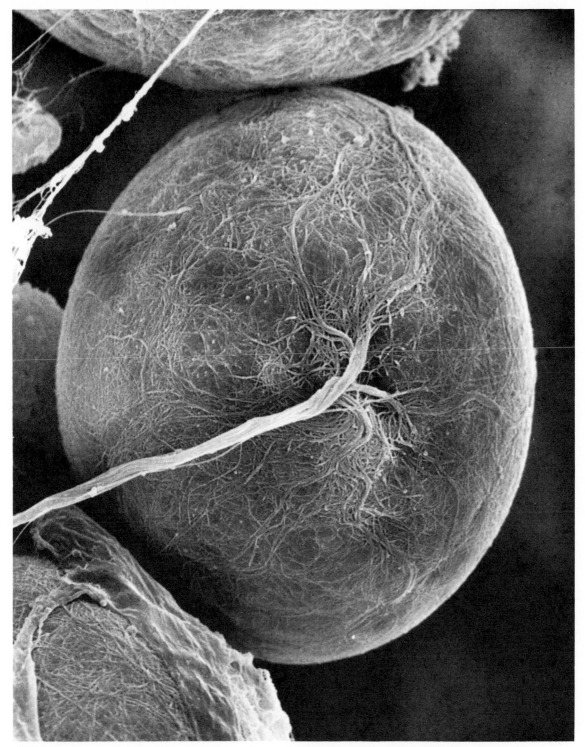

FIGURE 5-2 Scanning electron micrograph of adipocyte from rat thymus held by reticular fibers. ×5500. (Courtesy of L. Weiss)

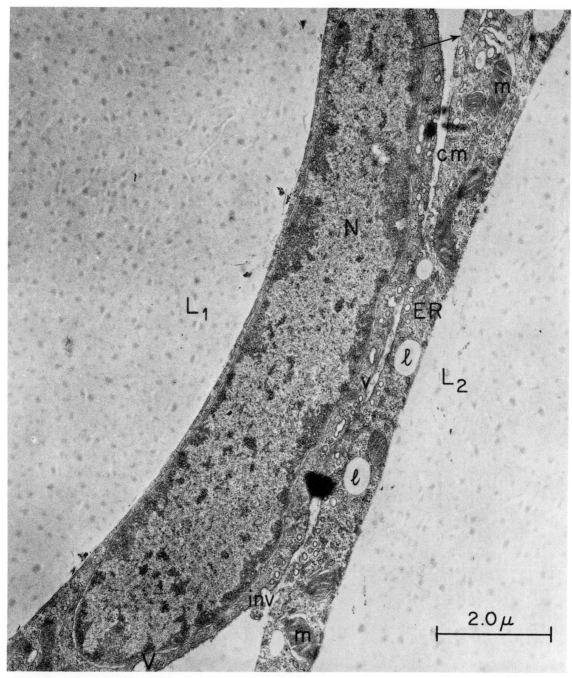

FIGURE 5-3 Isolated adipose cells incubated 60 min in KRB-albumin buffer in the presence of 1.0 μg epinephrine per ml. L, large, central lipid droplet; l, cytoplasmic lipid droplet; cm, cell membrane; m, mitochondrion; N, nucleus; V, vacuole; v, vesicle; inv, invagination; ER, endoplasmic reticulum; ↓, break in cell membrane. ×15,000. (From Cushman, Samuel W., Structure-function relationships in the adipose cell. I. Ultrastructure of the isolated adipose-cell, *J. Cell Biol.* **46:**326, 1970.)

tissue blood flow has been measured and shown to vary with the nutritional state and body weight of the animal. For example, blood flow per gram of tissue has been shown to increase during fasting in rats, dogs, and humans.

BROWN ADIPOSE TISSUE
MORPHOLOGY

The tissue is composed of loosely arranged lobules which become more compact with aging. The multi-

locular adipocytes vary in shape from round to polygonal or elongated. The most common state is polygonal, and the cells may reach 60 μm in diameter. The characteristic brown color of the tissue derives from its rich vascularization and the numerous mitochondria present in individual cells (Fig. 5-1).

When examined using the electron microscope, the plasmalemma of brown adipocytes is relatively free

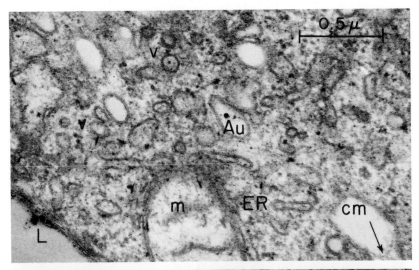

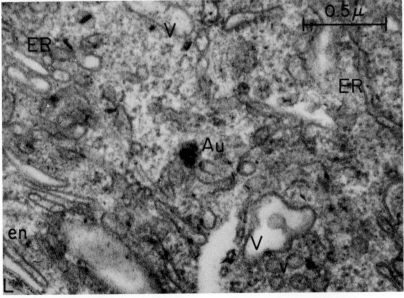

FIGURE 5-4 Isolated adipose cells incubated 240 min. in KRB-albumin buffer in the presence of 1000 μg colloidal gold per ml and in the absence of hormones. L, large, central lipid droplet; ER, endoplasmic reticulum; v, vesicle. Top: Au, single gold particle in small vacuole; cm, cell membrane; m, mitochondrion; ↓, electron dense debris. ×51,000. Bottom: Au, four gold particles in vesicle; V, vacuole; en, fenestrated envelope. ×51,000. (From Cushman, Samuel W., Structure-function relationships in the adipose cell. II. Pinocytosis and factors influencing its activity in the isolated adipose cell, *J. Cell Biol.*, **46**:342, 1970.)

of pinocytotic invaginations. A fine fibrillar network fills the narrow intercellular spaces. The mitochondria vary greatly in size and in shape, being round, oval, or filamentous. Lipid droplets within each cell may reach 25 μm in diameter, but they also show considerable size variation. Golgi structures are apparent, but rough endoplasmic reticulum and glycogen deposits are sparse (Fig. 5-6).

INNERVATION AND VASCULARIZATION OF BROWN ADIPOSE TISSUE

Brown fat differs from white fat in that the adipocytes themselves are directly innervated by sympathetic ad-

renergic neurons as are the blood vessels with which the brown fat is richly supplied. Bargmann et al. have demonstrated electron microscopically that paravascular nerves originating from the sympathetic nervous system innervate the interscapular brown fat of the rat. These neurons are nonmyelinated fibers, containing many microtubules with a central filament and some small mitochondria. In addition, their unmyelinated axons are found closely attached to adipocytes, frequently embedded in invaginations of the adipocyte plasma membrane. These terminal axons often contain synaptic vesicles, and it is proposed that these synaptic terminations on adipocyte membranes are the site of release of catecholamines. The existence of these "short adrenergic neurons" which directly innervate brown fat adipocytes has been confirmed by fluorescent histochemical studies of interscapular brown fat from immunosympathectomized rats. Derry

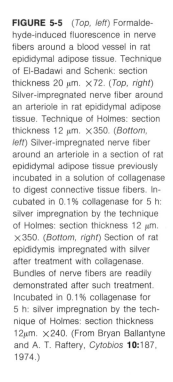

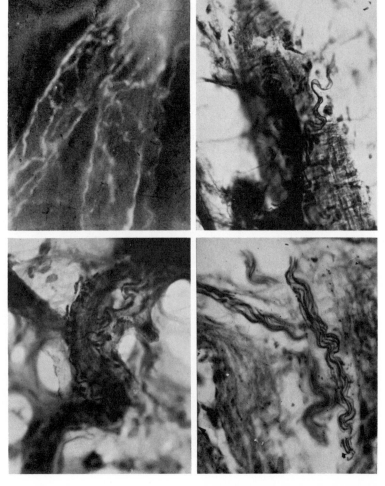

FIGURE 5-5 (*Top, left*) Formaldehyde-induced fluorescence in nerve fibers around a blood vessel in rat epididymal adipose tissue. Technique of El-Badawi and Schenk: section thickness 20 μm. ×72. (*Top, right*) Silver-impregnated nerve fiber around an arteriole in rat epididymal adipose tissue. Technique of Holmes: section thickness 12 μm. ×350. (*Bottom, left*) Silver-impregnated nerve fiber around an arteriole in a section of rat epididymal adipose tissue previously incubated in a solution of collagenase to digest connective tissue fibers. Incubated in 0.1% collagenase for 5 h: silver impregnation by the technique of Holmes: section thickness 12 μm. ×350. (*Bottom, right*) Section of rat epididymis impregnated with silver after treatment with collagenase. Bundles of nerve fibers are readily demonstrated after such treatment. Incubated in 0.1% collagenase for 5 h: silver impregnation by the technique of Holmes: section thickness 12μm. ×240. (From Bryan Ballantyne and A. T. Raftery, *Cytobios* **10:**187, 1974.)

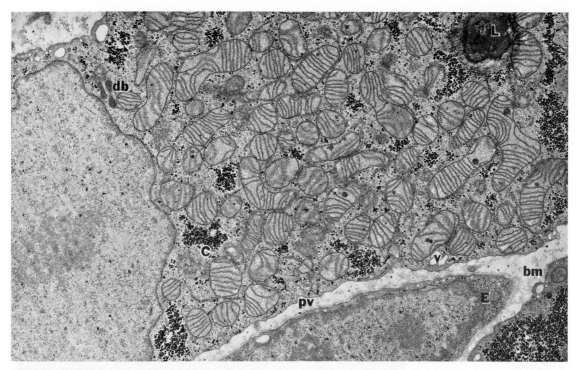

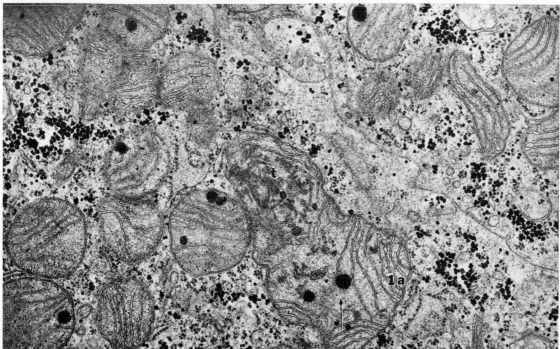

FIGURE 5-6 Top: Parts of adipocytes from a 20-day fetus. The cells have more cytoplasm and mitochondria are closer together. Their cristae are lamellar; the matrix is denser; and inclusions are more numerous and larger than in the 18-day fetus. Masses of glycogen particles (*G*) have accumulated. The cytoplasmic matrix contains fewer ribosomes. Pinocytotic vesicles (*pv*) and vacuoles (*v*) are more frequent. Lipid droplets (*L*) are larger. An endothelial cell (*E*) of a tangentially sectioned capillary is rich in ribosomes. A thin basement membrane (*bm*) envelops it. *db,* Dense bodies. ×13,000. Bottom: A large mitochondrion in an adipocyte from a 20-day fetus. Its complex inner structure comprises lamellar cristae (*la*), several material inclusions (*arrows*) of various sizes and densities, and a multitude of tubular elements (*t*). ×32,500. (From Elsi R. Suter, Fine Structure of Brown Adipose Tissue. Laboratory Investigation, *Res. Lab Plasma.* **21:**3, 1969, p. 246.)

and coworkers have shown in rabbits that these short fibers remain after the nerve supply to the blood vessels is removed either by immunosympathectomy or surgical denervation of the tissue (Fig. 5-7). Thus, these authors have proposed that the nerve fibers remaining after such treatment must be immunologically, as well as neurophysiologically, different from those which innervate blood vessels in the brown fat organ. Presumably, it is the short adrenergic neurons which provide the rapid thermogenic response of brown adipose tissue to cold stress.

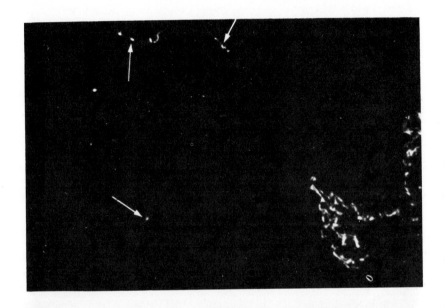

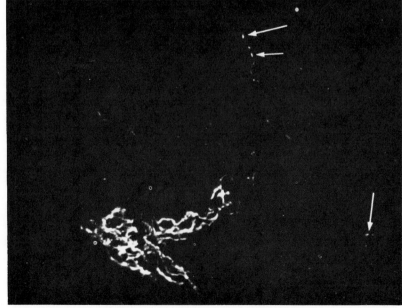

FIGURE 5-7 Top: Section of the interscapular brown fat pad of a 2000-g rabbit. Fewer nerves are seen in the parenchyma, and autofluorescence is barely visible. The nerve supply to the arteriole on the right is almost normal. Arrows show synaptic varicosities on nerve fibers. ×300. Bottom: Section of the dorsal brown fat pad of a 2000-g rabbit. There is practically no parenchymal innervation. The autofluorescence is decreased to the point of being difficult to photograph in the presence of the bright arterial nerves. The arteriole nerves look practically normal. Arrows show synaptic varicosities on nerve fibers. ×300. (From Derry et al., Brown and White Fat during the Life of the Rabbit. *Developmental Biol.* **27:**204–216, 1972.)

Unlike hematopoietic, muscle, or pancreatic beta cells for which functional correlates can be measured before the cells assume their characteristic morphology, there is no morphological or enzymatic marker for the precursor adipose cell. Most of the morphological criteria for identifying or counting adipocytes depend upon the presence of accumulated lipid within the cell after proliferation has ceased and cell DNA content is diploid. The earliest investigations into the development of adipose tissue were conducted by Fleming in 1871. He carried out extensive observations of adipose tissue and suggested that adipocytes were derived from mesenchymal cells. During the same period, Toldt (1870) hypothesized that adipocytes were specific cell types arising from nonmesenchymal origin. His hypothesis was based on the observation that developing fat globules had their own vascular system and were separate from surrounding connective tissue.

Controversy continued into the 1920s and 1930s. Evidence for the idea that adipocytes were modified fibroblasts was strengthened by the investigations of Clark and Clark utilizing rabbit-ear windows. They showed the appearance and apparent differentiation of fibroblasts into a lipid-laden signet-ring adipose cell. When the cell was depleted of lipid, it returned to fibroblast type. Such studies tended to give strong support to the theory of the adipose cell as a modified fibroblast. Evidence supporting Toldt's concept of adipose tissue as a distinct organ was presented by Wasserman and Hausberger. Wasserman (1926) demonstrated that distinct primitive organs of white adipose tissue existed in human embryos and were derived from reticuloendothelial tissue. Wasserman contended that fat tissue consisted of fat organs each of which derived from a single primordial cell. His theory was substantially strengthened by Hausberger's finding in 1938 that tissue taken from presumptive adipose tissue sites and transplanted to nonadipose tissue sites did differentiate into fat tissue and *not* into connective or other tissue types. The transplantation studies combined with the observation that adipose tissue arises in well-defined and not random areas in normal organisms still remains as some of the most convincing evidence that adipose tissue can be considered an organ.

The concept that adipocytes originate from a specific precursor cell in defined anatomical locations has found recent support in studies of cells cultured from mouse embryonic tissue and human subcutaneous adipose tissue. When adipocytes derived from human subcutaneous fat are placed in culture, they lose most of their lipid content and assume a fibroblast-like appearance. These "adipofibroblasts," however, show a pattern of enzymatic activity that differs from cultured human skin fibroblasts, although the two cell types are very similar in morphological appearance at the light-microscopic level. Furthermore, if the synthetic culture media is replaced with blood sera collected from obese humans, the adipofibroblasts reaccumulate intracellular lipid from the free fatty acid-rich serum, while skin fibroblasts do not (Fig. 5-8). Thus, although it remains to be clearly demonstrated that these cultured cells display all the enzymatic and hormonal properties one might expect to find in a preadipocyte, they are distinctly different from human skin fibroblasts.

Electron-microscope studies have now provided us with well-fixed samples of mature adipocytes, yet they have not been very enlightening in terms of elucidating a structural-functional relation that could be used to follow, or to identify unequivocally, the preadipocyte or adipogenic cells. At present, the clearest demonstrations of a functional marker for the preadipocyte have come from the work of Mohr and Beneke (1969) and Pilgrim (1971). Mohr and Beneke demonstrated the presence of an α-naphthyl acetate esterase in fibrocytic cells which did not yet have lipid accumulations. Since similar appearing cells were also glycogen-positive, they suggested that these cells were precursors to cells that later became osmophilic and still later assumed the appearance of mature adipocytes. The accumulation of glycogen has been shown to precede fat deposition in starved and refed rats and presumably occurs in the normal development and differentiation of adipose tissue. Pilgrim used these reactions to study the development of adipose tissue in pre- and early postnatal rat epididymal fat pads and found that the proliferative index measured by tritiated thymidine autoradiography was highest in esterase and glycogen-positive cells lacking lipid vacuoles. He suggested that these cells were preadipocytes. Nonetheless, there is still no clear-cut morphological or cytochemical marker that can be used to distinguish fibroblastlike cells that will become adipocytes from fibroblastlike cells that will not differentiate into adipocytes. There is disagreement among investigators about the relation of brown adipose tissue to white adipose tissue. During the course of normal adipocyte development, cells are multilocular before coalescence of the numerous small lipid inclusions into a single large droplet of triglyceride. Starvation and refeeding studies have also indicated that when white adipocytes deplete lipid, they become multilocular and look much like brown adipocytes. While it may be true that in some specific anatomical locations white adipose tissue appears where brown adipose tissue had previously existed, the reverse is not true; brown adipose tissue does not occur in all the anatomical locations that contain white adipose tissue. It seems likely, therefore, on both anatomical and functional bases that brown and white fat are fundamentally different.

POSTNATAL GROWTH OF ADIPOSE TISSUE

The postnatal growth of adipose tissue has been thoroughly studied in the rat. It has been firmly established that the size of the adipose tissue mass is a function of both the number of adipocytes and their size. During growth of the tissue mass, well-defined stages occur which are characterized by changes in the number of adipocytes brought about primarily by mitotic activity in precursor cells, that is, *hyperplastic* growth, or

change in the size of adipocytes brought about primarily by intracellular lipid accumulation, that is, *hypertrophic* growth. In the rat epididymal fat pad from birth until the fourth postnatal week, growth of adipose tissue is hyperplastic. From the fourth to the fourteenth week both hyperplasia and hypertrophy contribute to the enlargement of the adipose tissue mass, and from fourteen weeks until senescence, hypertrophic growth predominates. Therefore, influences early in postnatal life may affect both fat-cell number and size, whereas influences that occur later in life affect only fat-cell size.

The major pathological condition of adipose tissue, obesity, can also be described on the basis of cellularity changes, and the classification of obesity on these grounds has become well established. Both in humans, and in rodents, at least two forms of obesity based on adipose depot morphology have been proposed: (1) hyperplastic-hypertrophic and (2) hypertrophic. Furthermore, the hyperplastic-hypertrophic type has been suggested to occur primarily in early onset obesities (Fig. 5-9). Adult fat-cell hyperplasia

FIGURE 5-8 A. Freshly isolated adipose cells from the anterior abdominal wall of a 3-month-old child (×150). There is significant variation in the sizes of the cells from the same site. B. Adipocytes from a 2-month-old child; many of the cells have lost their intracellular lipids, others have much of the lipids still present, but all have changed to oval or fibroblast-like appearance. This culture was 17 days old (×100). C. Photomicrograph of the same cells as in B, 27 days after initial culture and 10 days after Figure B was taken. Practically all intracellular lipids have disappeared. These cells are termed adipofibroblasts in this study. (From Festus O. Adebenoio, *Pediat. Res.*, **9**:889–893, 1975.)

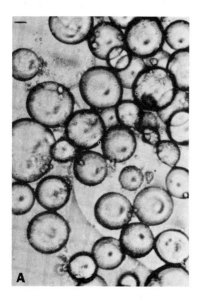
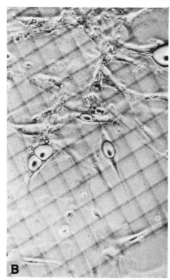
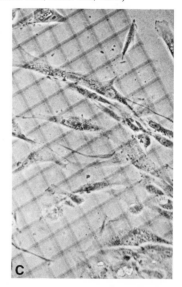

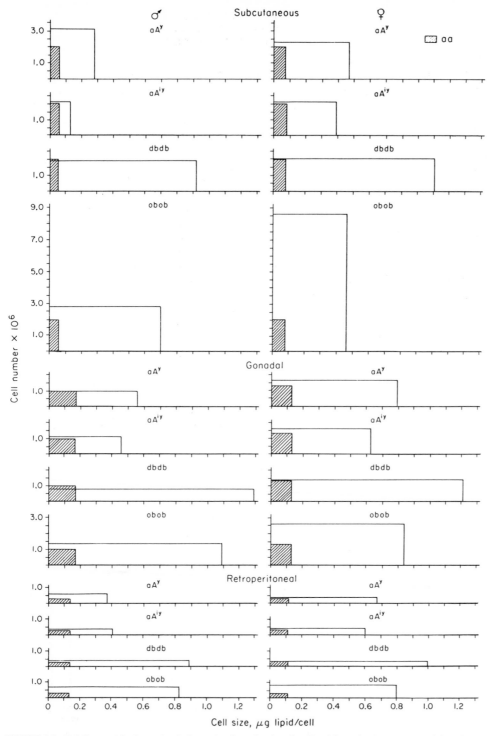

FIGURE 5-9 Relative contributions of cell size and cell number to adiposity of the subcutaneous, gonadal, and retroperitoneal depots in male and female mice of the strains *aA^y*, *aA^iy*, *dbdb,* and *obob*. (From P. R. Johnson and J. Hirsch, The Cellularity of Adipose Depots in Six Strains of Genetically Obese Mice, *J. of Lipid Research,* **13:**2, 1972.)

can be associated with early overnutrition or may, at least in genetically obese rats, be associated with an inherited and different pattern of cellular proliferation in the adipose depots. In children, the hyperplastic-hypertrophic form of obesity has been reported as early as 2 years of age. In hyperplastic obesity, the total number of fat cells may exceed by three- to fourfold the number found in the normal-weight adult. The exact developmental sequence of cellularity characteristics in the human is not yet known. However, it has been suggested that the human, unlike the rat, has both an early postnatal proliferative period and a prepubertal proliferative period. Whatever the developmental pattern, investigators agree that once formed, fat cells remain in the tissue throughout life with little or no removal or replacement. The adipocyte lipid is in a constant state of dynamic equilibrium, with lipogenesis and lipolysis being controlled by numerous stimuli, as will be discussed later. Weight reduction in humans and in the rat comes about when caloric restriction limits substrate availability to the adipocyte, inhibiting lipogenesis and enhancing lipolysis (fat mobilization). The morphological result of caloric restriction is a reduction in individual fat-cell size with no reduction in fat-cell number (Fig. 5-10).

In white adipose tissue, the major biochemical functions are associated with the deposition and mobilization of triglyceride lipid in response to caloric demands. The structural-functional correlates of lipid deposition and mobilization are not well understood, but the mechanisms for controlling the balance between the two are related to neuroendocrine secretions and to the nutritional status of the individual. In fact, the white adipocyte has become a favorite subject for study by endocrinologists who wish to unravel mechanisms of hormone action, since it is exquisitely sensitive to a number of hormones—for example, insulin, catecholamines, glucagon, ACTH, thyroxine, TSH, somatotrophin, all of which are essentially lipolytic except insulin, which inhibits lipolysis and promotes lipogenesis. The development by Rodbell (1964) of a technique for the isolation of intact white adipocytes has furthered the use of these cells for investigation of hormone binding and metabolic regulation. Most attempts to document the cytological and morphological changes in the white adipocyte that are related to biochemical function have been done in animals refed after a fast, have examined structural changes in the fasting animal, or have examined morphological change after hormone administration.

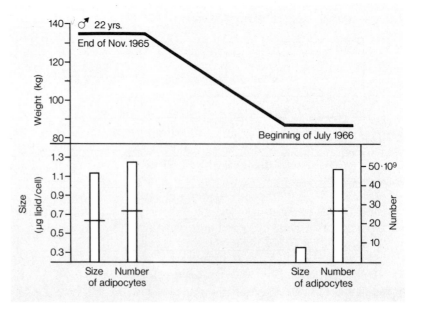

FIGURE 5-10 Adipose cell size and total adipose cell number before and after weight reduction. (From J. L. Knittle, Obesity and the Cellularity of the Adipose Depot, Triangle, *Sandoz Journal of Medical Science*, **13**:3, 57, 1974.)

The original light-microscopic observations were made by Clark and Clark in 1940 when they observed subcutaneous fat transplanted to a transparent rabbit-ear preparation. They observed that the unilocular signet-ring white adipocytes became multilocular and decreased in diameter as the cells were mobilizing lipid. This transition from unilocular to multilocular type while undergoing lipolysis has been repeatedly confirmed by other investigators in other tissue sites at the light-microscopic level.

In intact white adipose tissue of rats, morphological correlates of the fasting state can be detected after 24 h. At this time, there is a reported increase in the number of micropinocytotic invaginations, and pseudopodlike evaginations of the cytoplasm appear. However, there are no detectable changes in the size or the appearance of the unilocular fat droplets. After 48 h of fasting, the size of the unilocular lipid droplets decreases. At this point, some of the cells begin to assume a multilocular appearance. After 72 h of fasting, adipocyte morphology is distinctly altered (Fig. 5-11). Adipose cells are reduced in size and contain many and smaller lipid droplets. The plasmalemma surface becomes very irregular. In addition, the smooth endoplasmic reticulum appears to be proliferating and becomes more obvious than that seen in normal adipose tissue (Fig. 5-11). Some investigators have reported that fenestrated double-membrane envelopes are in close apposition to the lipid droplets and are more visible during fasting. Mitochondrial size and shape do not appear to be affected during fasting. With continued fasting, white adipocytes may become spindlelike and appear more like fibroblasts, containing few, if any, fat droplets. They may show further indentations of the cell surface and the size of the micropinocytotic vesicles may be enlarged, reaching 600 to 1000 Å. Some investigators have demonstrated that the smooth endoplasmic reticulum abundant in the fasted rat adipocyte appears to be continuous with the micropinocytotic invaginations at the surface of the cell. However, other investigators, although finding proliferation of smooth endoplasmic reticulum, have not been able to document the continuity between the smooth endoplasmic reticulum and the micropinocytotic invaginations. Jarret and Smith have suggested that the observed pinocytotic microvesicles are part of an alveolarlike interconnecting system with the cell surface, which functions to

increase surface area and thus facilitate cytoplasmic-surface interaction. Other, and much less well understood, cellular inclusions that have been described by various investigators are the complex vesiculated bodies and pentalaminar membranous structures described by Napolitano and Gagne (1963). These structures are spherical in shape, usually membrane-bound, and slightly larger than mitochondria. Within these vesiculated structures are a variety of granules

FIGURE 5-11 Portion of a mesenteric adipose cell from a 3-day fasted rat. Smaller lipid droplets (LL) are seen near the large central lipid droplet (L). Note the abundance of micropinocytotic vesicles (PV) and endoplasmic reticulum (ER). The external lamina (EL) is clearly visible, especially where it juts out beyond the plasma membrane. RNP, ribonucleoprotein particles. ×32,000. (From Bernard G. Slavin, The Cytophysiology of Mammalian Adipose Cells, *International Review of Cytology* **33**:1972.)

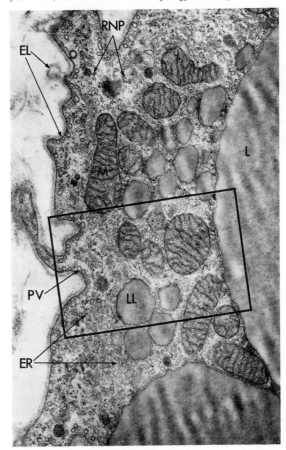

and vesicles of differing size and electron opacity. In the white adipose cell there seems to be no morphological change in the nucleus or the nucleolus except for, perhaps, the increased number of nuclear pores occasionally seen during fasts.

MORPHOLOGICAL CORRELATES OF FAT DEPOSITION

During the postulated development of an adipocyte, the cell goes from a fibroblast spindle shape with small lipid inclusions to a multilocular stage with larger but numerous lipid inclusions to a state of a single, large, lipid inclusion. This progression from multilocular to unilocular is thought to be associated with the normal process of lipogenesis and development. During development and during refeeding after a fast, it has been reported that glycogen is deposited in the cytoplasm prior to lipid filling. Napolitano has described the morphological changes that occur during development and presumably also during refeeding after a fast. This description has been modified in the light of more recent work (Fig. 5-12).

As the cell accumulates lipid, the following morphological changes have been noted. In fibroblast-type cells, visible osmophilic lipid droplets are first noted at one pole of the cell. The lipid droplets tend to coalesce at one pole and become progressively multilocular and then unilocular. At first, lipid droplets are found free in the cytoplasm, apparently morphologically unrelated to the organelles. As lipid accumulates, the plasma membrane shows several micropinocytotic vesicular areas and the external lamina elaborates. As lipid accumulates, there is a gradual reduction in the amount of endoplasmic reticulum and smooth-surfaced vesicles appear in abundance. Their origin is unclear. The amount of Golgi apparatus diminishes. At no time during the process does any specific organelle show intimate association with lipid droplets.

BIOCHEMICAL CORRELATES OF ULTRASTRUCTURE

Attempts to correlate biochemical function with ultrastructural changes have met with variable success. Hollenberg, Angel, and Steiner studied the subcellular distribution and composition of exogenously synthesized lipids in isolated white adipocytes. Their results

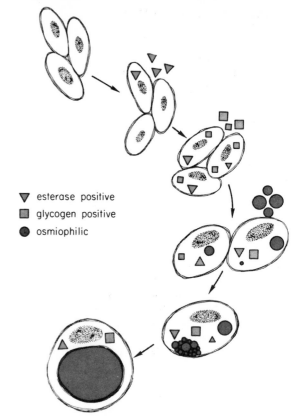

▽ esterase positive
◼ glycogen positive
● osmiophilic

FIGURE 5-12 A generalized schema for the development of an adipose cell. The sequential acquisition of esterase activity, glycogen deposition, and lipid accumulation is depicted as described in the text.

indicate that after a brief incubation of isolated fat cells with labeled glucose, acetate, or palmitic acid, more than 90 percent of the newly synthesized triglyceride was stored in the bulk lipid or unilocular lipid inclusion, indicating rapid intracellular transport and storage. However, if the relative specific activity of the organelles was monitored after cell fractionation, the order of highest specific activity of the organelle triglyceride was mitochondria, microsome, liposomes,[1] soluble supernatant, and bulk lipid. They consider that these experiments establish the structural

[1]"Liposomes are isolated as a floating fraction from adipose cell homogenates. They vary in diameter from 0.5 to 2 μm and contain neutral lipids. Each is surrounded by a single layer of electron dense membrane; dense osmophilic aggregates are associated with the limiting material. Some liposomes have a granular-appearing membrane. There are some structural similarities between liposomes and the morphology of chylomicra." (Hollenberg et al., 1970.)

correlates of the intracellular pools of lipid which are known to exist in adipose tissue, that is, a rapidly exchanging pool and a large-storage, slowly exchanging pool with less metabolically active lipids (Fig. 5-13).

Using isolated fat cells, Cushman (1970) has been able to demonstrate the uptake by micropinocytotic vesicles of radioactive colloidal gold and radio-labeled glucose (Fig. 5-3). The function of these micropinocytotic vesicles is yet to be established physiologically, but presumably they represent a mechanism for transport of large molecules. A study by Daikoku et al. (1973) utilized freeze-etched preparations of adipocytes in order to demonstrate structural alterations that correlate with metabolic state. In the normal rat, the cleaved surface of normal fat cells in freeze-etched preparation shows the thin smooth membrane and numerous globular structures that are described

as a lamellar phase. During fasting, this globular appearance disappears, and vertically arranged canalicular structures which are close to the surface of the lipid accumulation are observed. This conversion from globular to canalicular phase is also observed in the cleaved surfaces of fat cells that have been incubated with epinephrine (Fig. 5-14). Therefore, the work also suggests that the structural alterations in the lipid phase of the fat cell are related to the biochemical changes associated with lipid mobilization.

Although morphological correlates with changes in the cytophysiology of the white fat cell that have been reported to date are sparse, there are numerous reports that relate to the hormonal binding sites associated with the fat-cell plasmalemma. Both lipolysis and lipogenesis are regulated by hormones, and both lipolytic and antilipolytic hormones are believed to

FIGURE 5-13 Glyceride synthesis and storage in the adipose cell: structure-function correlation. (From: Hollenberg, Angel & Steiner, 1970, p. 847.)

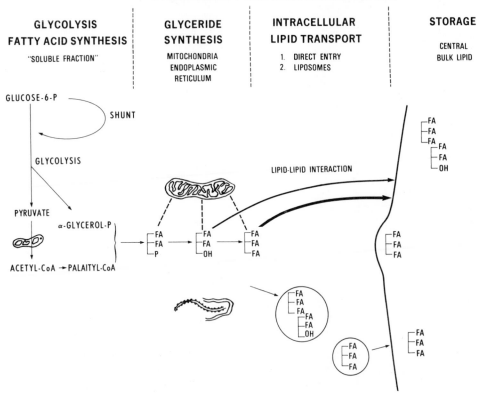

GLYCERIDE SYNTHESIS AND STORAGE IN THE ADIPOSE CELL:
STRUCTURE–FUNCTION CORRELATION

initiate their action by first binding with the adipocyte plasma membrane. Hormone-specific receptor proteins in the adipocyte plasma membrane bind with the hormone. The binding is often, if not always, followed by an activation or inhibition of the adenylate cyclase enzyme system in the membrane. Activation of adenylate cyclase results in an increase in the intracellular concentration of cyclic adenosine 3'5'-monophosphate (cyclic AMP) which mediates the intracellular action of the hormone, according to the "second messenger" hypothesis of Sutherland and Rall. For example, physiological concentrations of the catecholamines bind at β-adrenergic receptor sites in the adipocyte membrane, adenylate cyclase activity is stimulated, intracellular cyclic AMP concentration rises, and lipolysis proceeds at an elevated rate. While it is very clear that insulin binds to fat-cell membranes and that the resultant action of insulin on the fat cell is to stimulate lipogenesis and to inhibit lipolysis, the number, the nature, and the binding affinity of insulin receptors are all matters of great controversy. It has

FIGURE 5-14 A. Fat cell from normal adult epididymal tissue. Cytoplasm (*Cy*) with nucleus (*N*) is displaced to periphery. Lipid accumulation (*La*) appears to be granular. Arrows show globular structures found in cleaved surface. Fixed in 2.5% glutaraldehyde. ×12,000. B. A fat cell and its lipid accumulation from epididymal adipose tissue of a rat fasting for 3 days. The lipid accumulation (*La*) shows canalicular or cylindrical structures (arrows) instead of the granular appearance which has been seen in normal fat cells. *Cy* cytoplasm. Not fixed in 2.5% glutaraldehyde. ×3120. C. Fat cell from normal epididymal adipose tissue incubated in Krebs-Ringer butter without epinephrine (left) and with epinephrine (right). On left, the granular structure is prominent, but on right it has almost disappeared. Fixed in 2.5% glutaraldehyde. ×4800. (From Daikoku, Shigeo, et al., *Arch Hist. Jap.*, **35:**395, 1973.)

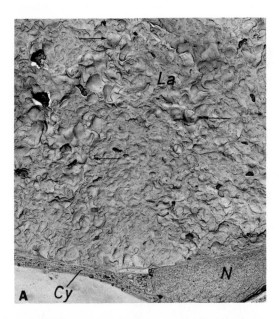

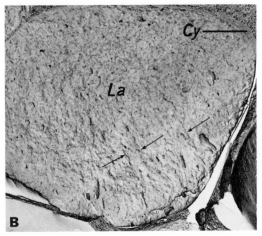

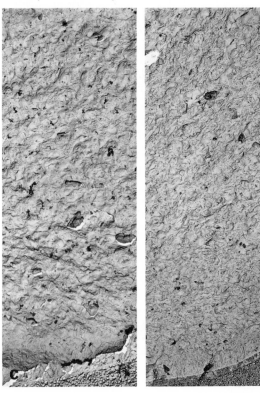

been variously reported that there are high-affinity binding sites ($K_D = 5 \times 10^{-11}$ M), low-affinity binding sites ($K_D = 5 \times 10^{-9}$ M), and as many as 30,000 and as few as 3000 insulin receptor sites per fat cell. Furthermore, it has been suggested that insulin inhibits cyclic AMP production by binding at an adrenergic receptor site as well as at its own specific receptor and that it can stimulate cyclic AMP accumulation under conditions of accelerated lipolysis. Regardless of what the specific kinetics of binding are and what the interaction with the adenylate cyclase system is, that insulin does bind to the surface of the adipocyte has been elegantly demonstrated by Jarett and Smith (1975) using covalently linked ferritin-insulin complexes. The ferritin-insulin complex provides an electron-microscopic marker for the insulin receptor and reveals that the receptor exists in association with the glycocalyx coating in the external surface of the intact adipocyte plasma membrane (Fig. 5-15). The fact that the insulin receptor is associated with the surface coat of the fat cell lends credence to other studies which suggest that the insulin receptor may be glycoprotein in nature. It has recently been demonstrated in addition to binding to cell-membrane receptor sites, insulin promotes microtubule assembly in isolated rat adipocytes (Fig. 5-16). Other stimuli such as oxytocin and high concentrations of glucose do not promote the assembly of microtubules. Since colchicine inhibits the insulin stimulation of lipid and glycogen synthesis in the fat cell but does not influence insulin stimulation of glucose oxidation, it was suggested that microtubule assembly may be important as part of the direct effect of insulin in inhibiting lipolysis and promoting lipogenesis. Nonetheless, with the possible exception of this microtubule assembly study and the freeze-etched preparations, the internal morphological correlates associated with hormone binding to the fat-cell surface have never been systematically documented.

A quantitative study of changes in the adipocyte plasma membrane under the influence of a lipogenic stimulus (insulin) or a lipolytic stimulus (glucagon or epinephrine) has been conducted using the freeze-fracture technique. Carpentier, Perrelet, and Orci (1976) reported that the number of intramembranous particles seen in the fractured faces of plasma membrane increased in membranes from white adipose cells that had been incubated with insulin, but decreased in preparations from cells that had been incubated with either glucagon or epinephrine.

Since these intramembranous particles, which

may be seen in both the P and E faces of a fractured plasma membrane (Figure 5-17) are believed to be membrane proteins (possibly hormonal receptors and/or membrane-bound enzymes), these data may be the first quantifiable morphological evidence of the modulation of membrane, and thus, cellular function by a hormone. In these same preparations, the number of membrane invaginations was increased by all three hormones as compared to untreated material, but the size and shape of all membrane structural components remained unaltered regardless of treatment.

CYTOCHEMISTRY OF BROWN ADIPOSE TISSUE

In addition to the differences in cell structure and tissue-sympathetic innervation that are seen between brown and white adipose tissue, there are several known functional differences. Some of these have been reviewed by Hull and Segall (1966). Perhaps the most striking physiological difference is that brown fat mobilizes little, if any, triglyceride in response to dietary restriction and increases triglyceride deposition very little in response to overfeeding. In contrast, brown-fat stores respond dramatically, both during development and in mature mammals (especially hibernators), to the demands of cold stress. White adipose tissue undergoes lipolysis and becomes depleted during a fast even at higher than normal environmental temperature. Brown adipose tissue, in contrast, rapidly mobilizes lipid when the animal is cold-stressed; but brown adipocytes may remain lipid-filled even when the animal is starved to death in a thermoneutral environment. The thermogenic properties of brown adipose tissue are thought to result from cyclic AMP modulation of norepinephrine stimulation. The noradrenergic stimulation results from neural innervation of individual fat cells and the subsequent activation of adenylate cyclase through adrenergic receptors in brown adipose tissue cell membranes.

Structure-function relationships in brown adipose tissue both during development and in response to stimuli are much more clearly documented than those in white adipose tissue. During the first few days of rat postnatal development, brown adipose tissue progressively loses cellular glycogen deposits, the multilocular

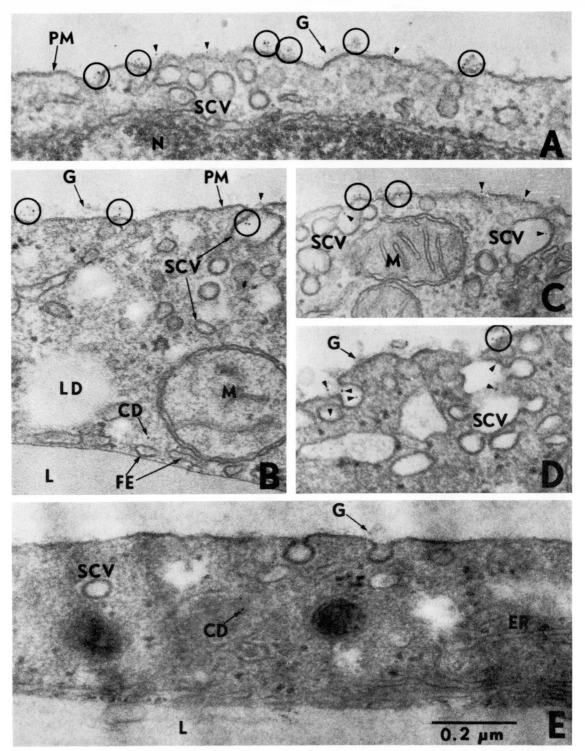

FIGURE 5-15 Intact adipocytes were isolated, incubated, and prepared for electron microscopy. In order to allow better visualization of ferritin-insulin molecules, sections were examined without staining. All micrographs were oriented with the plasma membrane toward the top of the figure, the central lipid depot to the bottom. Micrographs ×100,000. Scale bar equals 0.2 μm. PM, plasma membrane; G, glycocalyx; SCV, surface connected vesicles; N, nucleus; LD, cytoplasmic lipid droplet; CD, cytoplasmic density; M, mitochondria; FE, fenestrated envelope; L, central lipid depot; ER, endoplasmic reticulum. (From Leonard Jarett and Robert M. Smith, *Proc. Nat. Acad. Sci. USA*, **72:**9, 1975.)

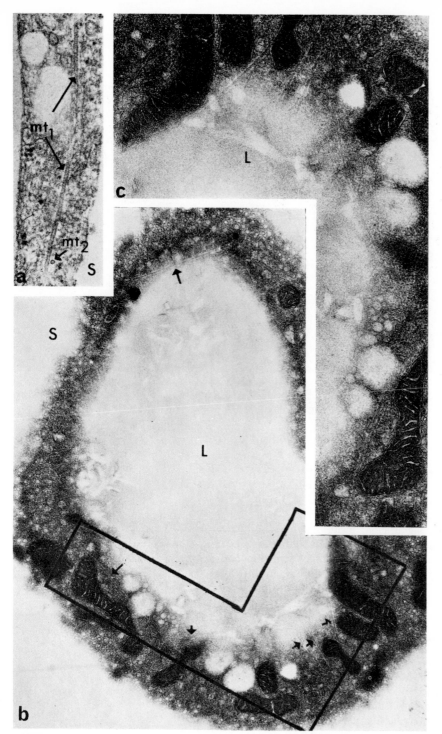

FIGURE 5-16 Sections of adipocytes fixed after incubation with 10 microunits of insulin per milliliter without glucose for 10 min. *S* is the extracellular space: *L* is the lipid drop within the fat cell. (a) Section through the central part of an adipocyte showing cytoplasmic envelope that surrounds lipid. Two microtubules (mt) lie nearly in the plane of section; another (mt_2) is transverse to it (×18,000). (b) Fairly thick section near one pole of a cell. Plane of section nearly tangent to lipid droplet. Arrows indicate some of the many microtubules in this section. The tubules appear to form a network tangent to the fat droplet (×18,000). (c) Enlargement of region of adipocyte outline in (b). Note electron-lucent region around each tubule (×30,000). (From D. Soifer et al., Insulin and Microtubules in Rat Adipocytes. *Science* **179:**269, 1971.)

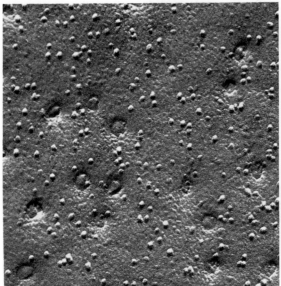
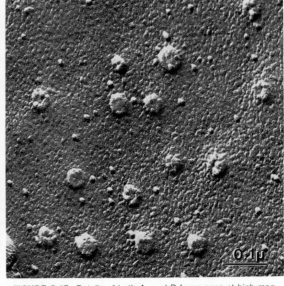

FIGURE 5-17 Details of both A- and B-faces seen at high magnification. The reverse appearance of the membrane invaginations as well as the unequal number of intramembranous particles are clearly evidenced. ×126,000. [Note that according to the new freeze-etching nomenclature (Branton D. et al., Science, **190**:54, 1975). A-face is now called P-face and B-face is called E-face.] (From Jean-Louis Carpentier, Alain Perrelet, and Lelio Orci, *J. Lipid Research*, **17**:335, 1976.)

lipid droplet diameter decreases, and dense bodies and cytolysosomes become more prominent. Major changes in mitochondrial ultrastructure are noted. Principally, the mitochondria swell and cristae are reoriented to a transverse configuration. Inclusions which are typically noted in the internal mitochondrial matrix in prenatal development and under thermoneutral conditions are decreased in number (Fig. 5-18). The ultrastructural changes presumably associated with lipid mobilization in cold stress can be produced both in vivo and in vitro by norepinephrine administration. The ultrastructural effects are blocked by the use of Trasicor (a β-adrenergic blocking agent) and mimicked by theophylline. Presumably, the effect of theophylline is to inhibit the intracellular phosphodiesterase leading to decreased degradation of cyclic AMP and consequently higher intracellular cyclic AMP levels. Therefore, theophylline administration leads to higher cellular lipolytic activity. Although there are many points about structural correlates of brown adipose tissue that remain to be established, it is

reasonable to assume that the process of neural integration and substrate mobilization reflected in the ultrastructural changes described above is highly likely to be correct.

FIGURE 5-18 A. Brown adipocyte from a newborn rat. Several mitochondria contain large matrix inclusions. In most of them a tubular substructure is visible. In filamentous mitochondrial profiles the cristae are oriented lengthwise. Two kinds of particles occur in the cytoplasmic matrix, the smaller less dense ones are ribosomes, the larger black-appearing ones are glycogen granules. ×24,500. B. Brown adipocyte from a 17-h-old rat. The mitochondrial matrix inclusions have disappeared, and in their place much smaller granular elements are visible. The mitochondria are somewhat larger and more nearly round. The cytoplasm contains only ribosomes, and no glycogen remains. ×24,500. (From Elsi R. Suter, *Specialia*, **15**:3, 1969.)

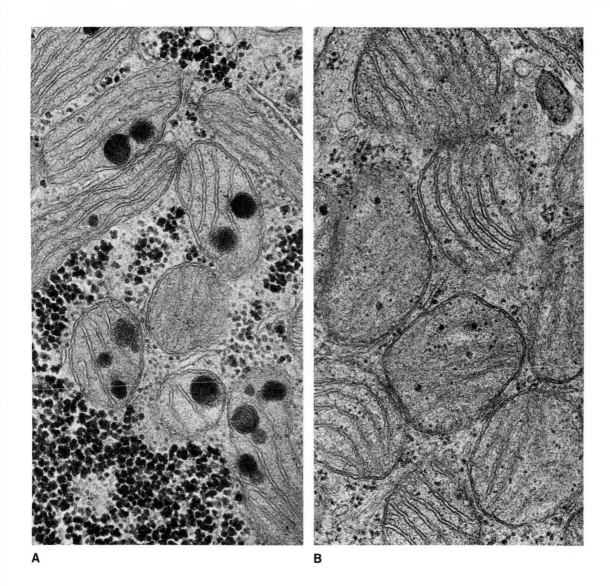

A

B

REFERENCES

ADEBONOJO, F. O.: Enzymatic Adaptations by Cultured Adipocytes of Human Infants and Children: Effect of Obese Serum on the Activities of Lactate-, Malate-, and Glucose-6-phosphate Dehydrogenases, *Pediatr. Res.,* **9:**889–893 (1975).

BALLANTYNE, B., and A. T. RAFTERY: The Intrinsic Autonomic Innervation of White Adipose Tissue, *Cytobios.,* **10:**187–197 (1974).

BARGMANN, W., G. V. HEHN, and E. LINDER: Veber die Zellen des braunen Fettgewebes und ihre Innervation. *Z. Zellforsch. Mikrosk. Anat.,* **85:**601–613 (1968).

CARPENTIER, J. L., A. PERRELET, and L. ORCI: Effects of Insulin, Glucagon and Epinephrine on the Plasma Membrane of the White Adipose Cell: A Freeze-Fracture Study, *J. Lipid Res.,* **17:**335 (1976).

CUATRECASAS, P.: Insulin-Receptor Interactions in Adipose Tissue Cells: Direct Measurement and Properties, *Proc. Natl. Acad. Sci. U.S.A.,* **68:**1264– (1971).

CUSHMAN, S. W.: Structure-Function Relationships in the Adipose Cell. I. Ultrastructure of the Isolated Adipose Cell, *J. Cell Biol.,* **46:**326–341 (1970).

CUSHMAN, S. W.: Structure-Function Relationships in the Adipose Cell. II. Pinocytosis and Factors Influencing Its Activity in the Isolated Adipose Cell, *J. Cell Biol.,* **46:**342–353 (1970).

DAIKOKU, S., Y. SHINOHARA, and Y. G. WATANABE: The Appearance of Lipid Cells in Freeze-etched Preparations, *Arch. Histol. Jap.,* **35:**395–401 (1973).

DERRY, D. M., E. MORROW, N. SADRE, and K. V. FLATTERY: Brown and White Fat during the Life of the Rabbit, *Dev. Biol.,* **27:**204–216 (1972).

DERRY, D. M., E. SCHONBAUM, and G. STEINER: Two Sympathetic Nerve Supplies to Brown Adipose Tissue of the Rat, *Can. J. Physiol. Pharmacol.,* **47:**57–63 (1969).

FAIN, J. N.: Insulin as an Activator of Cyclic AMP Accumulation in Rat Fat Cells, *J. Cyclic Nucleotide Res.,* **I:**359–366 (1975).

GLIEMANN, J., S. GAMMELTOFT and J. VINTEN: Insulin Receptors in Fat Cells. Relationship between Binding and Activation, *Isr. J. Med. Sci.,* **II:**656–663 (1975).

GREENWOOD, M. R. C., and J. HIRSCH: Postnatal Development of Adipocyte Cellularity in the Normal Rat, *J. Lipid Res.,* **15:**474 (1974).

HIRSCH, J. and J. L. KNITTLE: Cellularity of Obese and Non-obese Human Adipose Tissue, *Fed. Proc.,* **29:**1516 (1970).

HOLLENBERG, C. H., A. ANGEL, and G. STEINER: The Metabolism of White and Brown Adipose Tissue, *C.M.A. Journal,* **103:**843–849 (1970).

HULL, D., and M. M. SEGALL: Distinction of Brown from White Adipose Tissue, *Nature (Lond.),* **212:**469–472 (1966).

JARRETT, L., and R. M. SMITH: Ultrastructural Localization of Insulin Receptors on Adipocytes, *Proc. Natl. Acad. Sci. U.S.A.,* **72:**3526–3530 (1975).

JOHNSON, P. R., and JULES HIRSCH: The Cellularity of Adipose Depots in Six Strains of Genetically Obese Mice, *J. Lipid Res.,* **13:**2 (1972).

JOHNSON, P. R., L. M. ZUCKER, J. A. F. CRUCE, and JULES HIRSCH: The Cellularity of Adipose Depots in the Genetically Obese Zucker Rat, *J. Lipid Res.,* **12:**1706 (1971).

KONO, T., and F. W. BARHAM: The Relationship between the Insulin-binding Capacity of Fat Cells and the Cellular Response to Insulin, *J. Biol. Chem.,* **246:**6210 (1971).

MERKLIN, R.: Growth and Distribution of Human Fetal Brown Fat, *Anat. Rec.,* **178:**637–646 (1973).

MOHR, W., and G. BENEKE: Histochemische Untersuchungen der Enstehung von Fettzellen, *Virchows. Arch. B.,* **3:**13 (1969a).

NAPOLITANO, L.: The Differentiation of White Adipose Cells. An Electron Microscopic Study, *J. Cell Biol.,* **18:**663–679 (1963).

NAPOLITANO, L., and H. GAGNE: Lipid-depleted White Adipose Cells: An Electron Microscope Study, *Anat. Rec.,* **147:**273 (1963).

PILGRIM, C.: DNA Synthesis and Differentiation in Developing White Adipose Tissue, *Develop. Biol.,* **26:**69–76 (1971).

RENOLD, A. E. and G. F. CAHILL: Adipose Tissue, "Handbook of Physiology," Sec. 5, American Physiological Society, Washington, D.C., 1965.

ROBINSON, G. A., R. W. BUTCHER, and E. W. SUTHERLAND: "Cyclic AMP," Academic Press, Inc., New York, 1971.

RODBELL, M.: Metabolism of Isolated Fat Cells. I. Effects of Hormones on Glucose Metabolism and Lipolysis, *J. Biol. Chem.,* **239:**375 (1964).

SLAVIN, B. G.: The Cytophysiology of Mammalian Adipose Cells, *Int. Rev. Cytol.,* **33:**297–334 (1972).

SOIFER, D., T. BRAUN, and O. HECHTER. Insulin and Microtubules in Rat Adipocytes, *Science,* **179:**269–271 (1971).

SUTER, E.: The Fine Structure of Brown Adipose Tissue, *Lab. Invest.,* **21:**246–258 (1969).

SUTER, E. R.: The Fine Structure of Brown Adipose Tissue. I. Cold-induced Changes in the Rat, *J. Ultrastruct. Res.,* **26:**216–241 (1969).

SUTER, E. R., and W. STAUBLI: An Ultrastructural Histochemical Study of Brown Adipose Tissue from Prenatal Rats, *J. Histochem. Cytochem.,* **18:**100–106 (1970).

WASSERMAN, F., and T. F. MACDONALD: Electron Microscopic Investigation of the Surface Membrane Structures of the Fat Cell and of Their Changes during Depletion of the Cell, *Zeitsch. Zellforsch.,* **52:**778–800 (1960).

The Skeletal Tissues

LEONARD F. BÉLANGER

Skeleton is a Greek word which refers to the dry object of the sometimes equally dry anatomical lessons. To the gross anatomist, it is a bilaterally symmetrical series of jointed structures arranged along and around the vertebral axis. To the classical histologist, it consists of only a few types of microscopic entities—dense fibrous tissue, chordoid, cartilage, bone—which form complex functional units between themselves. To the physiologist and to the biochemist, these tissues, especially bone, represent an important reservoir of essential electrolytes which control many of the vital functions. To the pathologist and to the sociologist, the skeleton has revealed a great deal about the nutrition, customs, diseases, and even the religion of contemporary and historic man. To the anthropologist, the skeleton has been the most important—sometimes the only—record of the progressive evolution of ancient human beings and of the gradual growth of their brain. A few scholars of the vertebrate skeleton (Romer, 1946 and 1963; Urist, 1964; Tarlo and Tarlo, 1965; Urist and van de Putte, 1967; McLean and Urist, 1968; Hall, 1975; Moss, 1961, 1964, 1968) have in recent time brought to life the fascinating story of the origin of bone, its progressive adaptation, and its regulating mechanisms. Through them we have learned that the cartilaginous fish were not, as we believed, the earliest of vertebrates. One million years before them were the Ostracodermi, fishes with a dermal skeleton, a protective armor against dominant invertebrate predators (Romer, 1963). The loss of armor for better mobility and the subsequent development of the endoskeleton in soft-water teleosts, the synthesis of vitamin D, and the development of the branchial hormone-producing derivatives (thyroid, parathyroid, and ultimobranchial gland) are only a few aspects of this marvelous story.

MINOR VARIETIES

CHORDOID TISSUE

Chordoid tissue is an ancestral remnant in vertebrates. In humans, it is represented by only the embryonic notochord. This tissue consists of large, contiguous cells filled with fluid and forming in their ensemble a compartmented "water bag" that provides some structural support. There is practically no intercellular substance between the chordal cells.

DENSE FIBROUS TISSUE

This variety of connective tissue is generally not described in this chapter. However, the fact that it can become mineralized "by the addition of a new matrix to the collagen bundles" (Weidenreich, 1930; Johnson, 1960), as is the case with the turkey leg tendon, makes it a primitive form of skeletal tissue. The new matrix consists of polysaccharides and lipids in part (Johnson, 1960). A "chemical metaplasia" also occurs in the collagen bundles. The fibers become enlarged and lose their waviness and their staining properties are modified; eventually they become mineralized. In the turkey tendon, these changes lead to the adjacent formation of true cartilage or true bone. Thus, we learn that the occurrence of these two main forms of skeletal tissues was probably the result of persistent local conditions such as the quantity and quality of mucopolysaccharides in the matrix, the amount of oxygenation

and hydration, and possibly also some local mechanical irritant (Hall, 1970).

FIBROCARTILAGE

Special mechanical conditions seem to be provided by the large, mobile articulations. In some of the dense fibrous tendons and ligaments which surround them, a regularly occurring change leads to the formation of single rows of large, rounded cells surrounded by matrix rich in mucopolysaccharides (Fig. 6-1). These conditions are characteristic of cartilage, and the tissue in its ensemble is known as fibrocartilage.

CHONDROID

A primitive tissue commonly found in cyclostomes and other early vertebrates has been described as pseudocartilage, or chondroid. It consists of closely adjacent vesicular cells surrounded by a thin capsule rich in collagen fibers but poor in mucopolysaccharides.

CARTILAGE

DEVELOPMENT

Cartilage in the human embryo appears during the fifth week of life. Different inducers, such as the noto-

cord and cells migrating from the neural crest, have been proposed by the early embryologists. More recently, Anderson (1967) has shown that injections of cultured amnion cells can provoke the formation of

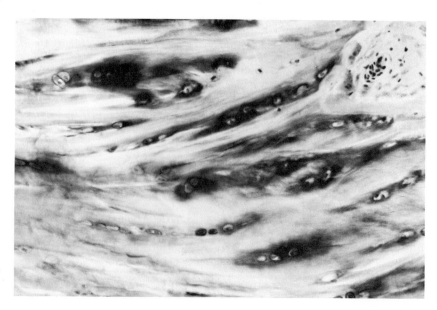

FIGURE 6-1 Fibrocartilage, knee joint of young chick. Wright stain. ×240.

heterotopic cartilage and bone. The mother tissue is, of course, the versatile and multitalented mesenchyme.

The first histologic evidence of the new tissue consists of variously shaped agglomerations of closely apposed rounded cells. These units or centers of chondrification at first resemble the chondroid of more primitive species. They will grow from then on by division of already differentiated cartilage cells (interstitial growth) or by addition of more mesenchymal elements at the periphery of the unit (appositional growth). After a time, an envelope, the perichondrium (Fig. 6-2, P), consisting of densely arranged flattened cells and fibers, will form around the unit, separating it from the mesenchyme. This envelope is not only a protective one but is also a growth regulator. Appositional development will occur from then on through cellular differentiation at the inner surface of the perichondrium.

The main property of cartilage resides in the ability of its cells to secrete a complex protein-polysaccharide mixture which gels as it accumulates in the intercellular matrix (Figs. 6-2 and 6-3), producing the solid yet resilient consistency characteristic of this tissue.

A variety of technical procedures and especially electron microscopy have revealed that fibrillogenesis goes on inside the cartilage masses as well as outside. In most cartilage units, the fibers are of the white

collagenic variety. These are optically homogeneous with the environmental amorphous matrix and consequently invisible by light microscopy (Figs. 6-2 and 6-3). This type of cartilage is known as hyaline.

A few cartilage pieces, however, such as those of the external ear, the auditory canal, the epiglottis (Fig. 6-4), and certain small laryngeal units, contain yellow elastic fibers. These are optically different from the fundamental substance and thus easily recognized in routinely stained preparations (Fig. 6-4).

ADULT CARTILAGE

Cells

In the appositional growth process, the new cartilage cells originate from the inner portion of the perichondrium. They are, at first, flattened elements (Fig. 6-2) which are progressively dispersed by their secretory activity that results in the production of the new hyaline matrix (Figs. 6-2 and 6-3). In routinely stained preparations where acid dyes such as eosin, phloxine B, and orange G are used in combination with the basic dye hematoxylin, the matrix which is proximal to the perichondrium is stained with the acid dyes and is described as acidophilic. The immature

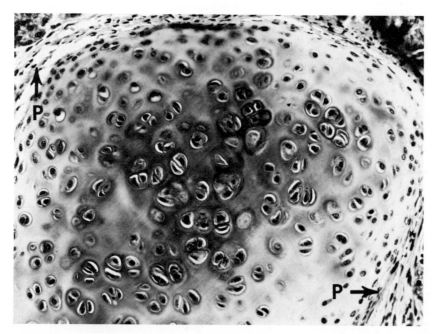

FIGURE 6-2 Hyaline cartilage, a part of the nasal choanae of a young cat; P, perichondrium; hematoxylin-phloxine-orange stain. ×240.

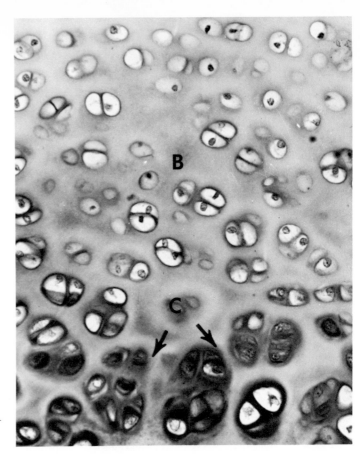

FIGURE 6-3 A portion of hyaline cartilage of a young cat; B, chondroblasts; C, chondrocytes. Hematoxylin-phloxine-orange stain. ×370.

FIGURE 6-4 A portion of the epiglottis cartilage of an adult man. The elastic fibers are quite prominent. H&E. ×370.

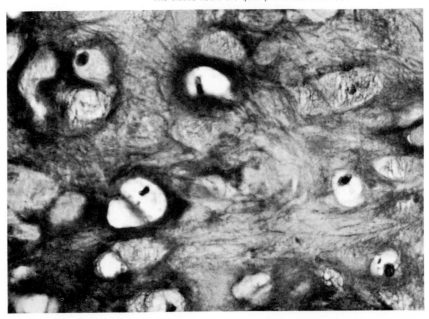

small cells in this peripheral area are sometimes referred to as chondroblasts (Figs. 6-2 and 6-3, B).

Farther inward, the cells are progressively larger and the matrix around them preferentially takes up the basic dye (Figs. 6-2 and 6-3, C). This difference in staining behavior has long been thought to be related to the progressive acquisition of secretory ability by the cartilage cell through the completion of its differentiation (chondrocytes).

At the light-microscope level, the cytoplasm of the chondrocytes exhibits progressive staining affinity for the acid dyes along with maturation. The adult cells often show accumulation of metaplastic masses of carbohydrates and lipids. Technical dehydration is mainly responsible for the shrunken, sometimes crenated appearance of these cells.

Viewed through the electron microscope (Fig. 6-5), the chondrocytes exhibit a membrane system "characteristic of cells responsible for discharge of protein secretion" (Davies et al., 1962); the rough endoplasmic reticulum and portions of the Golgi complex are prominent. Granular material (Godman and Porter, 1960; Anderson, 1967) (Figure 6-5) and fine nonperiodic filaments (Revel and Hay, 1963) have been identified within the enlarged vesicles of the Golgi complex (Anderson, 1967) (Fig. 6-5). The mitochondria are surprisingly abundant and apparently capable of "well-marked glycolysis" (Bywaters, 1937). The accumulation of intracytoplasmic glycogen is apparently related to senescence (Silberberg et al., 1964).

Ground Substance

Following the introduction of the integrated process of radioautography (Bélanger and Leblond, 1946), which allows the simultaneous visualization of tissue tracers and their photographic record (Fig. 6-6), dynamic histology has rapidly advanced. One of the early achievements was the demonstration of the role of the chondrocytes in mucopolysaccharide and protein secretion.

Radioactive sodium sulfate injected into young rats was thus found incorporated into a stable compound present in considerably greater proportion within the larger cells (Fig. 6-7) a short time after the treatment and subsequently into the surrounding matrix (Bélanger, 1954). The existence of a hyaluronidase-resistant sulfated fraction and its localization at the site of insertion of tendons and ligaments (Fig. 6-8) also was revealed by combining $^{35}SO_4$ radioautography with enzyme incubation (Bélanger, 1954).

ISOGENIC GROUPS, CAPSULE, LACUNA *Interstitial growth* occurs through division of adult chondrocytes. The result is manifested histologically by the presence of closely apposed large cells in groups of two or more located deep inside the cartilage piece (Figs. 6-2 and 6-3). These groups are called isogenic or are said to form nests because they are often surrounded by a common dense basophilic layer termed *capsule* by the early histologists. This term was motivated by the fact that the layer was considered as an outer wall of the chondrocyte. Inside the capsule, the often shrunken cartilage cell occupies a space called the *lacuna.*

The *capsule* is a pericellular zone of concentrated chondromucoprotein. The presence of sulfated mucopolysaccharides in that area has been revealed histochemically by Revel (1964) with his thorium reaction (Fig. 6-9).

The basophilia of the adult cartilage matrix is not always maintained. With age and a critical increase in size of the cartilage mass, centrally located areas of some cartilage pieces lose their basophilia. This is due to a decrease in the secretion of sulfated mucoprotein and also to the accumulation in the matrix of an *albuminoid* chemically related to keratin, a strongly acidophilic substance.

Collagen

Histologic procedures for staining cartilage have placed a great deal of emphasis on the mucopolysaccharides and the protein components of ground substance. However, the masked collagen forms an important component of this tissue: up to 40 percent of the dry weight is collagen.

Electron-microscope radioautographic studies of a collagen precursor, [³H] proline (Revel and Hay, 1963), have revealed the presence of this substance inside the endoplasmic reticulum of the chondrocytes and its rapid passage into the surrounding matrix. Apparently there are fibrils of different sizes in cartilage and also fibrils with a varying periodicity (Anderson, 1967; Fahmy et al., 1969) which may possess different physiologic properties.

Collagen fibers are said to be randomly distributed in the matrix. There are, however, local concentrations in the immediate vicinity of the lacuna (capsule). The same is true of elastic fibers (Fig. 6-4). In some cartilage pieces, an apparently organized net-

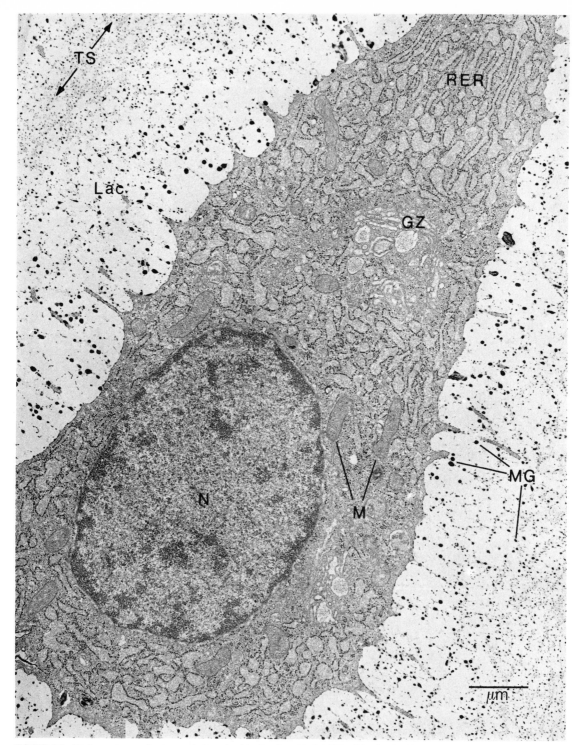

FIGURE 6-5 Electron micrograph of an early hypertrophic chondrocyte of rabbit epiphysis, showing a lacuna (Lac), matrix granules (MG), and a portion of transverse matrix septum (TS); GZ, Golgi apparatus; M, mitochondria; N, nucleus; RER, rough endoplasmic reticulum. (Courtesy of Dr. H. Clarke Anderson.)

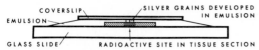

COVERSLIP
SILVER GRAINS DEVELOPED
IN EMULSION
EMULSION
GLASS SLIDE
RADIOACTIVE SITE IN TISSUE SECTION

FIGURE 6-6 Diagram representing the components of an integrated radioautograph.

work of fibers seem to radiate from a nutritional zone containing blood vessels to surrounding lacunae (*interlacunar network,* Fig. 6-10: Bélanger and Migicovsky, 1961).

Blood Vessels

Cartilage is essentially an avascular tissue. In contrast to most other tissues (another remarkable exception is the cornea), it has no capillary network of its own. It must draw its nutrition from fluids which are capable of diffusing through its matrix. The fluid content of this matrix is on the order of 75 percent of the fresh weight, a finding surprising to the morphologist.

It has been said that interstitial growth is stimulated by the need for the hinterland chondrocytes to increase their surface in order to maintain their oxygen supply from a progressively poorer environment as these cells become located farther away from the blood vessels. When interstitial growth is no longer possible, often the cells cannot maintain their normal metabolic activities; they then degenerate and die.

GROWTH AND MAINTENANCE FACTORS

Nutritional

Severe deficiency in the nutritional supply of protein precursors, minerals, and vitamins such as A, C, and D leads to abnormal growth and maturation of cartilage.

VITAMIN A There is very little information as yet available on the skeletal effects of vitamin A deficiency in human beings. Nevertheless, in birds, where Wolbach and Hegsted (1952) have studied this problem particularly well, the maturation of the epiphyseal cartilage was irregular and less extensive than normal. Mitotic activity was arrested, but continuous secretion associated with lack of maturation led to the formation of a broad zone of immature tissue.

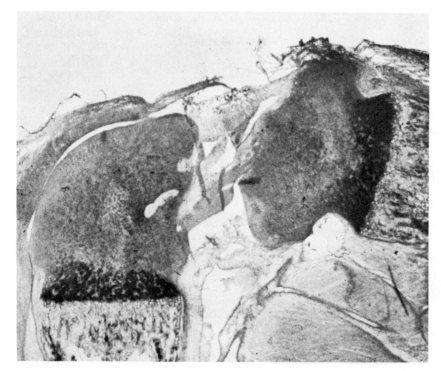

FIGURE 6-7 Radioautograph of $^{35}SO_4$ incorporation and synthesis into sulfated mucopolysaccharide by the cartilage cells. The label is located mostly in the large chondrocytes 2 h after administration. ×50.

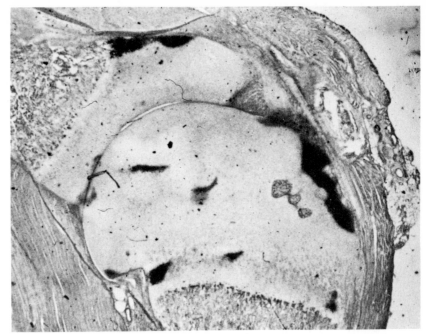

FIGURE 6-8 Radioautograph of $^{35}SO_4$ incorporated as sulfated mucopolysaccharide and secreted into the matrix. The section has been treated with hyaluronidase, which has removed the label except in sites of insertion of tendons and ligaments where presumably a hyaluronidase-resistant mucopolysaccharide is present. ×50.

FIGURE 6-9 Electron micrograph of a portion of mouse cartilage. The section has been stained with colloidal thorium to show the presence of acid mucopolysaccharides. A perilacunar concentration is apparent. ×10,000. (Courtesy of Dr. J. P. Revel and *Journal de Microscopie*.)

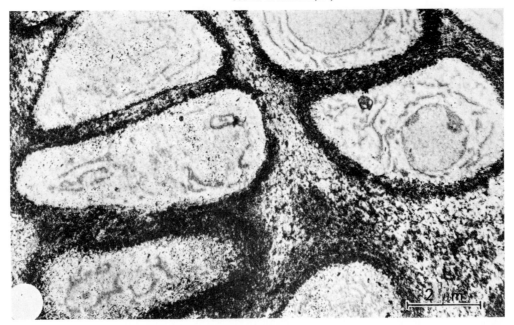

VITAMIN C This vitamin is apparently needed for the production if not for the maintenance of collagen (Ham and Elliot, 1938). According to Bourne (1956), it also has a role in the production of ground substance through its stimulation of the oxidative enzymes which preside over the oxidation of organic sulfur to sulfate as part of the process of chondroitin sulfate synthesis.

VITAMIN D Rickets ("die Englische Krankeit," Glisson, 1650) was a prominent disease of the Northern countries in days gone by. The use of cod-liver oil as a cure in human beings dates back to the end of the eighteenth century (Harris, 1956). However, the syn-

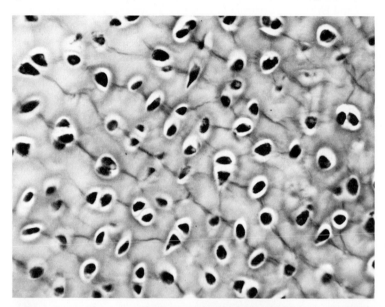

FIGURE 6-10 A portion of the articular cartilage of the tibia of a young chick, stained by the PAS reagent. The fibers of the interlacunar network are apparent. ×550.

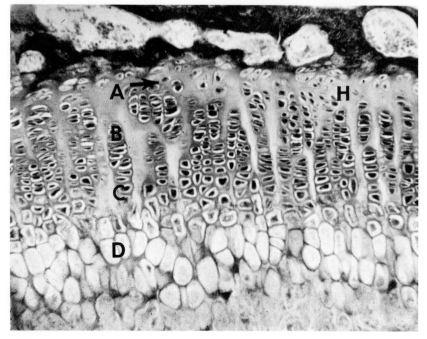

FIGURE 6-11 A portion of the epiphyseal plate of the tibia of a young rat. A, zone of resting or reserve cartilage; B, zone of young proliferating cartilage; C, zone of maturing cartilage; D, zone of calcifying cartilage. Toluidine blue stain. ×120.

thesis of vitamin D and its abundance in the liver of the teleost fish recall dramas of survival which occurred millions of years ago as the bony fishes migrated into mineral-poor ponds and streams (McLean and Urist, 1968).

The search for the intimate effects of vitamin D has "frustrated the efforts of so many for so long" (DeLuca, 1967) until this substance was recently recognized as involved in inducing the synthesis of enzymes "responsible for the formation of a calcium transport protein" (DeLuca, 1970). The role of vitamin D in skeletal formation has been a matter of considerable controversy. Investigations of collagen synthesis, hydroxylation of lysine residues on the collagen molecule, and maturation of the collagen fibrils have demonstrated that each of these processes occurs to a greater extent in vitamin D–rich as compared with vitamin D–deficient animals. However, the possibility that these changes are due to an improved calcium status is likely (Wasserman, 1975).

Hormones

Several hormones have an important role in the growth and maintenance of cartilage.

SOMATOTROPIN This is the growth hormone of the adenohypophysis, which is essential for the proper growth of cartilage and for the maintenance of the secretory activity of the chondrocytes. In a young rat surgically deprived of its hypophysis, the thickness of the epiphyseal plate of the long bones is most affected (Fig. 6-12). As compared with that of a normal littermate (Fig. 6-11), the cartilaginous plate is thinner, the cells are flattened and less numerous (Fig. 6-12), their mitotic activity decreases (Bois et al., 1963), and the matric looses its metachromasia (Fig. 6-12), an indication that its sulfated mucopolysaccharide content has considerably decreased. Treatment of an hypophysectomized animal with growth hormone fully restored the normal size, histologic appearance (Fig. 6-12), and mitotic (Bois et al., 1963) and secretory activity (Fig. 6-13) after 3 days.

THYROID The thyroid gland is apparently synergistic with the hypophysis in promoting normal skeletal growth (Turner, 1966). Removal of either the hy-

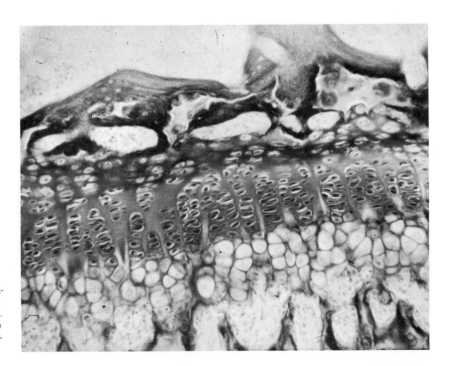

FIGURE 6-12 An area comparable to that of Fig. 6-11, but from an hypophysectomized littermate. The plate is thinner; the cartilage cells have practically stopped secreting. ×120.

pophysis or the thyroid in a young animal produces dwarfism. An exaggerated amount of growth hormone during the period of growth promotes gigantism. In the absence of the hypophysis, the thyroid hormone thyroxine promotes erosion of the cartilage and its replacement by bone.

MALE SEX HORMONE   Testosterone, the male sex hormone, is an anabolic factor and promotes protein synthesis. Thus, in principle, it favors cartilage growth. However, since it has been found to promote maturation at the same time (Silberberg and Silberberg, 1956; Joss et al., 1963), the net result is harmonious maintenance.

ESTROGENS   "Present knowledge concerning the relationship of estrogens to postfetal osteogenesis is obscure" (McLean and Urist, 1968). Fahmy et al., (1969) have recently observed that fibrillogenesis in cartilage is stimulated by this type of hormone.

CORTISONE   The antiinflammatory hormone of the adrenal cortex, cortisone apparently retards the maturation of cartilage and its replacement by bone at the epiphyseal plate. It interferes somehow with the me-

tabolism of the sulfated mucopolysaccharides (Kowalewski, 1958; Bélanger and Migicovsky, 1960).

DEGENERATION AND CALCIFICATION

When the chondrocytes can no longer maintain their production of sulfated mucoprotein, the water content of the matrix decreases and albuminoid appears as mentioned above. The matrix sometimes takes on a fibrous appearance ("asbestfaserung," amiantine degeneration) and precipitation of mineral salts occurs. These events add insult to injury: separated further from their vital supplies, the chondrocytes rapidly lose their glycogen reserves and soon degenerate and perish. These various episodes of cartilage degeneration are far less frequent in elastic cartilage than in the hyaline variety.

The electron microscope has revealed in recent time the vital participation of the cartilage cell in the early phase of mineralization (Anderson, 1967; Bonucci, 1967). Since these events are apparently

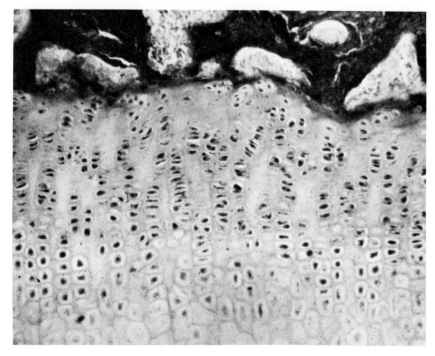

FIGURE 6-13 The epiphyseal plate of an hypophysectomized young rat treated with growth hormone. Growth and secretion have been resumed. ×120.

similar to what has been recorded with bone, they will be discussed later in this chapter.

REPAIR, TRANSPLANTATION, ANTIGENICITY, SELF-INDUCTION

The chondrogenic activity of the perichondrium is limited to the period of youth and active growth. When injury occurs in an adult cartilage piece, cells from the perichondrium proliferate but generally produce dense fibrous tissue which may then change slowly and only in part into cartilage.

Cartilage is considered a good candidate for transplantation in autografts and even in allografts. Because of their low metabolic activity in a normally avascular environment, chondrocytes, are well adapted to surgical transfer. However, the host is protected against their antigens, which cannot diffuse easily through the matrix. It seems from recent observations that cartilage antigenicity is very low at any rate (Peacock et al., 1960). But a cartilage allograft in the connective tissue of a young growing animal, even if it dies after a time, often induces a chondrogenic or osteogenic persistent reaction from the host (McLean and Urist, 1968).

BONE

ORIGIN

The sharks, which have an endoskeleton entirely composed of cartilage, have calcium deposits in the interior of their vertebrae which apparently are highly reactive and constitute a mineral bank of a sort (McLean and Urist, 1968). In the majority of modern fishes, in amphibians, and in terrestrial vertebrates, however, the organism depends for support and for storage of minerals on the ancestral armor tissue known as bone. Although in a few species such as the turtle, the exoskeleton or dermal type of bone persists, the dermal skeletal pieces have disappeared in most species and have been replaced by a well-developed internal bony framework, the endoskeleton. The endoskeleton is of mesodermic origin. It sometimes arises directly from the primitive cells of mesenchyme, as in the case of a small number of flat bones—membrane bones—located close to the surface. More often, bone is preceded in the embryo by a cartilage template which it replaces totally or partially; all the long bones arising through this replacement process are thus described as endochondral.

These traditional appellations have caused a great deal of confusion. It is now suggested that they be replaced by the following: (1) The bones of direct connective tissue origin could be called *mesenchymal bones*. (2) Those that arise by partial replacement of a prior cartilage anlage would then be known as *osteochondral complexes*.

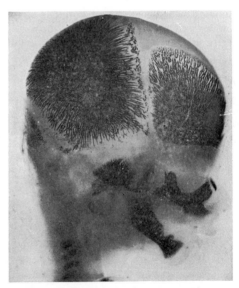

FIGURE 6-14 Head of a human embryo of $3\frac{1}{2}$ months' gestation. Stained with alizarin and cleared to reveal the trabeculae radiating from the centers of intramembranous ossification in the frontal and parietal bones. ×1.5.

BASIC STRUCTURAL COMPONENTS

Mesenchymal Bones

Mesenchymal bones arise at ossification centers (Fig. 6-14). These are areas in which the loosely arranged mesenchymal cells of the embryo are seen to increase in number through a local acceleration of the mitotic rate. The new cells soon show a modified microscopic appearance: they become enlarged and their cytoplasm shows an affinity for the basic dyes. Soon they will line up in single or double rows and as a result of a newly acquired secretory activity, a layer of modified intercellular substance will appear (Fig. 6-15).

BONE MATRIX New matrix called bone matrix contains densely arranged collagen fibers soon obliterated from the microscopic picture as they become embedded in amorphous ground substance rich in mucopolysaccharides. Also, mineral salts consisting mainly of a crystalline form of calcium phosphate known as hydroxyapatite almost immediately precipitate into the newly formed bone matrix.

The early bone histologists (Pommer, 1885) used to describe a zone of nonmineralized matrix, which they called osteoid, at the border of the bone matrix. Using the silver nitrate method of von Kossa to demonstrate microscopically the bone minerals, McLean and Bloom (1940), concluded that "the matrix may be

regarded as calcifiable as soon as the tissue is recognizable as bone." Current observations with the electron microscope have shown, on the other hand, that "there is a thin layer of $1\,\mu$ or less of uncalcified preosseous tissue, during the formation of bone even in animals with an optimum intake of minerals" (McLean and Urist, 1968).

OSTEOBLASTS The cells with the new osteogenic potential are called osteoblasts. These highly basophilic elements, closely apposed in an epithelial-like fashion (Fig. 6-15), show in the electron microscope a typical secretory development of the rough endoplasmic reticulum and the Golgi (Fig. 6-16). Sometimes large confluent vesicles are present at the apical pole of the cell (Fig. 6-16), which faces the new mineralized matrix.

OSTEOCYTES As subsequent rows of osteoblasts differentiate behind the original one, the new osteoblasts will start secreting and the cells of the first row will now be imprisoned in bone matrix which will segregate them generally as single cells in lacunae

FIGURE 6-15 Intramembranous bone formation in the maxilla of a cat fetus. Osteoblasts are aligned along a trabeculum of new bone. ×1200. (Noridez and Windle.)

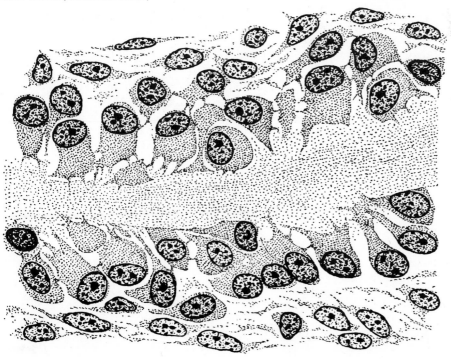

(Fig. 6-17), as was the case for cartilage. However, here there are two major differences. (1) The imprisoned cells, now called *osteocytes,* will rarely divide, so that growth of bone will be strictly by the appositional process. (2) The osteocytes will not be isolated in their lacunae. Through a large number of processes they will remain in close membrane contact with adjacent osteocytes and with the surface osteoblasts. The processes under normal conditions maintain their integrity inside channels known as canaliculi (Fig. 6-19).

In electron micrographs young osteocytes resemble osteoblasts. However, a gradual decrease in the amount of endoplasmic reticulum and a diminution in the size of the Golgi complex occurs (Jande and Bélanger, 1973) (Fig. 6-20). Fine filamentous processes appear under the plasma membrane. These extend into the processes, where they become the main constituents (Fig. 6-20). A few membrane-bound dark bodies also appear in the young osteocytes.

These are probably lysosomes; they will be discussed later. The pericellular space separating the plasma membrane of the osteocyte from the border of the lacuna is quite small at first (Fig. 6-20).

The processes of the osteocytes form a vast network of apparently branching individual units (Fig. 6-18), traveling inside matrix spaces called *canaliculi.* The processes of adjacent osteocytes are joined over an extended portion of their length by a structured organization which has been described as either a gap or a tight junction (Fig. 6-19). Eventually some of these processes reach out to the periphery of the nutritive spaces (Fig. 6-18), where presumably they all meet with the processes of lining osteoblasts, thus completing the vital network of the tissue.

TRABECULAE As more rows of primitive cells differentiate into osteoblasts and new bone is laid

FIGURE 6-16 Electron micrograph showing an osteoblast (B) immediately adjacent to the bone surface. Development of rough ER and Golgi is great compared with that in undifferentiated cells above. Almost no unmineralized bone is visible. ×6000. (Courtesy of Dr. Stephen B. Doty.)

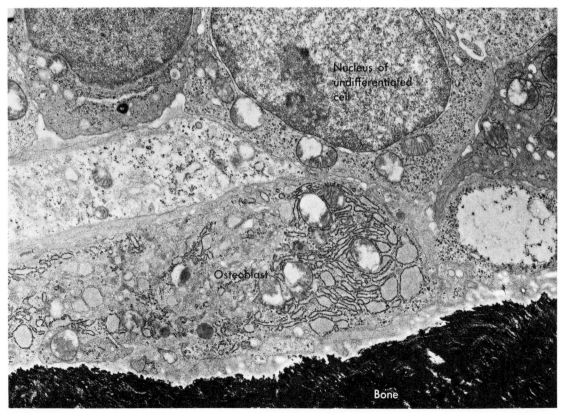

Nucleus of undifferentiated cell

Osteoblast

Bone

down, the new tissue will not grow into a uniform mass like cartilage, but spiderlike threads will radiate away from the centers of ossification (Fig. 6-14). These bone threads are called *trabeculae*. They are the units of mesenchymal or membranous bone.

BLOOD VESSELS A very interesting observation was made by Harris and Ham (1956) in their study of fracture repair and the conditions which made bone transplants viable. It had been known for some time that bone grafting, even in autotransplants, was a far more hazardous affair than cartilage transplantation. One important factor was the more critical requirement for blood circulation. As new layers of bone are being added to preexisting surfaces, "this must be accomplished . . . so that no bone cell is removed more than a fraction of a millimeter from a capillary" (Harris and Ham, 1956). In his textbook, Ham (1974) emphasizes this point: "In the experience of the author, trabeculae of more than one fifth of a millimeter

in thickness generally have blood vessels disposed in canals near their middles to provide the more deeply disposed bone cells with nourishment. Accordingly the thickness of solid trabeculae is limited."

OSTEOCLASTS When the growing trabeculae reach a critical thickness, when there is a need for the bone unit to adopt a special form in order to conform to regional requirements, or if something happens to the nutritional supply or to the regulating agents so that abnormal bone formation occurs, a new type of cell will enter the scene. This new cell will always appear at the periphery of the trabecula. Generally it will be located next to the bone surface itself. It is sometimes found half buried in indentations known as Howship's lacunae (Figs. 6-17 and 6-21). It is easily distinguished from adjacent osteoblasts or preosteoblasts: it is several times larger than these and contains several nuclei (Figs. 6-17 and 6-21). The cytoplasm of these multinucleated cells stains with either the basic

FIGURE 6-17 Osteoclasts. The large one is in a Howship's lacuna, on a trabeculum of fetal jawbone. Osteoblasts, osteocytes, osteoclasts, fetal jawbone. ×1200. (Nonidez and Windle.)

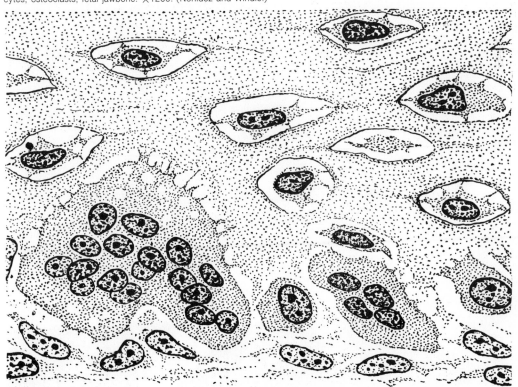

or the acid dyes, sometimes with both. On the surface which touches the bone, a *ruffled border* is seen; underneath it, the cytoplasm is frothy as if intense gas bubbling were occurring. The bone surface of the Howship's lacuna is also modified. It often shows patches of lower density in microradiographs. It is not surprising that Kölliker (1873) from the very beginning considered these cells as bone-destroying rather than bone-building elements and called them Ostoklast, which later became osteoclast, the bone-eating cell.

In recent times, electron microscopists have confirmed the classic status of these bone-eaters. The ruffled border was shown to be constituted by microvilli (Fig. 6-22A and B).

The intimate mechanism of osteoclastic resorption has recently been investigated by Bonucci (1974). Free crystals have been found between the ruffled border of the osteoclast and the bone matrix and even within the channels of the ruffled border (Fig. 6-22B).

They have apparently been produced by the breakdown of the calcified matrix. It seems that these crystals do not undergo great changes until they are taken up by the cell where they are gradually solubilized in the segregated medium of the cytoplasmic vacuoles (Fig. 6-22A).

Radioautography of a DNA precursor, [³H] thymidine, has revealed that a flow of new nuclei enters constantly into these cells as older nuclei degenerate (Bélanger and Migicovsky, 1963; Bélanger and Drouin, 1968). The new nuclei are apparently contributed by adjacent primitive cells which fuse with the osteoclasts. Once inside the osteoclast, the nuclei seldom divide but have a limited life-span of only a few days (Bélanger and Drouin, 1968), whereas the large multinucleated cells, capable of renewing their nuclei, seem to enjoy a very long life.

FIGURE 6-18 The osteocyte network as drawn by Virchow (1856). Cellular interconnections and the relationship between osteocytes and osteoblasts located in the osteonic canals (O.C.) were not recognized at that time, although the microscopy of these early days of histology was very thorough. (Courtesy Wild of Canada Ltd.)

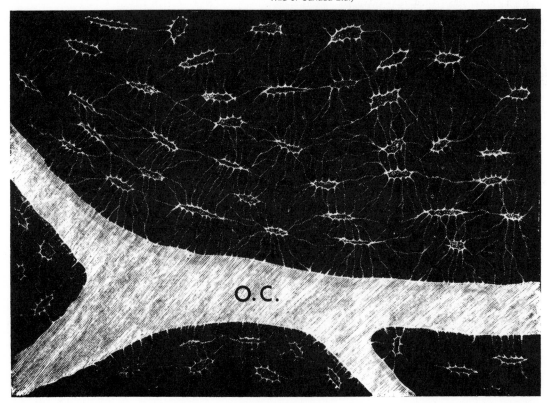

CANCELLOUS BONE, MARROW SPACES

Mesenchymal bone or trabecular bone is the original form of bone in the embryo. When considered as a tissue, it constitutes what is referred in anatomy textbooks as *cancellous,* or *spongy, bone.* This type of bone tissue represents the aggregate of mesenchymal bone even in adult life. In the more numerous osteochondral complexes which are the long bones, the trabecular, cancellous type of bone will represent a general embryonic condition. As the more adult type, known as *compact bone,* develops, the cancellous trabeculae will persist within the deeper regions of the

extremities (Fig. 6-23). In fresh preparations, these trabeculae are easily recognized by the honeycomb, spongy appearance of the bone and by the intense red color of the tissue in between. In the early days of cancellous bone, this new tissue seems to have an inducing influence on the immediately adjacent mesenchyme. In the highly protected little locular spaces between the branching trabeculae, the hematopoietic marrow will differentiate. The spaces then become known as *primary marrow spaces.* Cancellous bone will retain its hematopoietic red marrow throughout life.

FIGURE 6-19 Electron micrograph of an undemineralized section showing a canaliculus containing two overlapping osteocyte processes connected by a trilaminar tight junction, ×120,000. (Courtesy Dr. Randi Furseth.)

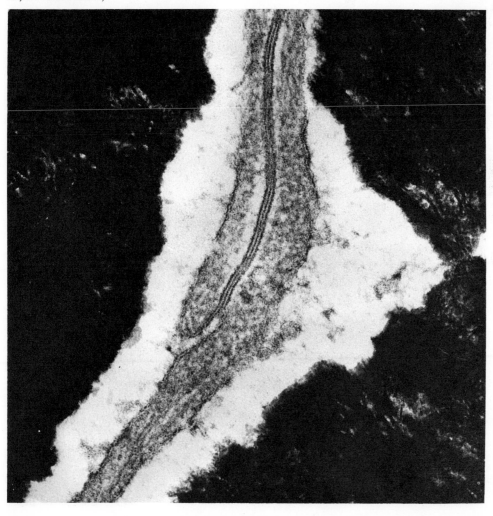

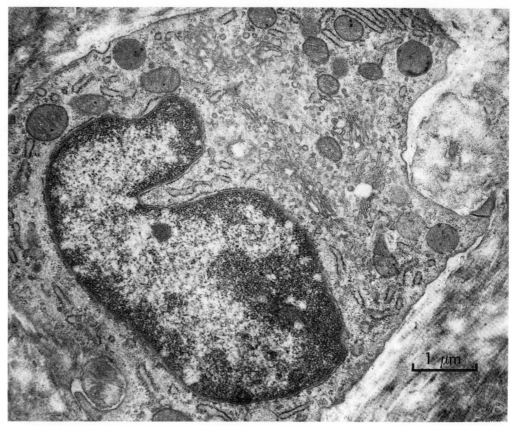

FIGURE 6-20 A young osteocyte showing endoplasmic reticulum, the Golgi complex, and lysosomes.

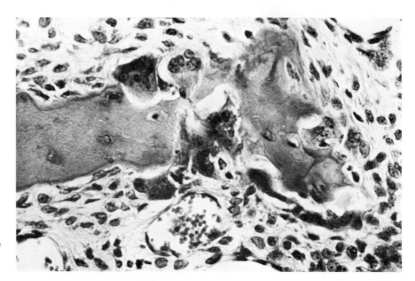

FIGURE 6-21 A portion of a trabecula from the jawbone of a horse which has been fed an exaggerated amount of phosphate for 30 weeks. The newly formed bone is fibrillar and poorly mineralized. The trabeculae are surrounded by a large number of osteoclasts. Wright stain. ×360.

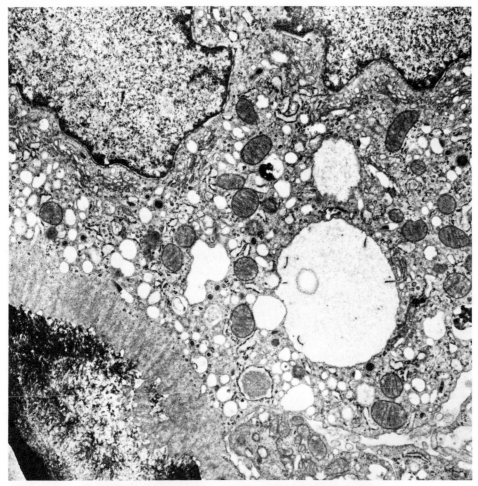

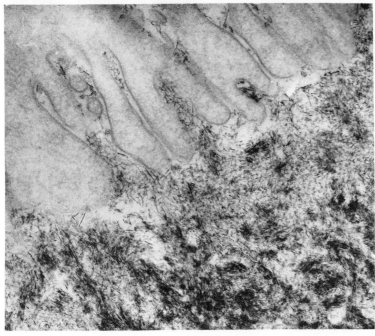

FIGURE 6-22 Top: Electron micrograph of a portion of an osteoclast showing the brush border (B) and a variety of intracellular constituents, such as vacuoles (V), lysosomes (L), mitochondria (M), the Golgi (G), and portions of the nucleus (N). ×6000. Bottom: Detail of the resorption zone and ruffled border of an osteoblast. The zone of resorption consists of loosened crystals distributed at random. Many are contained within channels of the ruffled border. Between the crystals, a granular and amorphous material can be seen. Unstained electron micrograph, ×96,000. (Courtesy Dr. E. Bonucci.)

PERIOSTEUM As each unit of mesenchymal bone becomes constituted and takes shape, as with the pieces of cartilage previously described, it becomes surrounded by a distinct membrane, the *periosteum.* Histologically it is possible to distinguish two regions in the periosteum, especially during the period of growth of the bone: an *outer portion,* made of tough, fibrous tissue; and an *inner region,* called the *cambium,* more loosely arranged and better vascularized, from which the bone-forming osteoblasts will differentiate.

THE OSTEOCHONDRAL COMPLEXES All the bones of the body are of mesenchymal origin. Nevertheless, most bones will develop around and eventually within a cartilage primordium. In some rare instances, as in the case of Meckel's cartilage of the lower jaw, the new tissue will completely replace the preexisting cartilage piece. In the majority of cases, the osseous tissue will replace the cartilage *only in part—* thus the term *osteochondral complex,* which is now

proposed for this variety, classically known as *endochondral bone.*

Ossification of the cartilage primordium begins very early. For instance, the human femur begins to ossify when the embryo is only 7 weeks old and 17 mm long. The general shape of the early embryonic femur closely resembles that of the adult. Its main features are the two extremities, the proximal and distal *epiphyses,* and the elongated, roughly cylindrical midpiece, the *diaphysis.*

The Diaphyseal Phase

PERICHONDRAL OSSIFICATION The cartilage primordium belongs to the hyaline variety. Although wider, the epiphyseal portions do not grow at the same rate as does the diaphyseal portion. In the latter, the newly formed cells align themselves in rows between which only a small amount of matrix forms (Fig. 6-24A). The first mature chondrocytes occupy the mid-diaphysis. They will rapidly degenerate (Fig. 6-22B),

FIGURE 6-23 Section of the upper end of the human femur and x-ray picture (right) showing weak area of neck. (Courtesy of Dr. William J. Tobin.)

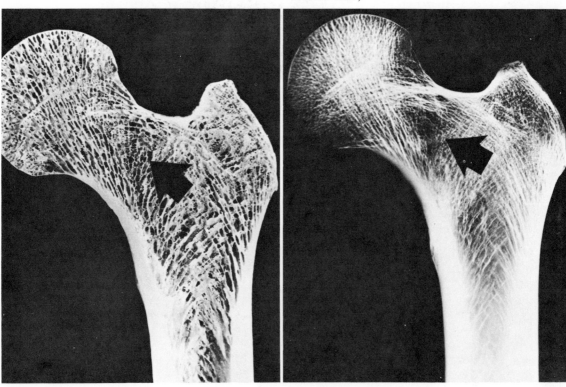

and the adjacent matrix will become mineralized. At this moment, the surrounding perichondrium changes its potential: from chondrogenic, it becomes osteogenic.

The initial bone deposition will be in the form of a *middiaphyseal ring* surrounding the area of cartilage degeneration and calcification. Some years ago, Lacroix (1949) postulated an induction effect from the modified cartilage in the form of a secretory product ("osteogenin") capable of influencing the perichondrial cells (or for that matter, connective tissue cells anywhere in the body) so that they would be programmed toward manufacturing bone. Further work has failed to reveal a specific inducer; it seems that a variety of chemical substances can trigger the phenomenon of bone growth. However, after an experimental program dating from 1965, Urist has shown that many of the tissues capable of bone induction—

calcified cartilage, bone, dentin—contained a substance now called bone morphogenetic protein (BMP) (Urist, 1973; Urist, Mikulski, and Boyd, 1975) and that lathyric bone in which collagen is poorly cross-linked and readily solubilized did not possess morphogenetic properties.

SUBEPIPHYSEAL BONE GROWTH As the initial peripheral bone ring enlarges by further perichondrial-periosteal conversion toward the epiphyses (Fig. 6-24C), the cartilage inside seems to accelerate its degeneration (Fig. 6-24C). Blood vessels (Fig. 6-24C and D) will invade the spaces created by the cartilage breakdown and will colonize the inner portion of the degenerating primordium, stretching their network

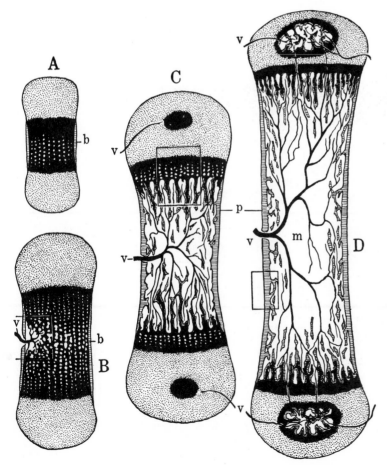

FIGURE 6-24 Diagrams of the ossification of a long bone. A. Early cartilaginous stage. B. Stage of eruption of the periosteal bone collar by an osteogenic bud of vessels. C. Older stage with a primary marrow cavity and early centers of calcification in the epiphyseal cartilages. D. The condition shortly after birth with epiphyseal centers of ossification. Calcified cartilage in all diagrams is black; b, periosteal bone collar; m, marrow cavity; p, periosteal bone; v, blood vessels entering the centers of ossification. (Nonidez and Windle.)

until they reach the subepiphyseal area where accompanying cells will turn into osteoblasts and lay down bone onto calcified remnants of cartilage matrix. The result will be a subepiphyseal bone colony in which the units will be linear, fragile, pencil-like outgrowths known as *spicules,* consisting of a small layer of bone investing an acellular, calcified cartilage core (Fig. 6-24C and D). While this subepiphyseal colony is being established, the peripheral periosteal growth continues (Fig. 6-24C and D). Since growth has originated at the middiaphysis, it is not surprising to find that the bone is thickest in that area, tapering down to the epiphyseal limits where a circular depressed area (notch of Ranvier) marks the zone of transition.

In normal vertebrate bones, the length of the subepiphyseal spicules and the thickness of the periosteal bone are constantly kept in check by osteoclasts which appear in the *central cavity.* This cavity, like the primary marrow spaces, will soon become filled with hematopoietic and adipose-rich *marrow* (Fig. 6-24D, m).

EPIPHYSEAL BONE CENTERS; ARTICULAR CARTILAGE; EPIPHYSEAL PLATE

The next major step in the establishment of a long bone is the development within the epiphyses of one or more ossification centers. This phenomenon is marked by the development of blood vessels which will occasionally penetrate the epiphyseal cartilage radiating toward its center (Fig. 6-24C and D, v). These apparently, hasten the degeneration and calcification of cartilage which precedes bone formation (Fig. 6-24C and D).

The epiphyseal bone centers will undergo limited growth only. Throughout life, in most instances, a cartilage vault will persist over this bone-marrow center and will take part in the mobile relationship with adjacent bone units; this permanent feature of the bone head is the *articular cartilage.*

FIGURE 6-25 A. Radioautograph of the head of the tibia of a young growing rat killed a few hours after injection of ^{32}P. The blackened areas of the photographic emulsion reveal the location of the radioactive phosphorus in the underlying section of the bone. The phosphorus is incorporated at the sites of active bone deposition. (Radioautograph by C. P. Leblond, G. W. Wilkinson, L. F. Bélanger, and J. Robichon, reproduced from a review by J. Gross et al., *Am. J. Roentgenol.,* **65:**443, 1951). B. Diagram interpreting the radioautograph. Black areas indicating the sites of incorporation of ^{32}P are found overlying the zone of provisional calcification in the epiphyseal cartilage, the trabeculae of the metaphysis, the endosteal surface of the conical portion, and the periosteal surface of the cylindrical portion of the shaft.
C. Diagram showing distribution of the radioisotope in the tibia of an animal killed several days after injection of ^{32}P. As a result of growth subsequent to the injection, the reactive material is now found in trabeculae well below the epiphyseal cartilage and in the interior of the compacta in the shaft. (B and C, after C. P. Leblond, G. W. Wilkinson, L. F. Bélanger, and J. Robichon, *Am. J. Anat.,* **86:**289, 1950).

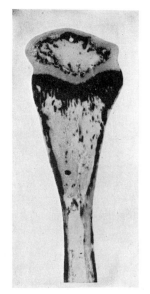

A

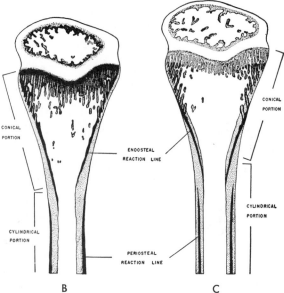

B

C

Underneath the epiphyseal bone center, cartilage will also remain, separating the epiphyseal bone colony. This cartilaginous disc is the *epiphyseal plate* (Fig. 6-24D; also Figs. 6-12 to 6-14). The epiphyseal plate will persist until the adult length for each individual bone has been reached. In the human species, the life-span of the epiphyseal plate is, on the average, 3 years shorter for the female than for the male. In the male, most of the plates have disappeared by the twentieth year.

THE METAPHYSIS: ENDOSTEAL BONE GROWTH

In the bony fishes and the amphibians, only periosteal bone develops. When a long bone of these early vertebrates is boiled and all organic matter is destroyed, a hollow, diaphyseal cylinder is the only thing that remains. In reptiles, birds, and mammals, the diaphyseal cylindrical shaft is united to the much wider epiphysis by a tapered conical portion (Fig. 6-25) known as the *metaphysis*. This strong and graceful additional supporting structure, akin to the capitals of columns in architecture, was developed at a time when the body lost the buoyancy of its original aquatic environment as the reptiles became the conquerors of the earth.

The metaphysis appears late in the embryo as it does in the history of bone. It grows through the establishment of an osteoblastic colony, probably originating from the subepiphyseal center. However, as

this *endosteal* colony has to cope with the problem of maintaining a relationship between a slowly expanding diaphysis and a rapidly enlarging epiphysis, metaphyseal growth must occur according to a *gradient* progressively accelerated toward the epiphysis. That this is actually the case has been demonstrated by radioautography (Leblond et al., 1950) (Fig. 6-25).

THE EPIPHYSEAL PLATE The role of the epiphyseal plate in controlling growth in length was recognized early in the eighteenth century by Hales (1727) and by Duhamel (1743a) through simple experiments in which metal implants above and below the plate of young animals became progressively separated, while two implants, both located below the plate, retained a constant relationship. Duhamel (1743b) apparently also recognized the mechanism of peripheral accretion as responsible for the increase in diaphyseal thickness. This observation was the result of intermittent feeding of madder, a plant which contains a red coloring agent that attaches itself to newly formed bone. Thus, red rings alternating with white and originating at the periosteal surface marked the period of madder-labeling in the growing bones. *Intravital color labeling* is still widely used in contemporary bone investigation. In the nineteenth century, intersti-

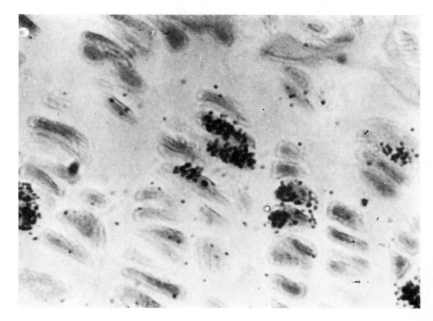

FIGURE 6-26 Radioautograph of [³H]thymidine incorporation into some of the cells of the proliferating zone of the epiphyseal plate of the tibia of a young rat. ×370.

tial metal implants were employed by John Hunter to demonstrate that interstitial growth does not exist in bone.

A variety of growth mechanisms have been observed in recent time by the use of x-ray (Fig. 6-23), a method which still yields considerable information in the case of individual children about their skeletal response to nutritional, hormonal, genetic, climatic, and even economic factors (Harris, 1933; Lacroix, 1949).

Endosteal accretion in the metaphysis and the existence of the growth gradient at that level have been revealed by *radioautography* of labeled bone precursors (Leblond et al., 1950) (Fig. 6-25).

Recently, alizarin, the bone-coloring substance extracted from the madder plant, has been found to fluoresce brightly in ultraviolet light. Other substances, such as antibiotic cyclines, porphyrin, and carotenoids, have the same property and have been utilized for bone labeling. Krook et al. (1970), using a triple *fluorochrome label* in dogs, have recently mapped the transit of the variously colored fluorescent lines in long bones of dogs over a period of 41 weeks. Such studies have led the authors to conclude "that these tissues are in a state of constant flow."

In the functional epiphyseal plate responsible for the growth in length of the osteochondral complex, four zones are described, extending from the epiphyseal side toward the subepiphyseal ossifying portion.

Zone of resting or reserve cartilage   These cells (Fig. 6-

FIGURE 6-27 Epiphyseal cartilage of a rat's tibia stained for alkaline phosphatase. Only traces of activity are found in the zone of proliferation, but a strong reaction occurs in the zone of calcification and in the osteoblasts covering the trabeculae of the metaphysis. Gomori method glycerophosphate substrate. ×200. (Courtesy of R. O. Greep.)

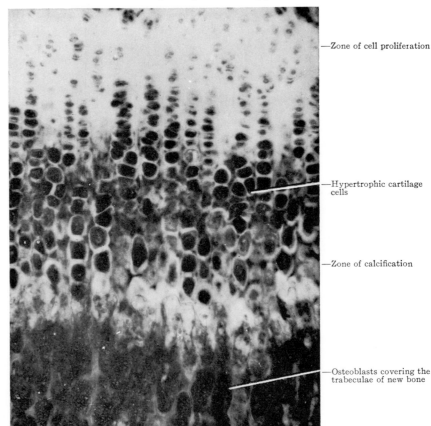

—Zone of cell proliferation

—Hypertrophic cartilage cells

—Zone of calcification

—Osteoblasts covering the trabeculae of new bone

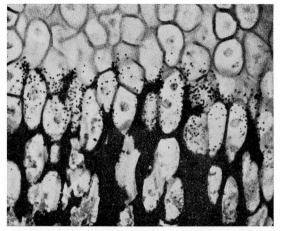

FIGURE 6-28 Section through the zone of calcification in the epiphyseal cartilage at the proximal end of the tibia of a 28-day-old normal rat. The granular deposits of bone salts are stained black. Undecalcified section; silver nitrate-hematoxylin-eosin. ×295. (F. McLean and W. Bloom, *Anat. Rec.*, **78:**357, 1940).

11A) consist of only a few rows of small cells, mostly immature and evenly distributed in the intercellular matrix.

Zone of young proliferating cartilage   The cells in this zone are bunched in linear piles like coins (Fig. 6-11B). In spite of the known function of this zone, mitotic figures are rare in routinely prepared specimens. However, when a DNA tracer such as [³H]-thymidine has been administered, radioactive, newly synthesized DNA, mostly located in the first few rows of cells in this zone, is revealed by radioautography (Fig. 6-26).

Zone of maturing cartilage   This area is thinner than the former one; the cells are larger (Fig. 6-11C), and they secrete and accumulate carbohydrates and lipids; they show a strong alkaline phosphatase activity (Fig. 6-27).

Zone of calcifying cartilage   This zone contains mainly degenerating and dead chondrocytes (Fig. 6-11D). The lacunae are considerably enlarged and the thin intercellular bands of matrix are calcified as demonstrated by the von Kossa procedure, whereby calcium phosphate is transformed into a silver phosphate from which a black silver precipitate is obtained by treatment with a reducing agent (Fig. 6-28).

SIGNIFICANCE AND FATE OF THE EPIPHYSEAL PLATE   Comparisons between bone radiographs taken at two successive periods of growth indicate clearly that with time the epiphyseal plate is displaced in relation to the diaphysis (Fig. 6-29). The distance between the two positions indicates the growth in length. It is also evident that in the meantime

the metaphysis has undergone a complex remodeling (Fig. 6-29) as the result of the teamwork of the bone-forming and bone-destroying cells.

The significance of the spicules hanging like stalactites from the epiphyseal plate is at first mysterious. However, comparative histology has revealed that in female birds these spicules grow to fill the entire marrow cavity (medullary bone) at the time when the large mineralized eggs are produced.

BLOOD VESSELS AND NERVES

The main artery—the *medullary*, or nutrient, artery—reaches the marrow cavity from the periosteum. It is accompanied by one or two veins. The branches of these vessels distribute themselves proximally and distally to reach all the nutritive spaces in the bone.

Little is known about lymphatics, but they have

FIGURE 6-29 Superimposed tracings of two radiographs of the tibial head taken 1 year apart. The epiphysis has become displaced upward by growth. The underlying metaphysis has undergone remodeling as indicated by the stippled areas. (Courtesy of Dr. Pierre Lacroix and Masson & Cie.)

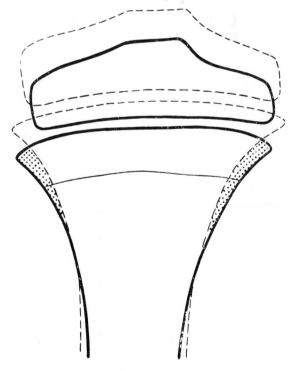

been seen accompanying the larger blood vessels (Goss, 1959). Recently, channels that were in striking contrast to the blood capillaries have been observed by Cooper (1972) in about 3 percent of the osteonic canals of immature dogs (Fig. 6-30). These are presumably the first intraosseous lymphatic capillaries reported. There was already indirect evidence of the existence of a lymphatic circulation in bone. "India ink injected into the peritoneal cavity can be traced across small cortical channels to the endosteal surface of

bone. Three or four percent of bone sarcomas metastasize to regional lymph nodes" (Cooper, 1972).

Nerves are abundant in the periosteum. Unmyelinated branches located in the depth of the small nutritive spaces have been observed recently through the electron microscope (Cooper et al., 1966).

FIGURE 6-30 An osteonic canal from the midfemoral shaft of an immature dog showing in the upper-right-hand corner a portion of a capillary wall with typical endothelial cells and surrounding basement membrane. The large channel in the center, presumably a lymphatic vessel, does not have a basement membrane and the fluid in its lumen consists only of precipitated protein. C, blood capillary; L, lymphatic capillary. ×10,000. (Courtesy of Dr. Reginald R. Cooper.)

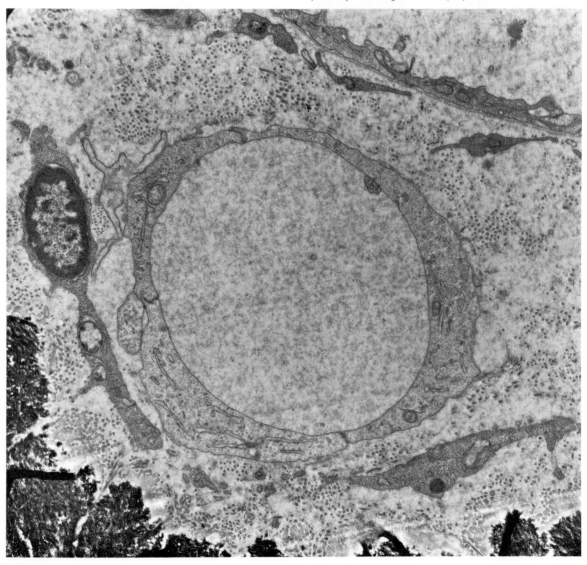

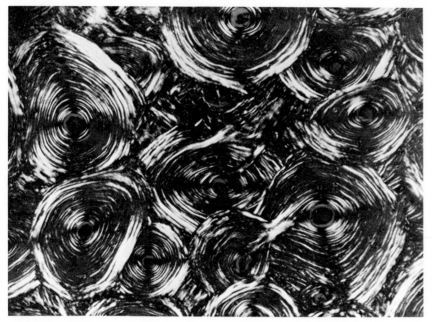

FIGURE 6-31 A portion of a nondemineralized cross section of the humeral diaphysis of a horse, photographed in polarized light. ×130. (Courtesy of Dr. Lennart Krook.)

COMPACT BONE: GROWTH AND REMODELING

As organisms have grown bigger and heavier, new stresses and strains have occurred in the bones, necessitating increased support. This need has apparently been met by the transformation of trabecular, spongy bone into compact bone (Amprino, 1965). As this operation begins in the young bone, a large number of osteoblasts appear in the nutritive spaces. These cells deposit at the border of the space concentric rings of new bone (lamellae) separated by narrow bands of less mineralized interlamellar substance. This operation continues until the nutritive space reaches a critical diameter of approximately 20 μm and then the growth ceases. The unit of the new compact bone is called an *osteon* (Figs. 6-31 and 6-32). The small, remaining nutritive space is now an *osteonic canal* (Figs. 6-31 and 6-32).

The original osteons are known as *primary oste-

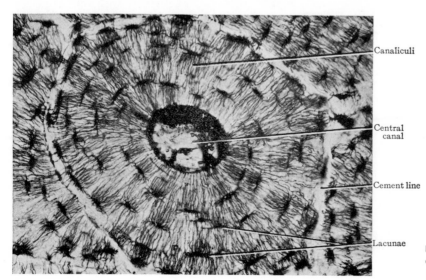

Canaliculi

Central canal

Cement line

Lacunae

FIGURE 6-32 Ground cross section of typical osteon of human femur. ×225.

ons. Since their nutritional support is apparently critical, some of this bone becomes necrotic. Nature responds by initiating *remodeling.*

According to Currey (1968), remodeling begins in areas of the osteons in which a considerable number of osteocytes are "in a bad way." Remodeling tunnels are filled with osteoclasts followed by blood vessels and connective tissue cells. These soon differentiate into osteoblasts that lay down new concentric lamellae, which constitute a group of *secondary osteons.* The remnants of the primary osteons are now represented by the filling substance between the secondary osteons and are described as *interstitial lamellae* (Fig. 6-31). Several successive orders of smaller and smaller osteons are thus formed until the bone acquires adequate strength. Then the growth of compact bone, dealing only with normal turnover, becomes very slow. Frost (1963) states that whereas remodeling is of the order of 200 percent per year in young children, this rate falls to 1 percent in the adult.

RESORPTION CAVITIES: OSTEOPOROSIS

In older people, a variety of conditions such as negative salt balance, sex hormone deficiency, hypercorticoadrenalism, thyrotoxicosis, or simply prolonged immobilization may cause an increased amount of bone resorption. In compact bone, this phenomenon is marked by the appearance of local resorption cavities (Fig. 6-33) and an overall remodeling resulting in a thinner diaphyseal cortex and a progressively enlarged marrow cavity (Duncan and Jaworski, 1970).

FIGURE 6-33 Microradiograph of a 200-μm-thick cross section of bone from a normal 19-year-old male. Secondary Haversian bone is actively replacing non-Haversian bone, which is seen on the periosteal (upper) surface. New low-density bone in Haversian systems appears gray, whereas high-density bone appears white and is seen largely in interstitial areas. ×57. (Courtesy of Dr. Jenifer Jowsey.)

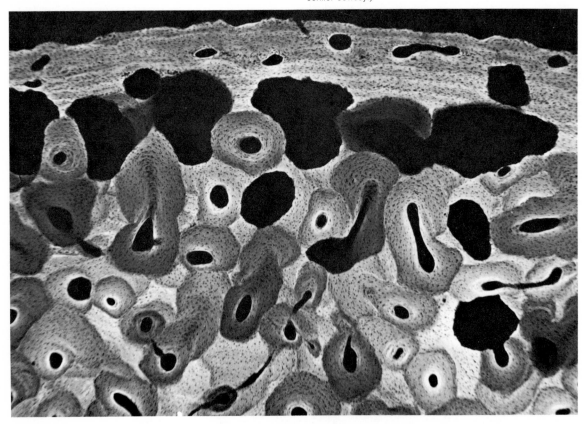

This phenomenon is clinically described as *osteoporosis.*

The early clinical diagnosis of osteoporosis is difficult because approximately 30 percent of bone mineral has to have been lost before it can be detected radiologically (Riggs et al., 1973). This disorder is not an inevitable accompaniment of the aging process. A recent study of elderly people has shown that 22 percent of women and 38 percent of men failed to lose bone over a period of 11 to 15 years (Adams et al., 1970).

THE LIFE CYCLE OF THE OSTEOCYTES; OSTEOCYTIC OSTEOLYSIS

The original observations of Baud (1962) and Bélanger et al., (1963) concerning the three phases in the life of the osteocytes and the phenomenon of *osteocytic osteolysis* have been confirmed in recent time by many investigators using a variety of procedures, such as alpharadiography (Bélanger and Rasmussen, 1968, Fig. 6-34), microroentgenography (Duriez and Flautre, 1973a, 1975; Duriez, 1974, Heuck, 1966, 1973, 1974; Remagen, 1973), bone densitometry (Henrikson and Wallenius, 1974; Krook et al., 1971; Whalen et al., 1973), differential osteocyte counts (Krempien et al., 1973), lacunar measurements (Baylink et al., 1973; Duriez and Flautre, 1973; Duriez, 1974; Liu et al., 1974; Meunier et al., 1971a, 1971b; Porte et al., 1972) and electron microscopy (Jande and Bélanger, 1973; Schulz et al.,

1973; Luk et al., 1974; Bonucci, 1975). The three phases have been recorded in the tibial diaphysis of young chicks and are illustrated in Fig. 6-35 and briefly described by Jande and Bélanger (1973) as follows:

In A, the young osteocyte is in the *formative phase.* It has the organelles related to bone matrix synthesis and secretion (endoplasmic reticulum and the associated ribosomes, Golgi complex, and mitochondria). The pericellular space (PCS) is occupied by a primary matrix (osteoid) formed by this cell.

In B, the osteocyte has attained its *resorptive phase,* characterized by the appearance of many lysosomes and by the decrease of the other organelles. The space surrounding the cell is now occupied by a flocculent material (FM), which is a breakdown product of the primary matrix. Peripherally, the mineralized interlacunar matrix (Fig. 6-36A, ILM) has been modified by the proteolytic activity of the cell (modified matrix, MM) and has lost some of its minerals.

In C, the osteocyte has reached senescence and shows signs of *degeneration* (vacuolization of the nuclear envelope, cytoplasm, mitochondria, and Golgi complex).

When resorption cavities such as those in Fig. 6-34 are examined under high power, their border often shows a characteristic pattern of enlarged and confluent lacunae (Fig. 6-37), the result of osteocytic osteolysis. The osteoclasts also frequently seen along

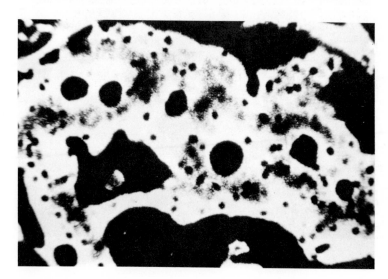

FIGURE 6-34 A portion of a cross section of the metaphysis of the tibia of a young rat. Several areas of osteocytic osteolysis show enlarged confluent lacunae surrounded by low-density matrix. Alpharadiograph. ×120.

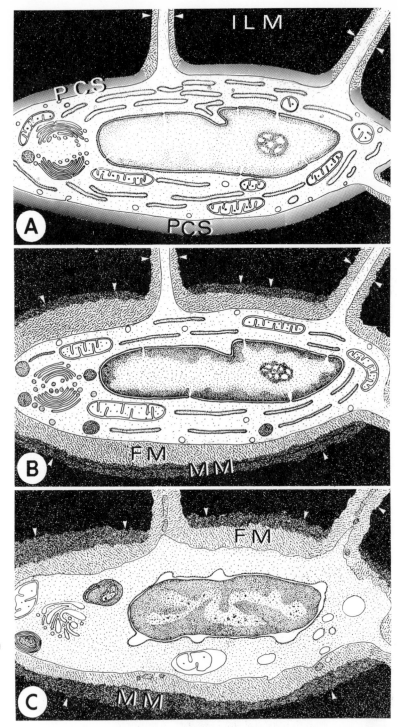

FIGURE 6-35 Schematic representation of three osteocytes seen in a cross section of the tibia of a young chick, from the periosteal surface inwards. A. Osteocyte in the formative phase. B. Osteocyte in the resorptive phase. C. Osteocyte in the degenerative phase. (Courtesy Dr. S. S. Jande.)

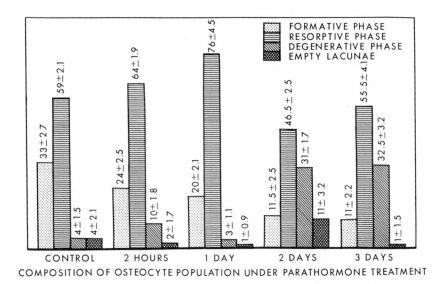

Bars in chart labeled:
FORMATIVE PHASE
RESORPTIVE PHASE
DEGENERATIVE PHASE
EMPTY LACUNAE

CONTROL: 33 ± 2.7, 59 ± 2.1, 4 ± 1.5, 4 ± 2.1

2 HOURS: 24 ± 2.5, 64 ± 1.9, 10 ± 1.8, 2 ± 1.7

1 DAY: 20 ± 2.1, 76 ± 4.5, 3 ± 1.1, 1 ± 0.9

2 DAYS: 11.5 ± 2.5, 46.5 ± 2.5, 31 ± 1.7, 11 ± 3.2

3 DAYS: 11 ± 2.2, 55.5 ± 4.1, 32.5 ± 3.2, 1 ± 1.5

COMPOSITION OF OSTEOCYTE POPULATION UNDER PARATHORMONE TREATMENT

FIGURE 6-36 Composition of the osteocyte population and the effect of hyperparathyroidism.

the border of resorption cavities are probably generated by the presence of the devitalized and modified bone matrix remaining after the last stage of the osteocyte cycle.

Both aspects of bone resorption, osteocytic osteolysis and osteoclasia, are governed by the calcium-controlling hormones parathormone and calcitonin.

FIGURE 6-37 Alpharadiograph of a demineralized section showing a portion of the border of a resorption cavity in the tibia of a horse which had been fed a diet rich in phosphate for 30 weeks. Several enlarged and confluent lacunae are indicative of an increase in osteocytic osteolysis preceding osteoclasia. ×370 (Courtesy of Dr. Lennart Krook.)

The relative composition of the osteocyte population in the tibial diaphysis of a young chick is illustrated in Fig. 6-36 (controls). As early as 2 h after the initiation of parathyroid treatment, the number of cells in the resorptive phase rose to a peak which is reached at 24 h. The second and third day after treatment showed a decline of this effect but an increase in the number of degenerating cells. Thus, osteocytic osteolysis is stimulated early and the cells are more rapidly worn out by their increased activity.

Bélanger and Rasmussen (1968) and more recently Bélanger and Copp (1972) and also Duriez and

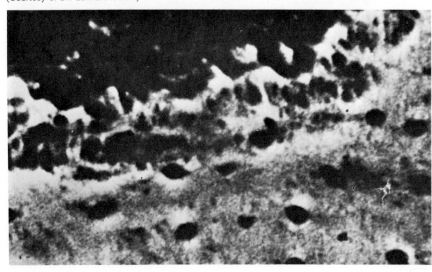

Flautre (1973a,b) have established that *calcitonin* inhibits the effect of parathyroid hormone on osteocytic osteolysis. Others such as Kallio et al. (1972) have shown a rapid morphological effect on the osteoclasts.

In a form of bone pathology known as Paget's disease, lines well stained by the penodic acid Schiff reaction and other stains for mucopolysaccharides form a typical pattern (Fig. 6-38A). These are known as *cementing lines*. It has been interesting to observe that in this disease, osteocytic osteolysis is also greatly increased (Bélanger et al., 1968) and much new bone is also being made in some places. In the latter areas, it appears that the cementing lines are remnants of modified matrix left over after the death of the osteocytes (Fig. 6-38B).

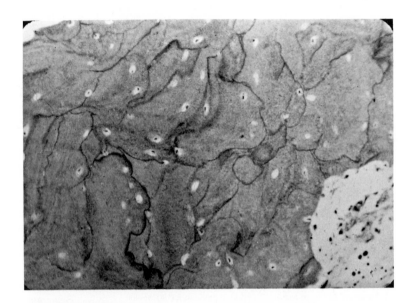

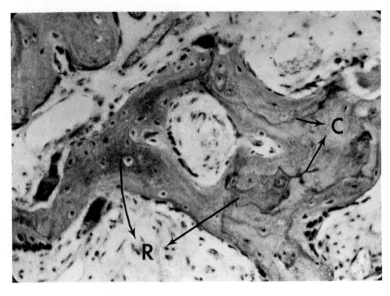

FIGURE 6-38 (Above). Typical mosaic pattern of cementing lines in advanced Paget's disease. Notice numerous empty lacunae. ×120. (Below). A portion of newly formed bone in the vicinity of the above: cementing lines (C) appear to be remnants of areas of osteolytic osteolysis (R). ×120.

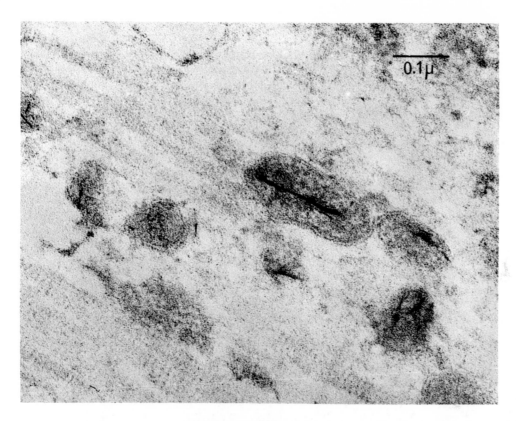

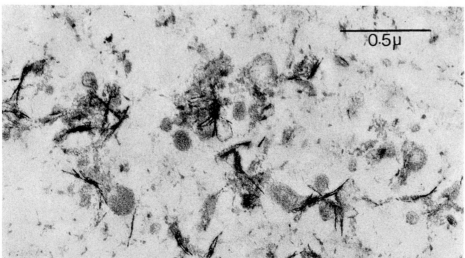

FIGURE 6-39 (Above). Matrix vesicles containing needlelike profiles of apatite in the osseous of 7-day chick femur, midshaft. The investing trilaminar membranes and the characteristic electron-dense homogeneous contents of matrix vesicles are quite clearly seen. Stained with lead only. ×152,000. (Courtesy Dr. H. Clark Anderson.) (Below). Upper calcifying zone of growth plate cartilage of weanling mouse tibia. With progressive normal mineralization, apatite accumulates at the surfaces of vesicles to form radial clusters of needles. Stained with lead and uranium. ×50,000. (Courtesy Dr. H. Clark Anderson.)

ULTRASTRUCTURAL EVENTS OF BONE MINERALIZATION

The events leading to mineral precipitation in the skeletal tissues and the factors favoring or inhibiting this phenomenon have been under intense scrutiny in recent times. A greater collaboration between morphologists, physiologists, and biochemists has led to considerable information. According to Hirschman and Dziewiatkowski (1966) "during or just preceding calcification, protein-polysaccharide or its protein component is lost or drastically altered." The relationship of collagen to mineralization is now known through the beautiful electron micrographs of Robin-son and Watson (1952), Jackson (1957), Glimcher et al., (1957) and Nylen et al., (1960): the crystals of hydroxyapatite in the form of little needles line themselves up along the collagen fibers, starting at the periodically repeated nodes.

The events preceding the collagen-crystal union and especially the contribution of the cartilage or bone-forming cells to mineralization have come to light through the discovery of the "calcification vesicles" (Anderson, 1967, 1969, 1973, 1975; Anderson and Reynolds, 1973; Bonucci, 1967; Ali et al., 1970). These matrix vesicles which have been seen near the cells possess a trilaminar border and oftentimes contain crystalline needles (Fig. 6-39A), closely resem-

FIGURE 6-40 Perifibrillar particles stained by ruthenium red, indicative of mucopolysaccharides (Courtesy of Drs. Reginald R. Cooper and Gerald Laros.)

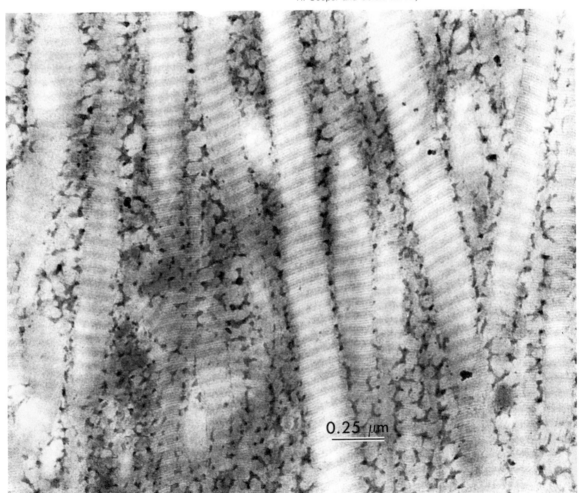

0.25 μm

bling hydroxyapatite crystals. Alkaline phosphatase is present, mostly as an exoenzyme in their immediate vicinity (Anderson, 1975). Crystalline needles have also been observed to form clusters in this extravesicular position (Fig. 6-39B) (Anderson, 1969).

The mechanism of transfer of the crystals to collagen is as yet unknown. The electron micrographs of Cooper and Laros (Fig. 6-40) indicate a potential role of mucopolysaccharides in this operation.

An intracellular phase of mineralization has also been postulated by several investigators: Kashiwa (1968) and Silberman and Frommer (1974) have shown histochemically, a concentration of calcium in

the osteoblasts. Talmage (1969) has produced evidence about the pumping activity of the cell system in the transit of cations. Baud (1962) and also Matthews et al., (1970) have revealed the presence of calcium salt in the mitochondria. The interrelationship between these interesting observations, have not yet been demonstrated. They have recently been summarized by Sayegh (1974) (Fig. 6-41) as a working hypothesis, in a discussion of the mineralization of deer antlers.

JOINTS

The site of union between two or more bones is called a *joint* or an *articulation*.

FIGURE 6-41 Schematic representation of the potential prevesicular events in mineralization. (Courtesy of Dr. F. S. Sayegh.)

SYNARTHROSES

Some of these joints which are quite rigid are called *synarthroses*. The inventory of the whole skeleton has revealed that the synarthroses represent a variety of histologic components: (1) The sutures of the skull

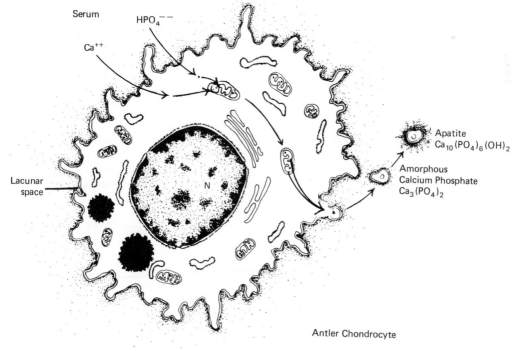

Serum

HPO_4^{--}

Ca^{++}

Lacunar space

N

Apatite $Ca_{10}(PO_4)_6(OH)_2$

Amorphous Calcium Phosphate $Ca_3(PO_4)_2$

Antler Chondrocyte

HYPOTHESIS
1. Extracellular Calcium concentration
2. Intracellular Calcium attraction
3. Calcium Phosphate formation in Mitochondria
4. Calcium Phosphate extrusion from Mitochondria

consist of dense fibrous tissue (Fig. 6-42) and are thus referred to as *syndesmoses.* (2) Between some of the bones of the face, cartilage is the unifying tissue. These pieces of cartilage, unlike the epiphyseal plate, show two or more calcifying surfaces. This type of joint is a *synchondrosis.* (3) When a synchondrosis eventually becomes completely ossified, it is then a *synostosis.* (4) In a few areas, such as between the mandibles or the pubic bones, the articulation consists of two plates of cartilage united by dense connective tissue. This type of joint is a *symphysis.* In certain species of mammals, there is considerable disparity between the size of the pelvic birth canal and the full-term fetus. In the free-tailed bat, the pelvic joint "stretches to more than 15 times its original length" (Crelin, 1969).

The *intervertebral disc* is a specialized type of symphysis. Between the cartilage plates covering adjacent vertebrae, the dense fibrous tissue encloses a space filled with semifluid material rich in hyaluronic acid. This is the *nucleus pulposus,* which provides increased resiliency for the spine and thus cushions the upper nerve centers against trauma. Ruptures of the intervertebral disc followed by herniation of the nucleus pulposus are common in this era of mechanized crafts of all sorts.

MOBILE JOINTS

Joints that allow great mobility of the bones are called *diarthroses.* They consist of a joint cavity, mobile surfaces and envelopes, the inner synovial membrane, and the outer protective components.

In the embryo, the *joint cavity* appears in an original *interzone* densely packed with mesenchymal cells (Fig. 6-43A). Early cleft formation is characterized by loosening of the cellular material in the interzone (Fig. 6-43B). This is followed by the appearance and coalescence of several *miniature spaces* (miniclefts, Fig. 6-43C). The end result is a single joint space (cavitation phase; Figs. 6-43D and 6-44). According to Drachman and Sokoloff (1966), the final modeling phase is dependent on skeletal muscle contractions occurring during the intrauterine life. A marked decrease in muscle activity would lead to fusion of the mobile joint (ankylosis) or deformity.

The *articular surfaces* of a diarthrosis consist of hyaline cartilage (Fig. 6-44) that normally persists throughout life. According to Mankin (1967), "there is

ample evidence" that this articular cartilage "differs considerably in basic structure, chemical composition and metabolism" from cartilage located elsewhere.

The articular surfaces decrease rapidly in thickness in young organisms, as shown by comparative studies of rabbits 2, 6, and 18 months old (Mankin, 1967). In the adult, four zones can be recognized in routine histologic preparations (Fig. 6-45): (1) at the surface, a narrow layer of flattened cells, called the gliding layer or *tangential zone;* (2) underneath, a *transitional zone* consisting of ovoid or rounded cells randomly distributed; (3) beneath this, cells arranged in short columns, the *radial zone;* followed by (4) the cone of calcified cartilage.

The articular cartilage matrix is 70 to 85 percent water. Collagen makes up 50 percent of the dry mass; the rest is a protein-mucopolysaccharide complex. The metabolism in articular cartilage is normally very low and the turnover of its components consequently slow.

The articular surfaces are naked (Fig. 6-47, AS). No limiting membrane of any kind has been seen even with the electron microscope (Cameron and Robinson, 1958).

The *synovial membrane,* the inner layer of the protective membranes, lines the joint everywhere except over the articular surfaces (Figs. 6-43D and 6-44, SM). It is somewhat like the cambium, being made of loose connective tissue (Fig. 6-44, SM) in which adipose cells are present in some areas. Elsewhere, such as at the site of attachment of the synovial membrane to the periphery of the articular cartilage, dense fibrous tissue is present (Fig. 6-44).

The surface cells of the synovial membrane are arranged in an epithelial-like fashion; when stretched, they appear squamous, but otherwise they look cuboidal. The surface cells sometimes undergo temporary outfolding. Some outward folds, however, are stable components called *villi* that are generally rich in capillary blood vessels. Infoldings of the surface form pediculated sacs called *bursae* which can become obstructed and distended with synovial fluid, causing discomfort.

The joint cavity is filled with *synovial fluid,* generally considered to be an exudate of the blood to which mucopolysaccharides, particularly hyaluronic acid, are added, probably through the secretory activity of the cartilage cells of the articular surfaces. The term *synovial* (G., *syn ovum*) refers to this viscous fluid, which reminded the ancients of egg white.

The outer covering of the diarthrosal joint is

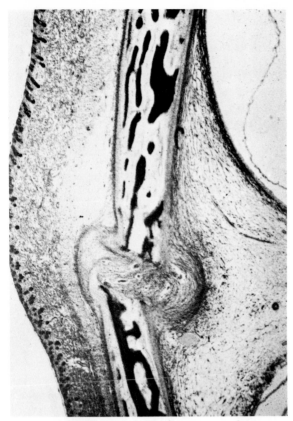

FIGURE 6-42 Section through the roof of a fetal calf skull showing the formation of a fibrous joint (syndesmosis). ×30.

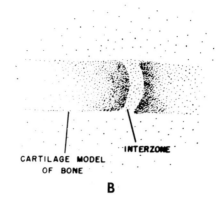

CARTILAGE MODEL
OF BONE

INTERZONE

B

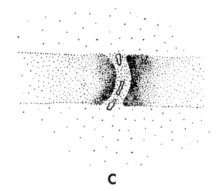

C

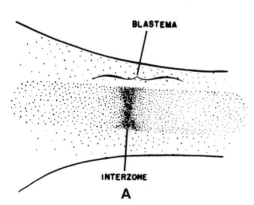

BLASTEMA

INTERZONE

A

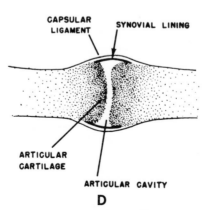

CAPSULAR
LIGAMENT

SYNOVIAL LINING

ARTICULAR
CARTILAGE

ARTICULAR CAVITY

D

FIGURE 6-43 Diagram showing the main steps in the development of a diarthrosis. A. Early limb formation showing the blastema, already segmented. B. The cartilage model of bone is well outlined and there is loosening of the cellular material in the interzone. C. Early cleft formation. Coalescence of the miniclefts has begun. D. Mature joint. The opposed articular surfaces are covered by articular cartilage, while synovial lining is present around the periphery of the joint. (Courtesy of Dr. D. B. Drachman.)

known as the *capsule* (6-44C). It is continuous with the outer periosteum and similarly composed of dense fibrous tissue. Cordlike thickenings of the capsule are called *ligaments*. They are sometimes made of fibrocartilage. Alpharadiography (Bélanger and Bélanger, 1959) has revealed particularly well their deep insertion in the articular cartilage (Fig. 6-46).

The *menisci* are also derivatives of the capsule found in some articulations, such as the knee joint. They are crescent-shaped discs of fibrocartilage attached marginally to the capsule and ending in a free edge inside the joint cavity (Fig. 6-47).

Arthritis, or joint disease, is a very widespread problem which has plagued man and beast of all ages, but mostly the elderly, through the centuries. There are more than 100 forms of arthritis, but they all have one thing in common: they all involve the connective tissues. A close relationship has been established recently between some of these disorders and the immune system.

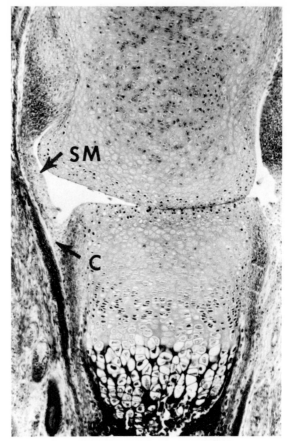

FIGURE 6-44 Intermetacarpal articulation, human fetus; SM, synovial membrane; C, capsule. Mallory stain. ×62.

REFERENCES

ADAMS, P., G. T. DAVIES, and P. SWEETNAM: Osteoporosis and the Effects of Aging on Bone Mass in Elderly Men and Women, *Q. J. Med.,* **39:**601 (1970).

ALI, S., S. W. SADJERA, and H. C. ANDERSON: Isolation and Characterization of Calcifying Matrix Vesicles from Epiphyseal Cartilage. *Proc. Na. Acad. Sci. U.S.A.,* **67:**1513 (1970).

AMPRINO, R.: Bone Structures and Functions, in W. Bargmann (ed), "Werkstatt der Anatomen," Georg Thieme Verlag, Stuttgart, 1965.

ANDERSON, H. C.: Electron Microscopic Studies of Induced Cartilage Development and Calcification, *J. Cell Biol.,* **35:**81 (1967).

ANDERSON, H. C.: Vesicles Associated with Calcification in the Matrix of Epiphyseal Cartilage, *J. Cell Biol.,* **41:**59 (1969).

ANDERSON, H. C.: Calcium Accumulating Vesicles in the Intercellular Matrix of Bone, In "Hard Tissue Growth, Repair and Mineralization," Excerpta Medica, Amsterdam, 1973.

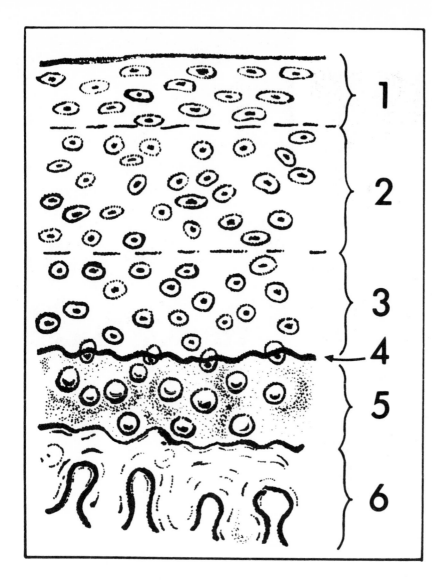

FIGURE 6-45 Artist's diagram depicting the four zones of adult articular cartilage. At the surface is a narrow layer of flattened cells called the gliding layer or tangential zone (1). Beneath this is the transitional zone (2) in which the ovoid to rounded cells are randomly distributed. Short irregular columns are noted deep to this in the radial zone (3), which is separated from the zone of calcified cartilage (5) by the "tidemark" (4), a thin, wavy basophilic line. The bone end plate below is mature cortical bone with well-defined Haversian systems (6). H&E. (Courtesy of Dr. H. J. Mankin.)

ANDERSON, H. C.: Formation and Calcification of Matrix Vesicles during Bone Development, 4th Panamerican Congress of Anatomy, 1975.

ANDERSON, H. C., and J. REYNOLDS: Calcium Accumulating Vesicles in the Intercellular Matrix of Bone, *Dev. Biol.,* **34:**211 (1973).

BAUD, C. A.: Morphology and Inframicroscopic Structure of Osteocytes, *Acta Anat. (Basel),* **51:**209 (1962).

BAYLINK, D., J. SIPE, J. WERGEDAL, and O. J. WHITTEMORE: Vitamin D-Enhanced Osteocytic and Osteoclastic Bone Resorption, *Am. J. Physiol.,* **224:**1345 (1973).

BÉLANGER, L. F.: Autoradiographic Visualization of the Entry and Transit of S^{35} in Cartilage, Bone and Dentine of Young Rats and the Effect of Hyaluronidase in Vitro, *Can. J. Biochem. Physiol.,* **32:**161 (1954).

BÉLANGER, L. F.: Observations on the Manifestations of Osteolathyrism in the Chick, *Am. J. Bone Joint Surg.,* **41B:**581 (1959).

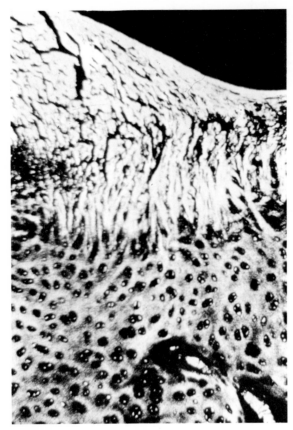

FIGURE 6-46 Ligament insertion into cartilage of articular surface. Notice deep penetration of dense fibrous tissue. Alpharadiograph. ×300.

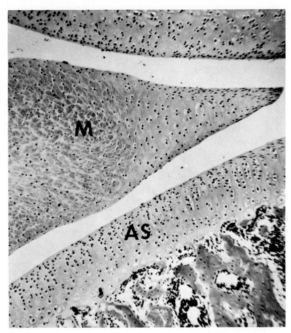

FIGURE 6-47 A portion of the knee joint of an adult rat. Notice the naked articular surfaces (AS) and the medial meniscus (M) made of fibrous tissue and cartilage. Hematoxylin-phloxine-orange stain. ×40.

BÉLANGER, L. F.: Osteocytic Osteolysis, *Calcif. Tissue Res.,* **4:**1 (1969).

BÉLANGER, L. F., and C. BÉLANGER: Alpharadiography: A Simple Method for Determination of Mass Concentration in Cells and Tissues, *J. Biophys. Biochem. Cytol.,* **6:**197 (1959).

BÉLANGER, L. F., and D. H. COPP: The Skeletal Effects of Prolonged Calcitonin Administration in Birds, under Various Conditions, in ''Calcium, Parathyroid Hormone and the Calcitonins,'' Excerpta Medica, Amsterdam, 1972.

BÉLANGER, L. F., and P. DROUIN: A Radioautographic Survey of the Formation and Fate of Connective Tissue Giant Cells in Selye's Granuloma Pouch, in G. Jasmin (ed.), ''Endocrine Aspects of Disease Processes,'' Warren H. Green Inc., St. Louis, 1968.

BÉLANGER, L. F., L. JARRY, and H. K. UHTHOFF: Osteocytic Osteolysis in Paget's Disease, *Rev. Can. Biol.,* **27:**37 (1968).

BÉLANGER, L. F., and C. P. LEBLOND: A Method for Locating Radioactive Elements in Tissues by Covering Histological Sections with a Photographic Emulsion, *Endocrinology,* **39:**8 (1946).

BÉLANGER, L. F., and B. B. MIGICOVSKY: Comparative Effects of Vitamin D, Calcium, Cortisone, Hydrocortisone and Norethandrolone on the Epiphyseal Cartilage and Bone of Rachitic Chicks, *Dev. Biol.,* **2:**329 (1960).

BÉLANGER, L. F., and B. B. MIGICOVSKY: Comparison between Different Mucopolysaccharide Stains as Applied to Chick Epiphyseal Cartilage, *J. Histochem. Cytochem.,* **9:**73 (1961).

BÉLANGER, L. F., and B. B. MIGICOVSKY: Histochemical Evidence of Proteolysis in Bone: The Influence of Parathormone, *J. Histochem. Cytochem.,* **11:**734 (1963).

BÉLANGER, L. F., and H. RASMUSSEN: Inhibition of Osteocytic Osteolysis by Thyrocalcitonin and Some Anti-growth Factors, in R. V. Talmage and L. F. Bélanger (eds.), ''Parathyroid Hormone and Thyrocalcitonin (Calcitonin),'' Excerpta Medica, Amsterdam, 1968.

BÉLANGER, L. F., J. ROBICHON, B. B. MIGICOVSKY, D. H. COPP, and J. VINCENT: Resorption without Osteoclasts (Osteolysis), in R. F. Sognnaes, (ed.), ''Mechanism of Hard Tissue Destruction,'' American Academy of the Advancement of Science, Washington, D.C., 1963.

BERNARD, G. W.: The Ultrastructural Interface of Bone Crystals and Organic Matrix in Woven and Lamellar Endochondral Bone, *J. Dent. Res.,* **48:**781 (1969).

BERNARD, G. W., and D. C. PEASE: An Electron Microscopic Study of Initial Intra-membranous Osteogenesis, *Am. J. Anat.,* **125:**271 (1969).

BOIS, P., and L. F. BÉLANGER, and J. LE BUIS: Effect of Growth Hormone and Amino-acetonitrile on the Mitotic Rate of Epiphyseal Cartilage in Hypophysectomized Rats, *Endocrinology,* **73:**507 (1963).

BONUCCI, E.: Fine Structure of Early Cartilage Calcification, *J. Ultrastruct. Res.,* **20:**33 (1967).

BONUCCI, E.: The Organic-Inorganic Relationships in Bone Matrix undergoing Osteoclastic Resorption, *Calcif. Tiss. Res.,* **16:**13 (1974).

BONUCCI, E.: Personal communication, 1975.

BOURNE, G. H.: Vitamin C and Bone, in G. H. Bourne (ed.), ''The Biochemistry and Physiology of Bone,'' Academic Press, Inc., New York, 1956.

BYWATERS, E. G. L.: The Metabolism of Joint Tissues, *J. Pathol. Bact.,* **44:**247 (1937).

CAMERON, D. A., and R. A. ROBINSON: Electron Microscopy of Epiphyseal and Articular Cartilage Matrix in the Femur of the Newborn Infant, *J. Bone Joint Surg.* [*Am.*], **40A:**163 (1958).

CLARK, I., and L. F. BÉLANGER: The Effects of Alterations in Dietary Magnesium on Calcium, Phosphate and Skeletal Metabolism, *Calcif. Tiss. Res.,* **1:**204 (1967).

COOPER, R. R.: Personal communication, 1972.

COOPER, R. R. and G. LAROS: Personal communication, 1972.

COOPER, R. R., J. W. MILGRAM, and R. A. ROBINSON: Morphology of the Osteon. An Electron Microscopic Study, *J. Bone Joint Surg.* [*Am.*], **48A:**1239 (1966).

CRELIN, E. S.: The Development of the Bony Pelvis and its Changes during Pregnancy and Parturition, *Trans. N.Y. Acad. Sci.,* (II) **31**(8):1049 (1969).

CURREY, J. D.: Biology of Hard Tissue, National Aeronautics and Space Administration SP-161 (1968).

DAVIES, D. V., C. H. BARNETT, W. COCHRANE, and A. J. PALFREY: Electron Microscopy of Articular Cartilage in the Young Adult Rabbit, *Ann. Rheum. Dis.,* **21:**11 (1962).

DELUCA, H. F.: Mechanism of Action and Metabolic Fate of Vitm. D, Vitm. Hormones, **25:**315 (1967).

DELUCA, H.: The Metabolism and Mechanism of Action of 25 Hydroxycholecalciferol, Franklin C. McLean Commemorative Workshop Conference on Cell Mechanism for Calcium Transfer and Homeostasis., Portsmouth, N.H., September 1970.

DRACHMAN, D. B.: Normal Development and Congenital Malformation of Joints, *Bull. Rheum. Dis.,* **19:**536 (1969).

245

DRACHMAN, D. B., and L. SOKOLOFF: The Role of Movement in Embryonic Joint Development, *Dev. Biol.,* **14:**401 (1966).

DUHAMEL, H. L.: Cinquiéme Mémoire sur les Os, dans Lequel on Se Propose d'Éclaircie Comment Se Fait le Crûe des Os Suivant leur Longeur. *Mem. Acad. Roy. Sci.,* **56:**111 (1743a).

DUHAMEL, H. L.: Quatrième Mémoire sur les Os, dans Lequel on Se Propose de Rapporter de Nouvelles Preuves qui Établissent que les Os Croissent en Grosseur par l'Addition de Couches Osseuses qui Tirent leur Origine du Périoste, *Mem. Acad. Roy. Sci.,* **56:**87 (1743b).

DUNCAN, H., and Z. F. JAWORSKI: "Osteoporosis. Tice's Practice of Medicine," vol. 5, chap. 52, Harper & Row, Publishers Incorporated, New York, 1970.

DURIEZ, J.: Les Modifications Calciques Péri-Ostéocytaires. Etude Microradiographique à l'Analyseur Automatique d'Images, *Nouv. Presse Médicale,* **3:**2007 (1974).

DURIEZ, J., and B. FLAUTRE: Effet de la Calcitonine sur l'Ostéogénèse. Etude en Microscopie de Fluorescence au Niveau du Tissu Osseux Spongieux Iliaque Normal de l'Homme et du Chien, *Nouv. Presse Médicale,* **2:**3103 (1973a).

DURIEZ, J., and B. FLAUTRE: Ostéogénèse, Activité Ostéocytaire et Clacitonine, *Acta Orthop. Belg.,* **39:**471 (1973b).

DURIEZ, J., and B. FLAUTRE: Fixation Calcique Péri-ostéocytaire sous Calcitonine. Etude Microradiographique à l'Analyseur Automatique d'Images dans Huit Cas d'Ostéogénèse Imparfaite, *Nouv. Presse Médicale,* **4:**97 (1975).

FAHMY, A., W. HILLMAN, P. TALLEY, and V. LONG: Fibrillogenesis in the Epiphyseal Cartilage of Adult Rats, *Am. J. Bone Joint Surg.,* **51A:**802 (1969).

FROST, H. M.: A Unique Histological Feature of Vitamin D Resistant Rickets Observed in Four Cases, *Acta Orthop. Scand.,* **33:**220 (1963).

FURSETH, R.: Tight Junctions between Osteocyte Processes, *Scand. J. Dent. Res.,* **81:**339 (1973).

GLIMCHER, M. J., A. J. HODGE, and F. O. SCHMITT: Macromolecular Aggregation States in Relation to Mineralization. The Collagen-hydroxyapatite System as Studied in Vitro, *Proc. Na. Acad. Sci. U.S.A.,* **43:**860 (1957).

GLISSON, F.: "De Rachitide," London, 1650.

GODMAN, G. C., and K. R. PORTER: Chondrogenesis, Studied with the Electron Microscope, *J. Biophys. Biochem. Cytol.,* **8:**719 (1960).

GOSS, C. M.: "Gray's Anatomy," 27th ed. Lea & Febiger, Philadelphia, 1959.

HALES, S.: "Statistical Essays," W. Innys, London, 1727.

HALL, B. K.: Differentiation of Cartilage and Bone from Common Germinal Cells: I. The Role of Acid Mucopolysaccharides and Collagen, *J. Exp. Zool.,* **173:**383 (1970).

HALL, B. K.: Evolutionary Consequences of Skeletal Differentiation, *Am. Zool.,* **15:**329 (1975).

HAM, A. W.: "Histology," 7th ed., J. B. Lippincott Company, Philadelphia, 1974.

HAM, A. W., and H. C. ELLIOTT: The Bone and Cartilage Lesions of Protracted Moderate Scurvy, *Am. J. Pathol.,* **14:**323 (1938).

HANCOX, N., and B. BOOTHROYD: Structure-Function Relationships in the Osteoclast, in R. F. Sognnaes (ed.), "Mechanisms of Hard Tissue Destruction," American Academy for the Advancement of Science, Washington, D.C., 1963.

HARRIS, H. A.: "Bone Growth in Health and Disease," Oxford University Press, London, 1933.

HARRIS, L. J.: Vitamin D and Bone, in G. H. Bourne (ed.), "The Biochemistry and Physiology of Bone," Academic Press, Inc., New York, 1956.

HARRIS, W. R., and A. W. HAM: The Mechanism of Nutrition in Bone and How it Affects its Structure Repair and Fate on Transplantation, in G. E. W. Wolstenholme and C. M. O'Connor (eds.), "Bone Structure and Metabolism," J. & A. Churchill Ltd., London, 1956.

HENRIKSON, P.-A., and K. WALLENIUS: The Mandible and Osteoporosis, *J. Oral Rehabil.,* **1:**67 (1974).

HEUCK, F.: The Osteolytic Action of the Osteocytes in Disorders of Bone Metabolism, Excerpta Medica, Amsterdam, 1966.

HEUCK, F. H. W.: Macro- and Microstructure of Bone in Osteoporosis, Excerpta Medica, Amsterdam, 1973.

HEUCK, F.: Microradiography (Report), *Verh. Dtsch. Ges. Pathol.,* **58:**114 (1974).

HIRSCHMAN, A., and D. D. DZIEWIATKOWSKI: Protein-Polysacchardie Loss during Endochondral Ossification: Immuno-chemical Evidence, *Science,* **154:**393 (1966).

JACKSON, S. F.: The Fine Structure of Developing Bone in the Embryonic Fowl, *Proc. R. Soc. Lond.* [*Biol.*], **B146:**270 (1957).

JANDE, S. S., and L. F. BÉLANGER: The Life Cycle of the Osteocyte, *Clin. Orthop.,* **94:**281 (1973).

JOHNSON, L. C.: Mineralization of Turkey Leg Tendon. I. Histology and Histochemistry of Mineralization, in R. F. Sognnaes (ed.), "Calcification in Biological Systems," American Academy for the Advancement of Science, Washington, D.C., 1960.

JOSS, E. E., K. A. ZUPPINGER, and E. H. SOBEL: Effect of Testosterone Propionate and Methyl Testosterone on Growth and Skeletal Maturation in Rats, *Endocrinology,* **72:**123 (1963).

KALLIO, D. M., P. R. GARANT, and C. MINKIN: Evidence for an Ultrastructural Effect of Calcitonin on Osteoclasts in Tissue Culture, in "Calcium, Parathyroid Hormone and the Calcitonins," Excerpta Medica, Amsterdam, 1972.

KASHIWA, H. K.: The Glyoxal BIS (2-hydroxyanil) Method for Differential Staining of Intracellular Calcium in Bone, in R. V. Talmage and L. F. Bélanger (eds.), "Parathyroid Hormone and Thyrocalcitonin (Calcitonin)," Excerpta Medica, Amsterdam, 1968.

KÖLLIKER, A.: "Die Normale Resorption des Knochengewebes und Ihre Bedeutung fur die Entsechung der Typischen Knochenformen," Vogel, Leipzig, 1873.

KOWALEWSKI, K.: Uptake of Radiosulphur in Growing Bones of Cockerels Treated with Cortisone and 17-ethyl-19-nortestosterone, *Proc. Soc. Exp. Biol. Med.,* **97:**432 (1958).

KREMPIEN, B., G. GEIGER, E. RITZ, and S. BUTTNER: Osteocytes in Chronic Uremia. Differential Count of Osteocytes in Human Femoral Bone. *Virchows Arch.* [*Pathol. Anat.*], **360:**1 (1973).

KROOK, L., L. F. BÉLANGER, P.-A. HENRIKSON, L. LUTWAK, and B. E. SHEFFY: Bone Flow, *Rev. Can. Biol.,* **29:**157 (1970).

KROOK, L., L. LUTWAK, P.-A. HENRIKSON, F. KALLFELZ, C. HIRSCH, B. ROMANUS, L. F. BÉLANGER, J. MARIER, and B. E. SHEFFY: Reversability of Nutritional Osteoporosis: Physicochemical Data on Bones from an Experimental Study in Dogs, *J. Nutr.* **101:**233 (1971).

LACROIX, P.: "L'Organisation des Os," Masson et Cie, Paris, 1949.

LEBLOND, C. P., G. W. WILKINSON, L. F. BÉLANGER, and J. ROBICHON: Radioautographic Visualization of Bone Formation in the Rat, *Am. J. Anat.,* **86:**289 (1950).

LIU, C. C., D. J. BAYLINK, and J. WERGEDAL: Vitamin-D-Enhanced Osteoclastic Bone Resorption at Vascular Canals, *Endocrinology,* **95:**1011 (1974).

LUK, S. C., C. NOPAJAROONSRI, and G. T. SIMON: The Ultrastructure of Cortical Bone in Young Adult Rabbits, *J. Ultrastruct. Res.,* **46:**184 (1974).

MANKIN, H. J.: The Structure, Chemistry and Metabolism of Articular Cartilage, *Bull. Rheum. Dis.,* **17:**447 (1967).

MATTHEWS, J. L., J. H. MARTIN, K. KUETTNER, and C. ARSENIS: The Role of Mitochondria in Intracellular

Calcium Regulation, Franklin C. McLean Commemorative Workshop Conference on Cell Mechanisms for Calcium Transfer and Homeostasis, Portsmouth, N.H., September 1970.

MATUKAS, V. J., and G. A. KRIKOS: Evidence for Changes in Protein-Polysaccharide Associated with the Onset of Calcification in Cartilage, *J. Cell Biol.,* **39:**43 (1968).

MCCLEAN, F. C., and W. BLOOM: Calcification and Ossification: Calcification in Normal Growing Bone, *Anat. Rec.,* **78:**333 (1940).

MCCLEAN, F. C., and M. R. URIST: ''Bone. Fundamentals of the Physiology of Skeletal Tissue,'' 3d ed., The University of Chicago Press, Chicago, 1968.

MEUNIER, P., J. BERNARD, and G. VIGNON: La Mesure de l'Élargissement Périostéocytaire appliquée au Diagnostic des Hyperparathyroidies, *Pathol. Biol.* (Paris), **19:**371 (1971a).

MEUNIER, P., J. BERNARD, and G. VIGNON: The Measurement of Periosteocytic Enlargement in Primary and Secondary Hyperparathyroidism, *Isr. J. Med. Sci.,* **7:**482 (1971b).

MOSS, M. L.: The Initial Phylogenetic Appearance of Bone. *Trans. N.Y. Acad. Sci.,* **23:**495 (1961).

MOSS, M. L.: The Phylogeny of Mineralized Tissues, *Int. Rev. Gen. Exp. Zool.,* **1:**297 (1964).

MOSS, M. L.: The Origin of Vertebrate Calcified Tissues, in T. Orvig (ed.), ''Current Problems of Lower Vertebrates Phylogeny,'' Almquist and Wiksell, Stockholm, 1968.

An Hypothesis for the Action of Vitamin D on Bone, *Nutri. Rev.* **26:**183 (1968).

NYLEN, M. U., D. B. SCOTT, and V. M. MOSLEY: Mineralization of Turkey Leg Tendon. II. Collagen-Mineral Relations Revealed by Electron and X-ray Microscopy, in R. F. Sognnaes (ed.), ''Calcification in Biological Systems,'' American Academy for the Advancement of Science, Washington, D.C., 1960.

PAUTARD, F. G. E.: A Biomolecular Survey of Calcification, in H. Fleisch, H. J. J. Blackwood, and M. Owen (eds.), ''Calcified Tissues,'' Springer-Verlag New York Inc., New York, 1966.

PEACOCK, E. E., JR., P. M. WEEKS, and J. M. PETTY: Some Studies on the Antigenicity of Cartilage, *Ann. N.Y. Acad. Sci.,* **87:**175 (1960).

POMMER, G.: ''Untersuchungen über Osteomalacie und Rachitis, nebst Beiträgen zur Kenntnis der Knochenresorption und Apposition in Verschiedenen Altersperioden und der Durchbohrenden Gefässe,'' Vogel, Leipzig, 1885.

PORTE, J. P. MEUNIER, J. BERNARD, and M. ROCHE: L'Ostéolyse Périostéocytaire dans l'Hyperparathyroidisme Expérimental induit par l'EDTA Influence de la Calcitonine, *Pathol. Biol.* (*Paris*), **20:**775 (1972).

REMAGEN, W.: The Bone Cell System: Form and Function, *Beitr. Pathol.,* **150:**1–10 (1973).

REVEL, J.-P.: A Stain for the Ultrastructural Localization of Acid Mucopolysaccharides, *J. Microsc.,* **3:**535 (1964).

REVEL, J.-P., and E. D. HAY: An Autoradiographic and Electron Microscopic Study of Collagen Synthesis in Differentiating Cartilage, *Z. Zellforsch. Mikrosk. Anat.,* **61:**110 (1963).

RIGGS, B. L., J. JOWSEY, P. J. KELLY, D. L. HOFFMAN, and C. D. ARNAUD: Studies on Pathogenesis and Treatment of Post-menopausal and Senile Osteoporosis, *Clin. Endocrinol. Metabolism,* **2:**317 (1973).

ROBINSON, R. A., and M. L. WATSON: Collagen-Crystal Relationship in Bone as Seen in the Electron Microscope, *Anat. Rec.,* **114:**383 (1952).

ROMER, A. S.: The Early Evolution of Fishes, *Q. Rev. Biol.,* **21:**33 (1946).

ROMER, A. S.: The ''Ancient History'' of Bone, *Ann. N.Y. Acad. Sci.,* **109:**168 (1963).

SAYEGH, F. S., G. C. SALOMAN, and R. W. DAVIS: Ultrastructure of Intracellular Mineralization in the Deer's Antler, *Clin. Orthop.,* **99:**267 (1974).

SCHULZ, A., K. DONATH, and G. DELLING: Zur Ultrastruktur in der Corticalis der Rattentibia, *Verh. Dtsch. Ges. Pathol.,* **57:**397 (1973).

SILBERBERG, M., and R. SILBERBERG: Steroid Hormones and Bone, in G. H. Bourne (ed.), "The Biochemistry and Physiology of Bone," Academic Press, Inc., New York, 1956.

SILBERBERG, R., M. SILBERBERG, and D. FEIR: Life Cycle of Articular Cartilage Cells: An Electron Microscope Study of the Hip Joint of the Mouse, *Am. J. Anat.,* **114:**17 (1964).

SILBERMAN, M., and J. FROMMER: Initial Locus of Calcification in Chondrocytes, *Clin. Orthop.,* **98:**288 (1974).

TALMAGE, R. V.: Calcium Homeostasis—Calcium Transport—Parathyroid Action. The Effects of Parathyroid Hormone on the Movement of Calcium between Bone and Fluid, *Clin. Orthop.,* **67:**210 (1969).

TARLO, B. J., and L. B. H. TARLO: The Origin of Teeth, *Discovery,* **26:**1 (1965).

TURNER, C. D.: "General Endocrinology," 4th ed., W. B. Saunders Company, Philadelphia, 1966.

URIST, M. R.: The Origin of Bone, *Discovery,* **25:**13 (1964).

URIST, M. R., and K. A. VAN DE PUTTE: Comparative Biochemistry of the Blood of Fishes, in P. W. Gilbert, R. F. Mathewson, and D. P. Rall (eds.), "Sharks, Skates and Rays," Johns Hopkins Press, Baltimore, 1967.

URIST, M. R.: Biologic Initiators of Calcification, in Isodore Zippin, (ed.), "Biological Mineralization," John Wiley & Sons, Inc., New York, 1973.

URIST, M. R., A. MIKULSKI, and S. D. BOYD: A Chemosterilized Antigen-Extracted Autodigested Alloimplant for Bone Banks, *Arch. Surg.,* **110:**416 (1975).

WASSERMAN, R.: Metabolism, Function and Clinical Aspects of Vitamin D, *Cornell Vet.,* 1975.

WEIDENREICH, F.: Das Knochengewebe, in W. von Möllendorff (ed.), "Die Gewebe, Handbuch der Mikorskopischen Anatomie des Menschen," Julius Springer, Berlin, 1930.

WHALEN, J. P., N. O'DONOHUE, L. KROOK, and E. A. NUNEZ: Pathogenesis of Abnormal Remodeling of Bones: Effects of Yellow Phosphorus in the Growing Rat, *Anat. Rec.,* **177:**15 (1973).

WOLBACH, S. B., and D. M. HEGSTED: Vitamin A Deficiency in the Chick, *Arch. Pathol.,* **54:**13 (1952).

Muscular Tissue

GERALDINE F. GAUTHIER

The function of movement in multicellular organisms is usually assumed by specialized cells, called muscle fibers, which contract upon appropriate stimulation. This property is also manifested by other structures such as cilia and flagella. These various motile systems have in common the ability to transform chemical into mechanical energy through the enzymatic splitting of ATP, and each possesses precisely arranged filamentous proteins. Comparable proteins have recently been implicated in motility in a wide variety of cell systems (see Pollard and Weihing, 1974). In muscle cells, filaments are oriented parallel to the direction of movement, and because of their precise arrangement, constitute the actual contractile machinery of the cell. In the vertebrate body, there are three types of muscle based on the appearance and location of their constituent cells: smooth, skeletal, and cardiac. All three types are composed of asymmetric cells, or fibers, with the long axis arranged in the direction of movement.

Smooth muscle, which is the simplest in appearance of the three types, consists of narrow and relatively short, tapering cells, each with a single centrally located nucleus. This type of muscle occurs in the walls of the viscera and hence is often referred to as *visceral* or *involuntary,* muscle. *Skeletal* muscle is associated, as the name implies, with the body skeleton. The cells are greatly elongated, and each contains numerous peripheral nuclei. Because of the conspicuous transverse striations of the individual cells, skeletal muscle is also referred to as *striated* muscle. It is controlled by the somatic nervous system and hence is often called *voluntary* muscle. *Cardiac* muscle is a highly specialized form of *involuntary striated* muscle found only in the heart and, in some species, in the walls of the pulmonary vein. It is similar to skeletal muscle in that the cells are transversely striated and multinuclear, but as in smooth muscle, the nuclei are centrally located.

In the descriptions which follow, emphasis will be placed on the appearance of muscle as it occurs in the mammal. Reference will be made to other vertebrate classes, however, particularly where information is otherwise limited. Discussion will be concerned with skeletal muscle in particular, since it has been the primary source of data concerning relationships between structure and function.

SKELETAL MUSCLE

GENERAL FEATURES

Skeletal muscle (Fig. 7-1) consists of long bundles of more or less parallel cells called *muscle fibers.* Cross-sectional dimensions (Fig. 7-7) vary from about 10 to 100 μm. In longitudinal section, these cells are clearly marked by transverse striations (Figs. 7-2 and 7-3), and nuclei are located just beneath the cell membrane, or *sarcolemma.* The fibers contain smaller parallel units

251

about 1 to 3 μm in diameter, the *myofibrils,* which are also transversely striated (Figs. 7-1 and 7-4) and are composed, in turn, of *myofilaments* that are visible only with the electron microscope (Fig. 7-5). The myofilaments are not transversely striated but are responsible for the striations because of their arrangement within the myofibril (Fig. 7-6).

Skeletal muscles are attached to bony structures by tendons, which are continuous with a connective tissue covering over the entire muscle, the *epimysium.* This outermost connective tissue extends into the muscle and surrounds bundles, or *fascicles,* of muscle fibers, forming the *perimysium,* which eventually divides into a delicate sheath of reticular fibers around each muscle fiber called the *endomysium.* Blood vessels and nerves follow these sheaths into the interior of the muscle, and a rich capillary network closely invests each muscle fiber.

Skeletal muscle fibers also contain a cytoplasm, or *sarcoplasm,* which occupies the limited space between the abundant myofibrils. Muscle fibers are conventionally depicted in longitudinal section, and

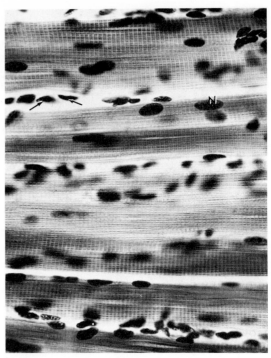

FIGURE 7-2 Longitudinal section of several skeletal muscle fibers (cat tongue). Each fiber is characterized by a transverse pattern of alternating dark A bands and light I bands, repeated along the length of the fiber. In certain areas, individual myofibrils can be recognized by their longitudinal orientation. Nuclei (N) are located at the periphery of the fibers. Angular structures (arrows) between fibers are distorted red blood cells present within capillaries, which closely invest individual muscle fibers. Iron-hematoxylin. ×560.

FIGURE 7-1 Longitudinal organization of skeletal muscle. Dimensions are based on rabbit psoas muscle. (From H. E. Huxley, in J. Brachet and A. E. Mirsky (eds.), "The Cell," vol. 4, Academic Press, Inc., New York, 1960.)

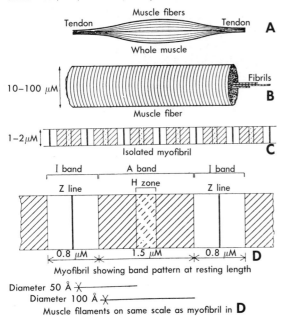

emphasis is usually placed on the myofibrillar component. However, mitochondria are usually conspicuous components of the sarcoplasm (Figs. 7-7 and 7-8). Interfibrillar mitochondria are arranged in pairs at regular intervals in relation to the banding pattern of the myofibrils (Figs. 7-3 and 7-4). These paired mitochondria, which are characteristic of mammalian skeletal muscle fibers in general, encircle the myofibrils at the level of the I bands (Fig. 7-28B). Their arrangement is readily visible in transverse sections of the muscle fibers (Fig. 7-9), where they appear as filamentous profiles. In longitudinal sections of the fibers (Figs. 7-3 and 7-4), these mitochondria are usually sectioned transversely and thus appear as elliptical profiles on either side of the Z line. In a tangential section through a myofibril, mitochondrial profiles extend transversely across the I bands (Fig. 7-29). In certain types of fibers, mitochondria also form more

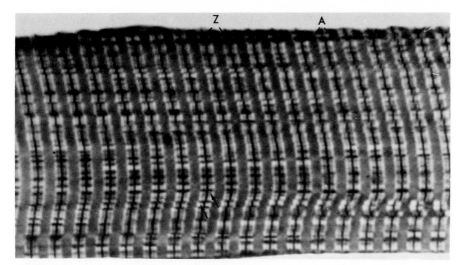

FIGURE 7-3 Longitudinal section of a single muscle fiber (guinea pig plantaris). The transverse banding pattern is clearly resolved, and part of a peripheral nucleus is visible at the upper left of the fiber. A bands are dark; I bands are light and are bisected by a very dark, narrow Z line. The precise alignment of paired mitochondria (arrows) in transverse rows over the I bands, on either side of each Z line, creates the impression of an additional interrupted dark band in this position. Toluidine blue. × 1,900.

FIGURE 7-4 Electron micrograph of a portion of a fiber (rat semitendinosus). Several myofibrils are present in this longitudinal section, and at least two sarcomeres are included in each myofibril. The regular arrangement of transverse bands in each myofibril gives rise to the banding pattern of the whole fiber seen with the light microscope (Fig. 7-3). Profiles of paired mitochondria (arrows) are present on either side of the electron-opaque Z line (see also Fig. 7-5). × 17,500.

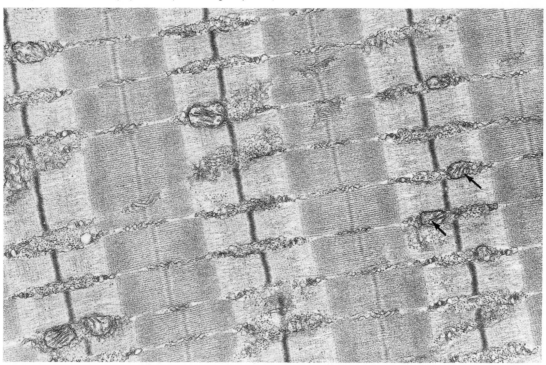

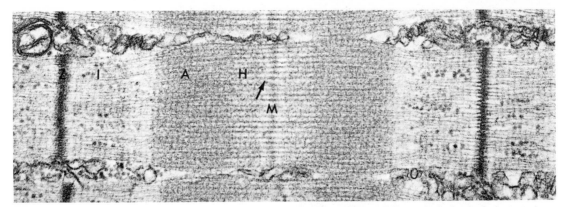

FIGURE 7-5 Single sarcomere from a preparation similar to that in Fig. 7-4. The conspicuous Z line marks the longitudinal extent of this structural and functional unit. The myofilaments, which compose the myofibrils, are visible, but their arrangement is more readily apparent in Fig. 7-6. All the major transverse bands can be seen in this micrograph, including the pseudo H band (arrow), which is often confused with the H band. Glycogen particles occur among the filaments of the I-band region. ×48,000.

FIGURE 7-6 Sarcomere from rabbit psoas muscle which has been glycerinated removing soluble components of the sarcoplasm. In this type of preparation, it is possible to discern the organization of myofilaments, which constitutes the ultrastructural basis of transverse banding in the myofibril. In the A band, there is a simple alternation of thick and thin filaments in this particular plane of section, and in the I band there are only thin filaments. The thick filaments extend to the limits of the A band, where their ends become tapered (arrow). The thin filaments extend from each Z line through both the I band and A band, but terminate at the H band. Bridgelike structures extend radially from the surfaces of the thick filaments. Six such structures are arranged in a helical pattern which is repeated every 400 Å along the thick filament (see Fig. 7-19). ×128,000. (From H. E. Huxley, 1957.)

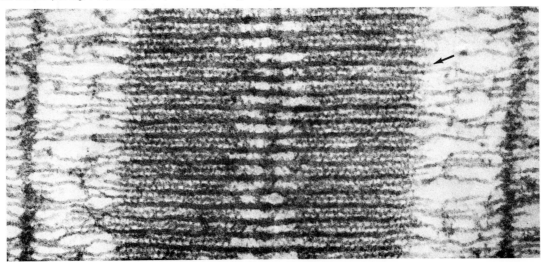

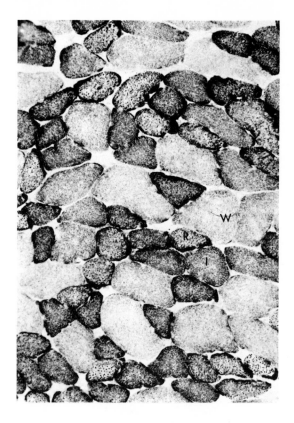

FIGURE 7-7 Transverse section of several muscle fibers (rat diaphragm), showing the localization of succinic dehydrogenase activity. Reaction product reflects the location of mitochondria. Small (red) fibers (R) are rich in mitochondria, especially along the periphery; large (white) fibers (W) have a low mitochondrial content; and intermediate fibers (I) have characteristics between the two. ×200.

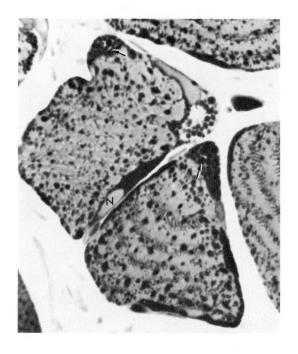

FIGURE 7-8 Transverse section of two red fibers (rat diaphragm), illustrating the distribution of mitochondria, which are stained darkly with toluidine blue. The myofibrils appear relatively unstained. Large circular profiles of mitochondria form conspicuous peripheral aggregations (arrows) at sites where enzymatic activity is demonstrated (Fig. 7-7) and are also abundant in the interior of the fibers. Nuclei (N) appear in negative image. ×1,200. (From G. F. Gauthier, 1970.)

continuous longitudinal rows and subsarcolemmal aggregations (Fig. 7-36), which are apparent in transverse as well as in longitudinal sections (Figs. 7-7 and 7-8).

The sarcoplasm also contains an elaborate membrane system, the *sarcoplasmic reticulum,* which surrounds individual myofibrils (Figs. 7-9 and 7-10). This system will be discussed in a later section. In addition, a Golgi apparatus is present in the perinuclear sarcoplasm. Glycogen, in the form of β particles, is abundant between myofibrils, particularly in the region of the I bands, and it occurs within the myofibrils as well (Figs. 7-5, 7-9, and 7-10). Lipid droplets are frequently closely associated with large mitochondria (Fig. 7-36). Both lipid and glycogen provide metabolic fuel for the contractile machinery.

The banding pattern of the skeletal muscle fiber reflects the ultrastructural oganization of each myofibril, and knowledge of this pattern is fundamental to an understanding of the mechanism of contraction. *The two largest bands are named according to their appearance in polarized light* (Figs. 7-11 and 7-12). Certain bands exhibit positive birefringence, which reflects a parallel arrangement of asymmetric subunits. These birefringent or anisotropic bands are called *A bands* and are bright when viewed with a polarizing

FIGURE 7-9 Electron micrograph of a transverse section (rat semitendinosus). The section passes through the I band and, therefore, through only the thin filaments which compose this part of the sarcomere. Braceletlike mitochondria (M) encircle individual myofibrils; these mitochondria appear as paired elliptical profiles on either side of the Z line in longitudinal sections of a muscle fiber (Figs. 7-3 and 7-4). In addition, profiles of the sarcoplasmic membrane systems (S) surround individual myofibrils, and clusters of glycogen particles (arrow) occur close to them. ×42,000.

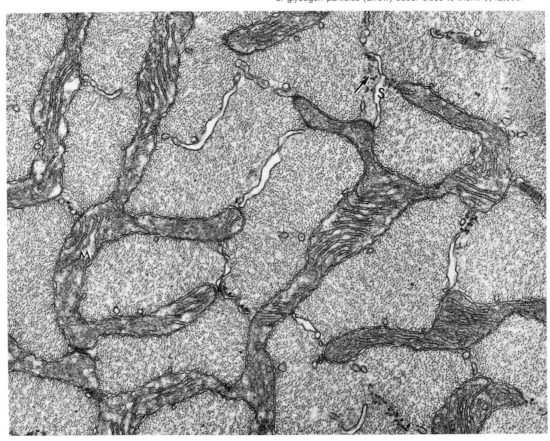

microscope (Fig. 7-12). They alternate with dark isotropic *I bands,* and the pattern is repeated along the
length of the myofibril. Each A band has a less birefringent central zone called the *H band,* and each I
band is bisected by a distinct *Z line.* The *M line* marks
the center of the H band, and in some instances (in
insect muscle, for example), an N line is apparent on
either side of the Z line. When viewed with phase-
contrast optics (Fig. 7-11) or with ordinary light after
staining with a cationic dye (Figs. 7-2 and 7-3), the
banding pattern appears reversed. That is, the A band
and Z line are basophilic or dark and the I and H
bands are light. This is also the usual appearance of
the various bands in electron micrographs (Figs. 7-4
and 7-5), but the appearance with polarized light is the

basis for the more widely used nomenclature. The
segment between two successive Z lines is called a
sarcomere (Fig. 7-5) and is approximately 2 to 3 μm
long, with the A band contributing about 1.5 μm and
each full I band, about 0.8 μm. This structural and
functional unit is repeated along the length of the
myofibril.

Biochemical analysis has revealed that the myofibril consists of a number of proteins. Two of these,
myosin and *actin,* account for most of the dry weight
of the myofibril. Their interaction in the presence of
ATP to form *actomyosin* is fundamental to myofibrillar
contraction. Two other proteins, *tropomyosin* and
troponin, play a regulatory role in the contractile
process. Troponin, in particular, inhibits the formation
of actomyosin when the calcium level is low (see
Cohen, 1975). It has been possible also to locate some
of these proteins within the sarcomere. If, for example,
myosin is extracted from a preparation of myofibrils,

FIGURE 7-10 Transverse section through the A-band region
(frog sartorius). Both thick and thin filaments are present, and
each thick filament is surrounded by six thin filaments, giving rise
to a precise hexagonal array. The presence of cross bridges im-
parts a rough surface to the thick filaments. Myofibrillar boundaries are marked by profiles of the sarcoplasmic reticulum (S) and
by glycogen particles (arrows). ×150,000. (From H. E. Huxley, *J.
Molec. Biol.,* **37:**507, 1968.)

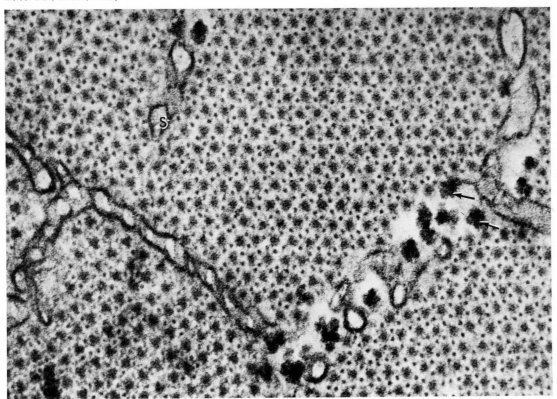

the density of the A band is diminished (Figs. 7-13 and 7-14), indicating that myosin is located in this region. The fluorescent antibody technique has become an increasingly useful tool for the localization of muscle proteins. An antibody to myosin, for example, is conjugated with a fluorescent dye, and this complex is allowed to interact with a preparation of myofibrils. The complex becomes bound to the site where myosin is located, and the fluorescence serves as a visual marker. The site of florescence, and therefore of myosin, is the A-band region of the myofibril (Figs. 7-15 and 7-16). By following similar procedures, actin can be demonstrated in the I band along with troponin and tropomyosin.

Ultrastructurally, the myofibril is composed of two major types of filaments, one type being thicker than the other (Figs. 7-6 and 7-10). When extracted myo-

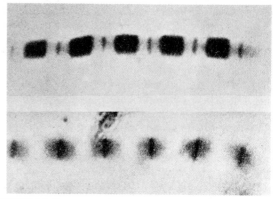

FIGURES 7-13 (upper) and **7-14** (lower) Single myofibril (glycerinated rabbit psoas) photographed with phase-contrast optics showing the appearance before (Fig. 7-13) and after (Fig. 7-14) extraction of myosin. Following removal of myosin, the density of the A band is decreased, but that of the I band and the Z line remains. (From J. Hanson and H. E. Huxley, 1955.)

FIGURES 7-11 (upper) and **7-12** (lower) A single isolated myofibril (glycerinated rabbit psoas), illustrating the banding pattern with phase-contrast optics and with polarized light. In the phase-contrast image (Fig. 7-11), the A band and Z line are dark and the I band is light. When viewed with polarized light (Fig. 7-12), the A band and Z line are bright and the I band is dark. (From J. Hanson and H. E. Huxley, 1955.)

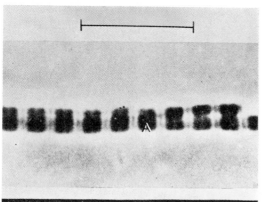

fibrils are examined with the electron microscope, loss of myosin is associated with loss of the thick filaments, which indicates that the thick filaments are composed largely of myosin. The thin filaments, on the other hand, are composed primarily of actin. In a classic ultrastructural study, H. E. Huxley (1957) demonstrated the exact arrangement of these filaments, which established the ultrastructural basis of the banding pattern and of the contractile mechanism as well. In the A band, thick (100-Å) filaments alternate with thin (50-Å) filaments (Figs. 7-6 and 7-10). The thick filaments are 1.5 μm long and extend only to the limits

FIGURES 7-15 (upper) and **7-16** (lower) Myofibril (chicken breast muscle) treated with a fluorescent antibody to myosin and photographed using phase-contrast (Fig. 7-15) and fluorescence (Fig. 7-16) microscopy. The site of fluorescence (antimyosin) in Fig. 7-16 corresponds to the dark (A band) in Fig. 7-15. (From F. A. Pepe, J. Cell Biol., **28**:505, 1966.)

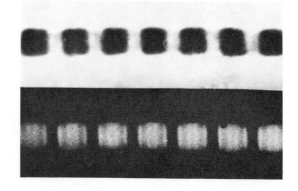

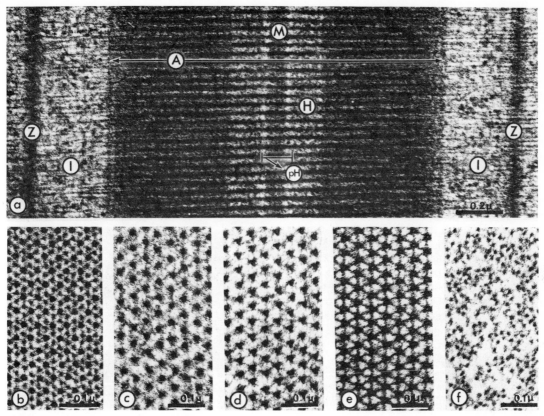

FIGURE 7-17 Single sarcomere (fish muscle) in longitudinal section (a), showing transverse banding pattern together with corresponding transverse sections through each of the bands. The A band (A) consists of both thick and thin filaments (b), the H band (H) and the bridge-free pseudo H band (pH), only of thick filaments (c and d, respectively). The M band (M) also contains only thick filaments, but conspicuous transverse extensions are present as well (e). In the I band (I) only thin filaments are present (f). (From F. A. Pepe, 1971.)

FIGURE 7-18 Diagrammatic interpretation of the organization of filaments giving rise to the transverse banding pattern. (From H. E. Huxley, 1969.)

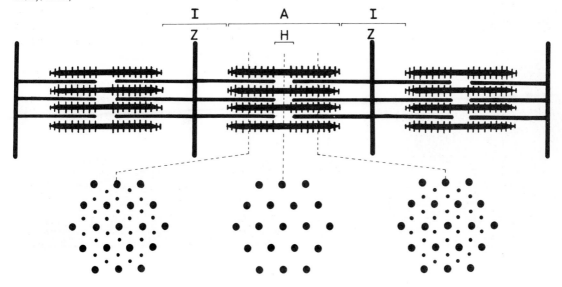

of the A band, where their ends become tapered. The thin filaments, however, extend from each Z line for a distance of 1 μm through the I band and into the A band. They are absent from the H band. The banding pattern is therefore the result of the presence or absence of overlap between the two sets of filaments (Figs. 7-6, 7-17, and 7-18). The A band, which is relatively dense when viewed with the light microscope, consists of both thick and thin filaments (Figs. 7-6 and 7-10). The less-dense I band consists only of thin filaments (Figs. 7-6 and 7-9), and the H band, only of thick filaments (Fig. 7-17a and c). The M line reflects the transverse extension of a series of projections from the centers of the thick filaments (Fig. 7-17a and e). The filaments are arranged, in transverse section, so that they appear as more or less circular profiles in a remarkably precise hexagonal pattern. In the A-band region, where the two sets of

FIGURE 7-19 Diagram illustrating the helical organization of cross bridges along the thick filament. The arrangement of six successive bridges corresponds to the 400-Å intervals observed in electron micrographs of sectioned muscle fibers. (From H. E. Huxley and W. Brown, *J. Molec. Biol.*, **30**:383, 1967.)

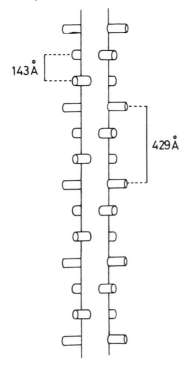

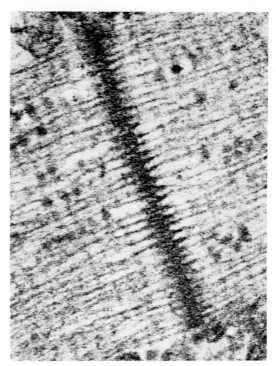

FIGURE 7-20 Appearance of the Z line in a longitudinal section of a myofibril (rat semitendinosus). Each I-band filament on one side of the Z line faces the space between two filaments on the opposite side, and there appear to be filamentous structures connecting these filaments obliquely within the Z line itself. ×117,000.

filaments overlap, each thick (myosin) filament is surrounded by six thin (actin) filaments (Figs. 7-10, 7-17b, and 7-18). In addition, a series of bridgelike structures extends radially from the thick filaments toward the thin filaments (Figs. 7-6, 7-10, 7-17b, and 7-18). There are six of these bridges arranged about each thick filament in a helical pattern that is repeated about every 400 Å along the length of the thick filament (Fig. 7-19). The absence of bridges from the center of the H band produces an area of lower density often confused with the H band itself; this is called the L band, or *pseudo H band* (Fig. 7-17a and d). The bridges, which are part of the myosin molecule, possess ATPase activity, and they play a major role in the interaction of actin and myosin during contraction (see below).

Perhaps the least-understood structural component of the myofibril is the Z line. The thin filaments composing the I band are arranged so that in longitudinal sections of the myofibril, each thin filament on one side of the Z line faces the space between two thin

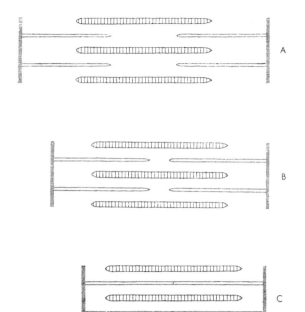

filaments on the opposite side, and connecting elements appear to run obliquely across the Z line, creating a zigzag appearance (Fig. 7-20). In myofibrils sectioned transversely, filamentous components in the region of the Z line form a tetragonal pattern. On the basis of studies of amphibian muscle, it is believed that each terminating I-band filament forms the apex of a pyramid whose base is a square formed by four I-band filaments from the opposite side of the Z line. The sizes of the pyramid are formed by the oblique structures composing the Z line itself. The arrangement in mammalian muscle is probably even more complex. The manner in which the I-band filaments terminate at the Z line is not clear; it is possible, for example, that they actually continue into the Z line. Evidence for the chemical nature of the Z line is conflicting also. Tropomyosin may be present along with other proteins, such as α-actinin. Both the chemical and structural composition of the Z line remains puzzling.

THE ULTRASTRUCTURAL BASIS OF CONTRACTION

Early observation with the light microscope showed that during contraction the length of the sarcomere was shortened. The I band in particular decreased in length, but there was no change in the length of the A band. The mechanism by which this occurs can be explained by the ultrastructure of the sarcomere. The extent to which the thick and thin filaments overlap accounts for the change observed with the light micro-

FIGURE 7-21 Diagram illustrating the manner in which the thin filaments of the I band may be pulled progressively toward the center of the A band during contraction, thereby decreasing the width of the I band (B and C) and eventually obliterating the H band (C). The sarcomere in B is at resting length, A is stretched, and C is contracted. (From H. E. Huxley, *Sci. Am.,* **199:**No. 5, 1958.)

FIGURE 7-22 Purified myosin, showing two examples of filaments aggregated at low ionic strength. Projections correspond to bridgelike structures seen in intact myofibrils (Fig. 7-6), and the bare central zone corresponds to the bridge-free pseudo H band. ×145,000. (From H. E. Huxley, 1963.)

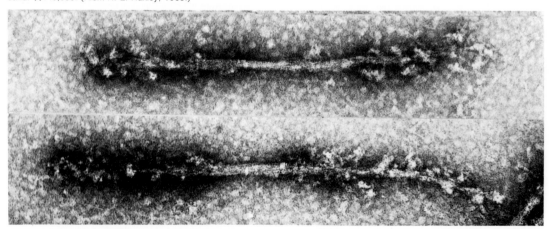

262

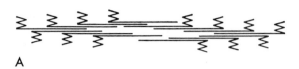

A

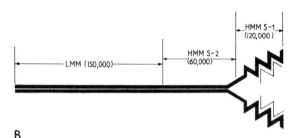

B

FIGURE 7-23A Diagrammatic interpretation of the arrangement of myosin molecules giving rise to the myosin filament, based on images such as those seen in Fig. 7-22. LMM units are parallel to the longitudinal axis of the filament, and HMM units extend at right angles from them. (From H. E. Huxley, 1963.)

FIGURE 7-23B Schematic representation of the myosin molecule. (From S. Lowey et al., *J. Molec. Biol.,* **42:**1, 1969.)

scope. X-ray diffraction data and direct observation with the electron microscope have established that as the sarcomere shortens, the thin filaments of adjacent I bands are pulled toward the center of the A band, thereby obliterating the H band and decreasing the width of the I band (Fig. 7-21). According to this so-called *sliding filament hypothesis* (Hanson and Huxley, 1955), the A band maintains its original length, since the thick and thin filaments themselves do not shorten. The detailed events that take place as

actin and myosin combine and chemical energy is converted to mechanical energy are not fully understood, but recent studies of the molecular basis of contraction are rapidly adding new information. The evidence suggests that the bridges move toward the actin filaments, engage them, and cause them to move along the myosin filament (see Huxley, 1969).

THE MOLECULAR CONFIGURATION OF THE MYOFILAMENTS

Myosin can be enzymatically cleaved into two fragments, referred to as light meromyosin (LMM) and heavy meromyosin (HMM). The former is believed to form the linear "backbone" of the myosin molecule, whereas the latter projects outward from this backbone at regular intervals. Arrangement of LMM units parallel to one another but in a slightly staggered fashion (Fig. 7-23A) would permit the HMM units to occur at intervals of about 400 Å, thereby accounting for the spacing of bridges observed with the electron microscope and the periodicity of skeletal muscle observed by x-ray diffraction (429 Å). Each visible bridge, therefore, reflects a single HMM unit. Electron micrographs of purified myosin confirm this arrangement. Such preparations consist of tapered filaments, approximately 100 Å in diameter and 1.5 μm long, each resembling intact A-band filaments with their bridge-like projections (Figs. 7-22 and 7-23A). Under certain experimental conditions, the molecules align with their HMM portions polarized toward either end of the filament, thereby leaving a bare zone that is equivalent to the bridge-free zone in the intact sarcomere. The

FIGURE 7-24 Purified F-actin showing the beaded appearance of several filaments and reflecting the helical arrangement of strands of G-actin monomers. ×525,000. (From J. Hanson and J. Lowy, 1963.)

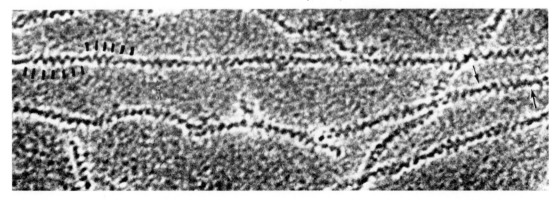

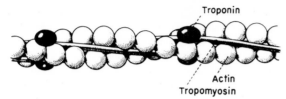

Troponin

Actin
Tropomyosin

FIGURE 7-25 Diagrammatic interpretation of the organization of actin, troponin, and tropomyosin to form the I-band filament. Globular monomers of G-actin are arranged in rows forming a two-stranded helix which corresponds to the structures visible in Fig. 7-24. (Courtesy of S. Ebashi.)

HMM fragment of myosin can be further cleaved into two proteolytic subfragments (see Lowey, 1971). One of these, HMM S-2, is attached in series with the LMM "backbone," forming the so-called "rod" portion of the molecule. The other subfragment, HMM S-1, or

FIGURE 7-26 Isolated thin filaments treated with S-1 subfragments of HMM. The bridgelike units have become attached to the thin filaments at regular intervals, reflecting the periodicity of F-actin. Note that the subunits project at an angle from the filaments and with a definite polarity, which is the same along the entire length of a given filament. ×180,000. (From P. B. Moore, H. E. Huxley, and D. J. DeRosier, 1970.)

"head" portion, extends at an angle with respect to the rod (Fig. 7-23B).

Preparations of pure actin consist of thin filaments with dimensions comparable to intact I-band filaments. Each filament consists of a two-stranded helix with a turn about every 360 Å. The periodicity of actin is therefore close to but not equal to that of myosin. The individual strands (F-actin) composing the helix are actually a linear array of globular units called G-actin (Fig. 7-24). Although the periodicity of actin is 360 Å, that of the I band itself is actually greater, approximately 400 Å. This most likely reflects the arrangement of troponin and tropomyosin in the I band. There is considerable evidence that the regulatory proteins are closely associated with actin in the thin filament. It is believed that tropomyosin occupies the groove formed by the twisted double standards of actin and that troponin is confined to more circumscribed sites along the filament (Fig. 7-25).

When pure HMM or HMM S-1 is added to a

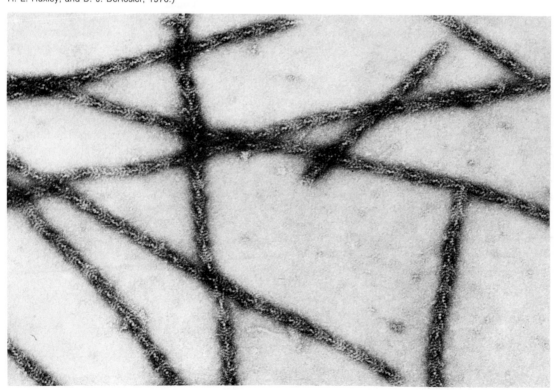

preparation of F-actin, the fragments attach precisely to the F-actin filaments (Fig. 7-26), and the complex has a 360-Å periodicity, which is characteristic of actin. This molecular interaction suggests that in whole muscle, the HMM or bridge portion of the thick filament makes physical contact with the thin filament at the start of contraction. The polarity of the attachment, moreover, is consistent with the ability of the filaments to slide in one specific direction. It is postulated that the HMM or bridge portion swings out radially toward an adjacent thin fialment while maintaining its base in the myosin filament (Fig. 7-27).

THE SARCOPLASMIC MEMBRANE SYSTEMS

Each myofibril is surrounded by an elaborate system of membranes aligned precisely with respect to the banding pattern of the myofibrils (Figs. 7-28A and B and 7-29). It is apparent that a relationship exists between the sarcoplasmic membranes and the conduction of the impulse leading to contraction. The complex arrangement of tubules and cisternae which compose this system is best understood in the relatively simple form that exists in certain amphibian muscles (Fig. 7-28A). A parallel array of tubules is oriented along the long axis of the myofibril. They extend along the full length of the A band and most of the I-band region of each sarcomere and fuse in the region of the H band to form a fenestrated cisterna. As the tubules approach the Z lines at each end of the sarcomere, they join to form greatly expanded *terminal cisternae*, which run parallel to each Z line. Each terminal cisterna is faced by an equivalent structure on the opposite side of the Z line. This membrane complex is referred to collectively as the *sarcoplasmic reticulum*. It is associated with a transverse membrane system which originates at the cell surface. Between two terminal cisternae a tubular element runs transversely at the Z line. It extends through the sarcoplasm and is continuous, with comparable tubules at the same level of adjacent myofibrils. These transverse

tubules compose the *T system*, which is separate from the sarcoplasmic reticulum. Two adjacent cisternae plus the intervening T tubule are referred to as a *triad*.

In mammalian skeletal muscle, the general arrangement of these two systems is similar except that triads are located, not at the Z line, but at the junction of the A and I bands (Fig. 7-28B). An additional network of tubules connects the teminal cisternae over the intervening I-band and Z-line regions (Fig. 7-29). In addition, the fused portion of the system over the H-band region may be either cisternal or tubular.

Although terminal cisternae and T tubules are separated from each other, they have a close apposition, which is, at some points, reminiscent of junctional complexes between certain epithelial cells. The membrane of each terminal cisterna is invaginated along the surface which faces the T tubule so that it appears "scalloped" in profile (Fig. 7-30). Between sites of invagination, the membrane of the terminal cisterna makes very close contact with that of the T tubule. However, this is not strictly comparable to an intercellular relationship (see Franzini-Armstrong, 1974).

Various kinds of evidence indicate that the T system is continuous with the plasmalemma of the muscle cell, a structural relationship which facilitates the inward conduction of the impulse that leads to contraction. Electron micrographs of certain fish muscles, for example, reveal a direct continuity between the T tubule and the sarcolemma (Fig. 7-31). In addition, when frog muscle fibers are immersed in a solution of ferritin, this electron-opaque protein is subsequently observed within the T tubule (Fig. 7-32), which suggests a functional continuity as well. The form and distribution of the T system would thus permit rapid distribution of a wave of depolarization from the cell surface deep into the interior of the fiber to each

FIGURE 7-27 Diagram illustrating a possible mechanism whereby a HMM bridge can make contact with a nearby thin filament to bring about a sliding of the filaments with respect to each other. The LMM unit remains as part of the thick filament itself, whereas the HMM portion swings out radially. The S-1 subfragment of the latter is thus brought into contact with the thin filament. (From H. E. Huxley, 1969.)

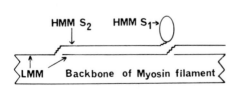

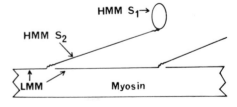

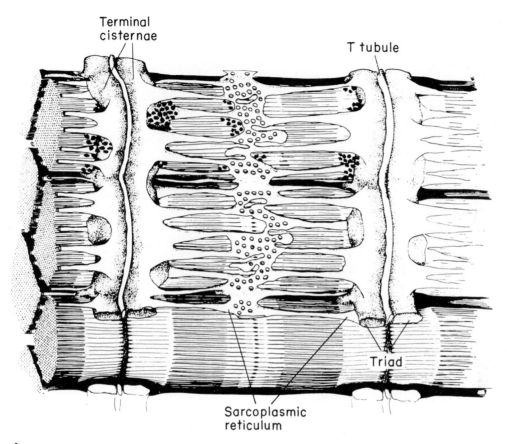

A

FIGURE 7-28A Three-dimensional model of the sarcoplasmic membrane systems and their relationship to myofibrils in the frog sartorius muscle. Note that triads (terminal cisternae of the sarcoplasmic reticulum plus the intervening T tubule) in this *amphibian* muscle, are aligned with the Z lines of the myofibrils. Compare with Fig. 7-29. (From L. D. Peachey, 1965.)

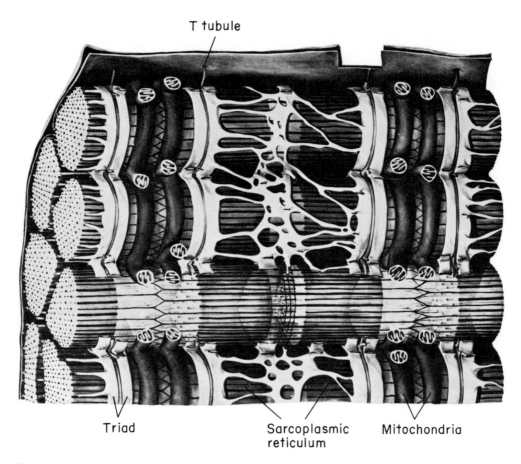

T tubule

Triad

Sarcoplasmic
reticulum

Mitochondria

B

FIGURE 7-28B Three-dimensional model of the sarcoplasmic membrane systems in the rat diaphragm. Note that triads in this *mammalian* muscle are aligned with the A-I junctions in close association with I-band mitochondria. (From H. Schmalbruch, ''Advances in Anatomy, Embryology and Cell Biology,'' **43:**No. 1, Springer-Verlag, Berlin, 1970.)

myofibril. Comparative physiologic studies have shown, in fact, that those muscle fibers in which the triads are located at the Z line can be made to contract by means of a stimulating electrode placed at the Z line, whereas those fibers in which the triads are located at the A-I junction can be made to contract only if the same electrode is placed at the A-I junction. The manner in which a stimulus is transmitted from the T system along the length of the myofibril is less clear, but the close apposition of the T system to the terminal cisternae of the sarcoplasmic reticulum suggests that these are sites of low resistance across which an electrical impulse could pass to the sarcoplasmic reticulum.

THE NEUROMUSCULAR JUNCTION

The plasma membrane of the muscle cell or sarcolemma is structurally equivalent to the plasma mem-

FIGURE 7-29 Electron micrograph showing tangential section of a single sarcomere (rat diaphragm). The sarcoplasmic reticulum extends over the A band and into the I band, and forms a tubular network in the region of the H band. Longitudinal tubules give rise to terminal cisternae closely associated with the transversely oriented T tubule (arrows). The triads, in this *mammalian* muscle, are located near the junction of the A and I bands. That part of the sarcoplasmic reticulum which connects with that of the succeeding sarcomere is not fully included in this plane of section. Portions of it are visible between paired I-band mitochondria (M), which are closely aligned with the triads. See also Fig. 7-30. × 42,500. (Courtesy of H. A. Padykula.)

brane of other cell types, and a typical basal lamina is applied to its outer surface. It is electrically polarized and, upon appropriate stimulation, usually by a nerve fiber, becomes depolarized, after which contraction of the muscle fiber ensues. Branches of each motor nerve fiber terminate at specic sites along the muscle fiber; these are called *neuromuscular junctions.* The relationship between nerve fiber and muscle fiber is intimate and complex (Figs. 7-33 to 7-35). At all points, the plasmalemmas of the two cells remain separate, but the surface of the muscle fiber invaginates to form a shallow trough, the *primary synaptic cleft,* which receives the nerve terminal, or *axonal ending.* The sarcolemma invagintes further to form numerous deep *secondary synaptic clefts,* or *junctional folds,* which greatly increase the surface area of the muscle fiber (Fig. 7-34). The axon loses its myelin sheath as it approaches the neuromuscular junction, and its basal lamina, together with that of the Schwann cell (see Chap. 8), becomes fused with that of the muscle fiber. This cell coat extends into the primary synaptic cleft, as a single layer, separating nerve fiber from muscle fiber. It enters each junctional fold and forms a coating over its inner surface. That portion of the muscle fiber which contributes to the neuromuscular relationship is referred to as the *muscle sole*

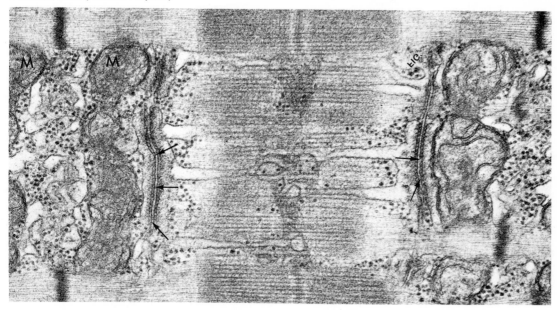

plate, or *motor end plate.* Nuclei and mitochondria are particularly abundant in this so-called junctional sarcoplasm. Cisternae of rough-surfaced endoplasmic reticulum and free ribosomes occur in this region also, perhaps in relation to synthesis of a receptor protein. The axonal ending is typically filled with vesicles (*synaptic vesicles*), that correspond to sites of the neurotransmitter acetylcholine. Mitochondria are present, but filaments and microtubules, characteristic of the more proximal part of the axon, are absent.

FIGURE 7-30 Single triad (rat semitendinosus). The membranes of both terminal cisternae (arrows) are "scalloped" along the surface that faces the T tubule (T). At the left, longitudinal tubules of the sarcoplasmic reticulum from the A-band region connect with one of the terminal cisternae. ×94,500.

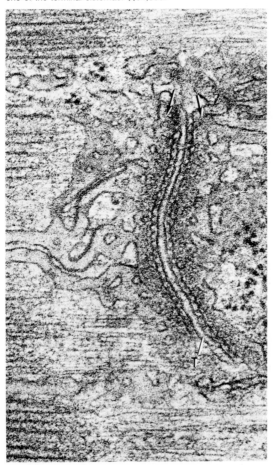

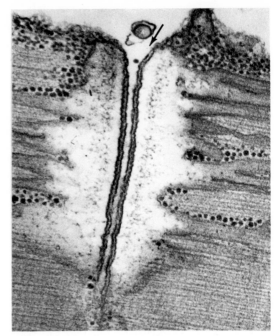

FIGURE 7-31 Single triad (fish muscle) illustrating the direct continuity between the membrane of the T system and the sarcolemma at the upper surface of the fiber (arrow). ×60,000. (From C. Franzini-Armstrong and K. R. Porter, 1964.)

Though myelin is absent from the axon at the neuromuscular junction, a Schwann cell remains closely associated with the axon and forms a covering over the junctional complex (Fig. 7-33). In this way, the axonal ending remains enclosed by the Schwann cell on one surface and by the muscle fiber on the other.

THE HETEROGENEITY OF SKELETAL MUSCLE FIBERS

It has long been known that skeletal muscles differ in their color, with certain muscles being redder than others when viewed grossly. The fibers composing an individual muscle differ also, and the resulting heterogeneity is especially conspicuous following histochemical procedures for localizing enzymatic activity (see Gauthier, 1971). Fibers differ, for example, in mitochondrial enzymatic activity, and this activity is, for the most part, inversely proportional to the cross-sectional dimensions of the fibers (Fig. 7-7). In the mammal, small fibers, which are rich in mitochondria,

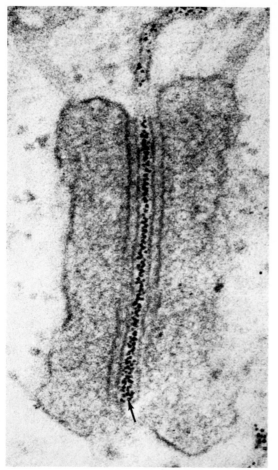

FIGURE 7-32 Triad from frog muscle fiber that had been immersed in a solution containing ferritin. Electron-dense particles of ferritin are present in the T system (arrow) but not in the sarcoplasmic reticulum, which suggests a functional continuity between the T system and the sarcolemma. ×178,200. (From H. E. Huxley, 1964.)

between myofibrils. The intermediate fiber is similar except that mitochondria tend to be smaller and their cristae less abundant than in the red fiber. Also, the Z line is noticeably thinner in the intermediate than in the red fiber. In the white fiber (Fig. 7-37), subsarcolemmal and interfibrillar mitochondria are sparse, and paired elliptical profiles at the I bands, which are present in all three fiber types, are the major form. The Z line in the white fiber is about half as wide as that of the red fiber. It is of interest that the red fiber, which is the smallest fiber, has the highest concentration of mitochondria, particularly at the cell surface. These features are consistent with a high rate of metabolic exchange.

Ultrastructural features of the neuromuscular junctions of red and white fibers indicate that differences exist also in the motoneurons serving these fibers. In the white fiber (Fig. 7-34), axonal vesicles are abundant and junctional folds are long and closely spaced. In the red fiber (Fig. 7-33), axonal vesicles are less numerous and junctional folds are relatively short and sparse. Experiments with cross innervation have shown that the microscopic distribution of fiber types as well as physiologic and biochemical properties of the muscles are altered when the nerve supplies are switched. It has been demonstrated also that stimulation of a particular motor neuron can bring about the cytochemical alteration of a single type of muscle fiber. It is evident, therefore, that the pattern of distribution of fiber types is under the influence of the nervous system, and these findings are consistent with the distinctive ultrastructural features of the muscle fibers and of their neuromuscular junctions. Physiologic data indicate that red muscles contract more slowly than do white muscles, so it has been assumed that the red fiber is a slow fiber. However, physiological properties attributed to individual fibers have been derived largely by extrapolation from measurements on whole muscles. These muscles, moreover, do not necessarily consist of typical red fibers. The functional significance of individual fiber types is only beginning to be understood. There is, for example, increasing evidence of chemical heterogeneity of individual myofibrillar proteins, and it is possible that differences in the protein composition of whole muscles are related to differences in the pattern of distribution of fiber types.

are prevalent in red muscles and are thus referred to as *red fibers*. Large fibers with a low mitochondrial content predominate in white muscles and are thus called *white fibers*. Fibers with characteristics between the two, but which superficially resemble red fibers, are also prevalent in red muscles and are called *intermediate fibers*. It is possible to distinguish these three types of fibers by their ultrastructural features also. In the red fiber (Fig. 7-36), numerous large mitochondria with closely packed cristae form conspicuous aggregations beneath the sarcolemma and longitudinal rows

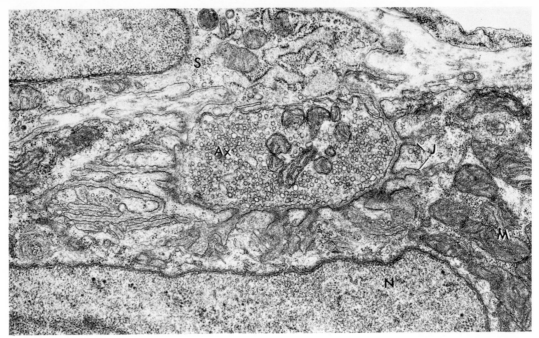

FIGURE 7-33 Neuromuscular junction of a red fiber (rat diaphragm). The axonal ending (Ax) is located in a depression of the surface of the muscle fiber (primary synaptic cleft), and the surface is further invaginated to form junctional folds or secondary synaptic clefts (J). Axonal vesicles and mitochondria are present in the axon. Part of a Schwann cell (S) covers the upper surface of the axon, and a nucleus (N) and mitochondria (M) are present in the sarcoplasm below the axonal ending. Structural organization is more readily apparent in the diagram in Fig. 7-35. ×22,500 (From G. F. Gauthier, 1970.)

FIGURE 7-34 Neuromuscular junction of a white fiber (rat diaphragm). Junctional folds are longer and more closely spaced than in the red fiber (Fig. 7-33), and axonal vesicles are more closely packed. ×24,000. (From H. A. Padykula and G. F. Gauthier, *J. Cell Biol.,* **46:**27, 1970.)

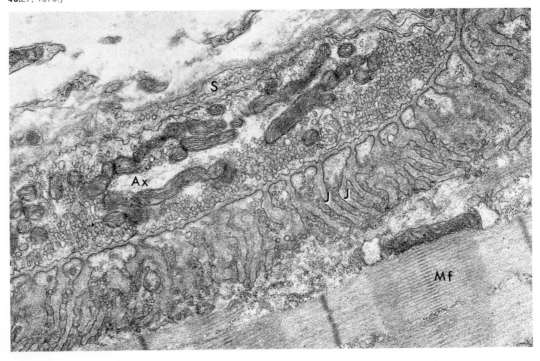

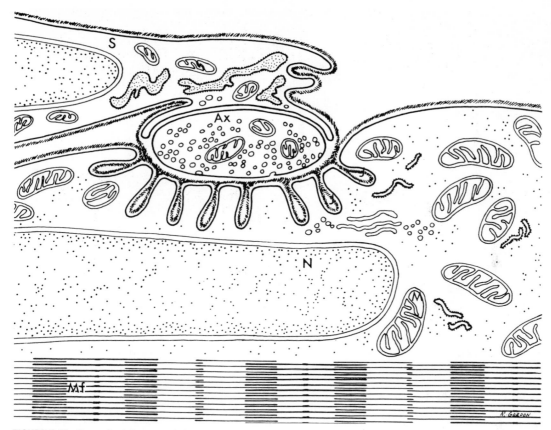

FIGURE 7-35 Generalized diagrammatic interpretation of the neuromuscular relationship. A Schwann cell (S) forms a covering over the axonal ending (Ax), and its basal lamina becomes fused with that of the muscle fiber, forming a coating which extends along the primary synaptic cleft and into each secondary synaptic cleft or junctional fold (J). Nuclei, mitochondria, free ribosomes, and rough endoplasmic reticulum occur characteristically in the junctional sarcoplasm.

CARDIAC MUSCLE

GENERAL FEATURES

The myocardium is composed of distinctive multinucleated striated fibers called *cardiac muscle fibers*. They are rich in mitochondria and are closely invested with an extensive capillary network. Although the nervous system is not required to initiate the heart beat, autonomic nerves are abundant. Nerve fibers appear to make contact with cardiac muscle fibers, but elaborate neuromuscular junctions such as those described for skeletal muscle fibers have not been observed.

Cardiac muscle is transversely striated; but unlike skeletal muscle, the fibers are branched and the nuclei are centrally located (Figs. 7-38 and 7-40). Bundles of myofilaments diverge as they approach the poles of the nucleus, leaving conical accumulations of sarcoplasm. Large mitochondria with closely packed cristae are abundant in the perinuclear sarcoplasm and form almost continuous longitudinal rows elsewhere in the fibers (Fig. 7-39). Paired I-band mitochondria, which are characteristic of skeletal muscle, are not present in cardiac muscle. The sarcoplasm is rich in glycogen and lipid (Fig. 7-39), which, as in skeletal muscle, constitute metabolic fuels for contractile activity.

There are no apparent differences in the basic

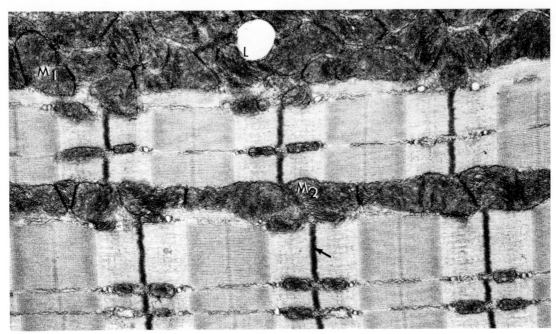

FIGURE 7-36 Longitudinal section of a typical red fiber (rat semitendinosus). Large mitochondria (M₁) with closely packed cristae are aggregated just beneath the sarcolemma and in longitudinal interfibrillar rows (M₂). The Z line (arrow) is relatively wide. Compare with Fig. 7-37, which is at the same magnification. × 16,500. (From G. F. Gauthier, 1970.)

FIGURE 7-37 Typical white fiber (rat semitendinosus). Subsarcolemmal and interfibrillar mitochondria are small and sparse. Paired mitochondria (M₃) at the I bands, which are characteristic of mammalian skeletal muscle in general, are the predominate form in the white fiber. The Z line (arrow) is about half as wide as in the red fiber (Fig. 7-36). × 16,500. (From G. F. Gauthier, *Z. Zellforsch,* **95:**462, 1969.)

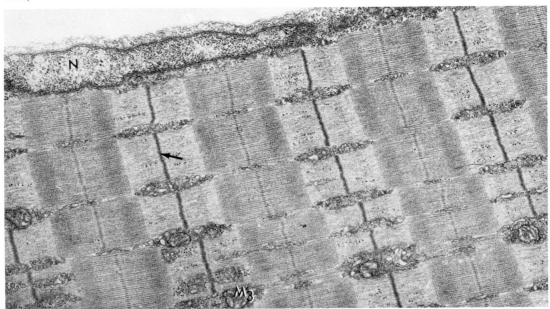

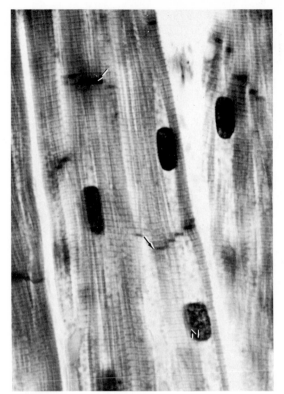

FIGURE 7-38 Longitudinal section of several cardiac muscle fibers. Nuclei (N) occupy a central position in these fibers, which are transversely striated. Bundles of filaments diverge as they approach the nucleus, leaving a conical region of sarcoplasm at each nuclear pole. Intercalated discs form conspicuous bands (arrows) which extend stepwise across the fibers, always at the level of a Z line. (H&E) ×1,200.

ultrastructural configuration of the contractile apparatus of skeletal and cardiac muscle fibers. The precise arrangement of thick and thin myofilaments produces a transverse banding pattern equivalent to that of skeletal muscle (Fig. 7-39). However, bundles of filaments are not aggregated transversely to form discrete myofibrillar units as in skeletal muscle fibers. The transverse continuity of myofibrillar material is interrupted only by the longitudinal rows of mitochondria and scattered profiles of the sarcoplasmic reticulum (Figs. 7-40 and 7-41).

THE SARCOPLASMIC MEMBRANE SYSTEMS

Both the sarcoplasmic reticulum and the T system are present in mammalian cardiac muscle. The sarcoplasmic reticulum is less abundant and less elaborate

than in skeletal muscle. An irregular network of tubules extends over the full length of the sarcomere, with no transverse specialization at the H band. Terminal specializations occur at the Z lines, that is, at a position comparable to that of the triads of amphibian skeletal muscle. However, the terminal cisternae are not so extensive or regularly arranged and thus make less-frequent contact with the transverse tubules (Fig. 7-42). This leads to the appearance of so-called dyads, or "couplings," where only one cisterna is apposed to a T tubule. The cisternae may also be apposed to the sarcolemma and, because of this relationship, are given the designation *subsarcolemmal cisternae*.

There are fewer T tubules in cardiac than in skeletal muscle, but they are larger in diameter (Fig. 7-42). The continuity of the T system with the sarcolemma is even more conspicuous than in skeletal muscle, and the basal lamina extends inward along with the membrane, forming a coating over the inner surface of the T tubule. The relationship between the cisternal membrane and that of the T tubule or the sarcolemma is similar to that observed in the triads of skeletal muscle, and this close relationship is believed to favor the transmission of an electrical stimulus carried by the T system.

INTERCELLULAR RELATIONSHIPS

Unlike skeletal muscle fibers, individual cardiac muscle fibers are associated in an end-to-end arrangement which produces the so-called intercalated discs at frequent intervals. The intercalated disc is a complex cell junction which consists of several transverse portions arranged stepwise at different levels across the fiber (Figs. 7-38 and 7-39). Two successive transverse portions are connected longitudinally by a continuation of the respective cell membranes, thereby creating a complete separation between cells. Therefore, contrary to early beliefs, the myocardium is not a syncytium. The transverse cell surfaces are elaborately interdigitated and, in longitudinal sections of the fibers, they have a characteristic undulating pattern (Figs. 7-39 and 7-43). The subsarcolemmal sarcoplasm contains dense masses of filamentous material into which the I-band filaments insert (Fig. 7-43). The appearance of the intercellular relationship at certain points is therefore similar to the desmosome or *macula adherens* observed in certain epithelia (see

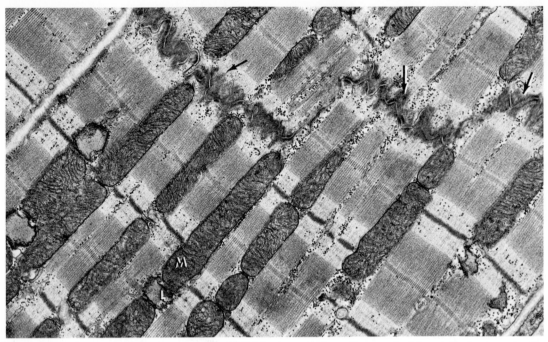

FIGURE 7-39 Electron micrograph of a longitudinal section from the ventricular papillary muscle of the cat. The transverse banding pattern is similar to that of skeletal muscle. Paired mitochondria are absent from the I bands, but large mitochondria (M) form almost continuous longitudinal rows, and lipid droplets (L) are closely associated with them. A transverse cell junction is arranged in the typical stepwise pattern that constitutes the intercalated disc. Parts of three transverse portions (arrows) of the intercalated disc are included in the section, together with the longitudinal portions that connect them. ×15,000. (From D. W. Fawcett and N. S. McNutt, 1969.)

FIGURE 7-40 Electron micrograph of portions of four fibers sectioned transversely (cat papillary muscle). The central position of the nucleus (N) is apparent in one of the fibers. Though discrete myofibrils are not apparent, the transverse continuity of myofibrillar material is partially interrupted by numerous large mitochondria (M). ×6,700. (From D. W. Fawcett and N. S. McNutt, 1969.)

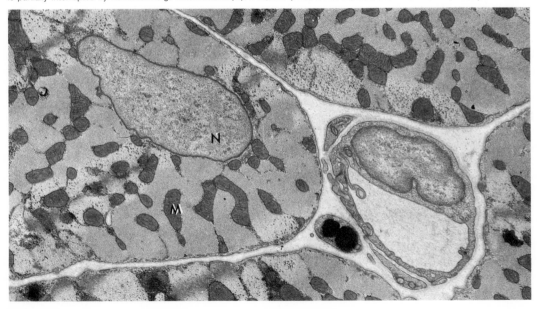

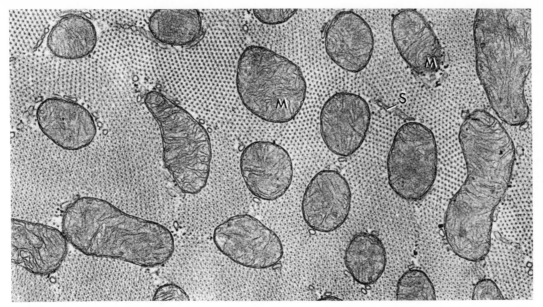

FIGURE 7-41 Transverse section similar to that in Fig. 7-40 showing the arrangement of myofilaments and sarcoplasmic organelles. The hexagonal array of thick and thin filaments is similar to that of skeletal muscle, but there is no organization into individual myofibrils. Transverse sections of longitudinal rows of mitochondria (M) and profiles of sarcoplasmic membranes (S) form a discontinuous boundary between masses of myofilaments. ×30,000. (From D. W. Fawcett and N. S. McNutt, 1969.)

FIGURE 7-42 Three-dimensional model of the sarcoplasmic membrane systems of cardiac muscle. The sarcoplasmic reticulum is less elaborate than in skeletal muscle. T tubules, on the other hand, are even more prominent than in skeletal muscle, and their membranes are clearly continuous with the sarcolemma. Note that they are located at the level of the Z line. (From D. W. Fawcett and N. S. McNutt, 1969.)

Subsarcolemmal cisternae

Mitochondrion

T-tubule

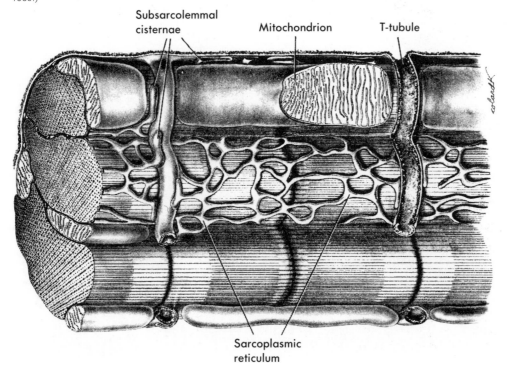

Sarcoplasmic reticulum

Chap. 3). In addition, the relationship may be more extensive than that of a typical desmosome, and is thus referred to as a *fascia adherens*.

At other sites, the intercellular space appears to be obliterated as in a typical tight junction or zonula occludens, but since this relationship is more circumscribed, it is referred to as a *macula occludens*. The longitudinal portion of the intercalated disc is continuous with the transverse portions. The longitudinal intercellular relationship is similar to the zonula occludens of epithelial cells, but is even more extensive, and thus constitutes a *fascia occludens*. Both the macula occludens and fascia occludens constitute the so-called nexus of cardiac and smooth muscle. Advances in the methodology of ultrastructure have revealed that a narrow intercellular space (about 18 Å) exists at the nexus; therefore it is more correctly described as a *close,* or *gap, junction* rather than a tight junction. The gap junction is believed to be a site of low electrical resistance. Since electrical coupling between cells is a fundamental property of both cardiac and smooth

muscle, the gap junction might constitute the structural basis for electrical transmission among cardiac- or smooth-muscle cells.

Most of the description above has been derived from the study of ventricular cardiac muscle, but atrial muscle shares many of the basic features. However, in the cat, at least, the atrial fibers tend to be smaller in diameter. The mitochondrial content tends to be even greater than in ventricular fibers, but T tubules are relatively sparse.

The origin and distribution of electrical activity leading to the characteristic rhythmical contraction of cardiac muscle reside in special forms of cardiac muscle fibers which compose the conducting system of the heart, namely, the SA node, AV node, and AV bundle. These fibers make contact ultimately with ordinary

FIGURE 7-43 Part of a single transverse portion of an intercalated disc. The cell membranes at the extremities of the two fibers included in the micrograph are continuous at the left (arrow) with part of a longitudinal segment of the intercalated disc. The cell membranes pursue a wavy course but remain parallel to each other throughout the intercalated disc. I-band filaments above and below appear to insert into the dense sarcoplasmic material adjacent to the cell membranes. ×70,000. (From D. W. Fawcett and N. S. McNutt, 1969.)

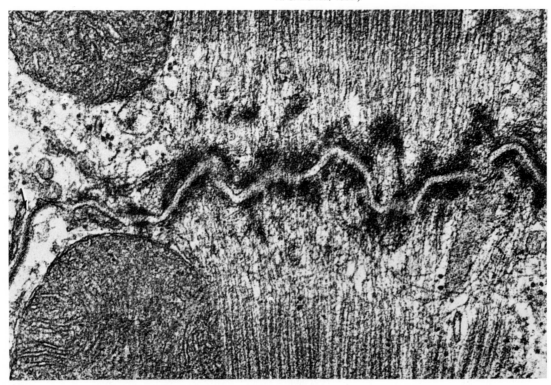

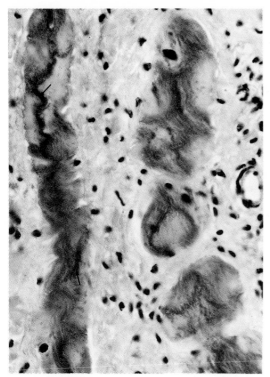

FIGURE 7-44 Section of ox heart including portions of several Purkinje fibers. The fiber at the left is sectioned longitudinally, and those at the right are sectioned transversely or somewhat obliquely. The fibers are large when compared with most ordinary cardiac muscle fibers (Fig. 7-38), and myofibrils (arrows) are relatively sparse. Most of the sarcoplasm is occupied by glycogen, which has been extracted from this preparation. (H&E) ×480.

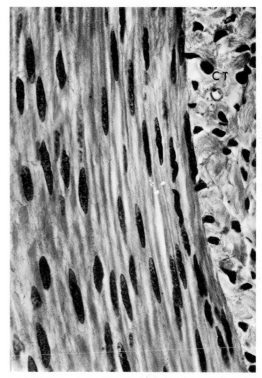

FIGURE 7-45 Transverse section of frog intestine showing the typical appearance of the circular layer of smooth muscle adjacent to connective tissue (CT) of the submucosa. The fibers are arranged circumferentially with their narrow tapered ends adjacent to the wider central regions of nearby fibers. Nuclei are centrally located. Cell boundaries are somewhat difficult to distinguish. (H&E) ×500.

cardiac muscle fibers. Nodal fibers tend to be smaller, but those of the AV bundle tend to be larger, than ordinary cardiac muscle fibers. The fibers of the AV bundle often acquire a distinctive appearance and may therefore be distinguished from ordinary cardiac muscle fibers. These special conducting fibers, or *Purkinje fibers,* are responsible for the final distribution of the electrical stimulus to the myocardium. Variable amounts of connective tissue separate the conducting

fibers from one another, and this differs from species to species. Myofibrillar material tends to be less abundant than in ordinary cardiac muscle fibers, but this too varies with the species. In some species, notably among the ungulates, Purkinje fibers are extremely large, and massive amounts of glycogen are accumulated in the sarcoplasm. Only scattered strands of myofibrillar material are apparent in these fibers (Fig. 7-44).

SMOOTH MUSCLE

GENERAL FEATURES

Smooth muscle plays a critical role in the maintenance of the caliber of the lumens of the viscera and certain blood vessels. Through the appropriate degree of contraction or relaxation of the component fibers,

physiologic processes such as digestion, respiration, and blood flow can be regulated. Accordingly, the fibers are arranged in characteristic directions, reflecting the functional activity of the organ (Fig. 7-45). Connective tissue, carrying blood vessels and autonomic nerve fibers, penetrates among individual

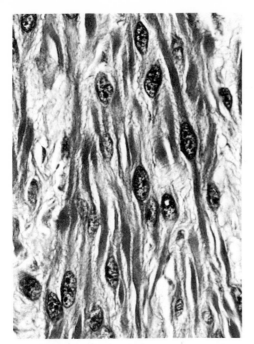

FIGURE 7-46 Longitudinal sections of several smooth-muscle fibers (lateral vaginal canal of the opossum). Because of the relative abundance of connective tissue in this bundle of smooth muscle, the cellular outlines are clearly distinguished. Nuclei occupy the broad central regions of these tapering fibers. (H&E) ×760.

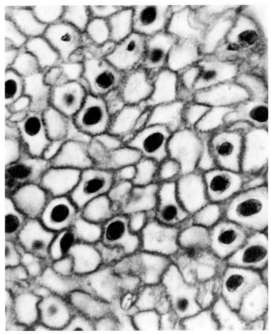

FIGURE 7-47 Transverse section of smooth-muscle fibers (stomach of the grasshopper mouse), which has been stained by the periodic acid–Schiff reaction and with hematoxylin. The carbohydrate component of the conspicuous basal lamina is stained, and this facilitates visualization of individual fibers. Note that the plane of section passes through the broad nuclear regions of only certain fibers and through the narrow tapered ends of others. ×1,200.

FIGURE 7-48 Electron micrograph of a longitudinal section of a smooth muscle fiber (ileum of a 13-day-old rat). Part of the centrally located nucleus (N) is included at the left. Mitochondria, a Golgi apparatus, and ribosomes are particularly abundant in the conical perinuclear region. The remainder of the fiber is occupied by thin filaments and by dense bodies (arrows) into which the filaments appear to insert. There are no transverse striations. ×17,220.

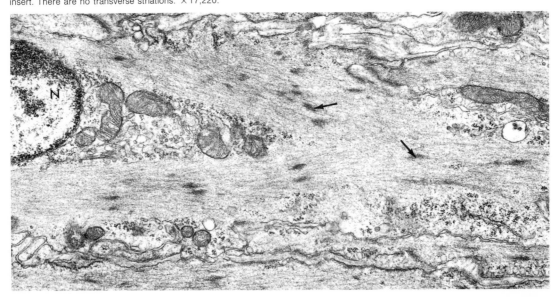

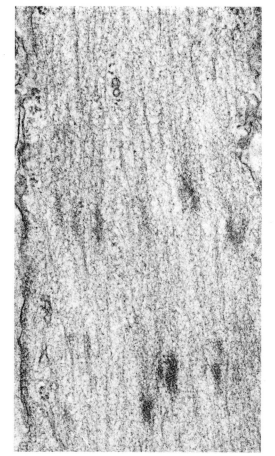

FIGURE 7-49 Longitudinal section similar to that in Fig. 7-48, illustrating the filamentous composition of the smooth-muscle fiber. There is an apparently homogeneous population of thin filaments with dimensions similar to those of actin filaments from striated muscle. Compare with Fig. 7-50. ×43,700.

fibers, but the amount of stroma varies among species and among the organ systems of a given species (for example, compare Figs. 7-45 and 7-46).

Smooth muscle fibers are narrow and tapering, and their length varies from about 20 μm in certain small blood vessels to 500 μm or more in the gestational uterus. The nucleus is centrally located, and there are no transverse striations (Figs. 7-46 and 7-47). A typical basal lamina is applied to the outer surface of the sarcolemma. In fact, when stained, the basal laminae facilitate the visualization of individual fibers (Fig. 7-47).

The arrangement of fibers is staggered so that the broad nuclear region of one fiber lies opposite the

narrow tapered end of an adjacent fiber (Fig. 7-45). A transverse section would therefore pass through the nuclear level of only certain fibers and through the tapered ends of those which intervene (Fig. 7-47). At various points, adjacent fibers form an intimate association, called a nexus, or gap junction, where electrical coupling is believed to be facilitated as described earlier.

The cytoplasmic organelles, which include mitochondria, Golgi apparatus, scattered profiles of rough endoplasmic reticulum, and free ribosomes, are confined, for the most part, to a conical region at each

FIGURE 7-50 Transverse section of smooth muscle from rabbit portal-anterior mesenteric vein. Both thick and thin filaments are evident in this preparation, although the spatial arrangement is different from that of striated muscle (Fig. 7-10). ×153,000. (From A. P. Somlyo et al., *Philos. Trans. R. Soc.,* 1973.)

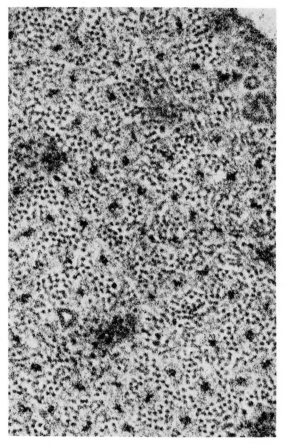

pole of the nucleus (Fig. 7-48). The remainder of the sarcoplasm is occupied by filaments which usually appear thin (Fig. 7-49). Characteristic dense bodies, into which the thin filaments appear to insert, are distributed throughout the sarcoplasm (Figs. 7-48 and 7-49).

THE ULTRASTRUCTURAL BASIS OF CONTRACTION

Much less is known about the mechanism of contraction in smooth muscle than in striated muscle. The absence of transverse banding has made application of the sliding filament model seem inappropriate. Although both myosin and actin can be demonstrated in smooth muscle by chemical procedures, conventional ultrastructural preparations ordinarily reveal a homogeneous population of thin filaments.

Under precisely controlled conditions, thick filaments can be prepared from homogenates of mammalian smooth muscle, and the ultrastructural appearance of these filaments closely resembles that of myosin fialments prepared from skeletal muscle. Also, thick filaments can be observed in ultrathin sections of smooth muscle fibers prepared under appropriate pH, temperature, and ionic conditions (Fig. 7-50). As in skeletal muscle, therefore, two types of filaments can be demonstrated. It has been suggested that in smooth muscle, myosin is labile, and that under conditions favorable for contraction, well-defined thick filaments are formed. It is thus likely that a sliding filament mechanism is operative in the contraction of smooth muscle as well as skeletal muscle.

REFERENCES

BÜLRING, E., and D. M. NEEDHAM (organizers): A Discussion on Recent Developments in Vertebrate Smooth Muscle Physiology, *Philos. Trans. R. Soc. Lond.,* B. [*Biol. Sci.*], **265:**1–231 (1973).

COHEN, C.: The Protein Switch of Muscle Contraction, *Sci. Am.,* **233** (5):36 (1975).

DEVINE, C. E., and A. P. SOMLYO: Thick Filaments in Vascular Smooth Muscle, *J. Cell Biol.,* **49:**636 (1971).

DEWEY, M. M., and L. BARR: A Study of the Structure and Distribution of the Nexus, *J. Cell Biol.,* **23:**553 (1964).

EBASHI S., M. ENDO, and I. OHTSUKI: Control of Muscle Contraction, *Q. Rev. Biophys.,* **2:**351 (1969).

FAWCETT, D. W., and N. S. MC NUTT: The Ultrastructure of the Cat Myocardium. I. Ventricular Papillary Muscle, *J. Cell Biol.,* **42:**1 (1969).

FRANZINI-ARMSTRONG, C.: Freeze Fracture of Skeletal Muscle from the Tarantula Spider, *J. Cell Biol.,* **61:**501 (1974).

FRANZINI-ARMSTRONG, C.: Studies of the Triad. I. Structure of the Junction in Frog Twitch Fibers, *J. Cell Biol.,* **47:**488 (1970).

FRANZINI-ARMSTRONG, C., and K. R. PORTER: Sarcolemmal Invaginations Constituting the T System in Fish Muscle Fibers, *J. Cell Biol.,* **22:**675 (1964).

GAUTHIER, G. F.: The Motor End-Plate, in D. N. Landon (ed.), ''The Peripheral Nerve,'' Chapman & Hall, Ltd., London, 1976.

GAUTHIER, G. F.: The Structural and Cytochemical Heterogeneity of Mammalian Skeletal Muscle Fibers, in R. J. Podolsky (ed.), ''The Contractility of Muscle Cells and Related Processes,'' Prentice-Hall, Inc., Englewood Cliffs, N.J., 1971.

GAUTHIER, G. F.: The Ultrastructure of Three Fiber Types in Mammalian Skeletal Muscle, in E. J. Briskey, R. G. Cassens, and B. B. Marsh (eds.) ''The Physiology and Biochemistry of Muscle as a Food,'' vol. 2, The University of Wisconsin Press, Madison, 1970.

HANSON, J., and H. E. HUXLEY: The Structural Basis of Contraction in Striated Muscle, in "Fibrous Proteins and Their Biological Significance," no. 9, Academic Press, Inc., New York, 1955.

HANSON, J., and J. LOWY: The Structure of F-Actin and of Actin Filaments Isolated from Muscle, *J. Molec. Biol.,* **6:**46 (1963).

HUXLEY, H. E.: The Mechanism of Muscular Contraction, *Science,* **164:**1356 (1969).

HUXLEY, H. E.: Evidence for Continuity between the Central Elements of the Triads and Extra-cellular Space in Frog Sartorius Muscle, *Nature,* **202:**1067 (1964).

HUXLEY, H. E.: Electron Microscope Studies on the Structure of Natural and Synthetic Protein Filaments from Striated Muscle, *J. Molec. Biol.,* **7:**281 (1963).

HUXLEY, H. E.: The Double Array of Filaments in Cross-striated Muscle, *J. Biophys. Biochem. Cytol.,* **3:**631 (1957).

KELLY, D. E.: Models of Muscle Z-band Fine Structure Based on a Looping Filament Configuration, *J. Cell Biol.,* **34:**827 (1967).

KELLY, R. E., and R. V. RICE: Ultrastructural Studies on the Contractile Mechanism of Smooth Muscle, *J. Cell Biol.,* **42:**683 (1969).

KELLY, R. E., and R. V. RICE: Localization of Myosin Filaments in Smooth Muscle, *J. Cell Biol.,* **37:**105 (1968).

KNAPPEIS, G. G., and F. CARLSEN: The Ultrastructure of the Z Disc in Skeletal Muscle, *J. Cell Biol.,* **13:**323 (1962).

LOWEY, S.: Myosin: Molecule and Filament, in S. N. Timasheff and G. D. Fasman (eds.), "Biological Macromolecules Series," vol. 5, pt. A, chap. 5, Marcel Dekker, Inc., New York, 1971.

MC NUTT, N. S. and D. W. FAWCETT: Myocardial Ultrastructure, in G. A. Langer and A. J. Brady (eds.), "The Mammalian Myocardium," John Wiley & Sons, Inc., New York, 1974.

MC NUTT, N. S., and D. W. FAWCETT: The Ultrastructure of the Cat Myocardium. II. Atrial Muscle, *J. Cell Biol.,* **42:**46 (1969).

MOORE, P. B., H. E. HUXLEY, and D. J. DE ROSIER: Three-dimensional Reconstruction of F-actin, Thin Filaments and Decorated Thin Filaments, *J. Molec. Biol.,* **50:**279 (1970).

PEACHEY, L. D.: The Sarcoplasmic Reticulum and Transverse Tubules of the Frog's Sartorius, *J. Cell Biol.,* **25** (3):209 (1965).

PEPE, F. A.: The Structural Components of the Striated Muscle Fibril, in S. N. Timasheff and G. D. Fasman (eds.), "Biological Macromolecules Series," vol. 5, pt. A, chap. 7, Marcel Dekker, Inc., New York, 1971.

POLLARD, T. D. and R. R. WEIHING: Actin and Myosin and Cell Movement, CRC *Crit. Rev. Biochem.,* **2:**1 (1974).

PORTER, K. R., and G. E. PALADE: Studies on the Endoplasmic Reticulum. III. Its Form and Distribution in Striated Muscle Cells, *J. Biophys. Biochem. Cytol.,* **3:**269 (1957).

ROBERTSON, J. D.: The Ultrastructure of a Reptilian Myoneural Junction, *J. Biophys. Biochem. Cytol.,* **2:**381 (1956).

SOMMER, J. R., and E. A. JOHNSON: Cardiac Muscle. A Comparative Study of Purkinje Fibers and Ventricular Fibers, *J. Cell Biol.,* **36:**497 (1968).

Nervous Tissue

EDWARD G. JONES and W. MAXWELL COWAN

DEVELOPMENT OF NERVOUS TISSUE

NEURAL INDUCTION AND THE FORMATION OF THE NEURAL TUBE

With the exception of the sensory epithelia and the associated ganglion cells of certain of the cranial nerves, all elements of the central and peripheral nervous systems are derived from a specialized region of ectoderm along the dorsal midline of the embryo. Initially, this zone is indistinguishable from the rest of the ectoderm, but under the inductive influence of the underlying notochord and the adjoining mesoderm, its cells become elongated and appear to be irreversibly determined to form neural tissue. In the human embryo, at about the 18-day stage, this specialized zone forms a slipper-shaped area immediately rostral to the *primitive knot,* or *Hensen's node,* and in transverse sections appears as a thickened and slightly depressed region dorsal to the notochord (Fig. 8-1). The central portion of this region is called the *neurecto-derm.* Interposed between it and the nonspecialized, or *somatic* ectoderm is a second specialized zone, the *neurosomatic junctional region.* The neurectoderm will form the *neural* (or *medullary*) plate from which the entire central nervous system is derived; the neurosomatic junctional region will give rise to the cells of the *neural crest* from which much of the peripheral nervous system (and a number of other tissues) will be formed.

With the progressive thickening of the epithelium of the neurectoderm, the lateral edges of the neural plate become increasingly elevated to form a *neural groove* bounded on either side by raised *neural folds* (Fig. 8-1). Toward the end of the third embryonic week the lips of the neural groove fuse together in the upper cervical region. From this region the process of fusion extends rostrally and caudally, converting the original neural plate into a *neural tube* (Fig. 8-1). For a time, the tube remains open at its rostral and caudal ends (the openings are termed the *anterior* and *posterior neuropores*), but with the closure of the neuropores (during the fourth embryonic week), it becomes completely closed off from the rest of the embryo. At the time of fusion of the folds of the neural groove, the cells of the neurosomatic junctional region become separated from both the somatic ectoderm and the neurectoderm and come to occupy a position along the dorsolateral aspect of the neural tube. This initially more or less continuous column of cells constitutes the *neural crest.* Subsequently, three vesicular swellings—termed the *prosencephalic, mesencephalic,* and *rhombencephalic* vesicles—appear in the rostral part of the neural tube; respectively they give rise to the forebrain, midbrain and hindbrain. The more caudal, unexpanded portion of the neural tube forms the spinal cord.

HISTOGENESIS IN THE NEURAL TUBE

Until shortly after its closure, the neural tube consists of a simple, columnar epithelium. However, as cell proliferation proceeds, the wall of the tube soon becomes converted into a *pseudostratified* epithelium, with nuclei at several levels, but with each cell retaining a basal cytoplasmic process in contact with the *basement membrane,* or *basal lamina,* which surrounds the neural tube and separates it from the adjoining mesodermal tissues. The luminal processes of the cells are ciliated and joined to each other by a series of *junctional complexes* (or, as they were formerly referred to, *terminal bars*). The epithelium as a whole is variously named the *germinal epithelium* or *neuroepithelium,* and as the *matrix* or *ventricular layer;* from it are derived both the neuronal and supporting elements of the central nervous system.

As Figs. 8-2 and 8-3 show, all the readily identifiable mitotic figures in the neuroepithelium are found along its ventricular or luminal border. This unusual appearance suggested to an earlier generation of embryologists that the wall of the neuroepithelium consisted of two distinct classes of cells: a population of *germinal cells* close to the lumen, which were thought to be the precursors of the neuronal elements of the nervous system; and a deeper population of nonneuronal *spongioblasts.* This view is now known to be erroneous, although the term spongioblast is sometimes still used, especially in neuropathology where, for example, certain tumors of the nervous system are known as *spongioblastomas.*

That the neuroepithelium is a pseudostratified epithelium was first recognized in 1931 by Sauer, who pointed out that all the cells of the neuroepithelium are of essentially the same type, and differ only in being at different stages of the cell cycle. This view was arrived at initially on cytological grounds, but it has been experimentally confirmed in several ways. Of these, the most convincing has been the analysis of cell proliferation in the neuroepithelium by tritiated [^{3}H]thymidine autoradiography.

FIGURE 8-1 The sequence of changes which lead to the formation of the spinal cord and the associated nerve roots from the neural plate and the adjoining neurosomatic junctional region.

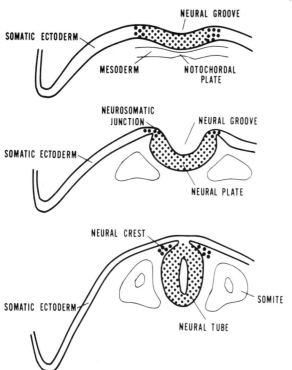
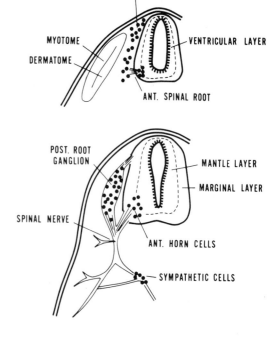

Within an hour or two after the administration of a small dose of [³H]thymidine, the label can be seen in autoradiographs of the neural tube, to have been incorporated into the DNA of cells whose nuclei lie in the basal or middle thirds of the neuroepithelium (Fig. 8-4). At this time all other nuclei in the epithelium appear unlabeled. However, if the autoradiographs are prepared at a later time, say 8 to 12 h after the administration of the isotope, *most* of the nuclei in the epithelium (including those in the later stages of mitosis—metaphase, anaphase, and telophase) will be labeled. This type of experiment not only demonstrates that *all* the cells in the neuroepithelium are capable of DNA synthesis (and hence, of mitosis) but also suggests that cell proliferation in the epithelium proceeds in the following characteristic sequence. Interphase cells in the neuroepithelium (that is, those in the G_1 *phase* of the cell cycle—see Chap. 1) are elongated with their nuclei in the upper or middle thirds of the epithelium (Fig. 8-2). As they enter the *S phase* of the next cycle, their nuclei come to lie, first, deeper within the epithelium; and then at progressively later times in this phase (which generally lasts about 8 to 12 h), the nuclei begin to migrate toward the luminal pole of the cell (Fig. 8-2). By the time the cell enters the G_2 *phase* of the cycle, its nucleus is close to the luminal margin, and the cell as a whole is beginning to round up, by withdrawing its basal process from the basal lamina (Fig. 8-2). The G_2 phase lasts no more than 1 to 2 h and leads directly into the *M phase,* or mid and late mitotic, phase of the cell cycle. Immediately prior to cytokinesis, the now more or less spherical cells appear to lose parts of their junctional complexes; this must be an extremely rapid process, because shortly after cytokinesis the two daughter cells resulting from telophase appear to have reconstituted the junctional

complexes. The entire M phase lasts about 1 h, and leads directly into the subsequent G_1 phase (which is of variable duration). During this phase the cells again become elongated, their nuclei descend, and their abluminal processes reestablish an association with the basal lamina (Fig. 8-2) prior to the next round of DNA synthesis. The changes in the morphology of the cells at different phases of the cell cycle has been strikingly confirmed by recent studies with the scanning electron microscope (Fig. 8-5).

The actual times taken for each phase of the mitotic cycle vary somewhat from region to region in the neural tube and with the age of the embryo. (At late embryonic stages the G_1 phase becomes progressively longer and the entire cycle may take as long as 48 to 96 h.) However, the pattern of DNA synthesis and the interkinetic migration of the nuclei of the neuroepithelial cells remain the same. The process of cell proliferation continues in this manner for a variable period of time in different regions of the neural tube. However, at some point DNA synthesis ceases in certain of the neuroepithelial cells. The time at which the first postmitotic cells appear can also be readily established by [³H]thymidine autoradiography, which has been used experimentally to establish the "dates of birth" of various classes of neurons. On completing their last mitotic division, one, or both, of the daughter cells become arrested in the G_1 phase of the cell cycle; and in this state the cells migrate out of the neuroepithelium and come to lie in a layer deep to the nuclei of the neuroepithelial cells. This newly formed layer of postmitotic cells is known as the *mantle zone* (Figs. 8-3 and 8-4); it is the growth of this layer that leads to

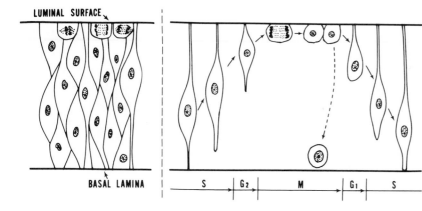

LUMINAL SURFACE

BASAL LAMINA

S | G₂ | M | G₁ | S

FIGURE 8-2 The pseudostratified character of the neuroepithelium and the pattern of interkinetic nuclear migration during the major phases of the cell cycle in the neuroepithelium.

the progressive expansion of the walls of the brain and spinal cord. The region of the neural tube between the developing mantle zone and the basal lamina is called the *marginal zone*. Initially this zone contains only the basal processes of the neuroepithelial cells, but it is soon invaded by the processes of the postmitotic cells in the mantle zone of the same area and by processes entering it from other parts of the nervous system.

We do not know what factor, or factors, bring about the cessation of DNA synthesis in certain cells while permitting it to continue for several further cell cycles in others. Nor is it known whether the two daughter cells of a terminal mitosis are both determined to form nerve cells (or *neurons*), or supporting cells (*neuroglial* cells), or if one cell may later be differentiated into a neuron and the other into a glial cell. At present only three generalizations seem justifiable. First, in most regions of the nervous system the first neurons and the first glial cells *seem* to be formed

at the same time. Second, glial cell proliferation generally continues for some time after all the neurons are formed, and indeed most glial cells retain the capacity for further division throughout the life of the organism. Third, the larger nerve cells are generated earlier than the smaller neurons in the same region. There is also some evidence that the positional information that determines to what sites the larger (projection) neurons will send their axons becomes fixed at the time of the last mitotic division. In view of the importance of the changes that occur in the neuroepithelial cells at the time they become postmitotic, it is somewhat surprising that they show so little morphological evidence of the establishment of the differentiated state. In the light microscope, the only indication that the cells have made this transition are (1) their location in the mantle zone, and (2) the fact that they appear more rounded and have rather more cytoplasm. In the electron microscope they can be seen to have lost their junctional complexes, but otherwise they display the same cytoplasmic organelles as the neuroepithelial cells.

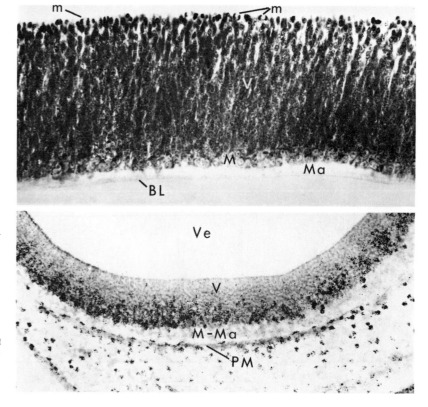

FIGURE 8-3 (Upper) A photomicrograph of the neuroepithelium of the chick optic tectum with the mitotic figures (m) confined to the luminal surface. Postmitotic cells (M) form a mantle or intermediate zone immediately above the marginal zone (Ma). BL, basal lamina. Thionin stain. ×465. **FIGURE 8-4 (lower)** An autoradiograph of the neuroepithelium a short time after the administration of [³H]-thymidine. Only the nuclei in the deeper part of the ventricular zone (V) are labeled, together with cells in the surrounding pia mater (PM). Ve, ventricle. ×93.

It is customary to refer to the cells of the mantle zone as *neuroblasts* (if they give rise to mature neurons) or *glioblasts* (if they form neuroglial cells). But since the neuroblasts can no longer divide, the suffix *-blast* (which is often used in cytology for a precursor cell) is inappropriate and the term *neuroblast* should be replaced by *young neuron*. The essential point is that the newly formed neurons and neuroglial cells are differentiated cells and the further changes which they undergo (including the growth and elaboration of their various processes and appendages) simply reflect their prior commitment to the neuronal or glial cell line.

The subsequent fate of these cells and their mature morphological appearance will be dealt with in a later section. With the notable exception of the last remaining neuroepithelial cells, which persist in the mature nervous system as the *ependymal cells* lining the ventricular system of the brain and spinal cord, all cells in the nervous system migrate, at least once, from the region in which they are generated to their definitive location. The details of the migratory process remain to be determined (at present it is thought to be similar to the migration of ameboid cells elsewhere), but one intriguing suggestion is that migrating neurons may be directed toward their terminal loci by the neighboring preformed neuroglial cell processes. Certainly, in many parts of the nervous system, the glial cells have long radially oriented processes (which may extend across most of the thickness of the expanding neural tube, or its derivatives) and the migrating neu-

rons are nearly always found in close association with such processes (Fig. 8-6). And in certain genetic disorders which are characterized by the early degeneration, or incomplete development, of the glial cells, the neurons in the affected regions fail to migrate in the normal manner.

SOME LESS-COMMON HISTOGENETIC PATTERNS

The pattern of cell proliferation, differentiation, and migration just described is typical of most regions of the central nervous system, but in certain regions a rather different sequence of events occurs. In the cerebral hemispheres a second proliferative zone appears immediately deep to the neuroepithelium. In this *subependymal* or *subventricular* layer (Fig. 8-7), glial proliferation (and possibly the proliferation of some classes of small neurons) persists for some time after the cessation of mitosis in the neuroepithelium. In the cerebellum, there is an early migration of a population of precursor cells (that is, true neuroblasts) from the neuroepithelium to form a second proliferative zone on the outer surface of the cerebellar cortex. In this layer (known as the *external granular layer*), cell proliferation continues for several weeks, the precursor cells giving rise to at least four different classes of neuron, including the enormous population of small

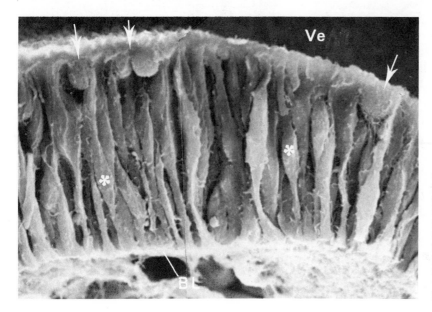

FIGURE 8-5 A scanning electron micrograph of the neuroepithelium to show the form of the interkinetic cells (marked by asterisks) and the dividing cells at the ventricular surface (Ve) marked by arrows. BL: basal lamina. ×1318 (R. M. Seymour and M. Berry, *J. Comp. Neurol.,* **160:**5, 1976; courtesy of Dr. M. Berry.)

FIGURE 8-6 A low-power electron micrograph of a migrating granule cell (right) in the developing cerebellar cortex. ×21,340 (P. Rakic, *J. Comp. Neurol.*, **141:**253, 1971; courtesy of Dr. P. Rakic.)

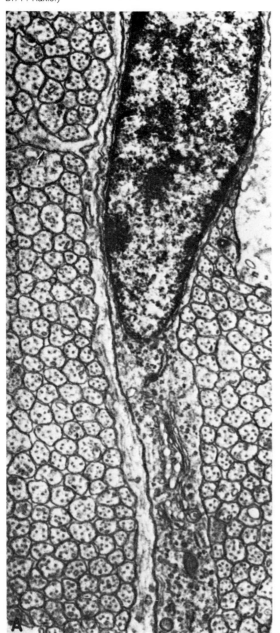

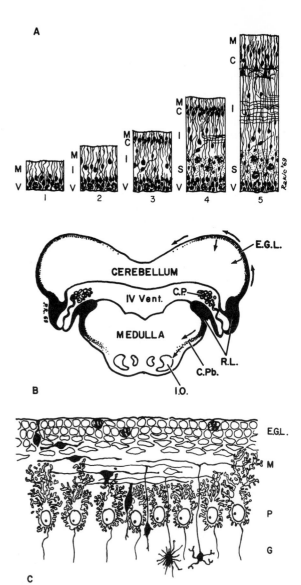

FIGURE 8-7 A. The progressive enlargement of the marginal and intermediate or mantle (I) zones of the neural tube at the expense of the ventricular or neuroepithelial (V) and subventricular (S) zones. B. The formation of the proliferative external granular layer (EGL) of the cerebellum from the rhombic lip (RL). Several of the nuclei of the brainstem are also formed from the rhombic lip (arrows). C. Proliferation in the external granular layer and the migration of the granule cells (G) of the cerebellar cortex. (Drawings by Dr. P. Rakic to illustrate various of his publications, from R. L. Sidman, ''The Neurosciences, Second Study Program,'' Rockefeller University Press, New York, 1970; courtesy of Dr. R. L. Sidman and Dr. P. Rakic.)

granule cells whose later migration is illustrated in Fig. 8-7.

As they migrate from the neuroepithelium, or from one of the secondary proliferative zones in the central nervous system, the differentiated neuronal and glial cell precursors either are ellipsoidal in shape or have a single leading process. Such cells are said to be *apolar* or *unipolar*, respectively. A small number of neurons in the vertebrate central nervous system persist into adult life as *unipolar neurons* (see Fig. 8-8), but the majority pass through a *bipolar phase*. Several different classes of bipolar neurons are seen in the mature nervous system (Fig. 8-8), but the great majority develop a number of processes and are collectively referred to as *multipolar neurons*. The development of the glioblasts is less well documented, and although it is formally convenient to divide them into two classes—astroblasts and oligodendroblasts (for the precursors of astrocytes and oligodendrocytes, which are the two main categories of supporting cell in the central nervous system)—there is little cytological distinction between them.

THE NEURAL CREST AND ITS DERIVATIVES

Whereas the neuroepithelium gives rise only to neurons, glial cells, and the modified columnar epithelium which forms the ependymal lining of the ventricles and the choroid plexuses (see below), the *neural crest* gives rise to an *extremely diverse range* of cells and tissues. Most of the nonneural derivatives are dealt with elsewhere in the appropriate chapters of this volume; they include:

1. The cells of the pia mater and arachnoid mater

2. Certain of the branchial cartilages and odontoblasts, and some of the cranial mesenchyme

3. Pigment-producing cells of the skin and subcutaneous tissues

4. Chromaffin tissue, including the chromaffin cells of the adrenal medulla

The neural derivatives include most of the sensory neurons of the cranial and spinal sensory ganglia; the postganglionic neurons of the sympathetic and parasympathetic ganglia; and the Schwann cells of the peripheral nervous system, including the sheath or satellite cells of the ganglia. At present we know little

about the factors that are responsible for this morphogenetic diversity, but it is clear that many of the cells of the neural crest are determined, at a very early stage in development, to follow one or another line of differentiation. The neuronal derivatives of the crest show almost the same range of morphological specializations as do the cells in the central nervous system. Most of the cells begin as *apolar* neuroblasts; those in the sensory ganglia associated with cranial nerves V, VII, IX, X, and XI and with the dorsal roots of spinal nerves become *bipolar* and then as the result of a coming together and fusion of the two processes become *secondarily unipolar* (and for this reason are sometimes referred to as *pseudounipolar* neurons) (Fig. 8-8). The sympathetic and parasympathetic neuroblasts generally become *multipolar,* with several dendritic processes and a single efferent process, or *axon*.

OTHER NEURAL DERIVATIVES

The sensory epithelia of certain of the cranial nerves, and the associated sensory ganglion cells, are derived either wholly or in part from specialized ectodermal thickenings, or *placodes*. The first of these is the nasal placode which gives rise to the olfactory epithelium in the upper part of the nose, including the olfactory receptors. The latter are modified bipolar neurons, with the shorter peripheral process or dendrite, being specifically adapted to respond to the presence of odoriferous molecules in the overlying mucous layer, and a longer central process (or axon) passing into the olfactory bulb. Parts of the trigeminal (Vth), facial (VIIth), glossopharyngeal (IXth), and vagal (Xth) ganglia are also formed from placodes. The thickened epithelial cells sink beneath the rest of the ectoderm and then proliferate and migrate toward clusters of neural crest cells which form the remaining parts of the ganglia. The *acousticovestibular placode* gives rise to the sensory epithelia of the internal ear, and to the bipolar ganglion cells of the *acoustic* (or *spiral*) ganglion, and of the *vestibular ganglion*. It is not known if the sheath cells in the trigeminal, facial, glossopharyngeal, or vagal ganglia are derived from the placodes or from the neural crest, but in the case of the acoustic and vestibular ganglia, it is quite clear that the placodal epithelium can form both neurons and sheath cells.

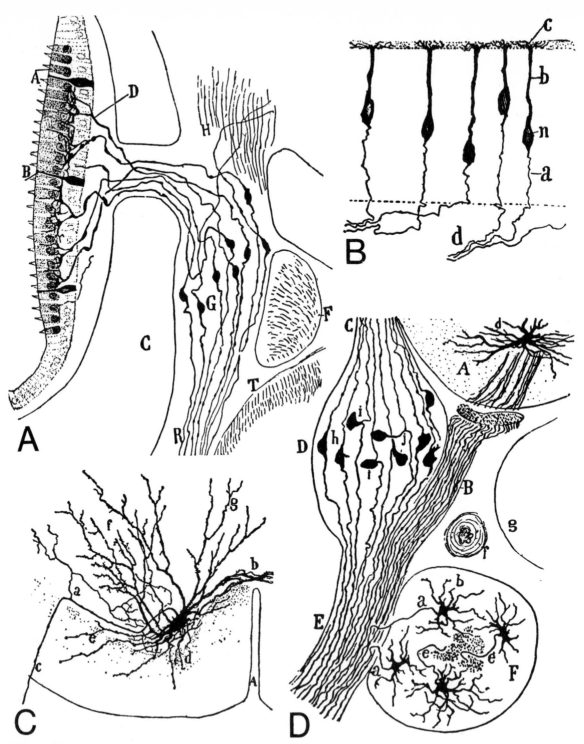

FIGURE 8-8 A variety of neurons stained by the Golgi method. A. Bipolar cells (G) of the vestibular ganglion in the mouse. Peripheral branches (D) innervate vestibular hair cells; central branches (R) pass centrally. B. Bipolar neurons in the olfactory mucosa with peripheral processes (b) and centrally projecting axons (a). C. A large multipolar neuron in the anterior horn of the spinal cord. D. Spinal ganglion cells at different stages in development from their early bipolar form (h) to the mature pseudounipolar form (j). A, spinal cord; B, ventral root; F, sympathetic ganglion. (S. Ramón y Cajal, ''Histologie du Système Nerveux de l'Homme et des Vertébrés'', 1909, Consejo Superior de Investigaciones Cientificas, Madrid, 1952.

THE STRUCTURE OF NEURONS AND NEUROGLIAL CELLS

The end result of the histogenetic sequence outlined above is the production of two classes of cells which together constitute the nervous tissue. These are the nerve cells, or *neurons,* and the supporting or *neuroglial* cells.

NEURONS

From a functional point of view, the most significant single feature of neurons is that they are surrounded by an *excitable membrane,* which under normal resting conditions is capable of maintaining a differential distribution of ions on either side of it. This membrane in turn gives rise to the so-called resting membrane potential of about 90 mV (inside negative), which under the influence of other nerve cells may be either partially or wholly depolarized or hyperpolarized. In addition, each neuron has a characteristic morphological structure. The final appearance of different classes of neuron may seem radically different (see Figs. 8-8 to 8-10), but all neurons have, in fact, an underlying similarity in form. The expanded part of the cell containing the nucleus is known as the *cell soma;* and in certain types of preparations, this is the only part of the neuron stained (see Fig. 8-11). However, when the cell is stained in its entirety (for example, by means of the Golgi method, see Figs. 8-12 to 8-15) the soma is seen to have extending from it one or more slender processes which may be of considerable length and highly branched. All the neurons illustrated in Fig. 8-9 possess two distinct types of processes: a number of *dendrites* and a single *axon.* The *dendrites* are drawn out of the soma in such a way that it is often difficult to define their exact point of origin; and they usually undergo several generations of branching, progressively narrowing in diameter as they do so. Together with the soma, the dendrites provide the main recipient surface of the nerve cell and it is upon these that the processes of other nerve cells mainly terminate at specialized regions of contact, called *synapses.* The totality of the influences (excitatory and inhibitory) exerted by other nerve cells at any instant in time determines the state of excitability of the neuron, and the soma-dendritic membrane can be regarded as an integrating mechanism which serves to sum these influences together.

Also arising from the soma (or less commonly from one of the dendrites) is a single process called the *axon.* This is usually thinner than the dendrites and when it arises from the soma, it usually does so at a clearly recognizable elevation, termed the *axon hillock.* Just beyond this elevation, the axon narrows over a length of a few microns, forming what is known as the *initial segment* of the axon. Beyond the initial segment it may initially increase in diameter somewhat, but as it passes to its destination, its diameter tends to remain relatively uniform until it reaches its terminal arborizations Though usually longer than the dendrites, the axon is of variable length and may terminate close to or at some considerable distance from the soma. Along its course, it may give off branches, the largest of which are termed *axon collaterals.* These may accompany the main axonal trunk or they may re-enter the area containing the parent cell, in which case they are referred to as *recurrent collaterals.* The axon and its branches are the main transmitting channels through which the neuron exerts its effect upon other nerve cells, or upon other tissues such as muscles and glands, usually by the relatively rapid conduction of nervous impulses.

The Shapes of Neurons

From the above it should be apparent that neurons exhibit what has sometimes been called a principle of *dynamic polarization;* that is, they possess what is essentially a receiving surface—the synaptic sites upon the dendrites and soma; an integrating mechanism—the somatic and dendritic membrane; an impulse initiating mechanism—the initial segment of the axon; and an impulse conducting process—the axon itself. Most neurons conform to this basic pattern of organization, though the overall shape of different nerve cells may vary considerably.

Perhaps the simplest class of neuron is that in which only a single process arises from the soma; such cells are commonly referred to as *unipolar neurons.* From the single connecting process, several branches are usually given off, some of which are mainly receptive and function as dendrites, while others are effector in action and together represent the branching axonal plexus of the cell. Neurons of this type are particularly common in invertebrates. In vertebrates, true unipolar neurons are rare, but the receptor cells of the retina may be regarded as unipolar neurons with short axonal processes.

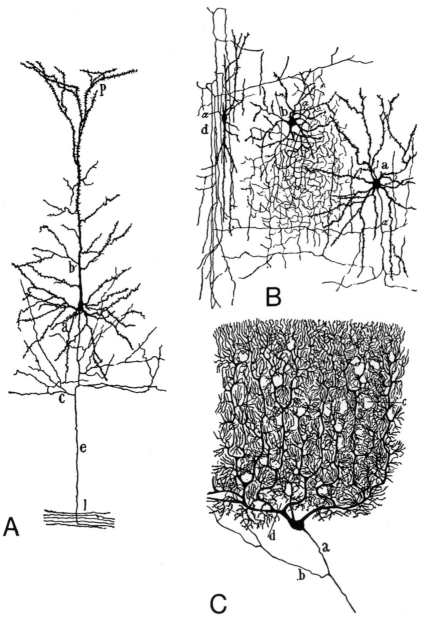

FIGURE 8-9 A. A pyramidal neuron from the cerebral cortex with a prominent apical dendrite (b), several basal dendrites (a), and a lengthy axon (e) which gives off a number of collateral branches (d) and enters the subcortical white matter. B. A variety of short axon (Golgi type II cells) in the cerebral cortex. a, stellate; b, ''spider web''; d, ''double bouquet.'' C. A cerebellar Purkinje cell with its extensive planar-arranged dendritic tree, axon (a) and recurrent axon collaterals (b). (S. Ramón y Cajal, Histologie du Système Nerveux de l'Homme et des Vertébrés, 1911; Consejo Superior de Investigaciones Científicas, Madrid, 1955.)

A second class of neuron which is also relatively uncommon in vertebrates, being found primarily in the retina and in the vestibular and acoustic ganglia of the inner ear, is the *bipolar neuron* (Fig. 8-8). Such neurons are relatively symmetrical with the axon (or central process) and a single dendritic (or peripheral) process arising from opposite poles of the ovoid or elongated soma. The dendrite may or may not branch profusely, and the axon may be short (as in the case of the retinal bipolar cells) or long (as in the case of the

vestibular and acoustic ganglion cells). A rather unique type of unipolar cell is that found in the dorsal root ganglia of the spinal nerves and in the sensory ganglia of certain of the cranial nerves (Fig. 8-8). These cells are actually derived from bipolar neuroblasts which in the embryo send a peripheral process out toward the ectodermal and mesodermal precursors of the skin and underlying tissues and a central process into the developing spinal cord or brainstem. As development proceeds, however, the two processes become approximated and eventually fuse, so that in the mature state the cells give rise to a single process which bifurcates into a proximal and distal process. These cells are thus referred to as *secondary,* or *pseudounipolar,* neurons. It should be noted, however, that both the central and peripheral processes resemble axons both in their structure and in their ability to conduct nerve impulses. These cells, therefore, lack dendrites.

FIGURE 8-10 A. A basket neuron from the cerebellum with its axon (c) giving off characteristic axonal baskets (a) surrounding adjoining Purkinje cells (A). B. Multipolar neurons with complex dendritic arborizations in the inferior olivary nucleus. (S. Ramón y Cajal, Histologie du Système Nerveux de l'Homme et des Vertébrés, 1909–1911; Consejo Superior de Investigaciones Cientificas, Madrid, 1952.)

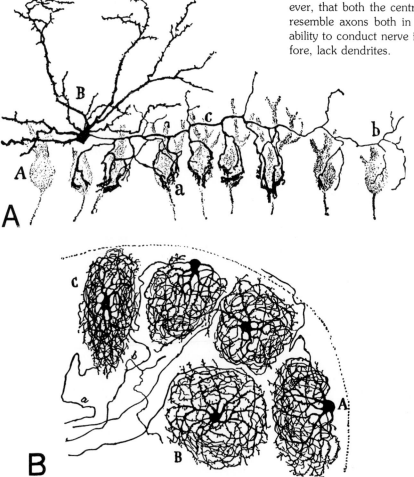

All other classes of neuron in the adult nervous system are essentially *multipolar neurons*. That is, the parent soma gives rise to more than one dendritic trunk. Most neurons have only a single axon, although rare cases with multiple axons have been described. In a few special cases to be described later, the cell may lack an axon altogether. Within the general category of multipolar neurons, many classes possess stereotyped shapes which are surprisingly constant from species to species and within any one species, from individual to individual. These have generally been given special names which either describe some aspect of their morphology or record the name of the investigator who first described them.

Perhaps the most typical multipolar nerve cells (Fig. 8-8) are the *motor cells*, or *motoneurons*, of the

FIGURE 8-11 Two motoneurons from a Nissl-stained preparation of the spinal cord of a cat. Note the large, angular Nissl bodies in the cytoplasm, the pale nuclei (N), the prominent nucleolus (Nu), and the extension of the Nissl material into the large dendrites (D). Several small glial cells (G) are also shown, and a small capillary (Cp). ×480.

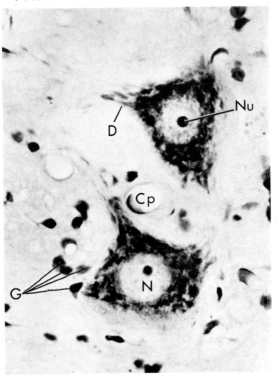

ventral horn of the spinal cord. The large somata of these cells customarily give rise to six or more large stem dendrites which radiate out in all directions from the perikaryon and branch into secondary and tertiary dendrites. Since the length of the stem dendrites is fairly uniform, the total *dendritic field*, (that is, the spatial volume occupied by all the dendrites together) is approximately symmetrical and when viewed three-dimensionally forms a round or ovoid figure enclosing the perikaryon. In some cases the dendritic fields are particularly symmetrical; and since the dendrites radiate more or less uniformly in all directions, these cells are termed *stellate neurons*. A true stellate cell would be one in which the dendrites of the cell arose at constant angles to one another from all sides of the soma and were of exactly equal length; few of the cells that are commonly termed stellate, such as those in the fourth layer of the cerebral cortex, have such uniform dendrites or spherical dendritic fields. More commonly, the field tends to be eccentric or flattened in one dimension, and such cells are called *spindle-shaped* or *fusiform*, etc.

Several examples of multipolar neurons which have been given special names are shown in Figs. 8-9 and 8-10. Some of these neurons have long axons which leave the territory of the cell soma, and each has a highly characteristic dendritic field. The *Purkinje cells* of the cerebellar cortex have only ascending dendrites directed toward the surface of the cerebellum, but these and their branches are all oriented in the plane at right angles to the long axis of the cerebellar folia so that the dendritic field has a very narrow profile when viewed from the side. The *pyramidal cells*, which are especially common in the cerebral cortex, are so named because of the pyramidal shape of their somata. From the base of the perikaryon, four or more branching *basal dendrites* extend laterally and downward; from its apex, an *apical dendrite* ascends toward the surface of the cortex giving off side branches along its course and commonly ending in a small spray of laterally directed branches. Another class of cells has a dendritic field in the shape of an inverted cone; these are the *mitral cells* of the olfactory bulb, so named because the shape of the cell soma was thought to resemble a bishop's miter.

An unusual class of small multipolar cell includes those which lack an axon altogether. These are most common in the retina, where they are referred to as *amacrine cells* (the Greek term *amacrine* means without an axon), and in the olfactory bulb, where they are referred to as *granule cells*. Although these cells lack

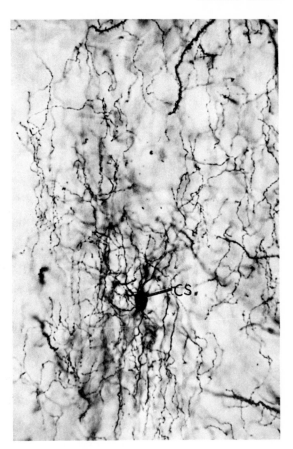

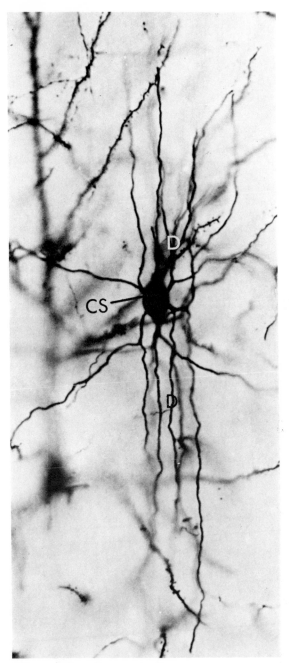

FIGURES 8-12 (left) and 8-13 (right) Photomicrographs of Golgi-impregnated cells from the cerebral cortex of a monkey. Note that the dendrites (D) ramify in all directions and that the cell on the right has an extensive locally ramifying axonal plexus. CS, cell soma. (8-12: ×303; 8-13; ×338.) (E. G. Jones, *J. Comp. Neurol.*, **160:**205, 1975.)

an axon, they are able to influence the activity of other nerve cells by means of unusual specializations of their processes which seem, unlike most dendrites, to have some of the characteristics of axons (Fig. 8-42).

In some instances the name given to a neuron is determined by the nature of its axonal ramifications. This is especially true of neurons with relatively short axons that break up into their terminal branches close to the parent cell soma. A well-known example is the *basket cell* of the cerebellar cortex, the axons of which give off sprays of small branches, which enclose the somata of adjoining Purkinje cells as though in a series of baskets (Figs. 8-10 and 8-30). The small cell from the cerebral cortex illustrated in Figs. 8-8 and 8-13, with its highly branched and intensely intertwined axon, was termed a spider-web cell by the great Spanish histologist Ramón y Cajal. The same investigator

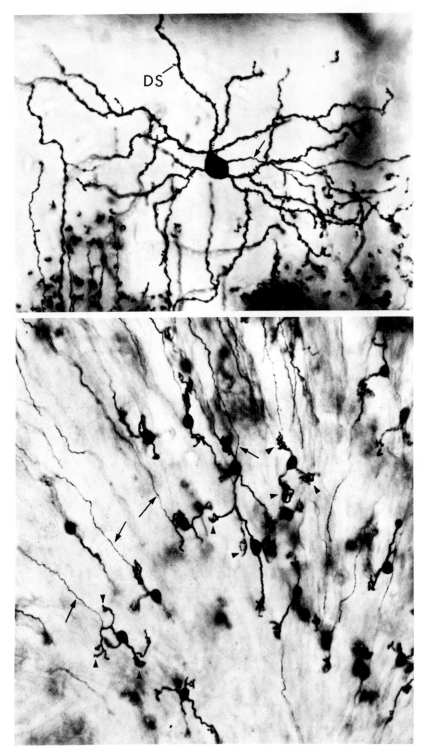

FIGURES 8-14 (upper) and 8-15 (lower) Photomicrographs of a stellate cell (upper) and several granule cells (lower) in a Golgi-stained preparation of the cerebellar cortex of a monkey. Arrows indicate axons. Arrow heads in Figure 8-15 indicate the terminal claws on the dendrites of the granule cells. Some of the axons of these cells arise from the dendrites. DS, dendritic spine. ×500.

referred to other cells of the type illustrated in Fig. 8-8 as double bouquet cells because of their long ascending and descending axonal systems. These two examples are of interest because they show that cells with essentially the same type of dendritic field (both would be called stellate cells) may give rise to systems of axon branches which are quite different.

These are merely three examples of cells whose axonal ramifications are very characteristic, but it is clear that the nature of a cell's axonal plexus may be just as characteristic as the shape of its dendritic field. And, as in the case of dendritic fields, it is possible to recognize certain basic types. Very shortly after his introduction of the stain upon which so much of our knowledge concerning the overall shapes of nerve cells depends, the Italian histologist Camillo Golgi pointed out that the majority of nerve cells fall into one of two classes, which have come to be termed Golgi type I and Golgi type II neurons. Golgi type I neurons have long axons which pass out of the region in which the parent cell soma is situated and terminate at some distance either in some other part of the nervous system or in some other tissue such as skin or muscle. The motoneurons of the spinal cord, the pyramidal cells of the cerebral cortex, and the Purkinje cells of the cerebellar cortex are all examples of Golgi type I cells. Golgi type II neurons, on the other hand, have short axons that ramify locally in the region in which the parent cell soma is situated and may not even extend much beyond the confines of its dendritic field (like the spider-web cell shown in Fig. 8-13).

Some idea of the significance of the Golgi classification may be grasped by considering, for example, any of the ascending sensory pathways of the nervous system. The long axoned cells are the main transmission lines conveying information from the periphery through various synaptic relay centers (nuclei) to the cerebral cortex. Short axoned cells are situated at each synaptic station, and these may bring an additional influence to bear upon the long axoned cell that projects its axon up to the next level. The Golgi type II cells, thus, serve as modulators of synaptic events in the long pathways of the nervous system. A common alternative term for these cells is, therefore, *interneurons*, since they are, in a sense, intercalated between any two links in a long pathway.

It should also be pointed out that the name applied to a particular type of nerve cell may vary depending upon the nature of the histological preparation in which it is observed. The names of the examples quoted above were derived from the *total*

appearance of the nerve cell—soma, dendrites, and axon—as seen in the silver impregnation method of Golgi. Unfortunately, some names are based on the appearance of the cells when stained by more routine histological techniques, that show only the cell somata. For example, the small stellate neuron of the cerebral cortex (Fig. 8-9) has been called a granule cell, but the same term has also been applied to quite different cells in the cerebellar cortex (Fig. 8-15), the dentate gyrus, the olfactory bulb, and certain other sites, even though their dendritic and axonal configurations are not at all comparable.

Factors Governing the Size and Shape of Neurons
Neurons differ a great deal both in size and shape. Possibly the smallest neurons in the mammalian central nervous system are found in parts of the hypothalamus. Such neurons have somata measuring little more than 3 to 4 μm in diameter and their axons and dendritic fields are comparably small. The largest cells are probably the giant pyramidal cells of the motor area of the cerebral cortex whose somata may measure as much as 120 μm in their largest dimension; and in addition to giving rise to a long, thick apical dendrite, their axons may be 50 cm or more in length. All sizes are to be found between these two extremes.

Two factors which appear to determine the size of a cell are (1) the number, length, and diameter of its processes, and (2) the number of synapses which it receives upon its surface. It is a useful generalization that neurons with the longest and thickest axons have the largest somata. In the case of one of the larger motoneurons in the lumbar or sacral parts of the spinal cord, for example, the axon may be almost a meter in length and 15 to 20 μm in diameter. It is clear that the greater part of the volume of the cell resides in the axon. As the axon itself appears to be incapable of synthesizing proteins and most other structural or functional constituents, the cell soma must maintain the appropriate amount of metabolic machinery to support the axon. The situation with regard to dendrites is probably comparable. In general, cells with long, thick, profusely branching dendrites also have large somata, and even though the dendrites possess certain synthetic capabilities, there is evidence that they, too, are in part maintained by the soma.

The number and length of the dendrites possessed by a particular cell seem to be related to the number of synaptic contacts which it receives from the axons of other cells. For example, the large motoneurons of the spinal cord which integrate activity from many diverse sources have been estimated to receive as many as 10,000 synaptic contacts, and the large Purkinje cells of the cerebellum may receive as many as 200,000. Small interneurons on the other hand have not only short axons of small diameter but also relatively few dendrites and probably receive far fewer synaptic contacts.

THE STRUCTURE OF NERVE CELL SOMATA

As well as providing a large surface area of membrane which may receive synaptic contacts from other neurons, the cell body, or soma, which contains the nucleus, is the trophic or nourishing center of the nerve cell. Before the structure of the soma is described, it may be useful to point out some of the functional characteristics of the nerve cell other than those concerned with the integration and transmission of nervous activity. Chief among these is the need to maintain itself and to provide various organelles and macromolecules to the terminals of its axon. This is achieved by the active synthesis in the soma of large amounts of protein, lipids, etc., and a highly efficient somatofugal transport system which enables it to deliver these metabolic products and organelles to the cell's processes. The probable structural basis for this transport system will be considered later. Here we shall deal primarily with the cytology of the cell nucleus and the surrounding perikaryon.

The Nucleus

The *nucleus* of most nerve cells is either spherical or ovoid in shape, and large relative to the size of the perikaryon;[1] and since a substantial part of the genome is continually being transcribed in keeping with the active synthetic state of the cell, it is euchromatic, that is, the nuclear chromatin is generally dispersed when seen in the electron microscope and the nucleus usually has a vesicular appearance when viewed with the light microscope (Fig. 8-11). The nuclear envelope, with its nuclear pores, is typical of

---

[1] At one time it was thought that the nuclei of many large neurons (for example, those of the pyramidal cells of the hippocampus and the Purkinje cells of the cerebellum) were tetraploid, but this appears to have been a result of a technical error in the measurement of the cells' DNA content.

that of all eukaryotic cells (Fig. 8-16). One, but sometimes two or even three, prominent nucleoli are present within the nucleus; their fine structure is also typical of that in other protein-synthesizing cells. Associated with the nucleoli may be one or more "satellites," of which the female sex chromatin (corresponding to the heterochromatic X chromosomes) is the best known (Fig. 8-17); indeed, this was first described in neurons by Barr. These so-called Barr bodies may be attached to the nucleolus, to the inner face of the nuclear membrane, or to both. Other nucleolar satellites, generally of relatively uncommon occurrence and uncertain significance, include the paranucleolar structure and the accessory body of Cajal. These commonly appear as tiny dense granules in the nuclei of neurons stained with reduced silver methods. Ultrastructurally, some of these structures resemble the nucleolus and may simply be detached nucleolar fragments. Other crystalline or filamentous intranuclear particles are occasionally seen, but these too are of unknown origin or significance.

The Perikaryon

Perhaps the most striking feature of the perikarya of neurons is the large amount of ribosomal material that they contain, indicative of the high rate of protein synthesis in these cells. In the electron microscope, the ribosomal material is mainly in the form of multiple stacks of rough endoplasmic reticulum, but a great many free ribosomes and polyribosomal rosettes are also present. These clustered masses of free and attached ribosomes are strongly basophilic, and when nervous tissue is stained with basic dyes and viewed in the light microscope, many neurons are seen to contain irregularly shaped clumps of intensely stained cytoplasmic inclusions; these are customarily called *Nissl bodies* after the German neurologist F. Nissl, who first applied aniline dyes to the study of the nervous system. Although the cytoplasm of all neurons is basophilic by virtue of their rich content of RNA, not all have distinct Nissl bodies. Such bodies can be seen particularly well in the large motoneurons of the spinal cord (Figs. 8-11 and 8-16) and in large dorsal root ganglion cells; smaller neurons merely show a diffuse, dustlike basophilia of their cytoplasm.

The *Golgi complex* is also prominent in all neurons, and at the electron microscopic level, it is commonly seen as several groups of flattened and dilated smooth-walled sacs and vesicles of variable size, usually near the nucleus but sometimes extending into the bases of the larger dendrites (Figs. 8-16 and 8-18). The reason for this well-developed Golgi complex is

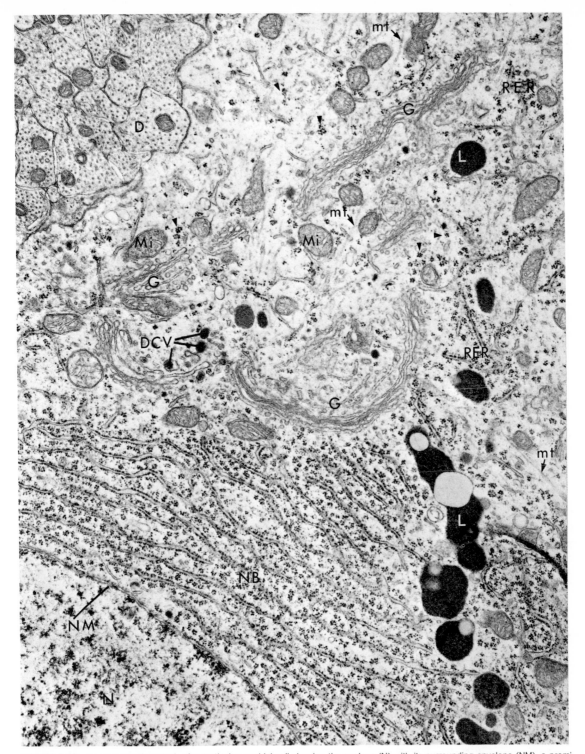

FIGURE 8-16 An electron micrograph of a cortical pyramidal cell showing the nucleus (N) with its surrounding envelope (NM), a prominent Nissl body (NB), several lysosomes (L), mitochondria (Mi), dense-core vesicles (DCV) and microtubules (mt). The cell has an extensive Golgi complex (G) and a good deal of rough endoplasmic reticulum (RER) and free ribosomes (arrow heads) outside the obvious Nissl body. In the upper-left corner there are several transversely sectioned dendrites (D) containing microtubules cut in transverse section. ×25,000.

incompletely understood; but by analogy with its appearance in other secretory cells it seems probable that it is engaged in the packaging of secretory products within membrane-bound vesicles. The most common vesicles found in neurons are the *synaptic vesicles,* which are present in large numbers in axon terminals and appear to contain the neurochemical transmitter agents that mediate synaptic function (see below). At present, it is not known to what extent these are produced in the perikaryon. In many sites, however, the cell bodies of some neurons contain variable numbers of membrane-bound dense vesicles that represent their main neurosecretory product or enzymes involved in its synthesis. In the perikarya of certain small neurons of the autonomic nervous system, for example, many dense-core vesicles about 600 to 800 Å in diameter are present in the perikaryon as well as in the axons and their terminals. These contain catecholamines which, when condensed with formaldehyde, cause the neurons to be intensely fluorescent when viewed in ultraviolet light (Fig. 8-19).

Neurosecretory products that act not as chemical transmitter agents at synapses but by being released into the general circulation are such polypeptide hormones as oxytocin and vasopressin, and the various

FIGURE 8-17 Nucleolus (Nu) and nucleolar satellite (arrow) from cortical neuron of a female rat. ×29,100.

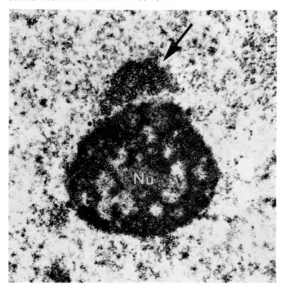

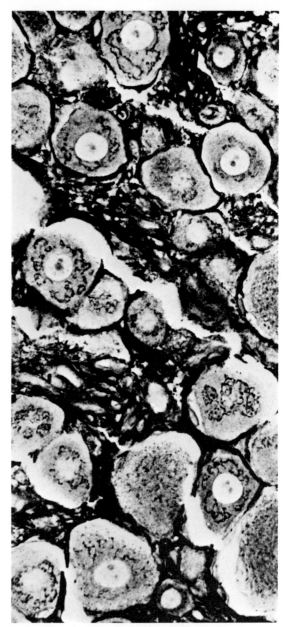

FIGURE 8-18 An osmic-acid-stained preparation of a spinal ganglion to show the reticular appearance of the Golgi apparatus. ×496.

hypothalamic-releasing hormones. These hormones are produced by the neurons in the hypothalamus and are transported in membrane-bound vesicles down their axons for release into the vicinity of the blood vessels of the neurohypophysis or the median eminence. The neurosecretory material is synthesized in the endoplasmic reticulum, packaged in the Golgi complex, and transported in large (around 1000 Å) membrane-bound, dense-core vesicles. Aggregations of these vesicles in the axons and their terminals may be selectively stained by means of the Gomori technique and visualized light microscopically as large granular masses called *Herring bodies.* Other neurons whose somata may contain large, membrane-bound granules are found in certain specialized portions of the ependymal lining of the central canal system of the brain, notably in the *subfornical organ.* Usually these can be visualized at the light microscopic level as large droplets or vacuoles.

As might be expected in metabolically active cells, *mitochondria* are also present in very large numbers in

neuronal perikarya (Fig. 8-16). They vary a great deal in size, density, and general configuration, but probably not more so in these than in other cells; and even though it has been claimed that differences in mitochondrial morphology are sufficiently marked to serve as useful bases for distinguishing different types of cell, at present this seems doubtful.

One of the most ubiquitous elements in neuronal perikarya are the large numbers of *microtubules* and *microfilaments* (or neurofilaments as they are sometimes referred to). Apart from the fact that they are found in all parts of the perikaryon, the microtubules (which have a diameter of about 250 Å) appear to be

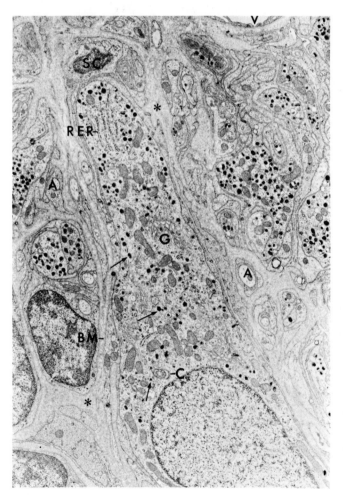

FIGURE 8-19 Electron micrograph of a catecholamine-synthesizing neuron from the nodose ganglion of a cat. Note the dense-core vesicles in the cytoplasm (marked by arrows). RER, rough endoplasmic reticulum; G, Golgi region; C, cilium; V, blood vessel. ×13,500. (M. A. Grillo, L. Jacobs, and J. H. Comroe, Jr., *J. Comp. Neurol.* **153:**1, 1974; courtesy of Dr. M. A. Grillo.)

identical to those in other cells (Figs. 8-16, 8-22, and 8-23). At present it is not known if neurofilaments (which have a diameter of about 100 Å) are identical to the larger microfilaments (Fig. 8-23) seen in other cells, and until their substructure and chemical composition have been adequately characterized, this will remain unsolved. Of course, both microtubules and neurofilaments are visible only at the electron microscope level. However, when neurons are stained with certain heavy metals (especially silver salts), thick, intertwined fibrillar strings up to 2 or 3 μm in diameter can be seen; these are known as *neurofibrils* (Fig. 8-29). It is currently thought that these represent metallic silver deposited upon bundles of neurofilaments; but in some cases, at least, the silver deposits may be around microtubules. As in the case of Nissl bodies, neurofibrils appear most distinctly in large neurons; in smaller cells the neurofibrillar methods give a diffuse staining of the cytoplasm, and because such cells contain substantial numbers of neurofilaments, at least part of the staining is probably associated with these organelles.

Lysosomes of various kinds are also to be found in neurons. These appear as dense, or multivesicular, bodies; they are usually closely associated with the Golgi complex and exhibit positive acid phosphatase activity. Their number varies from neuron to neuron and seems to increase with the age of the individual. It is probable that the yellowish pigment *lipofuscin*, which accumulates in neurons with advancing age, represents insoluble residues remaining from lysosomal activity. In the human brain, the yellowish lipofuscin pigment may build up with increasing age to the extent that it may occupy more than half the cross-sectional area of the soma of certain cells (Fig. 8-20). Its ultrastructural counterpart is a heterogeneous membrane-bound body composed of dense particles and lipid-filled vacuoles (Fig. 8-16). Other pigments occur naturally in certain groups of neurons. Perhaps the best known is the melanin of the nerve cells in the substantia nigra of the midbrain. The pigment seems to be absent in human infants, but by puberty it has reached its maximal development. The pigment is again enclosed in membrane-bound structures resembling lysosomes.

Neurons also frequently contain one or two typical centrioles, usually associated with a cilium that

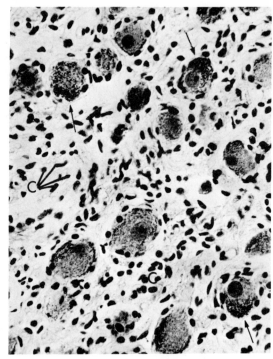

FIGURE 8-20 Lipofuscin granules (marked by arrows) in the cytoplasm of neurons in the human superior cervical ganglion. C. satellite Schwann cells. ×294.

may protrude for some distance from the cell surface. Their significance is quite obscure; it is possible that they simply reflect the epithelial origin of nerve cells.

THE STRUCTURE OF DENDRITES

In some respects, dendrites can be regarded as extensions of the cell soma, which is reflected in the fact that at both the light and electron microscopic level, it is difficult to define the point at which the soma ends and a dendrite begins. The dendrites appear as though they were "drawn out" from the soma, and most of the organelles typical of the perikaryon extend for considerable distances into the dendrites. Thus, the main-stem dendrites of larger neurons can usually be seen in material stained with routine neurohistological stains, since they often contain Nissl bodies or dispersed Nissl substance as distinct as that found in the soma (Figs. 8-11 and 8-26). At the electron microscopic level, considerable amounts of rough-surfaced endoplasmic reticulum, free ribosomes, and compo-

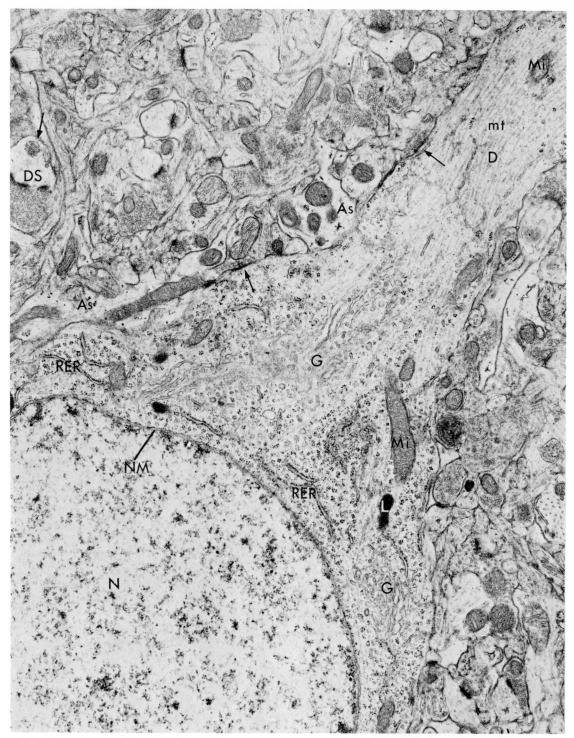

FIGURE 8-21 An electron micrograph of the apical portion of a pyramidal neuron from the cerebral cortex, with its apical dendrite extending toward the upper right corner. N, nucleus; NM, nuclear envelope; RER, rough endoplasmic reticulum; G, Gogi complex; L, lysosome; Mi, mitochondria; mt, microtubules; D, dendrite; As, astrocytic processes; Ds, dendritic spine with spine apparatus (arrow). The arrows in the cell soma mark the site of two synapses upon the surface of the neuron. ×15,000.

nents of the Golgi complex are often seen in the proximal portions of dendrites (Fig. 8-21).

As they extend away from the soma, the dendrites tend to taper and the successive generations of branches to which they give rise are always of smaller diameter than the parent trunk. In some neurons the dendrites appear to be beaded with irregular dilatations and constrictions. In some instances, this appearance may be artifactual; but in others, there is evidence that the beading may reflect the natural state of the dendrites.

As the dendrites extend away from the soma, the rough endoplasmic reticulum and other organelles become progressively diminished; and in the more peripheral dendrites, only small amounts of rough endoplasmic reticulum and free ribosomes are seen. The presence of ribosomal material is important, however, since it serves to distinguish, at the electron microscope level, dendrites from axons. But the most striking feature of dendrites is the presence of large numbers of microtubules and neurofilaments (Figs. 8-21 to 8-23). In general, these are much more conspicuous than in the soma and are more regularly aligned along the axis of the dendrite. The number of filaments and tubules seems to vary with the diameter of the dendrite and the distance from the soma. It is thought that some microtubules and neurofilaments may extend from the soma almost to the tips of the dendrites; as the dendrites branch, bundles of filaments and tubules diverge into the branches. The microtubules are thought to be involved in the transport of various materials including proteins and such organelles as mitochondria, from the perikaryon to the distal portions of the dendrites. By tracing the movement of labeled proteins following the injection of radioactive precursors into the soma, it has been possible to demonstrate "dendritic transport" with a rate of about 3 mm per h, which is comparable to that at

FIGURES 8-22 (left) and 8-23 (right) Electron micrographs of two transversely sectioned dendrites which contain saccules of smooth endoplasmic reticulum (SER), many microtubules, and neurofilaments (f). The dendrites are contacted by axon terminals (T) which form distinct synapses at the points marked by the large open arrows. The dendrites are surrounded by astrocytic processes (As) which also contain filaments (f). L, lysosome. The circled area shows an endocytotic vesicle thought to indicate retrieval of synaptic vesicle membrane from membrane of terminal. Fig. 8-22, ×38,600; Fig. 8-23, ×28,800. (A. J. Rockel and E. G. Jones, *J. Comp. Neurol.,* **147:**61, 1973.)

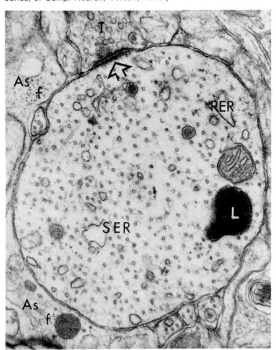

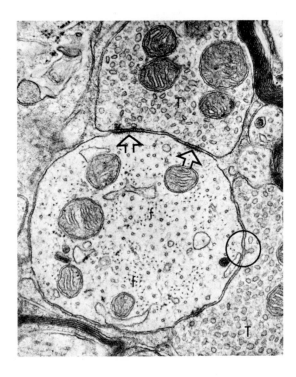

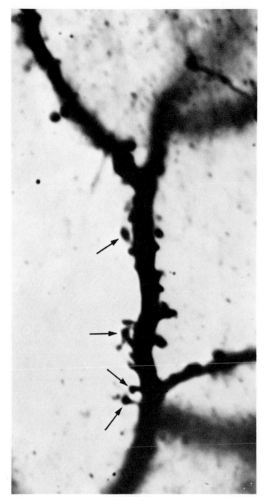

FIGURE 8-24 A high-power light micrograph of a portion of a dendrite of a cell in the inferior colliculus of a cat, stained by the Golgi method, to show the appearance of the dendritic spines (arrows). ×1800. (A. J. Rockel and E. G. Jones, *J. Comp. Neurol.,* **147:**11, 1973.)

which certain materials move down the axon; this transport is inhibited by drugs such as colchicine and vinblastine, which cause a breakdown of microtubules. The role of the neurofilaments is quite unknown.

Apart from their internal structure, one of the most distinctive features of dendrites is the presence upon their surfaces of synaptic contacts made by the axon terminals of other neurons. The structure and general distribution of synapses will be discussed elsewhere. At this point it is sufficient to note that all dendrites receive synaptic contacts at various points along their length. In addition, the dendrites of many

(but by no means all) classes of neurons possess multiple small protrusions known as *dendritic spines,* which are specialized for the reception of synaptic contacts.

As is seen in Golgi preparations, a typical dendritic spine is a pedunculated structure with an expanded tip, measuring 0.5 to 2 μm in diameter, and a narrow stalk 0.5 to 1 μm long (Fig. 8-24). In electron micrographs, the stalk can often be seen to contain one or more microtubules; but the expanded tip usually presents an amorphous matrix (Fig. 8-25), except at the point of synaptic contact where there is a considerable amount of electron-dense material attached to the postsynaptic membrane. In many spines, one or more smooth-walled vesicular or saclike structures are seen, often alternating with bands of electron-dense

FIGURE 8-25 Electron micrograph of a series of dendritic spines (DS), each contacted by an axon terminal (T). One spine contains a spine apparatus (SA). As, astrocytic cytoplasm. Cerebral cortex of rat. ×28,100.

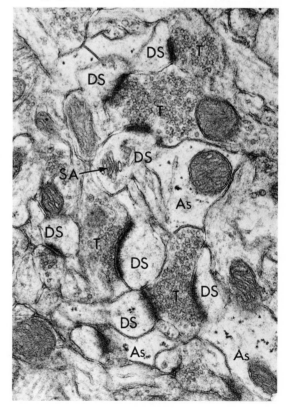

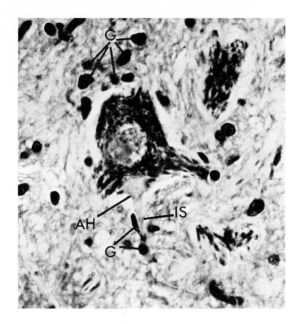

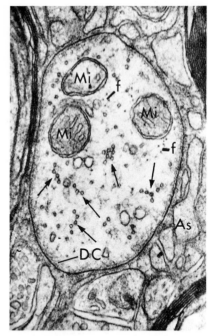

FIGURES 8-26 (left) and 8-27 (right) In a Nissl-stained preparation the axon hillock (AH) and initial axonal segment (IS) appear essentially unstained. An electron micrograph of a transversely sectioned initial segment shows a characteristic electron-dense undercoating beneath the axolemma (DC), and fasciculated clusters of microtubules (arrows). Mi, mitochondria; f, neurofilaments; G, glial cells; As, astrocytic cytoplasm. Fig. 8-26, motoneuron of cat, thionin stain, ×665; Fig. 8-27, electron micrograph from cat inferior colliculus, ×40,000.

material; these constitute a special organelle of unknown function called the *spine apparatus.*

On any given neuron, the spines may vary considerably in shape and size. Generally those situated most distally are the longest and may even be bifid; those near the soma are generally the smallest and are often simple, sessile protrusions of the dendritic surface, usually without a spine apparatus. There is also a fairly consistent relation between the number of dendritic spines and the distance from the soma; generally there are few or no spines on the proximal portions of the stem dendrites but their amount quickly increases to a maximum, maintained over the middle portion of the dendritic system, and then declines again toward the distal portions of the dendrites (Fig. 8-42). Although the significance of this characteristic spine distribution is difficult to assess, it is clear that, when present, the spines represent the principal synaptic surface on the dendrites. There is also some evidence that the dendritic spines may be labile structures in the sense that they may disappear after deafferentation or sensory deprivation and possibly with increasing age.

STRUCTURE AND FUNCTION OF AXONS

Whereas dendrites appear to be drawn out of the soma, the axon usually appears as a unique and sharply defined process. It generally arises from the soma as a conspicuous conical elevation called the *axon hillock* (Figs. 8-26 to 8-29), but it may also arise from the basal portion of a stem dendrite. The *initial segment* of the axon is commonly the narrowest portion of the process, and, like the axon hillock, has a number of distinctive morphological features. The most obvious feature of the axon hillock is the relative absence of free ribosomes and rough-surfaced endoplasmic reticulum, so that in Nissl-stained preparations it appears as a palely stained, triangular or fan-shaped area free of Nissl granules. In electron micrographs, the most obvious ultrastructural feature of the axon hillock is the presence of a large number of microtubules and neurofilaments which give the impression of streaming from the perikaryon into the initial segment. The extent of the initial segment is easiest to define in cells whose axons subsequently

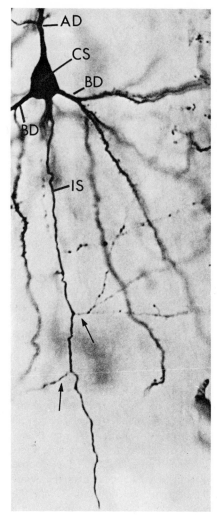

FIGURE 8-28 Pyramidal cell from the cerebral cortex of a monkey showing collateral branches (arrows) arising from initial segment of axon (IS). BD, basal dendrites; CS, cell soma; AD, apical dendrite. Golgi stain, ×700.

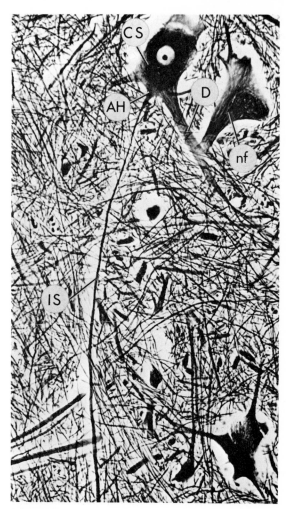

FIGURE 8-29 Motoneuron from spinal cord of a cat showing axon hillock (AH) and initial segment (IS). Dendrites (D) and cell soma (CS) contain neurofibrils best seen (nf) in part of second cell to right. Bodian stain, ×860.

acquire a *myelin sheath;* in these the segment reaches from the apex of the axon hillock to the commencement of the myelin sheath. It is characterized by the absence of ribosomes and rough-surfaced endoplasmic reticulum and by two special features (Fig. 8-27). First, the presence of an electron-dense "undercoating" beneath the plasma membrane (or axolemma as it has been called). The undercoat measures about 200 Å in thickness and is deficient only beneath the regions of synaptic contact that are sometimes made by the terminals of other axons on the initial segment.

The membrane of the initial segment generally has the lowest threshold of excitability, and is therefore commonly the site of initiation of the nervous impulse. To what extent the dense membrane undercoat serves to facilitate this is not known, but it is noteworthy that a similar dense undercoat is found at the nodes of Ranvier in myelinated axons (see below).

The second distinguishing feature of the initial segment is the fact that the microtubules passing through it are collected into small bundles within which the individual microtubules are linked at intervals to one or more of their neighbors by multiple small cross bridges best seen in cross sections of the initial segment. When seen in longitudinal sections, the electron-dense cross bridges resemble the rungs on a ladder, which in myelinated axons can be followed to the point at which the myelin sheath is acquired. In axons that do not acquire a myelin sheath, the fasciculation of the microtubules and the dense membrane undercoat cease at a comparable distance from the soma. To date, these two features of the initial segment seem to be peculiar to the central nervous system; they have not been found in neurons of the dorsal root ganglia or autonomic nervous system.

In addition to the microtubules, the axon contains a variable number of neurofilaments of unknown function (Fig. 8-63). They are commonly regarded as semirigid structures that provide a skeletal framework for the axon, but this has not been proven and other suggestions—for example, that they guide the axon toward its destination during the course of development—are dubious. It is known, however, that in cold-blooded animals the number of neurofilaments increases during cold adaptation, and in all animals their number increases after injury to the axon.

THE TERMINATIONS OF AXONS

Axons end by forming functional contacts with other nerve cells, muscle fibers, or gland cells. In the central nervous system the axon of a neuron terminates upon other nerve cells in the specialized junctions already referred to as synapses. As an axon approaches the region of the nervous system in which it terminates, it generally branches repeatedly; if it possesses a myelin sheath, the initial branches are myelinated, but as these approach the neurons with which they are destined to make synaptic contact, they usually branch again (Figs. 8-30 and 8-31), and the final branches are unmyelinated.[2]

---

[2] The individual branches that make up the terminal spray engendered by a long axon are commonly referred to as *telodendria* (singular, telodendron). This term, which means "branches at a distance," is often inappropriate if applied to the branches of a short, unmyelinated axon belonging to a Golgi type II neuron, for in the highly branched axonal plexus commonly engendered by such a cell, it is not possible to distinguish a major parent trunk much beyond the initial segment.

The appearance of the synapses in silver-stained preparations is very variable, but since they are usually in the form of tiny swellings on the axon branches, they are customarily referred to as synaptic *boutons* (or buttons) (Figs. 8-31 and 8-33). A synapse is therefore formed where a synaptic bouton comes into intimate association with a portion of the membrane of another nerve cell (commonly its soma or dendrites) and where, by means of a series of morphological specializations to be described below, the release of a neurochemical transmitter agent from the axon terminal can influence the conductance of the recipient (or *postsynaptic*) cell. Synaptic boutons may occur as swellings at the very ends of the terminal branches of an axon, in which case they are called *boutons terminaux*. Some axon terminals are exceedingly large and may cover a great deal of the surface of the postsynaptic cell, in which case they may be called *calyces,* or "baskets" (Figs. 8-10 and 8-30). Other synaptic contacts may occur at intervals along the length of a terminal segment of an axon or, in the case of a short axon, along most of its length. In this situation, they are usually referred to as *boutons en passant* (or *boutons de passage*) (Figs. 8-31 and 8-32). The term synapse was introduced by Sherrington in 1897, and even at that time there was good physiological evidence (based upon the direction of transmission of nervous impulses from cell to cell and the differential sensitivity of the junctional region to pharmacological agents such as nicotine) to show that this was a functionally specialized part of the nervous system. Morphological evidence about the nature of the synapse rested solely upon the knowledge that axonal boutons terminaux could be seen making contact with the somata and dendrites of nerve cells. It is only since the introduction of electron microscopy to the study of the nervous system that the structural correlates of synaptic activity have become fully understood.

A typical synapse in the central nervous system consists of a presynaptic element and a postsynaptic element in close association with one another at a region of membrane specialization, and separated only by a narrow extracellular cleft (Figs. 8-32 and 8-34). The commonest form of synapse in the central nervous system is one in which the presynaptic element is a synaptic bouton and the postsynaptic element a dendrite, and this type of synapse will be used to illustrate the general form (Fig. 8-35). The membranes of the pre- and postsynaptic elements are aligned to one another with a gap of only 200 to 300 Å between them and without any intervening tissue elements. The region of apposition between the axon terminal and the dendrite is usually somewhat more extensive than the region of membrane specializations that seems to constitute the active zone of the synapse. At the apparently active zone, the gap between the pre- and postsynaptic profiles, usually called the *synaptic cleft,* often becomes slightly wider than the 150 to 200 Å gap that separates other contiguous profiles in the nervous system, and may contain fine filaments or dense material derived from the outer coats of the membranes of the opposed pre- and postsynaptic membranes which are much more electron-dense than elsewhere. In addition to being denser, the membrane specializations appear thicker than the remainder of the dendritic or axonal membrane. This is because they each have attached to them a certain amount of electron-dense material that extends for a variable distance into the pre- and postsynaptic cytoplasm (Figs. 8-35 and 8-36). On the presynaptic side the material appears as a series of conical protrusions from the membrane. On the postsynaptic side, there is often a greater amount of dense material attached to the inner surface of the postsynaptic membrane; this is more homogeneous than on the presynaptic side and can extend for a considerable distance into the dendritic cytoplasm. The membrane thus appears "thicker" than that on the presynaptic side. In other words, the synaptic membrane specializations are

asymmetrical. There is good evidence that the pre- and postsynaptic membranes and their associated dense material have a protein composition different from that of the rest of the nerve cell membrane. One clear manifestation of this is the fact that they may be selectively stained in electron microscopic preparations with phosphotungstic acid.

The second distinguishing feature of a synapse is the presence in the presynaptic element of large numbers of clear-centered vesicles with diameters ranging from 400 to 600 Å. It is now generally accepted that these vesicles contain the neurotransmitter substances that are the basis of chemical synaptic action and for this reason they are called *synaptic vesicles.* The concentration of the vesicles is usually greatest near the presynaptic membrane specialization and many lie between the presynaptic-dense projections of the membrane. It is now generally accepted that as an action potential invades the axon terminal, synaptic vesicles fuse with special "release sites" in the presynaptic membrane between the dense projections and thence discharge their content of transmitter into the synaptic cleft. The transmitter then diffuses to the postsynaptic membrane where it interacts with special receptor molecules in the postsynaptic membrane which leads to a change in the membrane conductance of the postsynaptic neuron.

FIGURE 8-30 Basket cell axons (BCA) traversing molecular layer (ML) of cat cerebellum and descending to form terminal baskets over somata of Purkinje cells (PC). GCL, granule cell layer. Reduced silver stain, ×490.

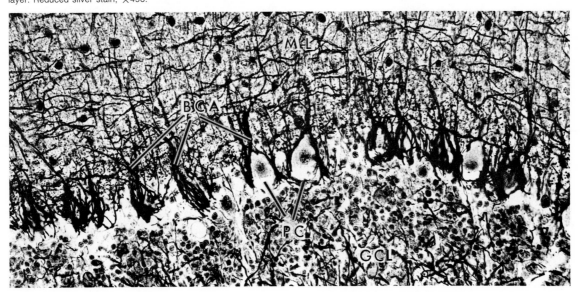

The only other elements that are consistent components of every synapse are mitochondria in the presynaptic process, their number varying with the size of the terminal (Figs. 8-32 and 8-34). In addition, a few sacs or tubules of agranular endoplasmic reticulum may be present and in some cases microtubules and neurofilaments also extend into the axon terminal. The neurofilaments if found in the presynaptic process are either diffusely scattered or occasionally aggregated in a single bundle which forms a loop or ring around a central cluster of mitochondria. In the latter case, neurofibrillar stains often show the axon terminals as ringlike boutons (Fig. 8-90).

From electrophysiological studies, it is known that synapses may be either *excitatory* or *inhibitory*, de-

pending on whether their activation drives the membrane potential of the postsynaptic neuron toward or away from its threshold level for firing nerve impulses. In chemical synapses these effects are usually mediated by different neurotransmitter agents, because as a general rule, an individual nerve cell releases only one kind of transmitter agent from its axon terminals. Certain transmitters that are known to have differing actions at different postsynaptic sites presumably do so because of differences in the postsynaptic receptors or in the properties of the postsynaptic membranes.

In parts of the vertebrate central nervous system, inhibition has often been found to involve Golgi type II

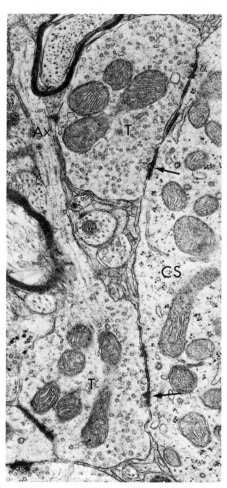

FIGURE 8-32 Electron micrograph showing preterminal axon (AX) and two terminal boutons (T) making synaptic contacts (arrows) on cell soma (CS) of a neuron in inferior colliculus of a cat. ×18,000. (A. J. Rockel and E. G. Jones, *J. Comp. Neurol.,* **147:**61, 1973.)

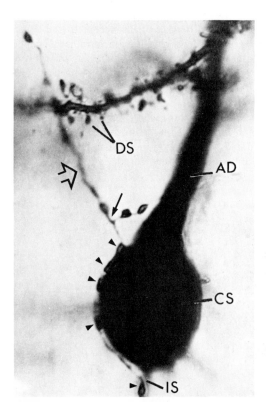

FIGURE 8-31 Terminal axon (open arrow) branching (arrow) and terminating as a series of end bulbs (arrow heads) on soma (CS) and axon initial segment (IS) of a pyramidal cell in the cerebral cortex of a monkey. AD, apical dendrite; DS, dendritic spines. Golgi stain, ×500. (E. G. Jones, *J. Comp. Neurol.,* **160:**205, 1975.)

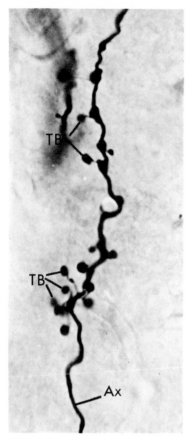

FIGURE 8-33 Terminal portion of an axon (Ax) in inferior colliculus of cat showing terminal boutons (TB). Golgi stain, ×1350. (A. J. Rockel and E. G. Jones, *J. Comp. Neurol.* **147**:11, 1973.)

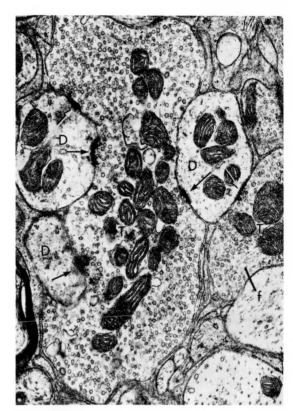

FIGURE 8-34 Electron micrograph from inferior colliculus showing two terminal boutons (T) of the type illustrated in Fig. 8-33. These make synaptic contacts (arrows) with small dendrites (D). One terminal contains a small cluster of neurofilaments (f). ×27,300. (A. J. Rockel and E. G. Jones, *J. Comp. Neurol,* **147**:61, 1973.)

neurons. Such neurons are, therefore, often referred to as *inhibitory interneurons.* Examples of such inhibitory interneurons are the basket cells of the cerebellum, and the Renshaw cells of the spinal cord. However, not all inhibitory neurons are of the Golgi type II variety; the Purkinje cells of the cerebellum have relatively long axons, but it is now known that they act to inhibit the cells of the deep cerebellar nuclei. Conversely, not all neurons with short axons are inhibitory in character; some (for example, the granule cells of the cerebellum) are clearly excitatory.

It has been evident for a long time that synapses in the central nervous system vary in their morphology. The earliest indication of this came from the work of E. G. Gray who noted in 1959, that in material fixed with osmium tetroxide and stained with phosphotungstic acid, synapses could, on the whole, be divided

into two categories on the basis of differences in the width of the synaptic cleft and the extent of the postsynaptic membrane thickenings. The typical axodendritic synapse described on page 309 is an example of what Gray referred to as a *type I synapse* (Fig. 8-38). The two characteristics of this type of synapse are a widening of the intercellular gap at the synaptic cleft to approximately 300 Å and a pronounced accumulation of dense material beneath the postsynaptic membrane. In aldehyde-fixed material the most striking feature of these synapses is the asymmetry in the pre- and postsynaptic membrane specializations and these contacts are now referred to as *asymmetrical synapses.* In Gray's second type of synapse (type II synapses, Fig. 8-37) the synaptic cleft is only slightly wider than the

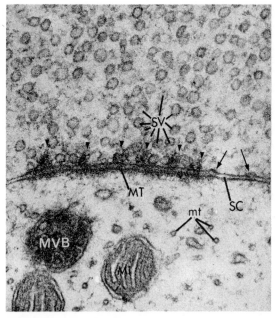

FIGURE 8-35 Electron micrograph of a synapse, showing synaptic vesicles (SV), presynaptic dense projections (arrow-heads) and possible sites (arrows) of incorporation of synaptic vesicle membrane into membrane of terminal. MT, membrane thickening; SC, synaptic cleft. Postsynaptic dendrite contains mitochondria (Mi), a multivesicular body (MVB), and microtubules (mt). ×57,400. (A. J. Rockel and E. G. Jones, *J. Comp. Neurol.,* **147:**61, 1973.)

normal intercellular gap (approximately 200 Å) and the postsynaptic membrane specialization is less marked. In aldehyde-fixed material, little or no dense material is seen attached to the deep surface of the postsynaptic membrane, and since the two apposed membranes appear equally "thick," such synapses are now usually referred to as *symmetrical synapses.*

Although the pre- and postsynaptic membrane specializations appear in single electron micrographs as linear structures, it should be pointed out that they are, in fact, fairly extensive plaquelike structures which may measure as much as 1×1 μm. The postsynaptic plaques of asymmetrical synapses are frequently perforated in one or more places, so that in a section passing perpendicularly through the plaque, the axon terminal appears to be associated with two or more postsynaptic "thickenings" (Fig. 8-34). Perforation of the postsynaptic plaques appears to be uncommon in symmetrical synapses.

Although to some extent the asymmetrical and the symmetrical synapses represent the extremes of a continuum, the majority of the synapses encountered can be readily placed in one or another of the two classes. The significance of this is emphasized by the observation that the synaptic vesicles in the presynaptic processes associated with the two classes may also differ. If nervous tissue is fixed in aldehyde-containing solutions with buffers of relatively high osmolality, then the synaptic vesicles in some axon terminals become "flattened," ovoid, or disc-shaped (Fig. 8-37), whereas those of other terminals retain the

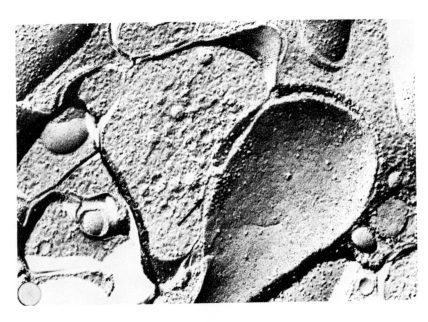

FIGURE 8-36 Freeze-etch preparation of a synaptic contact in cerebellum. Arrow indicates synaptic cleft. Note synaptic vesicles in terminal (left) and particles in postsynaptic membrane of Purkinje cell dendritic spine (right). ×79,000. (D. M. Landis and T. S. Reese, *J. Comp. Neurol.,* **155:**93, 1974; courtesy of Dr. T. S. Reese.)

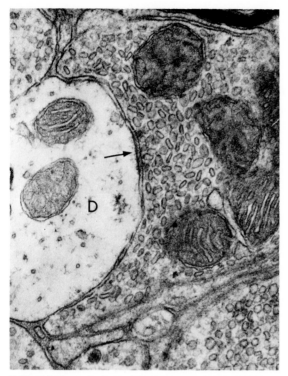

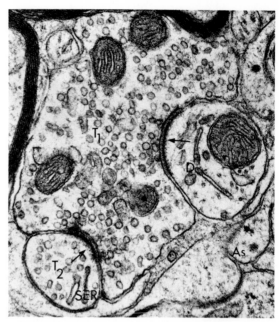

FIGURE 8-37 Flattened vesicle containing axon terminal making symmetrical synaptic contact (arrow) with a dendrite (D) in inferior colliculus of cat. ×36,000. (A. J. Rockel and E. G. Jones, *J. Comp. Neurol.*, **147**:61, 1973.)

FIGURE 8-38 Spherical vesicle containing terminal (T_1) making asymmetrical synaptic contacts (arrows) with a dendrite (D) and another axon terminal (T_2). Thalamus of cat. SER, smooth endoplasmic reticulum; As, astrocytic processes. ×35,200.

spherical form commonly seen after osmium tetroxide fixation (Fig. 8-38). Uchizono first noted that in the cerebellar cortex in which the functions of most synaptic contacts are known, this flattening of the synaptic vesicles occurs only in the terminals of known inhibitory neurons. Furthermore, since the synaptic vesicles in the terminals of the granule cell axons (which are known to be excitatory) remain spherical (S vesicles) under the same conditions of fixation, it was suggested that the presence of flattened (or F) vesicles in aldehyde-fixed material might serve as an identifying marker for inhibitory synapses and that spherical vesicles might always be associated with excitatory synapses. The subsequent association of flattenable synaptic vesicles with symmetrical membrane specializations and spherical vesicles with asymmetrical membrane thickenings, made first by Colonnier for synapses in the cerebral cortex, strengthened the idea that there was a close relation between vesicle morphology and functional synaptic type. The flattening of the synaptic vesicles is clearly an artifact induced by the high osmolality of the aldehyde fixative solutions, but in many

parts of the brain and spinal cord, the flattening is sufficiently consistent to provide a useful basis for the classification of synapses. However, it has become equally clear that the association of flattened synaptic vesicles and the presence of an inhibitory synaptic transmitter is not universal, and there are now several instances known in which the presynaptic process exerts an inhibitory influence but contains spherical vesicles. The mechanism responsible for the flattening of certain synaptic vesicles is not clear, but it presumably reflects either some basic differences in the vesicle membrane or possibly its content of synaptic transmitter. In some situations the vesicles which become flattened in aldehyde-fixed material are clearly of the same size as those which remain spherical, but others that become irregular in shape (or pleiomorphic) are distinctly smaller in diameter.

A third distinct class of synaptic vesicle has been recognized in axons that are known to release catecholamines or indolealkyl amines. This will be considered in greater detail in the section on the autonomic nervous system, but it may be noted here that the terminals of certain classes of aminergic neurons in the central nervous system contain small, spherical vesicles with electron-dense "cores" identical to those found in sympathetic nerve terminals (Fig. 8-39). These vesicles have diameters of 400 to 600 Å, with dense cores approximately 250 Å in diameter. In routinely fixed material the granular vesicles of these "G synapses" are not particularly prominent, since the material in the dense cores is not well retained. However, if the tissue is fixed in potassium permanganate or presoaked in the appropriate biogenic amine, the cores are seen to be present in the majority of the vesicles.

Such small dense-core vesicles are to be distinguished from a larger type that is found in small numbers in virtually every type of axon terminal throughout the nervous system. In this case, the spherical vesicle has a diameter of approximately 1000 Å and the core diameter of approximately 500 Å. One or more of these may be found in terminals containing small dense-core vesicles or clear vesicles, either spherical or flattened, and occasionally they are even found in the neuron soma. Their significance is unknown.

One final type of synaptic ending may be mentioned. These are most commonly found in the hypothalamus of vertebrates and in neurosecretory neurons of invertebrates. They contain very large dense-core vesicles (up to 2000 Å in diameter) which are clearly

FIGURE 8-39 Noradrenergic terminal (T) from tissue culture of rat superior cervical ganglion. Note large proportion of dense core vesicles demonstrated by soaking tissue in 10^{-5} M noradrenaline prior to fixation. Mi, mitochondrian. ×40,000. (Courtesy of Dr. M. I. Johnson.)

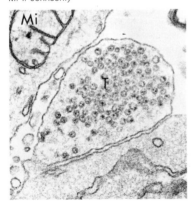

associated with the transport and release of various hormones (such as vasopressin or oxytocin). In the hypothalamus, secretory products appear to be elaborated in somata of distinct classes of neurons, "packaged" in the Golgi apparatus and then actively transported down the axons for release from the axon terminals either in the region of the median eminence or in the neyrohypophysis (see Chap. 27).

The site of formation of the clear and smaller dense-core vesicles is less certain. There is some evidence to suggest that they may be formed in the Golgi complex of the neuronal somata and that they are transported down to the terminals as part of the general "axoplasmic flow." This view is based partly on the known functions of the Golgi complex and partly on the fact that the neuronal somata usually contains considerable amounts of the appropriate neurotransmitter substance and of the enzymes involved in its synthesis. For example, the soma of neurons that release norepinephrine at their axon terminals contain quantities of norepinephrine and of the enzyme dopamine-β-hydroxylase, which serves to produce norepinephrine from the amine of dihydroxyphenylalanine (dopamine) (Fig. 8-40). On the other hand, smooth-walled, clear-centered vesicles are rarely seen in axons or in the somata of neurons, and since it is known that substantial amounts of most neurotransmitters can be synthesized in axon terminals, it is evident that many vesicles must be formed locally within nerve endings. Direct evidence for this comes from studies on the uptake of exogenous proteins by axon terminals (Fig. 8-41). If a histochemically identifiable marker such as the enzyme horseradish peroxidase is present in the extracellular space surrounding the terminals of an axon, it is rapidly taken up by the terminals in coated vesicles. At a slightly later stage, peroxidase-laden coated vesicles can be seen to fuse with the cisternae of smooth ER in the terminal and to lose their coats or shells, which appear to remain free in the terminal. Synaptic vesicles, containing horseradish peroxidase, are then budded off from the cisternae and are free to pass toward the presynaptic membrane, to fuse with it, and in the process to release the enzyme (and whatever transmitter may have been incorporated into the vesicles) into the synaptic cleft. If the terminal is subjected to repetitive stimulation, it can also be shown that as it becomes depleted of synaptic vesicles, the circumference is progressively enlarged. These experimental observations suggest that there is a continuous recycling of the synaptic vesicle membrane, with the vesic-

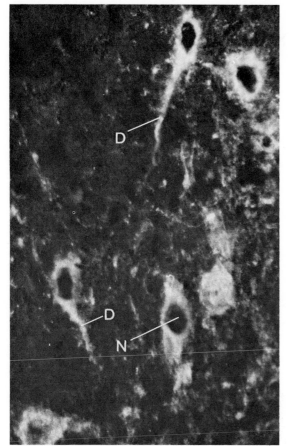

FIGURE 8-40 Noradrenergic neurons in locus coeruleus of a rat demonstrated by binding of a fluorescent-labeled antibody to enzyme dopamine-β-hydroxylase. D, dendrites; N, nucleus. ×950. (Courtesy of Drs. B. G. Hartmann and L. W. Swanson.)

ular membrane first becoming incorporated into the presynaptic membrane, then moving to one side of the presynaptic specialization and finally being returned to the interior of the axon terminal in the form of a coated vesicle.

The Distribution of Synapses

Axon terminals may make synaptic contacts with any portion of the surface of another neuron (Fig. 8-42). Although the majority occur on dendrites and perikarya, the axon terminals of one neuron may also contact the axon of another; and indeed the only parts of nerve cells that have never been seen to receive a synapse are those segments of an axon covered by a myelin sheath.

Synapses on dendritic spines are usually referred

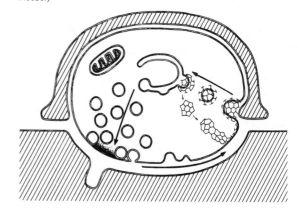

to as *axospinous synapses.* They are usually found on the expanded tips of spines, and each spine receives at least one. Since not all neurons possess spines on their dendrites, axospinous synapses are not always present; however, when they are present, they tend to be of the asymmetrical type and the weight of evidence points to their being excitatory in function. Synapses on the shafts of dendrites are referred to as *axodendritic synapses.* They may be either symmetrical or asymmetrical and their relative distribution and density depends on the type of neuron. The dendrites of some cells are covered with both types of synapse, whereas others have relatively few of one or the other type, and some have few of either type. Generally, the symmetrical synapses predominate on the larger dendritic trunks near the soma. Synapses on the perikaryon are referred to as *axosomatic synapses.* Again, their numbers and type vary from cell to cell; cells that receive few axosomatic synapses tend to have only symmetrical synapses upon the soma; those that receive many tend to have both types. Where a synapse is found on the initial segment of the axon or adjacent axon hillock of a neuron, it may be referred to as an *initial-segment synapse.* Because of the critical role played by the initial segment in impulse initiation,

FIGURE 8-41 Postulated mechanism for recycling of synaptic vesicle membrane at neuromuscular junction (J. S. Heuser and T. S. Reese, *J. Cell Biol.,* **57:**315, 1973). Vesicles discharge contents by exocytosis and membranes are incorporated into membrane of terminal; moving away from synaptic region, incorporated membrane is taken up as coated vesicle by endocytosis; joining smooth endoplasmic reticulum, it loses dense coat and is pinched off as new synaptic vesicle. (Courtesy of Dr. T. S. Reese.)

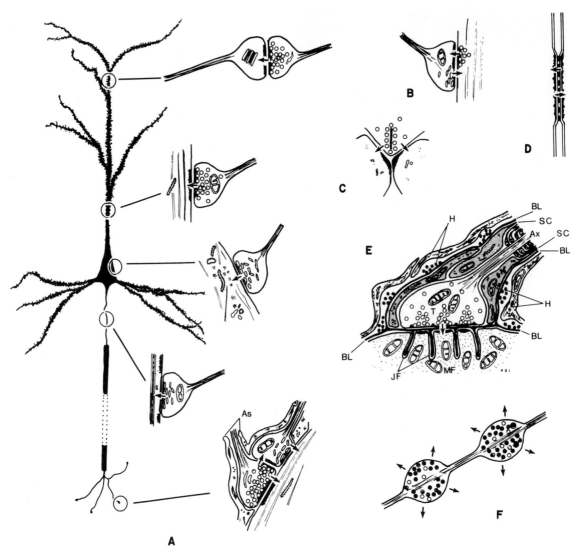

FIGURE 8-42 Types of synapse; arrows indicate direction of transmission. A. Types of synaptic contact received or made by pyramidal cell of cerebral cortex. From above, down: axospinous; axodendritic, axosomatic; initial segment synapse; axoaxonic and serial synapse. As, astroglial covering. B. Reciprocal synapse of olfactory bulb. C. Ribbon synapse of retina. D. Electrical (gap junction) synapse. E. Motor end plate. Ax, myelinated axon; BL, basal lamina; H, fibroblast processes and collagen bundles forming sheath of Henle; JF, junctional folds; MF, muscle fiber; SC, Schwann cell processes; T, axon terminal. F. Adrenergic terminal in sympathetic nervous system.

synapses located on or near it are in a unique position to influence the firing of the cell. It is significant therefore that wherever such synapses have been observed, they have invariably been of the symmetrical type, and it is generally assumed that they exert an inhibitory effect upon the postsynaptic cell. In some instances a terminal from one axon may form a synapse upon a terminal of another: this arrangement is called an *axo-axonic synapse*. Axo-axonic synapses appear to

be involved in the phenomenon of *presynaptic inhibition*, since their action tends to reduce the amount of transmitter released by the postsynaptic axon terminal. Occasionally axo-axonic synapses of this type are serially arranged so that one process is postsynaptic at one synapse and presynaptic (upon another process) at a second synapse. Such arrangements are referred to as *serial synapses*.

The remaining classes of synapses to be considered are all rather unusual and have been demonstrated in only a few sites in the nervous system. In some cases dendrites have been found to contain clusters of synaptic vesicles and membrane specializations indistinguishable from those seen in axon terminals; such processes are termed *presynaptic dendrites,* and since they usually contact other dendrites, the synapses they form are *dendrodendritic synapses.* Such dendrodendritic synapses have now been described in several sites such as the thalamus where they are of the symmetrical type, and the presynaptic dendrite usually contains flattened vesicles. A special type of dendrodendritic synapse has been found in the olfactory bulb between the dendrites of the mitral cells and the processes of granule cells. In this case the mitral cell dendrites form asymmetrical synapses (associated with spherical synaptic vesicles) upon the granule cell processes; and usually within a few microns of such a contact, the same granule cell process forms a *reciprocal synapse* upon the mitral cell dendrite. The granule cell processes usually contain flattened synaptic vesicles and form symmetrical synapses (which in this situation are known, from electrophysiological studies, to be inhibitory) upon the mitral cells. *Somatodendritic* and *somatosomatic* synapses have also been described in the optic tecta of certain amphibia and in the sympathetic ganglia of mammals; as the names suggest, the presynaptic element in both cases is the cell body of a neuron.

Another form of synapse is the so-called ribbon synapse, the best known examples of which are found in the retina. In these cases the axonal process of one type of cell makes synaptic contact with the juxtaposed processes of two other cell types. In the outer plexiform layer, the processes of receptor cells (rods and cones) are presynaptic to the processes of bipolar and

horizontal cells. In the inner plexiform layer, the axons of bipolar cells are presynaptic to the juxtaposed processes of ganglion and amacrine cells. These "triad" synapses are characterized by the presence in the presynaptic element of an electron-dense synaptic ribbon. The synaptic ribbon is invariably aligned perpendicular to the presynaptic membrane and the synaptic vesicles are gathered about it instead of aggregated at the presynaptic membrane. In the inner plexiform layer, the bipolar cell axon terminal forms a ribbon synapse as well as a conventional synapse with the ganglion cell dendrite (see Chap. 32).

All the synapses described so far are called chemical synapses because they act through the intermediary of a chemical synaptic transmitter. A final synaptic type, though infrequent in mammals, is very common in other vertebrates and in invertebrates; this is the so-called electrical synapse. In these synapses the pre- and postsynaptic elements are joined through low-resistance gap junctions so that the electrical activity set up in one cell readily spreads to the next cell without a significant delay. The gap junctions found between neuronal processes are identical to those found in other tissues in which electrical coupling occurs (see Chap. 3). In certain cases, an axon terminal may make both a conventional (chemical) and an electrical synapse with a postsynaptic element (usually a neuronal perikaryon or dendrite). The best-known example of such a mixed chemical and electrical synapse is in the ciliary ganglion of birds, but similar contacts have been found in the lateral vestibular nucleus and the mesencephalic nucleus of the trigeminal nerve of mammals.

NEUROGLIA AND OTHER SUPPORTING CELLS

Although neurons tend to dominate any microscopic section of nervous tissue, they form only a relatively small percentage of the total population of cells present in the section. In most regions they are far outnumbered by the generally smaller nonneuronal or supporting cells which in the central nervous system are collectively referred to as *neuroglial cells.* It has been estimated that such cells may account for more than one-half the total weight of the brain.

The supporting cells are characterized by their generally small size, their ubiquity, and their large numbers. Because of their small size, only their nuclei are seen in routine preparations (Figs. 8-11, 8-26, and 8-43). The nuclei vary in diameter from 3 to 10 μm, which is about the same size as the very smallest neurons. Where neuroglial cells have been counted, they outnumber neurons by as much as 10:1 to 50:1. They are found between neuronal somata and within fiber tracts. Unlike neurons, probably all supporting cells retain the capacity to proliferate under appropriate circumstances.

THE SUPPORTING CELLS
OF THE CENTRAL NERVOUS SYSTEM

Two main classes of supporting cell are recognized in the brain and spinal cord (Fig. 8-44). The first are the *astrocytes* and *oligodendrocytes,* sometimes known collectively as the macroglia. The second is a heterogeneous group of cells, including the *ependymal cells,* which form the epithelial lining of the choroid plexuses and of the ventricular system of the brain and the central canal of the spinal cord; a variety of vascular and perivascular cells; and cells commonly called *microglial* cells, which at one time were thought to be mesodermal rather than neurectodermal in origin but are now regarded as immature, or resting, glioblasts.

Astrocytes

As the name implies, astrocytes are star-shaped when demonstrated by heavy metal preparations that impregnate the whole cell (Figs. 8-45 and 8-46). A small, irregularly shaped cell soma gives rise to a number of processes of variable thickness, length, and branching pattern, which ramify between the perikarya and processes of nerve cells. Astrocytes situated near the surface of the brain or spinal cord commonly have one or more of their processes extending to the pial surface where they expand to form "end feet," which collectively form the so-called *glia limitans;* others have similar end feet on the walls of blood vessels. Two types of astrocyte have traditionally been recognized: *fibrous astrocytes* and *protoplasmic astrocytes.* Fibrous astrocytes (Figs. 8-44, 8-45, 8-52, 8-53), which are found predominantly in white matter, have long, slender, generally unbranched processes containing many delicate fibrils when stained with the usual metallic methods. Protoplasmic astrocytes are found predominantly in gray matter and have shorter, stouter, and much more highly branched processes which give to the cells a "fluffy" appearance (Figs. 8-46, 8-49, 8-52, 8-53). It is now recognized that the two types of astrocyte are in fact modulations in the form of a single cell type, the appearance of the cells apparently depending on their location and possibly on their metabolic state.

Although the full extent of individual astrocytes can be demonstrated only by the use of special metallic stains, it is more common to see them in routine neurohistological preparations; in such preparations generally only the nuclei of the cells are seen, since the

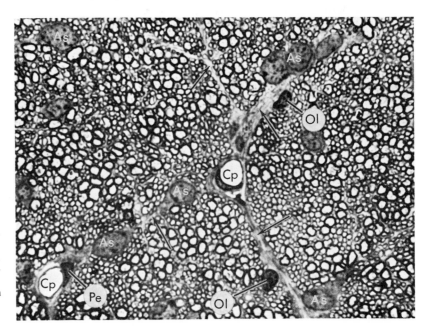

FIGURE 8-43 Cross section of monkey optic nerve showing myelinated axons, astrocytes (As), and oligodendrocytes (Ol). Septa (arrows) formed by astrocytic cytoplasm contain capillaries (Cp), one of which is associated with a pericyte (Pe). Toluidine-blue-stained plastic section. ×1620.

amount of perikaryal cytoplasm they contain is small and their cytoplasmic processes are thin. The nuclei are usually oval in shape, vesicular, and somewhat larger than the nuclei of oligodendrocytes (see below).

In electron micrographs, astrocytes are distinguished by their relatively organelle-free cytoplasm and their euchromatic nuclei (Figs. 8-54 and 8-55). Commonly the nucleus is oval and indented, and distinct nucleoli are not seen. Only a small amount of cytoplasm is usually seen around the nucleus in single sections; however, these give a very incomplete picture of the total extent of the cytoplasm, for several irregularly shaped cytoplasmic processes emanate from the perikaryon and often extend for considerable distances. As they do so, they give rise to branches and protrusions which align themselves along blood vessels or along the pial surface and insinuate themselves between the somata and processes of nerve cells and other glial cells. Some of these processes are stout and lengthy, but others are thin and sheetlike.

The cytoplasm contains few free ribosomes and little rough-surfaced endoplasmic reticulum. A Golgi complex is always present, and lysosomes and glyco-

gen granules are common. The most distinctive astrocytic organelles are the glial microfilaments which are similar in appearance and substructure to the neurofilaments of nerve cells (Figs. 8-51 and 8-54). Variably sized bundles of these microfilaments are found in the perikaryal cytoplasm and in most of the processes of all astrocytes. Such bundles of microfilaments clearly form the basis of the fibrils that are seen with the light microscope.

Two special types of modified astrocyte are known. One is the *Müller cell* of the retina, which is an elongated columnar cell extending across the thickness of the neural retina (see Chap. 32). Müller cells have expanded foot processes which form the inner and outer limiting membranes of the retina. The second type is the *Bergmann glial cell* of the cerebellum (Fig. 8-53). These have their somata at the level of the Purkinje cell layer and several ascending processes with short side branches that collectively envelop the Purkinje cell dendrites. Ultrastructurally, both the

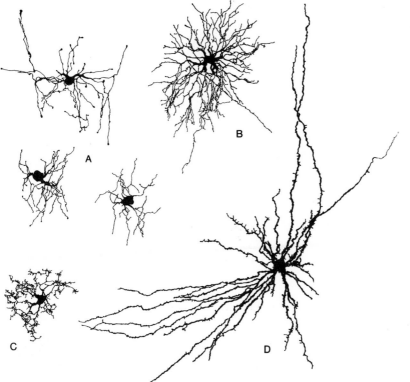

FIGURE 8-44 Camera lucida drawings at same magnification (×1065) showing oligodendrocytes (A), protoplasmic astrocyte (B), microglial cell (C) and fibrous astrocyte (D). Golgi stain, cerebral cortex of monkey.

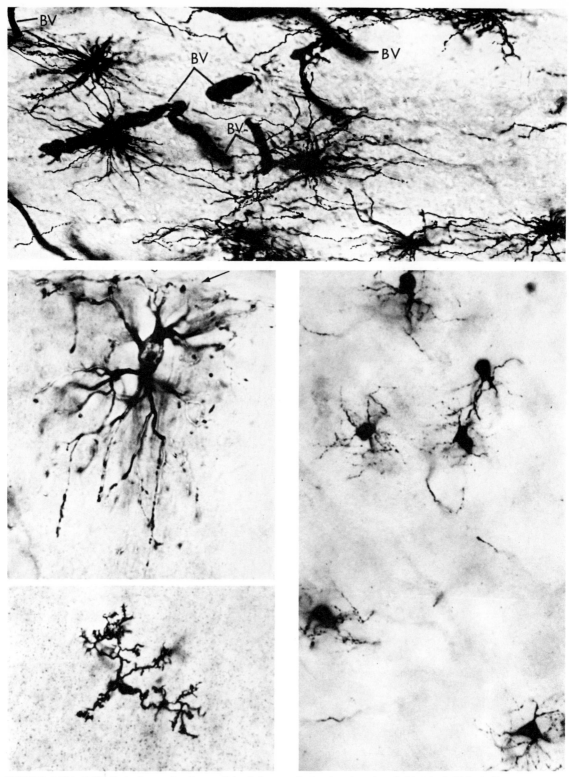

FIGURES 8-45 to 8-48 Photomicrographs of neuroglial cells from cerebral cortex of monkey, Golgi stain. **8-45 (top):** fibrous astrocytes; BV, blood vessels, ×990. **8-46 (middle left):** protoplasmic astrocyte; arrow: brain surface. ×1940. **8-47 (bottom left):** microglial cell, ×1746. **8-48 (right):** oligodendrocytes, ×1940.

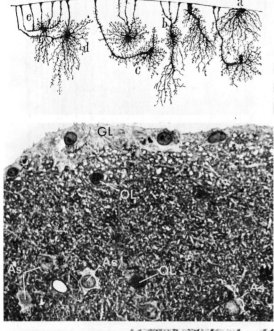

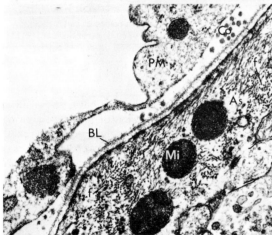

Müller and Bergmann glial cells closely resemble typical astrocytes found elsewhere in the nervous system.

The functions of astrocytes in the normal central nervous system are unknown, but there are some features about their distribution which are suggestive. First, as we have just seen, many of their processes are aligned at interfaces where the nervous system meets other tissues. Such interfaces occur at the surface of the brain and spinal cord where neural tissue abuts upon the meninges and along the walls of blood vessels within the central nervous system (Figs. 8-49 to 8-51, 8-56, and 8-57). The largest concentration of astrocytic processes is found beneath the pial surface where the processes of many astrocytic foot processes form the *glia limitans*. The outer surface of this zone of astrocytic processes is in contact with the *basal lamina* which encompasses the brain and spinal cord and is the derivative of the original basal lamina of the embryonic neuroepithelium (Fig. 8-51). Similarly, as the larger blood vessels enter or exit from the central nervous system, they are invariably separated from the neural tissues proper by the basal lamina and by a *perivascular space* which is continuous with the subarachnoid space surrounding the brain and spinal cord (Fig. 8-56). Again, the basal lamina is underlain by stacked astrocytic processes. As the vessels penetrate further into the brain or spinal cord, they progressively lose their muscle coats and the perivascular space becomes obliterated (Fig. 8-57). Finally the capillaries, deep within the substance of the brain or cord, are invested by a continuous basal lamina, which remains ensheathed by astrocytic end feet.

The presence of astrocytic processes at these interfaces suggested to earlier workers that they might serve as diffusional barriers and, in particular, that they might represent the morphological basis of the well-known blood-brain barrier. However, it is now clear that the intercellular spaces within the brain and spinal cord are in free communication with the subarachnoid space through channels between the astrocytic lamellae; and even though there are occasional gap junctions between adjoining lamellae, these do not prevent passage of even large molecules between the cerebrospinal fluid and the neural parenchyma. It is now evident that the bloodbrain barrier has as its structural basis occluding tight junctions between the capillary endothelial cells.

Astrocytes and their processes also divide the

FIGURE 8-49 (Upper) Protoplasmic astrocytes at surface of cerebral cortex in a Golgi preparation. (S. Ramón y Cajal, Histologie du Système Nerveux, 1909.)

FIGURE 8-50 (Middle) Protoplasmic astrocytes forming glia limitans (GL) at surface of cerebral cortex of monkey. Other astrocytes (AS) and oligodendrocytes (Ol) are more deeply situated. Toluidine blue stained plastic section. ×780.

FIGURE 8-51 (Lower) Electron micrograph showing cell process (PM) and collagen bundles (Co) of pia mater lying loosely on basal lamina (BL) of monkey cerebral cortex. Beneath basal lamina lie astrocytic processes (As) containing mitochondria (Mi) and many microfilaments (f). ×29,640.

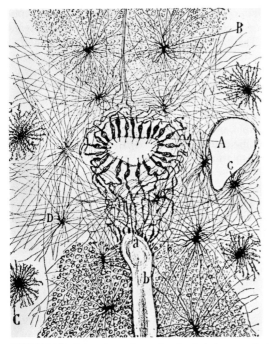

FIGURE 8-52 Astrocytes and ependymal cells in human spinal cord, Golgi stain. (S. Ramón y Cajal, Histologie du Système Nerveux, 1909.) Ependymal cell foot processes reach surface at "a."

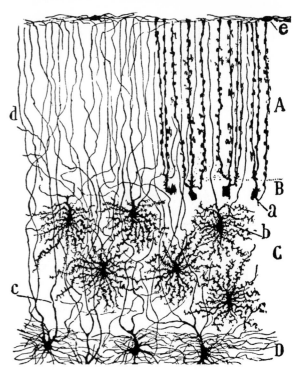

FIGURE 8-53 Astrocytes in human cerebellar cortex, Golgi stain. (S. Ramón y Cajal, Histologie du Système Nerveux, 1911.) a: Bergmann glial cells; b: protoplasmic astrocytes; c: fibrous astrocytes.

brain and spinal cord into sectors of varying distinctiveness, in some places such as the spinal cord and optic nerve (Fig. 8-43) actually forming septa. It has been suggested, therefore, that their major role is to provide a form of scaffolding, or structural support, upon which the neurons and their processes are assembled. It is doubtful that this could be their sole, or even principal, purpose, although it is possible that in some parts of the nervous system, they serve to isolate groups of neurons or, even commonly, groups of synapses, from their neighbors. It is perhaps noteworthy that the initial segments of most axons and the "bare" segments at nodes of Ranvier are usually ensheathed in astrocytic processes; in many situations, groups of axon terminals ending on a particular neuron, or part of a neuron, are often separated from the rest of the cells and their processes by an almost complete envelope of astrocytic processes. Such glial ensheathed synaptic aggregations are sometimes referred to as *glomeruli* (Fig. 8-42).

Electrophysiological studies have shown that some astrocytes undergo a slow depolarization during the repetitive activation of the neighboring nerve cells. This appears to be due to the uptake of excess potassium from the extracellular space which follows prolonged neuronal activity. The ability to serve as a "potassium sink" is extremely important, although it should be pointed out that at least some invertebrate neurons can be stripped of their glial ensheathment and yet continue to function for considerable periods of time.

Finally, as we shall see later, when we consider the response of the nervous system to injury, under various pathological conditions astrocytes play a key role in the removal of neuronal debris and in sealing off damaged brain tissue.

Oligodendrocytes

Oligodendrocytes are small neuroglial cells with relatively few processes. In common light microscopic preparations (Fig. 8-43) where only the nuclei are stained, they appear smaller, more irregular, and more deeply staining than those of astrocytes. Classically, two main types of oligodendrocyte are recognized: *interfascicular oligodendrocytes* and *perineuronal satellite cells* (Figs. 8-44 and 8-48). As the names suggest, interfascicular oligodendrocytes are found among the bundles of axons that constitute the white matter of the brain and spinal cord. Perineuronal satellite cells, on the other hand, are found in close association with the perikarya of neurons in areas of gray matter. Although the interfascicular form tends to be more elongated than the perineuronal satellite form, the two types are essentially similar.

In electron micrographs, the oligodendrocyte is recognized as a generally much denser cell than the astrocyte (Figs. 8-55 and 8-58). The nucleus is heterochromatic and the cytoplasm is filled with organelles, especially large numbers of free and attached ribo-

somes, the latter being associated with numerous short cisternae of endoplasmic reticulum. The Golgi apparatus is also extensive and mitochondria are present in considerable numbers. But perhaps the most striking cytoplasmic feature is the large number of microtubules which permeate the perikaryal cytoplasm and are abundant in the processes of the cell where they tend to be arranged in parallel arrays.

The close association of perineuronal satellite oligodendrocytes with neurons has suggested to some workers that they may be in some way involved with the maintenance of the metabolic state of the neurons with which they are associated. This has never been satisfactorily demonstrated, and at present only one function can be attributed with confidence to the oligodendrocytes. Oligodendrocytes, both interfascicular

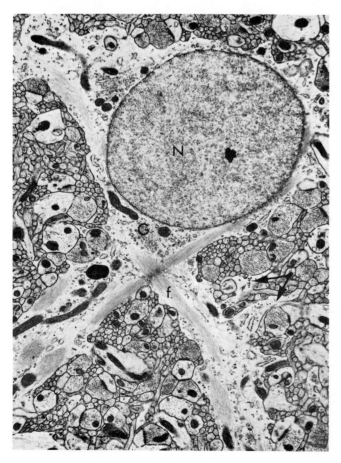

FIGURE 8-54 Electron micrograph of astrocyte from cerebral cortex of a cat. N, nucleus; f, microfilaments; G, Golgi complex; arrows, cell processes. ×8000.

and perineuronal, are the *myelin-forming* cells of the central nervous system (Fig. 8-59).

A myelinated axon acquires its sheath at the end of the initial segment, usually a few microns from the axon hillock, and the myelin sheath continues to near the region of termination of the axon (Figs. 8-60 and 8-61). In the light microscope the myelin sheath appears as an elongated tube that is interrupted at regular intervals along its length at what are termed the *nodes of Ranvier*. The segments of myelin between consecutive nodes of Ranvier are termed *internodal segments,* or *internodes.* The thickness of the myelin

FIGURE 8-55 Electron micrograph from spinal cord of a rat showing distinguishing features of neuron (N), astrocyte (As), and oligodendrocyte (Ol). Label is on nucleus in each case. ×15,000.

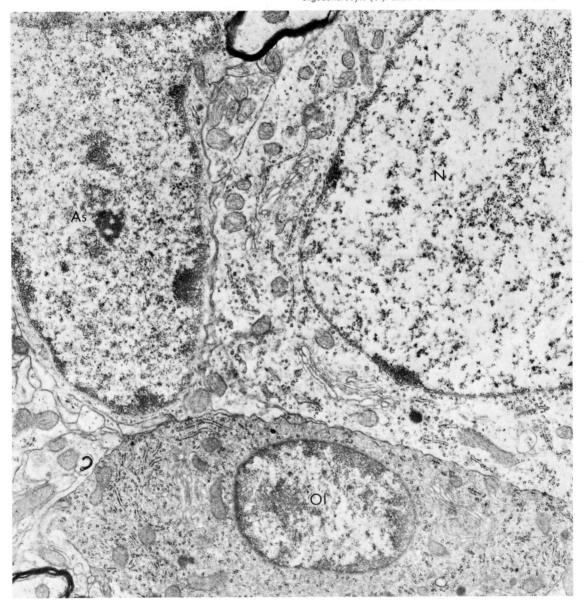

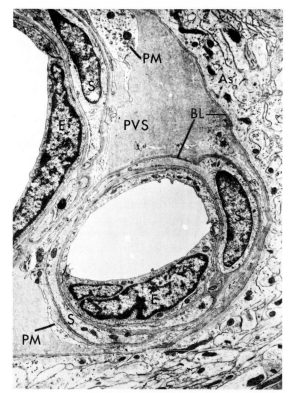

FIGURE 8-56 Electron micrograph of two blood vessels lying in perivascular space (PVS) as they enter cerebral cortex of cat. E, endothelial cells; S, smooth muscle cells; BL, basal lamina; PM, pia mater; As, astrocytic processes. ×8100. (E. G. Jones, *J. Anat., (Lond.),* **106**:507, 1970.)

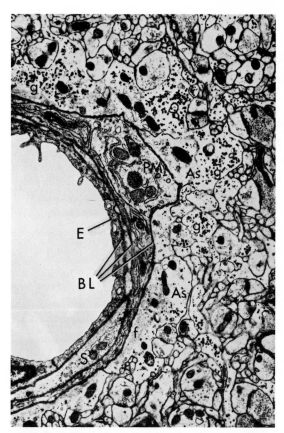

FIGURE 8-57 Electron micrograph showing small blood vessel with cell process of pia mater (PM) caught between it and basal lamina of brain. As, astrocyte foot processes containing microfilaments (f) and glycogen (g); BL, basal lamina; E, endothelial cell. Cat cerebral cortex, ×17,500. (E. G. Jones and T. P. S. Powell, *Philos. Trans. R. Soc. Lond.,* [Biol. Sci.], **257**:1, 1970.)

sheath and the length of the internodal segments are fairly constant for a given axon and have been found to be proportional to the diameter (or more strictly, the circumference) of the contained axon.

In the central nervous system, each internodal segment of myelin is formed by a cytoplasmic process of an oligodendrocyte wrapping itself around the axon in a spiral fashion (Figs. 8-58 and 8-59). As the process approaches the axon it becomes extremely attenuated, and this portion of the process is known as the *external tongue* (Fig. 8-60). As the process spirals around the axon, the cytoplasmic faces of its plasma membrane fuse to form what appears in section as a dense line some 25 to 30 Å thick. This is known as the *major dense line.* A myelin internode is made up of repeated wrappings or lamellae of the oligodendrocytic process and therefore appears as a regularly arranged, repeating series of major dense lines. These are separated from one another by an electron

lucent zone some 90 Å wide—referred to as the *intraperiod line*—that contains a faint line somewhat thinner than the major dense line. The intraperiod line is formed by the fused outer faces of the plasma membranes of adjoining wrappings of the oligodendrocytic process.

The outermost major dense line of a myelin internodal segment is directly continuous with the external tongue of the oligodendrocytic process. The innermost major dense line splits apart as it approaches its end to form a similar tongue of cytoplasm known as the *internal tongue.* The intraperiod line disappears as the inner and outer tongues emerge. The internal tongue is the leading edge, as it were, of the oligodendrocytic process. The thickness of a myelin sheath is determined by the number of wrappings of oligodendrocytic cytoplasm; therefore, in axons of increasing diameter, the number of major dense lines and intraperiod lines becomes progressively greater. It has been demonstrated that in myelinated axons, one lamella is added for approximately every 0.2-μm increase in axonal diameter. The great concentration of plasma membranes in the myelin sheath accounts for its high concentration of lipids and lipoproteins, which give it a high affinity for certain histological stains (Fig. 8-61) that are normally used for the demonstration of

fats and also accounts for its intense staining in electron-microscopic preparations.

Oligodendrocytes have several processes and, therefore, unlike Schwann cells in the peripheral nervous system (see below), can each form several internodal segments. It has been estimated that in the optic nerve of the rat, a single oligodendrocyte may give rise to as many as 40 or 50 internodal segments. If the portions of an oligodendrocyte that form myelin internodes could be unwrapped, they would appear as extensive flattened sheets roughly trapezoidal in shape. The total extent of the cell is therefore actually much greater than is shown in even the best specimen impregnated with metallic salts, for here the tenuous connections between the parent oligodendrocytic process and the myelin internodal segments are not visualized. Indeed, even in electron micrographs, clear

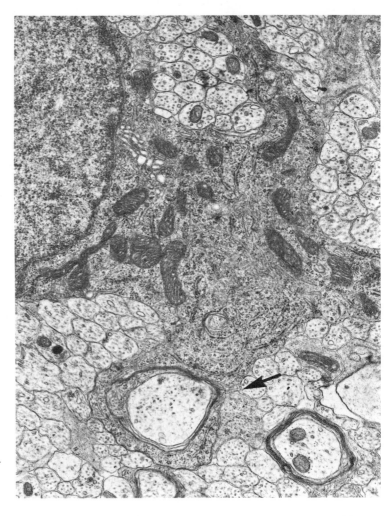

FIGURE 8-58 Electron micrograph of a myelin-forming oligodendrocyte in the developing optic nerve of a rat. ×12,450. (J. E. Vaughn, *Z. Zellforsch. Mikrosk Anat.*, **94:**293, 1969, courtesy of Dr. J. E. Vaughn.)

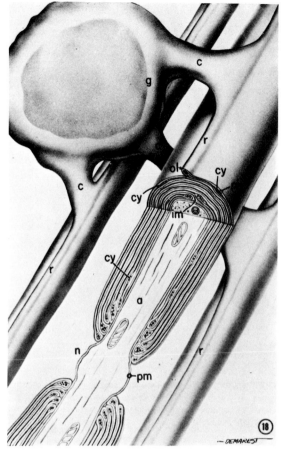

FIGURE 8-59 Schematic drawing of an oligodendrocyte forming internodes on three adjacent axons. r, outer tongue; n, node of Ranvier. (M. B. Bunge, R. P. Bunge, and H. Ris, *J. Biophys. Biochem. Cytol.*, **10:**67, 1961; courtesy of Drs. M. B. Bunge and R. P. Bunge.)

cytic covering and is usually separated from astrocytic processes by the 200 Å wide extracellular cleft seen between all processes in the central nervous system. The remainder of the axon is unchanged at the node, though occasionally a typical axon terminal may bulge from its side; and if a myelinated axon should branch, the branching always occurs at a node (Fig. 8-62). In such cases, three or more internodal segments come together.

As they approach a node, the edges of the spirally wrapped myelin lamellae separate at each major dense line and form a series of tonguelike processes. These, of course, contain oligodendrocytic cytoplasm; and microtubules and other organelles are usually seen in each tongue. The tongues of cytoplasm are best visualized in longitudinal sections where they collectively form the *paranodal region* of the myelinated fiber (Figs. 8-59 and 8-63). In the paranodal region, each tongue is in contact with the axolemma; thus the tongue arising from the most superficial major dense line adjoins the naked part of the axon at the node,

FIGURE 8-60 Electron micrograph of small myelinated axon in central nervous system showing inner and outer tongues of oligodendrocytic cytoplasm and major and minor dense lines of myelin sheath. ×161,000. (A. Hirano and H. M. Dembitzer, *J. Cell Biol.*, **34:**555, 1967. Courtesy of Dr. A. Hirano.)

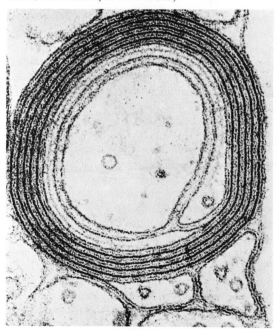

demonstrations of the continuity are limited to occasional fortuitous examples.

The "naked" portions of the axon at the nodes of Ranvier (Fig. 8-63) are highly specialized regions of high capacitance and low electrical resistance, responsible for the self-regenerative capacity of the conducted action potential. During the passage of an action potential, significant changes in membrane conductance occur almost exclusively at the nodes, so that the wave of depolarization leaps from node to node, a form of conduction known as "saltatory." The structure of the axonal membrane is modified at the node by the addition of a dense membrane undercoat similar to that seen at the initial segment. The outer surface of the membrane is free of any oligodendro-

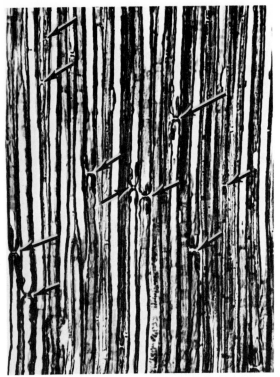

FIGURE 8-61 Osmium-tetroxide-stained longitudinal section of peripheral nerve of cat showing myelin sheaths and nodes of Ranvier (arrows). ×300.

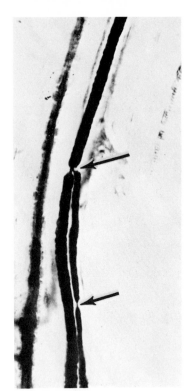

FIGURE 8-62 Gold-chloride-stained, teased preparation of myelinated nerve fiber branching at a node (upper arrow). Thinner branch has shorter internodal distance (to lower arrow). Muscle nerve of a marsupial. ×500.

whereas the tongue arising from the innermost major dense line is the deepest and lies farthest from the node. Because of the spiral nature of the myelin wrapping, the tongues are continuous with one another; and if they could be displayed three-dimensionally, they would appear as a helix spiraling around the paranodal segment of the axon.

The tongues of oligodendrocytic cytoplasm at the paranodal region are much more intimately associated with the axolemma than is the innermost myelin wrapping of the rest of the internodal region. At the paranodal region the gap between the tongues and the axolemma is reduced at intervals to a form of close junction in which the adjoining plasma membranes are separated by a gap no more than 20 to 30 Å wide. Within this gap, a series of regularly spaced, short, dense bands are seen extending from the axolemma to the oligodendrocytic tongues; these dense bands appear to form a continuous spiral around the internodal region with about 3 to 5 bands associated with each tongue. Despite the close proximity of the membranes of the oligodendrocyte tongues and the spiral bands,

there appears to be fairly free diffusion of ions and even larger particles between the axon and the innermost lamella of the myelin sheath, for electron-dense markers such as lanthanum can readily penetrate between them.

When first formed, all nerve fibers are unmyelinated. In the human embryo, myelination commences at about the fourteenth week of intrauterine life and accelerates in the last trimester of pregnancy. But a considerable amount of myelination occurs postnatally; and in some animals, such as the rat, which is born in a relatively immature state, the brain may be largely devoid of myelin at birth. In fiber pathways that normally myelinate after birth, the process of myelination is in general related to the functional maturation of the system of which the pathway forms a part. For example, in the human infant the myelination of the major descending pathways that control voluntary movements commences at birth and essentially all of the fibers have acquired a myelin sheath by the time of walking. Thereafter, no new internodal segments are added, but existing internodes increase in length as the brain and spinal cord grow and the nerve fibers elongate.

OTHER FORMS OF NEUROGLIAL CELL AND NEUROGLIAL CELLS IN PATHOLOGICAL STATES

For many years it has been known that in cases of injury or disease of the central nervous system, glial cells proliferate, become phagocytic, and are capable of forming a scar. The extent to which astrocytes and oligodendrocytes are involved in these three processes is still much debated, and the role of blood-borne and other macrophages is also uncertain. For some time it was believed that a specific class of cells, the so-called microglia, were the major source of phagocytes in the central nervous system. In light microscopic preparations, this cell is usually described as being the smallest of the glial elements, with a deeply staining, angular nucleus. When impregnated with heavy metal salts, it resembles a small oligodendrocyte, but with rather more spikelike projections from its slender processes

(Fig. 8-47). Microglia are said to be present in small numbers in the normal central nervous system. It was felt by the neuropathologist del Rio Hortega that they were mesodermal rather than neurectodermal in origin, and that they invaded the brain and spinal cord with the capillary network during the period of vascularization. In areas of neural damage, or during inflammatory disease processes, the microglial cells were said to proliferate and become actively phagocytic. As they ingest more and more debris, such as degenerating myelin, they enlarge and become globular in shape and filled with large vacuoles, lipid droplets, and other inclusions; They are then termed *compound granular corpuscles,* or *Gitterzellen.*

At the electron-microscopic level, microglia have proven extremely difficult to identify; and many workers, finding that virtually all glial cells can be fairly readily classified as either astrocytes or oligodendrocytes, would prefer to regard the resting microglial cell of conventional light microscopy as simply a variety of

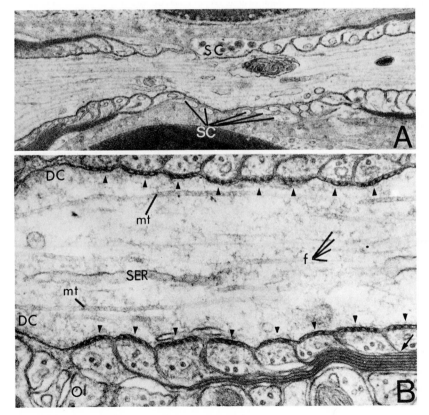

FIGURE 8-63 A. Electron micrograph of node of Ranvier in trigeminal nerve of rat. SC, Schwann cell processes. ×25,000. B, Electron micrograph of paranodal region of myelinated axon in inferior colliculus of cat. Arrowheads indicate dense bars joining tongues of oligodendrocytic cytoplasm to axon. Arrow indicates formation of major dense line. DC, dense undercoating of naked part of axonal membrane; f, neurofilaments; mt, microtubules; Ol, oligodendrocytic processes; SER, smooth endoplasmic reticulum. ×54,000.

oligodendrocyte. If this is the case, unless the vasculature of the nervous system is damaged, all the phagocytes in an area of neuronal death will be derived from astrocytes and oligodendroyctes. If the integrity of the vascular system is damaged, it is clear that extraneous cells may invade the damaged or diseased central nervous system. Many of these are blood-borne phagocytes, but some appear to be vascular pericytes associated with the walls of blood vessels, whereas others may be derived from the pia-arachnoid. In experiments in which the brain was subjected to heavy particle irradiation, it was found that the pericytes (Fig. 8-43) (which are normally surrounded by the basal lamina of the capillaries) can break through the basal lamina, invade the brain, and become phagocytic. The pericytes are thus regarded by some as being the source of microglial cells. Another possible source is the meninges, for the presence of infective agents or other foreign material in the subarachnoid space may cause many of the cells of the pia and arachnoid to detach themselves and to invade the brain, particularly by way of the perivascular spaces.

Several recent studies have led to the suggestion that there may be a third class of glial cell normally resident in the central nervous system that under the appropriate stimulus may proliferate and become the major source of phagocytic cells in pathological states. These cells are said to be more or less intermediate in fine structure between oligodendrocytes and astrocytes. The developing optic nerve is said to contain a considerable proportion of such cells, but their numbers decline as astrocytes and oligodendrocytes become more prominent. It has been claimed that they are a form of glial precursor cell derived from the neurectoderm, or the subventricular zone, which persists in small numbers into adulthood and retains the capacity to produce both oligodendrocytes and astrocytes. In regions of axonal degeneration, these precursor cells may become phagocytic and for this reason are regarded by some researchers as the source of the phagocytic microglia.

THE EPENDYMA AND THE CHOROID PLEXUS

The central canal system of the brain and spinal cord is lined by a layer of closely packed cuboidal or columnar epithelial cells known collectively as the

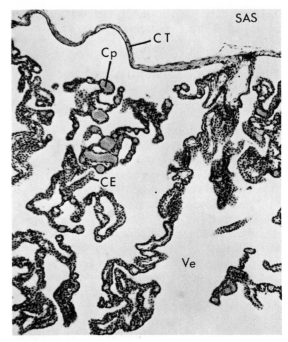

FIGURE 8-64 Choroidal tela (CT) and choroid plexus from fourth ventricle (Ve) of a cat. Cp, capillary; CE, choroidal epithelium; SAS, subarachnoid space. Hematoxylin and eosin stain, ×32.

ependyma (Fig. 8-52). These cells are the remnants of the embryonic neuroepithelium which retain their original position after the neuroblasts and glioblasts have migrated into the mantle layer. The ependymal cells have large numbers of microvilli at their luminal surfaces and commonly one or more cilia, although the distribution of cilia is patchy and large areas of the lining of the central canal system are devoid of cilia. The ependyma is only one cell thick, but its thickness varies because the constituent cells are of variable height in different regions. In parts of the third ventricle overlying the median eminence of the hypothalamus and over certain specializations of the ventricular walls, such as the subcommissural organ or the area postrema, the cells may be very attenuated and even absent. Elsewhere, they are tall and columnar. The apexes of the ependymal cells are bound to their neighbors by the usual junctional complexes, including close junctions and zonulae adhaerens. None of these, however, are occluding junctions (except in the modified ependymal lining of the choroid plexus) and solutes, and even moderately large protein molecules appear to be able to reach the brain parenchyma by passing between the cells; in this way the cerebrospinal fluid of the ventricular system can communicate freely with the intercellular spaces of the central nervous system.

Ependymal cells usually have a pronounced apical accumulation of mitochondria, but in most other respects their fine structure is reminiscent of that of astrocytes. Rough endoplasmic reticulum is not prominent and the cells contain bundles of microfilaments of 60 to 80 Å in diameter. Many ependymal cells have lengthy processes extending from their basal aspects. In the embryo, these commonly reach the surface of the developing brain and spinal cord; but in

the mature human brain, this arrangement is uncommon except in certain sites such as the anterior median fissure of the spinal cord, where the central canal is relatively close to the surface (Fig. 8-52).

In the four ventricles of the brain, the ependyma is modified to form the special secretory epithelium of the *choroid plexuses* (Figs. 8-64 and 8-65). The choroid plexuses are formed at regions where the *roof plate* of the developing neural tube becomes extremely

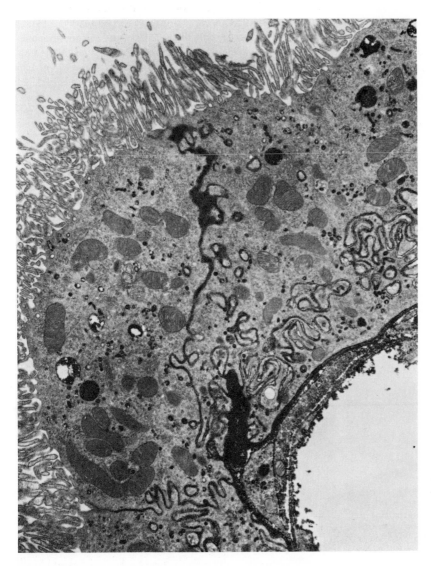

FIGURE 8-65 Electron micrograph showing choroidal epithelium of a mouse in an experiment in which the dense reaction product of the enzyme marker horseradish peroxidase passes freely from choroidal capillaries (lower right) and between choroidal epithelial cells but is prevented from reaching ventricle (top left) by occluding junctions at apexes of epithelial cells. ×13,000. (M. W. Brightman, *Prog. Brain Res.*, **29:**19, 1967; courtesy of Dr. M. W. Brightman.)

attenuated so that the ependyma and the overlying pia mater come into direct contact with one another over an area known as a *choroidal tela.* The portion of the pia mater entering into the formation of the choroidal tela becomes richly vascularized and this highly vascular tissue becomes invaginated into the ventricle as a mass of villouslike processes, collectively known as the choroid plexus. The line of invagination of the choroidal tela is known as the *choroid fissure.*

Electron micrographs of the choroid plexus reveal an essentially trilayered structure. (1) At the ventricular surface there is a row of closely packed, columnar ependymal cells with many microvilli but no cilia. The sides and bases of the cells are thrown into numerous interdigitating cytoplasmic processes, and near the apexes the cells are joined by zonulae adhaerens and true tight junctions (zonulae occludens) that encircle the cells so as to occlude the intercellular cleft. (2) The basal surfaces of these modified ependymal cells rest on a basal lamina continuous with that covering the

rest of the brain. (3) Deep to this is a thin connective tissue space containing free-lying pia-arachnoid cells, small irregular bundles of collagen fibers, and many small blood vessels. The endothelial cells lining the choroidal capillaries are highly fenestrated and the constituents of blood plasma, including proteins, can pass freely into the connective tissue spaces. However, these materials are prevented from reaching the ventricles by the apical tight junctions surrounding the epithelial cells. Thus, despite the permeability of the choroidal capillaries to plasma proteins, the cerebrospinal fluid under normal conditions contains little or no protein.

The secretion of cerebrospinal fluid is an active process requiring energy and can be readily inhibited by carbonic anhydrase inhibitors—and by ouabain, which blocks sodium transport. Moreover, it can continue in the face of an adverse pressure gradient, as in the case of an obstruction to its outflow (thus resulting in hydrocephalus).

Cerebrospinal fluid is produced in man at the rate of approximately 0.5 l/day. The fluid flows out into the subarachnoid space through the median and lat-

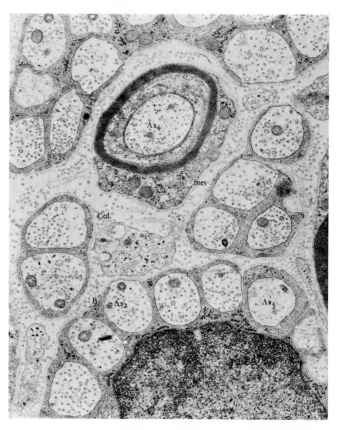

FIGURE 8-66 Electron micrograph of cross section of sciatic nerve of rat showing relation of Schwann cells and their processes to myelinated and unmyelinated axons. ×21,000. (A. Peters, S. L. Palay, and H. de F. Webster, "The Fine Structure of the Nervous System," Harper & Row, Publishers Incorporated, New York, 1970; courtesy of Dr. A. Peters.)

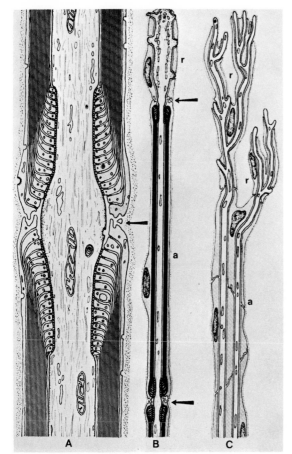

FIGURE 8-67 Schematic drawings of node of Ranvier in periph-eral nervous system (A), terminal portion of a myelinated sensory nerve fiber (B), terminal portion of two unmyelinated sensory nerve fibers (C), showing relation of axon to investing Schwann cells. (K. H. Andres and M. von Düring, Handbook of Sensory Physiology, vol. 2, Springer-Verlag New York Inc., New York, 1973; courtesy of Dr. K. H. Andres.)

eral apertures of the fourth ventricle and is absorbed primarily into the cranial venous sinuses through tufts of pia-arachnoid cells, called *arachnoid villi*, which protrude through the walls of the sinuses into the lumen.

SUPPORTING CELLS IN THE PERIPHERAL NERVOUS SYSTEM

The supporting cells of the peripheral nervous system are comprised of the *Schwann cells* associated with all peripheral nerve fibers and the capsular or satellite cells of the dorsal root and autonomic ganglia. They are all derived from the neural crest. Like their count-erparts in the central nervous system, all the periph-

eral supporting cells are small cells and cytologically they are unexceptional. The outer surface of their plasma membranes are always associated with a basal lamina.

Schwann Cells in Peripheral Nerve Trunks

The Schwann cells of peripheral nerve trunks are sometimes known as neurilemmal or sheath cells, because of the manner in which they enfold the con-stituent axons (Fig. 8-66). Every axon in the peripheral nervous system, from the dorsal and ventral roots to the most distal branches of the sensory or motor fibers, is surrounded over most of its length by a series of Schwann cells, and in the case of axons with a diameter greater than 1 to 2 μm each of these Schwann cells forms a single myelin internodal seg-ment (Fig. 8-67). In two respects the association of Schwann cells with peripheral axons differs from that between the supporting cells of the central nervous system and central axons: (1) unmyelinated axons in the central nervous system lack any form of ensheath-ment; and (2) whereas each Schwann cell forms only a single internodal segment, each oligodendrocyte may form 50 or more internodal segments and be associ-ated with a comparable number of axons.

Peripheral nerves have several coverings, of which the Schwann cell constituent of the axons is the most intimate. Outside this there are three connective tissue coats (Figs. 8-68 to 8-70): An *epineurium* made up of dense fibrous connective tissue encloses the entire nerve as in a sleeve. This covering is sufficiently thick to be sutured in operations involving nerve re-pair. Within the epineurium the axons of the nerve are formed into longitudinally running bundles, or *fas-ciculi*, of variable size. These fasciculi are also en-closed in a sleeve of moderately dense fibrous con-nective tissue called the *perineurium*. This is not a completely limiting sheath, however, since axons may leave one fasciculus to join another. Within the peri-neurium the axons and their associated Schwann cells are surrounded by a small amount of delicate, loose connective tissue known as the *endoneurium*. Gener-ally, a small number of blood vessels are also present, the so-called *vasa nervorum*, which penetrate the epineurial and perineurial sheaths and break up into a loose capillary plexus in the endoneurium.

Although Schwann cells are found along the length of peripheral nerve fibers, any short segment of the fiber is associated with only a single Schwann cell,

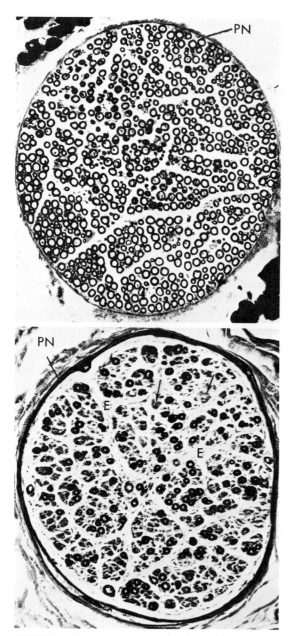

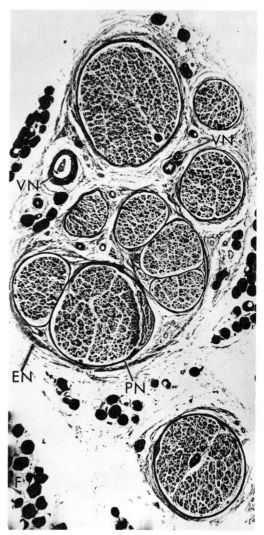

FIGURE 8-70 Cross section of small peripheral nerve consisting of several fascicles surrounded by epineurium (EN) and perineurium (PN). F, fat cells; VN, vasa nervorum. Osmium tetroxide stain, ×50.

FIGURE 8-68 (Upper) Cross section of a spinal ventral root of a cat showing bimodal myelinated fiber spectrum. PN, perineurium. Osmium tetroxide stain, ×125.

FIGURE 8-69 (lower) Cross section of a small cutaneous sensory nerve showing unmyelinated (arrows) as well as large and small myelinated fibers. E, endoneurium. Osmium tetroxide stain, ×166.

although there is some overlap between successive Schwann cells. To a greater or lesser degree, all fibers are invaginated into the Schwann cells. The line of the invagination, which commonly forms a narrow cleft leading from the endoneurium to the enclosed axon, is known as the *mesaxon* (Fig. 8-66) by analogy with the mesenteries of the alimentary canal. Schwann cells associated with unmyelinated fibers may invest as many as 20 such fibers, and surrounding the whole cell and the associated fibers is the basal lamina. Where one Schwann cell comes to an end, it is overlapped by the next cell in the chain of Schwann cells, and there is no gap comparable to the nodes of Ranvier of myelinated fibers. In the case of myelinated fibers, each Schwann cell is associated with only a single fiber.

Although the general form of myelin in the peripheral nervous system is identical to that found in the central nervous system, its mode of formation is rather different. In the peripheral nervous system the axon to be myelinated first becomes invaginated into the Schwann cell. Then one of the lips of cytoplasm adjoining the mesaxon appears to insinuate itself between the adjoining lip and the axon; and by the continued elongation of the lips of the mesaxon, a spiral wrapping made up of many lamellae is formed (Fig. 8-71). By the alternate fusion of the inner leaflets of the plasma membranes (belonging to the same lamella) and of the outer leaflets of the plasma membranes (belonging to adjoining lamellae), the major dense and intraperiod lines are respectively established. The exact manner in which the spiral wrapping occurs is uncertain, but there is some evidence from observations in tissue culture that at least in the initial phase the whole Schwann cell may rotate around the axon.

The innermost major dense line expands to form an inner tongue of Schwann cell cytoplasm, and the cleft formed by the associated separation of the innermost intraperiod line is usually referred to as the *inner mesaxon*. This is originally continuous with the initial line of invagination of the fiber, which constitutes the *outer mesaxon*. At the outer mesaxon, the outermost major dense line splits and becomes continuous with what is usually a substantial amount of Schwann cell cytoplasm—far greater than the small outer tongue of oligodendrocytic cytoplasm seen in the central nervous system. If the myelin sheath is seen in a longitudinal section or in a cross section near the middle of an internode, the nucleus of the Schwann cell will also be present; and, as in the case of unmyelinated fibers, the cell is surrounded by a basal lamina.

Nodes of Ranvier are present in myelinated peripheral nerve fibers, exactly as in the central nervous system (Fig. 8-63). The nodal portion of the axon has a dense membrane undercoat, and the Schwann cells of the two adjoining internodes form comparable tongues of cytoplasm in the paranodal regions. The spiral bands between the tongues and the outer leaflet of the axolemma are usually less distinct than in the central nervous system. However, the major difference between nodal regions in the central and peripheral nervous systems is that at peripheral nodes the nerve fiber is not completely bare; although devoid of a myelin sheath, the nodal segment is covered by large overlapping processes of Schwann cell cytoplasm derived from the cells that give rise to the two adjoining internodes, and the whole region is surrounded by a basal lamina.

Myelin internodes in the peripheral nervous system often show a series of small clefts or splittings running obliquely for some distance across the thickness of the myelin sheath. These are known as *Schmidt-Lanterman incisures*, or *clefts*, and they represent regions in which the major dense lines are separated over a short distance so that a small amount of Schwann cell cytoplasm is inserted into the myelin wrapping. Where the cleavage affects all lamellae, the cleft will form a helical wrapping around the sheath but commonly only a few adjacent major dense lines are affected.

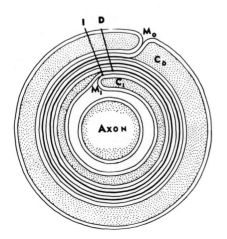

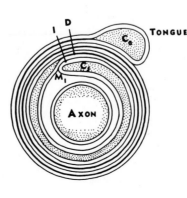

FIGURE 8-71 Schematic figure showing mode of formation of myelin in peripheral nervous system (left) and central nervous system (right). Ci, Co., inner and outer cytoplasmic leaflets; D, major dense line; I, intraperiod line; Mi, Mo, inner and outer mesaxon. (A. Peters, *J. Biophys. Biochem. Cytol.*, **7**:121, 1960; courtesy of Dr. A. Peters.)

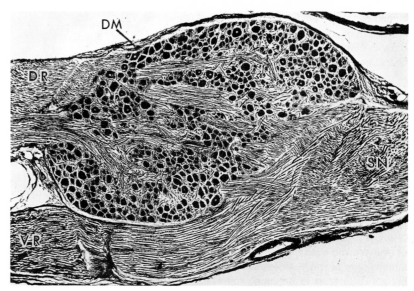

FIGURE 8-72 (Upper) Bodian-stained preparation of dorsal root ganglion of a cat showing covering of dura mater (DM), ventral root (VR), dorsal root (DR), and spinal nerve (SN). ×87.

FIGURE 8-73 (Lower left) Thionin-stained section showing dorsal root ganglion cells of varying size and enveloping Schwann (capsular) cells (Sc). ×480.

FIGURE 8-74 (Lower right) Higher-powered view of a part of Fig. 8-72, showing (arrows) coiled initial axon segments of ganglion cells. ×480.

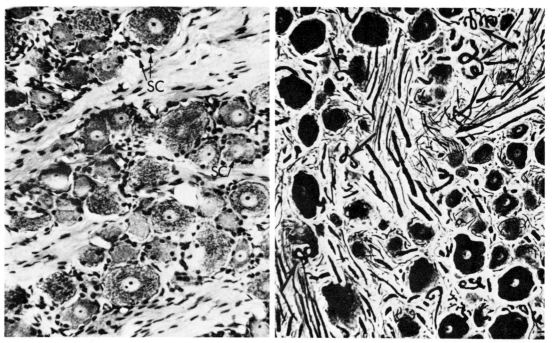

Supporting Cells in the Peripheral Ganglia

Supporting cells are found in large numbers in both dorsal root ganglia and in autonomic ganglia. In the dorsal root ganglia (Fig. 8-72) and in the sensory ganglia of certain of the cranial nerves, they tend to surround the pseudounipolar neurons and are, therefore, often referred to as *capsular* or *satellite cells* (Fig. 8-73). In autonomic ganglia, the investment of individual neurons is rarely so complete (Fig. 8-75), and most neurons are associated with a relatively small number of supporting cells.

The capsular cells are distinguished by their small size relative to the neurons and, in light micrographs, by their relative lack of cytoplasm. In electron micrographs they usually appear to be embedded in depressions in the ganglion cell cytoplasm, and the neurons may invaginate fingerlike extensions into the capsular cell. The cytoplasmic processes of adjacent capsular cells overlap to a variable extent, and the thickness of the capsular layer is usually proportional to the size of the ganglion cell. Since the cells are in most respects comparable to Schwann cells, it is not surprising that the entire "capsule" is invested by a basal lamina. No synapses are present in dorsal root ganglia, but in autonomic ganglia the capsule is deficient at several points for the passage of the terminal portion of the preganglionic axons which form synapses upon the cells. In some cases, capsular cells form myelin around the enclosed neurons. In mammals, this unusual situation is mainly confined to the ganglia of the vestibulocochlear nerve in which the somata of the bipolar cells commonly have a thin covering of loose myelin.

The capsular cells continue without interruption onto the initial segment of the axon, and portions of the same capsular cell may line both the perikaryon and the axon. In many animals, and particularly in man, the initial stem processes of the dorsal root ganglion cells, prior to their bifurcation into central and peripheral branches, are highly coiled, forming what is usually referred to as a *glomerular segment* (Fig. 8-74). The enveloping cells follow the contours of this convoluted structure and normally give rise to one or more myelin internodes just prior to the point of branching. The branching occurs, as always, at a node.

The Schwann cells continue along the central processes of the sensory ganglion cells to the spinal cord or brainstem. The point at which these cells disappear and the oligodendrocytes assume the responsibility for forming the myelin sheath of the cen-

tral process has not been studied intensively. The changeover appears to occur not at a sharp boundary line but over a long region of transition.

Schwann Cells in Degeneration and Repair of Peripheral Nerves

Degeneration of a peripheral nerve, secondary to a transection or some injury at a more proximal level, is always accompanied by reactive changes in the Schwann cells. The axons that are severed from their trophic center, the cell body, degenerate distal to a transection. This degenerative process is commonly known as Wallerian degeneration after the neurologist A. V. Waller, who first described it in 1850. It includes

FIGURE 8-75 Longitudinal section of otic ganglion of a dog showing neurons and intervening small nuclei of satellite Schwann cells. C, capsule. Hematoxylin and eosin stain, ×250.

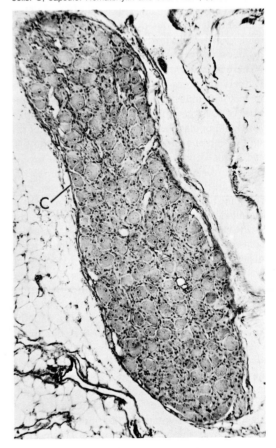

the whole distal portion of an axon and its terminal ramifications. Though the very earliest stages may be seen close to the severed end, the changes affect the whole distal portion more or less simultaneously. The earliest changes in the axon occur at the nodes of Ranvier and consist of swelling of the axon and disruption of mitochondria. Within a few hours the paranodal portions of the myelin sheath start to fragment and clefts resembling Schmidt-Lantermann incisures appear in large numbers in the internodes. This is followed by fragmentation of the whole myelin sheath, which appears in histologic preparations stained with normal myelin stains, such as osmium tetroxide, as a chain of ovoid or vesicular masses. These masses become denser and further fragmented and they and the fragments of degenerating axoplasm are phagocytosed by the Schwann cells and by macrophages that invade the degenerating section of the nerve from the bloodstream. These cells become filled with large heterogeneous dense bodies and vacuoles containing especially lipids derived from the further degradation of the myelin fragments.

There is hypertrophy of individual Schwann cells and a marked increase in their numbers. The proliferation may continue for as long as 3 weeks and the number of cells may increase to more than 10 times the original population. Clearly, large portions of the plasma membrane of the Schwann cell become disrupted in the course of fragmentation of the myelin sheath, but few actually appear to die. The proliferating Schwann cells seem to free themselves from their surrounding basal laminae, which remain as a series of longitudinally oriented tubes. Along these, the Schwann cells form a complexly interdigitated mass of cytoplasmic processes that together with the tubes of basal lamina material appear to guide the regenerating axonal sprouts proliferating into the degenerated distal segment from the proximal stump toward their target (Fig. 8-76). The extracellular compartments formed by the interdigitating Schwann cell processes and the basal laminae are often referred to as *Schwann tubes*.

As regeneration of the axons proceeds, the Schwann cells begin to become more orderly in their arrangement and gradually form linear arrays on the basis of the persisting tubes of basal laminae. Within these, the new axons become invaginated and thence remyelinated. The new myelin internodes are generally shorter and thinner than those in the normal nerve. The shortness is perhaps to be expected, in

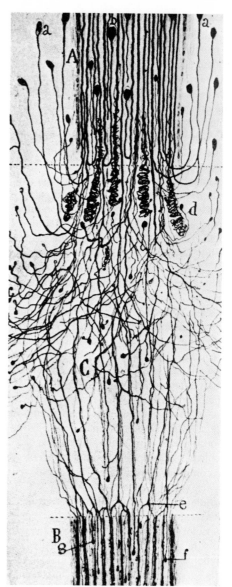

FIGURE 8-76 Some of the earliest degenerative and regenerative changes seen at the site of interruption of a nerve bundle. The proximal stump (A) shown in the upper part of the figure shows numerous retraction bulbs, convoluted spiral structures and newly formed axon sprouts, some of which have grown toward the Schwann tubes of the distal stump (B). (S. Ramón y Cajal, "Degeneration and Regeneration of the Nervous System," Hafner Publishing Company, Inc., New York, 1968.)

view of the marked proliferation of Schwann cells. It is uncertain, however, whether each of the newly produced Schwann cells forms an internode or becomes associated with a bundle of unmyelinated fibers or whether many die.

THE PERIPHERAL TERMINATIONS OF NERVE FIBERS

In the peripheral nervous system, the processes of the parent neurons either synapse with other nerve cells, as in the case of autonomic preganglionic neurons, or enter into a functional relationship with the cellular components of other tissues, as in the case of the dorsal root ganglion cells, or the motoneurons of the spinal cord and the autonomic postganglionic neurons. The structure of autonomic ganglia will be dealt with in another section. Here we will be concerned primarily with the peripheral terminations of dorsal root ganglion cells, of spinal motoneurons, and of autonomic postganglionic neurons.

The peripheral processes of dorsal root ganglion cells and of the cells in the comparable cranial ganglia terminate in association with connective tissues, epithelial tissues, or muscular tissues that in many cases facilitate the sensory transduction process leading to the discharge of action potentials in the nerve fiber and their propagation toward the central nervous system. The pseudounipolar ganglion cells are, therefore, *receptor* neurons and their peripheral terminals are specialized sensory receptors. Motoneurons in the spinal cord and brainstem and the autonomic postganglionic neurons are *effector* neurons and their axons terminate respectively upon skeletal muscle cells and in relation to smooth muscle or gland cells. In these cases, the peripheral terminal is an effector, or "motor," ending, comparable in its general structure and function to a central synapse, although the effect upon the target organ is, of course, to induce muscular contraction or glandular secretion.

THE STRUCTURE AND FUNCTION OF PERIPHERAL SENSORY RECEPTORS

The peripheral sensory receptors are concerned with the transduction of various forms of energy into neural activity which, if of sufficient intensity, results in the discharge of nerve impulses whose frequency and pattern constitute the neural code that is interpreted centrally as a sensory experience. Before describing individual receptors three general points should be made. (1) For the most part, the type or *modality* of sensation mediated by a particular axon is distinctive for each axon and its specification resides within the axon itself. As a rule, each axon is concerned with only one sensory modality. (2) The sensory transduction process occurs within the axon itself rather than in the specialized end formations which may be associated with it. (3) Not all activity in sensory receptors is consciously perceived; much of it is concerned with various reflexes and other adjustments to changes in the external or internal environment, of which the subject is often wholly unconscious. The use of the term *sensory* is synonymous with *afferent* and does not necessarily imply conscious *sensation.*

Sensory receptors are classified in several ways. Among the oldest is that of Sherrington, who spoke of (1) *exteroceptors,* specialized for the reception of stimuli on or beyond the surface of the body; (2) *interoceptors,* concerned with the reception of stimuli arising within the body itself; and (3) *proprioceptors,* which are a special group of interoceptors specialized for the reception of information about the position of the body, or its parts, in space; this group includes the receptors in the vestibular apparatus and those in muscles and joints. More recent physiological classifications tend to specify the nature of the stimulus that the receptors are equipped to deal with. Hence we may speak of *mechanoreceptors, thermoreceptors, nociceptors* (for pain), *chemoreceptors, photoreceptors* (in the retina), and so on.

A useful anatomical classification rests upon the fact that in most parts of the body, the terminal portions of the peripheral processes of cranial or spinal ganglion cells fall into the following three groups. (1) *Free nerve endings,* which in this case, are the terminal branches of the processes that lose all their coverings (including their Schwann cell investment) and end without specialization among the epithelial, connective tissue, or other cells of the innervated region (Fig. 8-67). (2) *Expanded tip endings,* which are found more especially in the skin. Here the terminal branches end in a series of bulbous expansions that make contact with the bases of domelike aggregations of specialized epithelial cells. (3) *Encapsulated endings,* in which the terminal axon ends inside a distinct connective tissue capsule in relation to either groups of connective tissue or muscle cells; such endings are apparently specialized for determining the direction or type of displacing force that acts upon the contained sensory nerve terminal. We shall follow this classification but will describe, for convenience, the sensory nerve terminals in relation to three main groups of tissues: skin and subcutaneous tissue, muscle and joints, and blood vessels and viscera.

SENSORY RECEPTORS IN THE SKIN AND SUBCUTANEOUS TISSUES

As the peripheral branches of a cutaneous nerve penetrate the subcutaneous tissues and approach the skin, they form an intricate plexus of interconnected bundles at the junction of the subcutaneous tissue with the dermis (Fig. 8-77). Several branches of a single nerve, and branches of different nerves, usually contribute to this *subcutaneous plexus*. From the subcutaneous plexus, branches pass to deep receptors, and many fine bundles of axons ascend to form a second *dermal plexus* beneath the epidermal ridges. From this plexus, terminal branches pass into the dermal papillae and into the epidermis. Unless otherwise specified, what follows refers to both hairy and nonhairy (glabrous) skin, but it should be noted that in addition to the sensory fibers, each plexus also contains sympathetic postganglionic fibers that supply the blood vessels, sweat glands, and arrector pili muscles of the skin.

Free Nerve Terminals

Free nerve terminals form the majority of the sensory receptors in the skin. All are derived from unmyelinated axons of small diameter (approximately 1 μm or

FIGURE 8-77 Schematic drawing showing innervation pattern of hairy skin. A. intraepithelial endings. B. Meissner corpuscles. C. Krause's end bulbs. D. Ruffini endings. E. endings associated with hairs. F. free endings. P, Pacinian corpuscle. (W. E. LeGros Clark, ''The Tissues of the Body,'' Oxford University Press, Fair Lawn, N.J., 1965.)

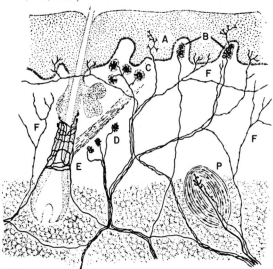

less) and a single fiber often branches profusely over a wide area. On approaching the deepest layer of the epidermis, the basal laminae of the Schwann cells fuse with that beneath the epidermis and the naked nerve fibers pass into the epidermis within deep invaginations of the epidermal cells. In this way they may penetrate the epidermis almost as far superficially as the stratum corneum. They display no obvious structural specialization, but there is evidence that different fibers are functionally specialized to respond to painful stimuli, to warmth or cold, and to mechanical displacement of the skin. Such receptors are connected to unmyelinated (Fig. 8-67) or finely myelinated axons in the peripheral nerve trunks.

Sensory Nerve Endings in Relation to Hairs

Hairs are associated with such a rich innervation that they should probably be considered as one of the more elaborate forms of sensory receptor. It has been estimated that at least 80 percent of the finely myelinated fibers in a cutaneous nerve may terminate in relation to hairs. It has also become clear that different categories of hair may be identified and that each type is associated with sensory nerve fibers that signal different types of information to the central nervous system. In what follows, we shall be concerned only with the generalities of this system and will not deal to any extent with the details of the different types.

Every hair follicle receives several fine unmyelinated axons, most of which are ultimately derived from thinly myelinated axons 1 to 5 μm in diameter in the peripheral nerve trunk. Others appear to be branches of thicker myelinated fibers with diameters up to 12 μm. A single parent fiber may branch many times and innervate several hundred follicles, so the *peripheral receptive field* from which the parent nerve fiber or its dorsal root ganglion cell can be activated may be very large. The various fibers innervating a single hair follicle form an encircling meshwork containing both longitudinally and circumferentially running branches. The complexity of the meshwork depends on the size and type of hair, but in every case it surrounds the greater part of the hair follicle as it traverses the dermis. Most of the terminal portions of the axons are enclosed in Schwann cells, but the ultimate portion is naked and embedded in the glassy membrane that forms the outermost covering of the follicle. The component nerve endings are thus in a position to be activated when the hair is deflected, and it has been shown that the majority of the nerve fibers distributed to hair follicles are activated only during movements of the hairs in one direction.

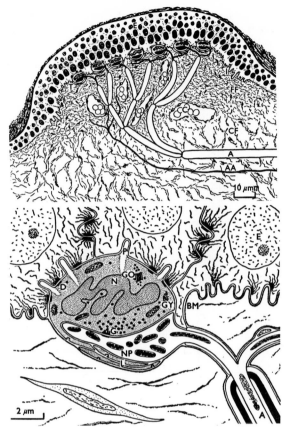

FIGURES 8-78 and 8-79 Schematic drawings of Merkel-type touch corpuscles from footpad of a cat. Merkel cell (indicated by shading in lower figure) contains granular vesicles (G) and is contacted by platelike axon terminal (NP). (A. Iggo and A. R. Muir, *J. Physiol.* (*Lond.*) **200**:763, 1969; courtesy of Professor A. Iggo.)

Nerve Terminals with Expanded Tips

Two kinds of sensory receptor with expanded nerve terminals are found in glabrous and hairy skin. The most distinctive of these in humans is the *Merkel's touch corpuscle* (Figs. 8-78 and 8-79). As a cutaneous nerve approaches one of these epithelial specializations, it gives rise to a number of unmyelinated branches that lose their Schwann cell covering and penetrate the basal lamina of the epidermis. Each terminal expands there to form a flattened disc or plate that is closely applied to a Merkel cell. The Merkel cell is a modified epidermal cell attached to the neighboring cells by desmosomes and having many flattened cytoplasmic protrusions which enclose the terminal discs of the nerve fiber. Where it is in close contact with the nerve ending, the Merkel cell contains many large, dense-core vesicles approximately

1000 Å in diameter. The nerve terminal itself does not contain vesicles. The myelinated nerves whose terminals end in Merkel's corpuscles are of large diameter (7 to 12 µm) and are usually excited by pressure applied directly to the touch corpuscles.

A simpler form of epithelial cell–nerve terminal complex, in which expanded terminals of an axon end in relation to normal basal epidermal cells, has been identified as a cold receptor. In these cases, the parent axons are myelinated and are about 1 to 6 µm in diameter; they are specifically activated by localized cooling of the epidermis over their terminals. No specialized receptors have yet been identified for the reception of warm stimuli.

Encapsulated Nerve Terminals

Although numerically in the minority, encapsulated receptors have tended to dominate descriptions of the innervation of the skin and subcutaneous tissues because of their large size and distinctive apperance. Three main types are usually recognized: *Pacinian corpuscles, Ruffini endings,* and *Meissner's corpuscles.* Others that are less distinct and not recognized by all authorities are *Krause's end bulbs* and *Golgi-Mazzoni corpuscles.* All these encapsulated endings are distinguished by the presence of a lamellated connective tissue sheath surrounding the nerve terminals. The form of the connective tissue ensheathment and of the nerve terminal is extremely variable but sufficiently characteristic for each type of receptor to be readily recognized. Each is innervated by a single myelinated axon, 6 to 12 µm in diameter, which is usually derived from a parent trunk that supplies many lamellated endings of the same type.

The Pacinian Corpuscle

This is one of the largest sensory receptors, often reaching a length of 1 mm. They are found in subcutaneous tissues deep to both hairy and glabrous skin and are especially numerous just beneath the dermis of the digits; they are also present in large numbers in the deep musculoskeletal tissues, especially in the periosteum and in the mesenteries of the peritoneal cavity. The capsule is ellipsoidal and made up of 30 or more concentric rings of flattened fibroblastlike cells that are continuous with the endoneurial sheath of the nerve terminating in the capsule (Fig. 8-80). The outer lamellae are essentially spherical, but the inner few layers are more or less semicircular in cross

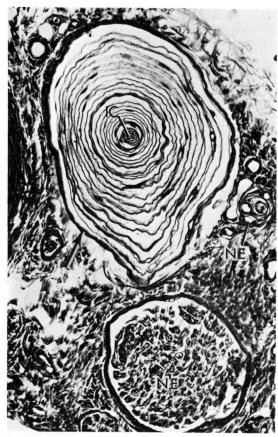

FIGURE 8-80 A hematoxylin-and-eosin-stained preparation of a Pacinian corpuscle showing its numerous concentric lamellae and inner core (IC) that contains the terminal part of the innervating axon, which is usually derived from a nearby nerve bundle (Ne). Arrow indicates capsule of Pacinian corpuscle. ×200.

FIGURE 8-81 This photomicrograph shows a myelinated nerve fiber (Ax) leaving a nerve bundle (Ne) to innervate a Pacinian corpuscle. The inner core of the corpuscle (IC) is clearly shown as are the naked terminal expansions of the nerve fiber (T). The outer capsular lamellae (OC) are lightly stained. Gold chloride stain. ×1000.

section. Each is formed by the overlapping processes of several cells and is separated from its neighbor by a fluid-filled space. The nerve fiber enters one pole of the capsule and its last one or two myelin internodes are usually contained within the capsule. However, the greater part of the axon within the sheath is unmyelinated. This part is straight and terminates near the

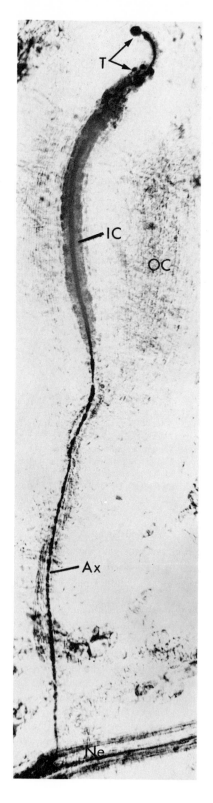

other pole of the corpuscle as a small spray of knob-like branches (Fig. 8-81). Like all other sensory nerve terminals, the axon endings display no unique structure at the electron-microscope level. The unmyelinated part of the axon is surrounded by multiple lamellae of flattened Schwann cells that are closely packed and form an *inner core* within the encircling fibrous connective tissue lamellae (the *outer core*). Pacinian corpuscles are exquisitely sensitive to mechanical displacement, but the enclosed nerve fiber is extremely rapidly adapting, so that the corpuscle can respond to vibratory stimuli up to about 400 per second. The capsule is not essential for the responsiveness of the terminal (since all the outer core and much of the inner can be removed without affecting the response of the nerve terminal to directly applied mechanical stimuli). However, it seems to serve as a mechanical filter, and its elastic components ensure that the nerve responds both when the stimulus is applied and when it is removed.

Meissner's Corpuscles

These are found in the dermal papillae of glabrous skin (Fig. 8-82). They are particularly common near the tips of the fingers and toes. The corpuscle is smaller (approximately 150 μm long) and more cylindrical than the Pacinian corpuscle. The flattened cells form the greater part of its mass and are arranged in multiple-stacked lamellae within a thin, fibrous connective tissue outer coat. The majority of the lamellar cells appear to be modified Schwann cells, and the unmyelinated terminal part of the axon appears to thread its way zigzag fashion among the lamellae to the superficial pole of the corpuscle. Commonly, more than one axon may enter a single Meissner's corpuscle, but it is not clear whether these are branches of the same or of different parent axons. Meissner's corpuscles appear to be sensitive tactile receptors usually activated by moving the epidermal ridges of the glabrous skin over a surface. Although they too are rapidly adapting, they seem to respond best to low-frequency stimuli (approximately 30 to 40 per second).

Ruffini Endings

Although once considered artifacts of metallic impregnation, these endings are now regarded as one of the commonest forms of slowly adapting mechanoreceptor (Fig. 8-83). They are elongated fusiform structures, up to 1 to 2 mm in length, and are found in the dermis of both hairy and glabrous skin, in subcutaneous tissues

and in joint capsules. They are the least highly lamellated of the encapsulated receptors and consist of a thin connective tissue capsule enclosing a fluid-filled space transversed by bundles of collagen fibers that often pass through the capsule and are joined to other collagen fibers in the dermis and adjacent tissues. A single myelinated axon, 5 to 12 μm in diameter, enters

FIGURE 8-82 Schematic drawing of a Meissner corpuscle showing linkage by tonofibrils to overlying epidermis. Ax, axons; pn, perineurial sheath; ra, receptor part of axons; SC, Schwann cells. (K. H. Andres and M. von Düring, Handbook of Sensory Physiology, Vol. 2, Springer-Verlag New York Inc., New York, 1973; courtesy of Dr. K. H. Andres.)

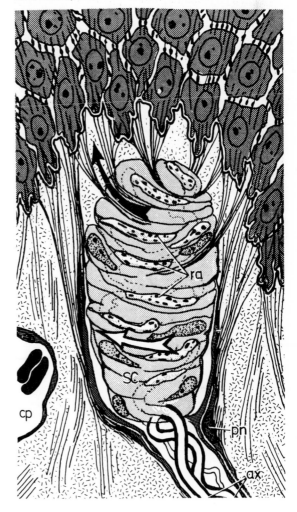

the capsular space, loses its myelin sheath, and breaks up into a large number of unmyelinated branches that intertwine with the collagen bundles. The receptors are activated by displacement of the surrounding connective tissues and they usually respond with a regular, sustained discharge to a maintained stimulus.

SENSORY RECEPTORS IN MUSCLES AND JOINTS

Sensory Receptors in Muscle

Skeletal muscles contain some of the most highly organized encapsulated sensory receptors, together with many free nerve endings (Fig. 8-84). The encapsulated endings are the *muscle spindles* and the *Golgi tendon organs*, both of which are to be considered *proprioceptors*.

Muscle Spindles

Muscle spindles are found in all human striated muscles but are occasionally absent from some muscles, such as the tongue, in other animals. Their numbers vary from muscle to muscle: in general, muscles that are capable of delicate movements and are subject to the highest degree of central nervous control contain the highest numbers of muscle spindles. For example, the eye muscles, the intrinsic muscles of the hand, and the neck muscles at the base of the skull that are responsible for the delicate postural adjustments of the

FIGURE 8-83 Camera lucida drawing of a gold-chloride-impregnated Ruffini ending in knee-joint capsule of a cat (S. Skoglund, *Acta Physiol. Scand.*, **36** (Suppl) **124:**1, 1956.)

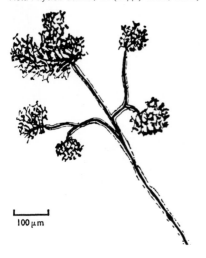

100 μm

head upon the spinal column contain a greater relative number of spindles than do such large muscles as the gluteus maximus and latissimus dorsi.

Each muscle spindle consists of an ovoid connective tissue capsule, about 1.5 mm long and 0.5 mm wide, enclosing a fluid-filled space (Figs. 8-85 and 8-86). This space is traversed from pole to pole by a bundle of special striated muscle fibers which are associated with specialized sensory and motor nerves. The capsule is composed of several circumferential lamellae of flattened fibroblasts (Fig. 8-86), joined to one another at intervals by desmosomes. At the poles of the spindle the lamellae are closely applied to the contained muscle fibers, but elsewhere they enclose a dilated *capsular space* containing tissue fluid, a little delicate endomysial connective tissue, and the neuromuscular apparatus of the spindle. The muscle fibers within the spindle are termed *intrafusal fibers* to distinguish them from the main contractile elements of the muscle, which are termed *extrafusal fibers*. The intrafusal fibers are much smaller, both in diameter and length, than extrafusal fibers, but their orientation is the same, so that the muscle spindles are said to be *in parallel* with the extrafusal fibers.

Each small bundle of intrafusal fibers contains from two or three up to twenty or more intrafusal fibers. In humans, and most mammals, they are of two types—a longer, somewhat thicker form which extends well beyond the poles of the spindle capsule, its ends being inserted into endo- or perimysial connective tissue; and a shorter, thinner form whose ends do not extend much beyond the poles of the capsule. Every spindle contains one or two of the thicker type and many more of the smaller type. Both types are striated over much of their length and have dark-staining, peripherally placed nuclei. As they approach the widest point of the capsular space (the "equator" of the spindle) they usually lose their striations. In the larger form of intrafusal fiber, there is a large central aggregation of nuclei in the equatorial region, and for this reason these fibers are known as *nuclear bag* fibers (Fig. 8-86). On each side of this central aggregation, the nuclei form a single row (the "myotube" region); and beyond this, they are progressively replaced by myofibrils and peripheral nuclei. Some nuclear bag fibers may enter a second spindle capsule at some distance from the first and give rise to a nuclear bag in the second as well. This arrangement constitutes a *tandem spindle*.

The smaller, shorter, and more numerous form of intrafusal fiber has only a single row of vesicular nuclei in its central nonstriated portion. It is thus known as a *nuclear chain fiber* (Fig. 8-86). Nuclear chain fibers have been found to be more rapidly contracting than nuclear bag fibers and they usually have a less-regular pattern of myofilaments with much intervening sarcoplasm and well-developed M lines. The nuclear bag fibers, on the other hand, have a more orderly array of myofilaments, less intervening sarcoplasm, and no M lines. Nuclear bag fibers seem to contract in a tonic fashion, and their activation is not associated with a propagated action potential. They therefore resemble the "slow" muscles of lower vertebrates. The contraction of nuclear chain fibers, on the other hand, is more twitchlike and is associated with propagated action

potentials. It is important to emphasize that because of the lack of myofilaments in the equatorial regions, the central parts of the intrafusal fibers are essentially noncontractile.

The sensory nerves to a muscle spindle enter through the capsule and terminate near the equatorial region of the intrafusal muscle fibers (Figs. 8-85 and 8-87). Every spindle receives a single, large, myelinated afferent fiber some 12 to 20 μm in diameter. This loses its myelin sheath close to the intrafusal

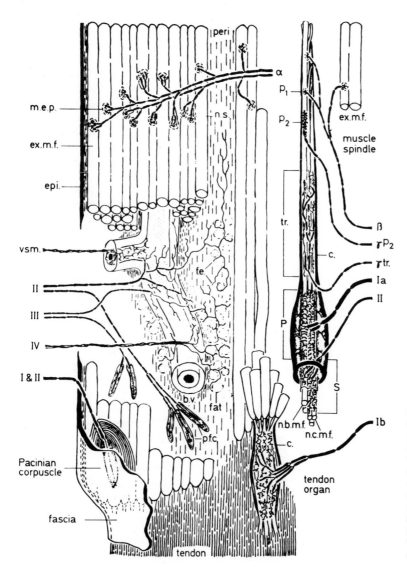

FIGURE 8-84 Schematic drawing showing pattern of innervation of skeletal muscle. Nerve fiber groupings indicated to left and right innervate structures shown. bv, blood vessel; fe, free endings; pc, Pacinian corpuscle; pfc, "Paciniform" corpuscles; vsm, vasomotor (sympathetic) endings. (D. Barker, "Handbook of Sensory Physiology," vol. III/2, Springer-Verlag, New York Inc., New York, 1974; courtesy of Professor D. Barker.)

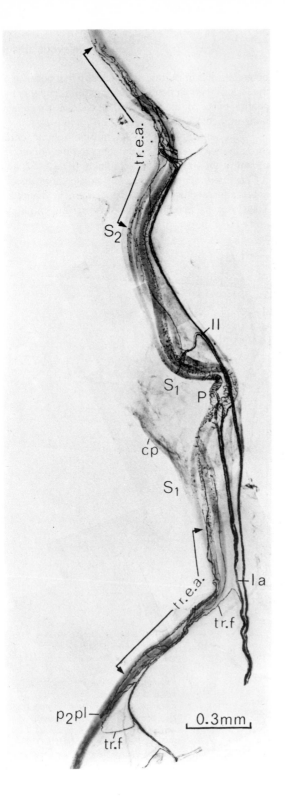

FIGURE 8-85 Silver-stained, teased, whole preparation of a muscle spindle from muscle of a cat. cp, capsule; P, primary ending; P₂pl, plate ending; S₁, S₂, secondary endings; Tr.e.a,tr.f., trail endings and trail fiber. (D. Barker, M. J. Stacey, and M. N. Adal, *Philos. Trans. R. Soc., Lond.* [*Biol. Sci.*], **258:**315, 1970; courtesy of Professor D. Barker.)

bundle and gives rise to several branches that end in a series of ribbonlike spirals which partially or completely encircle the central portion of each nuclear bag and nuclear chain fiber (Fig. 8-87). Electron microscopy shows that the terminal spirals and rings may be deeply invaginated into folds in the sarcolemma of the intrafusal fibers without any intervening basal lamina. The whole terminal complex is known as the *primary sensory ending* of the spindle and its parent fiber (which may supply primary endings to more than one spindle capsule) is usually referred to as a *group Ia afferent fiber*.

Many spindles, though not all, also receive one or more smaller (group II) afferent fibers, some 6 to 8 μm in diameter. These also lose their myelin sheath as they branch within the spindle capsule and form terminal spirals, rings, and sprays similar to those of the primary ending but predominantly on the nuclear chain fibers. This constitutes the *secondary sensory*

FIGURE 8-86 A muscle spindle in cross section showing the appearance of the connective tissue capsule (C), the capsular space (CS), two large nuclear bag intrafusal fibers (NB), and several smaller nuclear chain fibers (NC). The spindle as a whole is in parallel with the extrafusal muscle fibers (MF). Van Gieson stain, ×336.

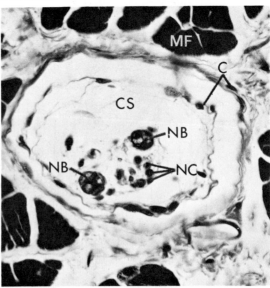

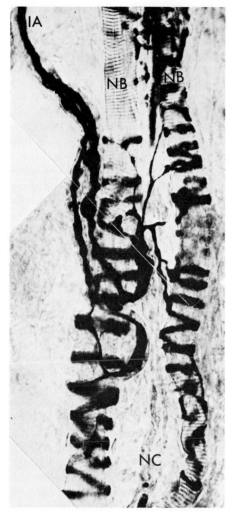

FIGURE 8-87 Group IA fiber terminating as spiral primary endings on two nuclear bag fibers (NB) in muscle spindle of a marsupial. Nuclear chain fibers (NC) do not appear to receive a primary ending in this methylene-blue-stained, teased preparation. ×400. (E. G. Jones, *J. Anat.* (Lond.), **100:**733, 1966.)

ending of the spindle. Both the primary and secondary endings of a spindle are activated by any stretching force acting on the muscle as a whole, which would tend to lengthen the intrafusal bundle. The primary ending responds most vigorously during the dynamic phase of the stretch, whereas the secondary endings are more responsive to maintained stretch. That is, the primary endings exhibit *dynamic sensitivity,* the secondary endings, *static sensitivity.*

The spindles are also innervated by a number of small motor nerve fibers which end on the striated portions of the intrafusal fibers near both poles of the capsule (Fig. 8-85). The parent nerve fibers are small, myelinated axons 2 to 8 μm in diameter that arise from a specific group of small motoneurons in the ventral horn of the spinal cord. These only innervate intrafusal muscle fibers and are known as γ *motoneurons,* or *fusimotor neurons;* the axons that provide the motor innervation to the spindle are, thus, termed γ *efferents,* or *fusimotor fibers.* Less commonly, some of the large α motor fibers that supply the extrafusal musculature also provide a branch to one or more intrafusal fibers in a neighboring spindle. Two types of motor nerve terminal are seen on the intrafusal fibers. Some are localized and closely resemble the motor end plates on extrafusal muscle fibers. Others are long, diffuse endings which ramify widely over the surface of the intrafusal fiber and make multiple *en passant* terminal contacts. The "plate" type of ending is found mainly on nuclear bag fibers, and the diffuse "trail" type, mainly on nuclear chain fibers; but both types can at times be found on the same fiber. Activity in the fusimotor fibers causes the intrafusal fibers to contract and thus effectively stretch the nonstriated part of the fiber that carries the sensory endings. This leads to a state of increased sensitivity of the sensory endings so that they discharge more readily and at increased rates, when the muscle in which they lie is stretched.

Golgi Tendon Organs

These receptors, which are found at musculotendinous junctions, consist of a thin, fibroblastic capsule which is filled with a number of large, collagenous fiber bundles continuous with those of the tendon in which the organ lies (Fig. 8-88). The whole complex may be about 1 mm long, and since a variable number (10 to 20) of extrafusal muscle fibers are inserted into the collagenous tendon slips that make up the greater part of the tendon organ, these receptors are said to be *in series* with the extrafusal fibers. This arrangement permits the sensory nerve fibers to be activated during both contraction and stretching of the relevant muscle.

Each tendon organ receives a single, large, myelinated sensory nerve fiber having a diameter of 12 to 15 μm; afferent fibers of this type fall within the group Ib class of muscle afferent (see below). The fiber loses its myelin sheath after entering the capsule of the tendon organ and gives rise to a number of longitudinally running unmyelinated branches which terminate in small sprays of naked terminals wrapped about, and insinuated between, the bundles of collagen fibers.

Sensory Receptors in Joints

The capsules and periarticular tissues of joints are richly endowed with proprioceptors that mediate the

FIGURE 8-88 Gold-chloride-stained, teased preparation of a Golgi tendon organ from myotendinous junction of a marsupial. Group IB fiber branches widely among tendinous slips (TS) attached to several skeletal muscle fibers (MF). ×80.

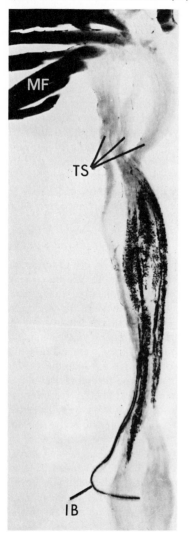

conscious awareness of movement and position (*kinesthesis*). The majority of receptors found in joints have already been described. There are many free nerve endings derived from both unmyelinated and finely myelinated parent fibers, some of which penetrate as far as the synovial membrane. The major type of encapsulated ending found in joint capsules is the Ruffini ending, but some Pacinian corpuscles are also present. In the ligaments associated with the joint capsule, Golgi tendon organs are not uncommon. The function of these different receptors in kinesthesis is not clear. The Ruffini endings seem to discharge in response to movement in one direction, and some show a substantial response when the joint is held in a fixed position. The small Pacinian corpuscles seem to respond only to movements. The role of the free nerve terminals is uncertain, but many are thought to be nociceptive.

SENSORY NERVE ENDINGS IN BLOOD VESSELS AND VISCERA

The walls of the larger blood vessels, and all the thoracic and abdominal viscera, contain a fairly rich complement of mechanoreceptors. In many regions nociceptors are also present and individual organs may have other special kinds of receptors that reflect their particular functions. Collectively, these receptors are termed *interoceptors*.

The majority of the interoceptors are free, or relatively poorly organized, nerve endings that ramify beneath and between epithelial cells and in the submucosal, muscular, and serosal coats of hollow viscera. The parent nerves are usually of small diameter (unmyelinated or thinly myelinated) and are distributed with the autonomic nerves. In some sites such as the mesenteries, encapsulated endings (and especially Pacinian capsules) are also seen.

The best-defined interoceptors are those associated with the aortic arch and with the carotid body and sinus. These monitor circulating-blood gas levels and blood pressure and mediate a variety of cardiovascular and respiratory reflexes. The receptors that are sensitive to changes in oxygen and carbon dioxide tension and blood pH are referred to as *chemoreceptors* and are found in the carotid body and in similar bodies on the arch of the aorta. Those sensitive to changes in blood pressure are referred to as *baroreceptors* and are found in the walls of the carotid sinus and aortic arch. Each has a rather similar structure consisting of glomerular aggregations of large globular cells (which are thought to be the actual receptors) upon which the highly branched afferent nerve fibers terminate. In the case of the chemoreceptors, the large cells are filled with dense-cored vesicles 1000 to 2000 Å in diameter and contain rich stores of catecholamines. Many arteriovenous anastomoses are also present and apparently serve to regulate blood flow through the carotid and aortic bodies. Free nerve endings are also found in the subendocardial layers of the heart, particularly near the valves and in the atrial walls close to the point of entry of the great veins.

In the hollow viscera of the alimentary and genitourinary tracts the free nerve endings appear to be excited mainly by distension of the viscus or by peristaltic or other muscular activity. In certain regions, groups of free receptor terminals in the epithelium are thought to be specifically excited by changes in intraluminal pH, by changes in glucose concentration, or by the presence of certain amino acids.

In the respiratory tract, free nerve endings in, and beneath, the epithelium of the larynx, trachea, and bronchi are sensitive to irritant particles and gases, and when stimulated evoke a coughing reflex. In the lungs themselves, the pulmonary stretch receptors are mainly free nerve endings associated with the smooth muscle of the bronchi. Their afferent fibers are myelinated and are among the fastest conducting interoceptive afferents. Other free endings in the interstitial tissue about the alveoli are thought to be sensitive to changes in the interstitial fluid, particularly those brought about by vascular congestion and irritant vapors.

THE PERIPHERAL TERMINATIONS OF EFFERENT NERVE FIBERS

Motor Nerve Fibers to Skeletal Muscle

Striated muscles are innervated by the axons of motor nerve cells (motoneurons) situated in the ventral horn of the spinal cord or in the motor nuclei of certain of the cranial nerves. Two classes of myelinated fiber are involved: (1) large fibers with diameters of 12 to 20 μm, commonly termed α motor fibers, which innervate the extrafusal muscle fibers; (2) thinner fibers, 2 to 8 μm in diameter, termed γ efferents, or fusimotor fibers, which innervate the intrafusal fibers of the muscle spindles. Since the latter have already been described, the following account will be concerned solely with the α fibers.

The α motor axons, which are among the largest in the peripheral nervous system, seldom branch before entering the muscle they innervate. However, they branch profusely in the muscle so that a single

parent axon may innervate anything from 1 or 2 muscle fibers to 500 or more. On the other hand, each muscle fiber is usually innervated by only one axon. A single motor axon and all the extrafusal fibers it supplies is referred to as a *motor unit.*

As the branches of an axon approach the muscle fibers they are to innervate, they lose their myelin sheaths; and covered only by their Schwann cell investment, they form specialized terminal formations known as *motor end plates* (Figs. 8-42, 8-89, and 8-92). Typically a motor end plate is made up of the dilated terminal portion of an α motor axon and its sheath, a junctional cleft, and a specialized portion of the underlying extrafusal muscle fiber. On the surface of the muscle fiber, the axon forms a number of interconnected terminal bulbs of varying size within a fairly circumscribed, round, or oval zone (Fig. 8-92). In the light microscope this zone appears slightly elevated since the terminal bulbs are overlain by Schwann cells and by the cells of the endoneurium which become continuous with the endomysium. This connective tissue layer, external to the Schwann cells, is referred to as the *sheath of Henle* (Fig. 8-42).

In electron micrographs the terminals resemble synaptic boutons, being filled with large numbers of clear vesicles approximately 400 Å in diameter, and many mitochondria. Fingers of Schwann cell cytoplasm cover the individual terminal bulbs and may penetrate between them and the muscle fiber (Fig. 8-91). The plasma membranes of the axon terminal and the underlying muscle fiber are separated by an extracellular cleft some 500 Å in width, which is filled with the basal lamina of the muscle fiber. The presynaptic membrane shows no distinctive specialization, but over the whole length of its approximation to the sarcolemma, the latter is thrown into a large number of folds which deeply invaginate the underlying sarcoplasm. Like the cleft, these infoldings are filled with basal lamina (Figs. 8-42 and 8-91).

The plasma membrane of the muscle fiber usually has a small amount of dense material attached to it along the crests between each infolding. This region thus resembles the postsynaptic specialization seen at central synapses and is thought to represent the "active site" of the neuromuscular junction. In the portion of the axon terminal immediately opposite each of the junctional folds, there is usually a ridge and a small accumulation of synaptic vesicles (Figs. 8-42, 8-91, and 8-93). During prolonged stimulation of a motor nerve, synaptic vesicles move toward these sites. The sarcoplasm beneath the nerve terminal is often referred to as the *sole plate* and is usually devoid of myofilaments but rich in free ribosomes, rough endoplasmic reticulum, and mitochondria. There is also an accumulation of nuclei in this region which are somewhat larger and more vesicular than other muscle nuclei; these are referred to as *sole plate nuclei*.

Motor end plates vary in structure, depending on the type of muscle in which they lie. In mammals, the motor end plates of *fast twitch muscles* have many long and often branched sarcolemmal infoldings. In *slow twitch muscles* the sarcolemmal infoldings are fewer and shallower; the axon terminals also contain fewer synaptic vesicles than do those ending on fast twitch muscles. True *slow muscles,* which do not show

FIGURE 8-89 (Upper) Gold-chloride-stained, teased preparation showing intramuscular nerve (NE) branching to supply motor end plates (MEP) on skeletal muscle fibers. Human intercostal muscle, ×69.

FIGURE 8-90 (Lower) Silver-stained, teased preparation showing motor axon (Ax) branching to supply diffuse multiterminal endings in slow muscle of a tortoise. Arrows indicate neurofibrillar rings, ×650.

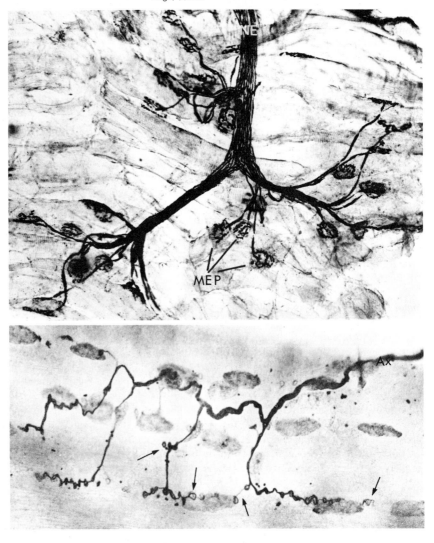

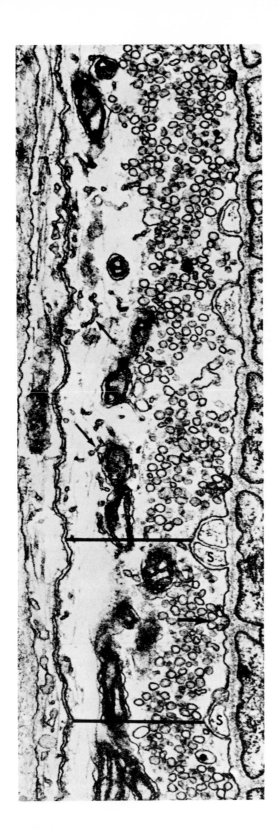

FIGURE 8-91 Electron micrograph of a frog neuromuscular junction. Terminal is separated by basal lamina from junctional folds of muscle fiber (to right). Schwann cell process covers it to far left and some Schwann cell processes (S) intervene between terminal and basal lamina. Small arrows indicate smooth endoplasmic reticulum. Large arrow indicates one of several aggregations of synaptic vesicles about a presynaptic density, site of active synaptic vesicle release. ×40,000. (J. E. Heuser and T. S. Reese, *J. Cell Biol.,* **5:**315, 1973; courtesy of Dr. T. S. Reese.)

propagated action potentials and which are capable of sustained, graded contractions, are not commonly found in mammals. When present (for example, in amphibians) they are characterized by diffuse, multiterminal (or *en grappes*) motor endings: the terminal motor axon spreads diffusely over much of the surface of the muscle fiber and gives off terminal bulbs at intervals (Fig. 8-90). Individual bulbs may be separated from one another by several hundred microns. Each of these bulbs contain synaptic vesicles and makes a contact in every way similar to a motor end plate, but there are no associated sarcolemmal infoldings.

THE PERIPHERAL TERMINATIONS OF AUTONOMIC NERVE FIBERS

The axons of the neurons in sympathetic and parasympathetic ganglia are extremely fine (approximately

FIGURE 8-92 Gold-chloride-stained preparation of two motor end plates from a human intercostal muscle. Dark bulbs are terminal contacts. ×1090.

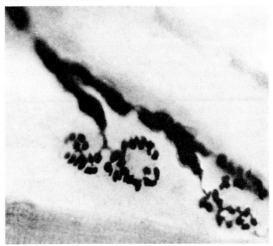

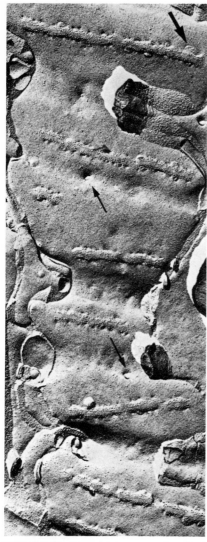

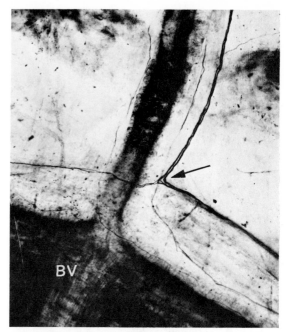

FIGURE 8-94 Silver-stained, teased preparation showing several unmyelinated axons accompanying a large blood vessel (BV). Arrow indicates point of bifurcation of certain fibers. ×490.

FIGURE 8-93 Freeze-fracture preparation showing surface of nerve terminal at a frog neuromuscular junction. Transverse ridges with membrane particles correspond to presynaptic regions indicated by large arrow in Fig. 8-91. Grooves between ridges correspond to regions occupied by Schwann cell processes. Arrows indicate presumed re-formation of synaptic vesicles by endocytosis. ×30,000. (J. E. Heuser, T. S. Reese and D. M. Landis, *J. Neurocytol.,* **3:**109, 1974; courtesy of Dr. T. S. Reese.)

1 μm) and in most cases unmyelinated. The postganglionic fibers of the sympathetic division of the autonomic nervous system are distributed in either peripheral nerves (which they join via the gray rami communicantes), plexuses associated with the larger blood vessels (Fig. 8-94), or the splanchnic nerves. In the autonomic plexuses of the abdominopelvic cavity,

sympathetic preganglionic fibers are distributed with the postganglionic fibers, since not all preganglionic fibers synapse in the sympathetic chain. Parasympathetic preganglionic fibers derived from the vagus are also found in the visceral autonomic plexuses.

Although the sympathetic nervous system is in general a diffusely distributed system, the density and diffuseness of the innervation varies from organ to organ. For example, the postganglionic axons supplying the sphincter pupillae muscle branch little before entering the iris and give rise to a relatively sparse terminal plexus within it, whereas those innervating the gut branch profusely and give rise to a widespread plexus in the gut wall. The terminal ramifications of sympathetic postganglionic fibers in an organ are referred to as the *sympathetic ground plexus*. This consists of a large number of fine, often interconnected, axons which ramify over the surfaces of smooth muscle and gland cells. At regular intervals each terminal branch has a series of bulblike expansions which are regions of transmitter release (Fig. 8-42).

At the electron-microscopic level, these bulblike expansions appear rather like synaptic boutons, since they contain large aggregations of synaptic vesicles and mitochondria. However, they are usually not in intimate contact with the underlying smooth muscle or gland cells and the characteristic pre- or postsynaptic membrane densities seen at central synapses are rarely present. In some organs such as the vas deferens and the sphincter pupillae, the terminal bulbs may approach to within 150 to 200 Å of the smooth muscle fibers and no Schwann cell processes intervene: in these sites it is possible that all or most muscle cells are contacted by at least one terminal bulb. In other sites, such as the gut, most terminal varicosities lie at some distance from the target cells and are thought to exert their effects by releasing their transmitters into the general intercellular space. Since smooth muscle cells are electrotonically coupled by means of gap junctions, the excitation of one cell rapidly spreads from cell to cell throughout the tissue.

The terminals of most sympathetic postganglionic axons release *noradrenaline* (*norepinephrine*), but some release *acetylcholine*. In the case of noradrenergic endings, the majority of the synaptic vesicles present are small (around 500 Å) and contain dense cores (Fig. 8-39). These dense cores are especially obvious if the tissue has been "loaded" with an analog of the transmitter, such as 6-hydroxydopamine, or by fixing it in potassium permanganate. A few larger, dense-core vesicles (approximately 1000 Å) are also found in adrenergic terminals. Both types probably contain noradrenaline and the final enzyme involved in its synthesis, *dopamine-β-hydroxylase.*

Cholinergic nerve terminals in the sympathetic system generally resemble the adrenergic terminals with the notable exception that the vesicles they contain are of the clear variety, comparable to those seen in motor nerve terminals in skeletal muscle. Although much less work has been done on the peripheral terminations of parasympathetic postganglionic fibers, they too appear to be of this type. Parasympathetic preganglionic fibers end in such sites as the sinoatrial and atrioventricular nodes and on the postganglionic neurons by means of clear vesicle containing terminals and with definite (asymmetric) pre- and postsynaptic membrane thickenings.

The walls of the alimentary tract possess extensive plexuses of nerve fibers that are derived partly from pre- and postganglionic sympathetic and parasympathetic fibers and partly from neurons that are intrinsic to the gut wall (see Chap. 18). These plexuses are concerned with maintaining the rhythmic peristaltic activity of the alimentary canal, although the intrinsic neuronal system is itself capable of maintaining this activity when the sympathetic and parasympathetic nerves are destroyed.

The two major plexuses of the gut wall are the

myenteric (or Auerbach's) *plexus,* which lies between the longitudinal and circumferential muscle coats, and the *submucosal* (or Meissner's) *plexus,* which lies in the submucosa. Each of these contains localized aggregations of moderately large, multipolar neurons which resemble those of the sympathetic and parasympathetic ganglia. The adrenergic nerve terminals in these plexuses are thought to be derived from sympathetic neurons situated in the sympathetic chain or in the ganglionated plexuses. These take the form of chains of bulbous terminals containing large numbers of small, dense-cored vesicles. Such terminals form axodendritic and axosomatic synapses upon the intrinsic neurons. Unlike adrenergic terminals elsewhere, definite membrane specializations are present. Other nerve terminals within the plexuses contain small, clear vesicles and also end axosomatically and axodendritically. These are thought to be the terminals of both sympathetic and parasympathetic cholinergic fibers. The intrinsic neurons themselves appear to have short axons that end as varicose, clear vesicle containing terminals among the smooth muscle cells adjacent to the plexus.

A third smaller plexus of fine nerve fibers is found in the gut wall at the level of the muscularis mucosae. This contains relatively few nerve cells and appears to be composed predominantly of sensory fibers whose finer branches ramify beneath the epithelium, sending naked terminal processes between adjoining epithelial cells. The sensory nerve fibers supplying the mucous membrane have their cell bodies of origin in the dorsal root ganglia, but they are distributed with the autonomic nerves and thus pass through the myenteric and submucosal plexuses en route to the mucosa.

THE FIBER SPECTRA OF PERIPHERAL NERVES

In the foregoing accounts of sensory, motor, and autonomic nerves and their terminations it has frequently been pointed out that different types of nerve endings are customarily supplied by axons whose diameter and degree of myelination are fairly constant for a particular category of ending. Since the diameter of an axon is closely related to its conduction velocity, fibers in a particular diameter range will also fall within a fairly constant range of conduction velocities. The range of fiber diameters in the nerve is known as the *fiber spectrum* of that nerve (Figs. 8-68 and 8-69), and

TABLE 8-1

FIBER TYPE	Aα		Aδ	C
	GROUP I	GROUP II	GROUP III	GROUP IV (UNMYELINATED)
Diameter (includes myelin sheath, where present)	5–20 μm 12–20 μm	5–12 μm	2–5 μm	0.1–1.5 μm
Conduction velocity	30–120 m/s 70–120 m/s	30–70 m/s	5–30 m/s	0.5–2 m/s
Receptor types	Primary endings in muscle spindles (IA) Golgi tendon organs (IB)	Secondary endings in muscle spindles Most other encapsulated endings Larger diameter mechanoreceptors and interoreceptors	Thermoceptors Nociceptors Smaller diameter mechanoreceptors and interoreceptors	
Other fiber types	α motor fibers, 12–20 μm		γ motor fibers, 2–8 μm Autonomic preganglionic fibers 1.5–4 μm (B fibers)	Autonomic postganglionic fibers; olfactory nerve fibers, 0.1–1 μm

because of the relation between diameter and conduction velocity, such a fiber spectrum also effectively indicates the range of conduction velocities in the fibers of that nerve.

On the basis of their diameters, conduction velocities, and certain other properties that need not concern us here, peripheral nerve fibers have been grouped into several classes. A summary of the two main classifications in current use is given in Table 8-1. The alphabetic classification into groups A, B, and C was made in the 1930s by Erlanger and Gasser and is based on the conduction velocities of mixed peripheral nerve fibers as revealed by the peaks of the compound action potentials recorded following electrical stimulation of the various peripheral nerves. Group A contains fibers with the fastest conduction velocities, and within it two subgroups are now identified. These (in order of decreasing diameter) are referred to as Aα and Aδ fibers. The B group is formed principally by autonomic preganglionic fibers, and the C group is composed of unmyelinated fibers (including both afferent fibers entering the spinal cord in the dorsal roots and autonomic postganglionic fibers).

A second classification, widely used by physiologists, was originally introduced to describe the afferent fibers in muscle nerves. Four groups of fibers were recognized on the basis of their diameters: groups I, II, III, and IV. This is perhaps the more useful classification (since it also takes into account the peripheral terminations of sensory fibers) but is less often applied to non-sensory nerves even though these can be made to fit into the scheme (Table 8-1).

SOME ASPECTS OF NEURONAL ORGANIZATION

Up to this point we have considered neurons more or less as isolated units, but after their migration from the neuroepithelium or the neural crest most neurons normally aggregate together with other similar nerve cells to form characteristic neuronal populations. Here we will consider some general principles of neuronal organization and indicate how the more common neural aggregates are constructed. The three most common types of neural aggregate are: (1) the ganglia of the peripheral nervous system, including the sensory ganglia associated with the cranial and spinal nerves, and the ganglia of the autonomic nervous system; (2) various cellular groups in the central nervous system, usually referred to as *nuclei;* and (3) cortical formations, also found in the central nervous system.

SENSORY GANGLIA

The cells of all the spinal ganglia (Fig. 8-72) and most of those in the sensory ganglia associated with many of the cranial nerves are derived from the neural crest. The cells of certain cranial nerve ganglia are derived from the associated placodal epithelia. The factors which lead to the segregation of the neural crest cells that give rise to the sensory ganglia from those that give rise to other crest derivatives are not known. After migrating to their definitive location, they aggregate together to form the presumptive ganglion. The key morphogenetic event—the coming together of cells of like kind—represents the first step in the formation of any neuronal population.

Subsequently, a high percentage of the neurons that were initially generated die, usually at about the time that the cells in the population as a whole make their synaptic connections. This *histogenetic cell death* appears to be a general feature of the formation of most neuronal populations in both the peripheral and central nervous systems: in all those that have been analyzed quantitatively, only about 30 to 60 percent of the cells survive to maturity. The factors responsible for the death of so many neurons are not known, but it is generally thought that the cells that die are unable to establish either the appropriate number or the appropriate type of synaptic or sensory connection.

At present the most complete accounts of the development of the sensory ganglia derive from the study of these structures in chick embryos. In these ganglia, distinct neuronal populations appear: initially a large-celled ventrolateral group of neurons (thought to be proprioceptive) arises, and somewhat later in development a smaller-celled dorsomedially located population is generated. Although at a later stage the topographic segregation of the two populations is obscured, they are clearly different. For example, following the early removal of a developing limb, the larger cells degenerate extremely rapidly, whereas the small-celled population usually persists for a much longer period. Conversely, the developing small-celled population appears to be particularly sensitive to the action of the neurotrophic protein commonly called

nerve growth factor (NGF). The precursors of this population and the postganglionic sympathetic neurons appear to be the only cells which actively proliferate under the influence of NGF. A process of *functional specification* of the ganglion cells must then occur. This determines not only the peripheral and central connections of the cells but also the sensory modality to which they will respond. The nature of this specification is poorly understood: it is not yet known whether it is an intrinsic property of the neurons themselves or if it is imposed upon them by the peripheral tissues they innervate. In the adult animal a number of different functional classes of ganglionic cell are present, corresponding to each of the various modalities of somatic sensibility, but with the exception of variations in size and in the relative amounts of Nissl material and other organelles that the cells contain, no distinct morphological differences exist within the population of ganglion cells. However, cells innervating closely adjacent peripheral receptive fields and projecting their central processes into the same dorsal root filament tend to lie together. This tendency for neurons which innervate a particular region to be closely related to each other topographically is one of the fundamental principles of neuronal organization and is found at virtually all levels of the nervous system. Throughout the somatosensory system, the arrangement is commonly referred to as *somatotopic organization,* reflecting the systematic central nervous mapping of the body surface; but comparable patterns of organization are found in the other sensory systems where the organizing feature is both topographic (for example, the retinotopic organization of the visual system) and functional (for example, the tonotopic organization of the auditory system).

Interestingly, both the large and small neurons in the sensory ganglia undergo chromatolysis (see page 363) when their peripheral processes are interrupted but not when their central processes are cut. The reason for this is not known, but it may be related to the observation that substantially more of the materials synthesized in the perikaryon are transported into the peripheral than into the central processes. Since impulse transmission in these sensory neurons seems to proceed directly from the peripheral to the central process (either without invading the soma or by invading it only after some delay), and inasmuch as there are no synapses on the perikaryon, it would appear that the principal role of the ganglion cell somata is trophic, in the sense that the soma serves primarily to maintain the integrity of the processes.

THE GANGLIA OF THE AUTONOMIC NERVOUS SYSTEM

The second major class of peripheral nerve cell aggregation is comprised of the ganglia associated with the sympathetic and parasympathetic divisions of the autonomic nervous system (Fig. 8-75). The structure of the para- and prevertebral sympathetic ganglia and the principal cranial and sacral parasympathetic ganglia is essentially the same. Certain of the ganglionic arrangements in the viscera (for example, the gut plexuses) are different and have already been briefly outlined.

Like the sensory ganglia, the ganglia of the autonomic nervous system are invested by a fairly dense fibrous connective tissue capsule which is continuous with the epineurium of the related pre- and postganglionic nerve trunks. Within the ganglia the nerve cells are surrounded by satellite cells which, like the neurons, are of neural crest origin. However, these ganglia differ from the sensory ganglia in two important respects. First, the neurons are all *multipolar,* usually with several dendrites of varying length as well as a single, usually unmyelinated, axon which passes out into the appropriate postganglionic trunk. Second, all the so-called principal ganglion cells (and these constitute the great majority of the neurons in each ganglion) receive synapses from the preganglionic fibers. These synapses are all cholinergic in type, and the great majority of them are distributed to the dendrites rather than to the cell soma. As a rule, each ganglion cell receives an input from several preganglionic fibers, and conversely each preganglionic fiber forms synapses with several neurons. There are exceptions to this pattern (for example, in the ciliary portion of the avian ciliary ganglion mentioned above, there is a one-to-one relation between preganglionic fibers and postsynaptic cells), but such exceptions are uncommon in the mammalian autonomic nervous system.

The ganglion cells themselves are not uniform in type. In most ganglia there is a class of principal cells which are relatively large, with ovoid or spherical nuclei and an abundance of rough endoplasmic reticulum. Those which are adrenergic (and these consti-

tute the majority of principal ganglion cells) contain large numbers of small, dense-core vesicles both in their somata and throughout their processes, but especially at the sites of presumed transmitter release from their axons. As we have seen, these dense-core vesicles contain the neurotransmitter noradrenaline (norepinephrine) and the last enzyme involved in its synthesis, dopamine-β-hydroxylase. The presence of these two substances provides the basis for two common methods for displaying postganglionic sympathetic fibers, namely, the Falck-Hillarp method in which the noradrenaline is condensed by formaldehyde vapor to form a highly fluorescent compound, and an immunohistochemical method, using a fluorescently labeled antibody to dopamine-β-hydroxylase (Fig. 8-40.)

In many sympathetic ganglia a second, smaller cell type is found which is intensely fluorescent when treated with formaldelyde vapor. These so-called SIF (small, intensely fluorescent) cells appear to be a class of *dopaminergic* interneurons, but their functional role remains to be determined. At their most numerous they constitute only a small percentage of the total number of ganglion cells. Their nuclei are smaller, often ellipsoidal or convoluted, and more heterochromatic than those of the principal cells. They contain many large, dense-core vesicles and are presynaptic to the principal cells, but they may also release their contents directly into the bloodstream (Fig. 8-19).

THE ORGANIZATION OF NEURONAL AGGREGATES IN THE CENTRAL NERVOUS SYSTEM

Compared with the relatively simple organization of peripheral neural aggregates, the central nervous system (CNS) presents a bewildering display of different neuronal patterns. No two regions of the CNS are identical in their organization, although from animal to animal within any species, and even between different species and different classes, homologous structures usually show a surprisingly consistent neural architecture. Only two of the more common patterns will be considered here. These are the so-called central *nuclei* and certain laminated or *cortical* structures. Each of these different types of neuronal aggregate can be readily recognized at a fairly gross level in preparations stained either by one of the Nissl methods or by one of the common methods for myelinated fibers; the analyses of neural organization at this level are referred to as *cytoarchitectonic* or *myeloarchitectonic* studies, respectively, and constitute an essential preliminary to any serious study of the central nervous system.

Central Cell Masses or "Nuclear Groups"

Collections of neurons of similar type in the CNS are usually referred to as nuclei (a term which should not be confused with the nuclei of individual neurons) (Figs. 8-95 and 8-96). The neurons in such nuclei are usually generated over a restricted period of time in a well-defined region of the neuroepithelium. From this region the postmitotic, but still immature, neurons migrate to their definitive location where they aggregate with other neurons of the same type. The factors responsible for this selective cell aggregation are not yet known, but are generally thought to involve the presence on the surfaces of the cells of certain cell type specific macromolecules (probably glycoproteins) which serve to "recognize" other cells of similar type. This does not imply that all the cells in a given nucleus are absolutely identical in structure or function. In fact, in nearly every center that has been carefully studied in adult animals, two or more distinct cell types have been found. One type, which we may again refer to as the principal cell, usually gives rise to the efferent axons which connect the cell mass to other parts of the CNS. These cells, therefore, have relatively long axons and are commonly the largest cells in the nucleus. Often, but not always, the afferent input to the nucleus ends upon the dendrites or somata of the principal cells. There is usually a second population of cells, commonly smaller than the principal cells, which are thought to serve as interneurons, being interposed either between the major source of afferents to the cell mass and the principal cells or between axon collaterals of some principal cells and other, adjacent principal cells. In the first case, they are usually excitatory in nature; in the second, inhibitory. Such small cells are generally Golgi-type II neurons with short, locally ramifying axons, but it has become evident in recent years that many of them may be axonless and act through "presynaptic dendrites."

"Cortical" and Other Laminated Structures

Where nerve cells are found on the surface of the brain, the region is referred to as a *cortex* (Figs. 8-97 and 8-98). Here the neurons are arranged in a series of superimposed layers with cells of similar type tending to occupy the same layer. As in the case of the nuclear masses, each cortical area is, in some re-

spects, morphologically distinct, so that no general account can be given that is applicable to all.

In the simplest types of cortex (like that in certain parts of the olfactory system and in the hippocampal formation), the principal cells have their somata arranged in a single, compact lamina, and their dendrites are regularly oriented in a second overlying layer. The various extrinsic inputs to the cortex terminate upon these dendrites and are so arranged that the afferents from different sources contact different segments of the dendritic tree (Fig. 8-99). Various interneurons, usually of an inhibitory kind, are found in a third, deeper layer and their axons usually terminate upon the cell somata or the proximal parts of the dendrites of the principal cell type. This type of spatial segregation of afferent inputs is most clearly seen in simple cortical areas such as this, but it may well be the case in most neurons which receive synapses from two or more sources. The output from such a cortex is represented by the collected axons of the principal cells, which generally enter a zone of subcortical white matter.

Most cortical areas are considerably more complex than this. For example, in all but a few regions of the cerebral cortex (the so-called neocortex) there are five superimposed cellular layers and a relatively cell-free outer zone, or molecular layer, just beneath the surface (Fig. 8-97). Within each cellular layer, there are often several different cell types, although for heuristic reasons it is convenient to regard them as belonging to only two major classes: *pyramidal cells* so called because of the pyramidal form of the cell bodies which lead superficially to a prominent ascending or apical dendrite; and nonpyramidal, or *stellate, cells,* whose dendritic arborizations lack the rigid organization of the pyramidal cell (see Figs. 8-8, 8-9, 8-12, and 8-13). The pyramidal cell bodies are generally found in layers II, III and V, and to a lesser extent in layer VI, and send their apical dendrites into supervening layers and their axons into the subcortical white matter. The nonpyramidal cells are found in all layers, but certain types are particularly concentrated in layer IV. Their axons are distributed within the cortex itself. Certain extrinsic inputs to the cortex (for example, those from the related thalamic nucleus) appear to terminate mainly upon the nonpyramidal cells in layer IV, whereas others (such as the commissural fibers from the cortex of the opposite hemisphere) end in layers I,

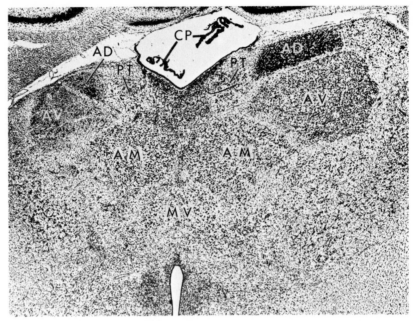

FIGURE 8-95 Frontal section of diencephalon of rabbit brain from which cingulate region of cerebral cortex was removed several weeks previously. Anterodorsal (AD) and anteroventral (AV) nuclei of left thalamus have undergone profound retrograde degeneration characterized by cell death and gliosis. Other nuclei (AM, Pt, MV) remain normal. CP, choroid plexus. Thionin stain. ×71.

FIGURE 8-96 Mamillary body of same brain as above, showing retrograde transneuronal degeneration of cells in left mamillary nuclei (MM) that project their axons to degenerated area of thalamus. Arrowheads indicate midline. Thionin stain. ×140.

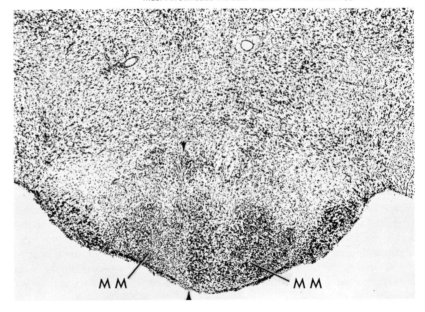

II, and III as well. These and other inputs are then relayed to the pyramidal cells in the other layers by nonpyramidal cells with vertical axons such as that shown in Fig. 8-9. The axons of the pyramidal cells, in turn, project to other regions of the brain. It has recently been found that the pyramidal cells in different layers project to different parts of the nervous system: generally the cells in layers II and III have been found

to project to other parts of the cerebral cortex, those in layer VI to the thalamus, and those in layer V to the brainstem, basal ganglia, and spinal cord. A second important principle that has emerged from recent studies of the sensory areas of the cerebral cortex is that interrelated cells are arranged into vertical columns or slabs perpendicular to the cortical surface and passing through all layers. In each column all the cells appear to subserve one sensory submodality, or some special feature of a sensory stimulus. Thus, in

FIGURE 8-97 (Left) Nissl-stained preparation of paravisual cerebral cortex of a monkey showing cell layers. ×66, WM.

FIGURE 8-98 (Right) Bodian-stained preparation of section adjacent to that shown in Fig. 8-97 demonstrating cellular and fiber lamination. ×66.

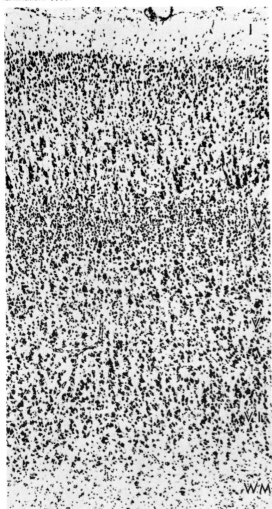

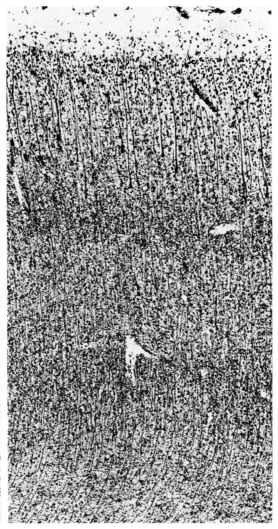

the somatosensory cortex the cells in one column may all respond to movement of a particular joint, whereas those in another column may all respond to light tactile stimulation of the skin. Similarly, in the visual cortex, cells in one slab will respond preferentially to stimulation of the left eye, whereas those in the adjoining slab will respond to stimulation of the right eye. And within either "eye-dominance column," as they have been called, all the cells in a single, narrow, vertical column may respond only to visual stimuli with a particular spatial orientation. In the case of the motor cortex, the cells of a column are all connected to the same group of spinal motoneurons.

The cerebral cortex can be subdivided into a number of different areas, each having its own distinctive structure. These so-called cytoarchitectonic fields differ from each other in the number, density, and arrangement of the cells and fibers in their various layers, and the boundaries between adjoining fields are occasionally remarkably distinct (Fig. 8-100). Most of these cytoarchitectonically distinct fields also have distinctive patterns of afferent and efferent connections, and in a number of cases it has been possible to show that functionally they are equally distinct. How

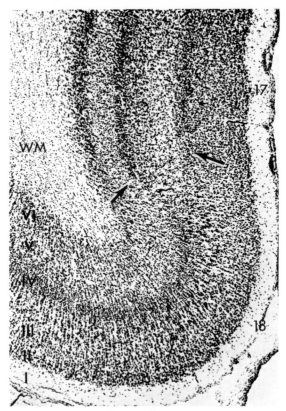

FIGURE 8-100 Junction of primary visual area (17) of monkey cerebral cortex with adjacent area (18). Arrows show region at which trilaminar layer IV of area 17 gives place to unilaminar layer IV of area 18. Latter area also has larger cells in layer III and layers V and VI are less distinct. Thionin stain. ×23.

FIGURE 8-99 Drawings of two types of pyramidal cell found in the mammalian hippocampus to illustrate the principle that afferents from different sources are usually spatially segregated upon the surface of complex neurons. Ent, Com, Sep, entorhinal, commissural, and septal afferents. (D. I. Gottlieb and W. M. Cowan, *Z. Zellforsch Mikrosk. Anat.,* **129:**413, 1972.)

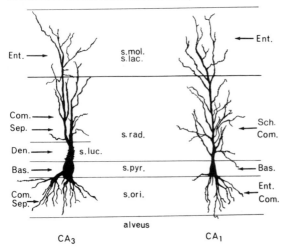

these striking differences are generated during the early development of the cortex is quite unknown. At present the only relevant evidence we have is that the cells in the different layers are generated at different times. The first-formed cortical cells are those which finally reside in the deepest lamina (layer VI) and those in the progressively more superficial layers are generated at successively later times. In addition, since many of the cells appear to display their characteristic functional properties shortly after the cortex is developed, it seems likely that the formation of their connections is genetically determined. But the "wiring pattern" seems also to be modifiable by environmental manipulation (for example, by depriving the visual cortex of its normal functional input from one eye).

THE REACTION OF NEURAL TISSUE TO INJURY

Since among animal cells, neurons are distinguished by the number and variety of their processes, considerable attention has been paid to the trophic relation between the nerve cell soma and its axonal and dendritic processes, and to the long-term consequences of neuronal injury. More than a century ago the English physiologist Augustus Waller formulated what is perhaps still the only "law" in neuroanatomy when he pointed out that when an axon is interrupted, the distal segment invariably degenerates. However, it is not only in this part of the axon that degenerative changes occur; in many neurons comparably severe changes can be seen in the perikaryon, and in several neuronal systems an atrophy, or even degeneration, can be observed in the neurons that are related synaptically to the injured nerve cells.

CHANGES AT THE SITE OF THE LESION

Following the uncomplicated interruption of an axon, there is a short period during which axoplasm leaks from the cut ends, since the axon appears to be in a state of some turgor owing to the continuous flow of axoplasm and axonal organelles. However, the leakage of axonal contents does not seem to be a serious matter, for within a short while there is a retraction of the axon and the axolemma appears to fuse over the severed ends and effectively seals them off. This is followed by a damming up of axonal material behind the fused membranes so that within 12 to 24 h there is a distinct swelling or dilatation of the axon. These swellings (which contain a variety of organelles, neurofilaments, vesicles of various kinds, mitochondria, and so forth, and stain deeply with most reduced silver methods) have been termed *retraction bulbs*. The subsequent fate of the retraction bulbs depends on whether or not regeneration occurs in the cut axon. In most, if not all, parts of the central nervous systems of higher vertebrates (including reptiles, birds, and mammals) no significant regeneration occurs, and within a day or two the proximal end of the severed axons degenerates at least as far back as the first collateral branch of the axon. In the peripheral nervous system (and to a lesser extent in the central nervous systems of fish and amphibians) numerous filopodia appear on the surface of the retraction bulb. Subsequently, large numbers of new axonal sprouts grow out from the bulb and make their way toward the distal segment of the nerve (Fig. 8-76).

At the site of the injury the supporting and certain other nonneural cells become activated and participate in the removal of the neuronal debris, in the formation of a "glial scar," and possibly also in the process of regeneration. In the central nervous system the cells principally involved in this "mopping-up operation" are the local astrocytes, which may be stimulated to proliferate and to become actively phagocytic. Oligodendrocytes and vascular pericytes also become reactive, and if there has been some damage to the neighboring capillaries, large numbers of blood-borne phagocytes (polymorphonuclear leukocytes and other macrophages) usually invade the tissue. Once the necrotic tissue has been phagocytosed, the glial cells initiate a vigorous repair process. Astrocytic processes either expand to fill the vacated area to form a dense "glial scar" which bridges across the traumatized zone or, if this is too large, they effectively seal off the damaged area as an encysted space. The oligodendrocytes, on the other hand, seem to be able to sequester large masses of cellular debris by forming myelin ensheathments around them. It is widely believed that these glial responses, and especially the formation of a glial scar, either prevent or seriously limit central neural regeneration.

In the peripheral nervous system, the Schwann cells show a similar prompt response by actively proliferating and phagocytosing the breakdown products of the neuronal degeneration. To what extent the reaction of the Schwann cells actually promotes regeneration is not known. To date, most attempts to demonstrate it experimentally have yielded equivocal results, but it is clear that they do form new sheaths for the regenerating axons.

THE REACTION IN THE DISTAL SEGMENT

In certain invertebrate nerves the surrounding sheath cells seem to be able to maintain the viability of the distal segment of a cut axon more or less indefinitely. But more commonly, and certainly in all vertebrates, the entire distal segment will, in time, undergo what is called *Wallerian degeneration*. However, the earliest changes seem to appear not close to the injury, as might be expected, but at the axon terminals.

Terminal degeneration, as it is usually called, takes several forms. The earliest changes, in the form of a swelling and possibly some loss of synaptic vesicles, can often be recognized within 12 to 24 h after axotomy. (The actual rate of appearance varies somewhat from system to system but, in general, appears to be a function of the distance of the nerve transection from the terminals: the closer to the terminals the axon is interrupted, the more rapidly the degenerative changes appear.) Subsequently, there may be a marked increase in the number of neurofilaments in the terminals, and a corresponding decrease in the number of synaptic vesicles (Fig. 8-101). The neurofilamentous hyperplasia (which is presumably a result of the polymerization of soluble filament precursor

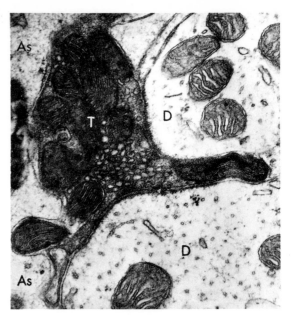

FIGURE 8-102 The electron-dense reaction in a degenerating axon terminal (T) which has been cut off from its cell soma. Note the dense clumping of the synaptic vesicles, the persistence of the postsynaptic membrane specializations on the dendrites (D), and the surrounding astrocytic processes (As). ×33,000. (E. G. Jones and A. J. Rockel, *J. Comp. Neurol.,* **147**:93, 1973.)

FIGURE 8-101 Electron micrograph showing proliferation of neurofilaments (f), reduction in synaptic vesicles (SV), and central clumping of mitochondria and lysosomes in an axon terminal following interruption of its parent axon. DA, degenerating axon. Inferior colliculus of cat. ×30,700. (E. G. Jones and A. J. Rockel, *J. Comp. Neurol.,* **147**:93, 1973.)

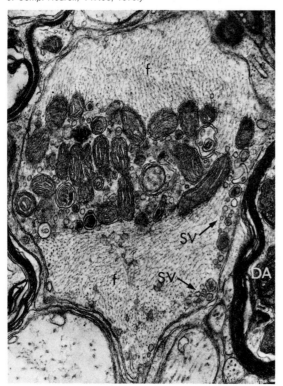

material in the axon) accounts for the increased argyrophilia of degenerating axon terminals; and since the filaments often appear as a tangled whorl around a central cluster of mitochondria and synaptic vesicles, in neurofibrillar preparations such degenerating terminals are often impregnated as ringlike structures. Later the whole terminal may become filled with filaments and, in silver preparations, appear as a swollen, degenerating end bulb.

A third reaction involves a progressive increase in the density of the axoplasmic matrix of the terminal and a concomitant loss of the remaining synaptic vesicles (Fig. 8-102). This "dark reaction" may occur as a primary response in certain nerve terminals or, in others, it may be secondary to the neurofilamentous change described above. The physicochemical nature of the axoplasmic change is unknown, but in time there is virtually a complete loss of synaptic vesicles and the mitochondria become increasingly dense and fragmented. A short while later the terminal appears to be "dissected" away from the postsynaptic membrane specialization and phagocytosed by the neighboring astrocytes; the engulfed fragments then resemble lysosomal dense bodies. Terminals undergoing this dense reaction are particularly susceptible to impregnation by certain silver methods, such as the Fink-Heimer modification of the Nauta technique (see the section on Methods Used in the Study of the Nervous System), a feature which makes these methods extremely useful for determining the sites of termination of neural pathways.

With the exception of the neuromuscular junction, the degeneration of most peripheral nerve terminations has not been carefully studied. In the case of the neuromuscular junction, the degenerative changes are essentially comparable to those at central neuronal synapses. However, because of the more favorable circumstances for experimental study, it has been easier to show that the cessation of transmission from nerve to muscle precedes the earliest morphological changes by several hours, and that the time required for transmission to fail varies directly with the length of the segment between the nerve section and the axon terminals.

Proximal to the terminals the axon—and in the case of myelinated fibers, the surrounding myelin sheath—seems to degenerate in a piecemeal fashion. Over most of its extent the axoplasm becomes progressively more electron-dense, the normally smooth contour of the axon becomes more and more irregular with fusiform swellings and constrictions every few microns along its length, and then it finally breaks up into numerous short fragments. This accounts for the characteristic fragmented appearance of degenerating nerve tracts which has been used to such good effect in tracing pathways in the central nervous system (Fig. 8-110). Concurrently, the myelin lamellae (where present) are drawn away from the axolemma and clefts appear between adjoining lamellae as the myelin sheath disintegrates. The fragmentation of the myelin sheath, and an alteration in its lipid composition, form the basis of yet another method for following neural pathways—the so-called Marchi technique. The signal for the disintegration of the myelin sheath, when its enclosed axon degenerates, is unknown, but the fact that it occurs so consistently suggests that there is normally a close—perhaps even trophic—relation between axons and the related myelin-forming cells.

DEGENERATIVE CHANGES IN THE PROXIMAL SEGMENT OF THE AXON

Depending on the reaction of the nerve cell soma, the axon proximal to the site of the transection may either degenerate completely or show only relatively minor

changes in the region adjoining the traumatized zone. Should the parent cell die (see below), the axon will degenerate in a proximodistal sequence starting near the initial segment. Since the appearance of the degeneration is essentially the same as that seen in the distal segment, it is now generally referred to as *indirect Wallerian degeneration* (or sometimes as retrograde fiber degeneration, although this is misleading since it may suggest that the degenerative change proceeds backward from the lesion to the cell soma).

In cases in which the cell body survives the injury, the axon appears to degenerate only as far back as its first collateral branch, proximal to the site of transection. In the absence of regeneration of the main portion of the axon, this collateral may become hypertrophied and function as the principal conducting channel of the neuron. Regeneration, when it occurs, may begin either from near the origin of this collateral or, more commonly, from the retraction bulb, as described above. The actual process of axonal regeneration appears to be identical to the initial outgrowth of the axon with the interesting difference that usually several (up to 50) sprouts grow out from the cut end of the axon. The great majority of these sprouts subsequently degenerate and only one or two actually grow into the distal stump of the nerve.

THE REACTION OF THE NERVE CELL SOMA TO AXOTOMY

Although it is commonly stated that the event termed *chromatolysis* is the characteristic response of nerve cells to interruption of their axons, a whole spectrum of reactions may in fact occur in the soma, from the death of the neuron at one end, to no discernible change at the other. The reason for this variability is unknown: it is widely believed that the presence of axon collaterals proximal to the nerve section is responsible for preserving the integrity of the soma, and that chromatolysis is essentially a regenerative response.

Chromatolysis This reaction is usually seen in motoneurons, in sensory ganglion cells, and in a number of large central neurons in the brainstem and spinal cord (Fig. 8-103). Characteristically it consists of a progressive breakdown of the Nissl material (from which the reaction gets its name), a tendency for the nucleus to become more and more eccentric (usually

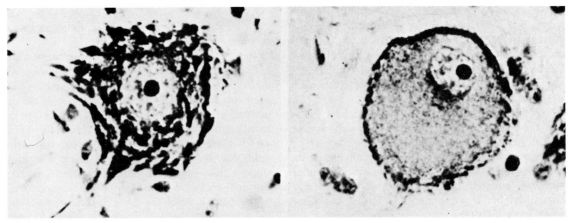

FIGURE 8-103 A normal motoneuron (left) and one showing advanced chromatolysis (right) following interruption of its axon. (D. Bodian and R. C. Mellors, *J. Exp. Med.,* **81:**469, 1945; courtesy of Dr. D. Bodian.)

FIGURE 8-104 (Left) Retrograde cell degeneration involving a wedge-shaped area extending through all layers of the lateral geniculate nucleus of a monkey after destruction of a small portion of the visual cortex. Thionin stain. (J. H. Kaas, R, W. Guillery, and J. M. Allman, *Brain Behav. Evol.,* **6:**253, 1973; courtesy of Dr. J. H. Kaas.)

FIGURE 8-105 (Right) Anterograde transneuronal degeneration in monkey lateral geniculate nucleus which has resulted in severe cell shrinkage in the neurons of layers 1, 4, and 6, following removal of the contralateral eye some months earlier. Thionin stain. ×20.

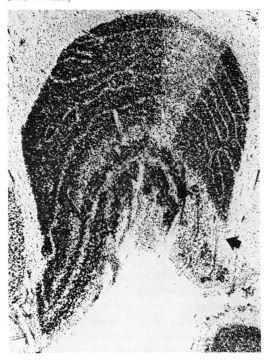

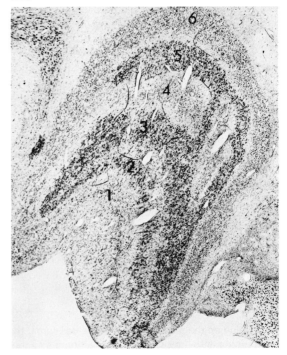

moving away from the axon hillock), and a variable amount of swelling of the perikaryon. In its fully developed state the cell appears globular, having lost its usual angular profile, with the nucleus pressing against the cell membrane and with only a narrow rim of Nissl material around the perimeter of the cell or in a "cap" over the nucleus. The whole process takes about 2 weeks to develop, and if the axon regenerates, the entire sequence of changes may be reversed over the next 4 to 6 weeks.

Cell death In many neural centers (such as the nuclei of the mammalian thalamus) and in the developing nervous system, axon section is followed within a few days by the death of the cell and its removal by glial action. The cytological changes vary from case to case, but characteristically the nucleus becomes increasingly pyknotic, the Nissl material is lost, and the perikaryon shrinks dramatically. In the adult nervous system these changes are accompanied by a marked glial proliferation (*gliosis*), which persists following the removal of the neuronal debris (Figs. 8-95 and 8-104). On the other hand, in embryos the neuronal death not only occurs more rapidly but is seldom accompanied by an obvious glial reaction (Fig. 8-106).

Other cellular reactions In some situations the neurons seem to persist more or less indefinitely after axon section, but in a shrunken, atrophied form. Whether this is because the cells have other axonal branches that escaped injury or because of some other reason remains to be determined. In still other cases, such as the large pyramidal neurons in the cerebral cortex, there may be no detectable reaction in the perikaryon even though the greater part of the axon has been amputated. In at least some instances the cell seems to be preserved by the hypertrophy of collateral branches given off close to the cell body.

TRANSNEURONAL (OR TRANSSYNAPTIC) DEGENERATIONS

In a few neuronal systems distinct degenerative (or atrophic) changes have been observed in the neurons that are synaptically related to those whose axons were interrupted. Depending on the direction of the transneuronal effects, they may be termed *anterograde* or *retrograde;* and in recent years it has been recognized that such effects may extend beyond the first synapse so that secondary, and even tertiary, transneuronal effects are recognized.

Anterograde Transneuronal Degeneration

The classic site for this type of change is the dorsal lateral geniculate nucleus of the mammalian thalamus which receives a substantial part of its input from the ganglion cells of the retina (Fig. 8-105). If an eye is removed, or if an optic nerve is cut, the related cells in the lateral geniculate nucleus undergo a progressive atrophy marked by the shrinkage of both the perikaryon and the nucleus, the loss of some Nissl material, and in adults, after many weeks or months, some degree of cell loss. In younger animals the changes occur more rapidly, are more severe, and if sufficient time has elapsed, may be associated with secondary changes in the neurons in the visual cortex upon which the geniculate cells project. The most commonly described secondary transneuronal change in the cortex is a loss of dendritic spines, but a generalized thinning of the cortex with a loss of cells in certain layers has also been described.

Whereas the transneuronal changes in the visual system are the best-documented examples of this form of degeneration, it is now known to occur in many regions in both the central and peripheral nervous systems. The causative mechanism has yet to be explained, but it is generally thought to be due either to the removal of some form of trophic substance passed from the pre- to the postsynaptic neuron or to the absence of appropriate functional activity in the postsynaptic cells.

Retrograde Transneuronal Degeneration

In some neural systems in which retrograde cell degeneration after axon section is particularly severe, such as the lateral geniculate and anterior nuclei of the mammalian thalamus, degenerative changes have also been observed in the cells which project to those nuclei (Fig. 8-96). Such retrograde transneuronal changes are significantly more severe in young animals and become progressively more marked with increasing survival after the initial lesion. And in the case of the anterior thalamic nuclei, it has been found in several species that if the primary lesion in the cerebral cortex occurs early enough, degenerative changes may be found not only in the mamillary nuclei (which project to the anterior thalamic nuclei) but also in one of the midbrain tegmental nuclei that sends its axons to the mamillary nuclei.

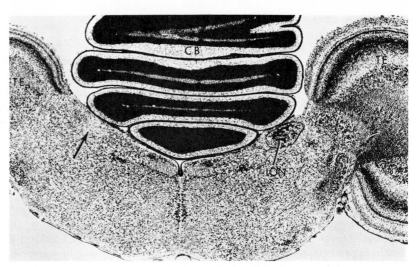

FIGURE 8-106 Neurons whose axons are unable to form synaptic connections during development degenerate completely as shown by the absence of the nucleus of origin of the centrifugal fibers to the chick retina (ION) after early removal of the contralateral eye in the embryo. In the region usually occupied by the ION, there is a complete cell loss on the side opposite the eye removal (arrow). Te, tectum. Thionin stain. ×28.

Why certain neural systems should show primary, or even secondary, retrograde transneuronal changes is not yet known; at present the only clue is that this type of degeneration is never seen unless there is marked cell loss in the initial retrograde degeneration. This suggests that there may be a two-way interaction between neurons that are synaptically related so that for the full growth and survival of a neuron it must both form an adequate number of synapses upon other neurons (or effector tissues such as muscle or gland cells) and also receive an adequate number of synaptic inputs from other neurons. Whether this is simply to maintain an adequate level of activity or to provide an adequate exchange of trophic materials remains to be determined.

METHODS USED IN THE STUDY OF THE NERVOUS SYSTEM

A wide variety of techniques is used for the study of the nervous system. We shall consider only those which are more commonly used. Broadly, the methods fall into two classes: (1) those based on the study of *normal* neural tissue, and (2) *experimental* methods.

METHODS FOR NORMAL NEURAL TISSUE

In the study of normal neural tissue, five groups of techniques are in common use.

The Nissl Method
The staining of the Nissl material within neurons, by any one of a number of basic aniline dyes, has been used for almost a century to identify the somata of individual neurons and to analyze the distribution of populations of neurons. Several of the illustrations (for example, Fig. 8-11, 8-100, and 8-106) in this chapter are of Nissl-stained preparations, and their use is essential for any cytoarchitectonic or cytological study of the nervous system.

Methods for Staining Nerve Fibers
These include a number of techniques which more or less selectively stain the sheaths of myelinated axons. Most of these involve some prior treatment of the tissue in a mordant such as potassium biochromate, which serves to stabilize the lipids of the myelin sheaths, and the subsequent staining of the pretreated

myelin with a basic dye such as hematoxylin. Figure 8-107 shows a preparation stained in this way. Because of its high affinity for lipids, osmium tetroxide also provides an extremely intense stain for myelin (Fig. 8-61). Axons themselves and dendrites can be stained by various *reduced silver methods*. The chemical basis for these methods is not well understood, but in a general sense they resemble certain photographic procedures in which silver salts are "developed" and the resulting metallic silver "fixed." Many of these methods involve a pretreatment of the tissue in a silver nitrate solution at high pH followed by a reduction involving an acidified formalin solution. This results in the deposition of "nuclei" of metallic silver around certain cellular organelles (for example, the nuclear membrane, nucleoli, and so forth) but especially around clusters of neurofilaments. As we have pointed out (page 302), this appears to be the basis for the light microscopic appearance of neurofibrils. These methods are sometimes called "neurofibrillar methods." Figure 8-29 is from a preparation of this kind.

The Analytic Methods

Because of the difficulty of analyzing preparations in which all the neuronal perikarya, or all the various processes, are stained, two invaluable methods were developed in the latter part of the last century. These are the *supravital methylene blue method* of Ehrlich and the *Golgi method*. These methods have two major advantages: first, they stain only a small percentage of the neurons in any one area (commonly less than 1 percent); and second, they commonly stain the cells in their entirety. As Figs. 8-12 to 8-15 show, in a preparation of this kind, individual neurons stand out strikingly against a relatively clear, unstained background, and usually the full extent of the perikarya, the dendrites (including dendritic spines), and the unmyelinated segments of their axons are displayed. The reason for the selectivity of these methods is not known, nor is the mechanism of the actual staining procedures. In the case of the Golgi method (which has been the more intensively studied and is currently the more widely used of the two methods), the tissue is commonly pretreated with potassium dichromate and then impregnated in a silver nitrate solution. This results in the deposition of silver salts throughout most of the interior of the neuron—excluding the various membranous components. Despite a certain capriciousness, these methods are extremely valuable for the study of dendritic organization, and at present are among the few that are useful for analyzing local neuronal circuitry.

Intracellular Labeling of Physiologically Identified Neurons

This recent development in neurobiology represents an especially powerful addition to the older analytic methods, since it permits the display of the full morphology of neurons whose functional properties have previously been defined electrophysiologically. Briefly, the method involves the introduction, through a micropipette, of a fluorescent dye, such as Procion yellow, or an opaque substance, such as a cobalt salt, or a histochemically demonstrable enzyme, such as horseradish peroxidase, into the cell (usually into the perikaryon), from which it diffuses or is actively transported into the dendrites and the initial portion of the axon. In suitably prepared sections and with the appropriate optics (fluorescence microscopy is needed to visualize cells filled with Procion yellow), the entire geometry of the cell can be readily demonstrated. Alternatively, the marker molecule can be iontophoresed up the axon, from the cut end, and subsequently precipitated in the perikaryon and dendrites. This approach has proved especially effective for labeling motoneurons in invertebrates. A recent variant of the intracellular labeling procedure involves the use of tritium-labeled precursors of certain macromolecules (such as [^{3}H]amino acids or [^{3}H]fucose) which are incorporated into proteins or glycoproteins and rapidly transported from the soma into the dendrites and axon of the labeled cell. After an appropriate interval to allow for the transport of the radioactive macromolecules, the distribution of the tritium label can be displayed autoradiographically.

Electron Microscopy

The introduction of the electron microscope to biology in the early 1950s added an entirely new dimension to neuroanatomical studies, not only because it offered increased resolution but, perhaps more importantly, because it displayed *all* the structures within the tissue being examined. In this respect it differs from all the other methods commonly used. One of its earliest contributions was the demonstration that there is no extensive "ground substance" in the brain and spinal cord as was formerly believed; rather, the CNS resembles most other ectodermal derivatives, with only narrow (200 Å) clefts between adjoining cells and their processes. In addition, it made possible, for the first time, the critical study of such structures as synapses and their associated organelles, the substructure of myelin sheaths, the form of nodes of Ranvier, and the ultrastructural counterparts of such neuronal organelles as Nissl bodies, neurofibrils, and so forth. The preparation of neural tissue for electron microscopy generally involves fixation by perfusion with a buffered solution of aldehydes (formaldehyde and glutaraldehyde are commonly used), postfixation in osmium tetroxide, and embedding in an appropriate plastic. Since the sections used are generally of the order of 600 to 1000 Å thick and the area available for study in any one section, usually only a few hundred square microns in extent, the amount of tissue that can be studied is rather limited. But within these limits the method is undoubtedly the most critical available to the neuroanatomist. In recent years this approach has been significantly extended by the development of techniques for preparing large numbers of serial sections, by the application of the electron microscope to tissue previously stained by some other method (such as the Golgi technique or after intercellular labeling with the dye Procion brown), and by the introduction of such special methods as freeze-etching, which permits the interior of membrane surfaces to be visualized. The use of the high-voltage electron microscope permits the study of sections as thick as 1 or 2 μm; this has been particularly valuable in the analysis of Golgi-impregnated material.

EXPERIMENTAL METHODS

While the examination of normal material is an essential prerequisite for all neuroanatomical studies, it is seldom possible in such material to determine the connections between groups of neurons which are separated by more than just a few hundred microns. For this, one must resort to experimental material which is basically of two kinds: the first is aimed at determining the *origin* of neuronal pathways, the second at mapping their sites of *termination*.

Retrograde Methods

For many years the method of choice for determining the origin of nervous pathways was based on the retrograde reaction seen in nerve cell somata following the interruption of their axons or the destruction of their synaptic terminals (for example, Figs. 8-95 and 8-104). This method was particularly successful in elucidating the origin of the motor divisions of the cranial nerves, the location of spinal motoneurons supplying various muscle groups and certain of the connections of the cerebellum, and most strikingly, in establishing the pattern of the projection of the various nuclei of the thalamus upon the cerebral cortex and corpus striatum. Unfortunately, as we have pointed out above, not all neurons show a clear-cut reaction to axotomy, and in these cases the method not only is of little value but has often proved to be misleading. Recently, a new "retrograde" method has been introduced which promises to be both more reliable and more generally applicable than the cell-degeneration

FIGURE 8-107 Several weeks after interrupting a fiber bundle, all the axons degenerate and are removed by the phagocytic action of glial cells. In this section of the human spinal cord in a case of tabes dorsalis, the fibers in the gracile funiculi (GF) have completely disappeared. (Weigert method, to show myelinated fibers.) AM, arachnoid mater; DR, dorsal root; VR, ventral root. ×9.

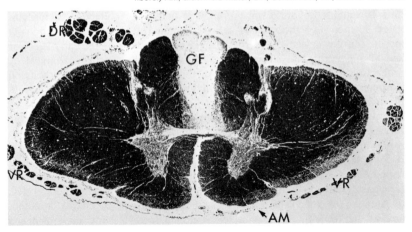

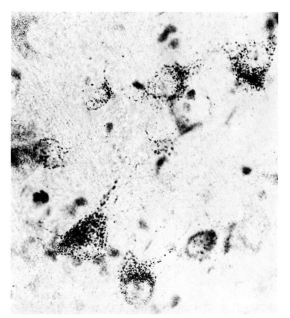

FIGURE 8-108 A group of neurons which have been labeled retrogradely with the enzyme marker horseradish peroxidase. Dark granules are reaction product in cell soma and dendrites. ×433. (E. G. Jones and R. Y. Leavitt, *J. Comp. Neurol.*, **154:**349, 1974.)

these changes have been described in the previous section, here we need only add that the methods most widely used at present are variants of a silver technique introduced by Nauta and Gygax in 1951 and commonly referred to as the *Nauta technique* (Figs. 8-109 and 8-110). This technique takes advantage of the increased argyrophilia of degenerating axons; and by critically suppressing the staining of the normal fibers, the degenerating axons and axon terminals can be displayed against a relatively clear background. Other reduced silver methods (for example, the *Glees method*) have been used from time to time, but in these both the normal and the degenerating neuronal processes are impregnated so it is extremely difficult to identify and follow the latter. Of course, the most critical method for identifying degenerating axons and presynaptic processes is by the use of the *electron microscope*. Indeed, this is the only method that enables one to confidently identify synaptic relationships; the presence of the various degenerative changes described in the previous section in a presynaptic profile (especially the enlargement or loss of synaptic vesicles, a proliferation of neurofilaments, or a marked increase in the electron density of the axoplasm) constitutes ineluctable evidence that the parent cell or its axon has been damaged.

An even earlier method was that introduced by Marchi in 1885. This was based on the increased affinity of disintegrating myelin sheaths for osmium tetroxide. However, since it was somewhat capricious and applicable only to myelinated pathways, the Marchi method is now only of historical interest. If a sufficiently long time has elapsed between the causative lesion and the fixation of the brain, the anterograde degeneration of the pathways in question may have proceeded to the point where all the fibers have been removed by glial action. In this case their former location can be identified, as it were negatively, by the absence of stainable fibers. Although this approach has little to commend it for experimental studies, it is still quite widely used in human neuropathology to follow the degeneration resulting from long-standing brain lesions (Fig. 8-107).

The second approach is based on the axonal transport of materials synthesized in neuronal somata and distributed along the length of the axons to their terminals. Most commonly various tritiated precursors, such as [³H]fucose or [³H]amino acids, are

approach. This new method is based on the uptake of exogenous marker molecules (such as the enzyme horseradish peroxidase (Fig. 8-108), the reaction product of which can be readily demonstrated histochemically) by axons, and especially by their terminals, and its transport back to the cell soma by the process of retrograde axonal flow. Although this method has been applied to the study of central neural pathways only since 1972, it has already proved to be invaluable in the study of such difficult problems as the origin of the various efferent projections from the cerebral cortex, the projection of different populations of retinal ganglion cells, and the connections of various nuclear groups in the thalamus and brainstem.

Anterograde Methods

The alternative approach is aimed at determining the site and pattern of termination of the axons arising from a given population of neurons. Three fundamentally different approaches to this problem have been used. The first is based on the anterograde degenerative changes seen in the distal portion of axons following their interruption or the destruction of their parent nerve cell bodies by an experimental lesion. Because

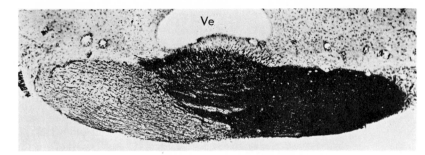

FIGURE 8-109 Degenerating axons become intensely argyrophilic, as seen in this photomicrograph of the optic chiasm of a guinea pig 6 days after removal of the left eye. Ve, ventricle. Nauta-Gygax method. ×78.

FIGURE 8-110 Silver-stained, degenerating axons ascending from the polymorph layer (PL) of the dentate gyrus through the granule cell layer (GCL) to end in a dense mass of terminal fragments in the deeper part of the molecular layer (ML). Fink and Heimer stain, marsupial brain after destruction of hippocampal commissure. ×194. (C. J. Heath and E. G. Jones, *J. Anat.,* Lond. **109:**253, 1971.)

FIGURE 8-111 Dark field photomicrograph from an autoradiograph demonstrating axoplasmically transported label in axon terminals in layers I and IV of the cerebral cortex following an injection of tritiated amino acids in the thalamus. ×165.

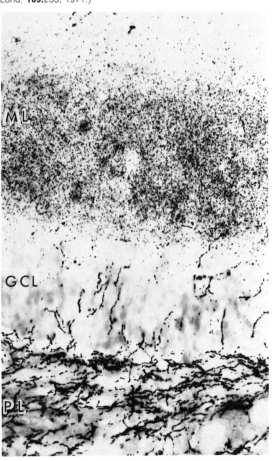

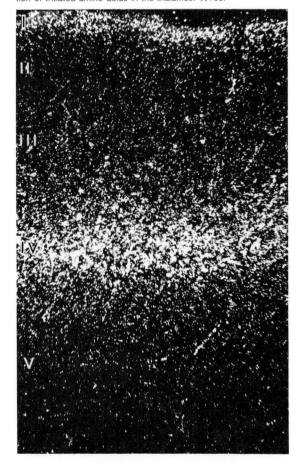

used. A concentrated solution of the labeled precursor is injected into the neuronal population whose connections are to be studied. The neurons in the immediate vicinity of the injection (but not axons passing through it) take up the precursor and incorporate it into certain macromolecules (such as proteins, glycoproteins, or glycolipids) which are then transported at various velocities down their axons. The presence of the labeled axons and axon terminals can then be identified in serial light microscopic autoradiographs (or electron-microscopic autoradiographs) of the relevant areas (Fig. 8-111). Since this method is based on an established physiological property of nerve cells and does not involve the destruction of the tissue being studied, it has a number of advantages over the degeneration methods and, in addition, appears to be somewhat more sensitive than the degeneration methods.

The third approach is aimed at identifying specific neural pathways which act by the release of certain identified neurotransmitters. These methods are based either on the inherent fluorescence of such biogenic amines as dopamine, noradrenaline and serotonin when exposed to formalin vapor or, in the case of

cholinergic and noradrenergic fibers, on the binding of fluorescent-labeled antibodies to the enzymes choline acetyltransferase and dopamine-β-hydroxylase which are, respectively, the key enzymes involved in the biosynthesis of acetylcholine and noradrenaline (Fig. 8-40). A somewhat different method in this category is based on the finding that neurons which release certain transmitter substances (such as γ-amino butyric acid or glycine) have a high-affinity uptake system for the transmitter. When exposed to a radioactively labeled solution of the transmitter, the neurons, and especially their axon terminals, take up the label in high concentrations; its presence in the cell or axon terminals can subsequently be demonstrated autoradiographically. Since their introduction in the late 1960s, these methods have proved extremely useful, both in the central and in the peripheral nervous system, and clearly presage the development of a new phase in neuroanatomical studies which should lead in time to a complete account of the "chemical architecture" of the brain and spinal cord.

REFERENCES

ANGEVINE, J. B.: Critical Cellular Events in the Shaping of Neural Centers, in F. O. Schmitt (ed.), "The Neurosciences Second Study Program," Rockefeller University Press, New York, 1970, pp. 62–72.

BARR, M. L., L. F. BERTRAM, and H. A. LINDSAY: The Morphology of the Nerve Cell Nucleus, According to Sex, *Anat. Rec.,* **107:**283–297 (1950).

BRIGHTMAN, M. W., and S. L. PALAY: The Fine Structure of the Ependyma in the Brain of the Rat, *J. Cell Biol.,* **19:**415–439 (1963).

BUNGE, M. B.: Fine Structure of Nerve Fibers and Growth Cones of Isolated Sympathetic Neurons in Culture, *J. Cell Biol.,* **56:**713–735 (1973).

BUNGE, R. P.: Glial Cells and the Central Myelin Sheath, *Physiol. Rev.,* **48:**197–251 (1968).

CHAN-PALAY, V., and S. L. PALAY: High Voltage Electron Microscopy of Rapid Golgi Preparations. Neurons and their Processes in the Cerebellar Cortex of the Monkey and Rat, *Z. Anat. Entwicklungs-gesch.,* **137:**125–152 (1972).

COOPER, J. R., F. E. BLOOM, and R. M. ROTH: "The Biochemical Basis of Neuropharmacology," Oxford University Press, New York, (1974).

CAJAL, S. RAMÓN Y: Histologie du Système Nerveux de l'Homme et des Vertébrés, 1909–1911; two volumes: Consejo Superior de Investigaciones Cientificas, Madrid, 1952, 1955.

CAJAL, S. RAMÓN Y: Histologie du Systéme Nerveux de l'Hoome et des Vertébrés, 1909–1911; two volumes: Oxford University Press, London, 1928.

GRAY, E. G.: Axo-somatic and Axo-dendritic Synapses of the Cerebral Cortex: An Electron Microscope Study, *J. Anat.* (*Lond.*), **93:**420–433 (1959).

GRAY, E. G., and R. W. GUILLERY: Synaptic Morphology in the Normal and Degenerating Nervous System, *Int. Rev. Cytol.,* **19:**111–182 (1966).

HEUSER, J. E., and T. S. REESE: Evidence for Recycling of Synaptic Vesicle Membrane during Transmitter Release at the Frog Neuromuscular Junction, *J. Cell Biol.,* **57:**315–344 (1973).

HEUSER, J. E., T. S., REESE, and D. M. D. Landis: Functional Changes in Frog Neuromuscular Junctions Studied with Freeze-Fracture, *J. Neurocytol.,* **3:**109–131 (1974).

HUBBARD, J. I. (ed.): "The Peripheral Nervous System," Plenum Press, New York, 1974.

IGGO, A. (ed.): "Handbook of Sensory Physiology," vol. 2, Somatosensory System, Springer-Verlag New York Inc., New York, 1973.

JONES, E. G., and T. P. S. POWELL: Morphological Variations in the Dendritic Spines of the Neocortex, *J. Cell Sci.,* **5:**509–529 (1969).

KUFFLER, S. W., and J. G. NICHOLLS: The Physiology of Neuroglial Cells, *Ergeb. Physiol.,* **57:**1–90 (1966).

NAUTA, W. J. H., and S. O. E. EBBESSON: "Contemporary Research Methods in Neuroanatomy," Springer-Verlag New York Inc., New York, (1970).

PALAY, S. L., and V. CHAN-PALAY: "Cerebellar Cortex. Cytology and Organization," Springer-Verlag New York Inc., New York, 1974.

PALAY, S. L., and G. E. PALADE: The Fine Structure of Neurons, *J. Biophys. Biochem. Cytol.,* **1:**69–88 (1955).

PALAY, S. L., C. SOTELO, A. PETERS, and P. M. ORKAND: The Axon Hillock and the Initial Segment, *J. Cell Biol.,* **38:**193–201 (1968).

PETERS, A., S. L. PALAY, and H. DE F. WEBSTER: "The Fine Structure of the Nervous System," Harper & Row Publishers, Incorporated, New York, 1970.

SHEPHERD, G. M.: "The Synaptic Organization of the Brain: An Introduction," Oxford University Press, New York, 1974.

SIDMAN, R. L: Cell-Cell Recognition in the Developing Central Nervous System, in F. O. Schmitt and F. G. Worden (eds.), "The Neurosciences Third Study Program." MIT Press, Cambridge, Mass., 1974, pp. 743–758.

UCHIZONO, K.: Characteristics of Excitatory and Inhibitory Synapses in the Central Nervous System of the Cat, *Nature,* **207:**642–643 (1965).

The Cardiovascular System

NICOLAE SIMIONESCU AND MAIA SIMIONESCU

The normal activity of cells requires a continuous equilibrium between the inflow of nutrient material and outflow of cell products and wastes. Unicellular organisms exchange such materials continually with the external medium by means of simple diffusion and various transport systems through their cell membranes. In multicellular organisms, the need for a mechanism to transport these substances to different parts of the body is met by the circulation of a fraction of the internal medium. This function is carried out in a specialized circuit of continuous and closed branching tubes (vessels), the *circulatory system*. In vertebrates, humans included, the body fluid is partitioned by semipermeable boundaries into four compartments: blood plasma, lymph, interstitial fluid, and intracellular fluid. For a human being weighing 160 lb, the circulating fluid amounts to approximately 17 l, and in a relatively steady state, it is distributed as follows: the blood plasma, is approximately 3 l; the lymph, approximately 3 l, and the interstitial fluid, approximately 11 l. An almost equal amount of fluid, approximately 15 l, is contained in cells. The blood plasma and the lymph circulate in a unidirectional flow in the blood circulatory system and the lymphatic circulatory system, respectively.

The *blood circulatory system* includes a muscular pump, the heart, and the blood vessels. (Together they are frequently referred to as the *cardiovascular system*.)

The *heart* is a modified blood vessel, specialized as a double pump for propulsion. Its right side receives blood from the whole body and this blood circulates through the lungs; its left side collects blood from the lung and distributes it to all other organs and tissues of the body. Vessels which carry blood to and from the lungs constitute the *pulmonary circulation*, whereas those which distribute and collect blood from the rest of the body form the *systemic circulation*. In both circulations, blood is pumped into and conducted through *arteries*, which by successive branching increase in number and decrease in caliber until they become *arterioles* that resolve into a network of *capillaries*. It is at the level of these fine vessels that the major exchanges between blood plasma and interestitial fluid take place. Blood returns via confluent *venules* and *veins* to the heart.

The *lymphatic circulatory system* carries lymph from tissue interstitia to the veins located at the base of the neck. This circulation drains the interstitial fluid and its movable cellular elements into the blindly ending *lymphatic capillaries*. The latter converge in various-sized *lymphatic vessels* (that are either provided or not provided with organized collections of lymphocytes, the *lymph nodes*), which return lymph to the blood venous system (see Chap. 14).

By ensuring the distribution of cell metabolites throughout all the tissues and cells, the circulatory system, in association with the nervous system, contributes to communication among, and integration of, all body constituents.

STRUCTURAL PLAN AND COMPONENTS

In the histogenesis of the blood circulatory system, one can postulate the influence of a genetic pattern as well as adaptive differentiations that modulate the basic organization of the system to meet various local functional requirements.

Physiological and biophysical conditions of the blood circulation are manifestly reflected in the tissue composition and structural organization of the cardiovascular system.

GENERAL FUNCTIONAL–STRUCTURAL CORRELATIONS

The blood is confined to a closed circuit of vessels lined by a thin layer of simple squamous epithelial cells, the *endothelium*. The latter is differentiated to fulfill the role of physical partition and semipermeable porous membrane between the blood and the interstitial fluid.

Propulsion of the blood is carried out by the heart, the muscular wall of which has become largely augmented and differentiated for intermittent contraction. During the systole, the heart ventricles eject the blood under considerable pressure into the large arteries, the aorta and pulmonary. On the account of the *elastic tissue* contained by their walls, the pressure at the level of these vessels is converted to a certain degree into increased wall tension; the tension is partially released during diastole, when the vessels passively contract. Hydrostatic pressure within the arterial system is thus maintained (at a lower level) during diastole, and the blood is conducted downstream.

The branches arising from the large arteries supply different parts of the body. The volume of the circulatory system is considerably larger than the blood volume, and the regional functional conditions vary. Therefore, to adjust the amount of blood to local metabolic requirements, a distributing system becomes necessary. This is accomplished by circularly or helically arranged muscle cells amply supplied in all *distributing,* or *muscular, arteries.* These vascular

smooth muscles can contract in response to nervous stimuli. As the vessels become smaller, the blood flow is progressively converted from an intermittent series of propulsions generated by the rhythmic contraction of the heart into a steady, continuous stream. This effect is primarily accomplished in elastic and muscular arteries.

Downstream, two mechanical conditions have to be met: (1) a relatively high hydrostatic pressure must be maintained in arteries to ensure sufficient quantities of blood to various organs and tissues; (2) the blood must be delivered into capillary beds under low pressure to protect the capillary wall, which is extremely thin to allow rapid and extensive exchanges through it. Both conditions are ensured in the smallest arterial ramifications, the arterioles, at the level of which relatively thick muscular layers have been differentiated. Smooth muscles of arterioles have the peculiarity of responding not only to nervous sympathetic impulses but also to metabolic stimuli expressing the local needs of the tissues (*autoregulation*). Owing to the factors just mentioned, about half the resistance to blood flow resides in arterioles that are the major regulators of blood flow.

At the level of capillaries, the speed, magnitude, and nature of the blood-tissue exchanges require a thin, semipermeable partition which is achieved by the reduction of the vascular wall to a single layer of flat cells, the endothelium. The exchanges occur also in the postcapillary (pericytic) venules, which have a comparable wall structure. In some tissues, the blood approaching the microvascular beds may bypass the exchange vessels (capillaries and pericytic venules) by using shunts, or *arteriovenous anastomoses,* that directly connect the arterioles with venules.

In the slightly larger venules at the beginning of the return circulation, the blood enters under a very low pressure and flows slowly. As a result, the veins exhibit larger lumina and thinner walls than the corresponding arteries. In their walls, connective tissue is more extensively used than the muscular tissue as structural material. The veins represent low-pressure vessels that are largely distensible and easily compressible. These properties pose particular problems for the venous circulation that are partially solved by special devices, *valves*. Owing to their distensibility, the veins play an important role as a variable blood reservoir (*capacitance vessels*). At normal hydrostatic pressure in human beings, the blood volume in the systemic veins is approximately four to five times greater than it is in the corresponding arteries.

TISSUE COMPONENTS

Three basic structural constituents may be recognized in the wall of the blood vessels: the *endothelium* (a specialized epithelial tissue), the *muscular tissue*, and the *connective tissue* with a large elastic component. Along the blood circulatory system, these tissues are unevenly distributed in the vascular wall.

The Endothelium

The sheet of thin squamous epithelial cells that lines the heart is called *cardiac endothelium*, and that lining the blood vessels is called *vascular endothelium*. The heart and the great majority of blood vessels (arteries, arterioles, capillaries of somatic tissues, venules, and veins) are provided with *continuous endothelium*. As opposed to the latter, in visceral capillaries the endothelium displays a relatively large number of small, transcellular openings called *fenestrae*; this endothelium is designated *fenestrated endothelium*. In organs in which extensive exchanges of relatively large particles (liver) or cells (spleen and bone marrow) take place between the vessel lumen and interstitia, large gaps occur; this is called *discontinuous endothelium*. As is the case with other epithelia, the endothelium rests upon a *basal lamina* that varies in thickness and continuity (Table 9-1). The endothelium and its basal lamina constitute the main *permeability barrier*, and the regional differences in their tightness and completeness impart a manifest porosity to the entire vascular wall. In some parts of the microvasculature, the endothelium is surrounded by satellite cells of still unknown function, the *pericytes*. In vessels in which smooth muscle cells exist in close vicinity with the endothelium, *myoendothelial* junctions occur.

The Elastic Elements

Two types of elastic structures may be found: (1) *isolated elastic fibers* dispersed within the layers of the

vascular wall, and (2) *elastic sheets*, organized either as separate units (*internal elastic lamina* and *external elastic lamina*) or as a system of concentric lamellae (*elastic lamellae*) developed in media of large arteries only (see Table 9-1). In the heart, a dense fibroelastic tissue forms the *cardiac skeleton*.

The Muscular Tissue

In the heart the muscular tissue is represented by a special type of *striated muscle cells* (*cardiac muscle*) that constitute the myocardium; in the wall of blood vessels, *smooth muscle cells* appear. The latter are encountered either (1) as organized concentric *layers* helically arranged (well developed in muscular arteries and arterioles) or (2) as longitudinally disposed *bundles* of muscle cells, intercalated with other structures in the vascular wall.

The Connective Tissue

Because of its diverse composition (collagen and reticular fibers,[1] fixed and wandering cells, ground substance), the connective tissue fulfills a complex role (see Table 9-1). Topographically, it is spread throughout the vessel wall with two especially large accumulations: beneath the endothelium, the *subendothelial layer*, and outside the tunica media, the *adventitial layer*. In both locations, the connective-tissue elements are interspersed with bundles of smooth muscle; in adventitia the connective tissue also houses the blood vessels, lymphatics, and nerves of the myocardium or those of the large vessels. An additional concentration of connective tissue is encountered in endocardium as the *subendocardial layer* (Table 9-1). The adventitial layer of connective tissue is relatively much thinner in the microvasculature than in large vessels. All cellular and fibrillar components of the cardiovascular wall are embedded in a highly hydrated gel-like matrix of glucosaminoglycans, which is the ground substance of the local connective tissue. The heart is covered by a coat of *mesothelial cells* representing the visceral leaflet of the pericardium.

---

[1] In light microscopy, special staining procedures reveal a network of relatively thin fibers, presumed to be a special form of collagen. In electron microscopy, the reticular fibers have not been clearly identified.

Functions of Segments of Tissues		Pump	Conducting Vessels	Distributing Vessels
	MORPHOLOGICAL EQUIVALENTS	HEART	ELASTIC ARTERIES	MUSCULAR ARTERIES
Physical partition; semipermeable barrier	ENDOTHELIUM	Continuous	Continuous	Continuous
	BASAL LAMINA	Thin, continuous	Thin, continuous; largely reticular	Thin, continuous; inconspicuous in small arteries
Contraction? phagocytosis	PERICYTES	Absent	Absent	Absent
Support; diffusion regulator medium; local vasoactive mediators; defense system	SUBENDOTHELIAL LAYER	Thick connective tissue, smooth muscle—subendothelial layer Subendocardial layer—loose connective tissue, conducting system, vessels, nerves	Thick connective tissue, smooth muscle (longitudinal)	Thick connective tissue, smooth muscle (longitudinal) at branching sites; thin or absent in small arteries
Elastic tension	INTERNAL ELASTIC LAMINA	Absent	Not distinct in light microscopy; distinct in electron microscopy	Prominent, fenestrated
	ELASTIC LAMELLAE	Dense, compact fibrous tissue (cardiac skeleton)	50 to 70 thick superposed lamellae	Present in large arteries; rare in small arteries
Active tension (contraction)	MUSCLE TISSUE heart = striated vessels = smooth	(Striated fibers; cardiac muscle)	Alternating but fewer than elastic lamellae	30 to 40 concentric layers
Elastic tension	EXTERNAL ELASTIC LAMINA	Absent	Not distinct as separate feature	Present in large arteries; thin or absent in small arteries
Support, vessels and nerves of the wall	ADVENTITIAL LAYER	Subepicardial layer—connective tissue vessels, nerves	Thin, connective tissue, smooth muscle (longitudinal) vessels, nerves	Thick, connective tissue, smooth muscle (longitudinal) vessels, nerves
Gliding surface	SEROSA	Mesothelial cells of visceral pericardium		

BASIC ORGANIZATION: LAYERED STRUCTURE (TUNICS)

The entire cardiovascular system follows a common plan of histological organization: the tissue components described above are arranged in concentric layers. As a result of particular local adaptations, some features of this basic plan are accentuated, reduced, or omitted; moreover, to meet some special local me-chanical or metabolic requirements, certain additional structures may be introduced. But, basically, the layered organization remains. For descriptive purposes, these concentric layers have been classified as three tunics, the boundaries of which are determined by convention. Considered from the lumen outward, tunics are the following:

Tunica intima, or simply the *intima,* contains, at most, the endothelium, the basal lamina (with peri-

Regulating and Resistance Vessels	Exchange Vessels		Returning and Capacitance Vessels		
ARTERIOLES	CAPILLARIES	PERICYTIC VENULES	MUSCULAR VENULES	VEINS	Tunics
Continuous	Continuous, fenestrated, or discontinuous	Continuous, (occasionally fenestrated)	Continuous	Continuous	TUNICA INTIMA heart = endocardium
Inconspicuous in arterioles >50 μm; present in terminal arterioles	Continuous; discontinuous or absent in sinusoids	Thin, continuous	Thin, continuous	Inconspicuous	
Absent	Present	Frequent (almost complete layer)	Rare	Absent	
Thin, connective tissue	Connective tissue (pericapillary space), variable	Thin, connective tissue	Thin, connective tissue	Thin, connective tissue	
Thin, fenestrated in arterioles >50 μm; absent in terminal arterioles	Absent	Absent	Absent	Inconspicuous or discontinuous in small veins; present in large veins	TUNICA MEDIA heart = myocardium
Absent	Absent	Absent	Absent	Absent	
1 to 2 layers	Absent	Absent	1 to 2 thin layers	Few, weak layers	
Not distinct	Absent	Absent	Absent	Absent	
Thin, connective tissue, nerves	Thin, connective tissue	Thin, connective tissue	Thick, connective tissue, nerves	Very thick, connective tissue, smooth muscle (longitudinal) vessels, nerves	TUNICA ADVENTITIA heart = epicardium

cytes), the subendothelial connective tissue, and the internal elastic lamina; in the heart the intima equivalent is the *endocardium*.

Tunica media, or *media*, is composed of muscular cells, elastic lamellae, and the external elastic lamina; in the heart the media is represented by the *myocardium*.

Tunica adventitia, or *adventitia*, contains the adventitial connective tissue with its various components; in the heart this outermost layer, together with the visceral pericardium, is called *epicardium*.

SEGMENTAL DIFFERENTIATIONS: CARDIOVASCULAR SEGMENTS

As previously mentioned, certain physiological conditions differentially prevail along the cardiovascular system. Accordingly, segmental specializations occur that are reflected in some relevant features that characterize each part of the system (Table 9-1). Several criteria (size, prominent structure, or function) have alternatively been used to define and classify these sequential segments, but each classification used is partially arbitrary and thus should not be taken rigidly. There are various transitional forms of vessels, one of which may be transformed with changing local conditions. The following classification will be used throughout this chapter:

Large vessels and their branches larger than 100 μm are visible with the naked eye and accordingly are considered as the *macrovasculature*. All blood vessels with diameters smaller than 100 μm may be seen only through the microscope. This is the case with the arterioles, capillaries, and their emerging venules as well as the arteriovenous anastomoses; together they are referred to as the *microvasculature*.

Blood circulatory system
- Heart
- Blood vessels
  - Elastic arteries (conducting arteries)
  - Muscular arteries (distributing arteries)
  - Arterioles
  - Capillaries
  - Venules
    - Pericytic
    - Muscular
  - Veins
    - Small and medium-sized
    - Large

THE BLOOD VESSELS

TISSUE COMPONENTS OF VASCULAR WALL

The layered structure of blood vessels undergoes segmental differentiations under the influence of the following two groups of functional factors. (1) *Mechanical factors*, primarily the blood pressure, act essentially on large vessels (conducting and distributing arteries and veins), determining the amount and arrangement of their elastic and muscular tissue constituents. (2) *Metabolic factors*, reflecting the local needs of the tissues, operate especially on the microvessels that are instrumental in blood-tissue exchanges, namely, the capillaries and the postcapillary pericytic venules. At this level, the only structural elements represented are the endothelium and its basal lamina. Unlike large vessels that occur as rather isolated anatomical entities, the capillaries and the pericytic venules appear structurally and functionally as part of the tissue they supply (Fig. 9-1).

ENDOTHELIUM

The lining of blood vessels consists of a single layer of flat cells measuring in their thinnest part from 0.1 μm (some capillaries and venules) to 1 μm (some large vessels) in thickness. As revealed by scanning electron microscopy, the endothelial surface may vary in ap-

pearance from smooth with longitudinal folds (aorta) to rough with aggregated fingerlike projections (approximately 300 nm wide $\times$ 3,000 nm long) that increase the surface area (pulmonary artery). The endothelial cells are linked to one another by *intercellular junctions* of two basic types: *occluding (tight) junctions* and *communicating (gap) junctions*.[2] As in other epithelia, the occluding junctions are presumably involved in the mechanical link between adjacent endothelial cells, and the control of permeability along the intercellular spaces. Communicating (gap) junctions represent the structure that allows direct two-way communication between cells. Each vascular segment has characteristically organized endothelial junctions that reflect various degrees of tightness and intercellular coupling along the vasculature (Table 9-2). The morphological evidence indicates that the endothelial junctions are generally more elaborate in arteries than in veins; the strongest junctional organization occurs in arterioles, whereas the loosest is found in venules; endothelial junctions of capillaries are structurally

---

[2] In the special case of the endothelium, the term *gap junction* is particularly confusing, since junctions open to a gap of 20 to 40 Å have been described as occurring instead of tight junctions of the capillary endothelium. Therefore, we use the term *communicating junction (macula communicans, maculae communicantes)*, which describes the macular geometry of the structure and relates to its main function so far established.

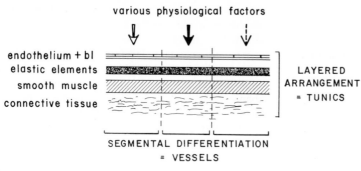

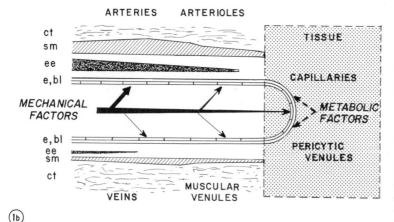

FIGURE 9-1 Diagrammatic representation of the functional factors associated with the layered organization and segmental differentiation of vessel wall. (*a*) Under the influence of various physiological conditions, the basic tissue layers of the vascular wall have undergone characteristic segmental differentiations. (*b*) The mechanical factors act primarily on the large vessels, whereas the metabolic factors are essentially related to the structural characteristics of the intratissular vessels (capillaries and pericytic venules especially) which are involved in the blood-tissue exchanges.

TABLE 9-2 SEGMENTAL VARIATIONS OF THE ENDOTHELIAL JUNCTIONS ALONG THE VASCULATURE (observations made on freeze-fracture preparations)*

	OCCLUDING JUNCTIONS		COMMUNICATING JUNCTIONS (Gap Junctions)
Vascular segments	Ridges/grooves predominantly with particles	Ridges/grooves predominantly without particles	
Arteries	2–4, continuous		Frequent, large, predominantly intercalated
Arterioles	2–6, continuous		Frequent, large, predominantly intercalated
Capillaries	2–5, continuous or staggered and quasi-continuous		Absent
Venules			
Pericytic		1–4, discontinuous	Absent
Muscular		1–5, discontinuous	Rare, small, isolated
Veins	2–5, continuous	1–4, discontinuous	Rare, small, predominantly isolated

* Adapted from Maia Simionescu, N. Simionescu, and G. E. Palade, *Thromb. Res.*, Suppl. II, **8**:247–256 (1976).

similar to the occluding junctions of the arterioles.

The endothelial cell is an approximately uniform repeating unit, polygonal in shape, about 10 to 15 μm wide by 25 to 50 μm long. The cells and their elongate prominent nuclei are oriented in the long axis of the vessel presumably arranged in longitudinal vector fields generated by shearing effects of the blood flow. The most characteristic feature is the presence of numerous, uniform (600 to 700 Å in diameter) infoldings of cell membrane called *plasmalemmal vesicles* (Palade). They are often referred to as pinocytotic vesicles. The term is questionable inasmuch as the vesicles are not engaged in true pinocytosis; in general, the endocytosis appears to be a secondary activity of the endothelial cells. Plasmalemmal vesicles are open either on the blood front or on the tissue front or they lie free in the cytoplasm of the endothelial cells; their fractional frequency in these three locations is almost even. As established for the capillary endothe-

lium, the fractional volume occupied by vesicles may amount to about one-third of the total cell volume. Vesicles are active in the transendothelial transport of some water-soluble molecules. They either can function as isolated units shuttling from one cell front to another or can fuse and form patent transendothelial channels (Fig. 9-22a). As suggested by the occurrence of transitional forms, the vesicles appear capable of forming fenestrae (Fig. 9-2). All these features—vesi-

FIGURE 9-2 Blood capillary: endothelium (rat tongue). Morphological modulations of plasmalemmal vesicles suggesting stages in the discharge process of vesicular contents. (a) Fusion of vesicular membrane with the cell membrane forming a five-layered structure. (b) Intermediary stage between (a) and (c) in the progressive elimination of membrane layers. (c) Vesicles on the blood front of the endothelium: the openings are provided with diaphragms (arrows) which display a central knob (arrowhead). ×240,000. (From G. E. Palade and R. R. Bruns, *J. Cell Biol.*, **37:**633, 1968). (d) Blood capillary (mouse intestinal mucosa): the attenuated part of the endothelium showing a channel (c) provided with two diaphragms (arrows), and a fenestra closed by a diaphragm (arrow). Note the presence of a central knob in each diaphragm (arrowheads). (From F. Clementi and G. E. Palade, *J. Cell Biol.*, **41:**33, 1969.)

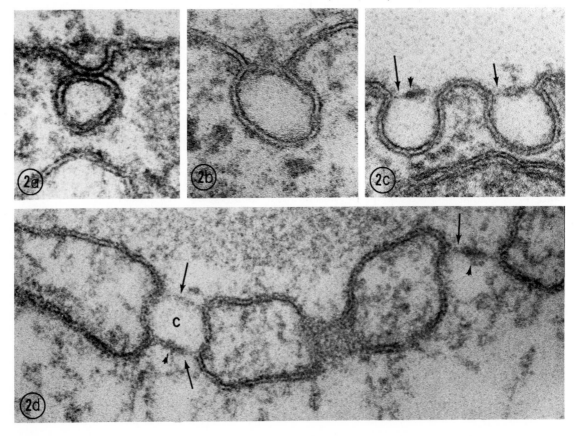

cles, channels, and fenestrae—represent different aspects of a common dynamic system. By their considerable aggregate inner volume, the vesicles may also represent a sort of transient and dispersed reservoir for plasma. In some capillaries, the endothelial cell displays several openings appearing either as uniform fenestrae or nonuniform large gaps (Fig. 9-22b and c) (see section on Capillaries).

Besides the nucleus, the endothelial cells contain the common set of *organelles:* rough endoplasmic reticulum, attached and free ribosomes, Golgi complex, a few mitochondria, a few cisternae of smooth endoplasmic reticulum, centrosphere regions with two centrioles, lysosomes (more frequent in arteries), multivesicular bodies, and glycogen. Thin and thick *filaments* are occasionally concentrated either in the junctional zone or at the albuminal cell membrane; the latter are sometimes in phase with similar extracellular fibrils. Indirect evidence (nuclear pinching and cellular shortening with intercellular gaps) suggests that in response to certain stimuli, the endothelial cells may contract. Peculiar rod-shaped granules, 0.1 μm thick on 3 μm long, consisting of several tubules (approximately 150 Å thick) embedded in a dense matrix, have been described by Weibel and Palade in arterial endothelia of human beings, rats, and amphibia and were later found in other vessels and other species as well. The significance of these organelles is unknown, but they are a reliable tag for the identification of isolated endothelial cells.

Qualitative *cytochemical* investigations revealed the presence in the endothelial cell of a relatively large spectrum of enzymes involved in activities such as anaerobic glycolysis, oxidative phosphorylation, and desulfation. Some enzymes are preferentially detected in plasmalemmal vesicles, for example, ATPase, nucleoside phosphatase, and 5'-nuceotidase (this localization is presumed to reflect the vesicles' involvement in the metabolism of some vasoactive substances). The catecholamine-sensitive adenyl cyclase found in both vesicles and junctions might be related to their participation in hormone transport. The endothelial surface is presumed to contain receptor sites for angiotensin.

The endothelium plays an important role in hemostasis as indicated by the localization of tissue factor (thromboplastin) on plasmalemma detected by using perioxidase-conjugated antibodies. Small vessels show more plasminogen activator than do large vessels and veins show more than do arteries. The antihemophilic factor VIII, and blood group substances A, B, and H were also detected in endothelium. En-

dothelial cells are able to synthesize and secrete sulfate mucopolysaccharides of heparin type as well as take up and utilize long-chain saturated fatty acids; the arterial cells can incorporate more labeled [^{3}H]-oleic acid than can the venous ones.

The endothelium is a slowly renewing population of cells that rarely divide (for example, the estimated life span of aortic endothelial cells in rabbit is 100 to 180 days). Endothelial cells of veins have a greater mitotic potential than those of arteries. Regeneration of damaged (for example, injury) or missing endothelium (for example, synthetic grafts) is assumed to occur from various sources such as circulating blood cells, fibroblasts, smooth muscle cells, adjacent endothelium, or undifferentiated cells from the subendothelial layers.

The surface of endothelium is different at the blood and tissue front. At the blood surface, the endothelial cell membrane is associated with a fuzzy coating 50 to 60 Å thick that usually extends into vesicles. This coat was called *endocapillary, or endoendothelial layer,* and by indirect evidence (staining with ruthenium red), it was assumed to consist of mucopolysaccharides or of an adsorbed film of fibrin. As in blood cells, the luminal surface of the endothelial cell is negatively charged, thus preventing intravascular aggregation and agglutination.

At the tissue surface, a rather amorphous matrix 300 to 500 Å wide separates the endothelium from the fine microfibrillar *basal lamina.* This is about 400 to 800 Å thick; and as in other epithelia, it is probably produced by the endothelium itself. The basal lamina is made up chiefly of type $\alpha 1$[III] and [IV]$_3$ collagen, and its inability to polymerize into striated fibrils may result from its high carbohydrate content. In renal glomerular capillaries, the basal lamina is fairly thick and has special chemical characteristics. Owing to its high content of collagen, the basal lamina can be digested by collagenase. After such treatment, endothelial cells from various vessels (human umbilical vein, animal arteries, and veins) can be isolated and grown in tissue culture for in vitro studies.

The endothelial cell may establish close apposition with the processes of neighboring *pericytes* (Figure 9-26). In vessels provided with an internal elastica, the endothelial cell may extend processes that penetrate the elastica and make close contact with the adjoining smooth muscle cells (*myoendothelial junction*) (Figs. 9-15 and 9-20).

VASCULAR SMOOTH MUSCLE

This tissue occurs in all vessels except capillaries and pericytic venules where its place is taken by pericytes, probably a variant of muscle cells. In contrast to other vertebrates, smooth muscle represents the only cellular element in the media of mammalian elastic arteries, and it is the prevailing component of muscular arteries and arterioles. Commonly, smooth muscle cells are frequent and arranged in helical layers in media, and are less numerous and usually longitudinally oriented in intima and adventitia. Additional muscle cells can appear in the intima during aging and under certain pathological conditions. Each cell is surrounded by the basal lamina it secretes and by various amounts of collagen fibers which may anchor the cell to neighboring elastic fibers (Figs. 9-3 and 9-4). Such attachments allow the transmission of the contracting force to the network of elastic fibers. Vascular smooth muscle cells are frequently held together by *communicating (gap) junctions* (Figs. 9-3 to 9-5), generally more frequent in arterioles and small arteries than in large vessels. These junctions may be instrumental in the conduction of impulses and transmission of information among cells. For the organization of smooth muscle cell in general, see Chap. 7. The vascular smooth muscle cells are smaller (25 to 80 μm) than the smooth muscle cells in other locations. The large population of *sarcolemmal vesicles* increases the surface area by approximately 25 percent. They are organized in characteristic longitudinal rows with vesicle-free areas in between (Fig. 9-6). The latter may correspond to regions of attachment of myofilaments and dense bodies. A salient component are the *lysosomes* that may accumulate cholesterol during the atheromatous process. Vascular smooth muscle cells behave phenotypically as fibroblasts during much of gestation; under various stimuli, they are capable of producing most components of vessel walls—elastic fibers, microfibrilar proteins, collagen, glucosaminoglycans, and more muscle cells. Like that of skeletal muscle, the activity of vascular smooth muscle is initiated by nervous stimuli. Not all cells have an *innervation;* excitation may spread between adjacent cells through communicating (gap) junctions. The distance observed between the unmyelinated axon and sarcolemma is larger than in the motor end plate of striated muscle (approximately 500 Å). Perturbations of the vessel wall (for example, mechanical stress, injury, ischemia, inflammation), drugs, hormones, etc., may stimulate migration into the intima and proliferation of smooth muscle cells, which, leads, in turn, to an *intimal thickening,* a characteristic feature of the atheromatous plaque. A similar change occurs in aging, but the media itself is not altered.

VASCULAR CONNECTIVE TISSUE

Elimination of muscle activity by treating aortic segments with potassium thiocyanate does not alter the static mechanical property of the media, which is, therefore, handled mainly by connective tissue components. These are present in the walls of the vessels in amounts and proportions that vary according to the local functional requirements and the interrelations with other tissues, especially the endothelium and smooth muscle.

Fibers

Elastic fibers secure the resilient rebound of the stretched vascular wall. Collagen fibers impart the tensile strength that supports and binds together coherent groups of other structural elements.

Elastic fibers are either *isolated* or, more frequently, in *sheets* of several micrometers in diameter. The sheets appear either as a single feature (internal elastic lamina, external elastic lamina, or the scattered elastic bundles of the adventitia) or as lamellae organized in a regular alternating pattern with the muscle cells throughout the entire media. These lamellae are extensively fenestrated and partially connected in a three-dimensional network. Two constituents have been recognized in elastic fibers: the amorphous-appearing *elastin,* which provides the elastometric properties of the fibers; and the *microfibrils,* the significance of which is less known (Fig. 9-4). Elastic fibers are oriented in different directions so that mechanical stresses are complexly balanced. The occurrence of elastic fibers along the vasculature is schematically tabulated in Table 9-1.

FIGURE 9-3 Smooth muscle cells of a tunica media of rat mesenteric artery; cells display frequent intercellular junctions (*mj*). Elastic elements appear either as isolated elastic fibers (*ef*) or wide elastic lamellae (*el*); microfibrils (*mf*) can also be detected. c, collagen; *sv*, sarcolemmal vesicles; G, Golgi complex; *ds*, dense segments of myofilaments (*m*). ×18,000.

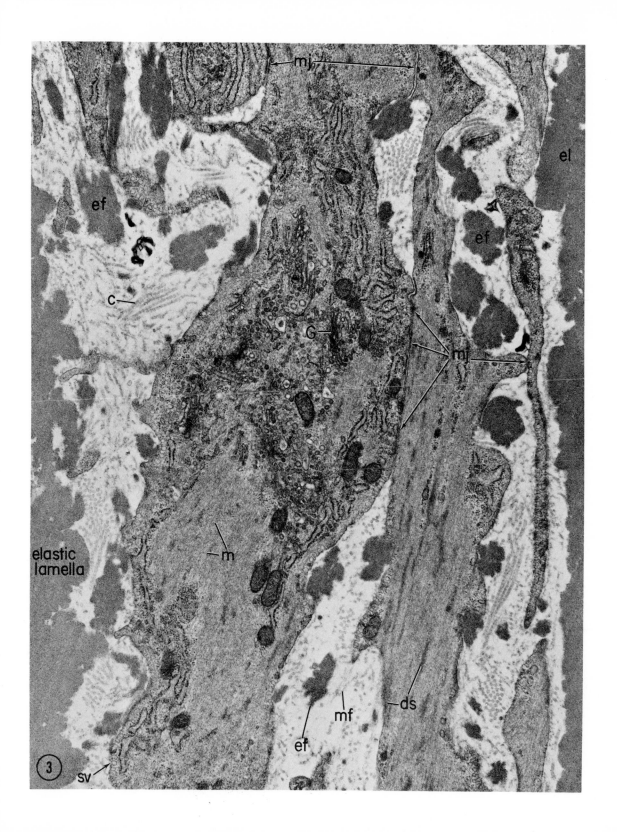

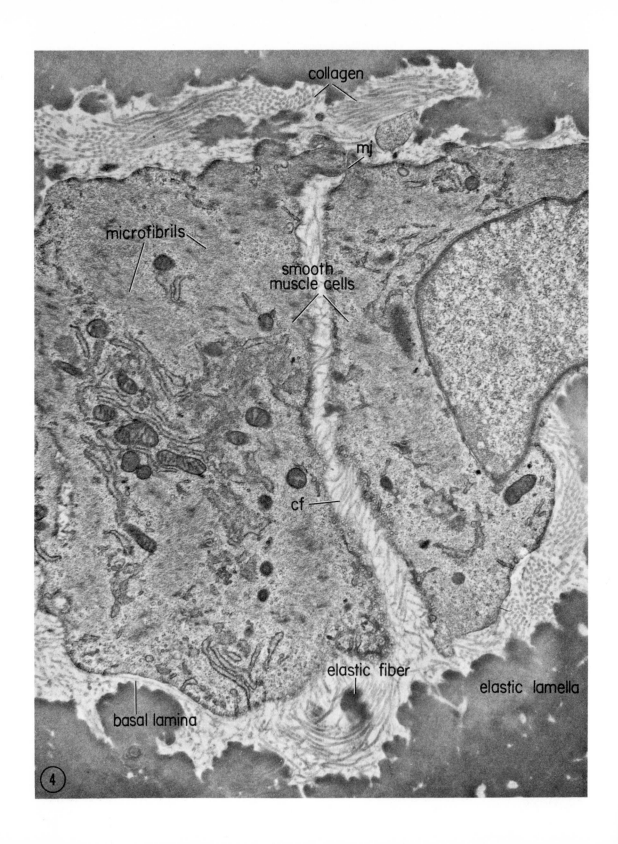

collagen

mj

microfibrils

smooth
muscle cells

cf

elastic fiber

elastic lamella

basal lamina

4

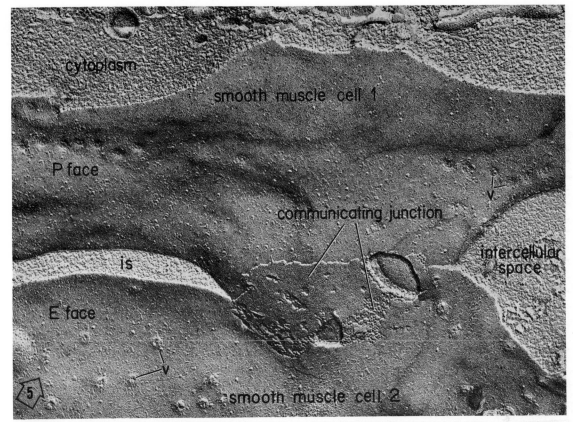

FIGURE 9-5 Freeze-cleaved preparation of aortic intima displaying a communicating (gap) junction between two adjacent smooth muscle cells. The junction appears as clusters of particles on the P face and as complementary pits on the E face. *is*, intercellular spaces; *v*, vesicle opening. ×75,000.

Collagen fibers are found throughout the vascular wall concentrated between muscle cells, in adventitia, and in some subendothelial spaces (Figs. 9-4, 9-10, and 9-22, respectively). In human aorta, collagen and elastin each represent 20 percent of the dry weight, whereas the vena cava contains about seven times more collagen (types I, III, and IV) than elastin. Preliminary information indicates that the collagen which prevails in arteries is collagen of type $\alpha 1$[III] characterized by smaller quantities of galactose or glucosylgalactose linked to hydroxylysine. Disorders in elastic and collagen metabolism are involved both in aging (increased cross-linking of collagen) and in major vascular disease such as atherosclerosis (ab-

normal pattern of elastin cross-linking) and arteriosclerosis) (increased collagen synthesis caused by a high proline-hydroxylase activity).

In diabetes, the thickening of endothelial basal lamina is presumed to be the result of a retardation in collagen degradation due to alteration in its glycosylation.

Ground Substance

Extracellular spaces of the vessel wall are occupied by a continuous but heterogeneous gel of proteoglycans. Some capillaries are surrounded by a relatively thin layer of ground substance; others can be considered embedded in the matrix gel, which may be responsible for the patency and apparent rigidity of capillaries under differential pressures in comparison with the distensibility of arteries and arterioles. The ground substance contains domains of different composition and hydration. The concentration of glucosamino-

FIGURE 9-4 Structural connections between two neighboring smooth muscle cells (the media of rat aorta), represented in this preparation by a narrow junction (*mj*) and frequent bridges of collagen fibers (*cf*). ×18,000.

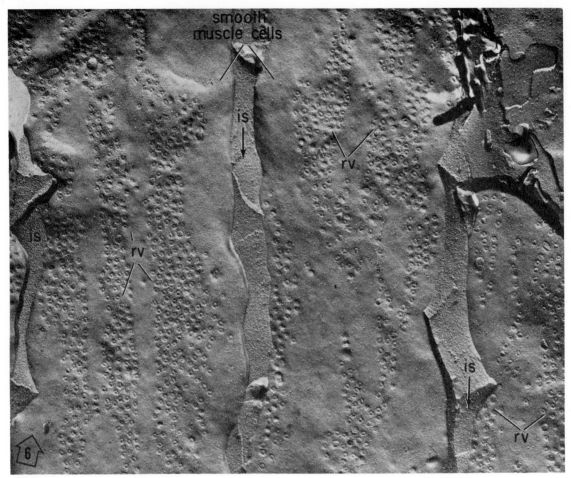

FIGURE 9-6 Replica of a freeze-cleaved sarcolemma of three adjacent smooth muscle cells of an arteriole. Vesicle openings are characteristically arranged in longitudinal parallel ribbons (*rv*) alternating with vesicle-free areas. Compare with Fig. 9-45. *is*, intercellular spaces. ×27,000.

glycans is higher in arterial than in venous tissue. In the former, chondroitin sulfate prevails; and in the latter, dermatan sulfate. The ground substance contributes to the physical properties of the walls of the vessels and is expected to affect diffusion differently from domain to domain and hence permeability across the wall.

Connective Tissue Cells

Located in the partition between internal medium and surrounding tissues and organs, the connective tissue cells of the vascular wall constitute a pluripotential system. In locations where the adventitia is continuous with the connective elements of the surrounding tissue, the boundary between the two compartments is arbitrary. This complex population is involved in the following important functions. (1) They play a part in the production, storage, and secretion of local *vasoactive mediators,* such as histamine and serontonin, primarily by the mast cells. (These are very frequently located along the microvasculature and their action seems to be particularly efficient on the pericytic venules.) (2) *Phagocytosis* is largely performed by *macrophages* almost constantly patrolling along the vessels. (3) Local *immunological reactions* may involve plasma cells and eosinophils. (4) *Secretion of connective tissue fibers* is carried out prominently by *fibroblasts,* which also represent a pluripotential pool for cell formation and local repair (for example, endothelial regeneration). In human beings, the main cellular component of the arterial adventitia are the fibroblasts, which are absent in the media.

NUTRITION OF THE VASCULAR WALL

Blood Vessels

The vascular wall is provided with its own nutrient vessels, called _vasa vasorum_. The extent of the intramural vascular bed is determined by (1) the tissue composition of the wall, (2) participation of the luminal blood in the supply of the wall, and (3) the wall compression under the blood pressure. In large vessels with well-developed media, the intima receives its nutrient material by diffusion from the luminal blood,

as does the microvasculature. On the adventitia (Fig. 9-7) and in some arteries, the outer layers of the media (in which tissue compression is lower than capillary blood pressure) are provided with vasa vasorum. The rest of the wall is nourished by diffusion. Vasa vasorum of veins are more abundant and penetrate much closer to the intima than do those of arteries.

Lymphatics

The lymphatic vessels are commonly encountered in the walls of large vessels in which they follow a distribution similar to that of the intramural blood supply. Lymphatics are more frequent and go deeper into the

FIGURE 9-7 Low-power electron micrograph of the adventitia of a muscular artery (rat mesenteric artery) showing some connective tissue constituents, vasa vasorum, and nerves. ×5000.

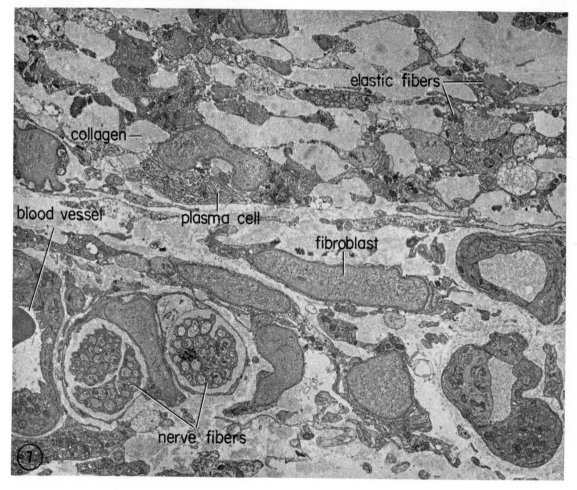

media of veins than arteries. The interstitial fluid circulates freely throughout fenestrated elastic lamellae. Favored by the prevailing blood pressure, both the interstitial fluids and the lymphatic flow go from within the wall outward.

Vascular Nerves

Except for capillaries and probably pericytic venules, all blood vessels have a relatively rich supply of nerves. Bundles or single nerve fibers are found in the adventitia (Fig. 9-7) and may extend their terminal processes into the media; a few of them can be traced as far as the intima. *Unmyelinated axons,* which are vasomotor (arising from the sympathetic ganglia), form plexuses in adventitia; and some of them end with fine knoblike terminations close to the muscle cells. A particularly rich innervation of the arterioles has been noticed. There is no accurate estimate of the ratio of nerve endings to muscle cells, and it is still questionable whether each muscle unit is innervated or whether the stimuli pass to neighboring muscle cells by other mechanisms. *Afferent myelinated* fibers (representing the dendrites of spinal or cranial ganglion cells) terminate in free sensory endings, found mostly in the adventitia. Small intraadventitial ganglia occur in aorta, coronary, coeliac, and mesenteric arteries. Sensory features are particularly well developed in some arteries: they are especially sensitive to pressure changes (*baroreceptors*) or to modifications in the chemical composition of the blood (*chemoreceptors*) (see under Special Sensory Tissues of Arteries).

ARTERIES

The dimensions of arteries and veins, unlike those of the microvascular components, are largely species-related and depend primarily on the total blood volume. In humans, despite their low number, the relatively large dimensions of arteries result in a blood volume of approximately 2 percent in the aorta and approximately 9 percent in the rest of the systemic arteries, whereas the pulmonary arteries contain almost 8 percent of the whole blood volume.

According to their prevalent tissue component, the arteries can be classified as *elastic arteries* and *muscular arteries* that continue the former.

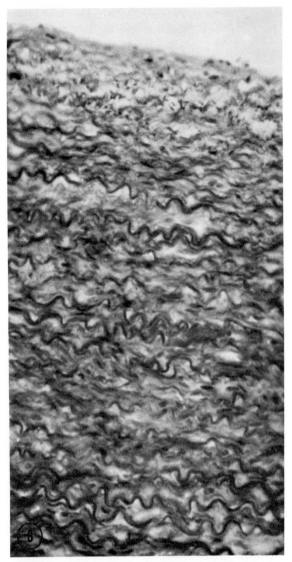

FIGURE 9-8 Photomicrograph of a cross section through the wall of human aorta. Elastic tissue has been darkly stained with resorcin fuchsin. Note the high frequency of concentric elastic lamellae. ×3000.

Elastic Arteries

Large vessels conducting blood from the heart to the muscular (distributing) arteries are characterized by a high content of elastic fibers, which justifies the name elastic arteries. To this category belong aorta, pulmonary, innominate (brachiocephalic), common carotid, subclavian (including its vertebral and internal thoracic branches), and common iliac arteries. In comparison with their large lumen, the wall is relatively thin, being less than one-tenth of the vessel diameter.

The *intima* is about 100 to 130 μm thick and represents approximately one-sixth of the wall thickness. The *endothelial* cells are rich in plasmalemmal vesicles and contain a variable amount of cytoplasmic filaments. The cells are extensively linked by a strongly organized combination of occluding (tight) junctions with closely intercalated communicating (gap) junctions (Fig. 9-11 and Table 9-2). The permeability characteristics of the arterial endothelium are not yet well defined, and conflicting observations have been reported, especially concerning a possible intercellular pathway for probe molecules as large as 50 to 60 Å (e.g., horseradish perioxidase). The vesicles appear to be active in the transendothelial transport of a large range of molecular species. The *basal lamina* is thin and of prominent reticular aspect. In humans, about

one-fourth of the total wall thickness is represented by the *subendothelial layer*. It contains loose connective tissue, elastic fibers oriented longitudinally, scattered fibroblasts, and a few elongated, mostly longitudinally running smooth muscle cells. The *elastica interna* is less distinct as a separate feature in light microscopy (Fig. 9-8); in electron microscopy, however, it appears as the first elastic lamella that merges with tunica media (Fig. 9-9).

The *media* is the thickest tunic: in humans it measures 500 μm and is essentially composed of 40 to 70 concentric elastic sheets, disposed 5 to 15 μm apart. Each sheet is 2 to 3 μm thick and consists of broad interwoven fenestrated bands and a few connecting bundles located between sheets (Fig. 9-10). The latter are interspersed with the ground substance in which lie elongated and branched smooth muscle cells bound to the adjoining elastic lamellae by micro-

FIGURE 9-9 Low-power electron micrograph of a portion of the wall of rat aorta in cross section. The vessel wall is formed by interspersed layers of elastic lamellae (*el*), and smooth muscle cells (*sm*). e, endothelium; A, adventitia; I, intima; M, media; vv, vasa vasorum; c, collagen. ×1000.

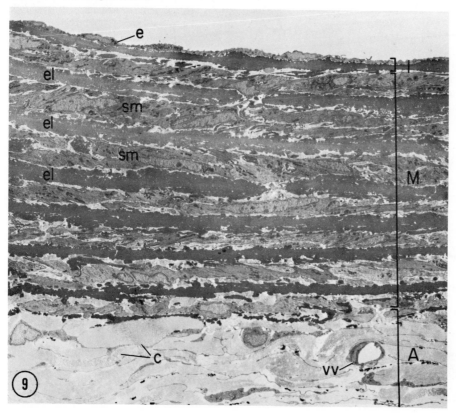

fibrils and collagen. (Types I, III, and IV are present in normal aortas.)

The *adventitia* is relatively thin and not highly organized. It contains bundles of collagen with longitudinal-helical courses, a few elastic fibers similarly arranged, fibroblasts, mast cells, and rare longitudinal smooth muscle cells (Fig. 9-10). The *elastica externa*, not always evident under light microscopic examination, appears at high magnification as a discontinuous lamella. The *vasa vasorum* and *lymphatics* are detected only as far as the outer half of the tunica media, sometimes accompanied by myelinated or non-myelinated *nerves*. The adventitia merges with the surrounding connective tissue. As they branch into smaller vessels, the structure of elastic arteries gradually changes to that characteristic of the muscular type.

Muscular Arteries

The general organization of the vessels that conduct blood to various regions and organs of the body is

FIGURE 9-10 Electron micrograph of an area of the outer part of the aortic media. Note the interspersed layers of smooth muscle cells (*sm*), which are the sole cellular component of this tunic, and the elastic lamellae (*el*). The outermost lamella represents actually the external elastic lamina (*ee*). *c*, collagen; *f*, fibroblast. ×6000.

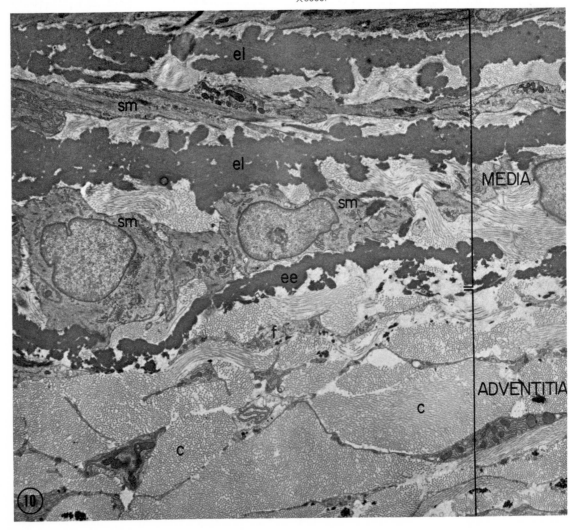

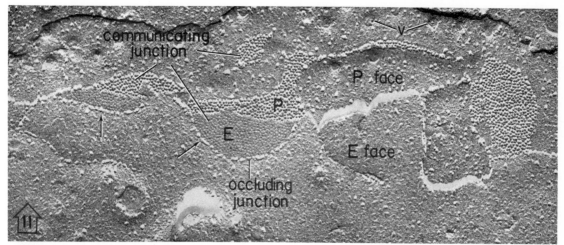

FIGURE 9-11 Endothelial junction complex of the aorta as revealed by freeze-fracture preparations. The cleavage plane exposes an occluding junction with large communicating (gap) junctions fitted within its meshes. On the E face (*E*), the grooves of the occluding junction (*arrows*) are marked by protruding, elongated particles, which tend to form continuous rows. *v*, openings of plasmalemmal vesicles. ×90,000. (From Maia Simionescu, N. Simionescu, and G. E. Palade, *J. Cell Biol.*, **86:**705, 1976.)

FIGURE 9-12 Longitudinal section through a muscular artery (rat external iliac artery). The vascular wall consists predominantly of layers of smooth muscle cells (*sm*) interspersed with discontinuous elastic lamellae (*el*). Note the conspicuous internal elastic lamina (*ie*). A, adventitia; e, endothelium; *rbc*, red blood cells; I, intima; M, media. ×600.

similar to that of elastic arteries, but the proportions of cell types and fibers are distinctive. The most abundant component is the muscular tissues (Figs. 9-12 and 9-13), the contraction and relaxation of which control the vascular lumen thus regulating the blood flow. The great majority of arteries belong to this category, with the exception of those mentioned as elastic arteries. The popliteal artery, in spite of its distal location as compared to the femoral artery, has predominantly an elastic structure. In humans the muscular arteries vary largely from 1 cm to 0.3 mm in diameter. Without any clear-cut boundaries, they are often arbitrarily subdivided into large, medium-sized, and small arteries, or only into the last two categories. In most cases, the

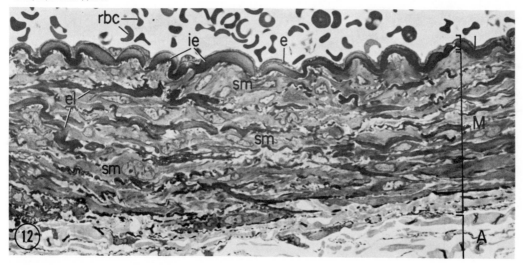

wall thickness represents one-fourth of the vessel diameter.

The *intima.* The *endothelium* is similar to that of elastic arteries. In small arteries, processes of the endothelial cells extend through the fenestrations of elastica interna and contact underlying smooth muscle cells (Figs. 9-14 and 9-15). Through the same openings, the ground substance of intima is in continuity with that of the media. Two types of junctions link the endothelial cells of muscular arteries: communicating (gap) junctions and occluding junctions that resemble those described in elastic arteries (Table 9-2). Junctions seem to undergo quickly reversible loosening or widening under various influences (diabetes, nicotine, epinephrine, angiotensin II, serotonin, and so forth). As a result, lipoproteins and other large molecules can be "trapped" by the vascular wall.

The *basal lamina* is thin and generally continuous in large arteries.

The *subendothelial layer* diminishes in thickness with the decreasing size of the vessel. It comprises collagen fibers and smooth muscle cells organized in longitudinal bundles in some specialized arteries (Fig. 9-14). At branching sites of some vessels (coronary, thyroid, renal, splenic, intracranial, nasal mucosa), protruding "intimal cushions" have been described. The *elastica interna* is generally prominent and fenestrated.

The *media* is mostly muscular, and in humans consists of 10 to 40 helical layers concentrically arranged. Their number can decrease to 3 to 4 in small arteries, being larger in the arteries of the lower extremities than in the upper ones. *Muscular cells* are surrounded by basal laminae and collagen fibers and are interspersed with isolated *elastic fibers or lamellae,* fenestrated and helically oriented (Figs. 9-13 and

FIGURE 9-13 Low-power electron micrograph of a cross section through a muscular artery (rat mesenteric artery). Note the predominant muscular content of the media, the relatively rare and largely fenestrated elastic lamellae, and the wide adventitia, only a part of which is presented in this area. ×1800.

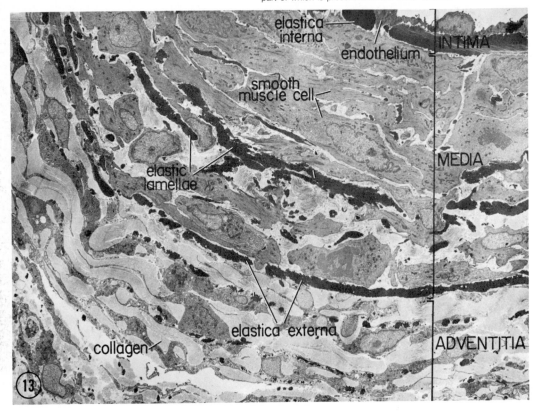

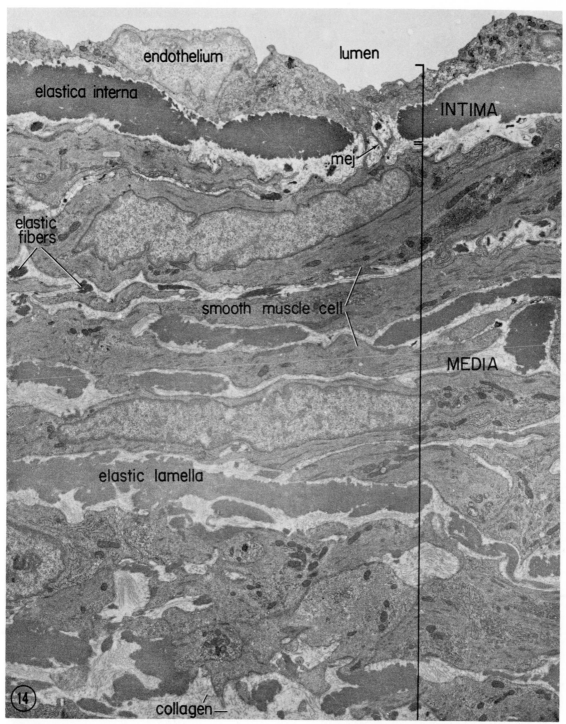

FIGURE 9-14 Muscular artery: detail of the inner part of the vascular wall. Through a fenestra of elastica interna, processes of the endothelial cell establish a myoendothelial junction (*mej*) with the adjacent smooth muscle cell belonging to the media. In the latter, the prevalent muscular tissue is interspersed with less frequent and discontinuous elastic lamellae. ×6000.

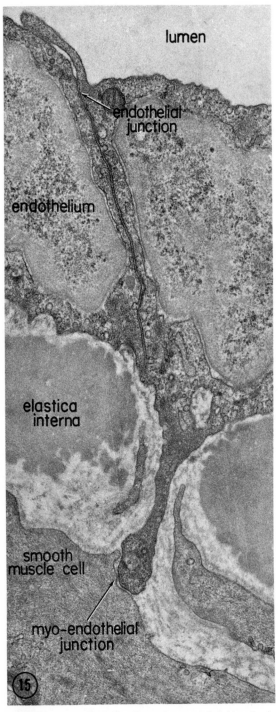

FIGURE 9-15 Endothelial junction and myoendothelial junction in a muscular artery. The latter occurs through a fenestra of the elastica interna. ×25,000.

9-14). The smooth muscles are the only cellular component of media (see Vascular Smooth Muscle, above).

The *adventitia* is thick with an inner dense and an outer loose part; it contains bundles of collagen and elastic fibers longitudinal or helically arranged, sparse fibroblasts, adipose cells, and a few longitudinal smooth muscle fibers.

The *elastica externa* is thin and discontinuous, especially in small vessels. The adventitia is provided with *vasa vasorum, lymphatics,* and *nerves* that penetrate to the external layers of media.

Transitional Segments of Arteries

The gradual transition from elastic to muscular arteries can be well recognized in the so-called arteries of mixed type (for example, axillary, carotid, common iliac arteries). In some places an abrupt structural change occurs: arteries with such short transitional segments are designated as arteries of hybrid type (for example, visceral branches of abdominal aorta). In their media, an internal muscular layer coexists over a certain distance with an external elastic layer.

Specialized Arteries

As a result of adaptations to local functional requirements, certain arteries display characteristic structural modifications: overall increase or decrease in the thickness of the vascular wall or particular development of either the muscular or elastic components.

An *overall augmentation* of the wall thickness occurs in the coronary arteries subjected to high pressure as well as in the arteries of the lower extremity in comparison with their analog in the upper limb. An overall reduction of the vessel-wall thickness is encountered in arteries protected by the skull from external mechanical forces (cerebral and dural arteries) and in regions of low blood pressure (arteries of the lung).

Well-developed bundles of *longitudinal muscle fibers* in both the intima and media are found in arteries subjected to repeated bending—carotid, axillary, common iliac, and popliteal arteries. Bundles of longitudinal muscle may be preferentially developed in the *intima* (occipital, palmar, uterine, penil arteries after puberty), *media* [penil arteries, splenic, mesenteric superior, renal and umbilical artery (the latter exhibits two layers, an inner longitudinal and an outer circular)], or in the *adventitia* (lingual, splenic, renal). *Cardiac muscle* extends into the wall of the roots of pulmonary artery and aorta.

Elastic components are relatively well developed

in arteries within the skull and in renal and popliteal arteries; the elastica interna is lacking in the umbilical artery.

Blood vessels, lymphatics, and nerves of arteries See Nutrition of the Vascular Wall, above.

Special Sensory Tissues of Arteries

Besides sensory endings dispersed within the wall of arteries, highly specialized tissues which monitor the blood by sensors particularly receptive to changes in blood pressure (*baroreceptors*) or in blood chemical composition (*chemoreceptors*) have been differentiated in certain regions of the arterial tree. In lower vertebrates, special vascular receptors are present in each of the branchial arch arteries; in human beings, such sensory organs are found in arteries that constitute persistent parts of the branchial arches.

As *baroreceptor,* the *carotid sinus* represents an enlargement at the bifurcation of the common carotid and of the origin of the internal carotid artery. At this level, the outer part of the thinned tunica media exhibits a rich network of large nerve endings. Most of them make contacts with the cells of adventitia. Pressure changes generate nerve impulses that are conducted by the glossopharyngeal nerve to the medulla. In addition to the carotid sinus, other similar but less easily recognizable areas have been described in the common carotid artery and great veins close to the heart. To an increase in blood pressure, the pressor-receptor mechanisms respond by an inhibition of heart action and by general vasodilation.

Chemoreceptors are primarily represented by the *carotid bodies* located at the bifurcation of each common carotid, and by the *aortic bodies.* On the right side, the aortic body lies in the angle between common carotid and subclavian; on the left, it is found on the aorta, medial to the origin of the subclavian artery. These small organs consist of cords and clumps of epithelial-like cells richly supplied with nerve endings and intimately associated with numerous fenestrated or sinusoid capillaries. Two types of parenchymal cells have been distinguished: the glomus cell, or *type I,* which occurs in clusters and contains many small vacuoles and secretory-type granules (rich in catecholamines and 5-hydroxytryptamine); and *type II cells,* which are free of granules. The function of these two categories of cells is still unclear. Changes in blood pH, oxygen, and carbon-dioxide tension generate nerve impulses that are conducted through the glossopharyngeal and vagus nerves to the central

nervous system, which initiates adequate respiratory and cardiovascular responses.

Age-related Changes in Arteries

The structural pattern of arteries, as described above, is gradually achieved through a continuous process of differentiation that extends to the age of 20 to 25 in humans (for example, the aorta is a muscular vessel at birth). Starting with middle age, a relative increase commonly occurs in elastic fibers, collagen, and mucopolysaccharides, with a concomitant reduction of smooth muscle and water content. This results in an overall stiffness, more pronounced in elastic than in muscular arteries; such a change is minimal or absent in small muscular arteries and arterioles. Each artery has its own way and schedule of differentiation and aging. At old age, regressive physiologic changes cannot be clearly distinguished from similar pathologic changes that lead to arterosclerosis or atherosclerosis. Modifications at the boundary between normal involution and pathologic condition include an increase in thickness of the vascular wall, an increase in the number of cross-linkages between collagen fibers, a relative decrease in endoplasmic reticulum of smooth muscle cells, a patchy, irregular thickening of the intima (by migration and proliferation of smooth muscle and accumulation of their products), a deposition of calcium salts and lipids in the media of muscular arteries, and a splitting of the elastica interna. The arteries most affected are the aorta, coronary, and brain vessels. It may thus be truly said that one is as old as one's arteries.

MICROVASCULATURE

The microvasculature is the connection site between arterial and venous circulation. Small arteries branch into tiny ramifications, the *arterioles,* which resolve into a fine network of *capillaries,* from which the blood is drained by emerging *venules* (Fig. 9-16). The blood can be also shunted from arterioles directly to venules via *arteriovenous anastomoses.* All these sequential segments of the terminal vascular bed which constitute the microvasculature[3] may be seen only through the microscope.

---

[3] According to other classifications, the microvascular system contains blood vessels below 500 μm diameter, the larger ones being assigned to the macrovascular system.

In mammals, the light microscope observations carried out in vivo under routine or special conditions (phase contrast, interference, fluorescence) have shown that the microvascular bed has a very complex architecture according to the nature and activity of the surrounding tissues to which the microvessels functionally belong. Usually the capillary bed is a network supplied by several arterioles and drained by multiple venules (mesentery). In some tissues (muscle), a terminal arteriole supplies groups, or "tufts," of capillaries. Besides the short arteriovenous anastomoses, some "preferential channels" that can shunt even earlier the true capillary network (for example, muscle) may also occur. The organization and the structure of the capillaries vary characteristically in the vascular beds of each organ (for example, the brain, heart, lung, liver, spleen, kidney, placenta, and so forth).

Various microvascular patterns are encountered: (1) a common sequence arteriole–capillary–venule; (2) a shunt, such as arteriole–arteriovenous anastomosis–venule (arteriovenous anastomoses can occur in a specific organ, the glomus); (3) a special pattern: capillaries–veins–capillaries [such vessels interposed between two capillary beds define a *venous portal system* (as in the liver and in the hypothalamo-hypophyseal complex)] or (4) a variant of the latter in which the sequence is: arteriole (afferent)–capillaries–arteriole (efferent)–capillaries, termed an *arterial por-*

tal system, or *rete mirabile* (renal glomeruli, pancreatic islands).

In humans, the microvasculature of the systemic circulation includes 10 percent of the blood volume: the corresponding figure for the pulmonary circulation is only 4 percent. The transition from macrovasculature to microvasculature is gradual and there is no general agreement about the limits between the two territories.

ARTERIOLES

The arterioles are the smallest arteries, the media of which is reduced to a single or double layer of muscle cells (Fig. 9-17a). The vessels' diameter, which is commonly less than 300 μm, may decrease in the proximity of capillaries to 75 to 30 μm, especially when this terminal part is provided with a muscular, sphincterlike structure (*precapillary sphincter area*) (Fig. 9-19). The wall thickness may be as much as one-half the inner diameter.

The *intima* includes endothelium, basal lamina, and a subendothelial layer. The endothelial cells are linked by strongly organized junctions basically similar to those found in arteries (Fig. 9-36a). Basal processes of the endothelial cells penetrate through fenestrae of the elastic lamina to form myoendothelial junctions with adjacent smooth muscle cells (Fig. 9-20). The *basal lamina* is thin, and less distinct in arterioles larger than 50 μm in diameter. The *subendothelial*

FIGURE 9-16 Photomicrograph of a microvascular unit in rat omentum. The arteriole branches into a network of capillaries that are collected by a venule. *fc*, fat cells. (From Maia Simionescu, N. Simionescu, and G. E. Palade, *J. Cell Biol.,* **67**:863, 1975.)

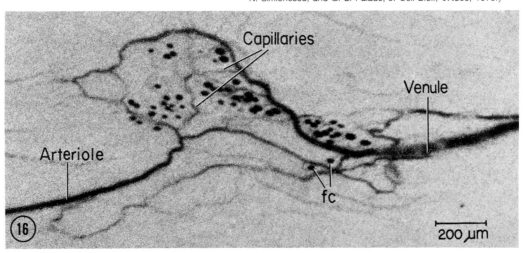

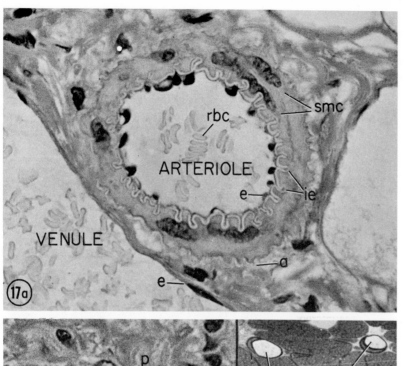

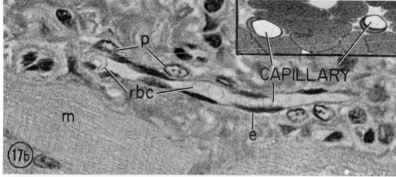

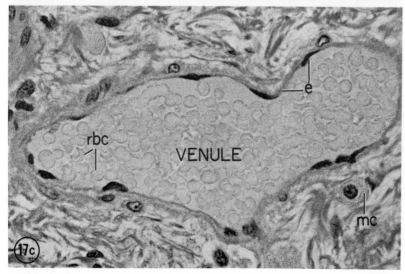

FIGURE 9-17 Photomicrographs of cross sections through an arteriole (a), capillaries (b, inset), and a venule (c), and of a longitudinal section through a capillary (b). *e*, endothelium; *ie*, internal elastic lamina; *m*, muscular fibers; *mc*, mast cell; *p*, pericyte; *rbc*, red blood cell. (a) ×600; (b) ×700; (b), inset, ×750; (c) ×500.

layer is usually thin and is composed of loose connective tissue and a few collagen and elastic fibers. The *internal elastica* is thin and fenestrated in arterioles larger than 50 μm; it disappears in the small terminal arterioles (except in the kidney, where it is present even in the terminal arterioles).

The *media* includes frequently one, rarely two (in large arterioles only), layers of smooth muscle cells helically arranged (Figs. 9-17 to 9-19). They are surrounded by basal laminae and collagen fibrils.

The terminal part of many arterioles (10 to 100 μm long), frequently called *metarteriole*, or the *precapillary sphincter area*, may have a cone-shaped lumen progressively reduced down to 5 μm (Fig. 9-19). Its media contains a few smooth muscle cells, some of them displaying myoendothelial junctions. The muscle contraction produces intermittent opening and closing of arteriolar-capillary communication, each phase of the relaxation-contraction cycle lasting 2 to 8 s. This activity induces intermittently new intra-capillary gradients of water and electrolytes. Sympathetic stimulation increases arteriolar resistance more than venular resistance. *Intima cushions* of the type described in arteries have also been found in some arterioles closely associated with the precapillary sphincters.

The *adventitia* is thin and composed of loose connective tissue with fibrilar elements and a few macrophages, mast cells (Fig. 9-18), plasma cells, fibroblasts, and unmyelinated nerve fibers.

CAPILLARIES

The terminal ramifications of the arterioles have been termed capillaries because Malpighi, who discovered them in 1661, called them "capilli" (hairs), having been impressed by their thinness. The term is restricted to vessels that consist only of endothelium, basal lamina, and a few pericytes. The inner diameter of blood capillaries ranges from 5 to 10 μm (Fig.

FIGURE 9-18 Low-power electron micrograph of a cross section through rat mesentery showing parts of the vascular walls of an arteriole, a capillary, and a venule. Note the frequency of mast cells closely associated with the vessels. *e*, endothelium; *ie*, internal elastica; *l*, vascular lumen; *sm*, smooth muscle cells. ×33,000.

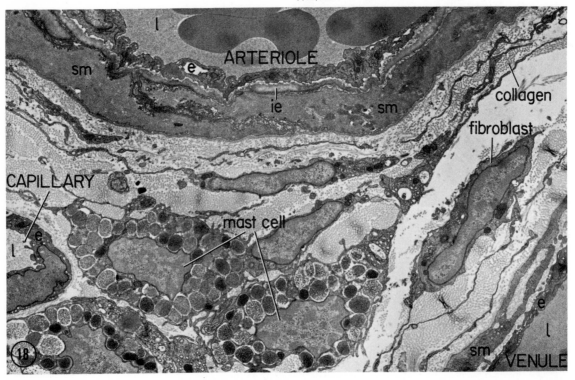

9-17b) and their average length is 200 to 1000 Å. Unlike the boundary between arterioles and capillaries, which is marked by the disappearance of the muscular tissue, the transition from capillary to venule is gradual and structurally less well defined. Capillary density in tissues reflects the magnitude of metabolic rates, especially the O_2 uptake. The transport of oxygen from plasma into cells is accomplished by diffusion. An increase in the diffusion distance is associated with a decrease in the oxygen pressure. This is particularly important in some tissues, such as the myocardium, in which even small increases in the diffusion distance may lead to a considerable cellular hypoxia. Capillary density can be estimated by different methods, one of them being that of counting numbers of capillaries in tissue sections. The frequency of capillaries per millimeter squared of tissue

yields significant differences between various tissues: for example, 2000 in myocardium, 600 to 1200 in skeletal muscle, 1000 in brain cortex, and only 50 in skin and connective tissue. These figures, however, may be affected by conditions of fixation (shrinkage, swelling). The figures for the capillary *surface* area vary from 0.9 to 2.4 m^2 per 100 cm^3 of muscle tissue or approximately 4 m^2 per 100 g tissue in the lung. For humans, the total surface area has been estimated at 60 m^2 in systemic capillaries and 40 m^2 in pulmonary capillaries. These values indicate that 1 ml of blood may be exposed to approximately 5000 cm^2 of capillary surface for exchanging materials through the thin (less than 0.5 μm) capillary wall. The capillary bed contains, however, only a small fraction of the blood volume: less than 8 percent.

The basic structure of blood capillaries is characterized by high simplification of tunics: *intima* is composed only of endothelium, basal lamina, and a few pericytes; *media* is virtually lacking; and *adventitia*

FIGURE 9-19 Low-power electron micrograph of cross-sectioned arteriole and precapillary sphincter (the adventitia of esophagus). Note the narrow lumen of the precapillary sphincter segment in contrast with its relatively thick layer of muscle cells (*smc*), and the presence of the basal lamina (*bl*) instead of the internal elastica (*ie*) occurring in the arteriole proper. Frequent nerve fibers (*) are located in the close vicinity of the vessel. *a*, adventitia; *e*, endothelium. ×4000.

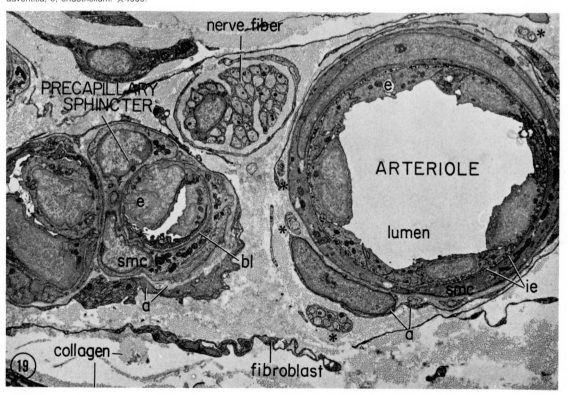

consists of a thin pericapillary layer of connective tissue continuous with that of the surrounding tissue (Figs. 9-17b and 9-21). The detailed structure of the layers varies from one capillary bed to another, reflecting local differentiations according to the nature and magnitude of blood-tissue exchanges. Based mainly on variations in the appearance and continuity of the endothelium and its basal lamina, as revealed by electron microscopy, three principal types of blood capillaries have been described: *continuous capillaries, fenestrated capillaries,* and *discontinuous capillaries (sinusoids)* (Fig. 9-22).

CONTINUOUS CAPILLARIES

They are characterized by a continuous endothelium similar to that found in the macrovasculature and a continuous basal lamina. This most common type of capillaries is found in muscular tissue (skeletal, cardiac, and smooth muscle), in connective tissue, in the central nervous system, and in the exocrine pancreas, gonads, and so forth. The endothelium is approximately 0.2 to 0.3 μm thick and is provided with a population of plasmalemmal vesicles 600 to 700 Å in diameter and of a high frequency (Table 9-3 and Figs. 9-22a and 9-23). A relatively thinner endothelium (approximately 0.1 μm) with fewer vesicles characterizes the capillaries of the central nervous system, lung and haversian systems of the bone. Plasmalemmal vesicles open on each front of the cell or are enclosed in the cytoplasm (Figs. 9-21 and 9-22a). In fixed tissues, the great majority appear as isolated units, but some of them can fuse and form patent transendothelial channels (Figs. 9-22a and 9-32). The intercellular clefts are of approximately 100 to 200 Å width, and are interrupted by occluding (tight) junctions (Figs. 9-21, 9-25 and 9-36). The appearance of the latter in thin sections varies from a close apposition to a complete fusion and an elimination of the outer leaflets of the neighboring cells. Open (20 to 40 Å)

FIGURE 9-20 Detail of the wall of a terminal arteriole showing the constituents of its tunics and the presence of two myoendothelial junctions (*mej*), and a rather unusual junction between two processes of the same muscle cell. ×25,000.

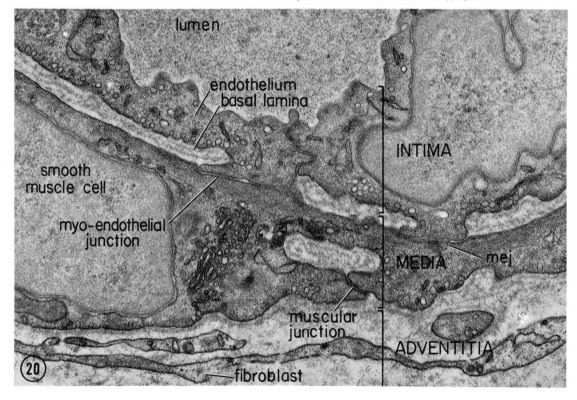

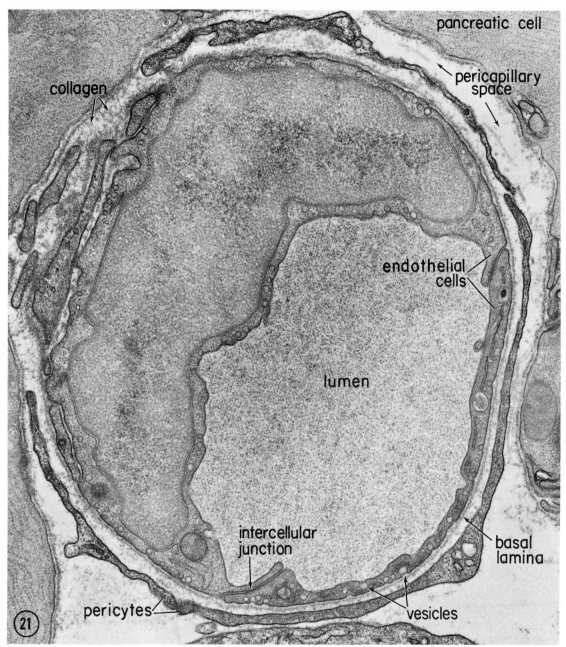

FIGURE 9-21 The most common feature of a blood capillary characterized by continuous endothelium and basal lamina (rat pancreas). In this case, the endothelial lining is formed by two cells held together by intercellular junctions of the occluding type. ×40,000.

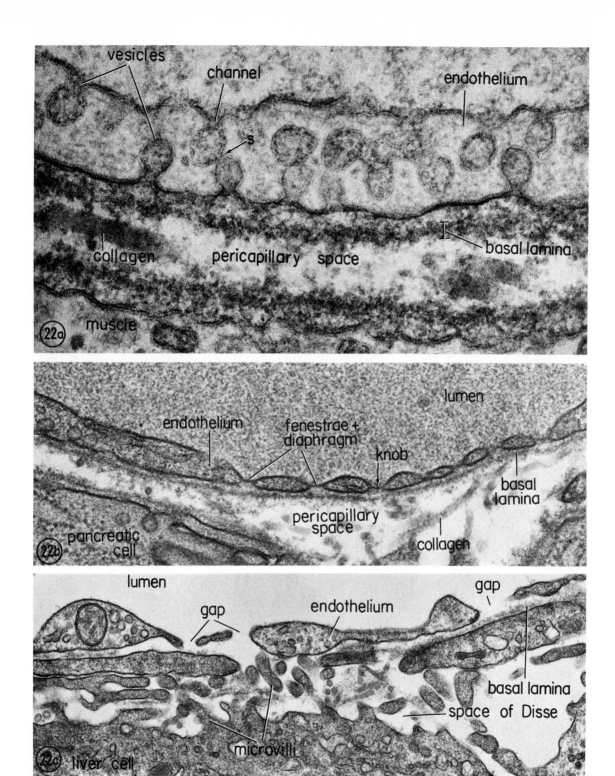

FIGURE 9-22 The three basic types of blood capillaries, different by the continuity of the endothelial cell and the basal lamina. a. continuous capillary. b. fenestrated capillary. c. discontinuous capillary (sinusoid). Rat diaphragm, pancreas, and liver, respectively. *s*, stricture. a, ×120,000; b, ×70,000; c, ×30,000.

TABLE 9-3 FREQUENCY OF VESICLE OPENINGS AND
FENESTRAE ON ENDOTHELIAL SURFACES*

TYPE OF CAPILLARY	Vesicular openings/μm^2		Fenestrae/μm^2
	Blood front	Tissue front	
Muscular			
Diaphragm	60	100	
Myocardium	70	110	
Visceral			
Pancreas	30	20	15
Jejunal mucosa	10	10	25

* Adapted from M. Simionescu, N. Simionescu, and G. E. Palade,
J. Cell Biol., **60**:128, 1974.

junctions have been occasionally encountered. There
is not enough information about the molecular organization at the surface of the cell-to-cell contact in this
system. In freeze-cleaved membrane, the occluding
junctions display an organization which is different
from that seen in other epithelia. Endothelial junctions
of blood capillaries consist of 2 to 4 strands of intramembranous particles; the strands are either continuous and connected or staggered (Fig. 9-36b). It
is difficult to ascertain whether they do or do not
form complete belts. Gap junctions seem to be absent
at this level.

Basal lamina is a continuous layer of approximately 200 to 500 Å thickness which appears as a
lightly matted feltwork of poorly resolved fibrils approximately 30 to 40 Å in diameter. This layer splits to
enclose the pericytes (or Rouget cells) that come into
close contact with the endothelial cell (Figs. 9-21 and
9-26). The basal lamina is inconspicuous in bone and
lymphoid tissue where the pericytes are very scarce as
well.

The adventitia is arbitrarily limited to the connective tissue components which may remain in close
association with the rest of the capillary wall when
experimental or pathologic interstitial edema occurs.
Such elements include fibroblasts, macrophages,
mast cells, collagen and elastic fibers, and ground
substance (Figs. 9-21 and 9-22). The amount and
nature of the adventitial connective tissue may influence both the vessel patency and the transcapillary
fluid exchanges.

FENESTRATED CAPILLARIES

The endothelium of these vessels is attenuated (approximately 0.06 to 0.1 μm) and exhibits several

transcellular circular openings, the fenestrae, with
a diameter of approximately 600 to 800 Å. All around
their periphery, the cell membrane of the blood front
is continuous with the cell membrane of the tissue
front. Therefore, the fenestrae cut across the endothelium without affecting the continuity of the plasmalemma of individual cells. Each fenestra is usually
closed by a thin single-layered diaphragm (approximately 40 to 60 Å), displaying a central knob about
100 to 150 Å in diameter (Figs. 9-2 and 9-22). The
chemical nature and the porosity of these diaphragms
are still unknown. It is assumed, however, that there is
not a hydrophobic barrier in these diaphragms. Their
frequency in some visceral capillaries is indicated in
Table 9-3. As revealed by the freeze-fracture preparations, the fenestrae can appear either randomly
distributed or in patches (Fig. 9-24).

The basal lamina is continuous. Fenestrated capillaries are found in the mucosa of the gastrointestinal
tract, endocrine glands, renal glomerular and peritubular capillaries, choroid plexus, ciliary body. In the
glomerular capillaries, the fenestrae are usually not
closed by diaphragms, and the basal lamina is almost
three times thicker than that of other capillaries and
plays a crucial role in the permeability characteristics
of the organ (see Chap. 22).

DISCONTINUOUS CAPILLARIES (SINUSOIDS)

These are thin-walled vessels with irregular caliber and
outline, molded on the neighboring epithelial cells.

The endothelium displays large gaps (up to thou-
sands of angstroms in diameter) and the basal lamina,
in most species, is either discontinuous or entirely
missing (Fig. 9-22c). Such capillaries are found in the
liver, spleen, and bone marrow; in each of these, the
sinusoids show local structural and functional peculi-
arities (for example, endothelial cells are phagocytic
in liver and much less so in spleen).

FUNCTIONAL-STRUCTURAL CORRELATES
IN CAPILLARY PERMEABILITY

The partition between plasma and interstitial fluid is
formed by four successive layers of various natures

FIGURE 9-23 Freeze-fracture preparation of a myocardium capillary. The cleavage plane exposes the P face of the blood front, breaks through the cytoplasm (*cy*) and continues on the E face of the tissue front of the same endothelial cell. Note the high frequency of vesicular openings (*v*). ×21,000. (From Maia Simionescu, N. Simionescu, and G. E. Palade, *J. Cell Biol.,* **60:**128, 1974.)

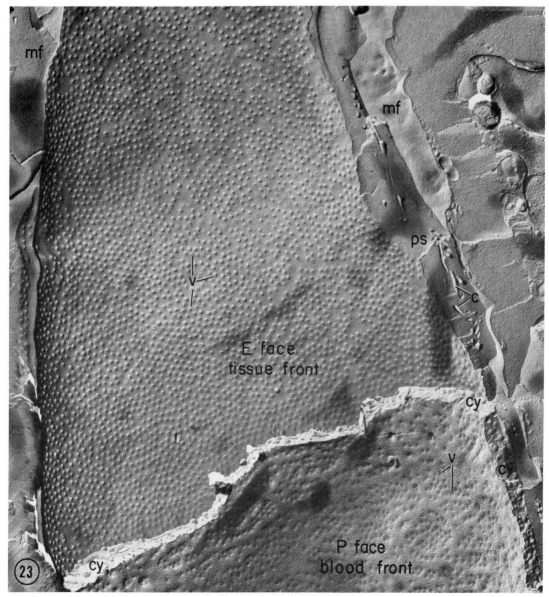

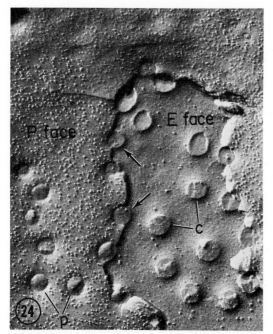

FIGURE 9-24 Freeze-fracture preparation of a fenestrated capillary (rat pancreas). The fenestrae appear as papillae (*p*) on the P face and as craters (*c*) on the E face of the cleaved membrane of the endothelial cell. Note the change in feature from crater to papilla for the fenestrae located along the fracture line through the endothelium (*arrows*). ×68,000. (From Maia Simionescu, N. Simionescu, and G. E. Palade, *J. Cell Biol.*, **60**:128, 1974.)

and functions (Fig. 9-27) as follows:

1. The endocapillary layer. On the luminal surface of endothelia, in some preparations, a thin (approximately 50 Å) coat of material can be seen. This is assumed to be either polysaccharide in nature or a deposition of fibrinogen within the outermost, immobile layer of plasma. This "unstirred" coat of still unknown composition might facilitate the stabilization and access of plasma molecules to the endothelial surface without being tormented by the blood flow.

2. The endothelium, main barrier; a thin space, filled with ground substance, mediates its contact with the next layer.

3. The basal lamina, and pericytes.

4. The adventitia (heterogeneous).

These layers form a functional and structural unit.

Comparing the blood circulation within the closed system of vessels with the invisible flow of water and dissolved substances across the vascular walls, we find that the latter is much greater. A submicroscopic circulation through the capillary wall is represented by the filtration-absorption phenomenon: water and solutes get out of plasma at the arteriolar end of capillary and enter back into it at the venular end. In addition to this, a more extensive fluid movement back and forth through the entire length of the capillary wall is carried out by diffusion which is practically independent of the rate and direction of the filtration-absorption flow.

The transcapillary exchanges are governed by the following driving forces acting on each side of capillary wall:

1. The hydrostatic pressure drives water out of the capillary

2. The osmotic pressure of plasma proteins draws water back into the capillary

3. Concentration gradients: molecules diffuse by themselves toward lower concentration

The hydrostatic pressure is higher than osmotic pressure at the arteriolar end of the capillary, but at its venular end, the osmotic pressure is predominant. As a result of these differences in the pressure, about 20 to 22 l of plasma water and solutes filtrate daily through the capillary walls. The magnitude of the exchanges by filtration alone is, therefore, too small to cover the metabolic requirements of the tissues. Work with isotopes has established, however, that in 24 h the water and solute molecules moving in and out of capillaries actually amount to approximately 80,000 l. Filtration carries small amounts of metabolites (for example, 20 g of glucose) into the tissues, insufficient to keep the cells alive. An extensive and effective exchange between plasma and tissues is accomplished by another mechanism, diffusion, which supplies cells with metabolites much in excess for a large margin of safety. Diffusion is possible owing to the high permeability of the endothelium: it is much higher than that of other cells, as well as other epithelia. Some aspects can be explained (permeability for lipid-soluble molecules), others require special adaptations to explain the high permeability for water and solutes and the unusual permeability for large water-soluble molecules. The latter could cross the endothelium only through some water-filled channels, or "pores."

Physiological experiments (Pappenheimer, Grotte) using molecules of graded size (dextrans) have indicated the presence of two types of pores:

Small pores: diameter, approximately 90 Å: frequency, 15 to 20 μm^2: aggregate area, 0.1 percent

Large pores: diameter approximately 500 to 700 Å: frequency, 1/15 to 20 μm^2

Unlike large pores, the small pores restrict diffusion with increasing molecular size. With the electron microscope, however, structures looking like true pores and displaying the exact dimensions and frequency postulated by the pore theory of capillary permeability have not been detected. To identify the structural equivalents of these two categories of pores, probe molecules of known dimensions have been used.[4]

The results obtained with such tracer experiments have brought out an almost general agreement regarding the equivalents of the two pore systems in fenestrated capillaries, as well as the structural equivalents of the large pores in continuous capillaries. The

location of the small pores in the continuous endothelium is still an unsettled issue.

In *fenestrated capillaries,* large probe molecules (100 to 300 Å in diameter) pass primarily through a fraction of the fenestral population which has been identified as the equivalent of the large pores (Fig. 9-28). Since molecules smaller than 90 Å diameter penetrate through all fenestrae (Fig. 9-29), the latter have been considered the equivalent of *small pores.* It is assumed

[4]Such molecules can be visualized with electron microscope either directly as individual particles (particulate tracers) as Ferritin (approximately 110 Å), dextrans (approximately 50 to 200 Å), and glycogens (approximately 250 to 300 Å), or indirectly through a reaction product (*mass tracer*) obtainable after histochemical reaction of such molecular species as horseradish peroxidase (approximately 50 Å), cytochrome C (approximately 33 Å) or hemepeptide (approximately 20 Å). All these molecules have peroxidatic activities. The former group has been used as a probe for the larger pores and the latter, primarily for the small pores.

FIGURE 9-25 Endothelial junctions in blood capillaries (rat diaphragm). (a) membrane fusion in which the outer leaflets are eliminated over a distance of ~80 Å (*arrow*). (b) fusion of the two outer membrane leaflets of the opposed cells (*arrow*). e, endothelial cell, *is,* intercellular space, *l,* capillary lumen, *ps,* pericapillary space. a, b, ×175,000. (From Maia Simionescu, N. Simionescu, and G. E. Palade, *J. Cell Biol.,* **67:**863, 1975.)

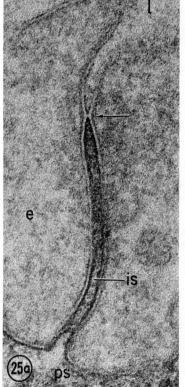
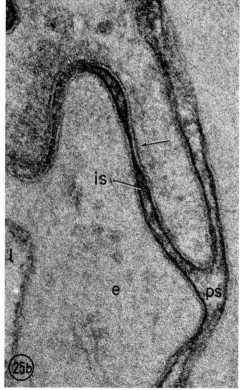

that the size-limiting structures are part of the fenestral diaphragms. For full agreement (predictions versus findings) a number of points, such as high frequency of fenestrae and the porosity of diaphragms, for example, remain to be reconciled.

In *continuous capillaries,* molecules larger than

100 Å cross the capillary wall only via plasmalemmal vesicles (vesicular transport) (Fig. 9-30), which have been recognized as the structural equivalent of the large pores provided that they open completely (full diameter) at loading or discharging. There is still disagreement concerning the main pathway followed by molecules smaller than 90 Å in diameter, that is, the small pores. According to some investigators, they are located in the intercellular junctions; according to others, plasmalemmal vesicles are involved in the passage of molecules of diameter larger than 20 Å.

FIGURE 9-26 Freeze-fracture preparation of a blood capillary (rat diaphragm). The endothelial cell is partially covered by a pericyte, the processes of which were in some places removed by the fracture exposing complementary depressions (*) left on the endothelium. Note the striking difference in the frequency of vesicular openings (v) between the endothelial cell and the pericytes. *mf,* muscle fiber; *c,* collagen; *ps,* pericapillary space. ×27,000. (From Maia Simionescu, N. Simionescu, and G. E. Palade, *J. Cell Biol.,* **60:**128, 1974.)

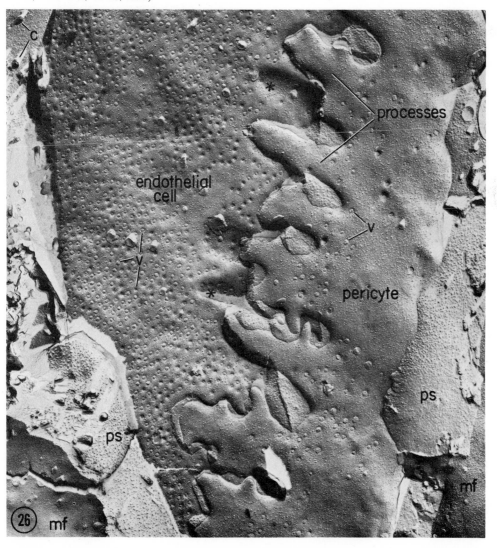

Recent work with small hemepeptides (MW, 1550 to 1900; diameter, 17 to 20 Å) favors a route through chains of vesicles which form patent transendothelial channels (simple or in chains) connecting the two endothelial fronts (Fig. 9-32). The size-limiting structure may be either the strictures at the fusion points of vesicles (diameter, approximately 80 to 100 Å) or diaphragms at their openings (Fig. 9-22a). According to these experiments and within the limitations of the methods used, the endothelial junctions are not permeable to molecules larger than 20 Å (Fig. 9-31). However, other investigators claim that at least some endothelial junctions are permeated by such tracers. This unsettled question requires more work, especially to clarify the size limit of the permeability of endothelial junctions to molecules smaller than 20 Å.

Similar findings were obtained also by back-dif-

fusion experiments in which the tracer was injected into interstitia from which they partially cross the endothelium to enter the blood. With the evidence so far in hand, the structural equivalents of the two pore systems are tentatively represented in Figs. 9-33 and 9-34. All important factors involved in transendothelial exchanges have already been mentioned: (1) the usual cell permeability, (2) the existence of intercellular flow (presumed in capillaries for some small molecules and water); (3) the structural equivalents of pores (Fig. 9-34). These various modes differ in relative importance from one capillary bed to another. At one extreme are the so-called blood-tissue barriers (brain, eyes, thymus, gonads): they are characterized by extensive tight junctions and few plasmalemmal vesicles, which indicates that these elements participate to a lesser extent in exchanges. At the other

FIGURE 9-27 Diagram representing the structural organization of the partition that mediates the transcapillary exchange between blood and tissues.

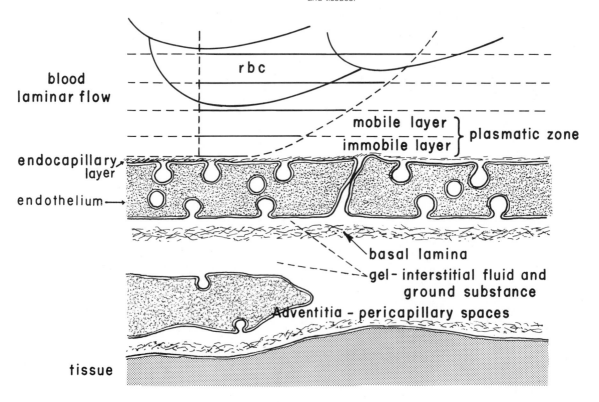

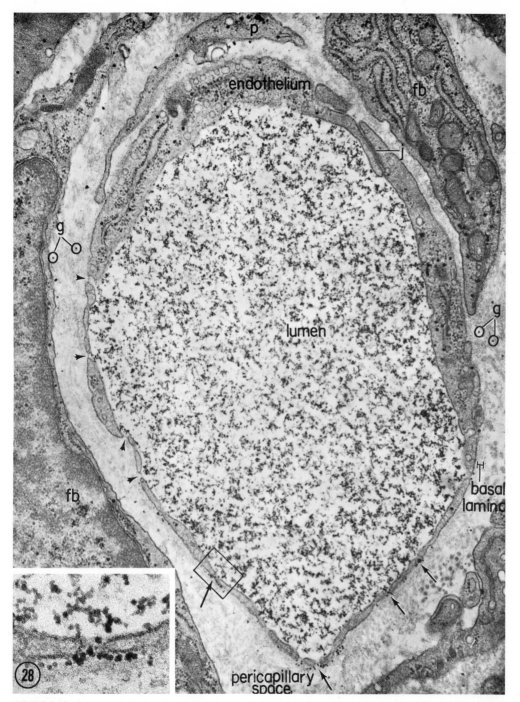

FIGURE 9-28 Fenestrated capillary (rat jejunal mucosa) 4 min after an intravenous injection of a tracer solution of shellfish glycogen. Tracer particles are in high concentration and even distribution in the lumen, and some of them have penetrated many endothelial fenestrae. Some fenestrae do not exhibit particles (*arrowheads*); at the level of others, the tracer is accumulated against the basal lamina (*arrows*). The intercellular junction (*j*) is free of tracer particles. *g*, individual particles in the pericapillary space. ×28,000; inset ×160,000. (From N. Simionescu, M. Simionescu, and G. E. Palade, *J. Cell Biol.*, **53:**365, 1972.)

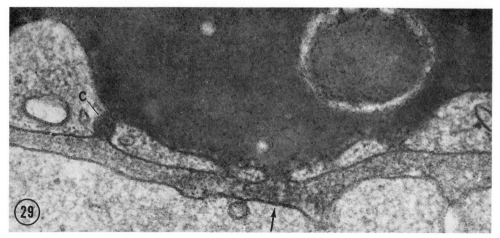

FIGURE 9-29 Blood capillary (mouse intestinal mucosa) 1 min 15 s after an intravenous peroxidase injection. In the pericapillary spaces the reaction product forms a gradient with its maximum opposite the fenestra (*arrow*) of the endothelium. *c*, channel. ×110,000. (From F. Clementi and G. E. Palade, *J. Cell Biol.,* **41:**33, 1969.)

FIGURE 9-30 Continuous capillary (rat diaphragm), 10 min after an intravenous injection of a tracer solution of shellfish glycogen. Tracer particles are present in the lumen and in vesicles open on the blood front or tissue front (*arrowheads*), or free in the cytoplasm (*double arrow*) of the endothelial cell. Some vesicles are closed by their diaphragms (*arrows*). ×94,000. (From N. Simionescu, M. Simionescu, and G. E. Palade, *Thromb. Res.,* Suppl. II, **8:**257, 1976.)

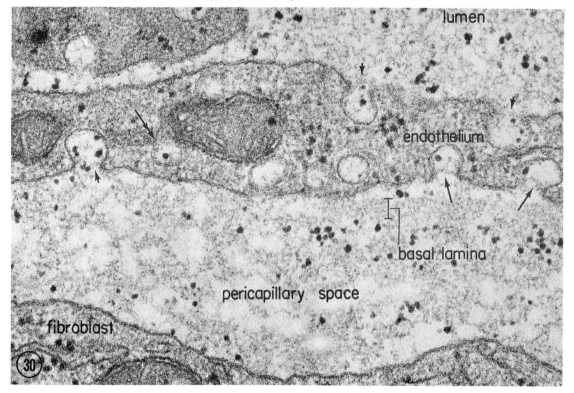

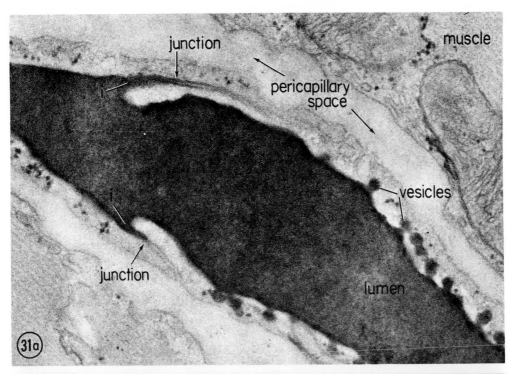

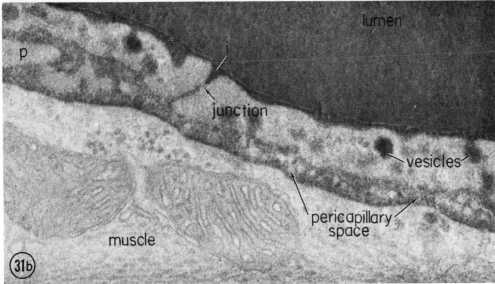

FIGURE 9-31 Blood capillaries of rat diaphragm after intravenous injection of a tracer solution of heme-octapeptide. a. 35-s post-tracer injection; the reaction product marks the infundibula leading to the endothelial junctions; the intercellular spaces beyond the junctions are free of reaction product, while many plasmalemmal vesicles are labeled. b. 60 s after tracer injection at the time when most vesicles are labeled (including those opened on the tissue front); the reaction product is present within the infundibulum (*i*) in the same concentration as in the capillary lumen, but shows a sharp stop at the level of tight junction. The intercellular space beyond this junction contains reaction product in concentration equal to that found in the adjacent pericapillary space. a, ×36,000; b, ×48,000. (From N. Simionescu, M. Simionescu, and G. E. Palade, *J. Cell Biol.*, **64:**586, 1975.)

412

extreme are the fenestrated or largely discontinuous capillaries which are freely and extensively permeable to molecules or particles larger than 700 Å (liver) or to cells (spleen and bone marrow).[5]

VENULES

The transition from capillaries to venules occurs gradually. The immediate postcapillary venules, ranging in diameter from 10 to 50 μm and in length from 50 to 700 μm, are characterized by the presence of pericytes

[5] In the kidney the process of filtration and absorption occurs in two distinct sets of capillaries (glomerular and peritubular capillaries, respectively) connected by the efferent arteriole.

(*pericytic venules*). They are drained by venules with diameter increasing from 50 to 200 μm, which contain in their media one or two thin layers of smooth muscle cells (*muscular venules*).

Pericytic Venules

The *intima:* The endothelium, 0.2 to 0.4 μm thick, is generally continuous, but occasionally a few

FIGURE 9-32 Transendothelial channels in muscle capillaries (rat diaphragm) from control animals (a) and after intravenous injection of heme-undecapeptide tracer solution (b). In (c) and (d), blood capillaries of rat cremaster after local interstitial injection of identical tracer solution. The channels are formed either by a single vesicle (c), by two fused vesicles (b and probably some of the features in d), or by a chain of more vesicles (a). Note that the plasma-lemma and the vesicle membranes are in continuity on both sides of the channels (*arrowheads*). a, ×150,000; b, c, d, ×200,000. (From N. Simionescu, M. Simionescu, and G. E. Palade, *J. Cell Biol.,* **64:**586, 1975.)

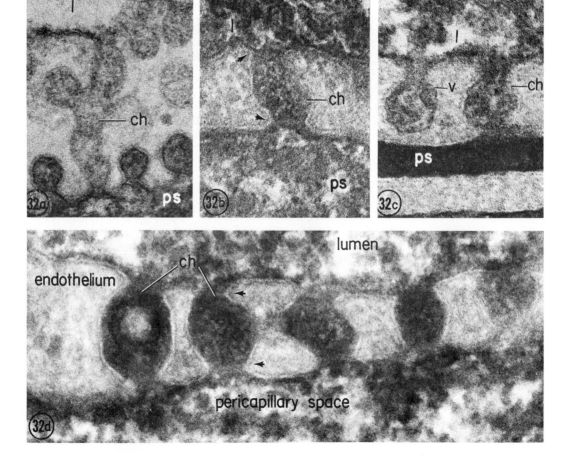

clusters of fenestrae may be encountered. The cells are joined by loosely organized intercellular junctions characterized in freeze-fracture preparations by discontinuous low-profile ridges and grooves frequently devoid of particles. They represent the loosest endothelial junctions encountered along the entire vascular system. Communicating (gap) junctions are usually missing (Table 9-2).

The venules seem to be particularly labile and sensitive to histamine, serotonin, and bradykinin, which induce the opening and leakage of their junctions (Figs. 9-37 and 9-38).

The basal lamina is thin and penetrated by pericytes which make an almost continuous layer and also establish frequent contacts of still unclear morphologic nature with the endothelium. The subendothelial layer is poorly developed as a thin coat of loose connective tissue.

A true *media* is lacking. In larger venules, the pericytes contain more cytoplasmic filaments and even dense bodies that make them resemble smooth muscle cells, to which they are assumed to be related.

The *adventitia* is relatively thin with few connective tissue fibrillar elements and scattered fibroblasts, macrophages, plasma cells, and mast cells. In lymph nodes, the venules may contain a relatively large number of lymphocytes within their walls.

Evidence is being accumulated that the immediately postcapillary venules play an important role in the blood-interstitial fluid exchanges. In contrast to capillaries, they are easily affected by extreme temperature, inflammation, and allergic reactions, to which they respond by opening the junctions for an augmented extravasation of water, solutes, and blood cells (Figs. 9-37 and 9-38).

Muscular Venules

These venules usually accompany arterioles, from which in sectioned specimens they are easily distinguished because of their thinner wall and irregular and collapsed lumen (Fig. 9-17c).

The *intima* displays a continuous endothelium slightly thicker than in pericytic venules. Two types of intercellular junctions have been found in these venules (Fig. 9-36c): (1) the occluding-type junctions, which are identical to those observed in pericytic venules (Table 9-2); (2) the communicating (gap) junctions, which may appear as rare, small, and isolated patches. A thin basal lamina is perforated only in areas of myoendothelial junctions. The scarce subendothe-

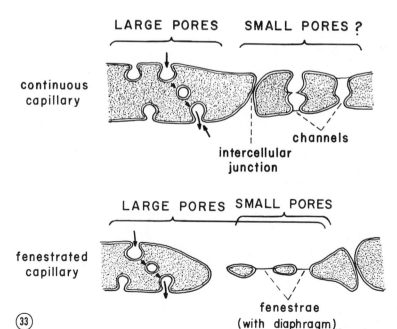

LARGE PORES SMALL PORES ?

continuous
capillary

intercellular
junction

channels

LARGE PORES SMALL PORES

fenestrated
capillary

fenestrae
(with diaphragm)

(33)

FIGURE 9-33 Diagram illustrating a tentative representation of the structural equivalents of the two pore systems in the endothelium of continuous and fenestrated capillaries.

lial layer is composed of connective tissue elements (Fig. 9-35).

The *media* is marked by the presence of one to two layers of flat smooth muscle cells (incomplete coat in venules of spleen and kidney). They are surrounded by basal laminae, little ground substance, a delicate network of collagen, and elastic fibers.

The *adventitia* is relatively thick (Fig. 9-35) and contains connective tissue elements among which thin flat fibroblasts, termed for this reason veil cells, are encountered. Unmyelinated nerve fibers occasionally occur.

ARTERIOVENOUS ANASTOMOSES

In certain regions, particularly those where the blood flow varies largely in time, many arterioles are directly connected to venules by short, coiled shunts, the arteriovenous anastomoses. These vessels have a thick wall, an average diameter of 12 to 15 μm, and may vary from 300 to 100 μm in length. Such shunts are frequent in the microvascular bed of the skin of the fingertips and toes, nail beds, lips, nose, intestinal tract, thyroid, and erectile tissue. Shunts also represent an essential part of the carotic, aortic, and coccygeal bodies. The latter consists of a group of coiled anastomoses arranged in a mass 2.5 mm wide and embedded in connective tissue. In the skin, the arteriovenous anastomoses are frequently convoluted and surrounded by a condensation of connective tissue, forming a glomus that contains also a part of the arteriole. The endothelium lies directly on a specialized muscular media, the cells of which are rather short and thick, forming a sphincter which in section resembles a stratified cuboidal epithelium (epitheloid cells). The adventitia of these anastomoses contains a large

FIGURE 9-34 Simplified diagram of the driving forces and mechanism involved in the pathway taken by plasma molecules across the capillary endothelium. (Left side: fenestrated endothelium; right side: continuous endothelium.)

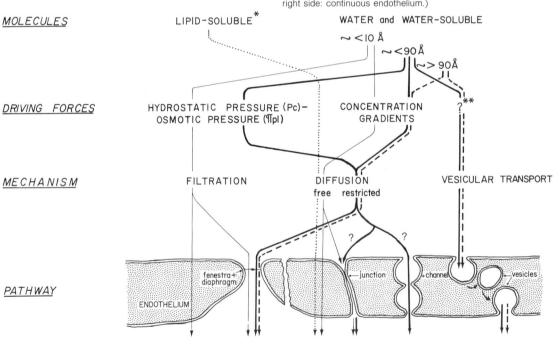

* except gases

** current thinking assumes that brownian movement of the vesicles through the cytoplasm is one of the forces involved

number of both myelinated and nonmyelinated nerve fibers.

VEINS

From venules, the blood is collected in veins of increasing size, arbitrarily classified as small, medium, and large. Unlike arteries, a correspondence between the size and structure in veins cannot be systematically established. In human beings and other mammals, the veins are very distensible and compressible as a result of the predominant elastic component of their vascular wall. In the systemic circulation, about 65 to 70 percent of the blood is contained in the veins (without counting the blood found in the reservoirs of the portal venous system, the liver, and spleen). In the pulmonary circulation, the figure is approximately 50 to 55 percent. The three basic tunics—media, intima, and adventitia—can be recognized in the wall of veins, although their boundaries are less distinct than in arteries. Roughly speaking, the veins of the upper

(supercardiac) regions of the body are essentially draining veins which return blood to the heart by gravity; their walls contain mostly elastic and collagen fibers. The veins of the lower (infracardial) regions of the body are predominantly propulsive veins which actively propel the blood to the heart by the contraction of their muscle fibers. The structure may be different in veins of the same caliber and even in separate regions of the same vein.

Small- and Medium-sized Veins

Small veins measure approximately 0.2 to 1 mm in diameter. The *intima* is formed by endothelium and a thin basal lamina. The *media* contains two to four layers of smooth muscle fibers interspersed between a thin network of elastic and collagen fibers (Fig. 9-39). The *adventitia* displays delicate bundles of collagen and elastic fibers longitudinally oriented and few fibroblasts and macrophages.

FIGURE 9-35 Cross section through a muscular venule exhibiting the tissue composition of the three tunics. Note the relatively wide adventitia. ×4600.

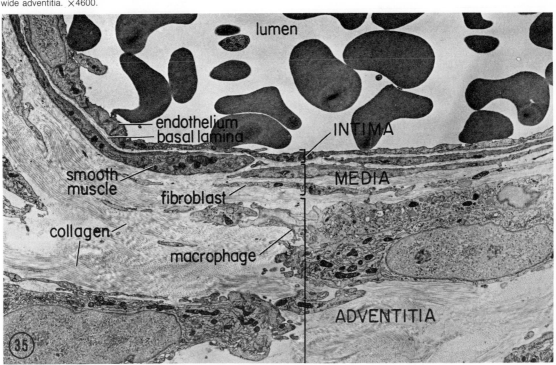

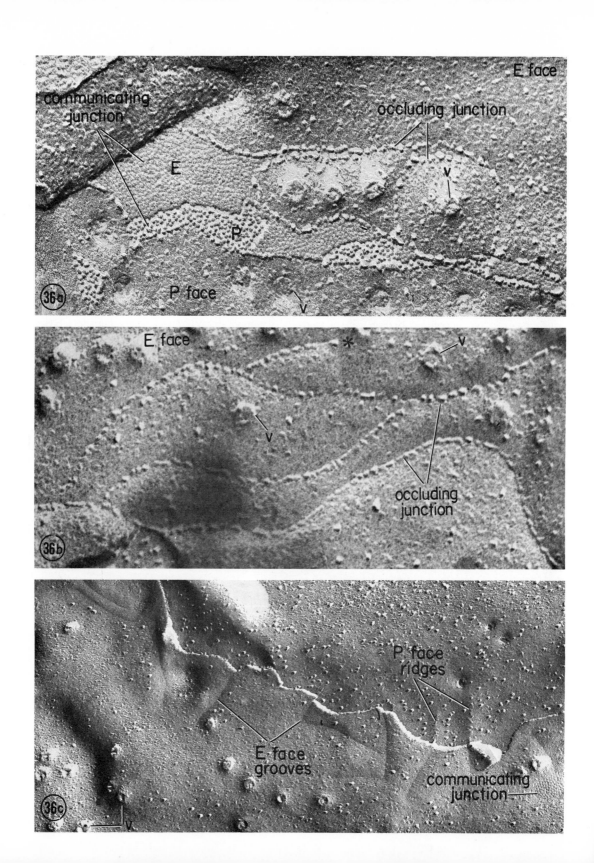

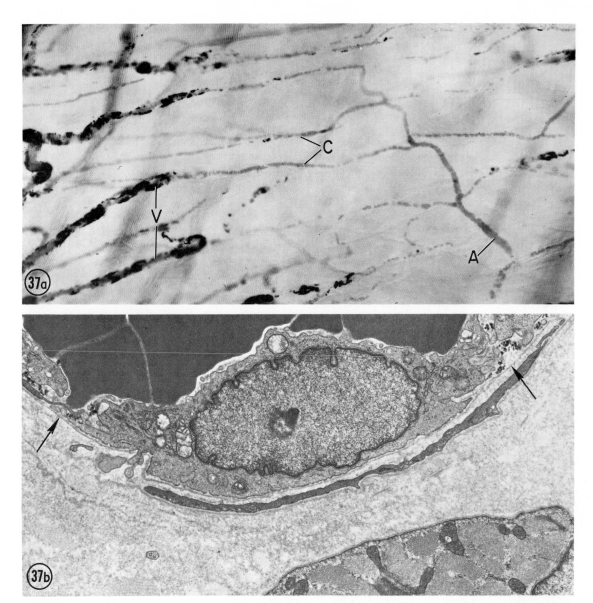

FIGURE 9-37 (a). The phenomenon of vascular labeling. Rat cremaster muscle, cleared in glycerine, 1 h after a local injection of histamine and an I.V. injection of colloidal carbon black. *A*, arteriole; *C*, capillaries. Carbon deposits occur almost exclusively in the venules. ×180. (From G. Majno, G. E. Palade, and G. I. Schoefl, *J. Biophys. Biochem. Cytol.,* **11:**607, 1961.) (b). Wall of a venule in a similar experiment as seen by electron microscopy. Note bulging endothelial cell with tight nuclear folds (suggestive of cellular contraction). Left arrow: gap between two endothelial cells. Right arrow: particles of carbon escaping along an intercellular junction. ×4100. (Courtesy of Drs. Isabelle Joris and G. Majno.)

FIGURE 9-36 The characteristic organization of the endothelial junctions in three segments of the microvasculature. a. arteriole: elaborate occluding junctions with intercalated large gap junctions. b. capillary: only occluding junctions are present, as branching or staggered strands. c. muscular venule: discontinuous, low-profile ridges and grooves usually devoid of particles (*arrows*) are seen on the P face and E face, respectively; also note a small, isolated communicating (gap) junction. *v*, vesicle openings. a, ×140,000; b, ×160,000; c, ×145,000. (From Maia Simionescu, N. Simionescu, and G. E. Palade, *J. Cell Biol.,* **67:**8, 1975.)

Medium-sized veins have a diameter that may vary from 1 to 10 mm. The wall thickness represents only one-tenth of the vascular diameter. With the exception of the main trunks, all named veins of the viscera and distal part of the extremities belong to this category.

The *intima* is rather thin, the endothelium being made up of short polygonal cells; some of them extend processes to form myoendothelial junctions with neighboring muscle cells. The basal lamina is thin. The subendothelial layer contains delicate collagen and scattered elastic fibers. The poorly defined elastica interna is found in veins which conduct blood against the force of gravity (lower limbs). The intima extends into the lumen pairs of semilunar folds, named valves, which are formed by a connective core covered on both surfaces by endothelium. These valves have their free margins directed toward the heart. The space between the concave aspect of the valve and the vein wall is called the sinus of the valve. At this level the venous wall is thick. Usually located just distally to the entry of a tributary vein, the valves help to prevent gravitational backflow of blood.

The *media* is thinner than in arteries of similar caliber: two to four circular layers of smooth muscle are separated by bundles of longitudinal collagen fibers interspersed with a delicate network of elastic fibers and a few fibroblasts (Fig. 9-40). The circumferential distensibility of the veins is owing in large measure to the circular-helical arrangement of muscle fibers. They are in close relation with the elastic fibers, which make a network with longitudinal cracks, and with the collagen fibers, which form another network in a crimped pattern. The changes in length are facilitated by the longitudinal orientation of some smooth muscle, elastic, and collagen fibers. The elastica externa is poorly defined.

The *adventitia* is thicker than the media and is composed of loose connective tissue with collagen and elastic fibers and smooth muscle cells frequently oriented longitudinally. Vasa vasorum, lymphatics, and unmyelinated nerves are consistently encountered.

Large Veins

In human beings, these veins are larger than 9 to 10 mm (external jugular, innominate, azygos, pulmonar, external iliac, renal, adrenal, superior mesen-

FIGURE 9-38 Cross section of a pericytic venule (rat omentum) 10 min after its exposure to air. Under these stressing conditions, large openings of some endothelial junctions occur. In this specimen, the open junction is occupied by a platelet and part of a red blood cell (*rbc*), both adhering to the subendothelial structures. *bl*, basal lamina; *ch*, chilomicrons. ×32,000.

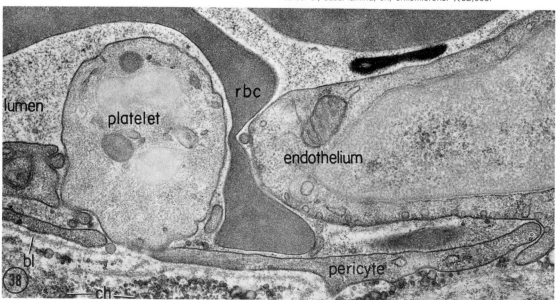

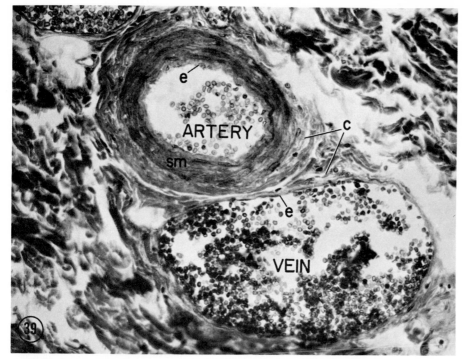

FIGURE 9-39 Cross section through small artery and vein. Note the difference in wall thickness between the two vessels. *e*, endothelium; *sm*, smooth muscle layer; *c*, collagen fibers. ×130.

FIGURE 9-40 Longitudinal section through a medium-sized vein (rabbit) showing the tissue composition of the three vascular tunics. The adventitia is only in part exhibited in this picture. ×4000.

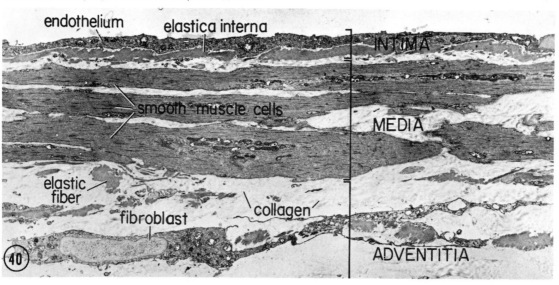

teric, splenic, portal, and vena cava). Their wall is extremely thin: one-twentieth of the vascular diameter.

The *intima* has the same configuration as in the medium-sized veins. The endothelial cells are linked together by two types of intercellular junctions: occluding junctions and communicating (gap) junctions. The latter are smaller and less frequent than those found in arteries (Table 9-2). Little is known about the permeability characteristics of the venous endothelium. Widening of the intercellular clefts has been observed after administration of angiotensin, serotonin, epinephrine, and bradykinin. The basal lamina is thin in comparison with the rest of the intima (45 to 70 μm thick), which contains loose connective tissue interposed with a network of collagen fibers, scattered elastic elements, and bundles of longitudinal muscle fibers. The elastica interna is largely fenestrated or fragmented.

The *media* is thin and in some areas of vena cava may be absent; otherwise the general organization is similar to that found in medium-sized veins, with few layers of muscle fibers. Rare processes of endothelial cells penetrate the elastica interna to establish myoendothelial junctions. Elastica externa is either poorly defined or is missing (Fig. 9-41).

The *adventitia* represents the greatest part of the wall. It contains loose connective tissue with thick bundles of elastic and collagen fibers longitudinally oriented; smooth muscle fibers display a similar arrangement, and in humans, they are numerous in vena cava inferior. Vasa vasorum and lymphatics are more developed than in arteries and can sometimes be traced as far as the intima. A rich nervous plexus is also encountered.

SPECIALIZED VEINS

Functional adaptations have introduced augumentation or reduction of structural elements especially in the muscular composition of some veins.

Veins rich in smooth muscle: longitudinally oriented muscle bundles may be encountered in all three tunics: in intima: internal jugular, veins of forearm, saphenous, popliteal, femoral, mesenteric, and uterine (of pregnancy); in media: limbs and umbilical; or in adventitia: veins of the abdominal cavity. In some regions of vena cava, the extreme thinning of media brings the longitudinal muscle of the adventitia in contact to intima. Cardiac muscle extends over a short distance in the adventitia of pulmonary veins and venae cavae.

Veins devoid of smooth muscle: Meningeal and dural sinuses, veins of retina, bones, splenic trabeculae, maternal placenta, and nail bed.

Blood vessels, lymphatics, and nerves of veins have been discussed previously (see page 387).

THE HEART

The heart is basically a segment of the vascular system, highly specialized as a pump made of striated muscle capable of spontaneous rhythmical contractions which propel blood through the blood vessels.

The heart displays the three basic tunics of a blood vessel, but a distinctive name has been given to each. The inner layer, homologous to the intima, is called the *endocardium*. The middle layer that corresponds to the media is termed the *myocardium* which is particularly differentiated and represents the main mass of the organ. The outer coat that represents the adventitia is called the *epicardium;* it also contains the visceral sheet of the serous pericardium. (See Table 9-1 and Fig. 9-42.) The endocardium lines separately the right and the left pairs of heart chambers and is continuous with the intima of the corresponding great vessels entering and leaving the heart. The atrial myocardium inserts on the upper aspect and the ventricular myocardium on the lower aspect of the annuli fibrosi of the cardiac skeleton. No morphological continuity occurs between these two parts of the myocardium, the only connection being the atrioventricular node of the conducting system of the heart. The epicardium behaves as a continuous coat that almost completely covers the heart and part of the roots of the large vessels.

ENDOCARDIUM

The endothelium is of continuous type similar to that encountered in large vessels and lies on a thin but

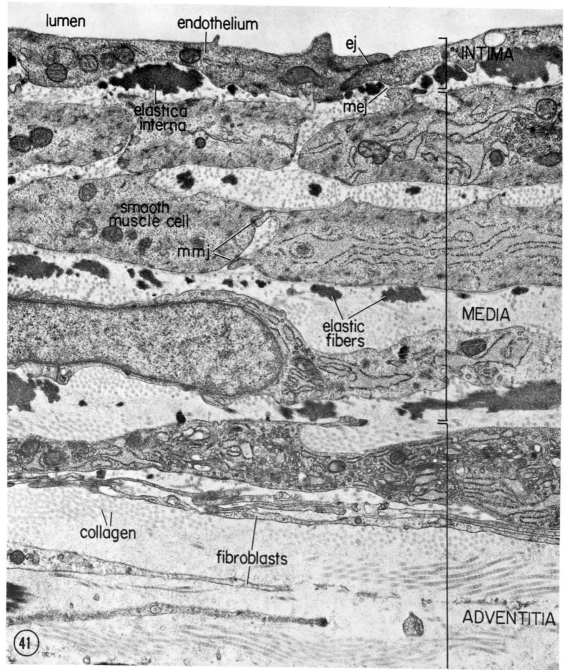

FIGURE 9-41 Cross section through the wall of a large vein (rat vena cava inferior). The elastica interna is discontinuous and largely fenestrated; a myoendothelial junction (*mej*) can be seen through one of such fenestrae. In this area, the media contains three layers of smooth muscle cells interspersed with rare isolated elastic fibers and bundles of collagen. The adventitia is only partially shown in this figure. ×15,000.

continuous basal lamina. Beneath the latter, the subendothelial layer of connective tissue is particularly dense in its inner part owing to a relatively large number of elastic and collagen fibers and smooth muscle cells. Closer and contiguous with the myocardium, additional loose connective tissue with collagen fibers marks the subendocardial layer: it contains small blood vessels, nerves, and, in ventricles, branches of the conducting system; it is continuous with the interstitial tissue of the myocardium (Fig. 9-43).

FIGURE 9-42 Cross section through the atrial wall of rat heart showing the three major tunics. Note the relative large thickness of both endocardium and epicardium. ×5000.

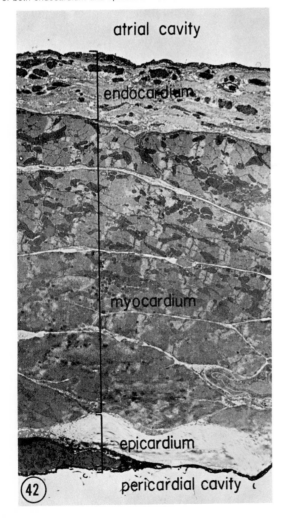

Cardiac Valves

Cardiac orifices are provided with valves consisting of folds of endocardium reinforced with a central flat sheet of dense connective tissue continuous with that of the fibrous ring from which they emerge. There are three atrioventricular valves (tricuspid valve) in the right homonym orifice and two (mitral valves) in its left counterpart. Near the base of these valves, sparse smooth muscle fibers, blood capillaries, and macrophages may exist. The free borders of the cusps are connected to the papillary muscles by several fibrous cords, the chordae tendinae. These restrain the valves from everting when the intraventricular pressure increases during systole. Orifices of the aorta and pulmonary artery have three semilunar valves each. At the middle of the free border, each cusp exhibits a small, ovoid thickening, the nodule. In the semilunar valves, the aspect toward the artery is strengthened with collagen and elastic fibers that withstand the backflow of blood when the valves close. The cardiac valves contain neither lymphatics nor nerves.

MYOCARDIUM

The middle tunic of the heart contains mainly three types of tissues: the myocardium proper, the impulse-conducting system of the heart, and the bulk of the cardiac skeleton. The entire wall is thinnest in atria and thickest in the left ventricle. Textbooks of anatomy should be consulted for the macroscopic and topographic description of these structures. The general histology and ultrastructure of the cardiac muscle and of the conducting system have been described in Chap. 7. The myocardium is arranged in layers and bundles of complex pattern which are embedded in connective tissue together with a large number of capillaries (Figs. 9-44 and 9-47). In atria, the muscles form a latticework and locally appear as prominent ridges resembling a comb (pectinate muscles) intercalated with relatively large amounts of collagen and elastic fibers connecting the endocardium and epicardium. In ventricles, the muscle bundles circumscribe the chambers in a complex, predominantly helical fashion. Superficial muscle layers surround both ventricles, whereas the deep layers encircle each ventricle and form in between the interventricular septum. A similar arrangement occurs in atria. Elastic fibers are scarce in ventricular myocardium. Most of the muscle fibers are inserted on the cardiac skeleton, mainly the fibrous rings (annuli fibrosi) which separate completely the muscle of atria from that of ventricles.

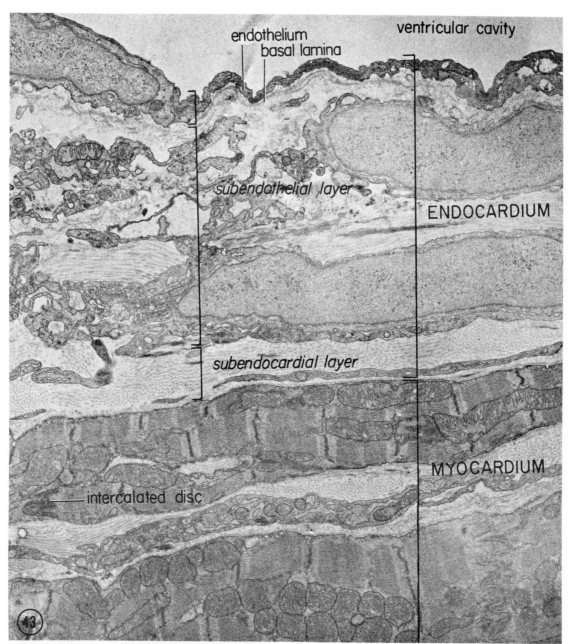

endothelium

basal lamina

ventricular cavity

subendothelial layer

ENDOCARDIUM

subendocardial layer

MYOCARDIUM

intercalated disc

FIGURE 9-43 Cross section through the inner part of the ventricular wall (rat heart). In addition to the endothelium and its basal lamina, the endocardium consists of a relatively large subendothelial layer and the subendocardial layer of loose connective tissue and collagen that continues with the interstitial spaces of the myocardium. ×9500.

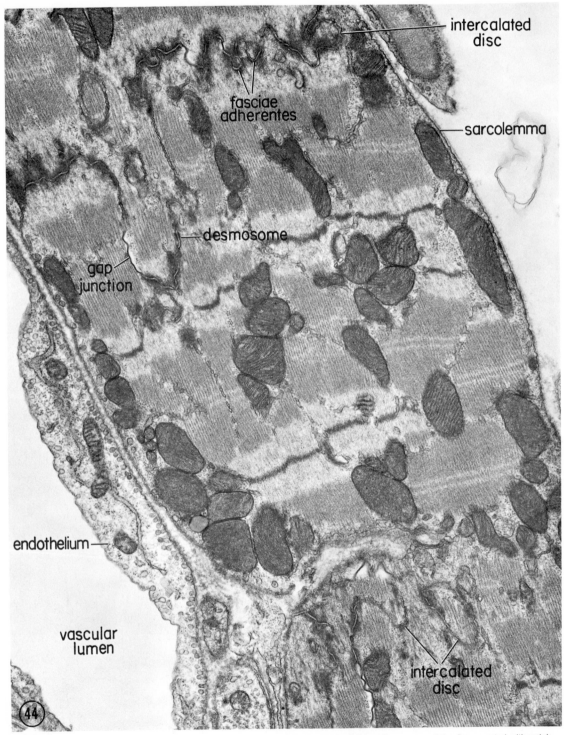

FIGURE 9-44 Longitudinal section of cardiac muscle (left ventricle) displaying on its full length a myocardial cell connected with neighboring myocytes by an intercalated disc at each end. Notice the three types of junctions in the latter. ×20,000.

Compared with the ventricular muscle cells, atrial cells are smaller, with a less elaborate T system (Fig. 9-45) and more frequent communicating (gap) junctions (Fig. 9-44), and contain numerous *granules* (Fig. 9-46) of unknown chemical composition. Some of these characteristics may contribute to a higher rate of conduction and greater intrinsic rhythmicity in atrial contractile cells than in those of ventricles. Physiological data suggest that ventricular myocardium has significant metabolic differences between its inner and outer layers. Connective tissue components surround the muscle cells as perimysium, continuous with the interfibrillar endomysium, that houses frequent fibroblasts. The latter may become very numerous in the focal repairs of heart injuries. The regeneration abilty of cardiac muscle itself is negligible.

FIGURE 9-45 Replica of freeze-cleaved sarcolemma of a cardiac muscle cell. Vesicle openings are organized in irregular clusters or appear randomly distributed. *Ts,* entry into a T system; *mf,* myofibrils in cross fracture. Compare with Fig. 9-6. ×26,000.

CONDUCTING SYSTEM

Mammals, humans included, possess a system of peculiar cardiac muscle cells specialized for initiating and conducting the rhythmical electrochemical impulses that generate the coordinated contraction and relaxation of the four chambers of the heart. This conducting tissue—called the *sinoatrial (SA) node*—is represented by a small mass (approximately 5×2 mm) that lies in the median wall of the right atrium close to the orifice of superior vena cava. From this pacemaker, the impulses spread through common cardiac muscle (although the possibility of some specialized conducting cells in atria is not ruled out) at a rate of approximately 1 m/s. The wave of excitation reaches another mass of conductive cells, the *atrioventricular (AV) node,* located on the right side of the interatrial septum. The

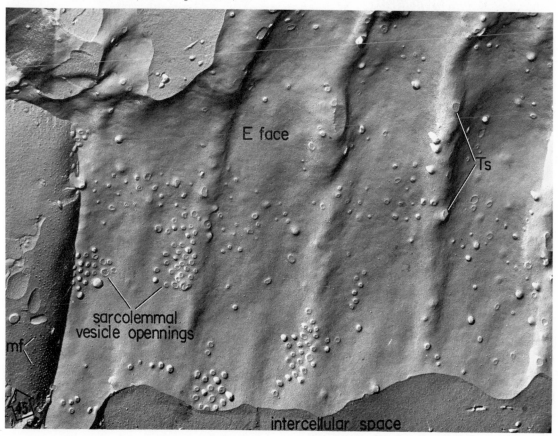

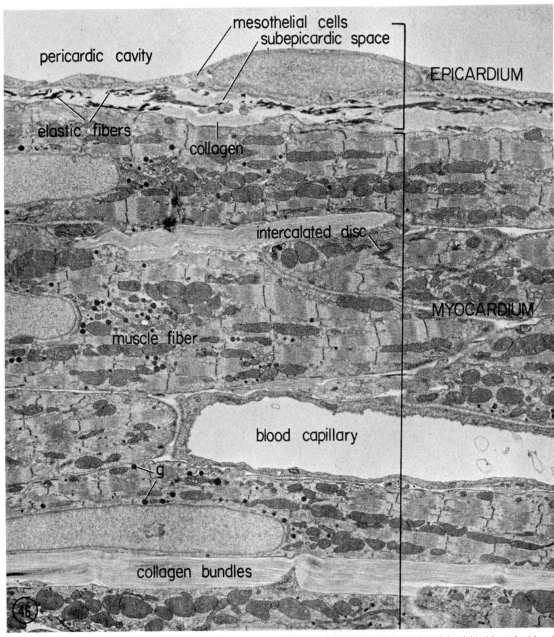

FIGURE 9-46 Longitudinal section of the right atrium of rat heart showing the general tissue organization of epicardium and myocardium. The atrial muscle cells contain characteristic granules (*g*); relatively large bundles of collagen occur in some regions of the atrial myocardium. ×6000.

slow conduction along the atrial fibers which contact the AV node induces a delay of 0.08 to 0.12 s, during which time the atrial contraction is completed. Leaving the AV node, the impulses pass rapidly (approximately 4 to 5 m/s) along an *atrioventricular bundle* (approximately 15 mm long by 2 to 3 mm wide) that passes into the interventricular septum and gives off a subendocardial branching trunk to each ventricle. Trunk ramifications, primarily described as *Purkinje fibers,* contact the ordinary muscle fibers. Three types of cells compose the conducting system of the heart: *nodal cells, bundle cells* (*Purkinje cells*), and *transitional cells* that connect with the myocardial cells (see Chap. 7). Bundles of conducting tissue are characteristically isolated from the surrounding myocardium by a sheet of connective tissue. The activity of the pacemaker system is regulated by complex feedback mechanisms involving nerves, baroreceptors, chemoreceptors, hormones, and so forth.

CARDIAC SKELETON

The fibrous base on which cardiac valves and muscle insert is inappropriately but customarily called the *cardiac skeleton.* Its main part consists of a mass of dense fibrous tissue organized in rings, the *annuli fibrosi,* which surround the atrioventricular canals and the origins of the aorta and pulmonary artery. Between the two groups of fibrous rings, additional masses of fibrous tissue constitute the *trigona fibrosa.* The upper part of the interventricular septum is represented by a fibrous partition, the *septum membranaceum.* Fibrous rings also contain elastic fibers and few adipocytes, whereas in the trigona fibrosa, islands of chondroid tissue may occur. During aging, these structures may become focally calcified.

EPICARDIUM

Its outermost coat is formed by the mesothelial cells of the visceral pericardium; their smooth, wet surface minimizes friction during heart contraction. Beneath a thin basal lamina, the subepicardial layer, composed of areolar connective tissue, elastic and collagen fibers, adipocytes, vessels, and nerves attaches the epicardium to the myocardium (Fig. 9-46).

INTRINSIC VESSELS OF THE HEART

The overall density of the blood microvascular bed is greater in myocardium than in skeletal muscle (see

Capillaries, page 398 and Fig. 9-47). The amount of blood passing through the coronary arteries is about 225 ml/min, representing approximately 4 to 5 percent of all the blood pumped by the heart. Unlike other parts of the circulation, coronary flow is greater during diastole than during systole. Myocardium capillaries are morphologically similar to skeletal muscle capillaries, but they are more permeable than the latter. The structural substrate of such differences is not clear. Controversial data suggest that macromolecules cross the endothelium of myocardial capillaries either through the intercellular clefts or via plasmalemmal vesicles. The frequency of the latter is remarkably high (Table 9-3). It has also been indicated that in regions with high oxygen tension such as subendocardial coat, capillaries are more permeable to probe molecules such as horseradish peroxidase than are the subepicardial capillaries.

Lymphatics are richly represented in myocardium. Small lymphatic capillaries (approximately 8 to 10 μm in diameter) originate near muscle fibers and endocardium and drain protein-rich fluid into the larger lymphatics of the epicardial coat.

INTRINSIC NERVES OF THE HEART

The heart receives numerous myelinated and unmyelinated nerve fibers of sympathetic and parasymphathetic (vagal) origin. They form plexuses in each major layer of the heart wall and many small ganglia occur in some of these (for example, subepicardial and perinodal networks). Sensory nerve fibers have their cell bodies either in the vagal or spinal ganglia (first to fourth pair). Nerve endings make myoneural junctions, presumably cholinergic, with the atrial myocardium. Sensory unencapsulated end organs (baroreceptors) associated with 4 to 9-μm-thick nerve fibers have been recently identified in the atrial endocardium. Despite many fine branches passing into the interstitia of ventricular myocardium, no neuromuscular junctions have been described in ventricles. At this level, the nerve processes lie within more than 200 Å of the sarcolemma, which does not exhibit any local specialization. The innervation, however, participates significantly in the complex mechanisms that regulate the heart's performance by making the adjustments necessary to meet the shifting circulatory needs of various organs and tissues of the body.

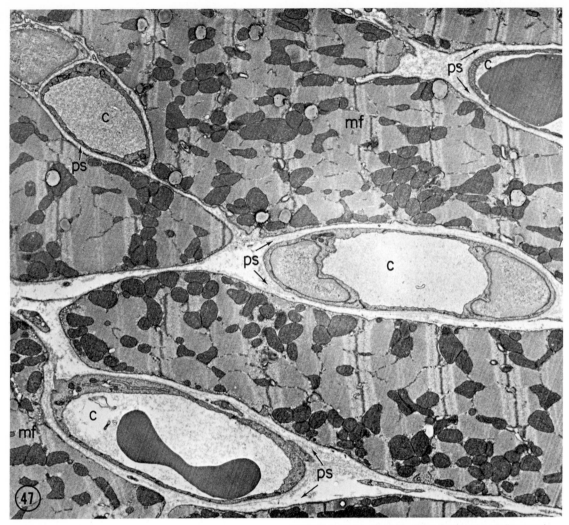

FIGURE 9-47 Longitudinal section through the cardiac muscle (guinea pig heart ventriculum) showing the general organization of muscle fibers (*mf*), the high frequency of blood capillaries (*c*), and the relative thinness of pericapillary spaces (*ps*). ×6000.

REFERENCES

Blood Vessels in General

BENNINGHOFF, A.: In W. von Möllendorf (ed.), "Handbuck der Microskopischen Anatomie des Merıschen," vol. 6, pt. I, p. 1, Blutgefässe und Herz, Springer Verlag, Berlin (1939).

KEFALIDES, N. A.: Isolation of a Collagen from Basement Membranes Containing Three Identical α-chains, *Biochem. Biophys. Res. Commun.,* **45:**226 (1971).

KRESSE, H., I. FILIPOVIC, A. ISERLOH, and E. BUDDECKE: Comparative Studies on the Chemistry and the Metabolism of Arterial and Venous Tissue. *Angiologica,* **7:**321 (1970).

MAJNO, G.: Two Endothelial Novelties: Endothelial Contraction; Collagenase Digestion of the Basement Membrane, F. Koller, K. M. Brinkhous, R. Biggs, N. F. Rodman, and S. Hinnom (eds.), in "Vascular Factors in Thrombosis," p. 23, F. K. Schattauer Verlag, Stuttgart, 1970.

ROSS, R., and P. BORNSTEIN: The Elastic Fiber. I. The Separation and Partial Characterization of Its Macromolecular Components, *J. Cell Biol.*, **40:**366 (1969).

SIMIONESCU, M., N. SIMIONESCU, and G. E. PALADE: Characteristic Endothelial Junctions in Different Segments of the Vascular System, *Thromb. Res.*, Suppl. II, **8:**247 (1976).

SMITH, U., J. W. RYAN, D. D. MICHIE, and D. S. SMITH: Endothelial Projections as Revealed by Scanning Electron Microscopy, *Science,* **173:**925 (1971).

SOMLYO, A. P., and A. V. SOMLYO: Vascular Smooth Muscle. I. Normal Structure, Physiology, Biochemistry and Biophysics, *Pharmacol. Rev.*, **20:**197 (1968).

WEIBEL, E. R. and G. E. PALADE: New Cytoplasmic Components in Arterial Endothelia, *J. Cell Biol.*, **23:**101 (1964).

WIGHT, T. N., and R. ROSS: Proteoglycans in Primate Arteries. I. Ultrastructural Localization and Distribution in the Intima, *J. Cell Biol.*, **67:**660 (1975).

ZELDIS, S. M., Y. NEMERSON, F. A. PITLICK, and T. L. LENZ: Tissue Factor (Thromboplastin): Localization to Plasma Membranes by Peroxidase-conjugated Antibodies, *Science,* **175:**766 (1972).

Arteries—Arterioles

BISCOE, T. J.: Carotid Body. Structure and Function. *Physiol. Rev.*, **51:**437 (1971).

GIACOMELLI, F., and J. WIENER: Regional Variation in the Permeability of Rat Thoracic Aorta, *Am. J. Pathol.*, **75:**513 (1974).

GOZNA, E. R., A. E. MARBLE, A. SHAW, and J. G. HOLLAND: Age-related Changes in the Mechanics of the Aorta and Pulmonary Artery of Man, *J. Appl. Physiol.*, **36:**407 (1974).

HÜTTNER, T., M. BOUTET, and R. H. MOORE: Studies on Protein Passage through Arterial Endothelium. I. Structural Correlates of Permeability in Rat Arterial Endothelium, *Lab. Invest.*, **28:**672 (1973).

RHODIN, J. A. G.: The Ultrastructure of Mammalian Arterioles and Precapillary Sphincters, *J. Ultrastruct. Res.*, *18:*181 (1967).

ROBERTSON, A. L., JR. and P. A. KHAIRALLAH: Arterial Endothelial Permeability and Vascular Disease. The "Trap Door" Effect, *Exp. Mol. Pathol.*, **18:**241 (1973).

SCHWARTZ, S. M., and E. P. BENDITT: Studies on Aortic Intima. I. Structure and Permeability of Rat Thoracic Aortic Intima, *Am. J. Pathol.*, **66:**241 (1972).

SCHWARTZ, S. M., and E. P. BENDITT: Cell Replication in the Aortic Endothelium. A New Method for Study of the Problem, *Lab. Invest.*, **28:**699 (1973).

SIMIONESCU, M., N. SIMIONESCU, and G. E. PALADE: Segmental Differentiations of Cell Junctions in the Vascular Endothelium. The Microvasculature, *J. Cell Biol.*, **67:**863 (1975).

SIMIONESCU, M., N. SIMIONESCU, and G. E. PALADE: Segmental Differentiations of Cell Junctions in the Vascular Endothelium. Arteries and Veins. *J. Cell Biol.*, **68:**705 (1976).

SIMIONESCU, N., S. DEMETRIAN, N. ABRAMESCU, and N. ABAGIU: Coussinets Endartériels des Artéres Segmentaires et Sous-segmentaires de la Râte chez l'Homme, *Arch. d'Anat. Pathol.*, **10:**215 (1962).

TRELSTAD, R. L.: Human Aorta Collagens: Evidence for Three Distinct Species. *Biochem. Biophys. Res. Commun.*, **57:**717 (1974).

WRIGHT, H. P.: Areas of Mitosis in Aortic Endothelium of Guinea-Pigs. *J. Pathol.*, **105:**65 (1971).

Capillaries

BENNETT, H. S., J. H. LUFT, and J. C. HAMPTON: Morphological Classification of Vertebrate Blood Capillaries, *Am. J. Physiol.*, **196:**381 (1959).

BRIGHTMAN, M. W., and T. S. REESE: Junctions between Intimately Apposed Cell Membranes in the Vertebrate Brain, *J. Cell Biol.*, **40:**648 (1969).

BRUNS, R. R., and G. E. PALADE: Studies on Blood Capillaries. I. General Organization of Muscle Capillaries, *J. Cell Biol.*, **37:**244 (1968).

BRUNS, R. R., and G. E. PALADE: Studies on Blood Capillaries. II. Transport of Ferritin Molecules across the Wall of Muscle Capillaries, *J. Cell Biol.*, **37:**277 (1968).

CLEMENTI, F., and G. E. PALADE: Intestinal Capillaries. Permeability to Peroxidase and Ferritin, *J. Cell Biol.*, **41:**33 (1969).

COPLEY, A. L., and B. M. SCHEINTHAL: Nature of the Endo-endothelial Layer as Demonstrated by Ruthenium Red, *Exp. Cell Res.*, **59:**491 (1970).

FARQUHAR, M. G.: Fine Structure and Function in Capillaries of the Anterior Pituitary Gland, *Angiology*, **12:**270 (1961).

FAWCETT, D. W.: Comparative Observations on the Fine Structure of Blood Capillaries, in Peripheral Vessels, *Int. Acad. Pathol. Monogr.* 4. Williams and Wilkins, Baltimore (1963).

GROTTE, G.: Passage of Dextran Molecules across the Blood-Lymph Barrier, *Acta Chir. Scand.*, Suppl., **211:**1 (1956).

KARNOVSKY, M. J.: The Ultrastructural Basis of Capillary Permeability Studied with Peroxidase as a Tracer, *J. Cell Biol.*, **35:**213 (1967).

KARNOVSKY, M. J.: Morphology of Capillaries with Special Reference to Muscle Capillaries, in Ch. Crone and N. A. Lassen (eds.), "Capillary Permeability," Alfred Bezon Symposium, II. p. 341, Academic Press, Inc., New York, (1970).

LANDIS, E. M., and J. R. PAPPENHEIMER: Exchange of Substances through the Capillary Walls, in W. F. Hamilton and P. Dow (eds.), "Handbook of Physiology," vol. II, sec. 2, p. 961, American Physiology Society, Washington, D.C. (1963).

LUFT, J. H.: Fine Structure of Capillary and Endocapillary Layer as Revealed by Ruthenium Red, *Fed. Proc.*, **25:**1773 (1966).

MAJNO, G.: Ultrastructure of the Vascular Membrane, in W. F. Hamilton, and P. Dow (eds.), "Handbook of Physiology," vol. III, sec. 2, p. 2293, American Physiological Society, Washington, D.C. (1965).

MAUL, G. G.: Structure and Formation of Pores in Fenestrated Capillaries, *J. Ultrastruct. Res.*, **36:**768 (1971).

PALADE, G. E.: Fine Structure of Blood Capillaries, *J. Appl. Phys.*, **24:**1424 (1953).

PALADE, G. E.: Transport in Quanta across the Endothelium of Blood Capillaries, *Anat. Rec.*, **136:**254 (1960).

PALADE, G. E.: Blood Capillaries of the Heart and other Organs, *Circ.*, **24:**368 (1961).

PALADE, G. E., and R. R. BRUNS: Structural Modulations of Plasmalemmal Vesicles, *J. Cell Biol.*, **37:**633 (1968).

RAVIOLA, E., and M. J. KARNOVSKY: Evidence for a Blood-Thymus Barrier using Electron Opaque Tracers, *J. Exp. Med.*, **136:**466 (1972).

REESE, T. S., and M. J. KARNOVSKY: Fine Structural Localization of a Blood-Brain Barrier for Exogenous Peroxidase, *J. Cell Biol.*, **34:**207 (1967).

SIMIONESCU, M., N. SIMIONESCU, and G. E. PALADE: Morphometric Data on the Endothelium of Blood Capillaries, *J. Cell Biol.*, **60:**128 (1974).

SIMIONESCU, N., M. SIMIONESCU, and G. E. PALADE: Permeability of Intestinal Capillaries. Pathway Followed by Dextrans and Glycogens, *J. Cell Biol.*, **53:**365 (1972).

SIMIONESCU, N., M. SIMIONESCU, and G. E. PALADE: Permeability of Muscle Capillaries to Exogenous Myoglobin, *J. Cell Biol.*, **57:**424 (1973).

SIMIONESCU, N., M. SIMIONESCU, and G. E. PALADE: Permeability of Muscle Capillaries to Small Heme-Peptides. Evidence for the Existence of Patent Transendothelial Channels, *J. Cell Biol.,* **64:**586 (1975).

SIMIONESCU, N., M. SIMIONESCU, and G. E. PALADE: Structural-Functional Correlates in the Transendothelial Exchange of Water-soluble Macromolecules, *Thromb. Res.,* Suppl. II, **8:**257 (1976).

WAGNER, R. C., P. KREINER, R. J. BARRNETT, and M. W. BITENSKY: Biochemical Characterization and Cytochemical Localization of a Catecholamine-sensitive Adenylate Cyclase in Isolated Capillary Endothelium, *Proc. Natl. Acad. Sci.,* **69:**3175 (1972).

Venules and Veins

AZUMA, T., and M. HASEGAWA: Distensibility of the Vein from the Architectural Point of View, *Biorrheology,* **10:**409 (1973).

BUCCIANTI, L.: Microscopie Optique de la Paroi Veineuse, *in Symp. Int. Morphologie Histochim. Paroi Vasculaire* (*Fribourg*), *1963,* pt. II, p. 211, S. Karger, Basel, (1966).

MAJNO, G., G. E. PALADE, and G. I. SCHOEFL: Studies on Inflammation. II. The Site of Action of Histamine and Serotonin along the Vascular Tree: A Topographical Study, *J. Biophys. Biochem. Cytol.,* **11:**607 (1961).

RHODIN, J. A. G.: Ultrastructure of Mammalian Venous Capillaries, Venules, and Small Collecting Venules, *J. Ultrastr. Res.,* **25:**452 (1968).

Heart

ABRAHAM, A.: "Microscopic Innervation of the Heart and Blood Vessels in Vertebrates Including Man," Pergamon Press, New York, (1969).

MCNUTT, N. S., and D. W. FAWCETT: Myocardial Ultrastructure, G. A. Langer and A. J. Brady, (eds.), in "The Mammalian Myocardium," John Wiley & Sons, Inc., New York (1974).

RAKUSAN, K.: Quantitative Morphology of Capillaries of the Heart. Number of Capillaries in Animal and Human Hearts under Normal and Pathological Conditions, *Meth. Achievm. Path.,* **5:**272 (1971).

Blood

LEON WEISS

The blood, in equilibrium with virtually every tissue, is one of the great homeostatic forces of the body. Blood distributes heat; carries respiratory gases, nutrients, and wastes; and flows through specific tissue sensors capable of reacting selectively to such factors as osmotic tension, pH, temperature, and the levels of certain hormones. The blood provides cellular transport among the hematopoietic tissues, the connective tissues, and other tissues and organs. The blood contains the agents, cellular and humoral, which control the effects of infections and tumors on the body. Thus it is a pervasive, regulative tissue playing a key role in maintaining the integrity of the body.

The blood is a fluid connective tissue composed of circulating cells and a liquid intercellular substance, the *blood plasma*. The blood is enclosed in blood vessels and flows through the body, propelled by the contraction of the heart, the recoil of the great vessels, the movement of muscles, the excursions of the lungs, and the force of gravity. Blood volume in the normal human adult is approximately 5 l.

Freshly drawn human blood is a red fluid of specific gravity 1.052 to 1.064. Standing only a short time it clots into a jellylike mass; but if clotting is prevented, the blood cells settle, leaving the plasma supernatant. Three layers may be observed in a column of sedimented or centrifuged blood (Fig. 10-1).

The lowermost layer, about 45 percent of the total blood volume, is red and consists of packed *erythrocytes*, or *red blood cells*. Above the erythrocytes is a thin gray-white layer, approximately 1 percent of the total blood volume, the *buffy coat*. It is formed of platelets and of *leukocytes*, or *white blood cells*, of which there are five types in human beings: lymphocytes, monocytes, polymorphonuclear neutrophils, polymorphonuclear eosinophils, and polymorphonuclear basophils. The uppermost layer is the plasma, a slightly alkaline, straw-colored, protein-rich fluid which constitutes the intercellular substance. The volume of packed blood cells is termed the *hematocrit*. It is evident that red cells far outnumber leukocytes. In fact, the normal blood red count is approximately $10 \times 10^6/mm^3$, and the white count $5 \times 10^3/mm^3$.

The mean numbers of the different leukocyte types per milliliter of circulating blood are

neutrophils	4400
eosinophils	200
basophils	5
lymphocytes	2500
monocytes	300

THE STRUCTURE OF BLOOD CELLS

LIVING BLOOD CELLS

Living blood cells may be studied in hanging drops, in tissue culture, in chambers of special design as ear chambers, or in such favorable places as the web of the toe, the tongue, or the mesentery in whole animals. Living cells may be studied unstained by phase-contrast microscopy or interference microscopy. Certain structures, moreover, may be selectively demonstrated by supravital staining. Our discussion, although applicable to many mammals, is directed primarily to

FIGURE 10-1 Blood before and after sedimentation. The volume of packed erythrocytes is almost 45 percent of the total blood volume. The leukocytes and platelets form a buffy coat, accounting for about 1 percent of the blood volume. The remainder of the blood is the supernatant plasma.

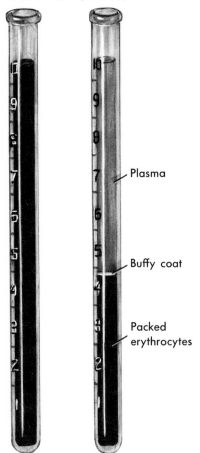

Plasma

Buffy coat

Packed erythrocytes

human blood [Figs. 10-2 to 10-4, 10-5 (color insert), and 10-8].

Unstained Blood Cells

Fresh red cells are orange-yellow in color without intrinsic motion. They are remarkably deformable, flexing, and twisting. Their biconcavity is striking, and they tend to aggregate into columns of cells similar to stacks of coins, called *rouleaux*. Rouleaux increase in size and frequency in certain diseases, notably those affecting plasma proteins. Their excessive presence may cause the blood to sludge within capillary beds of the body and interfere with efficient flow. Erythrocytes in hypertonic media lose water by osmotic pressure and shrink somewhat. The plasma membrane is thrown into folds, and the cells assume a burrlike or *crenated* appearance. In hypotonic solutions, on the other hand, water enters erythrocytes. Their hemoglobin is leached out and they become enlarged, virtually colorless structures, termed *ghosts*. The process, *hemolysis,* is used experimentally to obtain red cell membranes.

Living leukocytes are motile. As they move, they assume a characteristic polarization, with an active anterior end producing pseudopodia, a central portion containing the nucleus and the bulk of the cell, and a trailing, cytoplasmic tail. The tail is termed *uropod.* This configuration is best seen when leukocytes move over a flat surface and is obscured when they work their way through a clot or other three-dimensional matrix. Lymphocytes in motion give the appearance of a hand mirror; they show a round anterior nucleus surrounded by a rim of cytoplasm with the uropod trailing like a handle. The pseudopodia are delicate processes projecting forward in advance of the nucleus. The polymorphonuclear cells contain distinctive cytoplasmic granules; many of these can be seen as refractile structures in living cells. Platelets have little or no motility.

Chylomicrons and hemoconia are visible in fresh blood, especially with phase or dark-field microscopes. *Chylomicrons* are highly refractile fatty bodies about 1 to 3 μm in diameter. They increase considerably in number after a fatty meal. They are absent in most stained preparations of blood because they are soluble in alcohol, the fixative most commonly used. *Hemoconia* or blood dust are tiny particles of diverse origin—fragments of blood and endothelial cells, par-

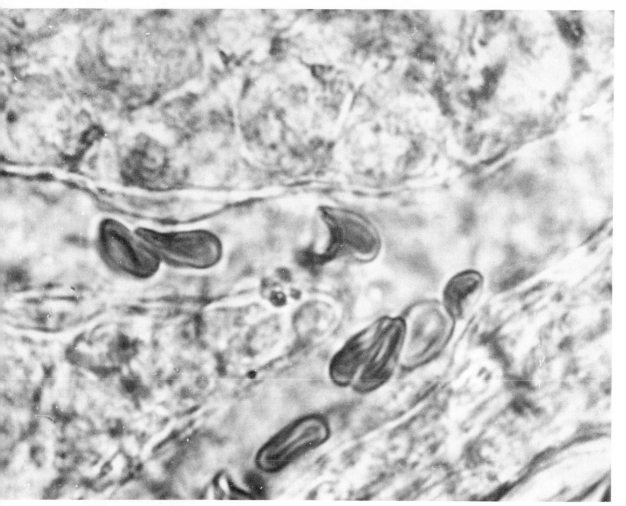

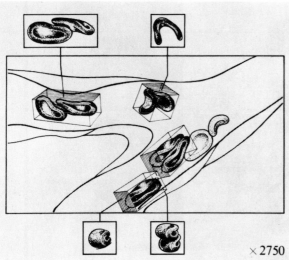

×2750

FIGURE 10-2 Deformation of erythrocytes in venule with an explanatory diagram illustrating Brånemark's interpretation of the mode in which each red cell has been stretched, bent, and twisted. Intravital photomicrogram of a human microvessel in connective tissue. ×2750. (From P-I. Brånemark, "Intravascular Anatomy of Blood Cells in Man," S. Karger AG, Basel, Switzerland, 1971.)

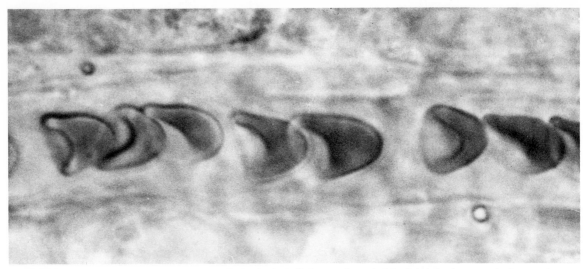

FIGURE 10-3 Deformation of human erythrocytes flowing in single file in a small venule. Intravital photomicrogram of a human micro-vessel. ×3000. (From P-I. Brånemark, "Intravascular Anatomy of Blood Cells in Man," S. Karger AG, Basel, Switzerland, 1971.)

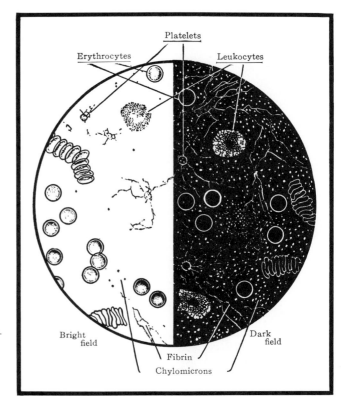

FIGURE 10-4 Fresh blood with chylomicrons. Right half of the field is under dark field; left half, under bright field. (Courtesy of S. H. Gage and P. A. Fish and the Wistar Institute of Anatomy.)

ticles of ingested material, etc. Since optimum visualization depends on the Tyndall effect, they are seen best in dark field rather than by transmitted light.

Supravitally Stained Blood Cells

It is possible to stain organelles in the living state and to observe them in the surviving cells (Fig. 10-5, color insert). Mitochondria are revealed selectively by their ability to maintain *Janus green B* in its oxidized or colored state. The granules of each of the polymorphonuclear leukocyte cell types take up the dye *neutral red,* which is a pH indicator that can differentiate by color the cytoplasmic granules of neutrophils, eosinophils, and basophils. Neutral red may also stain

FIGURE 10-6 Techniques of preparing blood smears on cover glass and slide. *Cover-glass method.* (1) A drop of blood is placed on one cover glass (a) by touching the surface of the glass to a drop of blood welling from a nick in a fingertip. (2) A second cover glass (b) is placed directly upon the first. (3) The drop of blood spreads out by capillary action between the cover slips. (4) As the drop reaches its maximal spread, the cover glasses are separated by pulling them apart in a sliding motion in a plane parallel to the surface of the glasses. In the process each cover slip bears a smear of blood. *Slide method.* A. A drop of blood is placed near the edge of a slide lying horizontally. A short edge of a second slide is placed across the first slide at an angle of about 30° and drawn backward so that the drop of blood is caught in the angle of the two slides. B. The drop spreads out in the angle. C. The second slide is drawn over the horizontal one. D. The blood is pulled over the surface of the horizontal slide and distributed as a smear. While more difficult to make, cover-slip smears are superior in affording a more random distribution of leukocytes than slide smears, permitting more accurate differential counts.

phagocytic and other vacuoles. A rosette of neutral-red-stained vacuoles characteristically surrounds the centrosome in monocytes, but supravital staining, once actively prosecuted by Florence Sabin and her students in an effort at delineating certain hematopoietic cell types, is now scarcely used. A most important exception, however, is the supravital staining of freshly produced erythrocytes, termed *reticulocytes,* by brilliant cresyl blue, new methylene blue, or some other suitable basic dye.

THE STRUCTURE OF BLOOD CELLS IN ROMANOVSKY-STAINED SMEARS

The structure of blood cells as observed in blood smears stained with Romanovsky-type stains is invaluable in research and clinical practice.

Blood smears are made quickly and easily (Fig. 10-6) by spreading a drop of blood on a slide or a cover slip in a layer one cell thick. Blood smears are air-dried and may be examined unstained by phase-contrast microscopy or stained with a variety of methods.

Romanovsky-type stains are complex dye mixtures designated *neutral stains.* In addition to ionized

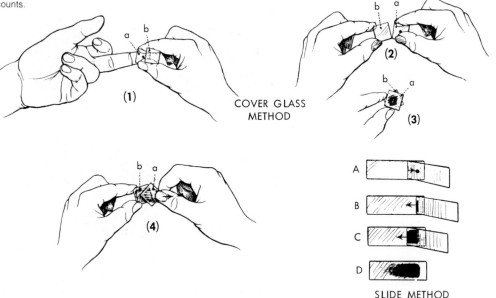

(1)

COVER GLASS METHOD

(2)

(3)

(4)

A

B

C

D

SLIDE METHOD

dyes—eosin⁻, methylene blue⁺, and the oxidation products of methylene blue, the azures⁺—these dyes contain neutral dye salts represented by nondissociated eosinates of methylene blue and the azures. Variants of Romanovksy stains, which include the Wright stain, and Giemsa's, MacNeil's, Leishman's, and May-Grünwald's mixtures, differ in the manner of oxidation of methylene blue to the azures.

Erythrocytes are round or slightly oval in outline. Their diameter is fairly constant for an individual, ranging in humans from 6.5 to 8.0 μm. They bind eosin and are deeply stained around their thicker periphery but the color gradually becomes very faint in their thin central zone (Fig. 10-7, see color insert).

Polymorphonuclear neutrophils, approximately 12 to 15 μm in diameter, contain a prominent nucleus segmented into three to five lobes joined by thin, sometimes invisible, strands. Chromatin is coarse and entirely heterochromatic. Nucleoli are absent. The cytoplasm is stained a faint pink and contains a moderate number of azurophilic granules.

Eosinophils, 12 to 15 μm in diameter, often contain a trilobed nucleus with two large lobes joined by a strand of chromatin from which a third small lobe hangs. The chromatin is heterochromatic. The cell is dominated by striking eosinophilic granules. These are large, closely packed, circular in outline, uniform in size, and stained a deep bright red or orange. They tend not to overlie the nucleus.

Basophils measure 12 to 15 μm in diameter. Their nuclei contain two or three lobes, often less distinctly segmented than those in neutrophils or eosinophils. Chromatin is heterochromatic, and no nucleoli are evident. Cytoplasmic granules are most prominent, deeply stained a metachromatic red-violet. Well preserved granules are nearly spherical and rather uniform in size. But they may be quite variable in size and shape because they are difficult to preserve and some of the granule's contents are extracted during fixation and staining. The granules of basophils may overlie and obscure the nucleus.

Lymphocytes vary in size. Although their size distribution falls on a bell-shaped curve, they are often grouped as small, medium, and large. The smallest, 5 to 8 μm in diameter, may be smaller than erythrocytes (Fig. 10-8). In small lymphocytes the nucleus fills almost the entire cell. It is round or slightly indented, heterochromatic, and without visible nucleoli. It is surrounded by a thin rim of basophilic cytoplasm containing a few small granules. The cytoplasm is typically stained a deep, clear blue. Large lymphocytes, up to 15 μm in diameter, have proportionally more cytoplasm. Their nucleus is often flattened or

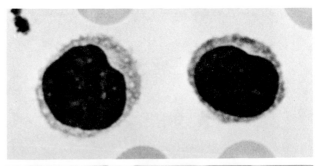

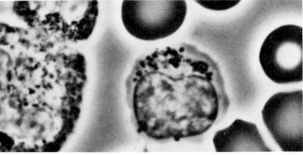

Figure 10-8 Lymphocytes of human blood. A. Blood film has been fixed and stained with Wright's stain. Two small lymphocytes are present. B. Small blood lymphocyte is seen in a phase-contrast photomicrograph. ×2400. (From the work of G. A. Ackerman.)

indented, and the chromatin tends to be less completely heterochromatic than that of smaller cells. Nucleoli may be visible.

Monocytes, 12 to 18 μm in diameter, may be among the largest of the white blood cells. The nucleus is often horseshoe-shaped but may show only a slight indentation. A subtle but important point of identification is that the chromatin of monocytes forms a lacy, delicate network, in contrast to the coarse chromatin of lymphocytes. Nucleoli, as a rule, are not visible. Monocyte cytoplasm is abundant and gray or blue in color. It may contain very many fine particles which impart a "dusty" character. A prominent centrosome lying in the nuclear indentation or *hof* may be present.

Blood platelets are ovoid bodies, 2 to 4 μm in size, that tend to clump, often in groups of two or three, occasionally into large, irregular masses. Platelets contain a central blue granular zone, the *granulomere,* and a lighter peripheral zone clear of granules, the *hyalomere.*

A few dead or dying leukocytes are always present in the blood. Degenerated cells are more fragile than normal ones and, in part because of mechanical stress in preparing the smear, they may extend over a relatively large area and appear reticulated or spongy, often with parts torn. Their capacity to bind dye is reduced. Their nuclei may be pycontic. Some dead cells retain their morphology so poorly that they are simply called *smudge cells.*

ELECTRON MICROSCOPY OF BLOOD CELLS

Erythrocytes contain a uniformly granular density representing hemoglobin. Some ferritin may be present. Ribosomes, mitochrondria, ER, Golgi, and lysosomes are absent in mature cells. Clear small vesicles may be present. Peripheral bands of microtubules occur in inframammalian erythrocytes but are absent in human cells.

FIGURE 10-9 Human erythrocytes; scanning electron micrograph. ×10,000. (From F. M. M. Morel, R. F. Baker, and H. Wayland, *J. Cell Biol.,* **48:**91, 1971.)

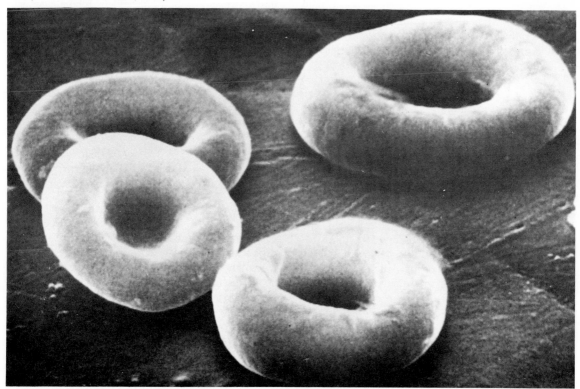

The plasma membrane is trilaminar by conventional electron microscopy (Fig. 1-24), but contains many discrete structures after freeze-fracture etch (Fig. 1-26). In the scanning electron microscope their biconcave shape is striking (Fig. 10-9).

Neutrophils[1] possess two types of granules which are bounded by a membrane and number, in total, about 200. *Primary, type A* granules, corresponding to the azurophilic granules of light microscopy, account for about 20 percent of the granules. They are large (approximately 0.4 μm), dense, and homogeneous when well fixed. Often some extraction occurs during processing, however, leaving less dense, irregular structures. Approximately 80 percent of the granules are *secondary, type B.* They are smaller (less than 0.3 μm) and less dense than primary granules and may contain a crystalloid (Fig. 10-10).

Mature eosinophils have large (0.6 to 1.0 μm), spherical, dense, membrane-bounded granules which contain an angular, very dense, tightly lamellated crystalloid (Figs. 10-11 and 10-12).

When well fixed, the specific granules of basophils are membrane-bounded structures about 0.5 μm in diameter (Fig. 10-13) which may contain granular material, myelin figures, lucent zones, and crystalloids. A few nonspecific granules may also be present.

Lymphocytes (Figs. 10-14 and 10-15) contain a number of lysosomes and small- to moderate-sized Golgi complexes. They may contain polyribosomes and some profiles of smooth ER, but unless undergoing transformation or proliferation, they possess little rough ER. Receptors on their surface may be visualized by EM cytochemistry.

Monocytes contain moderate numbers of lysosomes, several prominent Golgi complexes, and rough ER. The centrosome is large and may be surrounded by microtubules.

Platelets (Figs. 10-16, 10-17, and 10-13) possess a plasma membrane which dips into the cytoplasm to form an extended series of deeply penetrating canaliculi. Electron-microscopic markers such as thorium

dioxide placed in the plasma have ready access to the canaliculi. A variety of membrane-bounded granules are present. A group 0.5 to 1.5 μm in diameter is very dense, similar to certain synaptic vessels, and appears to contain serotonin. In addition, a moderate number of lysosomes occur. A band of microtubules runs about the periphery beneath the plasma membrane. These may well be a microskeletal system necessary to maintain the platelets' lenticular shape. Microfilaments, approximately 50 Å in diameter, lie among the microtubules and extend to the inner surface of the plasma membrane (Figs. 10-17 and 10-18). These are likely contractile, represent actin, and have been termed *thrombostenin.*

CYTOCHEMISTRY OF BLOOD CELLS

A great deal of chemical information may be inferred about blood cells from their appearance in Romanovsky-type preparations, such as the strongly anionic character of eosinophilic granules and the cationic metachromatic nature of basophilic granules. But by the use of selective or specific cytochemical reagents, this information may be extended. Ribonucleic acid may thus be disclosed in the cytoplasm of lymphocytes, monocytes, and occasionally in other cell types by showing that their basophilia is abolished by pretreatment of the cells with ribonuclease. Erythrocytes are positive in tests for hemoglobin. The azurophil granules of neutrophils are lysosomal in nature and are therefore positive for acid phosphatase, esterase, and other lysosomal-associated enzymes. The specific granules contain a cytochemically demonstrable peroxidase. Erythrocytes contain *spectrin,* a filamentous, apparently contractile protein associated with the inside of the plasma membrane and likely related to actin.

Without difficult-to-apply methods for cell surface markers, T and B lymphocytes look alike. B lymphocytes, which are precursors to plasma cells, antibody-producing cells, have approximately 150,000 molecules of antibody on their surface which can be shown by fluorescent antibody techniques or other immunocytochemical methods (Fig. 1–7). T lymphocytes lack readily demonstrable surface antibody. Their antigen receptors, whose existence can be inferred by the capacity of T lymphocytes to couple specifically with antigen, have not yet been demonstrated cytochemically or, in fact, by other techniques. T lymphocytes can be demonstrated cytochemically by means of cer-

---

[1] The term *neutrophil* designates the human cell. In rabbits and certain other species, the secondary granules are often eosinophilic and relatively large. To distinguish these cells from the true eosinophils, they are termed *pseudoeosinophils.* The generic term, embracing this cell type regardless of species and staining reaction, is *heterophil.* By electron microscopy, heterophils of rabbits (pseudoeosinophils) and of human beings (neutrophils) are remarkably alike.

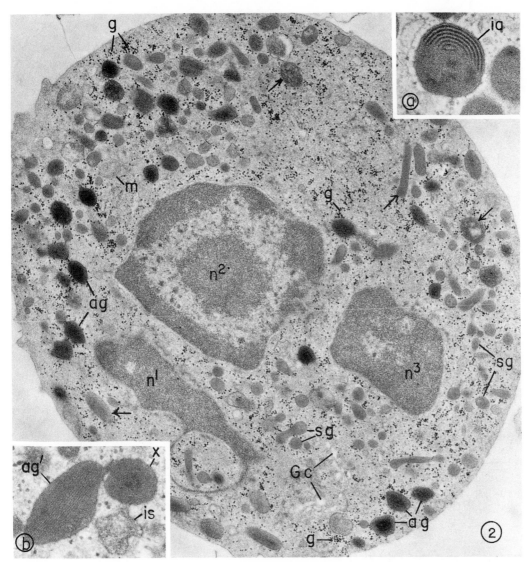

FIGURE 10-10 Mature human polymorphonuclear neutrophil (PMN). Several lobes of the nucleus are present (n^1 to n^3), and numerous granules, as well as glycogen (g), are scattered throughout the cytoplasm. A few mitochondria (m) and a small Golgi complex (Gc) are also visible. Some of the granules present are large and dense (ag), whereas others are small and less dense (sg). However, many granules are intermediate in size and density. Elongated forms, including football and dumbbell shapes, are also present (arrows). The insets depict internal structure within the large, dense (azurophilic) granules. Inset a shows a spherical granule (ia) containing concentric half-rings. Inset b illustrates the crystalline lattice with periodicity of approximately 100 Å which is commonly seen in football or ellipsoid forms (ag'). A cross section (X) of the ellipsoid form and an immature specific granule (is) are also present in this field taken from a PMN myelocyte. The sequence of development of these cells together with additional electron micrographs (Fig. 11-17) is presented in Chaps. 11 and 12. a. ×45,000; b. ×45,000 (From D. F. Bainton, J. L. Ullyot, and M. G. Farquhar, *J. Exp. Med.,* **134:**907, 1971.)

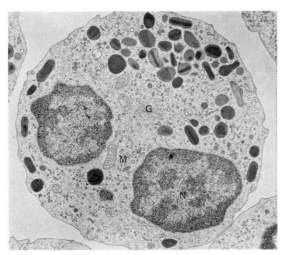

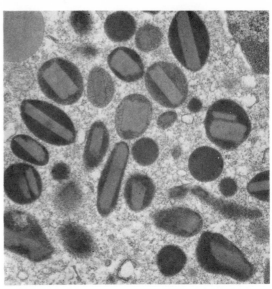

FIGURE 10-11 Eosinophil obtained from the peripheral blood of a normal subject. Fixed with glutaraldehyde and osmium tetroxide. Note that the granules have an electron-dense "core" and a less electron-dense "matrix." N, bilobed nucleus; G, Golgi body; M, mitochondria. ×7742. (From D. Zucker-Franklin, *Adv. Intern. Med.*, **19:**1, 1974.)

FIGURE 10-12 Eosinophil granules treated with phosphotungstic acid during dehydration. Note that the electron density of the core and matrix is reversed. ×27,160. (From D. Zucker-Franklin, *Adv. Intern. Med.*, **19:**1, 1974.)

tain substances present in T lymphocyte plasma membranes. Thus the mouse T lymphocytes contain a Θ antigen in their cell surface which can be revealed by an anti-Θ-antibody conjugated to ferritin or other tracer recongizable by electron microscopy.

The pronounced eosinophilia of the eosinophilic granule is a result of a high concentration of the amino acid arginine, which bears a strongly cationic, terminal guanidinium group (pK $>$ 11). The eosinophilic granules also contain lipid, being reactive both with sudan black B and with methods for phospholipid, and a number of enzymes, a prominent one being myeloperoxidase which can serve as a marker. The intense metachromatic basophilia of the specific granules of

the basophils is owing to heparin, a strongly anionic, sulfated mucopolysaccharide. These granules also contain histamine and, in rodents, serotonin. They are positive in the PAS reaction, indicative of the presence of 1,2 glycol groups (Chap. 2). The staining reactions of basophilic granules are similar or identical to those of mast cell granules. Lymphocytes may show no distinctive cytoplasmic reactions except the presence of cytoplasmic RNA. Monocytes contain lysosomes and therefore show reactions for acid phosphatase and other lysosome-related enzymes. Platelet thrombostenin can be demonstrated cytochemically (Fig. 10-17). Platelets contain glycogen and a number of enzymes which can be demonstrated cytochemically.

FUNCTIONS OF BLOOD CELLS

ERYTHROCYTES

Erythrocytes transport the respiratory gases oxygen and carbon dioxide between pulmonary alveoli and the tissues. In alveoli the partial pressure of oxygen exceeds 100 mmHg, whereas in systemic venous blood coming from the tissues it is approximately 40 mmHg.

Venous blood also carries carbon dioxide at a pressure of almost 50 mmHg, far greater than that in alveoli. As a result, oxygen diffuses through the alveolar wall into erythrocytes where it is loosely bound by the heme of hemoglobin. At the same time, carbon dioxide leaves the plasma and hemoglobin where it travels as a bicarbonate and carbaminohemoglobin and diffuses into the alveoli. Oxygenated blood has an oxygen tension of about 96 mmHg, whereas in the tissues the tension is only about 35 mmHg.

When oxygenated blood reaches capillaries, oxygen dissociates from the hemoglobin and diffuses through the plasma and capillary wall and out into the surrounding tissues. As a result, the oxygen tension drops from 96 percent in arterial blood to 64 percent

in venous blood. At the same time, carbon dioxide diffuses from the tissues into the plasma and into erythrocytes.

The iron of hemoglobin must be maintained in a ferrous form in order to transport oxygen. The oxidized form, *methemoglobin,* is incapable of respiratory functions. Erythrocytes contain an enzyme, *methemoglobin reductase,* which reverses the oxidation of ferrous hemoglobin into methemoglobin. The energy required for the maintenance of reduced hemoglobin is derived from glycolysis.

Erythrocytes are highly differentiated cells. They may be viewed as sacs, bounded by plasma membrane, containing hemoglobin. The hemoglobin constitutes about 33 percent of the weight of the cell and is in so concentrated a solution that it approaches the

FIGURE 10-13A Electron micrograph of a normal human basophil leukocyte. This cell was taken from a person who suffered from allergic rhinitis on exposure to grass pollen, but not on exposure to ragweed pollen. When an aliquot of washed blood cells was incubated in vitro with a ragweed extract, there was no release of histamine and the basophils looked normal as shown here. The cell surface is smooth, showing only small ridges (R), pockets (P), and vesicular protrusions (V). One platelet is adherent to the cell surface (Plat). The cytoplasm contains many typical basophilic granules (G), which vary in size and shape. Also shown are the polymorphous nucleus (N), four mitochondria (M), the Golgi apparatus (Go), the two centrioles (C) and a coated vesicle (C.V). ×15,000.

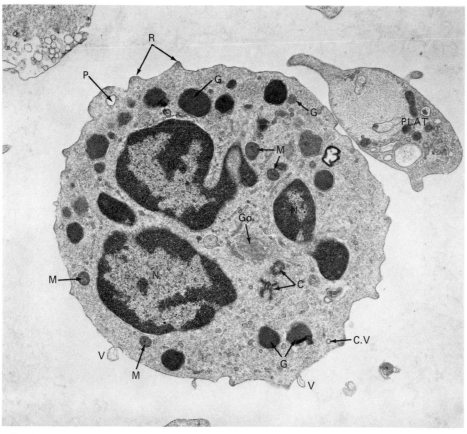

A

crystalline. Mature erythrocytes, without nucleus, ribosomes, and mitochondria, have lost their capacities for protein synthesis and aerobic metabolism. They depend upon glycolysis for energy, most of which is used to maintain hemoglobin in the reduced state and maintain proper internal ion concentration. Mature erythrocytes have lost the capacity to synthesize new membrane.

The parceling of hemoglobin into small anucleate corpuscles is a mammalian characteristic. Hemoglobin occurs in some invertebrates as a high-molecular-weight plasma protein. As a result the blood is quite viscous. In inframammalian vertebrates and certain invertebrates, hemoglobin occurs within rather large nucleated cells which require relatively large capillaries. They are, moreover, less efficient than anucleated mammalian corpuscles for gaseous exchange. The small size and biconcave shape of mammalian erythrocytes make the interior of the cell quite accessible to oxygen and carbon dioxide. In flow, the central biconcavity is commonly drawn out and the erythrocyte

FIGURE 10-13B Electron micrograph of a degranulated human basophil leukocyte. This cell was taken from the same donor as that shown in Fig. 10-13A. In the same experiment, an aliquot of washed blood cells was incubated in vitro with a grass extract. Secretion of more than 95 percent of the histamine in the cells resulted and the basophils appeared degranulated as shown here. The cell surface is irregular, showing numerous projections of variable appearance (Pr). Other leukocytes and platelets (Plat) are adherent to the surface of the basophil. No basophilic granules can be seen in the cytoplasm, but a large membrane-bounded cavity (C) is evident which contains residual granular material and communicates widely with the exterior (Ext). Further residual granular material can be seen at the cell surface (Resid). Also shown are the polymorphous nucleus (N), three mitochondria (M), and cisternae of smooth endoplasmic reticulum (ER). ×15,000. (From R. Hastie, D. Levy, and L. Weiss, *J. Lab. Investigation,* in press.)

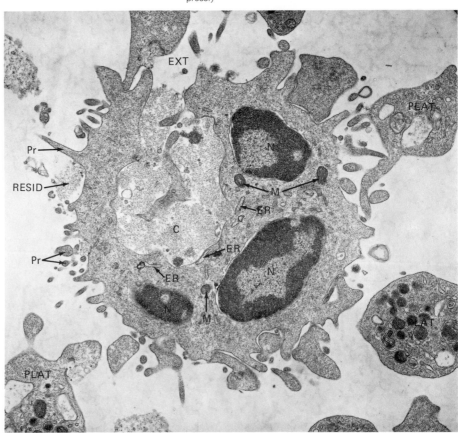

B

circulates in the shape of a cone, apex forward (Fig. 10-13).

NEUTROPHILS

The major function of neutrophils is to destroy bacteria and other infectious agents which penetrate the body. Neutrophils are necessary to life: an individual without them or with impaired neutrophils dies of infection. By and large, any microorganism which is phagocytized by a neutrophil is killed. Microorganisms resisting phagocytosis by neutrophils must be contained by antibodies or other cells. The tubercle bacillus is a major exception—it survives phagocytosis by

neutrophils and must be contained by the monocyte-macrophage system.

The chemotropic movement of neutrophils toward bacteria is influenced by polypeptides or small molecular weight compounds which are released by bacteria, diffuse into the surrounding tissue, interact with the leukocyte membrane, and attract the phagocyte (Fig. 10-19). There are, moreover, host factors, such as complement and the kinins (see below), which are released in an inflammatory response induced by bacteria or other agents which attract neutrophils. The movement of neutrophils toward the bacteria and their

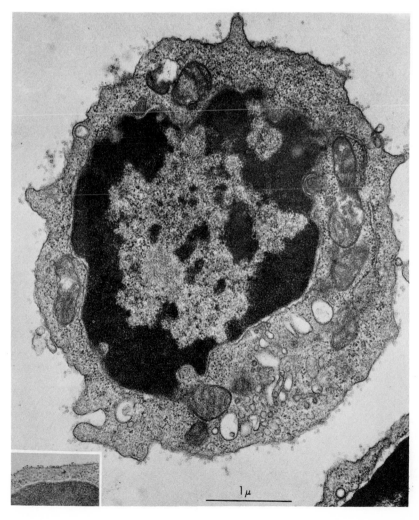

FIGURE 10-14 Electron micrograph of mouse B lymphocyte. The antibody receptors on the surface of this cell have been revealed by an antibody to the mouse antibody receptors prepared in a rabbit (rabbit anti-mouse immunoglobulin, RAMG). The RAMG has been linked to a large hemocyanin molecule, and this molecule, which looks like a little box under the electron microscope, serves as a label indicating the presence of the mouse antibody receptors. Note that the label is distributed rather uniformly over the surface of the B lymphocyte. This preparation was labeled at a temperature of 4°C. At this temperature the antibody receptors, which are mobile, are fixed in their uniform distribution on the cell surface. At higher temperatures, after being linked with RAMG, the antibody receptors would move to one pole of the cell and concentrate there—a phenomenon known as *capping*. In the inset, at the same magnification, is a portion of another mouse B lymphocyte treated in the same way, except that ferritin, an iron-bearing compound is conjugated to the RAMG. The disposition of ferritin, visualized as dense particles, indicates the distribution of antibody receptors on the surface of the mouse B lymphocyte. (From M. Karnovsky, *J. Exp. Med.*, **136**:907, 1972.)

1μ

subsequent phagocytosis depends upon the presence of microtubules beneath the plasma membrane which permit cellular asymmetry and microfilaments which are necessary for cytoplasmic movement. Phagocytosis of bacteria may require a surface against which the microorganisms can be pinioned. Often bacteria suspended in a fluid-filled body cavity escape phagocytosis. As Murphy points out, neutrophils can walk but not swim. Certain antibodies which enhance phagocytosis are termed *opsonins*. Neutrophils do not require the presence of opsonins to be phagocytic, but their plasma membrane contains surface receptors which bind certain opsonins and thereby facilitate phagocytosis.

Phagocytosis by neutrophils, and other granulocytes, is associated with fusion of lysosomes and other

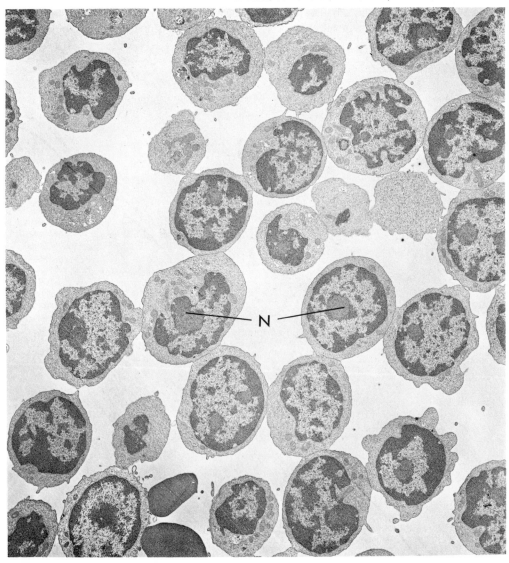

FIGURE 10-15 Lymphocytes of a rat. These cells have been isolated from the spleen. Many of them contain nucleoli (N). ×5000. (From L-T. Chen, A. Eden, V. Nussenzweig, and L. Weiss, *Cell Immunol.*, **4:**279, 1972.)

cytoplasmic granules with phagosomes (see full discussion of phagocytosis in Chap. 4). In neutrophils, the smaller specific granules usually fuse first with the phagosome, often within 30 s of its formation. Later, the azurophil granules may combine with the phagosome. As in macrophages, the fused phagosome and membrane-bounded granules remain contained in a membrane-bounded vesicle, the phagolysosome or heterolysosome, which protects the cell against the enzymes and other agents in the vesicle. Oxygen consumption is increased in phagocytosis. Adenosine triphosphate (ATP) is rapidly depleted by phagocytosis and is regenerated by glycolysis. It undoubtedly plays a role in phagosome formation and other membrane movements associated with phagocytosis.

Azurophil granules are lysosomal in character and thereby contain acid hydrolytic enzymes as DNAse, acid phosphatase, esterase, lipase, etc. In addition, they contain *lysozyme*, an enzyme complex

which hydrolyzes glycosides in the cell wall of bacteria. Azurophil granules also contain a *myeloperoxidase* which complexes with H_2O_2 and permits the production of an activated oxygen, which is bacteriocidal. The specific granules also contain lysozyme, as well as *lactoferrin,* a protein which has an affinity for ferric iron. Lactoferrin has a bacterisotatic action, since bacteria require this iron and lactoferrin makes it unavailable to them. The specific granules also contain cationic compounds rich in arginine and lysine, which are bacteriocidal. These granules, moreover, can generate lactic acid, peroxides, iodides, chlorides, fatty acids, and lecithins, all of which appear to have an inhibitor or killing action on microorganisms. For a comprehensive treatment of the neutrophil, consult Patrick Murphy's monograph.

Eosinophils and basophils are phagocytic and share many antimicrobial properties with neutrophils. The phagocytic system of neutrophils, eosinophils, and basophils has been termed the *microphage system,* to distinguish it from the *macrophage system* (see Chap. 4).

FIGURE 10-16 Human lymphocyte. A motile lymphocyte contains a moderate number of membrane-bounded granules. Note the microvilli on the cell surface. It is likely that the lymphocyte is moving to the left, advancing with its nuclear pole. The cell assumes a hand-mirror configuration. The tail of cytoplasm has been termed a *uropod.* ×9200. (From the work of G. A. Ackerman.)

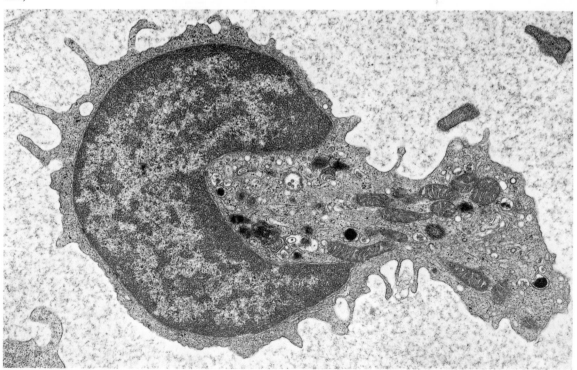

448

Certain fundamental properties of the neutrophils and other leukocytes are evident in the process of inflammation. If certain stimuli, often foreign substances such as chemical irritants or bacteria, are applied to the body or enter it, a series of reactions is initiated which constitute inflammation. Inflammation is largely a vascular and connective tissue phenomenon. The ground substance is depolymerized and becomes more liquid. Capillaries and venules supplying the affected area become dilated, increasing the blood supply to the part and hence its temperature. The permeability of the vascular wall is increased, and plasma pours into the surrounding connective tissue, causing swelling and increased pressure on local nerve endings. Macrophages, eosinophils, mast cells, and other connective tissue cells in the locale respond. Circulating polymorphonuclear leukocytes, monocytes, and lymphocytes escape through the capillary and postcapillary venular wall in great numbers and

move into the site. If the irritants are bacteria they are phagocytized—to a degree dependent upon their virulence and the resistance of the host. Leukocytes, largely neutrophils, die after a short time as a result of bacterial action, change in environmental pH, and an inherently limited life-span. Dead and dying leukocytes, in aggregate yellowish in color and often creamy or somewhat granular in consistency, are called *pus*. These are the events that underlie the swelling, redness, pain, and warmth of a boil or carbuncle.

The ancients recognized these characteristics of inflammation: *tumor, rubor, dolor,* and *calor.* They constitute the cardinal clinical features of the process. As the acute phase of inflammation subsides, macrophages come on the affected zone and clear some of

FIGURE 10-17 Platelet enmeshed in a fibrin clot from human blood. The platelet has a peripheral clear area, the hyalomere, and a central area containing mitochondria, ribosomes, and lysosomes, the granulomere. The platelet contains some glycogen, which is here selectively stained with lead, as minute granules. The fibrin forms an interlacing network which is in intimate contact with the platelet plasma membrane. ×32,000. Compare with Figs. 10-18 and 12-16.

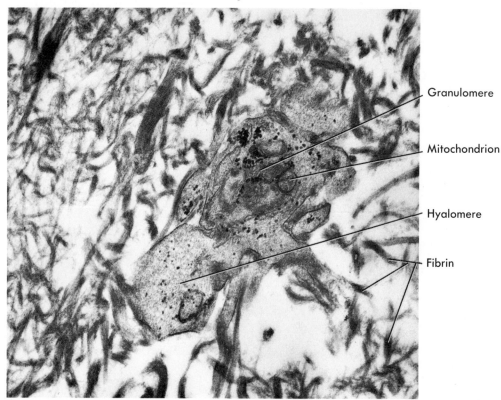

Granulomere

Mitochondrion

Hyalomere

Fibrin

the cellular remnants and persisting irritants by phagocytosis and the release of lytic enzymes. Although local macrophages participate in these reactions, in most instances of inflammation of any intensity, most of the macrophages come from circulating monocytes that leave blood vessels, move to the site of inflammation and, as they do, undergo transformation into macrophages which quickly become indistinguishable from resident macrophages of the connective tissues. These incoming phagocytes, at the outset smaller than some of the resident cells, have been termed *polyblasts*. Macrophages may, in some instances, accumulate and form nodules or *granulomata*. Indeed, there is a group of diseases, which includes tuberculosis and brucellosis, characterized by such accumulations of macrophages and identified as granulomatous diseases.

Eosinophils and basophils, like the neutrophils, are phagocytic. They appear, in addition, to play a more selective role in inflammation, especially in relation to immune reactions (see succeeding sections).

There are systems of polypeptides and proteins, many of them enzymes, which are complexly interrelated in the phenomena of blood coagulation, inflammation, and immunity. The *complement* system consists of at least 10 plasma components which, when activated, react sequentially or in a cascade. The consequences of this sequential action are multifold.

Components of complement may, in conjunction with certain antibodies, termed *lysins,* induce cell lysis. Other components induce the release of histamine from mast cells and basophils (see below), are chemotactic for neutrophils, enhance phagocytosis, induce smooth muscle contraction, and may initiate the coagulation of blood. The *kinins* are another plasmal system whose precursors are the prekallikreins. Intermediate compounds in the kinin sequences, as the kallikreins, are chemotactic for neutrophils and induce activation of the Hageman factor (see below). One product of this group of substances is the nonapeptide *bradykinin,* which is a potent agent, equivalent to histamine in inducing increased capillary permeability and the contraction of vascular and other smooth muscle. This system too is tied to the coagulation of blood. A central element in these humoral sequences is the *Hageman factor,* a plasma globulin which is capable of converting prekallikreins to active form and of both initiating blood coagulation and inducing lysis of the blood clot, *fibrinolysis.* Other humoral substances, *prostaglandins,* have inflammatory effects. These include the induction of pain, fever, and muscular contraction. (The salutory effects of aspirin appear to be largely owing to antiprostaglandin actions).

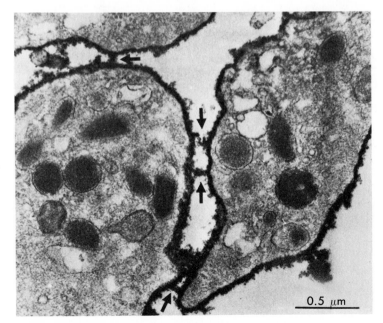

FIGURE 10-18 Platelets of human blood. Immunohistochemical localization of thrombostenin on the platelet surface and interplatelet bonds (arrows). (From F. M. Booyse and M. E. Rafelson, Jr., *Seri. Haematol.,* **4:**152, 1971.)

0.5 μm

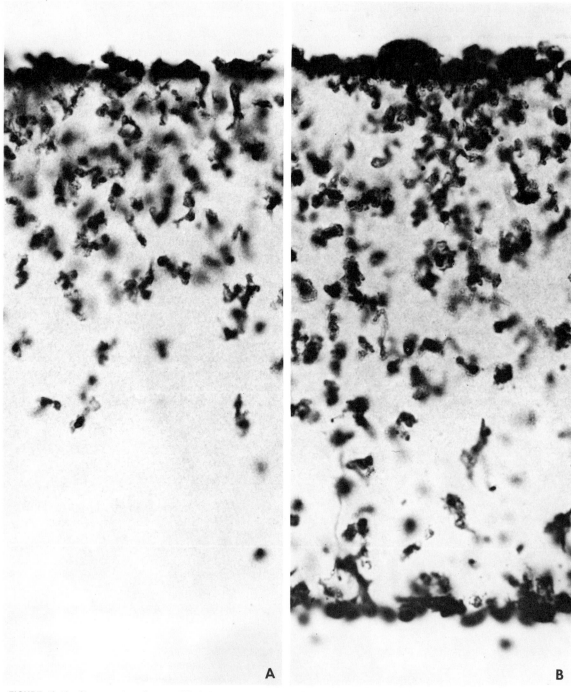

FIGURE 10-19 Chemotropism of neutrophilic leukocytes of the rabbit. Sagittal section of a millipore filter whose top surface has been layered with neutrophils. The bottom surface of A has been covered with serum alone. In B, however, a chemotropic substance has been applied to the bottom surface and the cells have migrated from the upper surface, through the filter, to the bottom surface. (From R. Snyderman, H. Gewurz, and S. E. Mergenlagen, *J. Exp. Med.,* **128:**259, 1968.)

Finally, in addition to the lysins, many antibodies facilitate phagocytosis. These are termed *opsonins*.

Phagocytosis has been emphasized as central to the antimicrobial activity of granulocytes. Their antimicrobial effects may be demonstrated without phagocytosis. Through the release of granules, akin to secretion, or the dissolution of the whole granulocyte, many powerful compounds are released. Where many granulocytes infiltrate and lyse, host tissue, as well as bacteria, may be damaged. The disease *gout* may depend upon such a process.

There are a number of syndromes in which heterophil granule formation or release is impaired. These conditions—which include chronic granulomatous disease of childhood, Chediak-Higashi syndrome, myeloperoxidase deficiency—interfere with the individual's ability to handle microorganisms and may be so severe as to result in death.

BASOPHILS

Basophils are phagocytic. Since they carry hydrolytic enzymes within their granules, they undoubtedly share antimicrobial features of heterophils. The granules contain *heparin* and *histamine.* Heparin is a sulfated mucopolysaccharide responsible for the metachromatic basophilia of the granules. It is an anticoagulant of blood and disperses lipid. Histamine, formed by the decarboxylation of the amino acid histidine, *serotonin,* which occurs in rodent basophil granules, and *slow reacting substance* (SRS) are vasodilating agents inducing increased vascular permeability. Unlike histamine, whose effects are prompt and transient, SRS acts in a more sustained fashion following a latent period. Serotonin is a peptide. SRS is lipid, possibly related to the fatty acid hormones known as the prostaglandins. Thus the granules of basophils contain certain very powerful vasoactive mediators which, on release, can induce widespread effects so severe as to induce vascular collapse. The granules of mast cells are similar to those of basophils, and the two cell types may be considered part of the same system. These granules may well be discharged following a variety of stimuli, and they may play a critical part in nonspecific inflammation. However, a specific type of degranulation does occur. Certain antigens, in the course of a distinctive immune response, for reasons unknown, induce the production by plasma cells of a distinctive class of antibody, immunoglobulin E (IgE), which quickly becomes fixed to the cell surface of basophils and mast cells. Thus, loaded with IgE, the basophils

and mast cells remain apparently undisturbed. But when the antigen which induced the formation of IgE reenters the body, it combines with the cell surface-bound IgE. The cells undergo acute degranulation, releasing histamine and the other mediators. The reaction may be localized to certain shock organs such as the skin (the so-called Prausnitz-Küstner reagenic response) and the lungs (as bronchial asthma); or it may be widespread and severe, as in the anaphylactic response following a bee sting or an injection of penicillin in allergic individuals.

EOSINOPHILS

Eosinophils, like neutrophils, are motile phagocytic cells containing lysosomelike specific granules. They therefore possess antimicrobial properties. The basic proteins and the considerable peroxidase in eosinophilic granules contribute additional bacteriocidal properties. Eosinophils have been described as having an affinity for antigen-antibody complexes.[2] They are attracted to these complexes and engulf them. Antigen-antibody complexes, though often inactive themselves, are capable of initiating a train of events with far-reaching effects. For example, antigen-antibody complexes bind *complement,* and as a result induce cellular lysis. By phagocytizing and inactivating antigen-antibody complexes, eosinophils may suppress or dampen the responses set in motion by such complexes.

In the horse and perhaps other animals, moreover, eosinophils are characteristically attracted to mast cells and basophils or, specifically, to the histamine that these cells release. There may be a type of balance or pairing off of eosinophils which mute allergic inflammatory responses and basophils and mast cells which excite them.

Certain processes drive the percentage of circulating eosinophils to more than 90 percent of the circulating leukocytes. These are parasitic infestations of muscle of which *trichinosis* is the paradigm. Evidence exists that extracts of trichina worms induce a class of lymphocyte to stimulate the marrow to produce eosinophils. Eosinophils accumulate in allergic

---

[2] The antigen-antibody complexes considered here are free, not cell-bound, as in the IgE system. The antibody involved here, moreover, is IgG or IgM, not IgE.

reactions, perhaps called there by the action of histamine and other mediators. In the pulmonary tissues in bronchial asthma, where eosinophils collect in great number, characteristic crystals—Charcot-Leyden crystals—occur. These are probably derived from the dense core or crystalloid in the eosinophilic granule.

It has recently been established that eosinophils have a central function in the control of certain parasitic diseases, as schistosomiasis. The parasites, on invading the host, induce the production of what appears to be a distinctive antibody. This antibody potentiates the action of eosinophils, causing them to exert a powerful antiparasitic action which can eliminate the parasites. This action can be aborted by an antieosinophilic antibody which destroys eosinophils. An antineutrophilic antibody and an antimonocytic antibody have no effect on the antiparasitic action.

LYMPHOCYTES

Lymphocytes are the cell types central in the immune system. The expressions of immunity are the consequences of interactions between lymphocytes and macrophages and other ancillary cells. These interactions depend upon receptor molecules lying in the plasma membrane and the release of chemical mediators which affect both the releasing cells and other cells.

The idea of immunity is rooted in infectious disease. If an individual survives a bout with infectious disease he may thereafter be resistant or immune to that disease. There is implicit in this concept both *specificity*—for the individual has resistance to the disease he has survived and not to others—and *memory*—because the immunity is long lasting, "remembered" for many years, even lifelong. The concept of immunity has become broadened in recent years. It is a means of recognizing genetic relatedness. Thus, an animal will mount an immune attack against foreign protein or tissue, but not against his own, or genetically identical, tissue. The immune system is very sensitive in recognizing even slight differences between what is native to an individual and what is foreign, what is "self" and what is "nonself," and in reacting against nonself. An intriguing speculation is that cancer represents a mutation which an individual's immune system recognizes as nonself and therefore reacts against it. The development of cancer as a disease may thus represent a failure of the immune system to control an essentially foreign process. Indeed, when an individual's immune system is suppressed by x-rays or other means, there is a great increase in the incidence of cancer. In some cases, the immune system may lose the distinction between self and nonself and mount an attack on the host's own tissues. This process, identified as *autoimmune disease,* is the basis of such clinical diseases as rheumatic fever, certain types of thyroid disease and hematologic disease, and diverse other diseases.

Two major expressions of immunologic activity are *humoral immunity* and *cellular immunity.*

Humoral Immunity

The basis of humoral immunity is the secretion of antibody by lymphocytes and plasma cells and the diffusion of the antibody throughout the blood plasma, lymph, and other fluids of the body. The large-scale secretion of antibody is triggered by an antigen (Ag). Antigens are particulate or colloidal substances, typically foreign to the host, which may be *immunogenic* (that is, capable of inducing an immune response). *Antibodies* (Ab) are proteins, for the most part gamma globulins. They are classified as *immunoglobulins* (Ig) and are of several types. IgM is a large molecule (molecular weight of approximately one million) and is typically, in humans and many animals, the first produced in an immune response. It is too large to cross the placenta. As an immune response proceeds, IgM production wanes and is succeeded by IgG, a smaller (molecular weight approximately 160,000), more efficient, higher-affinity antibody capable of crossing placenta. IgG accounts for most of the antibody in serum, and in *secondary responses,* in most animals; that is, in responses occurring after reintroduction of antigen, IgG is the immunoglobulin produced. It is, therefore, the antibody associated with memory. IgA is a secretory immunoglobulin produced in the respiratory tract in lymphatic tissues associated with the gut (GALT), the genitourinary tract, and places where a mucous membrane separates the body from the environment. It is produced by plasma cells and lymphocytes beneath the epithelium and then passes through the epithelium which secretes it into the lumen of the vicus. As it passes through the epithelium, two molecules of IgA (which in molecular configuration resemble IgG) are "dimerized" by a protein *secretory piece,* synthesized, and added by the epithelial cells. This dimerization may make the antibody more resistant to breakdown in the lumen of the gut or other viscera where it operates. IgE is the class of immunoglobulin, termed *homotropic,* that becomes affixed to the surface of mast cells and basophils. IgD has not been well defined, as yet.

Humoral immunity may be transferred from an immune to a nonimmune animal by the transfer of serum (which contains antibody) or by the transfer of antibody-producing cells.

Immunoglobulins, for the most part, are pro-

duced by *plasma cells.* These are, in essence, unicellular glands, containing the organelles associated with the synthesis and secretion of protein, namely, nucleoli, rough ER, and Golgi. They are free cells, concentrated in lymphatic tissues (as lymph nodes and spleen) but found in connective tissues throughout the body. They measure 10 to 20 μm in diameter. Plasma cells will vary in appearance, depending on phases in their life cycle (Fig. 10-20). In almost every phase, however, they have an ample cytoplasm with rough ER, the cisternae of which contain antibody. This antibody can be revealed by special stains. Their Golgi apparatus is large, lying in the cytocentrum, and is concerned with "packaging the antibody" and synthe-

FIGURE 10-20 Phagocytic polymorphonuclear heterophil of the rabbit. This cell, harvested from the peritoneal cavity, has ingested zymosan particles (Z). The specific granules of the heterophil discharge their content of hydrolytic enzymes into the phagocytic vacuole. The granule moves toward the phagocytic vacuole; its membrane fuses with the membrane of the vacuole (arrows); and the contents of the granule enters the phagocytic vacuole. ×30,000. (D. Zucker-Franklin.)

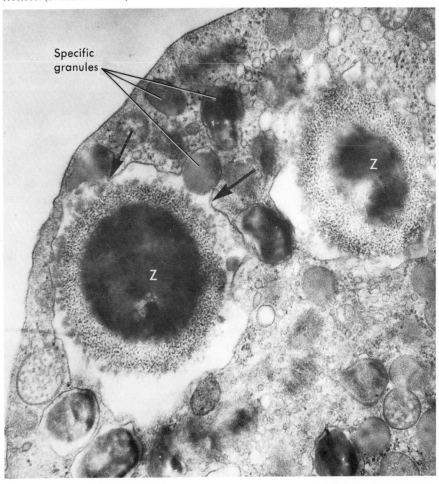

Specific granules

sizing and affixing a carbohydrate moiety to the protein antibody. The nucleus tends to lie eccentrically, displaced by the large cytocentrum. The precursors of plasma cells are B lymphocytes. These lymphocytes circulate in the blood and lie in characteristic loci in spleen, lymph nodes, and other lymphatic tissues. They are indistinguishable by Romanovsky staining and by most techniques, from the other major class of lymphocytes, T lymphocytes; but they can be recognized by special immunocytochemical methods. The surface of B cells is covered with molecules of immunoglobulin of the IgM type. These molecules lie in the plasma membrane of the cell, free to move about in the plane of the membrane, with their Ag-combining sites free to react. Their presence can be revealed by immunocytochemical reagents, which depend upon making, as a reagent, an antibody to the surface immunoglobulin (an antibody to an antibody). The reagent antibody is then labeled in order to be recognized by light microscopy (a fluorescent label) or by electron microscopy (an electron-dense label as *ferritin* or *peroxidase*, which can be made to yield a dense product). The labeled antibody reagent can now be used to react selectively with the antibody on the surface of B lymphocytes (or with the antibody within plasma cells) and thereby reveal these cells in sections or smears of tissue. (See Fig. 1-7 and discussion in Chap. 2.) The molecules of immunoglobulin which are so revealed on the surface of the B lymphocyte number about 150,000. Although they may move about over the surface, they tend to be rather uniformly dispersed. The B lymphocyte thus synthesizes enough antibody to coat its surface with some spilling into the immediate environment. These antibody molecules appear to act as receptors for antigen and are essential for the development of the immune response. B lymphocytes probably function in the following fashion. An antigen enters the body and is distributed rather selectively by the lymphatic apparatus to sites of B cell concentration (see Chaps. 13 and 14). Here it will "find," or "select," B cells whose surface antibody fit determinants on the antigenic surface, and the antigen will then link or form complexes with some of the surface immunoglobulin molecules. These linked surface complexes move to one pole of the cell and are then interiorized by pinocytosis. This linking initiates the differentiation of the B lymphocytes into plasma cells. It is a change which is associated with two proc-

esses. The first is differentiation, signified by the acquisition of antibody containing rough ER and other characteristics of plasma cells. The other is proliferation, the result of which is that from an antigen-activated B lymphocyte a clone of plasma cells (as well as additional B lymphocytes which do not differentiate) is produced. The rate of proliferation, moreover, is quite high, mitoses occurring every 6 h for a number of cellular generations. B lymphocytes may be long-lived cells, their life-span measured in months and even in years. Plasma cells, on the other hand, likely live only 2 weeks or thereabouts.

The conversion of B lymphocytes to plasma cells holds the key to several features of the immune process. The process is highly specific; only those antigens which fit sterically with the already produced surface immunoglobulin can trigger the conversion. It is thus a process of *selection* rather than, as had been thought, one of *instruction* wherein an antigen could choose any immunologically competent lymphocyte and "instruct" it to make an antibody against it. The role of antigen is, therefore, to stimulate the differentiation of B cells and induce high-level antibody formation.

Another feature of the process is the change from IgM to IgG production. The receptor immunoglobulin on the B cells is IgM (and IgD), and IgM is the first antibody produced. But as the lymphocytes differentiate into plasma cells, IgG is produced and the production of IgM is phased out. The basis of memory and of a heightened secondary response lies in the increased number of B lymphocytes as a result of the proliferation of the antigen-triggered B lymphocytes. Now there is a larger pool of B lymphocytes which provide memory and are the basis of a heightened response on reintroduction of antigen. (As will be evident from the discussion below, T cells may also be the basis of memory.) Specificity, memory, and heightened secondary response are thus inherent in the process. Humoral immunity is an efficient reaction because clusters of antibody-producing cells in strategic locations (see below) produce antibodies in prodigious quantity, and these antibodies diffuse through the fluids of the body and provide protection against foreign material which enters or originates in the body.

Many antigens, particularly those having a polymeric or repeating structure, can directly induce the transformation of B cells into plasma cells. But most cases of antibody production appear to be T-cell-dependent. The sequence is this: a T cell recognizes and combines with antigen by means of receptors on its surface. The T cell then moves to an appropriate B cell, perhaps with the help of a macrophage (see below), and presents the antigen to the Ig receptors on the B cell. Or the T cell may liberate microhumoral substances which activate the B cells. If the Ag or specific substance is presented in an appropriate pattern to the B cell, the cell is "turned on" and undergoes proliferation and differentiation to plasma cells. But Ag may be presented in such a manner by the T cell as to "turn off" the B cell and abort antibody formation. Thus, while Ab formation requires B cell differentiation, it is in most instances the consequence of cellular interactions, wherein T cells and B cells act sequentially. T cells modulate the immune response since they may induce or suppress antibody formation by B cells.

Finally, macrophages have a place in the process of antibody formation. They may process antigen, making it immunogenic. When sheep erythrocytes are given to mice and elicit an immune response, they must be broken up into colloidal or small-sized particles. Macrophages do this. In addition, macrophages may hold antigen on their surface for long periods of time and present it to T and B cells. This is an important function, since antigen otherwise is quickly eliminated from the body. Macrophages may eliminate excess antigen from the body. Curiously, Ag in very high (or very low) concentration causes the immune system to be unresponsive—a type of immune paralysis or tolerance. By phagocytizing a proportion of Ag in the body and thereby destroying it or isolating it from immunocompetent cells, macrophages may reduce the level of antigen to immunogenic levels. Finally, macrophages may play a physical role in bringing T and B cells into association, thereby permitting their interactions.

Cellular Immunity

In contrast to humoral immunity, which by the dispersion of antibody molecules has systemic scope, cellular immunity depends upon immunologically competent cells working over short range in restricted sites. The process may indeed be widespread, because of the migratory capacity of the competent cells and the multiplicity of sites. Cellular immunity depends upon T-lymphocytes (or T cells). Like B cells, they are circulating lymphocytes. In the blood of most mammals, T lymphocytes account for approximately 35 percent of the circulatory lymphocytes and B cells for the most of the remainder. T cells may be identified by surface receptors. It is a matter of controversy whether T cells bear surface immunoglobulin. If they

do, it is present in much smaller amounts than B cells (perhaps only about 700 molecules per cell surface), and it cannot be demonstrated immunocytochemically as in the case with B cells. There are functional immune response (Ir) genes in immunologically competent cells and a number of investigators believe that a low molecular weight factor with antigen-specific receptors may be produced by the Ir genes and move to the cell surface as antigen receptors. While there is controversy with respect to their nature, it must be emphasized that T cells do have receptors on their surface which can recognize antigen and react with it. As with B cells, moreover, these receptors are narrowly specific for antigen: T cells capable of reacting with albumin will not reaction with, say, globulin. It is possible, moreover, to demonstrate a number of distinctive substances on the surface of T cells; and even though the function of these substances is not known, they serve as markers. Antibodies to these substances may be prepared and, when suitably labeled, are the basis of immunocytochemical tests for the detection of T cells. In practice, to define these cell surface markers and to prepare antibodies against them, concentrations of T cells are injected into a suitable animal to raise antibodies, these antibodies are absorbed on possible contaminating cells and B cells and macrophages, and an anti-T-cell antibody is thereby refined and made more specific. By this means the theta (θ) *antigen* has been recognized on mouse T cells, and distinctive markers have been found on T cells of other species.

Cellular immunity appears to depend upon the specific interaction of antigen and T cell. If so stimulated, the T cell proliferates, forming a clone, and a number of cells in this clone synthesize and release low molecular weight compounds termed *lymphokines*. The T cells and antigen may interact near the site of introduction of antigen or in lymph node, spleen, or other lymphatic tissue if the antigen is carried there. The activated T cells will be distributed throughout the body, including sites of antigen concentration where they release their lymphokines and exert their effects locally.

Among the lymphokines are a macrophage migration inhibitory factor (MIF), chemotactic factors for basophils, lymphotoxins, and nonspecific cellular toxins. About a dozen lymphokine activities have been characterized. MIF is particularly important because it induces macrophages in the vicinity of the antigen–T-cell reaction to remain and to function there instead of moving away. Cellular immunity can thus be visualized as a complex process initiated by the *specific* reactions of T cells with antigen. But consequent to that, lymphokines are released which react nonspecifically. In contrast to the widespread effects of humoral immunity in which millions of antibody molecules are produced and released to circulate through the fluids or humors of the body, cellular immunity depends on sensitized cells reaching loci of antigen, reacting with them, and releasing lymphokines which act over a short distance. The events of cellular immunity, moreover, take longer to manifest themselves. For this reason, cellular immunity has been classified as a *delayed hypersensitivity* in contrast to the *immediate sensitivity* mediated by antibody. Examples will make the distinction clear. A classic type of cellular immunity occurs in tuberculosis, as the *tuberculin reaction*. A *purified protein derivative* (PPD) of tubercle bocilli is injected into the skin of an animal infected with tubercle bacilli and therefore sensitive to many antigens in the tubercle bacilli, including PPD. The site of injection is first apparently unreactive, and then in 6 to 8 h redness and induration (hardness) appear. The reaction builds to a peak in 24 to 48 h and then subsides. It may consist only of redness and some swelling, but if severe, it can be painful and lead to necrosis. The basis of the reaction is that circulating lymphocytes sensitive to the PPD (having surface receptors for the PPD) pass the site where tubercle bacilli lie, react there with the PPD, and liberate lymphokines. These immobilize local and passing macrophages and other lymphocytes, induce inflammation, and cause some cell damage and death. Despite the fact that sensitized lymphocytes initiated the process, the major cell types present and effecting the reaction are monocytes and macrophages. Indeed, of the lymphocytes present, a large portion accumulate nonspecifically so that sensitized lymphocytes are in the minority. The result is a lesion which, microscopically, consists of relatively few lymphocytes and large numbers of macrophages clustered together in an inflammatory site. This process takes some time to develop—hence the designation delayed hypersensitivity. The term cellular immunity emphasizes the local cellular reaction.

Among other examples of cellular immunity are the rejection of foreign tissue grafts, for example, skin, heart, or kidney. In contrast, an example of humoral antibody-mediated immunity is the *Arthus reaction*. Here, an antigen is injected into the skin of an individual who is immunized against that antigen and carries circulating antibody to it (antibody that had been produced by plasma cells). Within minutes after injection, the site is inflamed: red, painful, hot, and hard. The events were initiated by a complexing of injected antigen and circulating antibody at the site. The Ag-Ab complex combines with complement and other serum factors and cause some local injury, inducing inflammation with accumulation of large numbers of neutrophils. The immune responses associated with basophils and mast cells are immediate types of hypersensitivity associated with humoral antibody (see discussion above).

It is evident from the discussion above that lymphocytes are central in the immune response. In summary, B lymphocytes are precursors to plasma cells. They synthesize antibody and underlie humoral antibody production. T lymphocytes are the basis of cellular immunity. In addition, they may regulate humoral antibody production. T lymphocytes may be necessary to permit B lymphocytes to mount a humoral response—or, contrariwise, to suppress B cell differentiation and forestall a humoral response. It is becoming evident that there are subclasses of T cells which may account for the diverse reactions of this class of cells. Among the subpopulations of T cells is a group responsible for immunological memory and rejection of grafts and another group concerned with regulation of the immune response.

The Development of Immunologic Competence

At birth most mammals are immunologically inactive, both because their capacities to produce antibody and to participate in delayed hypersensitivity are not fully developed and because the placental barrier has shielded them, at least in part, from foreign material. In this period the newborn is protected against many infectious diseases by maternal antibodies, which cross the placental barrier and circulate in the body. Such transplacental transfer of antibody is a passive type of immunization. Within a few days of birth, however, the newborn's own immunologic mechanism becomes active. It is a matter of great theoretical significance that if a foreign substance is introduced into an animal before it is immunologically competent, that is, before the concept of self develops, and that substance persists, it becomes a part of self and antibodies are not produced against it. It thus is possible to give neonatal rabbits a powerful antigen, bovine serum albumin, and these animals will not elaborate antibody against this antigen if it persists in the body, despite the fact that they become immunologically competent. This phenomenon is of clinical significance in some cases of twinning, where fraternal twins of different blood types are tolerant of one another's blood because of some prenatal mixing.

A type of immunologic unresponsiveness may be induced in mature individuals by damaging the lymphatic tissue with x-ray or radiomimetic drugs. Advantage is taken of this phenomenon in the treatment of patients requiring transplants of kidneys or other tissue. To facilitate the acceptance of the graft, the patient is subjected to whole-body radiation or radiomimetic drugs at doses calculated to suppress immunologic competence.

Lymphocytes have been cast as hematopoietic stem cells by the monophyletic school of blood formation. The evidence for the existence of stem cells and their possible lymphocytic nature is presented in Chap. 11.

MONOCYTES

Circulating monocytes are the direct precursors of macrophages. Accordingly their functions are dis-

cussed in Chap. 4, dealing with Connective Tissues.

PLATELETS

Platelets have diverse functions that relate to endothelium and to blood clotting. They may release clot-inducing factors which they adsorb from serum or synthesize. Contrariwise, they may release a fibrinolysin which dissolves clots. Containing these functionally antithetic substances may permit platelets to nicely control the proper development and lysis of clots. Further, platelets are required for clot retraction. Indeed the degree of clot retraction may be used as an assay of platelet function.

Platelets contain serotonin and other vasomotor agents which, on release, induce vascular contraction. Normal vascular competence depends upon sufficient levels of circulating blood platelets. The normal level is 200,000 to 400,000/mm^3. If platelets drop below 60,000/mm^3, blood seeps out of the vessels, resulting in hemorrhage, or *purpura*. In fact, platelets are necessary for the maintenance of normal endothelial structure. When platelets are reduced to purpuric levels, the endothelium becomes attenuated, stretched and fenestrated. When platelets are restored, the endothelium returns to normal.

REFERENCES

See reference list at the end of Chap. 11.

The Life Cycle of Blood Cells

LEON WEISS

ORIGIN AND DEVELOPMENT OF BLOOD CELLS

This chapter treats the development, distribution, life-span, and destruction of blood cells. Blood cells are produced in specialized centers called *hematopoietic tissues*. Erythrocytes and granulocytes evolve from precursor cells by a series of profound cytologic transformations. The changes associated with lymphocytes and monocytes are less marked. Blood cells normally are released to the circulation only when sufficiently mature. They circulate within blood vessels but may be withdrawn from the circulation and remain pooled within certain vascular beds. They may leave blood vessels and enter the connective tissues, where they function, undergo transformation into other cell types, or are destroyed. Or, apparently unchanged, they may reenter the circulation, often via lymphatic vessels. Blood cells have a predictable life-span, and when they die, some of their components are reutilized in the manufacture of new cells.

SITES OF PRODUCTION OF BLOOD CELLS

The major postnatal hematopoietic organs are bone marrow, spleen, lymph nodes, and thymus. Prenatally hematopoiesis also occurs in the yolk sac and liver.

With the exception of the thymus, which has both entodermal and mesenchymal components, the major hematopoietic organs in mammals consist of specialized reticular connective tissues of mesenchymal origin. They contain a stroma made of reticular cells and fibers, and blood and lymphatic vessels, nerves, capsule, and trabeculae. Free cells include the blood cells and their precursors, macrophages, plasma cells, and other cells of the connective tissues.

PRENATAL HEMATOPOIESIS

Hematopoiesis in the human embryo begins in the second week of life, extraembryonically, in the wall of the yolk sac. Small nests of hematopoietic cells, largely erythroblastic (that is, productive of erythrocytes), lie in the mesenchyme. Most of these nests are surrounded by incomplete or isolated segments of developing blood vessels. These foci constitute *blood*

459

islands. Later the segments of vessels enlarge and coalesce, form a confluent network within the wall of the yolk sac, connect to the systemic intraembryonic vessels by means of the vitelline vasculature, and become part of the circulation. Most hematopoietic foci in the yolk sac are enclosed by endothelium, but some hematopoiesis is extravascular. Carried in the blood or by direct migration of cells, hematopoietic cells of yolk-sac origin become distributed through the embryo.

By the sixth week of embryonic life in human beings, hematopoietic foci appear in the liver. The liver is established as the major hematopoietic center (Figs. 11-1 and 11-2). Again, erythropoiesis dominates. Myelopoiesis (the production of granulocytes) is minor, but there is moderate production of platelets and macrophages.

Primitive and *definitive* erythroblasts are produced in embryos. There is a shift from the first to the second, which tends to occur at about the time that hematopoiesis shifts from yolk sac to liver. In the mouse, primitive erythroblasts are produced only in the yolk sac and definitive erythroblasts are produced in the liver. In rabbits, guinea pigs, and cats, on the other hand, great numbers of definitive erythroblasts are produced in the yolk sac. In human beings, mod-

erate numbers of definitive erythroblasts are produced there. Primitive erythroblasts are relatively large cells with a large euchromatic nucleus. Definitive erythroblasts are smaller cells with a small heterochromatic nucleus. Definitive erythroblasts, unlike primitive erythroblasts, lose their nuclei near the end of their maturation cycle and become anucleate erythrocytes. It is likely, moreover, that the definitive erythroblast is responsive to the hormone *erythropoietin* and the primitive erythroblast is not. Associated with the shift from the earlier to the later erythroblast is a shift in the chain structure of hemoglobin: from fetal (HbF) to adult (HbA and HbA_2).

Virtually all hepatic hematopoiesis is extravascular, occurring amidst the hepatic parenchymal cells.

On a minor level, hematopoiesis goes on in the spleen parallel to that in the liver. Hematopoiesis, largely erythropoietic, becomes established in the spleen in the third fetal month and, in human beings, fades in the fifth. In mice, splenic erythropoiesis occurs throughout life, as does thrombopoiesis (platelet production).

Bone marrow appears in the clavicle in the second month of human fetal life and, with the increased formation of bone, becomes more extensive. It becomes the dominant hematopoietic organ in the latter half of gestation and throughout postnatal life, the site where all of the blood cells except T lymphocytes are produced. A high concentration of hematopoietic

FIGURE 11-1 Liver of a fetal mouse. A light micrograph of 1-μm section of epon-embedded 11-day fetal mouse liver (gestation 21 days, 057B1/6J strain). Sinuses (S), endothelium of sinuses (En), and cords of hepatic parenchymal epithelium and differentiating erythroid cells (HP) are noted. Within the sinuses circulate nucleated red cells of the primitive, yolk-sac series. They are darkly stained because of their high hemoglobin content. Within the parenchymal cords the erythroblasts of the definitive erythroid lineage are observed as relatively distinct, rounded cell types. Between them, often vacuolated, are processes of the hepatocytes. ×780. (From the work of R. A. Rifkind.)

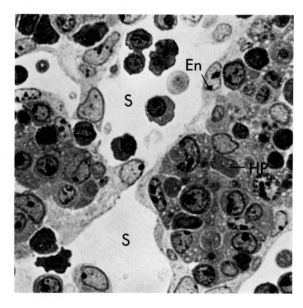

stem cells is maintained there, moreover. Streams of cells emanate from the marrow to circulate and populate other tissues.

A more restricted lymphatic type of hematopoiesis occurs in the thymus. From the second month of gestation, it produces T lymphocytes and may also contribute to mast cell formation.

The spleen and lymph nodes receive and begin to stock T cells from the thymus as early as the second fetal month in humans. But only in the first postnatal weeks are the stocks large. Thus, in the definitive layout of hematopoiesis which emerges in the late fetal period and becomes established in the weeks after birth, the bone marrow is the central hematopoietic organ. Its capacity for sequestering hematopoietic stem cells far exceeds that of any other organ. In human beings it produces all the erythrocytes, granulocytes, monocytes, and platelets. It supplies B lymphocytes or their precursors to the spleen, lymph nodes, and other lymphatic tissues. The spleen and lymph nodes are primarily traps or filters wherein cells

FIGURE 11-2 Electron micrograph from a preparation similar to that in Fig. 11-1. A sinus endothelial cell is seen (top right, En). Three early erythroblasts are seen within the cord (Pro). Hepatocytes (Ep) are distinguished by their content of endoplasmic reticulum and extended contours. The erythroblasts show minimal ER, many free ribosomes, few mitochondria, and a rounded, compact contour. Hematopoiesis (definitive cell line) is predominantly, if not exclusively, an extravascular event. By day 12 reticulocytes may be observed which then pass across the endothelial border and enter the circulation. ×5000. (From the work of R. A. Rifkind.)

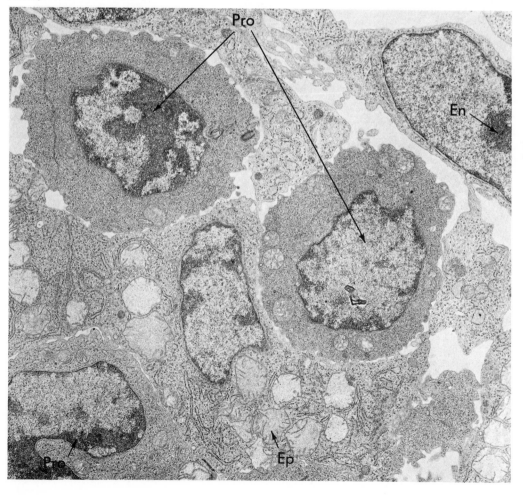

and materials from the blood and lymph are sequestered and permitted to interact. Thus, they trap monocytes released from the marrow and lymphocytes released from both marrow and thymus; and with antigens trapped from the blood (spleen) and lymph (lymph nodes), they permit the sequential cellular interactions which result in an immune response.

The liver is inactive hematopoietically in humans after birth. It reserves its potential for hematopoiesis, however, and in cases of failure of the marrow, hematopoiesis may be resumed there, a phenomenon termed *extramedullary hematopoiesis.*

SCHOOLS OF HEMATOPOIESIS

Sharply divergent views have been held regarding the hematopoietic potential of the earliest of the hematopoietic cells. These views have been codified in the *monophyletic* and *polyphyletic schools of blood formation.*

The monophyletic school considered the earliest recognizable precursor of blood cells, termed *hemocytoblasts,* capable of differentiating into any blood cell type. Further, it held that the lymphocyte and the hemocytoblast were equivalent cells. In other words, the lymphocyte was considered a multipotential stem cell.

The complete polyphyletists recognized a separate stem cell for each of the blood cell types, that is, a stem cell for erythrocytes, another for granulocytes, another for lymphocytes, and another for monocytes. The most strongly presented polyphyletic position evolved into a "dualist" position in which two precursor cell types were recognized: a primitive white cell that can produce granulocytes, lymphocytes, and monocytes; and an endothelial cell, lining a collapsed sinusoid or an intersinusoidal capillary, that can produce erythrocytes and megakaryocytes.

But the essence of the struggle between monophyletists and polyphyletists revolved around the capacity for differentiation of lymphocytes. The polyphyletists regarded these cells as an end stage incapable of further differentiation. The monophyletists regarded them as capable of differentiating into the other blood cells.

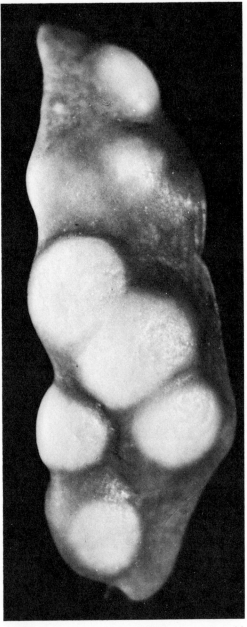

FIGURE 11-3 Splenic nodules. This spleen was removed from an animal given lethal irradiation and then a "rescuing" injection of bone marrow cells. The marrow cells circulated to the irradiated spleen where they remained, proliferated, and formed these macroscopic colonies. It is likely that each of these colonies is a clone (see text). (From the work of J. Till and E. McCulloch.)

The monophyletic and polyphyletic positions outlined above were developed and hardened almost a half century ago. We must now consider whether, by more recent evidence, a hematopoietic stem cell, *defined as a cell capable both of differentiating into any of the blood cells and of maintaining itself by mitotic division,* exists. If it exists, moreover, what is its relation to lymphocytes?

Experiments within the past 15 years by Ford, Barnes, and their associates and by Till and McCulloch and their associates strongly indicate that a hematopoietic stem cell exists (Figs. 11-3 to 11-6). Their work depends on observations of cells which bear distinctive chromosomal markers (revealed in the metaphase karyotype) and are injected into irradiated hosts. Their data and conclusions result from the following type of experimental model.

After lethal irradiation (that is, more than 900 rads) a mouse dies with a profound depletion of all its blood cells (pancytopenia). Death may be averted if such an irradiated mouse is given a suspension of living bone marrow cells from another mouse. Animals so treated survive and in early stages of recovery show in their spleen, against a background of radia-

tion-induced devastation, grossly visible nodules which represent small colonies of proliferating hematopoietic cells. The cellular composition of these colonies varies, but significant numbers contain erythroblasts, myeloblasts, megakaryocytoblasts, and cells of lymphoid character—in short, precursors of all the blood cells. There is direct and indirect evidence that each of these colonies, including those with multiple cell types, is a clone, that is, is derived from a single cell. Such a cell, termed a *CFU* or *CFC* (*colony-forming unit* or *colony-forming cell*) by Till and McCulloch, would clearly fit the definition of a stem cell.

The direct evidence for the existence of stem cells is obtained by irradiating the donor marrow cells severely, *but not lethally,* to induce chromosomal damage. This chromosomal damage occurs in a widespread, unpredictable way and typically results in unique or highly distinctive abnormal karyotypes. When such irradiated donor cells, containing uniquely damaged karyotypes, form splenic colonies in lethally irradiated recipients, Becker, Wu, Till and McCulloch found that different hematopoietic cell types within a given colony bore the same distinctive karyotype. This

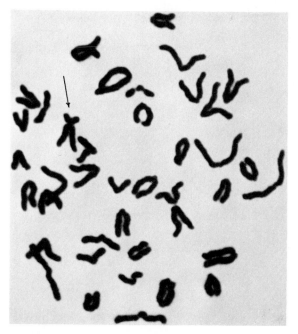

FIGURE 11-4 ''Unique'' mouse karyotype. The clonal nature of the splenic colonies exemplified in Fig. 11-3 is revealed by distinctive or unique karyotypes in the donor marrow cells. These karyotypes are induced by lightly irradiating the donor cells (see text). Arrow points to the distinctively damaged chromosomes which serve as a marker. (From the work of W. T. Wu, J. Till, and E. McCulloch.)

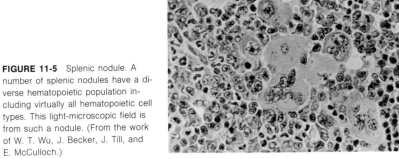

FIGURE 11-5 Splenic nodule. A number of splenic nodules have a diverse hematopoietic population including virtually all hematopoietic cell types. This light-microscopic field is from such a nodule. (From the work of W. T. Wu, J. Becker, J. Till, and E. McCulloch.)

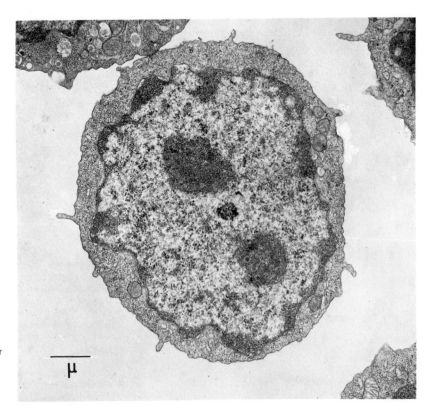

FIGURE 11-6 Candidate stem cell. There are no obvious morphological signs indicating cellular differentiation. The cytoplasm is rich in free ribosomes. ×15,130. (From the work of Van Bekkum et. al., *Blood,* **38:**547, 1971.)

reveals that different blood cell lines, such as erythrocytes, granulocytes, and platelets, can originate from the same cell. Indirect evidence supporting the clonal nature of splenic colonies includes the existence of a linear relation between the number of nucleated donor cells and the number of splenic colonies without an initial threshold, and the resemblance of the radiation survival curve of colony-forming cells to that of single cells in tissue culture or tumor transplants.

More differentiated cell types derive from the CFC. These include the precursor of erythroblasts, a cell sensitive to the action of erythropoietin (the hormone stimulating erythropoiesis), the *erythropoietin responsive cell* (ERC). There is, in addition, a myelopoietic precursor.

In addition to the experimental work of the Till and McCulloch group, the occurrence in human myelogenous leukemia of the Philadelphia chromosome, an abnormal chromosome revealed in karyotype analysis, suggests the presence of a cell of more restricted potential than stem cells because this abnormal marker may be found in every cell type except lymphocytes.

The greatest concentration of stem cells in the adult, as determined by splenic colony assay, is in the bone marrow. The total number in the marrow of the mouse may be 40,000 cells. In contrast, the mouse spleen may have only 2000. The vastly greater capacity of the marrow relative to the spleen to restore an irradiated recipient is explicable by its twentyfold superiority in stem-cell content. Even its relatively high content of stem cells does not represent, for the marrow, a high concentration; in the mouse it is 1 per 10,000 nucleated cells.

In the mouse, approximately 10 stem cells are present in each milliliter of blood; this is a concentration of approximately 1 per 1,000,000 nulceated blood cells, one one-hundredth the concentration in the marrow.

Stem cells circulate in the fetus and occur in fetal liver and marrow. At the time of the decline in hepatic hematopoiesis, the number of circulating stem cells is unusually high, suggesting large-scale hematopoietic movement to the marrow.

Although no direct evidence of the structure of the stem cell exists, there is strong indirect evidence that it is quite similar to lymphocytes in structure, even though many investigators eschew that term, preferring to call it a *candidate stem cell*. The indirect evidence is garnered from an experiment of the following sort as carried out by Van Bekkum and his colleagues. They used the Till and McCulloch model counting spleen colonies as an index of the number of stem cells. The number of stem cells in the bone marrow suspension is greatly increased by destroying hematopoietic cells capable of division in the donor by treatment with vincristine, a drug which acts similar to x-rays. (Stem cells divide only infrequently). The number of stem cells is further increased by subjecting the marrow suspension to density gradient centrifugation and obtaining a stem-cell-rich fraction. By these methods, the stem cell concentration in the marrow may be increased by a factor of 40 or more, as shown by spleen colony assay. In proportion to the increase in stem cells is the presence of a cell type, the *candidate stem cell,* which is lymphocytic in appearance. (See Fig. 11-6.)

THE LIFE CYCLE OF ERYTHROCYTES

DEVELOPMENT

The formation of an erythrocyte requires profound progressive changes in the nucleus and cytoplasm of its precursor cell. The nucleus becomes smaller and increasingly heterochromatic. It then becomes markedly polarized in the cell and breaks away leaving the anucleate erythrocyte. After becoming rich in polyribosomes, the cytoplasm synthesizes and accumulates hemoglobin and then loses its ribosomes, mitochondria, and many other structures characteristic of cytoplasm in general. There is thus a transformation of a nucleated cell endowed with most organelles into a biconcave, hemoglobin-containing, anucleate disc carrying enzymes necessary for the maintenance of functional hemoglobin and for anerobic energy production (glycolysis).

ERYTHROPOIETIN

Erythropoiesis is regulated by *erythropoietin*, a glycoprotein hormone of molecular weight 70,000. Erythropoietin is produced by interaction of precursor compounds synthesized in the kidney. It is not entirely dependent on the kidney for its production, however, since it is produced after nephrectomy. Erythropoietin drives erythropoietin-responsive cells (ERC) to differentiate into erythroblasts. In the fetus, moreover, it is active in the hepatic phase of hematopoiesis but not on the yolk sac.

There is some evidence that erythropoietin may also induce reticular cells in the bone marrow which clothe the outside surface of the vascular sinuses to move away from the wall and permit red cells to cross the wall of the sinuses and enter the circulation (see Chap. 12).

DIFFERENTIATION

Basophilic erythroblasts, the first of the cells in the erythroid line recognizable as erythroblasts, are free cells approximately 15 μm in diameter. They are rich in cytoplasmic ribonucleoprotein, visible under the electron microscope as polyribosomes, and contain little hemoglobin, and a relatively small heterochromatic nucleus. In Romanovsky preparations, hemoglobin binds the anionic dye eosin, since its protein globin is strongly cationic. The phosphate ion of RNA binds the cationic dyes methylene blue and the azures.[1] Accordingly, in early stage erythroblasts with little hemoglobin, the cytoplasm is stained deeply with basic dyes. In late stages of development, on the other hand, with little ribonucleic protein and abundant hemoglobin, the cytoplasm is stained deeply with anionic or acid dyes. Therefore, early erythroblasts are termed *basophilic erythroblasts,* and late erythroblasts are called *orthochromatic erythroblasts.* (The term *normoblast* is commonly applied to orthochromatic erythroblasts.) In stages intermediate between these, the hue of the cytoplasm represents a combination of the colors of the acid and basic dyes and the cells are therefore termed *polychromatophilic erythroblasts* [Figs. 11-7 (color insert) to 11-9].

By electron microscopy, the cytoplasm of erythroblasts contains polyribosomes, a density due to hemoglobin, ferritin, and scanty endoplasmic reticulum (ER). Polyribosomes are abundant. Those in basophilic and early polychromatophilic erythroblasts contain the largest number of ribosomes. By the orthochromatic stage, the polyribosomes are considerably reduced both in concentration and ribosomal number.

The density of the cytoplasm, due to hemoglobin, increases throughout maturation. Ferritin is present in these cells at every stage, and its presence in certain cells without evidence of hemoglobin may mark those cells as erythropoietin-sensitive erythroblast precursors (ERC). Ferritin is a storage form of iron, a protein linked to micellar iron and capable of holding as many as 2500 iron atoms. It may be scattered as single molecules that have a characteristic structure under the electron microscope or collected in large, membrane-bounded aggregates termed *siderosomes.* Erythroblasts may often display ferritin at their surface, sometimes in invaginations suggesting pinocytosis. It has been stated that ferritin passes into erythroblasts as a source of iron directly used in hemoglobin formation. But a clearly defined form of utilizable iron is transported by a special iron-binding globulin, *transferrin,* and ferritin in erythroblasts may, instead, simply represent excess or storage iron. In basophilic erythroblasts a slight to moderate amount of rough ER is present, but this rapidly becomes scanty. One or more Golgi complexes occur in basophilic erythroblasts, but again these become quite small and disappear by the orthochromatic phase. Mitochondria diminish in number and size in polychromatophilic cells. A few remain in orthochromatic erythroblasts and are absent in mature erythrocytes. Few lysosomes are present in erythroblasts.

The nucleus of basophilic erythroblasts, relative to other hematopoietic cells, is small and heterochromatic. It contains several nucleoli and conspicuous nuclear pores. With maturation, the nucleus becomes smaller, anucleolate, more pronouncedly heterochromatic, and more nearly spherical. At the time of nuclear loss, erythroblasts become markedly polarized, with the nucleus at one pole of the cell and the bulk of cytoplasm at the other. The cells break in two, and the nuclear-containing fragment is often rapidly phagocytized. A *free* nucleus is not released; it is surrounded by a very thin rim of hemoglobinized cytoplasm.

The loss of a nucleus converts an erythro*blast* to an erythro*cyte.* Nuclear loss occurs near the end of erythroblast maturation, near the orthochromatic stage. The nucleus may be lost at earlier stages, resulting in polychromatophilic or even basophilic *erythrocytes.* Then further maturation may proceed in the anucleate cell. In fact, even in orthochromatic

---

[1] Cationic dyes are termed *basic dyes* by histologists. Tissue components binding basic dyes are termed *basophilic.* See Chap. 2.

erythroblasts some ribosomes are present. (See discussion of reticulocytes below.)

The cell diameter decreases as erythroblasts mature into erythrocytes. Basophilic erythroblasts may

FIGURE 11-8 Polychromatophilic erythroblasts, bone marrow, of the rat. Two polychromatophilic erythroblasts press against different points of the endothelium (end) of vascular sinuses of the marrow. The erythroblasts are marked polarized. The cytoplasm, at one pole, contains ribosomes and mitochondria as well as hemoglobin. The nuclear pole is surrounded by a thin rim of hemoglobinized cytoplasm. The nuclear pole will be detached and phagocytized, and the cytoplasmic pole will become a reticulocyte. ×40,000. (From L. Weiss, *J. Morph.*, **117:**467, 1965.)

measure about 15 μm in diameter. The diameter of erythrocytes is about 7.5 μm. The relatively constant size of erythrocytes makes them useful in gauging the size of other structures in histologic sections.

Reticulocytes

A freshly produced erythrocyte, that is, one which has just lost its nucleus, always contains some ribosomes.

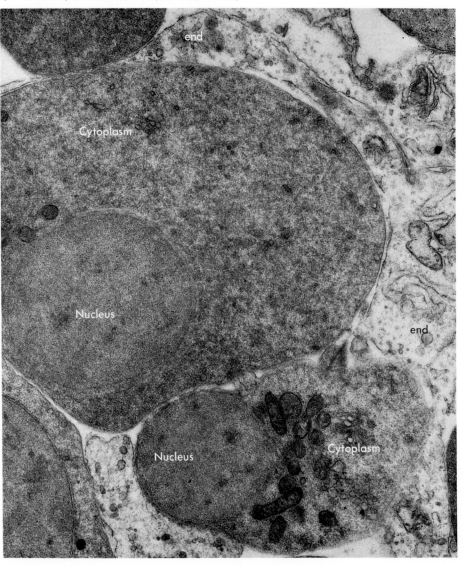

Less than 1 percent of human erythrocytes have enough ribosomes to be classed as *polychromatophilic* or *basophilic* as determined by their appearance in a blood film stained with a Romanovsky-type stain. A more sensitive method for revealing ribonucleoprotein in such newly produced erythrocytes is *supravital staining*. The technique consists of mixing a drop of freshly drawn blood with a drop of brilliant cresyl blue or other suitable dye and making a smear of the mixture. The residual ribonucleoprotein appears as a striking blue web or reticulum. These smears may be counterstained with a Romanovsky stain in the usual manner and the blue web will be superimposed on a pink erythrocyte. Such supravitally stained cells, termed *reticulocytes*, constitute about 2 percent of circulating erythrocytes. The enhanced sensitivity of supravital staining over conventional Romanovsky staining in demonstrating the small amount of ribonucleoprotein of freshly produced erythrocytes lies in the dispersion of ribonucleoprotein. In supravital staining, ribosomes are clumped into masses (the reticulum) visible by light microscopy. In the air-dried, methanol-fixed material of Romanovsky staining, the ribonucleoprotein of new erythrocytes remains, in most cells so finely dispersed that it is below the limit of resolution of the light microscope.

Unfortunately, the fibroblastic stroma of hematopoietic organs is fabricated of cells termed *reticular cells*, which form a meshwork termed *reticulum* or

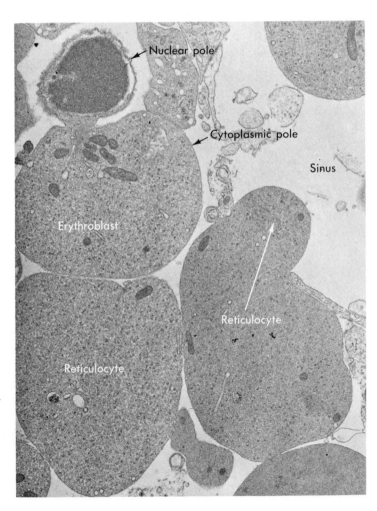

FIGURE 11-9 Bone marrow from a mouse. A reticulocyte is apparently passing across the wall of a sinus, through an aperture (arrow). An erythroblast is sharply polarized. Its nucleus, surrounded by a thin rim of cytoplasm, at the upper pole; its cytoplasm at the lower pole. The poles will probably separate with the formation of a reticulocyte. This process typically occurs at the wall of a vascular sinus. Reticulocytes contain some polyribosomes and, often, a few mitochondria, in addition to hemoglobin. ×12,000. (From the work of J. Chamberlain, R. Weed, and L. Weiss.)

reticular meshwork. These terms are occasionally confused with the term *reticulocyte* designating the freshly produced erythrocyte described above.

KINETICS

The erythroid cells in human beings may be divided into four categories: nucleated cells of the marrow, marrow reticulocytes, circulating reticulocytes, and circulating mature erythrocytes. The size of each of these classifications, as determined by Donahue, Gabrio, and Finch, is as follows:

ERYTHROID CELLS	NUMBER OF CELLS PER KILOGRAM OF BODY WEIGHT
Erythroblasts	5.59×10^9
Marrow reticulocytes	5.73×10^9
Circulating reticulocytes	3.22×10^9
Circulating mature erythrocytes	309.0×10^9

The bulk of this population circulates. The marrow has a population of reticulocytes as a ready reserve somewhat greater than the number in the blood, and equal to the number of erythroblasts.

It is possible to calculate the turnover rate of circulating erythrocytes, since the number of erythrocytes in the blood is constant and known and the life-span of erythrocytes (see below) is about 120 days. In a 70-kg man, the turnover rate being 0.83 to 1.0 percent daily, 17.9 to 21.6×10^{10} erythrocytes are produced each day and the same number destroyed. Further, the mean life-span of marrow reticulocytes is 36 to 44 h and that of the circulating reticulocytes approximately 25 h. The time required for erythroblasts to double by mitotic division is 36 to 44 h. Thus the total marrow turnover time is about 72 to 88 h from erythroblast to mature erythrocyte.

LIFE-SPAN

Erythrocytes display no clear morphologic changes as they age. But they gradually become more mechani-

cally fragile. They become unable to maintain their hemoglobin in a reduced, functional state, and the activity of certain enzymes, such as glucose-6-phosphate dehydrogenase, declines. The change that triggers the destruction of an erythrocyte is not known. Relatively few erythrocytes are destroyed at random; instead, about 120 days after a human red cell is released into the bloodstream, it is withdrawn from the circulation and destroyed.

The life-span of erythrocytes may be determined by several methods. Radioactive chromium tagging of erythrocytes, using ^{51}Cr, is now most commonly employed. A few microliters of washed red cells are mixed with a solution of $Na_2{}^{51}CrO_7$ and then reinjected into the subject from whom the blood was taken. The ^{51}Cr adheres tenaciously to hemoglobin without appreciably damaging the cells. Life-span is estimated by the persistence of circulating radioactivity.

DESTRUCTION

The macrophage system, notably in the spleen, liver, and bone marrow, plays a major part in the destruction of aged or damaged erythrocytes. Erythrocytes destined for destruction are withdrawn from the circulation, sequestered for short but variable periods, and then phagocytized. The hemoglobin is quickly degraded. The iron enters a labile pool from which it may be transferred by *transferrin* to the marrow, where it is reutilized in the production of new hemoglobin for new erythrocytes. Iron is stored as ferritin or hemosiderin, as discussed above. The labile iron pool exchanges with ferritin, which is present in erythroclastic tissues. The non-iron-containing portion of hemoglobin undergoes alteration to the bile pigment *bilirubin*.

THE LIFE CYCLE OF POLYMORPHONUCLEAR LEUKOCYTES

DIFFERENTIATION

In the formation of granulocytes from myeloblasts, the cytoplasm progressively acquires granules and the nucleus becomes flattened, indented, and then lobu-

lated [Fig. 11-7 (color insert), and 11-10 to 11-17]. A granulocyte precursor more differentiated than the CFU exists, demonstrable by plating marrow suspensions in soft agar. Clones, predominantly of granulocytic cells, form in 7 to 10 days.

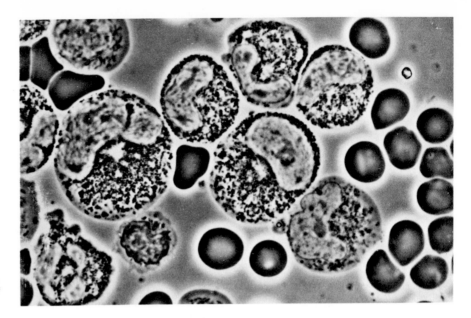

FIGURE 11-10 Human bone marrow cells. This field contains myelocytes together with erythrocytes. ×1300. (From the work of G. A. Ackerman.)

FIGURE 11-11 Human bone marrow cells. Myelocytes are present in this electron micrograph. Cells 1 to 4 are early myelocytes; 5 and 6, late. ×9200. (From the work of G. A. Ackerman.)

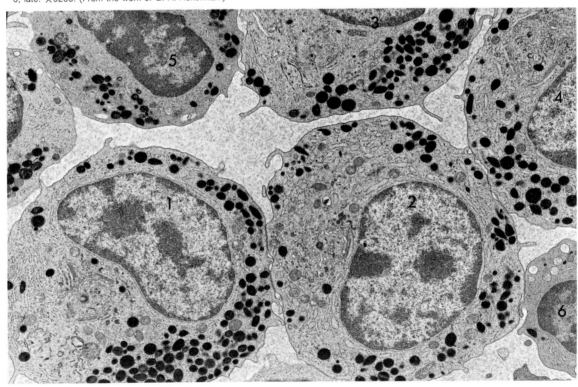

Leukopoietin, the leukocytic counterpart to erythropoietin, has not been characterized, but its existence has been postulated.

The first recognizable precursor of the granulo-

cytes is the myeloblast, a relatively small cell (approximately 10 μm in diameter) containing, in Romanovsky-stained smears, a large nucleus rich in euchromatin, three to five nucleoli, and a granule-free basophilic cytoplasm.

In the cytoplasm the first clear evidence of differentiation in Romanovsky preparations is the appearance of a few granules in the cytoplasm. Gradually cytoplasmic basophilia decreases and more and more granules accumulate until the full complement is attained.

Neutrophils produce two types of granules—a large azurophil primary granule and then a small definitive or secondary granule barely resolvable by light

FIGURE 11-12 Diagrammatic representation of the polymorphonuclear neutrophil (PMN) life cycle and stages of PMN maturation. The myeloblast has a large oval nucleus, large nucleoli, and cytoplasm lacking granules. It is followed by two granule-producing stages: the promyelocyte and the myelocyte. During each of these stages a distinct type of granule is produced: azurophils (solid black), formed only during the promyelocyte stage, and specific granules (light forms) produced during the myelocyte stage. The metamyelocyte and band forms are nonproliferating, non-granule-producing stages which develop into the mature PMN. The latter is characterized by a multilobulated nucleus and cytoplasm containing primarily glycogen and granules. The times indicated for the various compartments were determined by isotope-labeling techniques. (From D. F. Bainton, J. L. Ullyot, and M. G. Farquhar, *J. Exp. Med.,* **134:**907, 1971.)

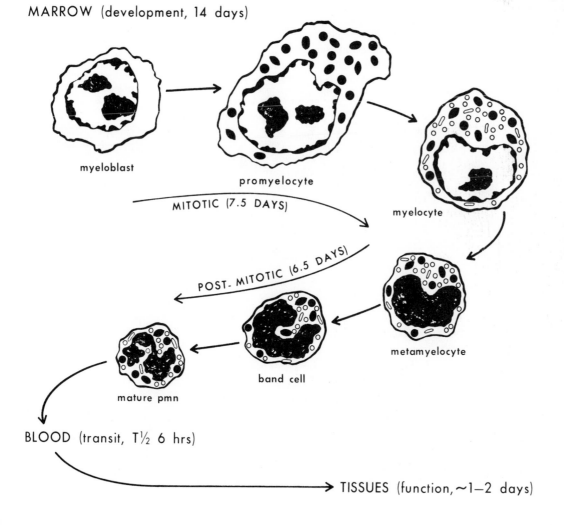

MARROW (development, 14 days)

myeloblast

promyelocyte

MITOTIC (7.5 DAYS)

myelocyte

POST-MITOTIC (6.5 DAYS)

metamyelocyte

band cell

mature pmn

BLOOD (transit, T½ 6 hrs)

TISSUES (function, ~1–2 days)

microscopy (see discussion of electron microscopy below). Basophilic and eosinophilic granules may usually be definitively recognized soon after they appear, although initially the latter may be somewhat basophilic or fail to bind eosin avidly. In adult neutrophils the hyaloplasm is usually slightly acidophilic. The hyaloplasm of circulating basophils and eosinophils may be slightly basophilic or appear to bind no dye.

The first nuclear changes are subtle, consisting of condensation of chromatin and some loss in its fine texture. Then the nucleus begins to flatten on one side and then becomes more and more deeply indented until it is markedly lobulated, the lobes connected only by slender threads of nuclear material. Two- to five-lobed nuclei are produced. Nuclear configuration in the circulation ranges from slight indentation to marked lobulation. A neutrophil with slight nuclear flattening and only primary granules in the cytoplasm is a *promyelocyte*. A cell with a flattened or indented nucleus and both primary and secondary granules is a *myelocyte*. When nuclear indentation becomes suffi-

ciently advanced to give the nucleus a U, V, or T shape, the cells are called *metamyelocytes* or *juvenile cells*. Further indentation results in nuclear lobes, the early stages of which have been termed *band forms*. Finally, when nuclear segmentation is marked and clear lobes formed, *mature granulocytes* exist. Metamyelocytes and more mature forms may be normally present in human circulating blood. Nuclei of eosinophils are often bilobed but may show a small median lobe. Nuclear polymorphism of basophils is not pronounced.

Nuclei of netrophils usually have three to five lobes. It had been thought that the degree of nuclear

FIGURE 11-13 Human polymorphonuclear neutrophil (PMN); early myelocyte reacted for peroxidase. The nucleus (n) with its prominent nucleolus (nu) occupies the bulk of this very immature cell. The surrounding cytoplasm contains a few azurophilic granules (ag), a large Golgi complex (G), several mitochondria (m), scanty rough endoplasmic reticulum (er), many free polysomes (r), and a centriole (ce). All the azurophilic granules (ag) appear dense, since they are strongly reactive for peroxidase. The granule-producing apparatus [the perinuclear cisterna (pn), rough endoplasmic reticulum (er), and some of the Golgi cisternae (Gc)] is also reactive, although less so than the granules. ×21,000. (Legend and figure from D. F. Bainton, J. L. Ullyot, and M. G. Farquhar, *J. Exp. Med.*, **134:**907, 1971.)

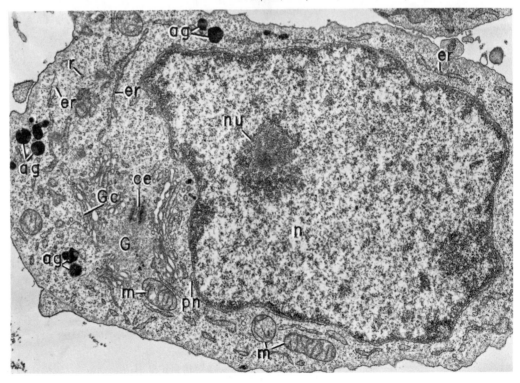

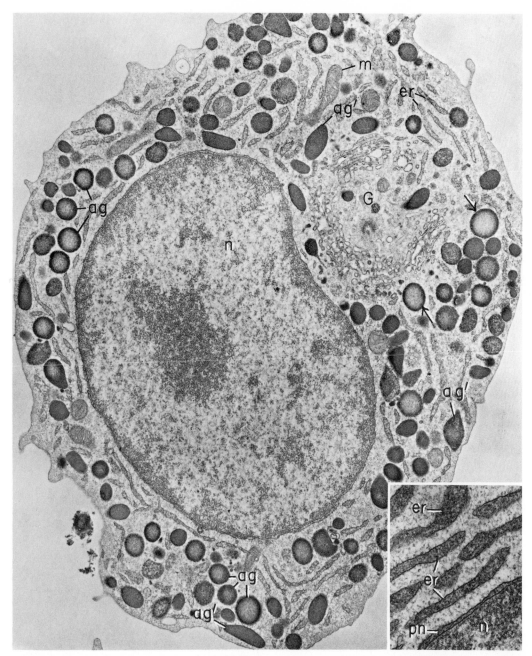

FIGURE 11-14 Human polymorphonuclear neutrophil (PMN); early myelocyte, reacted for peroxidase. This cell is the largest (approximately 15 μm) of the neutrophilic series. It has a sizable, slightly indented nucleus (n), a prominent Golgi region (G), and cytoplasm packed with peroxidase-positive azurophilic granules (ag). Note the two general shapes of azurophilic granules, spherical (ag) or ellipsoid (ag'). The majority are spherical, with a homogeneous matrix, but a few ellipsoid forms containing crystalloids are also present. Many of the spherical forms (arrows) have a dense periphery and a lighter core, owing presumably to incomplete penetration of substrate into the centers of granules. Peroxidase reaction product is visible in less concentrated form within all compartments of the granule-producing apparatus [endoplasmic reticulum (er), perinuclear cisterna (pn), and Golgi cisternae]. No reaction product is seen in the cytoplasmic matrix, mitochondria (m), or nucleus (n). The inset depicts a portion of another promyelocyte at higher magnification, showing to better advantage flocculent deposits of peroxidase reaction product in the rough ER (er) including the perinuclear cisterna (pn). ×15,000; inset, ×34,000. (From D. F. Bainton, J. L. Ullyot, and M. G. Farquhar, *J. Exp. Med.,* **134:**907, 1971.)

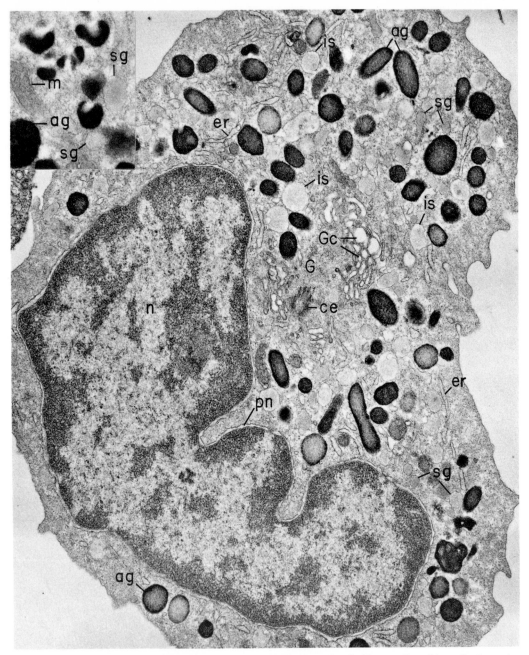

FIGURE 11-15 Polymorphonuclear neutrophilic (PMN) myelocyte, human peroxidase reaction. At this stage the cell is smaller (approximately 10 μm) than the promyelocyte (see Fig. 11-14), the nucleus is more indented, and the cytoplasm contains two different types of granules: (1) large, peroxidase-positive azurophils (ag) and (2) the generally smaller specific granules (sg), which do not stain for peroxidase. A number of immature specifics (is), which are larger, less compact, and more irregular in contour than mature granules, are seen in the Golgi region (G). The inset, a portion of a myelocyte, depicts a cluster of peroxidase-positive granules, most of which are smaller and more pleomorphic than the surrounding specifics (sg) and azurophils (ag). These are presumed to represent azurophil variants, since they appear during the promyelocyte stage. ×20,000; inset ×41,000. (From D. F. Bainton, J. L. Ullyot, and M. G. Farquhar, *J. Exp. Med.*, **134:**907, 1971.)

polymorphism was directly related to the age of the cell. It is now known that this is not the case. Mature neutrophils are released from the marrow to the circulation with about three to five lobes and live their entire life-span with their initial number. Certain diseases, as pernicious anemia, are characterized by hypersegmented nuclei containing six or more lobes. In mature granulocytes, the nucleus is markedly heterochromatic, its chromatin almost glassy in appearance. Nucleoli persist in granulocytes for only a very short time following nuclear indentation. Pinacyanol may be used as a supravital nuclear stain, but

FIGURE 11-16 Higher-power view of the Golgi region of PMN myelocyte similar to the cell shown in Fig. 11-15. As in the preceding figure, peroxidase reaction is seen in azurophils (ag) but not in specific granules (sg). The stacked, smooth-surfaced Golgi cisternae (Gc) are oriented around the centriole (ce). Note that the outer cisternae have a content of intermediate density (arrows) which is similar to the content of the specific granules. The images are less suggestive than in the rabbit, but they are compatible with the view that specific granules arise from the convex face of the Golgi complex in both species. ×33,000. (From D. F. Bainton, J. L. Ullyot, and M. G. Farquhar, *J. Exp. Med.*, **134**:907, 1971.)

nuclear detail is not rich. Cytoplasmic granules are stained with neutral red, and the earliest granules, often masked by cytoplasmic basophilia in Romanovsky-type stains, are visible. The character of the granules may be told by their staining reaction, size, and distribution. Mitochondria, present in the myeloblast in considerable number, become reduced in number and size until, in the mature cell, few are present, and they are not readily visible. Ameboid movement, activity of the plasma membrane, and movement of cytoplasmic granules appear in metamyelocytes. The inability of granulocytes to move until they are nearly mature favors the release of only mature cells to the circulation.

Knowledge of granule production has been provided by the electron-microscope studies of Bainton, Ullyot, and Farquhar (1971) and of G. A. Ackerman (Figs. 11-12 to 11-17). The human *myeloblast*, the first recognizable cell in the sequence of maturation, is

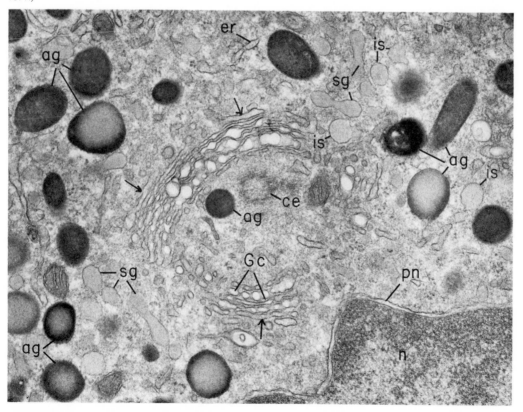

a relatively small cell (approximately 10 μm) without granules. The cytoplasm has many free polyribosomes and mitochondria. Annulate lamellae may be seen.

The *promyelocyte* in humans is larger (approximately 15 μm) than the myeloblast and contains peroxidase-positive granules which correspond to the azurophilic granules of light microscopy. A large Golgi complex and moderate amounts of rough ER are present. The granules are of two main shapes. The majority are round, approximately 500 nm in diameter, and contain flocculent material at first and dense, homogeneous material on maturation. Less common are football-shaped forms, approximately 300 × 900 nm, which frequently contain crystalline inclusions. The Golgi cisternae, the perinuclear space, and the rough ER—which constitute the secretory apparatus of the promyelocyte—often contain peroxidase-positive material, which is precursor to the azurophilic granules. Promyelocytes actively divide.

The *myelocyte* is smaller than the promyelocyte.

The nucleus flattens and indents. The cell has a prominent Golgi complex and mixed population of granules, including newly produced peroxidase-negative granules as well as the peroxidase-positive azurophilic granules of the promyelocyte. The new granules are the specific ones; they are spheres; approximately 200 nm in diameter, or rods, approximately 130 = 1000 nm, with homogeneous low-density content. These granules appear to form at the outer convex surface of the Golgi, in distinction to the azurophilic granules which are produced at the inner concave surface. Myelocytes actively divide.

The *metamyelocyte* (juvenile cell), band form, and mature neutrophil are nondividing cells which no longer produce granules. The Golgi is small and inactive. The nucleus is lobulated or segmented, and a mixed population of granules is present, numbering approximately 200 to 300 per cell. The ratio of definitive to primary granules is approximately 3 or 4:1.

The polymorphonuclear leukocytes of the blood are similar to the later marrow stages.

The primary or azurophilic granules are lysosomal; they contain myeloperoxidase, as indicated

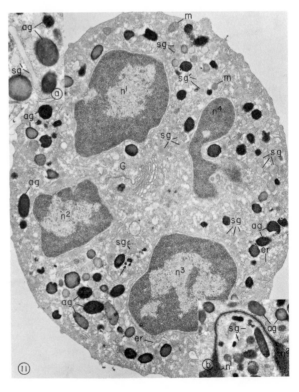

FIGURE 11-17 Human polymorphonuclear neutrophil (PMN), reacted for peroxidase. The cytoplasm is filled with granules; the smaller peroxidase-negative specifics (sg) are more numerous, azurophils (ag) having been reduced in number by cell divisions after the promyelocyte stage. Some small, irregularly shaped azurophilic granule variants are also present (arrow). The nucleus is condensed and lobulated (n¹ to n⁴), the Golgi region (G) is small and lacks forming granules, the ER (er) scanty, and mitochondria (m) few. Note that the cytoplasm of this cell has a rather ragged, moth-eaten appearance because the glycogen, which is normally present, has been extracted. The insets depict portions of the cytoplasm of mature PMN reacted for peroxidase. Inset (a) demonstrates that the peroxidase-positive azurophils (ag) can be easily distinguished from the unreactive specifics (sg). Note that one of the specifics is quite elongated (approximately 1000 μm). Inset (b) illustrates the narrow connection between two lobes (n₁ and n₂) of the PMN nucleus. Inset, specimen preparation as in Fig. 11-15. ×21,000; inset (a), ×36,000; inset (b), ×14,000. (From D. F. Bainton, J. L. Ullyot, and M. G. Farquhar, *J. Exp. Med.*, **134**:907, 1971.)

above, acid phosphatase, β-galactosidase, 5'-nucleotidase, and other enzymes characteristic of lysosomes. The secondary or definitive granules lack these acid hydrolytic enzymes. They contain a variety of compounds (see Chap. 10) many of which are known to have bacteriocidal properties.

Eosinophilic granules show little change on maturation, save the development of a crystalloid element. These granules are unusually rich in arginine, containing the strongly cationic guanidinium group which accounts for the marked eosinophilia of the granule. They contain a myeloperoxidase, which is somewhat different from that of the heterophil's primary granule, acid phosphatase, and alkaline phosphatase activity. They are, thus, complex granules with some lysosomal character.

Basophilic granules may show virtually no change on development.

Important physical and functional changes are associated with the maturation of neutrophils. Some are schematized in Fig. 11-18.

KINETICS AND DISTRIBUTION

Although the bulk of the erythroid complex is in the circulation, as Donahue, Gabrio, and Finch have shown, granulocytic forms in the bone marrow far outnumber those in the circulation. The table below indicates the numbers of different stages of granulocytes.

A ready reserve of adult granulocytes and metamyelocytes of about 5×10^9 cells per kg body weight is in marrow. This represents more than 16 times the number of circulating cells. Counting all marrow granulocytes, the ratio of cells in marrow to those of the blood is 38:1.

Studies of the distribution and kinetics of leukocytes have been carried out with radioactive tags. A useful one is diisopropyl fluorophosphate, the phosphate being radioactive ($DF^{32}P$). $DF^{32}P$ couples irreversibly with esterases. Experiments with this tracer have shown that there are two pools of granulocytes in blood vessels. The first is a circulating pool; the second, a marginating pool. The latter consists of cells within blood vessels lying out of flow or marginated against the walls. The marginated pool may be mobilized very quickly. It is likely that granulocytes leaving the bloodstream do not return. The two major sources of ready-reserve granulocytes, therefore, are those in the marrow and those in marginated pools.

Granulocytes remain in the circulation for only hours, in the neighborhood of 8 to 12 h in human beings. They appear, moreover, to leave the circulation at random, without regard to age.

The model shown below, modified from the work of Mauer, Athens, Warner, Ashenbrucker, Cartwright, and Wintrobe, indicates the relationship of the several granulocyte components.

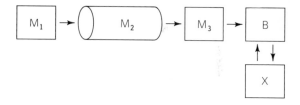

M_1 = pool of mitotically active cells in the marrow, including myeloblasts and myelocytes

M_2 = maturation phase, from which cells are not normally released until mature

M_3 = storage pool of mature granulocytes in marrow

B = granulocytic pool in blood

X = marginating cells in equilibrium with B

FATE

Mature granulocytes are end forms, incapable of further differentiation or of mitotic division. Their brief sojourn in the blood is but a fraction of their potential

GRANULOCYTE	NUMBER PER KILOGRAM OF BODY WEIGHT
Circulating	0.3×10^9
Total marrow granulocytes	11.4×10^9
Segmented forms	1.6×10^9
Band forms	3.6×10^9
Myelocytes	2.6×10^9
Metamyelocytes	2.7×10^9
Adult granulocytes	2.5×10^9

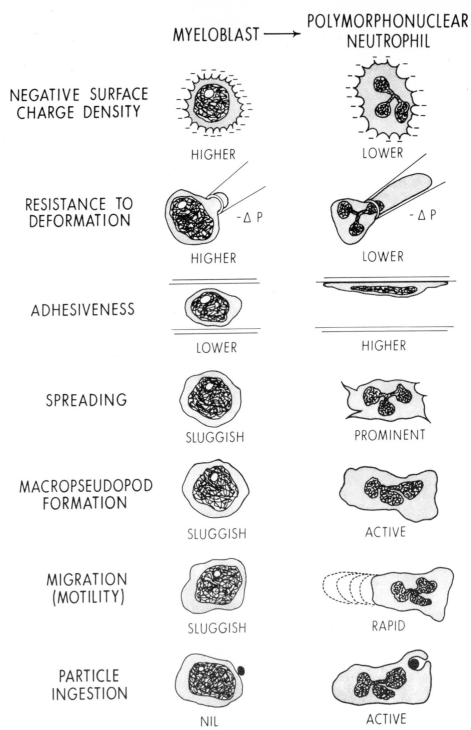

FIGURE 11-18 Physical and functional changes in polymorphonuclear neutrophils during maturation. (From M. Lichtman and R. Weed, *Blood,* **39:**301, 1972.)

life-span. In tissue culture, for example, neutrophils may survive for more than a week. Since extravascular granulocytes fail to return to the blood, we may conclude that 8 to 12 h after release to the blood from the marrow, granulocytes enter the connective tissue spaces. They die there or leave the body. A small number of granulocytes die in the bloodstream, as indicated by their reaction to supravital dyes; that is, they are nonselectively stained throughout.

MONOCYTES

Monocytes are circulating blood cells having a life cycle which includes *promonocyte, monocyte, macrophage, epithelioid cell* and *multinucleate giant cell* stages. The life cycle of monocytes is presented in Chap. 4 on the Connective Tissues.

THE LIFE CYCLE OF LYMPHOCYTES

It has been difficult to establish a life cycle for lymphocytes because they lack such markers as pigment, specific granules, or polymorphous nuclei by which it has been possible to establish life cycles of red cells and granulocytes. But by the use of sophisticated modern techniques, as light- and electron-microscopic autoradiography and cytochemistry, thymectomy, and other ablation procedures and sensitive immunological methods, it has recently been possible to establish the elements of lymphocytic life cycles.

Lymphocytes originate in the bone marrow from hematopoietic stem cells. With regard to the life cycle of T lymphocytes, stem cells leave the marrow and enter the circulation and reach the thymus. They penetrate the capsule and then, at the periphery of the cortex, begin to undergo differentiation toward T lymphocytes. They proliferate, and as they mature they move deeper into the thymic cortex. At the same time, they bear certain markers on their cell surface. In mice, for example, developing T lymphocytes bear a marker antigen, TL, on the cell surface. It has been estimated that as many as 90 percent of the proliferating differentiating precursors of T lymphocytes die in the thymus, but this figure has been disputed. T lymphocytes are released from the thymus through blood vessels and perhaps lymphatics, from the deep part of the cortex, and from the corticomedullary junction. These cells bear distinctive surface markers. In the mouse, one valuable marker has been the θ antigen in the cell surface. The function of this antigen is not known, but it serves to identify the lymphocyte as a T

lymphocyte. Other surface antigens or markers are being recognized. These cells are long-lived, small lymphocytes capable of years of life in humans and 16 or more weeks of life in the rat. They are migratory cells which circulate and recirculate through blood, lymph, and characteristic compartments in the spleen, lymph nodes, and other lymphatic tissues. Subclasses of T lymphocytes are now being recognized. (See discussion of Lymphocytes and Immune Response in Chap. 10).

B lymphocytes also originate from the marrow as stem cells. In birds, the *bursa of fabricius,* a cloacal lymphoepithelial organ is the locus to which stem cells migrate from the marrow and begin their differentiation into B cells. The counterpart of the bursa of fabricius has been sought in mammals but has not been definitively identified. It may well be that B cells are produced in bone marrow. As indicated in Chap. 10, the distinguishing characteristic of B cells is that they contain on their surface approximately 150,000 molecules of antibody, which serves as a receptor substance. B cells have a life-span of 6 or more weeks in the rat, and likely at least several months in humans. They circulate and recirculate through blood, lymph, spleen, lymph nodes, and other antibody-producing lymphatic tissues. When appropriately stimulated, as discussed in Chap. 10, B cells differentiate into *plasma cells,* unicellular antibody-producing glands (Figs. 11-19 and 11-20). Plasma cells have a life-span of approximately 2 weeks. B cells and T cells are migratory cells and their pathways facilitate meeting antigen in the process of clonal selection. In peripheral lymphatic tissue, such as spleen and lymph nodes, they are compartmentalized in characteristic patterns. Recirculating T and B cells seldom divide. The major basis by which division is induced is by meeting antigen under appropriate circumstances. There are, moreover, certain plant lectins such as phytohemogglutinin and pokeweed agglutinin which can induce in vitro proliferation in lymphocytes. This type of tissue-culture-induced proliferation facilitates making karyotype analysis of T and B cells.

The small lymphocytes of the blood are made up of lymphocytes of the B and T types. They include, of course, not only cells directly released from the bone marrow and the thymus but cells which have passed through spleen and lymph nodes or proliferated there and continue to circulate and recirculate.

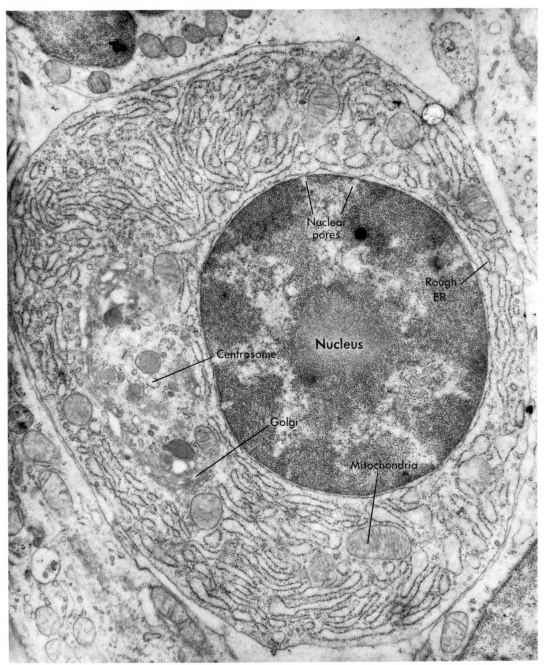

FIGURE 11-19 Plasma cell. Note the clumped chromatin, eccentric nucleus, prominent cytocentrum, and granular endoplasmic reticulum. Compare with light micrograph, Fig. 11-7.

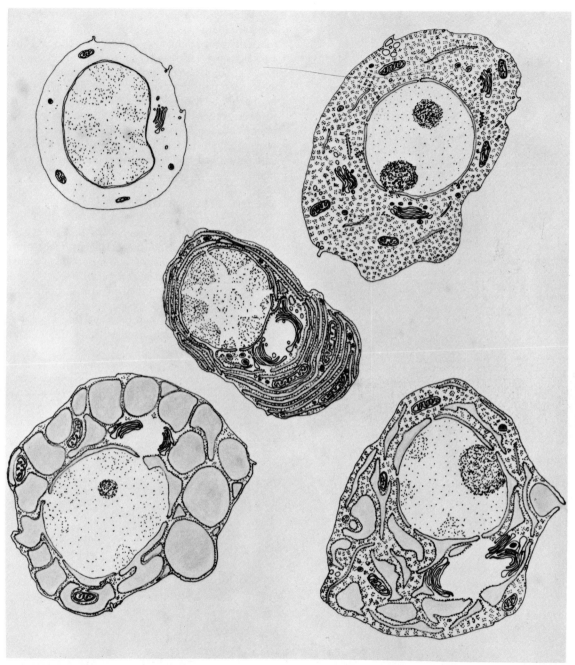

FIGURE 11-20 In this schematic view several stages of the life cycle of plasma cells are shown. At the upper left is a plasma cell precursor, lymphocytic in form. The upper right-hand cell is a "blast" form. It has polyribosomes, segments of RER, nucleoli, nuclear pores, and other cellular elements indicative of protein synthesis. Antibody may be present in the perinuclear space and in the lumen of the RER. The lower cells, right and left, are clearly plasmacytic, of intermediate or transitional character. They have dilated perinuclear spaces and dilated ER, both containing antibody. Indeed, the continuity of the outer nuclear membrane and the ER is shown. The cell in the center is the classic small plasma cell, displaying polarized nucleus and cytoplasm, distribution of heterochromatin in chunks along the inner nuclear membrane, prominent cytocentrum including Golgi and centrioles, and deeply basophilic or pyroninophilic (= RNA) cytoplasm. This cell is a near terminal form, past the peak of antibody production. The intermediate cells turn out most of the antibody. (From L. Weiss, "The Cells and Tissues of the Immune System," Prentice-Hall, Inc., Englewood Cliffs, N.J., 1972.)

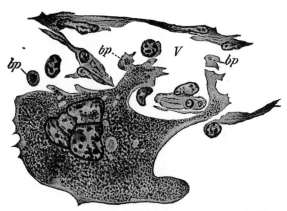

FIGURE 11-21 Megakaryocyte from the bone marrow of a kitten, showing pseudopodia or platelet ribbons extending into a blood vessel (V) and giving rise to blood platelets (bp). (From J. H. Wright, *J. Morphol.*, **21**:263, 1910.)

What is the significance of lymphocyte size? A number of large lymphocytes of the blood may result from antigenic stimulation of small lymphocytes and constitute the early stages in an immune response. There are undoubtedly lymphocytes stimulated in the wall of the gastrointestinal tract, for example, which are carried by lymphatics into the blood. The mitotic response to this stimulation may cause the development of medium or large lymphocytes. These cells will likely reach a lymphatic tissue within a short time after stimulation and remain there to continue their reactions.

THE LIFE CYCLE OF PLATELETS

Platelets originate as portions of the cytoplasm of giant cells, *megakaryocytes*. In human beings, megakaryocytes are largely restricted to the marrow. In rodents, they may also be found in the spleen.

A megakaryocyte may measure more than 100 μm in diameter. Its nucleus is a large, twisted, lobulated structure. It may be polyploid, degrees of ploidy up to 64n being regular. (See Chap. 1 for discussion of polyploidy.)

FIGURE 11-22 Platelet ribbons in bone marrow of rat; scanning electron micrograph. Platelets may be discharged singly or in ribbons which separate into individual platelets in the circulation. The ribbons may display beaded segments, each segment representing a platelet. Note that one ribbon is emerging into the lumen of a vascular sinus (arrow) through the endothelium (see Chap. 12). ×1980. (From the work of L.-T. Chen and L. Weiss.)

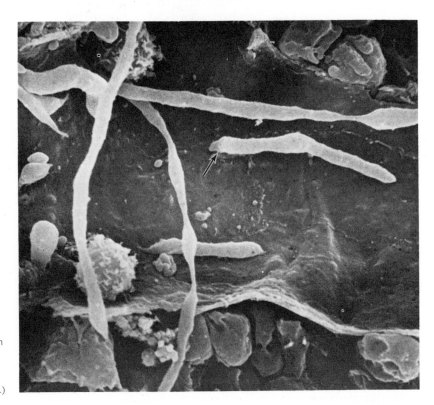

The abundant cytoplasm is divisible into three zones. The perinuclear zone contains Golgi, rough ER, polyribosomes, and some granules—in short, most of the organelles associated with a cell in large-scale protein, granule, and membrane synthesis. The intermediate zone consists of putative platelets demarcated to varying degrees of completeness by smooth ER. The outermost zone resembles ectoplasm; it is finely granular and contains packets of microfilaments but is largely free of organelles [Figs. 11-7 (color insert), 11-20 to 11-24, 12-3 to 12-5 and 12-11]. While these zones are typical, megakaryocytes may be found in which the entire mass of cytoplasm is demarcated into platelets.

FIGURE 11-23 Electron micrograph of a megakaryocyte in human bone marrow. The nucleus is large and polymorphous. The cytoplasm contains granules of varying density and small mitochondria. The arresting cytoplasmic characteristic is the extensive smooth-surfaced endoplasmic reticulum which loculates platelet zones in the peripheral cytoplasm. (See Fig. 11-24.) Later the platelets will separate from the megakaryocyte and become free circulating structures. ×9300. (From the work of I. Berman.)

A megakaryocyte forms platelets by the confluence of the vesicles or channels of membrane which demarcate them. Megakaryocytes sit against the outside surface of vascular sinuses in the marrow, delivering platelets through mural apertures directly into the vascular lumen. They may deliver individual platelets or ribbons of platelets (as tickets unwinding from a spool) which subsequently separate as individual platelets in the lumen of the vascular sinuses (Fig. 11-21).

Megakaryocytes originate from stem cells. The first morphologically identifiable precursor of megakaryocytes is a large cell 25 to 40 μm in diameter with a large oval or spherical nucleus and a cytoplasm containing ribosomes and other organelles, but without hint of platelet formation. This cell may be designated a *megakaryocytoblast.* It undergoes DNA repli-

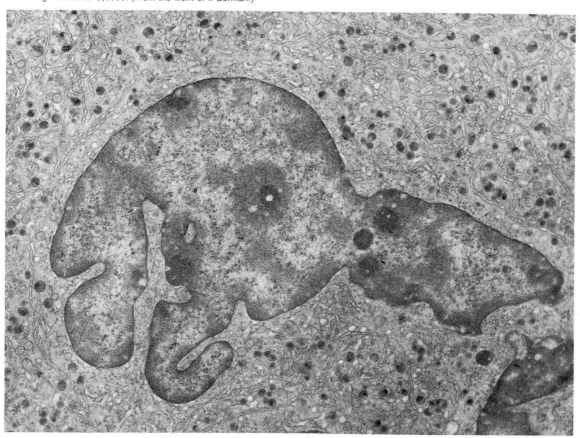

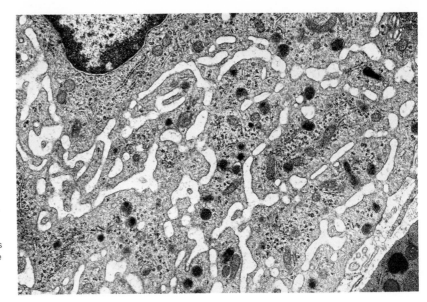

FIGURE 11-24 Electron micrograph of megakaryocyte in rat bone marrow. A portion of the nucleus and central cytoplasm is at the upper margin. Most of the peripheral cytoplasm is clearly demarcated into platelet zones. ×10,500.

cation to its final level of ploidy before the nucleus becomes polymorphous. In a population of megakaryoblasts, dependent somewhat on the species, ploidy varies from 2n to 64n. In general, both the nuclear and cytoplasmic sizes of the megakaryocyte are proportional to the degree of ploidy.

Circulating platelets, in humans, have a life-span up to about 10 days, determined in labeling experiments. The curve of labeled platelets decreases considerably in 6 to 8 days and tails off in about 10. It is likely that platelets are utilized randomly, that is, without reference to age.

It is quite likely that the number and size of circulating platelets are regulated by a hormone, *thrombopoietin*. The site of production and the nature of the hormone are not known. Its presence is inferred from the thrombopoietic activity of serum from individuals with low blood platelet levels (*thrombocytopenia*). Thrombopoietin may stimulate the conversion of certain stem cells into the megakaryocytic line and may, as well, induce an acceleration in maturation of megakaryocytes. As a result of such maturation, the number and size of megakaryocytes, and the size of platelets, are increased.

REFERENCES

ARCHER, G. T.: Motion Picture Studies on Degranulation of Horse Eosinophils during Phagocytosis, *J. Exp. Med.,* **118:**276 (1963).

ASHBY, W.: Determination of Length of Life of Transfused Blood Corpuscles in Man, *Blood,* **3:**486 (1948).

BAGGIOLINI, M., J. G. HIRSCH, and C. DE DUVE: Further Biochemical and Morphological Studies of Granule Fractions from Rabbit Heterophil Leukocytes, *J. Cell Biol.,* **45:**586 (1970).

BAINTON, D. F., J. L. ULLYOT, and M. G. FARQUHAR: The Development of Neutrophilic Polymorphonuclear Leukocytes in Human Bone Marrow. Origin and Content of Azurophil and Specific Granules, *J. Exp. Med.,* **134:**907 (1971).

BLOOM, W., and G. W. BARTELMEZ: Hematopoiesis in Young Human Embryos, *Am. J. Anat.,* **67:**21 (1940).

COHN, Z. A., and J. G. HIRSCH: The Isolation and Properties of the Specific Cytoplasmic Granules of Rabbit Polymorphonuclear Leukocytes, *J. Exp. Med.,* **112:**983 (1960).

COHN, Z. A., and S. I. MORSE: Functional and Metabolic Properties of Polymorphonuclear Leukocytes. I. Observations on the Requirements and Consequences of Particle Ingestion, *J. Exp. Med.,* **111:**667 (1960).

CRADDOCK, C. G., JR., S. PERRY, L. E. VENTZKE, and J. S. LAWRENCE: Evaluation of Marrow Granulocytic Reserves in Normal and Disease States, *Blood,* **15:**840 (1960).

DE BRUYN, P. P. H.: Locomotion of Blood Cells in Tissue Culture. *Anat. Rec.,* **89:**43 (1944); **95:**177 (1946).

DONAHUE, D. M., B. W. GABRIO, and C. A. FINCH: Quantitative Measurements of Hematopoietic Cells of the Marrow, *J. Clin. Invest.,* **37:**1564 (1958).

EBERT, R. H., A. B. SANDERS, and H. W. FLOREY: Observations of Lymphocytes in Chambers in the Rabbit's Ear, *Br. J. Exp. Pathol.,* **21:**212 (1940).

FOWLER, J. H., A. M. WU, J. E. TILL, E. A. MC CULLOCH, and L. SIMINOVITCH: The Cellular Composition of Hemopoietic Spleen Colonies, *J. Cell Physiol.,* **69:**65 (1967).

GILMOUR, J. R.: Normal Haemopoiesis in Intrauterine and Neonatal Life, *J. Pathol. Bact.,* **52:**25 (1941).

HIRSCH, J. G., and Z. A. COHN: Degranulation of Polymorphonuclear Leukocytes Following Phagocytosis of Microorganisms, *J. Exp. Med.,* **118:**1005 (1960).

HOWELL, W. H.: The Life History of the Formed Elements of the Blood: Especially the Red Corpuscles, *J. Morphol.,* **4:**57 (1890).

ISAACS, R.: The Physiological Histology of Bone Marrow, *Folia Haematol (Leipz),* **40:**395 (1930).

JOFFE, R. H.: The Reticuloendothelial System, in H. Downey (ed.), "Handbook of Hematology," vol. 2, Paul B. Hoeber, Inc., New York, 1938.

JORDAN, H. E.: The Evolution of Blood-forming Tissues, *Q. Rev. Biol.,* **8:**58 (1933).

KINDRED, J. E.: A Quantitative Study of the Hematopoietic Organs of Young Adult Albino Rats, *Am. J. Anat.,* **71:**207 (1942).

MAHMOUD, A. A. F., K. S. WARREN, and P. A. PETERS: A role for the Eosinophils in Acquired Resistance to Schistosoma Mansoni Infection as Determined by Antieosinophil Serum, *J. Exp. Med.,* **142:**805 (1975).

MAXIMOW, A. A.: The Lymphocytes and Plasma Cells, in E. V. Cowdry (ed.), "Special Cytology," vol. 2, Paul B. Hoeber, Inc., New York, 1932.

METCHNIKOFF, E.: "Lectures on the Comparative Pathology of Inflammation," trans. F. A. and E. H. Starling, Paul, Trench, Trübner and Co., London, 1893.

MIKLEM, H. S., C. E. FORD, E. P. EVANS, and J. GAR: Interrelationships of Myeloid and Lymphoid Cells: Studies with Chromosome-marked Cells Transfused into Lethally Irradiated Mice, *Proc. R. Soc. Lond.,* [*Biol.*], **165:**78 (1966).

MURPHY, P.: "The Neutrophil," Plenum Publishing Co., New York, 1976.

RAMSEY, W. S.: Locomotion of Human Polymorphonuclear Leukocytes, *Exp. Cell. Res.,* **72:**489 (1972).

SABIN, F. R.: Bone Marrow, *Physiol. Rev.,* **8:**191 (1928).

SABIN, F. R.: Studies of Living Human Blood Cells, *Bull. Hopkins Hosp.,* **34:**277 (1923).

SIMINOVITCH, L., E. A. MC CULLOCH, and J. E. TILL: The Distribution of Colony-forming Cells Among Spleen Colonies. *J. Cell Comp. Physiol.,* **62:**327 (1963).

SPITZNAGEL, J. K., F. G. DALLDORF, and M. S. LEFFELL: Characterization of Azurophil and Specific Granules Purified from Human Polymorphonuclear Leukocytes, *Lab. Invest.,* **30:**774 (1974).

WEISSMAN, G., and G. A. RITE: Molecular Basis of Gouty Inflammation: Interaction of Monosodium Urate Crystals with Lysosomes and Liposomes, *Nature* [New Biol.], **240:**167 (1972).

WRIGHT, J. H.: The Histogenesis of Blood Platelets, *J. Morphol.,* **21:**263 (1910).

WU, A. M., J. E. TILL, L. SIMINOVITCH, and E. A. MC CULLOCH: Cytological Evidence for a Relationship between Normal Hematopoietic Colony-forming Cells and Cells of the Lymphoid System, *J. Exp. Med.,* **127:**455 (1968).

WU, A. M., J. E. TILL, L. SIMINOVITCH, and E. A. MC CULLOCH: A Cytological Study of the Capacity for Differentiation of Normal Hematopoietic Colony-forming Cells. *J. Cell Physiol.,* **69:**177 (1967).

Comprehensive References

BESSIS, M.: "Living Blood Cells and their Ultrastructure," Trans. R. I. Weed, Springer-Verlag OHG, Berlin, 1973.

WILLIAMS, W. J., E. BEUTLER, A. J. ERSLAV, and R. W. RUNDLES: "Hematology, (McGraw Hill Book Company, New York, 1972.

WINTROBE, M. M.: "Clinical Hematology," 6th ed., Lea & Febiger, Philadelphia, 1967.

DOWNEY, H. (ed.): "Handbook of Hematology," 4 vols., Paul B. Hoeber, Inc., New York, 1938; reprinted by Hafner Publishing Company, Inc., New York, 1966.

GORDON, A. S.: "Regulation of Hematopoiesis," 2 vols., Appleton Century Crofts, New York, 1970.

STOHLMAN, F.: "Symposium on Hemopoietic Cellular Proliferation," Grune & Stratton, Inc., New York, 1970.

WEISS, L.: "The Cells and Tissues of the Immune System," Prentice-Hall, Inc., Englewood Cliffs, N.J., 1972.

YOFFEY, J. M., and F. C. COURTRICE: "Lymphatics, Lymph and Lymphoid Tissue," Harvard University Press, Cambridge, Mass., 1960.

Bone Marrow

12

LEON WEISS

Contained within the bones of the body, the marrow is a richly cellular connective tissue specialized in the production of blood cells and their delivery to the circulation. In human beings the marrow originates in the second month of intrauterine life within the clavicles, the first bones to ossify, and it expands with the maturation of the remaining bones (Fig. 12-1). The scapulae, innominate bones, occipital bones, ribs, and vertebrae contain marrow in the third fetal month. When it first appears, the marrow is concerned with the growth and modeling of bone, and it maintains its osteogenic functions throughout life. Secondarily, it assumes hematopoietic functions, and it becomes so active in the production of blood cells that in the latter half of fetal development and throughout postnatal life, the bone marrow is the major hematopoietic tissue. It possesses a distinctive stroma capable of preferentially trapping and holding hematopoietic stem cells. In human beings, virtually all erythrocytes, granulocytes, platelets and monocytes are normally produced in the marrow. It is likely that B lymphocytes are made there as well. Of the blood cells only T lymphocytes are not produced in the marrow. These differentiate in the thymus from stem cells released from the marrow (see Chap. 13).

STRUCTURE OF BONE MARROW

GROSS CHARACTERISTICS

On gross examination, bone marrow may be red, indicating active hematopoiesis, or yellow, indicating an hematopoietically inactive marrow (Fig. 12-2). The red color of marrow is owing to the hemoglobin of erythrocytes and their precursors. The major cell type in yellow marrow is fat cells, which impart a yellow color. Red and yellow marrow may be interconvertible, at least to a limited degree.

In neonatal human beings all the marrow is red. Fat begins to appear in the shaft of the long bones in the fifth to seventh years, and by the eighteenth year almost all the marrow of the limbs is yellow. Patches of red marrow persist only about the joints. Hematopoietic marrow in adults is virtually restricted to the skull, clavicles, vertebrae, ribs, sternebrae and pelvis. The bone marrow accounts for 3.4 to 6.0 percent of adult body weight, or about 1,600 to 3,700 g.

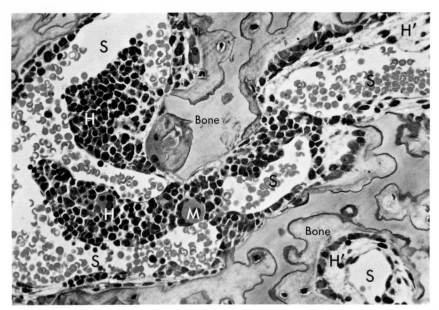

FIGURE 12-1 Bone marrow from central femur of human fetus, 200 mm crown rump length (22 weeks' gestational age). The marrow tissue occurs in the spaces within bone. In the adult the bone will be removed from much of the center of the shaft of the femur, remaining only to form a cortical shell. The marrow will therefore become a solid cylindrical plug of tissue. The marrow contains large, thin-walled vascular sinuses (S) containing blood. Outside the sinuses lie the hematopoietic compartments. Some of these (H) are filled with hematopoietic cells. Note the large megakaryocyte (M) characteristically set on the outside wall of the sinus (see text). In some sites, the hematopoietic compartments have not yet filled with hematopoietic cells but contain a primitive fibrous connective tissue (H'). × 1000. (From L-T. Chen and L. Weiss.)

FIGURE 12-2 Normal adult human bone marrow. A. Red marrow rich in hematopoietic cells. B. Yellow marrow rich in fat cells. (The fat has been extracted by embedding reagents and is represented by clear oval spaces.) C. Marrow intermediate to A and B in the proportion of hematopoietic and fat cells. ×400.

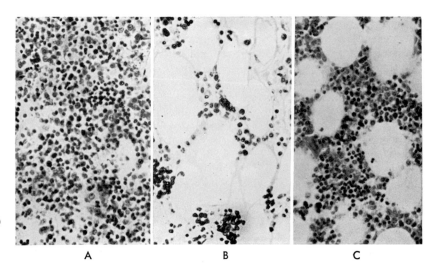

A

B

C

The marrow lies entirely within bone, reached by blood vessels and nerves which pierce its bony housing. Particularly at the end of long bones, the internal surface of bone may be ridged with shelves and spicules of bone, the *trabeculae,* which protrude into the marrow cavity. In many places, the internal surface of the bone may be quite smooth and the marrow cavity quite large. When trabeculae are present, they divide the marrow space into small bony locules which communicate with one another. The internal surface of bone is lined with endosteum, which is composed of osteoblasts and osteoclasts.

ARTERIAL VESSELS

There may be multiple, small penetrating arterial twigs or a major vessel, the *nutrient artery,* that enters the marrow at about midshaft in long bone. It sends branches called *central longitudinal arteries,* which run in the central longitudinal axis of the marrow to the diapheses. In addition, arterial branches enter the marrow from the epiphyseal ends. The central longitudinal arteries send out many slender radial branches which run radially through the marrow toward the encasing bone. They connect with venous sinuses throughout the marrow cavity (see below). Many small arterial vessels actually enter the bone where they may become part of osteones. But some of these vessels may curve back toward the marrow and either in the bone or out again in the marrow cavity open into venous sinuses.

VENOUS VESSELS

The vascular sinuses of marrow, the first vessels in the venous system, are thin-walled vessels 50 to 75 μm in diameter which anastomose richly. In long bones, they run radially and empty into the *central longitudinal vein* which runs in company with the major arteries (Figs. 12-3 and 12-4).

The continuity of arterial vessel with venous sinus has been demonstrated in the living circulation, by vascular injection and by scanning electron microscopy. Thus the circulation in the bone marrow is closed. Brånemark (1959) immobilized the thigh of an anesthetized rabbit, exposed the femur, and planed down the bony cortex until it was reduced to coverslip thickness, while leaving the marrow intact and little disturbed. Through a highpower light microscope with the light coming from above (epi-illumination) and passing through the planed-down bone, he observed direct connections between arterial and venous vessels in the living circulation. Irino and his colleagues found such connections between arterial vessels and venous sinuses in their SEM studies of methacrylate casts of the marrow vasculature.

The large, prominent system of sinuses, together with the far less evident arteries, constitute the *vascular compartment* of the marrow. The remainder of the marrow lies between these vessels as irregular cords and constitutes the *hematopoietic compartment* (Figs. 12-3 to 12-6). In red marrow, this compartment is filled with hematopoietic cells arranged upon a stroma. Hematopoiesis is most active in the periphery of the marrow. Some fat occurs near the center around the great vessels. In yellow marrow, virtually all the hematopoietic compartment is fatty. Some megakaryocytes may be present and vascular sinuses are reduced in number and size.

THE STRUCTURE OF
VASCULAR SINUSES

Vascular sinuses are the means of cellular exchange between the hematopoietic tissue and the circulation. The sinus wall is crossed by cells in transit. In its fullest development, the wall has three layers—endothelium, basement membrane, and adventitia (Figs. 12-5, 12-7, and 12-8).

The endothelium is a thin, simple layer of flat cells connected to one another by circumferential *zonulae adherens* (see Chap. 3). Endothelial cells contain many small vesicles, microfilaments, microtubules, some ribosomes and lysosomes, and small Golgi complexes (Figs. 12-8 to 12-10). Adventitial cells normally cover most of the outside surface of the endothelium. In the femoral marrow of the rat more than 60 percent is covered. When the level of cell passage across the sinus wall is heightened experimentally, however, adventitial cover may be reduced to less than 20 percent. Adventitial cells branch into the surrounding hematopoietic cords forming a spongework upon which hematopoietic cells are arranged (Fig. 12-10). The adventitial cells have been classified as *reticular cells,* a branched fibroblastic cell which elaborates argentophilic reticular fibers and

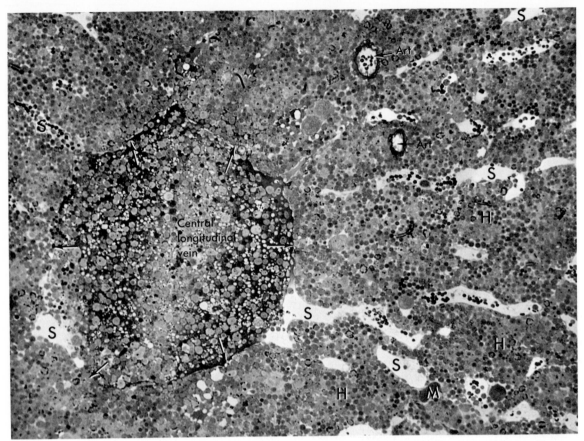

FIGURE 12-3 Rat bone marrow. This is a cross section of the marrow showing the relationships of major structural elements. The central longitudinal vein and branches of the nutrient artery (Art) are cut in cross section. The lumen of the vein is filled with cells: its wall is indicated by arrows. The sinuses (S) constitute a thin-walled radial system of venous vessels running into the vein. They are cut in longitudinal section. They are separated by hematopoietic compartments (H) containing the developing blood cells packed together. Megakaryocytes (M) lie characteristically against the outside wall of a sinus. ×750. (From L. Weiss, *J. Morph.,* **117:**481, 1965.)

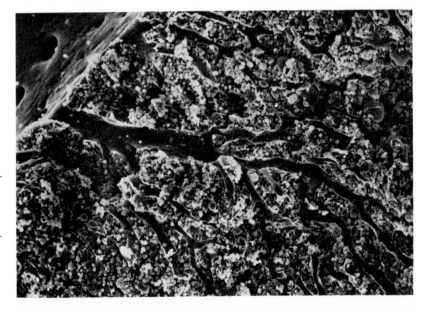

FIGURE 12-4 Rat bone marrow. This is a scanning electron micrograph of the cut surface showing a system of vascular sinuses originating at the periphery of the marrow (right side of field) and draining into a large vein (left upper corner). The large vein has several apertures in its wall, representing the entry of tributary venous sinuses. Hematopoietic tissue lies between the vascular sinuses. ×800. (From L. Weiss. *Anat. Rec.,* **186:**161, 1976).

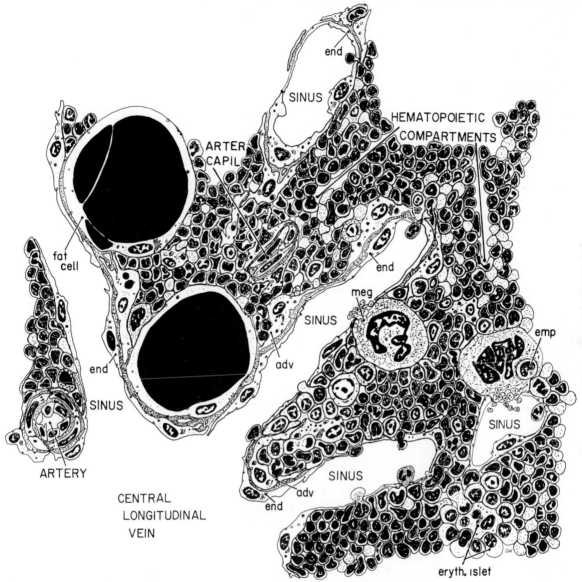

FIGURE 12-5 Bone marrow, schematic view of cross section near central longitudinal vein. Several sinuses drain into the central longitudinal vein. The sinuses are cut along their long axis, the vein, in cross section. A portion of the nutrient artery (Art) is present as is an arterial capillary. Hematopoietic cells lie between the sinuses, constituting the hematopoietic compartment. Where hematopoiesis is relatively quiet, the wall of the sinus and of the central longitudinal vein is trilaminar consisting of endothelium (end), a basement membrane, and adventitial cell (adv). The adventitial cell may become voluminous, encroaching upon the hematopoietic space and thereby displacing hematopoietic cells. The increased volume of the adventitial cell may be due to a gelatinous change wherein its cytoplasm becomes rarefied, presumably due to hydration. If this change is widespread, the marrow may become grossly white and gelatinous. A second and more common basis for large bulk of adventitial cells is fatty change, where they become fat cells. Contrariwise, when hematopoiesis is active the hematopoietic compartment is large and packed with myelocytes, erythroblasts, and megakaryocytes. The sinus wall becomes thin, reduced to an endothelial layer alone as the adventitial cells are displaced or lifted from the wall by infiltrating hematopoietic cells. Apertures appear in the endothelium, moreover, as maturing hematopoietic cells cross the sinus wall and enter the sinus lumen. Megakaryocytes characteristically lie against the outside of the sinus wall, discharging platelets into the lumen through an aperture. Occasionally the cytoplasm of megakaryocytes is entered by other cell types which remain visible and later leave the megakaryocyte. The phenomenom is known as emperipolesis (emp). Erythroblasts tend to be present in clusters near the sinus wall. Erythroblastic islets (see text) may be present. Granulocytes usually develop near the center of the hematopoietic space. Lymphocytes occur throughout the marrow. Macrophages are common, and mast cells, plasma cells, and other connective tissue cells are also present.

forms a spongework, or meshwork, characteristic of spleen, lymph node, and other hematopoietic tissues, as well as bone marrow.

This meshwork has been termed a reticular meshwork. The clearest function of this meshwork is that it supports the free, or migratory, hematopoietic cells. The fibroblastic cells of this meshwork may play a role in sorting out the free hematopoietic cells into their characteristic locations (see following section). The reticular cells may, as has been shown in a number of differentiating cellular systems involving fibroblastic cells, induce differentiation, namely, the differentiation of stem cells into blood cells.

Reticular cells may, under certain circumstances, appear to be swollen, quite voluminous, and "empty" in appearance, probably owing to marked water uptake. If this change is large scale, the marrow may become grossly white and gelatinous. Adventitial cells, moreover, may become fatty and if this change is large scale the marrow is yellow or fatty (Figs. 12-11 and 12-12). A major consequence of gelatinous or fatty change in reticular cells is that the volume for hematopoiesis is decreased with the change of the reticular cell from a slender branched cell to a large round cell. Gelatinous or fatty marrows, therefore, are inactive hematopoietically. As discussed above, certain marrow is normally yellow, notably in the appendicular skeleton, but following exposure to certain toxins or for unknown reasons normally hematopoietic marrow may become fatty with a resultant aplastic anemia.

Other functions have been ascribed to reticular cells. They have been regarded as phagocytes, the so-called fixed macrophages of the reticuloendothelial system. In fact, they are normally but slightly phagocytic. They have been characterized as stem cells, but recent work (presented in Chap. 11) indicates that they are not.

FIGURE 12-6 Rabbit bone marrow. Two sinuses (S), each having very thin walls, are present in this light-micrographic field. A megakaryocyte (M) lies against the outside wall of one of the sinuses. Portions of three fat cells (fat) are present; the one on the right lies against the wall of a sinus in an adventitial position. The hematopoietic compartment contains many granulocytes along the lower margin of the field. × 1200.

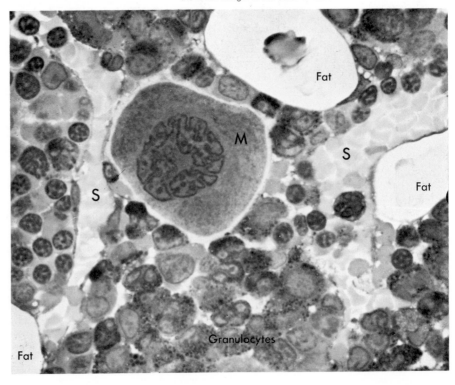

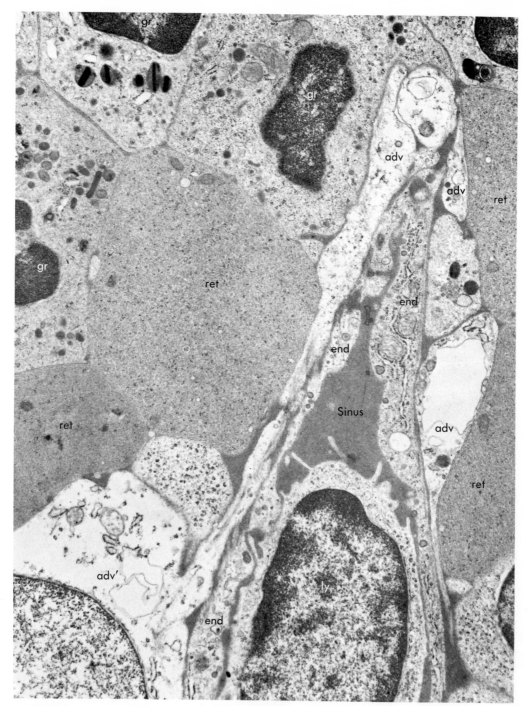

FIGURE 12-7 Rat bone marrow. A sinus is present, closely surrounded by hematopoietic cells. The lumen of the sinus contains a lymphocyte (ly). Its wall consists of endothelial (end) and adventitial (adv) layers. At the lower left corner of the field, the cytoplasm of an adventitial cell (adv') is voluminous and extends into the surrounding hematopoietic space. Reticulocytes (ret) and granulocytes (gr) surround the sinus. ×15,200. (From L. Weiss, *Blood,* **36:**189, 1970.)

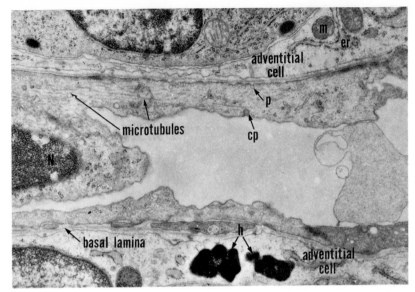

FIGURE 12-8 Rat bone marrow. A segment of vascular sinus shows an endothelium rich in microtubules and containing uncoated and coated pits (p and cp). The nuclear (N) portion of the endothelium protrudes into the lumen. Adventitial cells containing dense inclusions (h), mitochondrial (m), and endoplasmic reticulum (er) lie on the outside surface of the basal lamina. ×11,700. (From F. Campbell, *Am. J. Anat.*, **135:**521, 1972.)

FIGURE 12-9 Rat bone marrow, erythroblastic islet. A macrophage lies amid a cluster of red cells (E). It sends a system of slender branching cell processes which enclose the surrounding red cells and reach to the wall of a vascular sinus on the upper right. (This tissue was perfused and the cells, as a result, separated from one another thereby revealing the extensive branching of the macrophage clearly.) ×7300. (From L. Weiss, *Anat. Rec.*, **186:**161, 1976.)

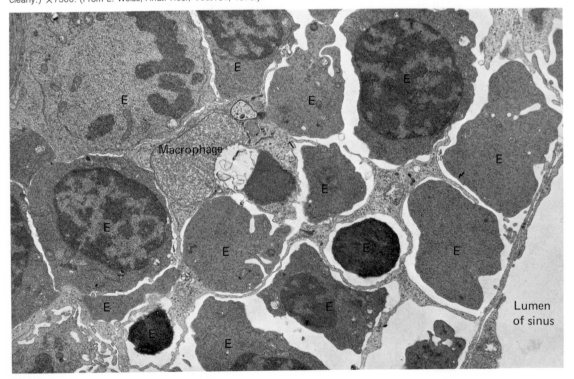

The marrow lacks lymphatic vessels. Indeed, lymphatic vessels are absent from sites in the spleen, liver lobule, and other places served by blood vascular sinuses. Nerves in bone marrow are associated with the vasculature and would appear vasomotor.

THE HEMATOPOIETIC COMPARTMENT

The hematopoietic tissue lying between the vascular sinuses consists, in hematopoietic marrow, of cords of hematopoietic cells and macrophages supported by a reticular meshwork. It contains mast cells, plasma cells, and other connective-tissue cell types. The relative numbers of nucleated marrow cells, as determined in smear preparations, are given in Table 12-1. Although their distribution may, on first view, appear

FIGURE 12-10 Rat bone marrow, scanning electron micrograph. A vascular sinus opens at the lower margin. The outside surface of its endothelium (End) is clothed by a reticular cell in adventitial position (Adv) in the vascular wall. The adventitial cell branches into the surrounding hematopoietic tissue. On the left a branch (Adv Process) partially envelopes an hematopoietic cell (Hemat. Cell). On the right, two hematopoietic cells (Hemat. Cells) bearing microvilli press against the outside surface of the vessel. Cells appear to develop microvilli preparatory to passage across the vascular wall into the lumen. ×4000. (From L. Weiss, *Anat. Rec.,* **186:**161, 1976.)

TABLE 12-1 RELATIVE NUMBER OF NUCLEATED CELLS IN NORMAL BONE MARROW

	RANGE	AVERAGE
Myeloblasts	0.3–5.0	2.0
Promyelocytes	1.0–8.0	5.0
Myelocytes		
Neutrophilic	5.0–19.0	12.0
Eosinophilic	0.5–3.0	1.5
Basophilic	0.0–0.5	0.3
Metamyelocytes ("juvenile" forms)	13.0–32.0	22.0
Polymorphonuclear neutrophils	7.0–30.0	20.0
Polymorphonuclear eosinophils	0.5–4.0	2.0
Polymorphonuclear basophils	0.0–0.7	0.2
Lymphocytes	3.0–17.0	10.0
Plasma cells	0.0–2.0	0.4
Monocytes	0.5–5.0	2.0
Reticular cells	0.1–2.0	0.2
Megakaryocytes	0.03–3.0	0.4
Pronormoblasts	1.0–8.0	4.0
Erythroblasts (basophilic, polychromatophilic, and acidophilic)	7.0–32.0	18.0

random, there is a pattern to the arrangement of hematopoietic cells.

Megakaryocytes lie tight against the adventitial surface of vascular sinuses (Figs. 12-3, 12-5, 12-6, 12-15 and 12-16). They lie over endothelial apertures

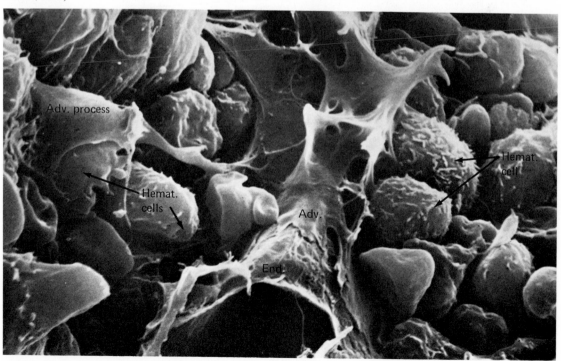

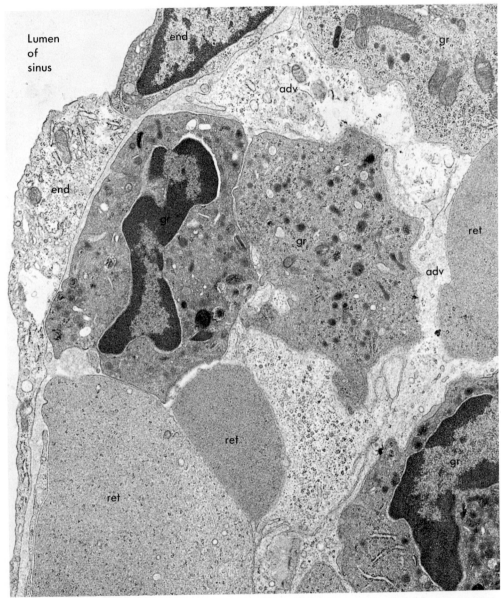

FIGURE 12-11 Rat bone marrow, vascular sinus. The lumen and the endothelium (end) of a sinus run along the left margin of the field. An adventitial cell (adv) is displaced from the wall by two granulocytes (gr) and two reticulocytes (ret). Thus the endothelium and its subjacent basement membrane are the only elements separating the late-stage hematopoietic cells from the lumen. The field also contains other reticulocytes and granulocytes. ×15,000. (From L. Weiss, *Blood,* **36:**189, 1970.)

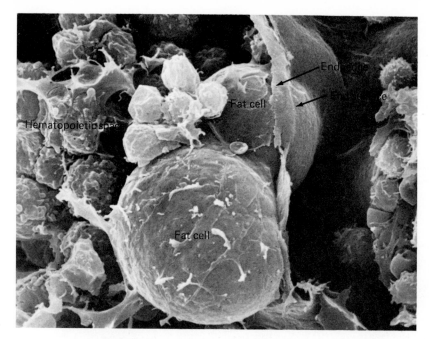

FIGURE 12-12 Rat bone marrow, scanning electron micrograph. A sinus lies at the right, with the luminal surface of its endothelium (End. Surface) and the torn edge of its endothelium (End. Edge) on view. The adventitial reticular cells have become fatty (Fat Cell) and extend into the hematopoietic space, occupying space that would otherwise be available for hematopoiesis. ×4050. (From L. Weiss, *Anat. Rec.*, **186:**161, 1976.)

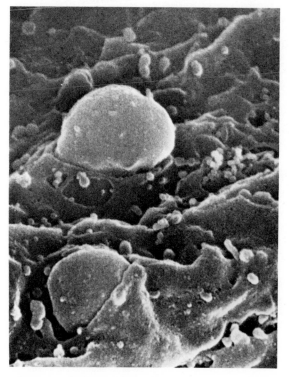

FIGURE 12-13 Rat bone marrow, scanning electron micrograph. This is a view of a vascular sinus on its luminal surface. Two cells are passing through the endothelium, likely entering the lumen of the sinus and the circulation. The upper cell is constricted as it squeezes through the endothelium. The lower one has a cowl of endothelium about it as it appears to emerge. ×3000. (From L. Weiss and L-T. Chen, *Blood Cells*, **1:**617, 1975.)

In the figure labels: End. edge, End. Surface, Fat cell, Hematopoietic space, Fat cell

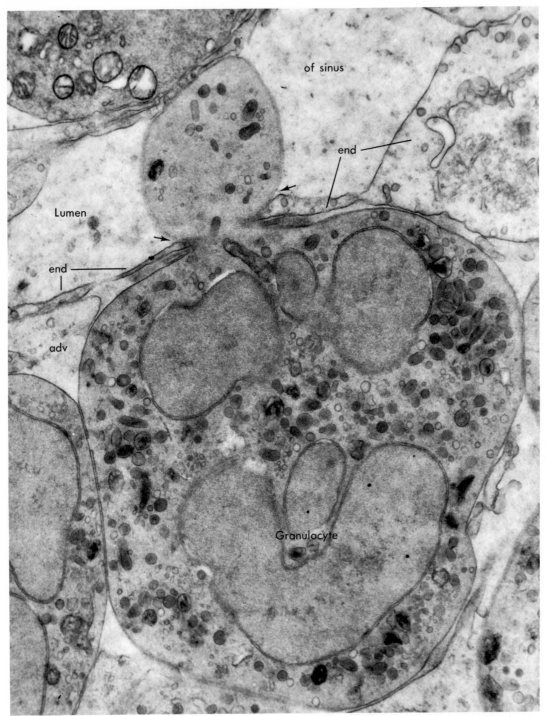

FIGURE 12-14 Rat bone marrow. A portion of a sinus, its lumen labeled, is at the top of the field. The wall of the sinus consists of endothelium (end), or lining cells, and adventitial cells (adv). A large granulocyte occupies most of the field. It lies almost entirely outside the sinus in the hematopoietic space and extends a process through an aperture (arrows) in the wall of the sinus and into the lumen. This granulocyte is crossing the wall of the sinus and will enter the circulation in the sinus. ×29,000. (From L. Weiss, *J. Morphol.* **117:**467, 1965.)

in the wall, moreover, and discharge platelets through the aperture into the lumen. Platelets may be discharged singly or in strips. By lying over an aperture in the sinus wall, the megakaryocyte efficiently delivers platelets into the vascular lumen and by its large size both resists being swept into the circulation and prevents vascular leakage.

Erythrocytes are produced near sinuses. As erythroblasts mature to the point where nuclear polarization is marked, they press against the sinus wall (Figs. 12-8 and 12-9). The cytoplasmic pole typically pushes into the adventitial surface of the wall. Nuclear and cytoplasmic poles separate and the cytoplasmic portion, now a reticulocyte, remains at the wall preparatory to passing through the endothelial cytoplasm and into the lumen of the sinus. The nuclear pole, surrounded by a thin rim of cytoplasm is phagocytized. In fact, there appears to be an obligatory relation between macrophages and developing erythroblasts in mammals. The macrophage lies in the center of an *erythroblastic islet*, its cytoplasm extending out and enclosing the surrounding erythroblasts (Fig. 12-13). There may be two (or more) circlets of erythroblasts in an islet, all partially enveloped by the macrophage. The outer tier of erythroblasts consists of more mature cells than the inner tier.

Granulocytes are typically produced in nests, somewhat away from the vascular sinus. On maturation, at the metamyelocte stage, they become motile and move toward the sinus and exit.

Lymphocytes tend to lie in rather compact clusters surrounding small radial arteries.

DELIVERY OF BLOOD CELLS TO THE CIRCULATION

The passage of maturing blood cells into the circulation requires the displacement of adventitial cells of

the vascular sinuses away from the vascular wall (Fig. 12-13). These adventitial cells may be under the control of erythropoietin in the case of the movement of erythrocytes across the sinus wall. After displacement of the adventitial cell, developing blood cells penetrate the basement membrane and the endothelium, squeeze through the wall, and enter the lumen of the vascular sinus (Fig. 12-14). Leukocytes appear to do this without association with other cell types. In the case of the red cells, the macrophage of the erythroblastic islet may interact with the adventitial cells and endothelium to facilitate passage. The aperture through which a developing blood cell passes occurs in the endothelial cytoplasm rather than between endothelial cells. It appears to develop in relation to cell passage and is absent otherwise.

Hematopoiesis in the marrow is almost entirely extravascular, yet some hematopoietic maturation normally occurs intravascularly. Perhaps the best example is that of the reticulocyte becoming a fully mature erythrocyte. The separation of platelet strips into individual platelets within sinuses is another example. Even in unstimulated marrow, moreover, erythroblasts and myelocytes may lie within the lumen of sinuses and undergo final maturation there or elsewhere in the circulation.

Some few cells not commonly considered blood cells may normally be found in the circulation. Thus, megakaryocytes, macrophages, and even some endothelial cells are found in blood in small numbers as are hematopoietic stem cells.

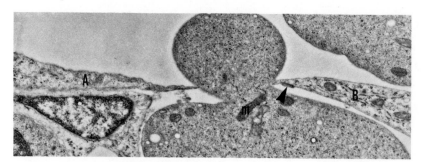

FIGURE 12-15 Rat bone marrow. Two lining cells, A and B, are joined at the tight junction (arrowhead). A reticulocyte is passing through an aperture in the endothelium. It contains a mitochondrian labeled m. Note that the aperture in the endothelium through which the reticulocyte is passing does not occur between endothelial cells (the site of the junction) but through their cytoplasm. ×11,500. (From F. Campbell., *Am. J. Anat.*, **135**:521, 1972.)

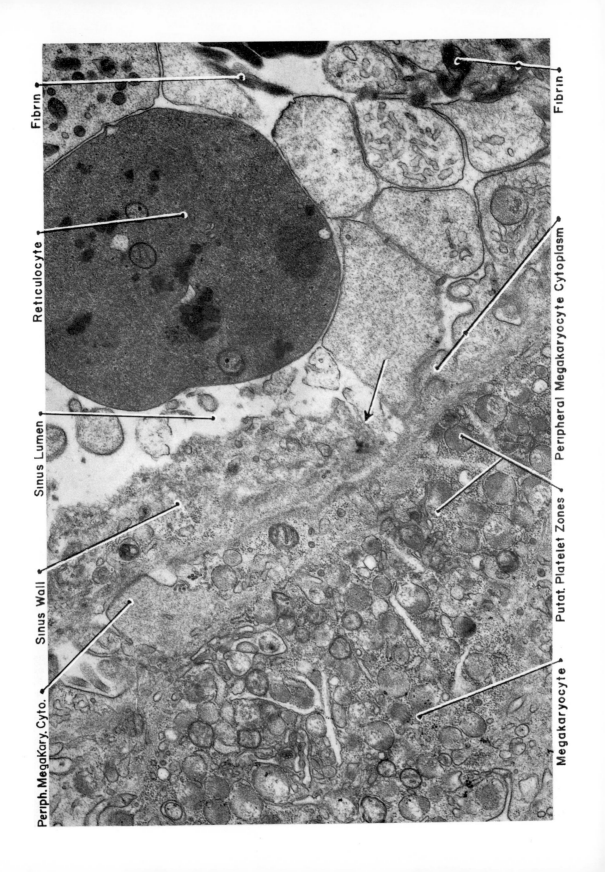

Fibrin

Fibrin

Reticulocyte

Peripheral Megakaryocyte Cytoplasm

Sinus Lumen

Putat. Platelet Zones

Sinus Wall

Periph.MegaKary. Cyto.

Megakaryocyte

FACTORS AFFECTING THE CELLULAR COMPOSITION OF BONE MARROW

PATHOLOGY OF THE BONE MARROW

In certain pathologic states the marrow may become hyperplastic. Yellow marrow may be replaced by hematopoietic tissue and normal hematopoietic tissue replaced by abnormal tissue. After severe hemorrhage, yellow marrow may quickly give way to red. In *leukemia*, abnormal leukocytes may be produced to the exclusion of normal red and white cells and may crowd the normal cells out. There are leukemias which correspond to the different white blood cell types as lymphocytic leukemia, monocytic leukemia, and so forth. A related malignancy of bone marrow is *multiple myeloma*. Here, the marrow is crowded with invasive myeloma cells, which represent abnormal plasma cells derived, in all likelihood, from abnormal B lymphocytes. The abnormal, or incomplete, antibody produced in certain myelomas has invaluably added to the elucidation of normal antibody structure. In *polycythemia*, there is a hypertrophy of the erythroblastic mass, but here the number of leukocytes and megakaryocytes may also be markedly increased, and the fat is displaced from the marrow. So intense may erythropoiesis be in certain anemias that the internal surface of the bone is eroded and the trabeculae become reduced in size and number. Despite this considerable increase in erythropoiesis, the number of circulating erythrocytes is quite severely reduced since the erythrocytes are markedly defective cells with considerably shortened life-spans.

There is a congenital, hemolytic anemia in the deer mouse which appears similar to a congenital hemolytic anemia in children. In contrast to aplastic anemias (see below) these marrows are hypercellular and markedly erythroid. The cortex and trabeculae of bone may be so thinned by the expansion and erosion of marrow in some of these anemias and, notably, in multiple myeloma and in leukemia, that fractures of bone may occur after slight trauma.

Contrarily, hematopoietic marrows may become hypoplastic inactive. Doan (1922) studied avian marrow reduced to a fatty state by starvation. He observed the rapid resumption of hematopoiesis after feeding. Many chemicals are toxic to marrow. Lead and benzene are industrial hazards capable of producing a severe depression of bone marrow termed *aplastic anemia*. Certain toxins are selective or may be controlled; for example, the *nitrogen mustards*, derivatives of the ill-reputed mustard gas, are used therapeutically to suppress or destroy an abnormal bone marrow. Aplastic anemia may be genetically determined and some animal models are providing insight into the mechanism. In the W/W^v strain of mouse, there is an aplastic anemia due to deficiency in hematopoietic stem cells. The S1/S1^d mouse strain, on the other hand, develops an aplastic anemia despite a normal number of stem cells because of a defect in marrow stroma or vasculature. There is a rare human condition, the *Diamond-Blackfan syndrome* of congenital aplastic anemia which would appear to correspond to the anemia in the S1/S1^d mouse. Hormonal imbalance from unchecked production of calcitonin may result in bony overgrowth and reduction in the volume of the marrow cavity. Malignant tumors may metastasize to bone marrow and create aplastic marrows by suppressing or displacing normal marrow tissue. In some instances, vascular sinuses may become widely dilated with blood, encroaching upon hematopoietic tissue and, paradoxically, conferring a brilliant red color upon a tissue which has become hematopoietically inactive.

FIGURE 12-16 Rat bone marrow. This field shows the typical relationship of a megakaryocyte to a sinus. The peripheral cytoplasm of the megakaryocyte, incompletely segmented into putative platelets by ER, is on the left. The peripheral cytoplasm may be granular or swollen and relatively free of organelles. The megakaryocyte abuts the outside surface of a sinus wall, which consists only of endothelium. The wall is defective with an aperture present in the lower third of the field, beginning at the arrow. The megakaryocyte cytoplasm protrudes through this aperture into the sinus lumen. Here incipient platelets, fully formed except for an attachment to the megakaryocyte, as well as detached platelets, may be seen. These platelets are somewhat swollen and lack lysosomes and ribosomes. Several do contain a complex branching system of ER, the canaliculi (see text). The platelets lie upon strands of fibrin and show the changes associated with platelets in clots. A reticulocyte also lies within the lumen of the sinus. ×20,000. (From L. Weiss, *J. Morphol.*, **112:**467, 1965.)

REFERENCES

BLOOM, W., and G. W. BARTELMEZ: Hematopoiesis in Young Human Embryos, *Am. J. Anat.*, **67:**21 (1940).

BRÅNEMARK, P. I.: Vital Microscopy of Bone Marrow in Rabbit. *Scand. J. Clin. Lab. Invest.* (Suppl. 38), **11:**1 (1959).

CAMBELL, F.: Ultrastructural Studies of Transmural Migration of Blood Cells in the Bone Marrow of Rats, Mice and Guinea Pigs, *Am. J. Anat.*, **135:**521 (1972).

DOAN, C. A.: The Capillaries of the Bone Marrow of the Adult Pigeon, *Bull. Johns Hopkins Hosp.*, **33:**222 (1922).

DONAHUE, D. M., B. W. GABRIO, and C. A. FINCH: Quantitative Measurement of Hematopoietic Cells of the Marrow, *J. Clin. Invest.*, **37:**1564 (1958).

FLEIDNER, T. M.: Research on the Architecture of the Vascular Bed of the Bone Marrow of Rats, *Z. Zellforsch Mikrosk. Anat.*, **45:**328 (1956).

FLEIDNER, T. M., W. CALVO, et al.: Morphological and Cytokinetic Aspects of Bone Marrow Stroma, in F. Stohlman (ed.), "Hematopoietic Cell Proliferation," Grune and Stratton, New York, 1970.

GILMOUR, J. R.: Normal Haemopoiesis in Intrauterine and Neonatal Life, *J. Pathol. Bact.*, **52:**25 (1941).

HUGGINS, C., and B. H. BLOCKSOM: Changes in Outlying Bone Marrow Accompanying a Local Increase of Temperature with Physiological Limits, *J. Exp. Med.*, **64:**253 (1936).

LICHTMAN, M. A.: Cellular Deformability during Maturation of the Myeloblast. Possible role in Marrow Egress, *N. Engl. J. Med.*, **283:**943 (1970).

WEISS, L.: The Hematopoietic Microenvironment of the Bone Marrow: An Ultrastructural Study of the Stroma in Rats, *Anat. Rec.*, **186:**161–184 (1976).

WEISS, L.: "The Cells and Tissues of the Immune System," Prentice-Hall, Englewood Cliffs, N.J., 1972.

WEISS, L.: The Histology of the Bone Marrow, in A. S. Gordon (ed.), "Regulation of Hematopoiesis," vol. 1, p. 79, Appleton-Century-Crofts, New York, 1970.

WEISS, L.: Transmural Cellular Passage in Vascular Sinuses of Rat Bone Marrow, *Blood,* **36:**189 (1970).

WEISS, L.: The Structure of Bone Marrow. Functional Interrelationships of Vascular and Hematopoietic Compartments in Experimental Hemolytic Anemia, *J. Morphol.*, **117:**467 (1965).

WEISS, L., and L-T. CHEN: The Organization of Hematopoietic Cords and Vascular Sinuses in Bone Marrow, *Blood Cells,* **1:**617 (1975.)

WICKRAMASINGHE, S. N.: "Human Bone Marrow," Blackwell Scientific Publications. Ltd., Oxford, 1975.

ZAMBONI, L., and D. C. PEASE: The Vascular Bed of Red Bone Marrow, *J. Ultrastruct. Res.*, **5:**65 (1961).

The Thymus

13

LEON WEISS

The human thymus is a lymphatic organ, pyramidal in shape, located in the superior mediastinum dorsal to the sternum. It achieves its greatest absolute weight, approximately 40 g, at puberty. The base of the thymus rests upon the pericardium; the pulmonary vessels, aorta, and trachea are dorsal to it. It is bilaterally symmetric, consisting of halves that meet in the midline except at the apex, which extends into the neck and diverges about the trachea. The thymus is derived from the epithelium of the third branchial pouch. Lymphocytes enter the epithelial rudiment, and the definitive thymus is a *lymphoepithelial* organ.

The thymus produces the T lymphocytes of the body from stem cells which emigrate from the bone marrow. The stem cells enter the thymus, and presumably under the influence of the epithelial cells, undergo differentiation into T cells. A great deal of cell death appears to be associated with this proliferation and differentiation. The surviving T cells are released to circulate and recirculate through the body stocking T-cell zones in lymph nodes, spleen, and other peripheral lymphatic tissues. These zones, accordingly, have been termed *thymic-dependent zones*. T-cell-dependent functions of the immune system, therefore, depend upon the thymus. Yet the adult thymus may be removed and T-cell functions may remain unimpaired for considerable periods because of the fullness to which T-cell stocks are built up in such peripheral lymphatic organs and the long life of T cells. The thymus does not itself participate in immune reactions. Its influence depends primarily upon production and release of T lymphocytes. The thymus, like the bone marrow, is therefore classified as a *central immune organ*.

The thymus is also required for the development of lymphatic leukemia in certain strains of mice and other animals. The thymus is sensitive to the effects of hormones, notably cortisone and related hormones of the adrenal cortex which cause a marked depletion in thymic lymphocytes. The thymus may play a role in mast cell differentiation.

The thymus develops early relative to the remaining lymphatic organs. Unlike the spleen and lymph nodes, it is well developed at birth. Before puberty, the thymus is a rounded, fleshy organ of some prominence. After puberty, it begins a remarkable involution or atrophy, its parenchyma being replaced by fatty and fibrous tissue until in old age it may be a shriveled, fibrous cord lying barely recognizable in the fat of the superior mediastinum. Despite postpubertal involution, the thymus remains a functional organ well into adulthood.

The thymus is divided into lobes and lobules by septae which extend into the organ from the surrounding connective tissues. The lobules are broad, roughly rectangular in outline, and 0.5 to 2.0 mm in length. Each lobule is divided into a peripheral zone relatively rich in lymphocytes, the *cortex,* and a central zone relatively rich in epithelial cells, the *medulla* (Figs. 13-1 and 13-2)

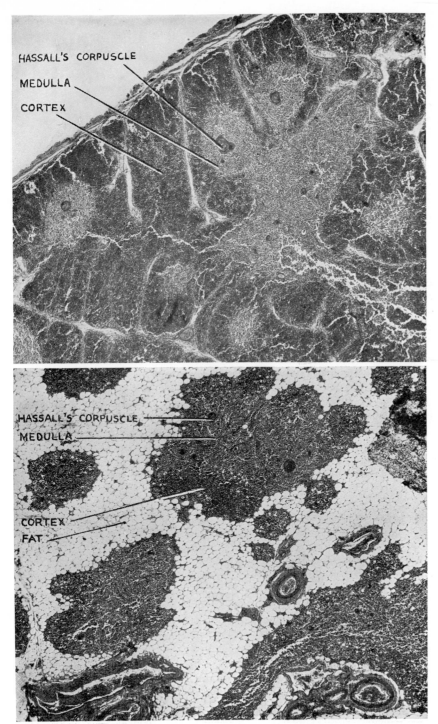

FIGURE 13-1 Human thymus before and after involution. The tissue in the upper micrograph is from a 4-year-old individual; the lower, from a 72-year-old person. Note the lobular pattern in the upper micrograph. The medulla is a branching structure. The cortex surrounds the lobular projections of the medulla. A thin fibrous capsule is present, Artefactitious cracks are present in the section. Involutional changes are evident in the lower micrograph. The cortex is markedly diminished, and the organ is fatty. The blood vessels display thickened sclerotic walls. Note, however, that the medulla has suffered relatively little change. ×30. (Preparations provided by B. Castleman.)

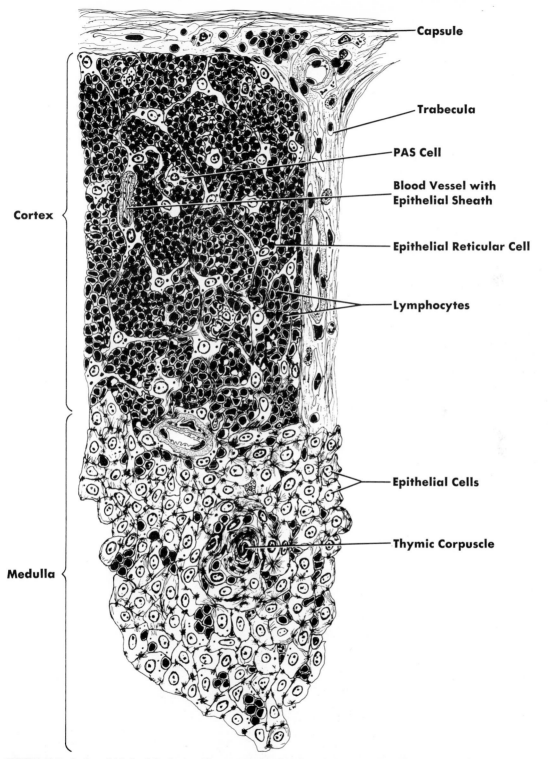

Capsule

Trabecula

PAS Cell

Blood Vessel with Epithelial Sheath

Epithelial Reticular Cell

Lymphocytes

Cortex

Epithelial Cells

Thymic Corpuscle

Medulla

FIGURE 13-2 Portion of lobule of the thymus. The cortex is heavily infiltrated with lymphocytes. As a result, the epithelial cells become stellate and remain attached to one another by desmosomes. The medulla is closer to a pure epithelium, although it too is commonly infiltrated by lymphocytes. A large thymic corpuscle, consisting of concentrically arranged epithelial cells, is figured. The capsule and trabeculae are rich in connective-tissue fibers (mainly collagen) and contain blood vessels and variable numbers of plasma cells, granulocytes, and lymphocytes. (From L. Weiss, ''The Cells and Tissues of the Immune System,'' Prentice-Hall, Inc., Englewood Cliffs, N.J., 1972.)

STRUCTURE OF THYMUS

MAJOR CELL TYPES

Epithelial Cells

Epithelial cells in the thymus may assume several forms. They line the walls of cysts as a simple cuboidal or columnar mucous ciliated epithelium. These structures probably represent remnants of branchial epithelium. They may be present in humans and are conspicuous in dogs and guinea pigs. A major group of thymic epithelial cells is in intimate association with lymphocytes. This epithelium consists of cells attached to one another by desmosomes. Lymphocytes in masses infiltrate the epithelium and separate these epithelial cells, but the latter remain attached to one another by their desmosomes with the result that they assume a branched or stellate appearance. The tips of these branches bear the desmosomes and are the points of intercellular attachment. The cells thereby form a meshwork which superficially resembles that of the mesenchymal reticular cells of the cords of spleen and lymph nodes. They have been called reticular cells. In recognition of their epithelial character, they will be designated here as *epithelial reticular cells*. (Figs. 13-4, 13-6, 13-12, and 13-14). In the interstices of their meshwork lie the lymphocytes that separate them. This meshwork is a cytoreticulum largely free of reticular fibers and of the intercellular substance associated with mesenchymal reticulum. It must be noted, however, that some mesenchymal reticulum exists in the thymus. As will be discussed below, this is associated for the most part with septa and blood vessels.

The epithelial-reticular cells are large, branched cells with large nuclei, prominent nucleoli, and voluminous eosinophilic cytoplasm. By light microscopy their epithelial nature may be suspected but not ascertained. In electron micrographs, these cells show tonofilaments, desmosomes, and cytoplasmic inclusions, some of which suggest a secretory function. In addition, they contain moderate but variable concentrations of ribonucleoprotein, moderate numbers of mitochondria, and a well-developed endoplasmic reticulum and Golgi apparatus.

Another major group of epithelial cells form thymic corpuscles. Here the epithelial cells may be swollen or flattened, tightly wound upon one another, and degenerated.

Lymphocytes

Thymic lymphocytes are small, medium, and large (Figs. 13-2 to 13-5). Like lymphocytes elsewhere, thymic lymphocytes are spherical cells with basophilic cytoplasm containing free ribosomes but scanty endoplasmic reticulum. Small thymic lymphocytes are somewhat smaller than small lymphocytes of other lymphatic organs; and while in the thymus, they may bear distinctive surface antigens, as the TL antigen in the mouse, which can serve as markers.

Other Cells

Macrophages are invariably present in large number within the thymus, scattered among the lymphocytes and epithelial cells of cortex and medulla. Some macrophages in the cortex (see below) may form a unit with closely surrounding proliferating lymphocytes.

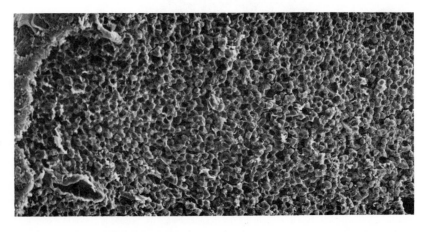

FIGURE 13-3 Rat thymus cortex, scanning electron micrograph. The capsule is on the left. The cortex is quite uniform in appearance, consisting of small lymphocytes closely arranged on a meshwork of epithelial-reticular cells. A number of blood vessels are evident. ×230. (From the work of L.-T. Chen, B. W. Wetzel, and L. Weiss.)

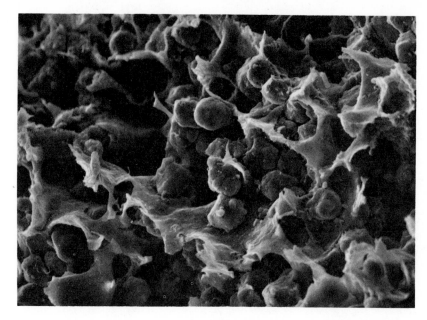

FIGURE 13-4 Rat thymus cortex, scanning electron micrograph. Many cortical lymphocytes have been washed away revealing the broad branchings of the epithelial-reticular cells. Note that some of the lymphocytes remain, lying upon the epithelial-reticular cells. ×5700. (From the work of L.-T. Chen, B. W. Wetzel, and L. Weiss.)

FIGURE 13-5 Thymus of a mouse, medulla. Several large epithelial cells are present. Their cytoplasm contains deeply stained inclusions. Many lymphocytes closely surround the epithelial cells. Compare with Fig. 13-6. PAS-hematoxylin stain. ×1300.

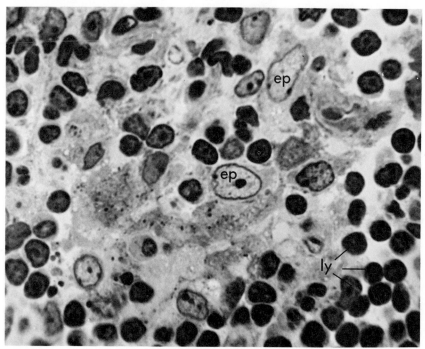

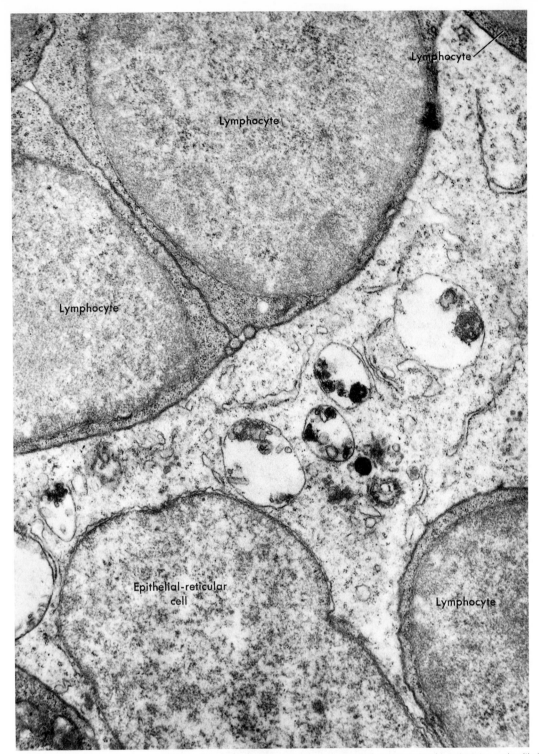

FIGURE 13-6 Electron micrograph of the cortex of rat thymus, showing a characteristic relationship of lymphocytes and epithelial-reticular cells. The lymphocytes are present in clusters. Their nucleus is spherical, their cytoplasm scanty and rich in ribonucleoprotein but poor in endoplasmic reticulum and mitochondria. The epithelial-reticular cells are larger cells. The nucleus is less dense and may contain a moderately sized nucleolus. The cytoplasm is voluminous, extending between lymphocytes as slender cytoplasmic processes, and contains distinctive multivesicular vacuoles, some ribonucleoprotein, and some endoplasmic reticulum. These epithelial cells may be rich in cytoplasmic filaments. ×33,000.

Such macrophages, which contain phagocytized lymphocytes in heterolysosomes stained in the periodic acid Schiff reaction, have been termed *PAS cells* (Fig. 13-2). The PAS cell is in some respects similar to the macrophage and the erythroblastic islet (see Chap. 12) and the macrophages of germinal centers which account for the "starry sky" pattern (see Chap. 9). Fat cells are prominent in aged thymus. Mast cells are always present in the capsule and septa and occasionally in the parenchyma of the organ; involuted thymuses may contain great numbers. A few plasma cells may be found scattered in the thymus.

Other blood cells and connective tissue cells may be found in variable but usually small numbers.

CAPSULE

The thymus is enclosed by a thin, well-defined capsule of dense white connective tissue variably rich in macrophages, plasma cells, granular leukocytes, mast cells, and fat cells (Figs. 13-1 to 13-3). Connective tissue continuous with the capsule dips into the organ

FIGURE 13-7 Thymus of a human being 20 years of age. Lymphocytes are concentrated in the cortex. They are present in the medulla as well but are scattered loosely among epithelial-reticular cells. A large, multicentric thymic corpuscle is present in the medulla. The interlobular septum is slender and contains lymphatic vessels, blood vessels, and nerves. × 200. (Preparation from B. Castleman.)

separating the lobes and lobules and forms *septa*. Blood vessels, efferent lymphatic vessels, and nerves run in the capsule and septa. The connective tissue continues into the organ, forming a perivascular cuff. (See discussion of blood vessels and Fig. 13-11.)

MEDULLA

The medulla is a broad, branched mass of tissue which forms the central part of the thymus (Figs. 13-1 and 13-2). The branches of the medulla provide the lobar and lobular patterns of the organ. The medulla is rich in epithelial cells.

Relative to the cortex (see below), there are few lymphocytes in the medulla so that the epithelial cells are not widely separated and therefore not as markedly branched as those in the cortex. They are therefore rather typically epithelial in appearance.

The medulla contains many large blood vessels from which collagenous and reticular fibers radiate and thread between epithelial cells.

Variable numbers of plasma cells, mast cells, eosinophils, and melanocytes are present in the medulla, usually near blood vessels.

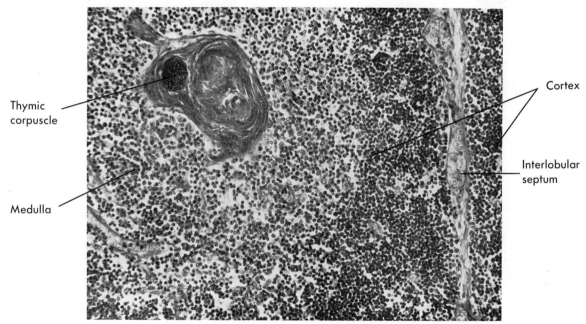

Thymic corpuscle

Medulla

Cortex

Interlobular septum

Thymic Corpuscles

Thymic corpuscles, or *Hassall's corpuscles,* are organizations of epithelial cells unique to the medulla of the thymus (Figs. 13-2 and 13-7 through 13-9). They typically consist of epithelial cells rather tightly wound about one another in a concentric pattern. The central cells are prone to become swollen, keratinized, calcified, and necrotic and may undergo lysis, leaving a cystic structure. The peripheral epithelial cells in a thymic corpuscle blend into the cytoreticulum. Thymic corpuscles may be well over 100 μm in diameter and are subject to considerable variation. They are well developed in human beings and guinea pigs but poorly developed in mice.

The essential changes in epithelial cells which signify a conversion to thymic corpuscles are hyalini-

zation of cytoplasm and swelling of nucleus and cytoplasm. Tonafilaments are markedly developed and desmosomes numerous. Small corpuscles may consist of a few cells or even of only one cell. As more cells contribute to a corpuscle, its concentric pattern evolves. Thymic corpuscles become larger with age. They may eventually become huge, multiform structures.

The function of thymic corpuscles is unknown. They may have immunologic functions. They have been regarded as degenerated structures.

FIGURE 13-8 Thymus of a mouse. A. Electron micrograph of a small corpuscle. By light microscopy this would probably appear as a unicellular corpuscle. Note the large swollen nucleus and the similarly degenerated cytoplasm. The epithelial cells surrounding the large central cell are arranged circumferentially, with desmosomes present at their cell membrane. (From Fig. 5, P. Kohnen and L. Weiss. *Anat. Rec.,* **148:**29, 1964.) B. Tracing of the corpuscle shown in A. Desmosomes are at d; cytoplasmic filaments at f. × 4000.

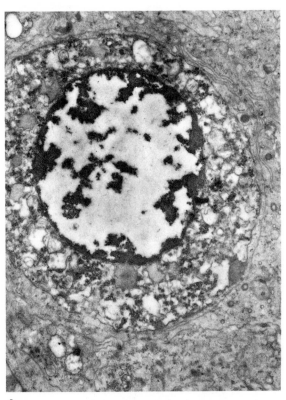

A

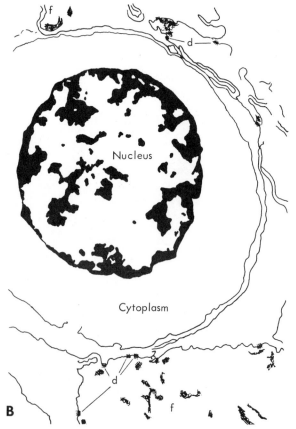

B

The cortex is a thick layer of lymphocytes and epithelial cells which lies upon the medulla and follows its contour. In the preinvolutional thymus, numerous lymphocytes lie between epithelial cells, separating and obscuring them. The epithelial-reticular cells are highly branched and form a cellular meshwork (Figs. 13-2, 13-4, 13-6, and 13-14).

It is likely that stem cells released from bone marrow enter the subcapsular cortex of the thymus

and move toward the medulla as they differentiate into T lymphocytes. There is considerable lymphocyte death in this process and many macrophages, including PAS cells, are present.

BLOOD VESSELS OF THE THYMUS

Major arterial vessels, branches of the subclavian artery, enter the medulla through septa. There are many arterial branches in the medulla. The blood supply of the cortex is derived from arterioles which run along the junction of cortex and medulla. From these vessels, arterial capillaries run outward to the capsule. They return as venous capillaries and venules to drain into veins running in company with the arterioles in the corticomedullary junction. These veins drain into

FIGURE 13-9 Thymus of a guinea pig. A. Electron micrograph of a thymic corpuscle. There is a small compressed central cell (labeled R in the accompanying tracing). Note the concentrate pattern of the cells. The inner cells have droplets, probably keratohyaline droplets. Cytoplasmic filaments and desmosomes contribute to this corpuscle. A portion of an epithelial cell in the cytoreticulum in the right upper corner contains intracytoplasmic vacuoles. (From Fig. 1, P. Kohnen and L. Weiss, *Anat. Rec.,* **148:**29, 1964.) B. Tracing of the corpuscle shown in A. Desmosomes are at d; cytoplasmic filaments at f, and intracytoplasmic vacuoles at c. R is degenerated nucleus. ×5000.

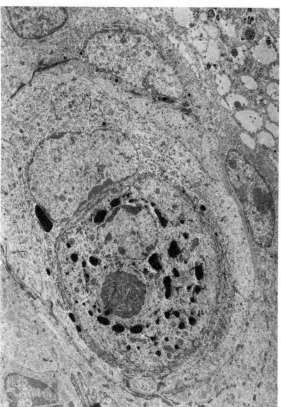

A

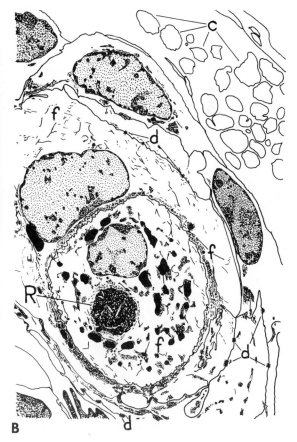

B

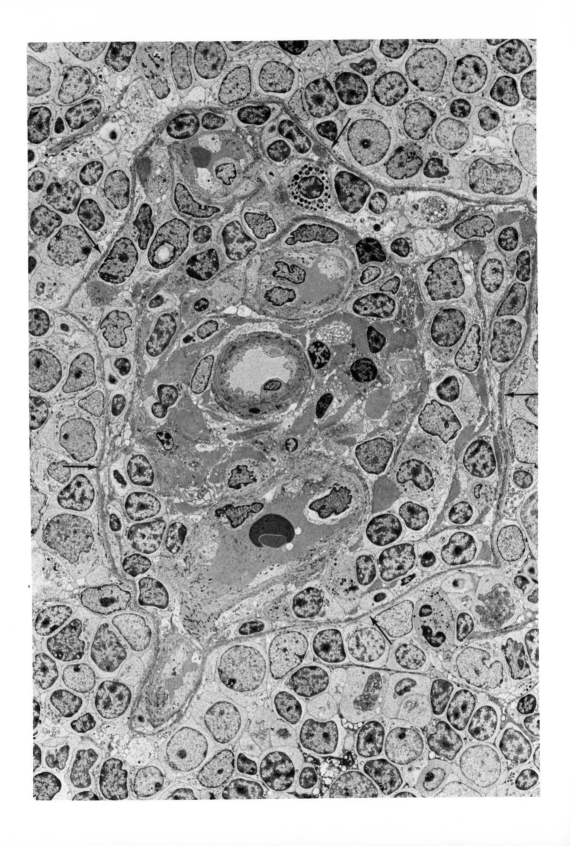

medullary veins, most of which empty into the innominate vein.

Capillaries may be but 4 to 6 μm in outside diameter. Epithelial-reticular cells envelop capillaries and larger vessels, particularly in the cortex of the thymus, thereby constituting the most peripheral cell of the vessel wall. These cells extend cytoplasmic processes outward between perivascular lymphocytes. Epithelial-reticular cells in thymic vessels thus occupy a position similar to that of the glial cells investing blood vessels in the central nervous system. They constitute an element in the *blood-thymus barrier* (Figs. 13-10 through 13-14) just as glial cells contribute to the *blood-brain barrier.*

Raviola and Karnovsky have shown, after the injection of peroxidase and other tracer substances visualized by electron microscopy, that the blood-thymus barrier is quite tight in most of the cortex. But in the juxtamedullary cortex, in the region of the cortical venules, the barrier is imperfect and tracer substances escape into the thymic parenchyma (Figs. 13-12 and 13-13).

The vasculature in the human thymus, as described by Bearman, Bensch, and Levine, is surrounded by a collar of connective tissue which, in turn, is enclosed by a layer of epithelial-reticular cells. Two distinct basal laminae are present in this perivascular envelope. One lies beneath the endothelium and the other lies against the vascular surface of the epithelial-reticular cells. The width of the perivascular connective tissue space varies with the caliber of the blood vessel, being greater in larger vessels and virtually absent in capillaries. In the larger vessels this space is traversed by large numbers of reticular fibers. It contains eosinophils and other granulocytes, plasma cells, mononuclear cells, and other connective tissue cells. Thus, many of the connective tissue cells lie in the thymus; in fact, they lie in the perivascular connective tissue and are excluded from the lymphoepithelial portion of the organ by the continuous barrier of epithelial-reticular cells and their basal laminae. The thymic lymphocytes are thereby separated from the vascular lumen by (1) endothelium (and in arteries and veins, a muscular coat); (2) endothelial basal

lamina; (3) a perivascular connective tissue collar of variable width with variable cell content; (4) basal lamina of epithelial-reticular cells; (5) a layer of epithelial-reticular cells.

LYMPHATIC VESSELS

There appear to be no afferent lymphatic vessels. Several groups of efferent vessels leave from the medulla and septa and drain into mediastinal lymph nodes.

NERVE SUPPLY

The capsule of the thymus is moderately rich in small myelinated and unmyelinated nerves from the vagus, cardiac plexus, first thoracic ganglion, and ansa hypoglossi. Vasomotor fibers enter the organ with blood vessels.

DEVELOPMENT

The human thymus develops bilaterally from the distal portions of the third branchial pouch. There may be a small contribution from the fourth. The thymic rudiment in human embryos of 10-mm crown-rump length (CRL) is a slender, tubular prolongation which extends caudad and mediad. It reaches into the mediastinum just caudal to the thyroid and parathyroid rudiments. The tip of the prolongation proliferates, becoming bulbous. The intermediate portion, constituting the connection to the pharynx, vanishes, leaving the proliferating terminal bulb free in the mediastinum at 35 mm CRL.

The epithelial thymic rudiment becomes surrounded by a layer of mesenchyme. Soon after, lymphocytes are found in the midst of the epithelium. Lymphocytes and epithelial cells proliferate; and when the embryo is 40 mm CRL, the lobular pattern is achieved. Thymic corpuscles begin to appear at 60 to 70 mm.

The development of the thymus outstrips that of the remaining lymphatic organs. The thymus is rather fully developed prenatally. Only postnatally do the spleen and lymph nodes attain such development.

The thymus may fail to develop normally. Swiss-type agammaglobulinemia in human beings is associated with defective thymic development. Among the

---

FIGURE 13-10 Human thymus, near the border of the cortex and the medulla. An arteriole with several branches is surrounded by a perivascular connective tissue space limited by epithelial-reticular cells (arrows). ×1850. (From R. M. Bearman, K. G. Bensch, and G. D. Levine. *Anat. Rec.,* **183**:485, 1975.) See Fig. 13-9.

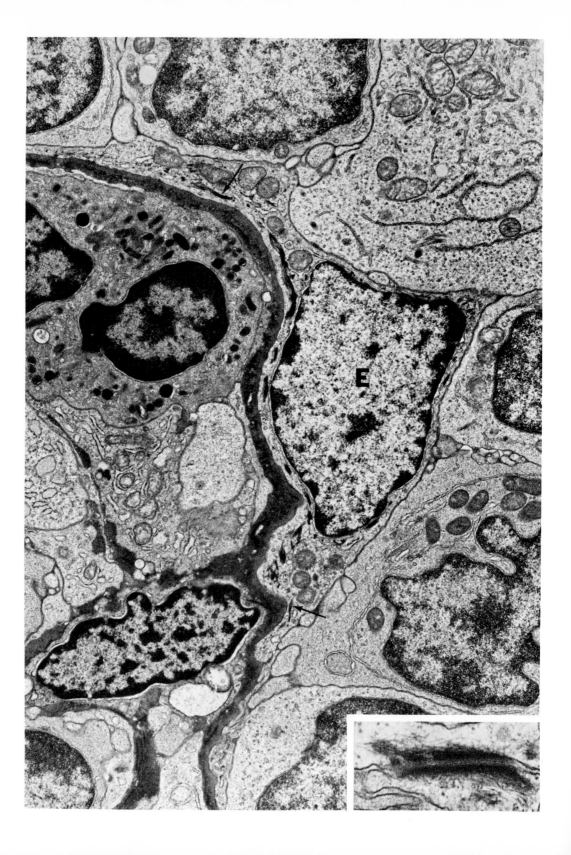

FIGURE 13-11 Human thymus, a higher magnification of the border of the perivascular space and the thymic parenchyma. An epithelial-reticular cell (E) delineates the space, which is to left of the cell. The epithelial-reticular cell contains prominent tonofilaments (arrows). ×16,500. Inset. Desmosome between two epithelial-reticular cells. ×50,000. (From R. M. Bearman, K. G. Bensch, and G. D. Levine, *Anat. Rec.,* **183**:485, 1975.)

consequences of this thymic deficiency are vulnerability to fungal and other infections and disorders in delayed hypersensitivity (see below). A valuable animal model in which the thymus fails to develop is the nude (nu/nu) mutant mouse. It shows immunologic deficiencies which neatly delineate T- from B-cell functions.

INVOLUTION OF THE THYMUS

Involution, the process of atrophy and depletion, is accelerated after puberty and consists primarily of a decrease in thymic weight and a conspicuous loss of cortical lymphocytes and often their replacement by fat, and an increase in size and a slight increase in number of thymic corpuscles. The septa show a proportionate increase in width as the lobules atrophy (Fig. 13-1). But the age-associated wasting of the organ has been perhaps unduly stressed, since the thymus remains substantive and functional in adulthood. The normal pattern of involution may be telescoped by a precipitous involution associated with disease, so-called accidental involution. The thymus in infants who die suddenly is occasionally large and has been considered causative in their deaths, a condition designated *status thymicolymphaticus;* but it is likely

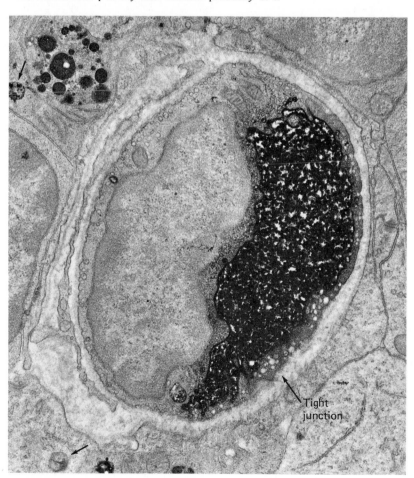

FIGURE 13-12 Mouse thymus, capillary in cortex. Horseradish peroxidase has been injected as a tracer. Very little of this low-molecular-weight (approximately 40,000) protein escapes the capillary lumen. Note that it fails to penetrate the junction between endothelial cells. The small amount of horseradish peroxidase that leaves the vessel is phagocytized by perivascular macrophages (arrows). Compare with vascular permeability in the medulla (Fig. 13-13). ×21,200. (From E. Raviola and M. J. Karnovsky, *J. Exp. Med.,* **136**:466, 1972.)

Tight junction

that this state represents simply a normal organ undiminished by accidental involution.

The thymus is at its greatest relative size at birth and at its greatest absolute size at puberty. The figures in Table 13-1, taken from Hammar's work, represent average weights of the thymus at different ages in human beings. Note that the weight of the organ diminishes in adulthood. Lymphatic tissue throughout the body suffers a decrease with age, but in the thymus the process is more marked.

TABLE 13-1 AGE AND THYMUS WEIGHT

AGE, YEARS	WEIGHT, G
Newborn	13.26
1–5	22.98
6–10	26.10
11–15	37.52
16–20	25.58
21–25	24.73
26–35	19.87
36–45	16.27
46–55	12.85
56–65	16.08
66–75	6.00

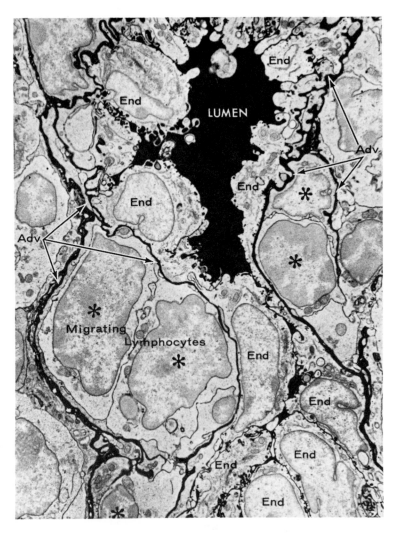

FIGURE 13-13 Mouse thymus, postcapillary venule in medulla. Horseradish peroxidase has been injected as a tracer. In less than 5 min there has been an impressive leakage, staining the endothelial basal lamina and the adventitia (Adv) with the same intensity as the plasma in the lumen of the vessel. Note the irregular endothelium (End) bearing many pinocytotic vesicles containing the peroxidase tracer. The thick connective tissue adventitial layer (Adv) is traversed by migrating lymphocytes (asterisks) which are likely moving toward the lumen and into the circulation. Compare with Fig. 13-11. ×7100. (From E. Raviola and M. J. Karnovsky, *J. Exp. Med.*, **136**:466, 1972.)

The thymus is present in every vertebrate. Thymuses in all mammals are remarkably alike, although such variations as differences in development of thymic corpuscles exist. Thus, thymic corpuscles are large and well developed in human beings and guinea pigs, but small and few in number in mice and rats.

FUNCTIONS OF THE THYMUS

LYMPHOCYTE TURNOVER

The mitotic rate of thymic lymphocytes is high, equaling that of those proliferating focuses in germinal centers of spleen or lymph nodes mounting antibody responses. Despite its high mitotic rate, the thymus normally contains no germinal centers. Despite the high rate of proliferation of its lymphocytes, moreover, the thymus depends upon outside sources for lymphocytes. Indeed, it is startling to consider that more

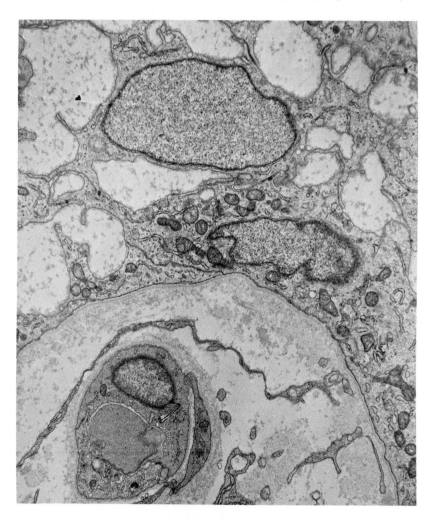

FIGURE 13-14 Hyman thymic cortex involution. A capillary at the bottom of the field lies in a perivascular space and is surrounded by an atrophic cortex. Lymphocytes have dropped out and the epithelial-reticular cells that remain form a fluid-filled meshwork. Note the desmosomes connecting the epithelial-reticular cells. ×1700. (From the work of G. D. Levine.)

than 90 percent of the lymphocytes within the thymus may die within a few days. In fetal life the thymus is supplied by stem cells produced and released into the circulation by the liver. When hematopoiesis moves to the marrow, that tissue becomes the source of thymic lymphocytes, a function it maintains throughout life.

The lymphocytes released from the thymus are distinctive in having a specific surface antigen—in mice, the theta (θ) antigen. These T cells enjoy a long life and circulate and recirculate in distinctive pathways through lymphatic tissues (excluding the thymus), blood, and lymph. They occupy distinctive sites in spleen and lymph nodes. See Chap. 12, 14, and 15.

The development of the spleen, lymph nodes, and other lymphatic tissue is dependent on the thymus. Following neonatal thymectomy, these organs are considerably diminished in size owing to a lack of small T lymphocytes (Fig. 13-15). The level of small lymphocytes in the blood may be reduced 60 percent or more and that in the lymph to an even lower level. Immunological deficiencies are associated with this lymphocytic depletion (see below).

As discussed below, thymectomy in adult individuals is not followed by such morphologic and immunologic deficiencies.

THYMIC HUMORAL FACTOR

It is likely that the thymus elaborates a humoral factor which stimulates conversion of stem cells to T lymphocytes. The evidence depends heavily on neonatal thymectomy. Thus a newborn mouse thymectomized at birth becomes deficient in both lymphocytes (Fig. 13-15) and immunologic capacity. By grafting with a thymus from a litter mate, however, such deficiencies are averted. If a thymectomized newborn mouse is supplied with a thymus grafted into his peritoneal cavity but wrapped in a cell-tight envelope fabricated of a millipore filter, the treated animal will have a partial restoration of his lymphocytes and suffer no immunologic deficiencies. In short, a factor which stimulates lymphocytic production sufficiently to allow normal immunological function appears to be escaping the millipore envelope. This preparation has largely substituted for the thymus. Further support for a thymic humoral factor comes from experiments in which thymectomized immunologically deficient female mice, on becoming pregnant, are found to have

their immunologic competence restored, even though placental arrangements preclude cellular transfer from fetus to mother. A substance, termed *thymosin,* has been extracted from the thymus and appears to promote a differentiation of T cells. There are strong inferences that epithelial reticular cells elaborate this factor.

IMMUNOLOGIC FUNCTIONS

The thymus possesses a fundamental immunologic role dependent on its production and release of T lymphocytes. This role is best revealed after neonatal thymectomy. The lymphocytic depletions which follow this procedure are associated with major immunologic deficiencies. Most consistently there is an impairment in delayed hypersensitivity or cellular immunity. Thus after thymectomy in the newborn, homografts (a graft from a genetically different animal but one within the same species, as mouse to mouse but not within the same inbred mouse line) may persist indefinitely instead of being rejected. In addition, there is interference with antibody production against those antigens (as foreign erythrocytes) that require the cooperation of T cells. These deficiencies can be fully corrected by thymic grafts.

Thymectomy in adults is attended by no such clear-cut change because the extrathymic tissues and circulation are already stocked with T cells. A significant reduction in splenic and lymph nodal weight occurs after thymectomy in adult rats, for example, although 6 to 8 weeks are required for the change. However, if adults are thymectomized and then irradiated to deplete the stores of T cells in their lymphatic tissue, a neonatal picture emerges.

ROLE OF THE THYMUS IN LEUKEMIA

In certain strains of mice and other animals, the incidence of leukemia is high. For example, 60 to 80 percent of mice of the AKR strain develop leukemia by their second year. In addition to a genetic predisposition, the presence of a virus and of the thymus is required for the appearance of leukemia. In high-leukemia strains of mice, the virus is transmitted transplacentally with the result that it is distributed in virtually every tissue of every individual. Thymectomy prevents the occurrence of the disease. The role of the thymus in unknown. Normally the mitotic rate of thymic lymphocytes is three to five times that of lym-

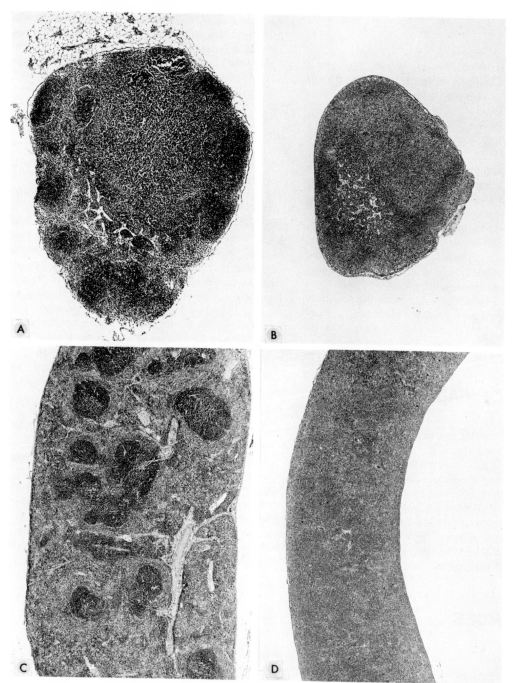

FIGURE 13-15 This plate illustrates the dependence of the lymph nodes and spleen upon the thymus. The tissues are taken from C57BL mice. A. Lymph node of 8-week-old mouse sham-operated at birth. ×32. B. Lymph node of 8-week-old mouse thymectomized at birth. ×32. C. Spleen of 7-week-old mouse sham-operated at birth. ×32. D. Spleen of 7-week-old mouse thymectomized at birth. ×32. Thymectomy is followed by a decrease in size of the lymph nodes and spleen, due primarily to depletion of small lymphocytes (T cells). (From the work of J. F. A. P. Miller.)

phocytes elsewhere. In leukemic strains, the mitotic rate in the preleukemic period may exceed that of nonthymic lymphocytes by a factor of 7 to 10.

MAST-CELL DIFFERENTIATION

There are strong hints that the thymus may play a role in the differentiation of mast cells. Ginsburg and Sachs showed that in tissue cultures of thymus there was large-scale differentiation of mast cells. Combs confirmed these cells as mast cells by both histochemistry and electron microscopy. The Ishizakas demonstrated that IgE receptors appeared on these cells at about the time granules began to appear. They also showed that thymus cells, undergoing transformation into mast cells, were not T cells. There thus exists the possibility that in addition to supporting the stem cell to T-cell differentiation that the thymus may support a stem cell to mast-cell differentiation. The differentiation to

granulated mast cells need not occur in the thymus in the intact animal. The conversion may be begun, the early mast cell released, and the differentiation completed (that is, granules developed), with the mast cells dispersed widely throughout the body. It is well known, moreover, that the thymus may become rich in mast cells, especially after involution.

INFLUENCE OF HORMONES

Following the administration of certain adrenocortical hormones, the thymus undergoes massive involution. The process primarily affects the cortex, as large numbers of lymphocytes are damaged and die. Macrophages in great numbers become mobilized and ingest these lymphocytes. The picture resembles that of acute involution. Indeed, it is possible that acute involution is mediated by adrenocortical secretion. Sex hormones may elicit similar responses in the lymphatic system, but they are not so pronounced as those of the adrenal cortex. Adrenocorticotropic hormone affects the thymus through the adrenal cortex. Growth hormone induces growth of the thymus.

BURSA OF FABRICIUS

The bursa of Fabricius is a lymphoepithelial organ in birds which originates as a dorsal epithelial diverticulum of the cloaca. It becomes infiltrated by lymphocytes. It resembles the thymus, in being a gut-derived epithelial structure intimately associated with lymphocytes. In the bursa, however, unlike the thymus, the epithelial diverticulum retains connection with the cloaca and forms follicles. The lymphocytes are organized about the follicles. The bursa involutes markedly on sexual maturation. Indeed its development

may be entirely suppressed by applying male sex hormones to the shell of embryonated eggs.

Birds possess a pharyngeal thymus and exhibit a division of labor between bursa and thymus which is of great theoretical importance. The thymus receives stem cells from the bone marrow and induces their differentiation to T cells. The bursa receives stem cells from the bone marrow and induces their differentiation to B cells. The letters T and B, in fact, derive from Thymus and Bursa.

REFERENCES

ARNASON, B. G., and C. WENNERSTEN: Role of the Thymus in Immune Reaction in Rats. II. Suppressive Effect of Thymectomy at Birth on Reactions of Delayed (Cellular) Hypersensitivity and the Circulating Small Lymphocyte, *J. Exp. Med.*, **116:**177 (1962).

BEARMAN, R. M., K. G. BENSCH, and G. D. LEVINE: The Normal Human Thymic Vasculature: An Ultrastructural Study, *Anat. Rec.*, **183:**485 (1975).

CHAPMAN, W. L., JR., and J. R. ALLEN: The Fine Structure of the Thymus of the Fetal and Neonatal Monkey (*Macaca mulatta*), *Z. Zellforsch. Miknosk. Anat.*, **114:**220–223 (1971).

CLARK, S. L., JR.: The Thymus in Mice of Strain 129/J, Studied with the Electron Microscope, *Am. J. Anat.*, **112:**1–33 (1963).

CLARK, S. L., JR.: The Intrathymic Environment, In A. J. S. Davies and R. L. Carter (eds.) ''Contemporary Topics in Immunobiology,'' vol. 2, ''Thymus Dependency,'' Plenum Press, New York, 1973.

DEFENDI, V., and D. METCALF (eds.): ''The Thymus,'' Wistar Institute Press, Philadelphia, 1964.

DOWNEY, H.: Cytology of Rabbit Thymus and Regeneration of Its Thymocytes after Irradiation; with Some Notes on the Human Thymus, *Blood,* **3:**1315 (1948).

GINSBURG, H., and L. SACHS: Formation of Pure Suspensions of Mast Cells in Tissue Culture by Differentiation of Lymphoid Cells from the Mouse Thymus, *J. Natl. Cancer Inst.,* **31:**1 (1963).

GOOD, R. A., and A. E. GABRIELSEN (eds.): ''The Thymus in Immunobiology: Structure, Function, and Role in Disease,'' Paul B. Hoeber, Inc., New York, 1964.

GOOD, R. A., and B. W. PAPERMASTER: Phylogeny of the Immune Response, *Fed. Proc.,* **20:**26 (1961).

HAAR, J. L.: Light and Electron Microscopy of the Human Fetal Thymus, *Anat. Rec.,* **179:**463–476 (1974).

HARRIS, J. E., and C. E. FORD: Cellular Traffic of the Thymus: Experiments with Chromosome Markers. I. Evidence That the Thymus Plays an Instructional Part, *Nature* (*London*), **201:**884 (1964).

HARRIS, J. E., C. E. FORD, D. W. H. BARNES, and E. P. EVANS: Cellular Traffic of the Thymus: Experiments with Chromosome Markers. II. Evidence from Parabiosis for an Afferent Stream of Cells, *Nature* (*London*), **201:**886 (1964).

HIROWAKA, K.: Electron Microscopic Observation of the Human Thymus of the Fetus and the Newborn, *Acta Pathol. Jap.,* **19:**1–13 (1969).

HWANG, W. S., T. Y. HO, S. C. LUK, and G. T. SIMON: Ultrastructure of the Rat Thymus. A Transmission, Scanning Electron Microscope, and Morphometric Study, *Lab. Invest.,* **31:**473–487 (1974).

ISHIZAKA, T., H. OKUDAIRA, L. E. MAUSER, and K. ISHIZAKA: Development of Rat Mast Cells in vitro. I. Differentiation of Mast Cells from Thymus Cells, *J. Immunol.,* **116:**747–754 (1976).

JANKOVIC, B., B. H. WAKSMAN, and B. G. ARNASON: Role of the Thymus in Immune Reactions in Rats. I. The Immunologic Response to Bovine Serum Albumin (Antibody Formation, Arthus Reactivity and Delayed Hypersensitivity) in Rats Thymectomized or Splenectomized at Various Times after Birth, *J. Exp. Med.,* **116:**159 (1962).

JOLLY, J.: La Bourse de Fabricus et les organes lympho-èpithèliaux, *Arch. Anat. Microbiol,* **16:**363 (1915).

KINDRED, J. E.: A Quantitative Study of the Hematopoietic Organs of Young Albino Rats, *Am. J. Anat.,* **67:**99 (1940).

KOHNEN, P., and L. WEISS: An Electron Microscopic Study of Thymic Corpuscles in the Guinea Pig and the Mouse, *Anat. Rec.,* **148:**29 (1964).

KOSTOWIECKI, M.: Development of the So-called Double-walled Blood Vessels of the Thymus, *Z. Miknosk Anat. Forsch.,* **77:**401–431 (1967).

LEVEY, R. H., N. TRAININ, and L. W. LAW: Evidence for Function of Thymic Tissue in Diffusion Chambers Implanted in Neonatally Thymectomized Mice, *J. Natl. Cancer Inst.,* **31:**199 (1963).

LEVINE, G. D., J. ROSAI, R. M. BEARMN, and A. POLLIACK: The Fine Structure of Thymoma, with Emphasis on its Differential Diagnosis. A Study of 10 Cases, *Am. J. Path.,* **81:**49–86 (1975).

LINNA, J., and J. STILLSTROM: Migration of Cells from the Thymus to the Spleen in Young Guinea Pigs, *Acta Path. Microbiol. Scand.,* **68:**465 (1966).

MANDEL, T.: Ultrastructure of Epithelial Cells in the Cortex of Guinea Pig Thymus, *Z. Zellforsch. Miknosk. Anat.,* **92:**159–168 (1968).

MANDEL, T.: Ultrastructure of Epithelial Cells in the Medulla of the Guinea Pig Thymus, *Aust. J. Exp. Biol. Med. Sci.,* **46:**755–767 (1968).

MANDEL, T.: Differentiation of Epithelial Cells in the Mouse Thymus, *Z. Zellforsch. Miknosk. Anat.*, **106:**498–515 (1970).

METCALF, D.: The Thymus: Its Role in Immune Responses, Leukaemia Development and Carcinogenesis, in "Recent Results in Cancer Research," no. 5, Springer-Verlag OHG, Berlin, 1966.

MILLER, J. F. A. P.: Effect of Neonatal Thymectomy on the Immunological Responsiveness of the Mouse, *Proc. R. Soc. Lond. [Biol.]*, **156:**415 (1962).

MILLER, J. F. A. P., A. H. E. MARSHALL, and R. G. WHITE: The Immunological Significance of the Thymus, *Adv. Immunol.*, **2:**111 (1962).

MOORE, M. A. S., and J. J. T. OWEN: Experimental Studies on the Development of the Bursa of Fabricius, *Dev. Biol.*, **14:**40 (1966).

MOORE, M. A. S., and J. J. T. OWEN: Experimental Studies on the Development of the Thymus, *J. Exp. Med.*, **126:**715–733 (1967).

OSOBA, D., and J. F. A. P. MILLER: The Lymphoid Tissues and Immune Responses of Neonatally Thymectomized Mice Bearing Thymic Tissues in Millipore Diffusion Chambers, *J. Exp. Med.*, **119:**177 (1964).

PARROTT, D. M. V., M. A. B. DE SOUSA, and J. EAST: Thymus-dependent Areas in the Lymphoid Areas of Neonatally Thymectomized Mice, *J. Exp. Med.*, **123:**191 (1966).

PEREIRA, G., and Y. CLERMONT: Distribution of Cell Web-containing Epithelial Reticular Cells in the Rat Thymus, *Anat. Rec.*, **169:**613–626 (1971).

RAVIOLA, E., and M. J. KARNOVSKY: Evidence for a Blood-Thymus Barrier Using Electron-opaque Tracers, *J. Exp. Med.*, **136:**466–498 (1972).

ROSAI, J., and G. D. LEVINE: "Tumors of the Thymus," second series, "Atlas of Tumor Pathology," A. F. I. P., Washington, D.C., (1975).

SAINTE-MARIE, G., and C. P. LEBLOND: Thymus-cell Population Dynamics, in R. A. Good and A. E. Gabrielsen (eds.), "The Thymus in Immunobiology," p. 207, Paul B. Hoeber, Inc., New York, 1964.

SAINTE-MARIE, G., and F. S. PENG: Emigration of Thymocytes from the Thymus. A Review and Study of the Problem, *Rev. Can. Biol.*, **30:**51–78 (1971).

TAKATSU, K., and K. ISHIZAKA: Reagenic Antibody Formation in the Mouse: VIII Depression of the On-going IgE Antibody Formation by Suppressor T-cells, *J. Immunol.*, **117:**1211–1218 (1976).

TORO, I., and I. OLAH: Penetration of Thymocytes into the Blood Circulation, *J. Ultrast. Res.*, **17:**439–451 (1967).

TRAINEN, N., and M. SMALL: Thymic Humoral Factors, *Contemporary Topics in Immunobiology*, **2:**321 (1973).

VAN HAELST, U. J. G.: Light and Electron Microscopic Study of the Normal and Pathological Thymus of the Rat. I. The Normal Thymus, *Z. Zellforsch. Miknosk. Anat.*, **77:**534–553 (1967).

VAN HAELST, U. J. G.: Light and Electron Microscopic Study of the Normal and Pathological Thymus of the Rat. III. A Mesenchymal Histiocytic Type of Cell, *Z. Zellforsch. Miknosk. Anat.*, **99:**198–209 (1969).

WAKSMAN, B. G., B. G. ARNASON, and B. D. JANKOVIC: Role of the Thymus in Immune Reactions in Rats. III. Changes in the Lymphoid Organs of Thymectomized Rats, *J. Exp. Med.*, **116:**187 (1962).

WEISS, L.: Electron Microscopic Observations on the Vascular Barrier in the Cortex of the Thymus of the Mouse, *Anat. Rec.*, **145:**413–437 (1963).

WEISS, L.: "The Cells and Tissues of the Immune System," Prentice-Hall, Inc., Englewood Cliffs, N.J., 1972.

WEISSMAN, I. L.: Thymus Cell Migration, *J. Exp. Med.*, **126:**291 (1967).

WOLSTENHOLME, G. E. W., and R. PORTER (eds.): "The Thymus: Experimental and Clinical Studies," A Ciba Foundation Symposium, Little, Brown and Company, Boston, 1966.

Lymphatic Vessels Lymph and Nodes

14

LEON WEISS

LYMPHATIC VESSELS

Lymphatic vessels make up a network of channels which originate in connective tissue spaces as anastomosing capillaries. The capillaries flow into larger collecting vessels, and the largest and most proximal lymphatic vessels empty into systemic veins in the base of the neck. Like blood vessels, lymphatic vessels are a system of endothelial-lined tubes of varying diameter which carry cellular elements suspended in a fluid intercellular substance. Unlike blood vessels, they do not form a continuous circular system but originate in the connective tissue spaces and carry their contents, called *lymph,* in only one direction, toward the base of the neck. The major function of lymphatic vessels is to recover fluids that escape into the connective tissue spaces from blood capillaries and venules and return them to the blood. In amphibians the lymphatic wall is thickened in certain places by muscle to form lymph hearts which help to propel lymph. In mammals, dense collections of lymphocytes develop as *lymph nodes,* often in sites corresponding to lymph hearts. The propulsive function is lost and lymph now percolates through the lymph nodes, as it moves toward the veins. Lymph nodes filter the lymph, add lymphocytes to the efferent lymph, and produce antibodies.

Lymphatic vessels from all the body except the right side of the head, neck, and thorax drain into the *thoracic duct,* the main lymphatic vessel of the body, which empties into the left *innominate vein.* Lymphatic vessels draining the upper right portion of the body form several trunks which separately enter the great veins at the right side of the base of the neck, or these trunks may join the *right lymphatic duct.*

DISTRIBUTION

Lymphatic capillaries are most numerous in the connective tissues beneath body surfaces. The skin; the mucous membranes of the gastrointestinal, respiratory, and genitourinary tracts; and subserous tissues are rich in lymphatics. Beneath the skin and mucous membranes, lymphatic capillaries are often arranged in superficial and deep plexuses (Figs. 14-1 to 14-3), each of which is more deeply placed than blood capillaries. Large areas in the body, however, are not supplied with lymphatics. The central nervous system contains none. The spleen has lymphatic vessels in its capsule, trabeculae, and white pulp, but not in red pulp. The bone marrow contains no lymphatic vessels. Striated muscle may contain lymphatic vessels only in the perimysium. The structures within the globus oculi are without lymphatic drainage. Within the liver, lymphatic capillaries reach only into the perilobular spaces and do not extend into the liver lobule. In the liver, spleen, and bone marrow, those loci supplied by venous sinusoids lack lymphatics: the sinusoids subserve lymphatic functions.

STRUCTURE

Lymphatic capillaries may reach up to 100 μm in diameter. Their walls are made of flattened endothelial cells (Figs. 14-4 to 14-6). The endothelial cells are attached to one another along their perimeter by zonulae adherentes. The contiguous cells may typically overlap in flaplike fashion. Fine *anchoring filaments* run from perivascular bundles of collagen and attach to the outer surface of the endothelium. In inflammation, in which the tissue pressure surrounding these vessels may build up considerably with the accumulation of inflammatory fluids, these anchoring filaments pull on the vessel wall like a guy rope on a tent and help keep lymphatic channels open (Fig. 14-6).

FIGURE 14-1 Lymphatic vessels of a dog. Superficial and deep vessels in the wall of the stomach as viewed from the surface. ×30. (From Teichmann.)

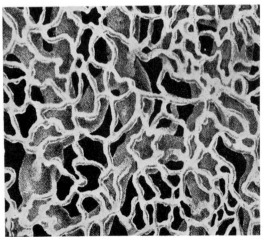

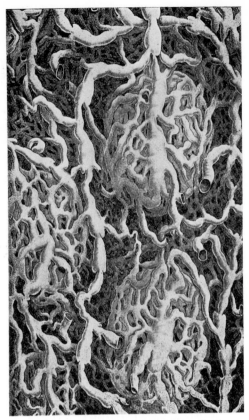

FIGURE 14-2 Lymphatic network in the human appendix as viewed from the surface. Note the enlargement of vessels over the lymphoid nodules and in the valves in the larger vessels. ×40. (From Teichmann.)

Unlike blood capillaries, lymphatic capillaries have no basal laminae or very poorly developed ones. The endothelium forms a complete layer in most sites. In some instances—for example, the *lacteals,* lymphatic capillaries in the villi of the intestine—small apertures are present.

Collecting vessels are slender, thin-walled vessels structurally similar to veins but without clearly defined mural layers. In conformity to the pattern seen in arteries and veins, three coats, or tunics, are present: *tunica intima, tunica media, and tunica adventitia* (Figs. 14-7 and 14-8). Even in the best-developed lymphatic vessel, the *thoracic duct,* however, it is difficult to delineate these layers as clearly as in veins. The fibers of the intima and adventitia run longitudinally; those of the media are circular. Nerves are present in larger vessels (Fig. 14-9). Lymphatic vessels anastomose with one another and tend to travel in

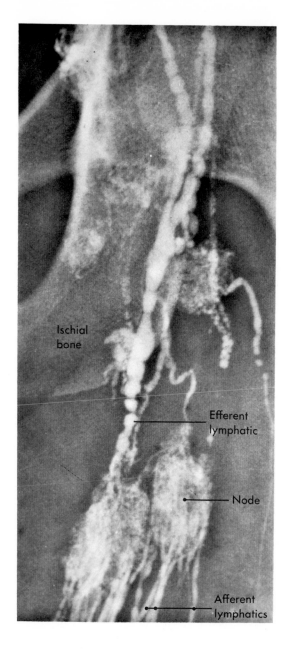

Ischial
bone

Efferent
lymphatic

Node

Afferent
lymphatics

FIGURE 14-3 Lymphogram of human inguinal lymph nodes and lymphatics. A radiopaque dye was injected into the lymphatic vessels in the thigh. It is carried by afferent lymphatic vessels into the draining lymph nodes of the inguinal region. The dye flows through the nodes and enters its efferent lymphatic vessels. The dye will continue centrally through the lymphatic system and eventually flow into the veins at the base of the neck. This lymphogram is an x-ray of the inguinal region some minutes after the injection of dye. Against the background of the soft tissues of the thigh and the pelvic bones. the lymphatic vessels and nodes are visualized. Note the large number of slender afferent lymphatics. The nodes are oval, the dark zones within them representing lymphocytes and other cells around which the dye flows. The efferent lymphatics have a wide caliber. The beaded appearance of the largest vessel is due to the presence of valves.

FIGURE 14-4 Skin of guinea pig. A lymphatic capillary is present in the dermis. A small blood-filled venule is nearby. (From D. Chou and L. Weiss, in L. Weiss, ''Cells and Tissues of the Immune System,'' Prentice-Hall, Inc., Englewood Cliffs, N.J., 1972.)

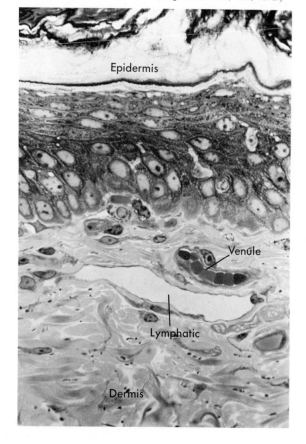

Epidermis

Venule

Lymphatic

Dermis

company with veins. Veins may be girdled in a web of lymphatics. A characteristic of collecting channels is that lymph nodes are inserted along their course in the path of lymph flow. Lymph must pass through the lymph node and is then once again channeled by a lymphatic vessel. It is likely that no lymph reaches the venous system without flowing through at least one node.

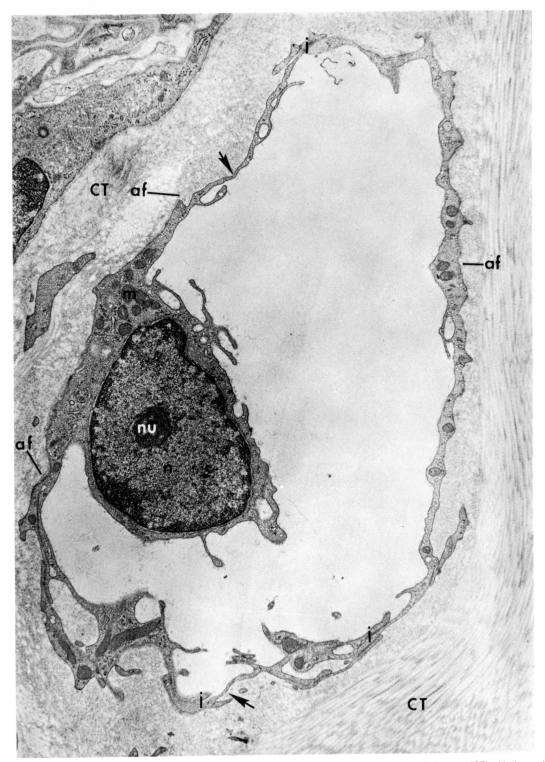

FIGURE 14-5 Cross section of lymphatic capillary. A close association of the surrounding interstitial elements (CT) with the capillary wall is maintained by numerous anchoring filaments (af) which appear as a network of small filaments in this low-power micrograph. The extreme attenuations (arrow) achieved by the endothelium are illustrated in various regions of the capillary wall. The nucleus (N) with its nucleolus (nu) protrudes into the lumen, and several intercellular junctions (j) are observed. Mitochondria (m) occur in the perinuclear regions and also throughout the thin cytoplasmic rim of the endothelial wall; ×11,000. (From the work of L. Leak and J. Burke.)

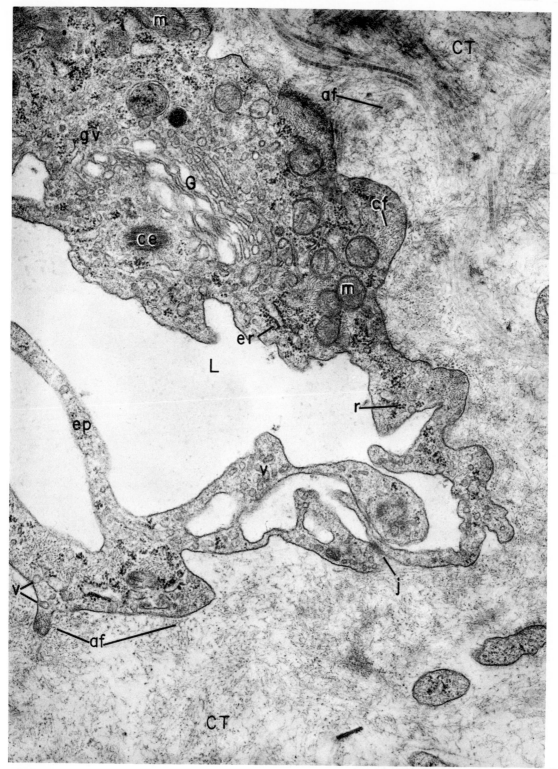

FIGURE 14-6 Lymphatic capillary. In this electron micrograph, the wall of a lymphatic capillary lies in its connective tissue bed. The lymphatic endothelium contains mitochondria (m), a Golgi complex (G), Golgi vesicles (gv), ribosomes (r), rough ER (er), a centriole (ce), luminal endothelial processes (ep), and pinocytotic vesicles (v). Anchoring filaments (af) are present. (From the work of L. Leak and J. Burke.)

The thoracic duct, largest of the lymphatic vessels, is 4 to 6 mm in diameter. Its wall is stouter than those of other lymphatic channels, especially in its most dependent portion. An internal elastic membrane is present. The thoracic duct is supplied by blood vessels and nerves which penetrate its adventitia and media, disposed much as the vasa vasorum and nerves of blood vessels.

Valves are a conspicuous feature of collecting vessels (Figs. 14-3 and 14-7). Valves consist of paired projections which originate from opposite endothelial surfaces and extend into the lumen. The base of a single valve cusp takes up approximately 180° of circumference so that the entire circumference of the vessel wall provides attachment for a valve. Occasional tricuspid valves are found. The cusps are formed as folds of the endothelium. A few connective tissue fibers and even muscle fibers extend between the folded endothelial surfaces of the cusps from the subendothelial tissue. The cusps project into the lumen in the direction of lymph flow and appear to be

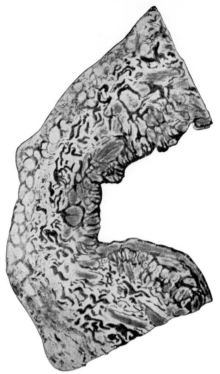

FIGURE 14-8 Portion of the wall from the upper part of the thoracic duct of a human adult. Weigert's resorcinfuchsin and picroindigo carmine. (From the work of Kajava.)

FIGURE 14-7 Lumbar lymphatic trunk of a human adult. A valve is present. Weigert's resorcinfuchsin and picroindigo carmine. (From the work of Kajava.)

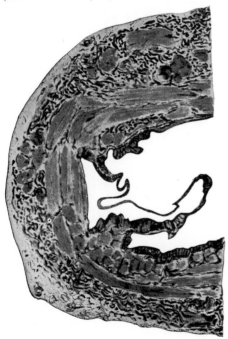

the most importat factor in controlling the direction of flow. A valve in each of the great lymphatic channels at its junction with the systemic veins prevents the gurgitation of blood into the lymphatic system. Valves are also responsible for the beaded appearance of lymphatic vessels, since the vessel is relatively constricted at the attachment of the base of the valve and dilated beyond.

ORIGIN AND REPAIR

Lymphatic channels appear in the human embryo at the age of 6 weeks. They originate independently of veins, connecting to them secondarily (Fig. 14-10).

After being damaged, lymphatic capillaries can regenerate by proliferation of endothelium of the remaining viable lymphatics. The process is similar to but slower than that of blood capillaries. Visualizing lymphatics by intradermal injection of dyestuffs, McMaster observed the regeneration of lymphatics across an incision in the skin of the rabbit in 7 to 10 days (Fig. 14-11).

The primary function of the lymphatic vessels is the return to the blood of material that has escaped the blood. The walls of blood capillaries and venules are semipermeable membranes which permit the diffusion of small-molecular-weight materials through their walls and retain larger molecules (proteins, certain fatty complexes, etc.) and the cellular elements of the blood (see Chap. 9). A considerable amount of plasma protein does escape blood vessels, however.

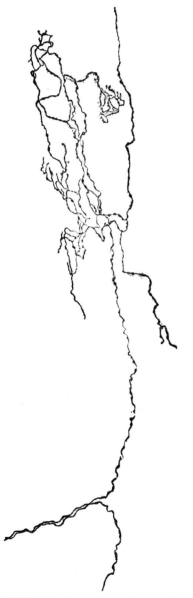

FIGURE 14-9 Nerve fibers in the adventitia of the thoracic duct of a dog. Methylene blue. (From the work of Kytmanof.)

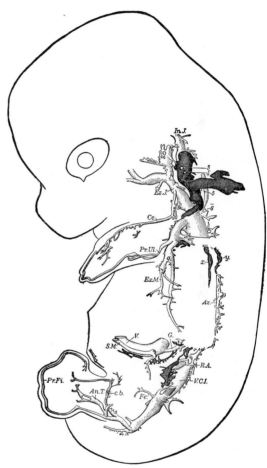

FIGURE 14-10 Lymphatic vessels and veins in a rabbit of 14 days, 18 h, 14.5 mm. The lymphatics are heavily shaded; x, a vessel along the left vagus nerve; y, along the aorta. The large jugular lymph sac is in contact with the internal jugular vein. In J, it passes to the junction of the external jugular (Ex J) and subclavian veins, the latter being formed by the union of the primitive ulnar (Pr Ul) and external mammary veins (Ex M). The mesenteric sac is in front of the vena cava inferior (VCI) and below the renal anastomosis (RA). Other veins include Az, azygos; V, vitelline; G, gastric; SM, superior mesenteric; etc. The figures indicate the position of the corresponding cervical nerves. ×11.5. (Lewis.)

This protein bathes the connective tissues and represents a normal, essential exchange between blood and the connective tissues. At least a part of this protein-rich fluid is absorbed into lymphatic capillaries and returned to the blood. The importance of the conservation of plasma protein is shown by the following case report from Crandall, Barker, and Graham (1943).

A 30-year-old woman was shot in the left side of the neck, 1 hour before admission to the hospital. The left internal jugular vein was ligated 2 days after admission. During the operation straw-colored fluid steadily welled up in the wound so that the skin was not closed. After this operation the dressings were rapidly saturated with this fluid and, for the next 6 weeks, a ceaseless leakage of what was unquestionably thoracic duct lymph continued. The patient at once took the regular hospital diet and, after she had eaten, the leaking fluid became milky. But she lost weight at the rate of 5 lb a week, and her plasma protein fell to 3.5 gm per 100 ml in just a month. A diet high in protein brought this to 4.6 gm per 100 ml in 13 days, but weight loss continued. Accordingly, in a second operation the thoracic duct was ligated and the wound closed. For 2 weeks after this ligation, the patient had cramps after eating but she gained 16 lb in a month and was discharged free of complaints. The concentration of protein in the lymph ranged from 3.19 to 5.28 gm per 100 ml.

The movement of plasma protein out of blood vessels into the surrounding connective tissues and back into blood by way of lymphatics should be regarded as an important physiological process and not as leakage due to defective vessels. This is the means by which hormones, antibodies, enzymes and other macromolecules interact with the cells and intercellular matrix of the body.

Lymphatic vessels absorb fat, especially neutral fat, from the intestine. The patient reported in the above case history was given olive oil stained with Sudan IV. Approximately 1-1/2 hr after the ingestion of the labeled olive oil, the dye appeared in the thoracic duct lymph.

In the resting state, probably 95 percent of the volume of thoracic duct lymph comes from the liver and intestine. The greater portion of protein in thoracic duct lymph originates in the liver.

FACTORS CONTROLLING ABSORPTION INTO LYMPHATIC CAPILLARIES

The permeability of lymphatic vessels increases greatly under certain mild conditions. Pressure sufficient to obstruct the flow of lymph results in an increase in permeability before visible dilation of the lymphatic. Stroking with a blunt wire or scratching the skin without breaking the epidermis causes an immediate great increase in lymphatic permeability. Warming the ears of mice to 43°C increases permeability. Similar reactions have been observed in the lymphatics in the skin of human beings. Histamine causes an increase in lymphatic permeability. Thus, the permeability of lymphatic endothelium may be greatly enhanced by phenomena which occur normally or, at most, represent but a slight departure from the normal. Such increased permeability may commonly permit the en-

FIGURE 14-11 Successive stages in the growth of a lymphatic vessel (lym) in the tail of a tadpole (*Rana palustris*). bv, blood vessel; n, nucleus of the lymphatic vessel. ×135. (From the work of E. Clark.)

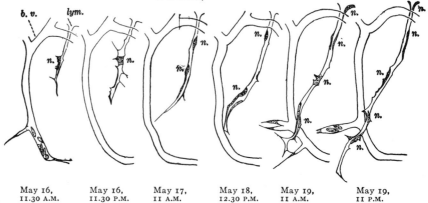

May 16, 11.30 A.M.	May 16, 11.30 P.M.	May 17, 11 A.M.	May 18, 12.30 P.M.	May 19, 11 A.M.	May 19, 11 P.M.

trance of large-sized materials into lymphatic capillaries.

Pinocytotic vesicles appear active in the transport of particles across the lymphatic endothelium. Cells in passage appear to pass between endothelial cells and not through them.

MOVEMENT OF LYMPH

Although larger lymphatic vessels respond to certain drugs, such powerful vasoconstrictor agents as epinephrine or pituitrin probably do not affect the caliber of lymphatic capillaries. Lymphatic capillaries are highly elastic structures, and have been distended by one-third without rupture. Coordinated contraction of the smooth muscle of the lymphatic wall produces propulsive movements.

Remitting compression of lymphatic vessels by

surrounding structures (particularly muscles and pulsating blood vessels), respiratory movements, propulsive actions of the lymphatic walls, and the force of gravity (in the lymphatics, above termination of the thoracic duct) are the major forces promoting lymph flow. The direction of flow is controlled primarily by lymphatic valves.

The rate of lymph flow varies considerably. Trypan blue injected into the hind foot of a dog reaches thoracic duct lymph in seconds.

The volume of lymph poured into the bloodstream is considerable. In a resting human patient, the rate of lymph flow from the thoracic duct averages 0.93 ml per min or 1.38 ml per kg per h (range 3.9 to 0.38). Flow was increased by the ingestion of food or water or by abdominal massage.

LYMPH NODES

Lymph nodes are encapsulated structures ranging in size from a few millimeters to more than a centimeter in their largest dimension, and generally ovoid in shape (Figs. 14-2, 14-3, and 14-12 to 14-14). They are present in the path of collecting lymphatic vessels, and through them lymph flows toward the junctions of lymphatics and veins. Lymph nodes attain their fullest development in mammals. In birds they occur in a rudimentary form, consisting of loosely organized lymphoid tissue lying alongside rather than across the lymph stream. In fishes, amphibians, and reptiles there are lymph hearts but no lymph nodes. In mammals, lymph hearts appear transiently in the embryo but disappear with the development of nodes.

The bases of the extremities, the neck, retroperitoneal areas in the pelvis and abdomen, and the mediastinum are sites especially rich in nodes.

STRUCTURE

A lymph node consists of capsule, reticulum, lymphocytes, other free cells, blood and lymphatic vessels, and nerves (Figs. 14-12 to 14-14).

The *capsule* is composed of dense collagenous connective tissue with some muscle. It presents a broad convex surface and, at one aspect, a deep indentation, the *hilus* or *hilum*. Afferent lymphatic

vessels pierce the convex surface of the capsule and empty into the node. Lymphatic vessels leave at the hilus, and blood vessels enter and leave there. The inner capsular surface is irregular. *Trabeculae* project into the node.

The *reticulum* of a lymph node is a delicate meshwork, occupying the space enclosed by the capsule and trabeculae (Fig. 14-15). Lymphocytes and other free cells of the node lie in this meshwork, and fine blood vessels and lymphatic sinuses are supported by it. The reticulum, as in the spleen, is composed of reticular fibers and reticular cells. The reticular cells are large, branched fibroblastic elements which form a meshwork, the *cellular reticulum*. They evidently elaborate the reticular fibers which lie upon their surface and form a branching fibrilar meshwork: the *fibrous reticulum*. The proportion of filaments to ground substance in reticular fibers varies from place to place in the node. The fibrous reticulum accounts for the argyrophilia of the reticulum and its capacity to stain in the PAS reaction.

Lymphocytes are the most conspicuous of the free cells lying within the reticular meshwork. In the peripheral parts of a node they are tightly packed, forming a blanket of cells and thereby creating the *cortex* of the node. Central to the cortex and extending to the hilus is the *medulla*, where lymphocytes and

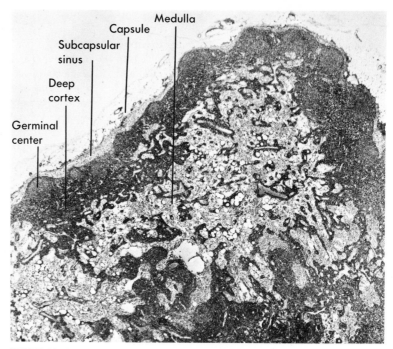

Germinal
center

Deep
cortex

Subcapsular
sinus

Capsule

Medulla

FIGURE 14-12 Lymph node of a human being. Giemsa stain. ×30.

FIGURE 14-13 Lymph node injected with india ink. The sinus system is well outlined. ×10.

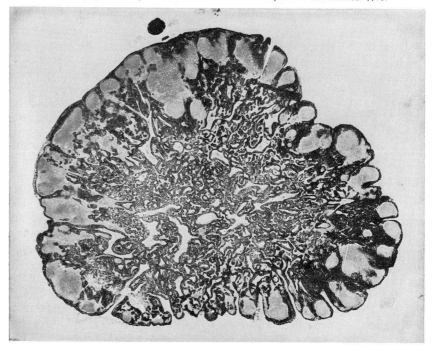

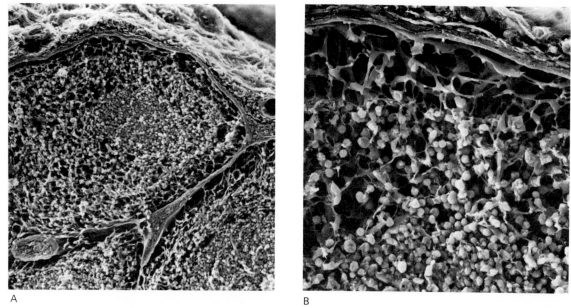

A   B

FIGURE 14-14 A. Popliteal lymph node; dog; scanning electron micrograph of cut surface of cortex. The capsule is prominent, and trabeculae extend from it into the node. Both the subcapsular sinus and the radial sinuses, which run along the trabeculae, are criss-crossed by the processes of reticular cells and reticular fibers. A germinal center, consisting of compactly organized cells, lies within a lymphatic nodule. ×111. B. A higher magnification showing details of capsule, subcapsular sinus, mantle zone of secondary lymphatic nodule and germinal center. ×370. (From S. Irino, T. Ono, K. Hiraki and T. Murakami, *Blood and Vessel,* **5:**595, 1974, in Japanese.)

FIGURE 14-15 A. Popliteal lymph node; dog; scanning electron micrograph of cut surface of medulla. Trabeculae lie in the parenchyma, surrounded by lymphatic sinuses whose lumen is crisscrossed by a reticular meshwork. Medullary cords are also present. ×110. B. A higher magnification showing a cell-packed medullary cord surrounded by a lymphatic sinus. ×358. (From S. Irino, T. Ono, K. Hiraki, and T. Murakami, *Blood and Vessel,* **5:**595, 1974, in Japanese.)

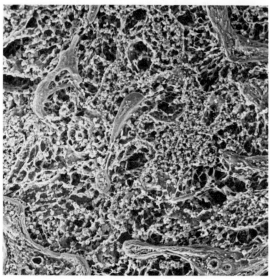

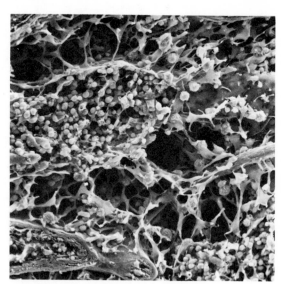

A   B

other cells are grouped in branching cords, the *medullary cords* (Figs. 14-12, 14-14, and 14-16).

Lying within the cortex at its periphery are concentrations of lymphocytes that form nodules which tend to be sperical or ovoid. (The term *follicle* has been used interchangeably with *nodule*.) Nodules may consist of a rather uniform population of tightly packed small lymphocytes. These nodules are termed *primary nodules*. But nodules may contain a central zone consisting of larger lymphoid cells and macrophages, which is relatively lightly stained because the larger cells have more voluminous pale-staining cytoplasm and an euchromatic nucleus which stains less densely than the heterochromatic nuclei of small lymphocytes. This central zone is termed a *germinal center*, and nodules which develop a germinal center are termed *secondary nodules*.

The presence of lymphatic nodules in the superficial cortex of lymph nodes establishes several cortical zones:

1. Internodular cortical tissue

2. A deep part of the cortex between the nodules and medulla. The deep cortex has been termed the *tertiary cortex* (Fig. 14-12).

Most of the cells in the cortex and medulla (except the germinal centers) are small lymphocytes. Those in the primary nodules are B cells, for the most part. Those in the tertiary cortex are predominantly T cells. (See Figs. 14-23A and 14-23B). Germinal cen-

FIGURE 14-16 Lymph node of rat. This axillary lymph node has been perfused arterially by alcion blue and then sectioned and cleared to reveal the vasculature. Arteries (A) exhibit dense staining. Arteriovenous communications (AVC), cortical and medullary capillary areodes (arrows), and the high endothelial post capillary venules (PCV) are shown in the preparation. ×47. (From A. O. Anderson and N. D. Anderson, *Am. J. Path.*, **80**:387, 1975.)

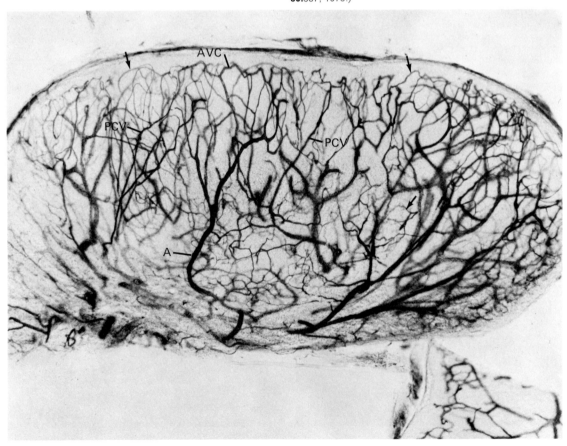

ters represent sites of B-cell differentiation and high-level antibody formation. They contain T cells and macrophages, as well as differentiating B cells. Plasma cell formation is initiated there but few plasma cells are present in germinal centers. As plasma cells mature, they tend to leave the germinal center and move into the medulla.

The medullary cords are rich in plasma cells, macrophages and lymphocytes.

VASCULAR SUPPLY

Lymphatic Vessels

Collecting lymphatic vessels pierce the capsule. They are afferent vessels carrying lymph from the connective tissue spaces or from a more peripheral lymph node. They empty into a large *subcapsular sinus,* which lies directly beneath the capsule and is coextensive with it. *Cortical sinuses* run radially from the subcapsular sinus, passing between cortical lymphocytes, often along trabeculae. These become *medullary sinuses* as they pass between the medullary cords and converge toward the hilus. There they become confluent with the *efferent lymphatic channels* leaving the node (Fig. 14-13).

The sinuses within a node are lined by reticular cells, which provide a rather irregular surface. Indeed, processes of these cells crisscross the lumen, undoubtedly causing retardation and turbulence in lymph flow.

Blood Vessels

Blood vessels enter the node at the hilus. Arterioles reach the cortex through trabeculae and break up into a rich capillary plexus. These vessels group into venules, tributaries of veins which run from cortex to medulla and then leave the node via the hilus. *Postcapillary venules* lie in the paranodular and tertiary cortex. These are distinguished by a high endothelium, cuboidal or even columnar. The wall of these vessels is often infiltrated with small lymphocytes (Figs. 14-13 and 14-16 to 14-18). As shown by Gowans, Marchesi, and Knight, using radioactively labeled cells and autoradiography, these lymphocytes pass from the blood into the parenchyma of the node. They pass between endothelial cells deeply indenting their lateral walls as they cross the endothelium. These vessels represent a major pathway through which small lymphocytes, both T cells and B cells, enter a node (Figs. 14-18 to 14-22). A few small blood vessels enter the node from the convex surface of the capsule. Some

unmyelinated nerves enter the node at the hilus. They run with blood vessels and are probably vasomotor.

Other Lymphatic Tissue

In addition to such discretely organized tissue as lymph nodes and spleen, other lymphatic tissue exists; the wall of the alimentary tract is infiltrated with it. Some tissue, such as Peyer's patches in the lamina propria of the small intestine and the tonsils in the pharynx, is well demarcated (Fig. 14-19), whereas in the appendix and, indeed, the remainder of the gut, lymphatic tissue infiltrates the lamina propria and extends into other layers without clear limits. The respiratory and urinary tracts are often less markedly infiltrated.

The lymphatic tissue lying beneath the epithelia of the gut, respiratory, urinary, and other tracts works in conjunction with the epithelia to produce a distinctive dimeric antibody, immunoglobulin A (IgA), or secretory immunoglobulin, which is secreted into the lumen that the epithelium faces on. (See discussion in Chap. 10 on Lymphocytes and Immunology.)

Lymphocytes, it will be remembered, are migratory cells. They may enter virtually any site and with appropriate stimulation set up loci of lymphatic tissue.

DEVELOPMENT AND DECLINE OF LYMPH NODES

Lymph nodes appear in the human embryo during the third month of life (Figs. 14-24 and 14-25) along the course of lymphatic channels. At sites of lymph node development lymphatic vessels display a richly plexiform character and are termed *lymphatic sacs.* Lymphocytes aggregate about the network of vessels. The complete development of lymph nodes is not realized until some weeks postpartum, for not until this time do cortex and medulla clearly differentiate and germinal centers appear.

Lymphatic tissue undergoes decline or involution with age. The thymus begins a dramatic involution at about the time of puberty; the aging of lymph nodes and spleen is more gradual and the changes are subtle.

Regression in lymph nodes begins shortly after puberty, the period during which they reach their maximal development. Hellman found that the lymph node mass of rabbits decreased in size after puberty but that certain nodes underwent a transient secondary growth period in adulthood. In old rabbits lymph

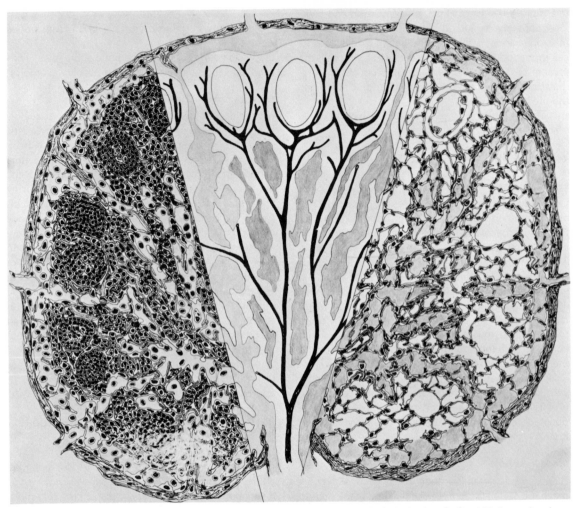

FIGURE 14-17 Three aspects of the structure of a lymph node are presented in this schematic drawing. On the right, the meshwork fabricated of reticular cells and fibers is depicted, the reticular cells in nucleated outline and the fibers in stipple. The subcapsular sinus and the radial sinuses are shaded. Afferent lymphatics penetrate the capsule, emptying into the subcapsular sinus. This sinus is coextensive with the capsule and is crisscrossed by reticular fibers. Radial sinuses, also crisscrossed by the reticulum, run from the subcapsular sinus toward the hilus, where they converge into large efferent vessels (see Figs. 14-2 and 14-3). The reticular meshwork is specialized to form the fixed elements or the scaffolding of the lymphatic nodules, the perinodular cortex, the tertiary cortex, and the medullary cords. In the central panel, the distribution of veins is shown against the outline of cortex, medulla, and lymphatic sinuses (closely drawn after the work and illustrations of Guy Sainte-Marie). The postcapillary venules and the terminal twigs originate about the cortical lymphatic nodules, as well as deep to the nodules. In the third panel, on the left, the reticulum loaded with lymphocytes and other free cells is drawn. The reticular meshwork becomes masked by the crowds of lymphocytes. The endothelium of the sinuses is incomplete on that aspect of the sinuses which abut masses of lymphatic tissue. (From L. Weiss, ''The Cells and Tissues of the Immune System,'' Prentice-Hall, Inc., Englewood Cliffs, N.J., 1972.)

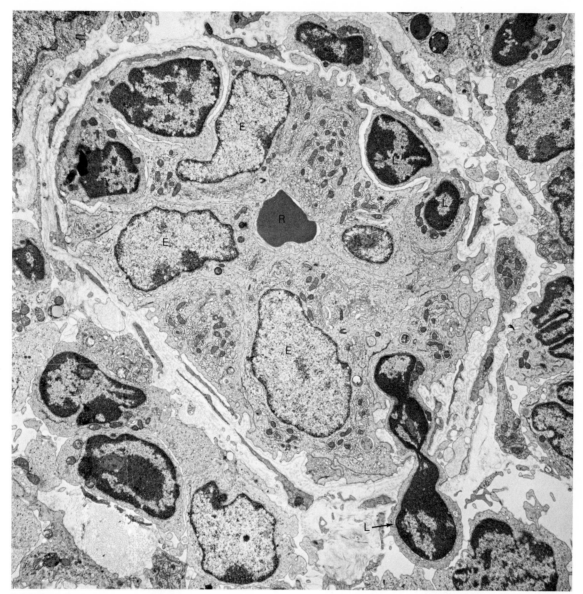

FIGURE 14-18 Postcapillary venules, mouse lymph node. The vessel has a high endothelium containing lightly euchromatic nuclei (E). The lumen is small and contains an erythrocyte (R). The wall of the venule is infiltrated by a number of lymphocytes whose nuclei are heterochromatic and thus dense (L). Note that one lymphocyte, its protoplasm beaded, appears emerging from the venule and entering the perivascular lymphatic cortex (L→). ×1200. (From the work of G. D. Levine.)

FIGURE 14-19 A. Postcapillary venule; rat lymph node; scanning electron micrograph. Many lymphocytes lie upon the endothelium, presumably about to penetrate between endothelial cells and through the wall of the venule, into the surrounding cortex. Preparatory to crossing the wall, the lymphocytes appear to develop microvilli. ×563. B. At higher magnification, a lymphocyte is seen lying upon the endothelium. The lymphocyte's microvilli appear to probe the endothelial surface. ×1760. (From the work of A. O. Anderson and N. D. Anderson, *Immunology,* in press.)

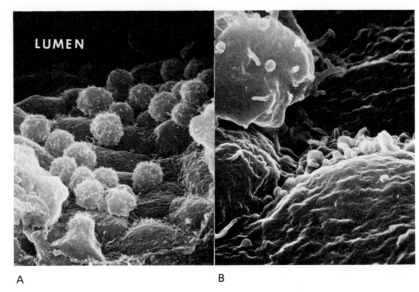

A

B

FIGURE 14-20 Postcapillary venule in a mesenteric lymph node 15 min after the initiation of a transfusion. Labeled cells have penetrated the endothelium of the vessel but have not yet migrated into the node. L, lumen of the vessel. Exposure, 28 days. Methyl green–pyronin stain. ×1200. (J. L. Gowans and E. J. Knight, *Proc. R. Soc. Lond.* [*Biol.*], **159:**257, 1964.)

FIGURE 14-21 Autoradiographs of thoracic duct cells which had been incubated in vitro with tritiated adenosine for 1 h at 37°C. Exposure, 14 days. Leishman stain. ×2250. (From J. L. Gowans and E. J. Knight, *Proc. R. Soc. Lond.* [*Biol.*], **159:**257, 1964.)

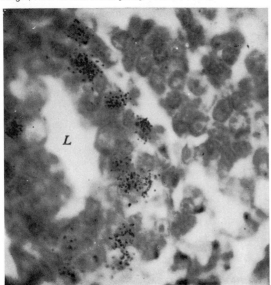

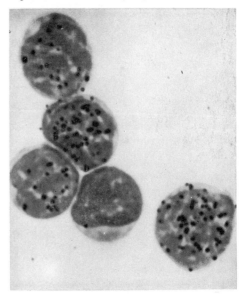

nodes were reduced to approximately one-half size. Lymph nodes, however, retain the capacity to enlarge in response to appropriate stimuli throughout life. The histologic picture in aging lymph nodes consists of absence of germinal centers and reduction in the numbers of lymphocytes with thinning of cortex and medullary cords. Fat appears under the capsule, especially at the hilus and in the septa. In humans, even moderate degrees of fatty or connective tissue replacement of lymphatic tissue are seen only in advanced age. Indeed, Krumbhaar states that most nodes go on to 60 years with but little atrophy.

FIGURE 14-22 Postcapillary lymph node, artist's reconstruction. The high endothelium and the infiltration of the wall by lymphocytes are shown. (From the work of A. O. Anderson and N. D. Anderson.)

FUNCTIONS OF LYMPH NODES

Filtration and Phagocytosis

Lymph nodes constitute extensive filtration beds which prevent the systemic distribution of infectious and other agents. Thus popliteal lymph nodes receive and filter lymph from the sole of the foot and dorsum of the leg. The reticular meshwork crisscrossing the sinuses and the parenchyma constitutes a mechanical filter. Flow in these large vascular spaces is quite slow with many eddies. Macrophages may abound in these sinuses and the conditions of flow favor phagocytosis of particulate materials carried into the node. As mac-

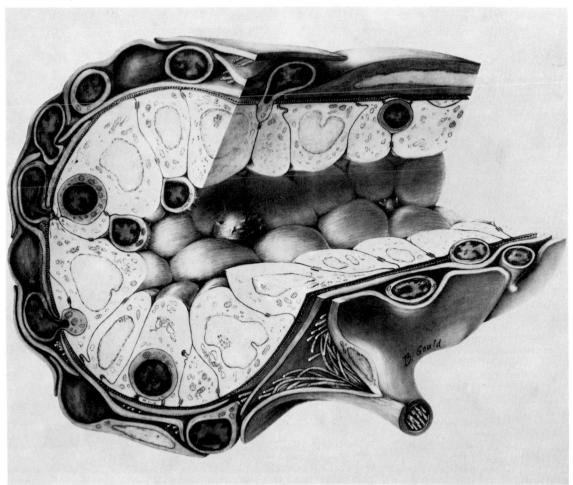

rophages increase in volume consequent to phagocytosis, their bulk further impedes flow through the node and further enhances phagocytosis. Lymph nodes produce antibodies and other substances which help to immobilize and agglutinate or lyse bacteria and cells, facilitating filtration and phagocytosis. The filtration power of lymph nodes has been demonstrated by

Drinker, Field, and Ward (1934): 5 ml of a serum-broth culture containing 600 million colonies per ml of hemolytic streptococci were perfused at the efferent lymphatic vessels. Cultures of effluent lymph contained 4.5 million colonies per ml, indicating 99 percent filtration.

Thus both mechanically, by the arrangement of reticulum, and biologically, by action of its phagocytes and production of antibodies and other factors, lymph nodes are very effective filters. The efficiency of filtra-

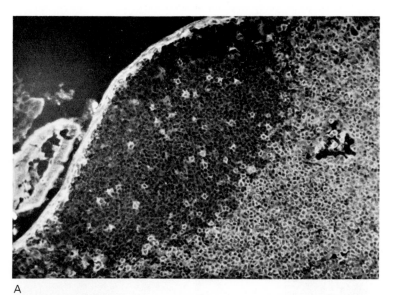

A

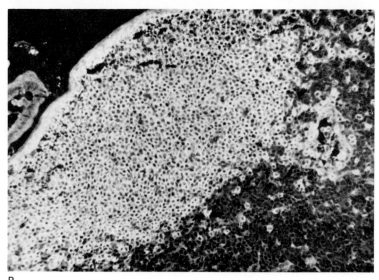

FIGURE 14-23 Lymph node, mouse. Distribution of T and B lymphocytes as revealed by fluorescence immunocytochemistry. The T and B cells are specifically stained in these frozen sections by antibodies to the surface of T and B cells, respectively. The antibody is conjugated to a fluorescent marker, visible by fluorescence microscopy. In Fig. 14-23A, the lymphatic nodules in the cortex are largely unstained, while the deep or tertiary cortex is deeply stained, indicating it as the site of concentration of T lymphocytes. Note that the postcapillary venule (V) is stained. In Fig. 14-23B, the cells of the lymphatic nodules are deeply stained, indicating that B lymphocytes are concentrated there. Note that the postcapillary venule (V) is also stained, as are some cells in the tertiary cortex. This demonstrates B cell traffic from the postcapillary venule toward the lymphatic nodule. (See Fig. 15-28 for distribution of T and B lymphocytes in the spleen.) (From I. L. Weissman, *Trans. Rev.*, **24:**159, 1975.)

B

tion makes lymph nodes vulnerable to disturbances in the regions they drain. If the nodes fail to destroy infectious agents or malignant cells which they concentrate from the regions they drain, the nodes may serve as new foci and facilitate the spread of disease through the body.

THE PRODUCTION AND RECIRCULATION OF LYMPHOCYTES

The lymphocytes within lymph nodes are both circulating lymphocytes and lymphocytes which are produced in the node. The proportion of newly produced lymphocytes to those in the recirculation pool varies from species to species, but recirculating cells in antigenically unstimulated animals are preponderant.

Recirculating lymphocytes are small. They enter the node through its arterial vessels, pass through capillaries, and reach the postcapillary venules. They then pass through these venules and lie in the paranodular cortex, particularly the tertiary or deep cortex

(Figs. 14-17 to 14-19). They remain there for variable periods of time and then migrate to the medulla. They leave the node through efferent lymphatics. Lymphocytes may also enter the node through afferent lymphatics—especially if the node is central, receiving lymphocytes from more peripheral nodes. Transit time through a node is 3 to 5 h in rodents. The recirculating lymphocytes reach the veins at the base of the neck through the system of lymphatic vessels. Once in the bloodstream they circulate and, in time, again reach a lymph node and repeat the cycle. Both T and B cells recirculate. After they cross the wall of the postcapillary venule (Figs. 14-18 through 14-22) and enter the lymph node cortex, they move in different directions: B cells out to the nodules, T cells down to the tertiary cortex and to the internodular cortex. Because the tertiary cortex is depleted of T cells after thymectomy (see Chap. 13), it is characterized as *thymic depend-*

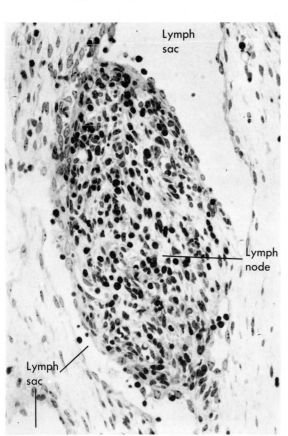

FIGURE 14-24 Lymph node of a human fetus. 57-mm crown-rump length (12 weeks gestational age). Lymph nodes develop in relationship to a plexus of lymphatic vessels, the lymph sacs. The lymph node consists of a loose connective tissue which becomes infiltrated by lymphocytes. At this stage, the ovoid shape of the node, its moderate content of lymphocytes, and its relationship to lymphatic vessels are evident. Toluidine blue. ×250. (From the work of R. P. Bailey.)

ent. Following thoracic duct cannulation with loss of T cells, there is depletion of the tertiary cortex. It is possible, moreover, to demonstrate the distribution of T and B lymphocytes in lymph nodes (Figs. 14-25a and b) and in spleen (Figs. 15-28a and b) by immunofluorescent reagents applied to tissue sections. Gowans and his associates first (1964) traced the pathways of recirculating lymphocytes in the rat by the use of small lymphocytes obtained from the thoracic duct, labeled with tritiated adenosine, and injected intravenously. At different times after the injection of lymphocytes, tissues were fixed and embedded and sectioned and autoradiographs were prepared. Passage of lymphocytes across the postcapillary venule was documented by electron microscopy (Figs. 14-17 to 14-19).

Large lymphocytes do not recirculate. Most injected large lymphocytes migrate from the blood into the wall of the gut and appear to remain there.

Immunologic Functions

The lymph node is an immunologic structure highly specialized in the production of antibodies and in cellular immune responses to antigen coming from the region it drains. Thus antigen introduced into the foot pad elicits an antibody response in a popliteal lymph node. This responsiveness of the lymph node to regional influences complements that of the spleen, which produces antibodies to blood-borne antigen.

That lymphatic tissue produces antibody was shown by McMaster and Hudack (1935), who injected antigen into the ears of rats and recovered antibody from the draining lymph nodes before it could be detected elsewhere. Two antigens were injected, one

FIGURE 14-25 Lymph node, human fetus, 200-mm crown-rump length (22 weeks gestational age). A (left). The node is an oval structure, considerably infiltrated by lymphocytes. The capsule and subcapsular sinus are well defined. Cortex and medulla have not yet differentiated, however. B (right). An enlargement of the boxed area in A. Toluidine blue. ×450. (From the work of R. P. Bailey.)

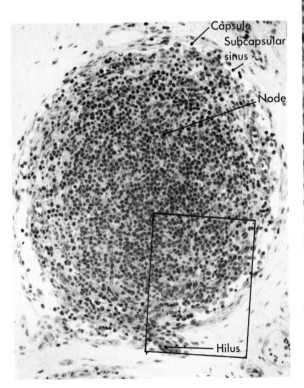

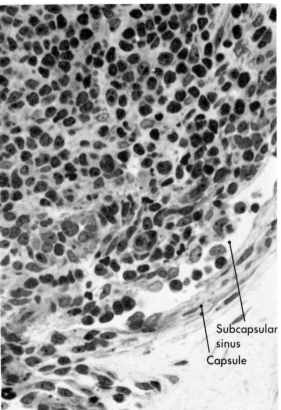

in each ear, and the antibody to each of the antigens was first detected in the homologous node.

On initial administration of antigen, a primary immune response follows which varies with the character of antigen, dose, and route of administration. With particulate antigens, phagocytosis is one of the earliest responses. The antigen is engulfed in the sinuses and in the medullary regions most conspicuously. But rather rapidly, antigen becomes concentrated about the primary nodules at the interface of T- and B-cell zones. Some of the antigen is free, some is phagocytized, and some seems to be held on the surface of large cells—macrophages and perhaps reticular cells. Later, the antigen may penetrate the nodule and after it has disappeared from other sites remain affixed to local macrophages or dendritic reticular cells near and within the nodules. Antigen thus held would appear able to interact with T and B cells as they move and sort out in the cortex of the node. This process would enhance the phenomenon of clonal selection.

Antibody-producing cells appear first in the cortex in small clusters of cells and then they apparently migrate to the medulla, where they tend to accumulate in large numbers within the medullary cords. It is in the cords that the fully differentiated B cells, the plasma cells, accumulate. After the initial cortical response, antibody production is often taken up in germinal centers. As determined histochemically and by assay of isolated portions of lymphatic tissue, antibody production here is intense. A given germinal center appears to produce antibody against only one antigen.

On subsequent exposure to antigen (the secondary response), germinal centers dominate the response. They are large, synthesize antibody very actively, and expand at such a rate as to blur their margins. Over a period of weeks, the cells synthesizing antibody in the germinal center die or are dispersed and the titer of antibody begins to fall.

REFERENCES

ANDERSON, A. O., and N. D. ANDERSON: Studies on the Structure and Permeability of the Microvasculature in Normal Rat Lymph Nodes, *Am. J. Pathol.*, **80:**387 (1975).

CLARK, S.: The Reticulum of Lymph Nodes in Mice Studied with the Electron Microscope, *Am. J. Anat.*, **110:**217 (1962).

COONS, A. H., E. H. LEDUC, and J. M. CONNOLLY: Studies on Antibody Production. I. A Method for the Histochemical Demonstration of Specific Antibody and Its Application to a Study of the Hyperimmune Rabbit, *J. Exp. Med.*, **102:**49 (1955).

CRANDALL, L. A., S. B. BARKER, and D. G. GRAHAM: A Study of the Lymph Flow from a Patient with Thoracic Duct Fistula, *Gastroenterology*, **1:**1040 (1943).

DOWNEY, H.: The Structure and Origin of the Lymph Sinuses of Mammalian Lymph Nodes and Their Relations to Endothelium and Reticulum, *Hematologica (Pavia)*, **3:**31 (1922).

DRINKER, C. K., M. E. FIELD, and H. K. WARD: The Filtering Capacity of Lymph Nodes, *J. Exp. Med.*, **59:**393 (1934).

DRINKER, C. K., G. B. WINSLOCKI, and M. E. FIELD: The Structure of the Sinuses in the Lymph Nodes, *Anat. Rec.*, **56:**261 (1933).

GOWANS, J. L., and E. J. KNIGHT: The Route of Recirculation of Lymphocytes in the Rat, *Proc. R. Soc. Lond.* [*Biol.*] **159:**257 (1964).

GOWANS, J. L., D. MC GREGOR, and D. COWEN: Initiation of Immune Responses by Small Lymphocytes, *Nature (Lond.)*, **196:**651 (1962).

HAN, S.: The Ultrastructure of the Mesenteric Lymph Node of the Rat, *Am. J. Anat.*, **109:**183 (1961).

LEAK, L. V., and J. F. BURKE: Ultrastructural Studies on the Lymphatic Anchoring Filaments, *J. Cell Biol.,* **36:**129 (1968).

LEAK, L. V. and J. F. BURKE: Fine Structure of the Lymphatic Capillary and the Adjoining Connective Tissue Area, *Am. J. Anat.,* **118:**785 (1966).

LEAK, L. V., and J. F. BURKE: Studies on the Permeability of Lymphatic Capillaries during Inflammation, *Anat. Rec.,* **151:**489 (1965).

MARCHESI, V. T., and J. L. GOWANS: The Migration of Lymphocytes through the Endothelium of Venules in Lymph Nodes: an Electron Microscope Study, *Proc. R. Soc. Lond.* [*Biol.*], **159:**283 (1964).

MC MASTER, P. D., and S. HUDACK: The Formation of Agglutinins within Lymph Nodes, *J. Exp. Med.,* **61:**783 (1935).

MOE, R.: Electron Microscopic Appearance of the Parenchyma of Lymph Nodes, *Am. J. Anat.,* **114:**341 (1964).

MOE, R.: Fine Structure of the Reticulum and Sinuses of Lymph Nodes, *Am. J. Anat.,* **112:**311 (1963).

ORTEGA, L., and R. MELLORS: Cellular Sites of Formation of Gamma Globulin, *J. Exp. Med.,* **106:**627 (1957).

PARROTT, D. M. V., M. A. B. DE SOUSA, and J. EAST: Thymic Dependent Areas in the Lymphoid Organs of Neonatally Thymectomized Mice, *J. Exp. Med.,* **123:**191 (1966).

PECK, H. M., and N. L. HOERR: The Effect of Environment Temperature Changes on the Circulation of the Mouse Spleen, *Anat. Rec.,* **109:**479 (1951).

WEISS, L.: ''The Cells and Tissues of the Immune System,'' Prentice-Hall, Inc., Englewood Cliffs, N.J., 1972.

WEISSMAN, I. L.: Development and Distribution of Immunoglobulin-Bearing Cells in Mice, *Trans. Rev.,* **24:**159–176 (1975).

YOFFEY, J., and F. COURTICE: ''Lymphatics, Lymph, and Lymphoid Tissue, Harvard University Press, Cambridge, Mass., 1956.

The
Spleen

LEON WEISS

The human spleen is a highly vascular hematopoietic organ located in the left upper quadrant of the abdomen and weighing approximately 150 g in adults. It receives blood from the splenic artery and drains into the portal venous system. The spleen may be best understood as a discriminatory filter, consisting of specialized vascular spaces through which blood flows. The foundation of its structure and its filtration capacities is a reticular meshwork fashioned of reticular cells and reticular fibers (see discussion under Bone Marrow and Lymph Nodes). There is no element of the blood, cellular or plasmal, which the spleen may not affect. It monitors the red blood cells in the circulation and destroys or modifies imperfect ones. It removes other blood cells when damaged or aged. It sequesters monocytes from the blood and facilitates their transformation into macrophages and holds them as splenic macrophages which act in antibody formation and other splenic functions. It traps T and B cells from the blood and antigen and sorts them into compartments, permitting them to interact with macrophages and antigen in immune responses. It stores as many as a third of the platelets of the body in a ready reserve. In certain species, it can also function as a reservoir for erythrocytes and granulocytes, capable of delivering them rapidly to the blood when needed. The adult spleen is not essential to life. In some abnormal conditions, it may, in fact, eliminate circulating cells with such avidity that it must be removed to save life.

STRUCTURE OF THE SPLEEN

CAPSULE AND TRABECULAE

The spleen in man is enclosed by a capsule of dense, white connective tissue, a few millimeters in thickness. From the internal capsular surface, a rich branching network of trabeculae subdivides the organ into communicating compartments several millimeters in each dimension (Fig. 15-1). The capsule contains relatively little muscle and is therefore incapable of the profound contraction exhibited by the muscular capsule of the spleen in dogs and cats. The capsule is deeply indented at the medial aspect of the organ, the *hilus,* where it is penetrated by blood vessels, lymphatic vessels, and nerves. Arterial vessels branch into the trabeculae and from there enter the *pulp* or parenchyma of the organ. Veins and lymphatics also run in the trabeculae, entering from the pulp.

SPLENIC PULP

The tissue enclosed within the capsule, the splenic pulp, is a reticular connective tissue (Figs. 15-2 to 15-7). Most of the pulp is typically red, owing to the presence of blood, and is designated the *red pulp*. The red pulp is made up almost entirely of two kinds of structure: large, branching, thin-walled blood vessels, *splenic sinuses* (or *sinusoids*), and thin plates or partitions of cellular tissue which lie between the sinuses, *splenic cords*. The red pulp is a site of storage and "tests" the viability of red blood cells. Lying in the splenic pulp, surrounded by red pulp, are clusters of lymphocytes which are grossly visible as gray-white zones. They consititute the *white pulp* of the spleen. The white pulp may assume two formations. One is a cylindrical form, which surrounds the major arterial branches of the splenic pulp as *periarterial lymphatic sheaths*. Within the periarterial lymphatic sheaths may lie spherical or oval clusters of lymphocytes termed *lymphatic nodules*. The white pulp of the spleen is the site of initiation of immune responses. In highly im-munologically active spleens, the white pulp may account for well over half the volume of the spleen. In most instances, however, it occupies perhaps 20 percent or less of the volume. The splenic pulp at the junction of the white pulp and the red pulp is designated the *marginal zone*. It is the site where much of the blood brought into the spleen is released and the processes of filtration and sorting are initiated.

BLOOD FLOW

The pattern of blood flow in the spleen will be outlined as a preliminary to consideration of the structure of white pulp, marginal zone, and red pulp. Blood enters the spleen by way of splenic arteries, passing through the hilus. The splenic artery branches into the trabeculae as *trabecular arteries,* which turn out of the trabeculae and enter the periarterial lymphatic sheaths, where they are known as *central arteries*. As the central artery travels through the periarterial lymphatic sheath, it sends out many branches. Some supply lymphatic nodules within the sheath. Most travel to the periphery of the sheath, however, and terminate in the marginal zone. The central artery runs out into the red pulp and usually terminates in the

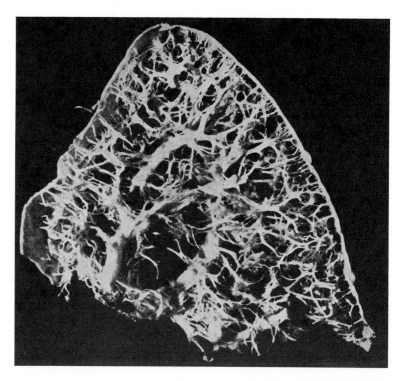

FIGURE 15-1 Human spleen. The trabecular framework and capsule remain after the pulp has been digested away by 1 percent sodium carbonate. ×4. (From the work of Schleicher.)

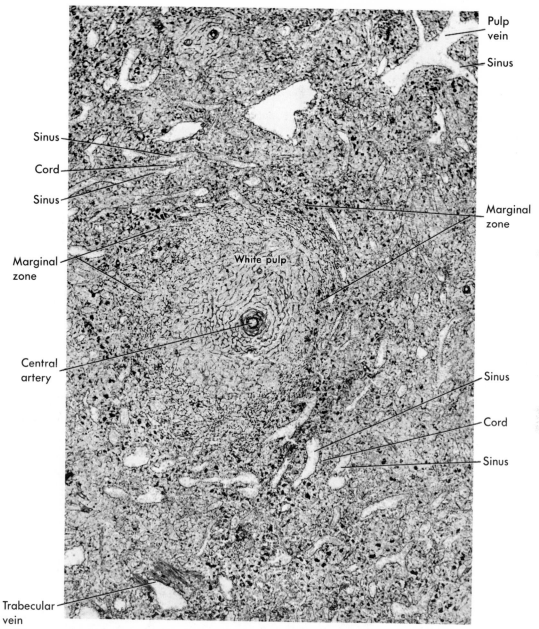

Pulp vein

Sinus

Sinus

Cord

Sinus

Marginal zone

Marginal zone

White pulp

Central artery

Sinus

Cord

Sinus

Trabecular vein

FIGURE 15-2 Spleen of a rat. The extracellular reticulum is stained by the PAS reaction. The white pulp contains a darkly outlined central artery. Note the circumferential pattern of the reticulum of white pulp. A marginal zone surrounds the white pulp and contains a relatively dense meshwork of reticulum and many darkly stained cells. Beyond the white pulp and marginal zone lies the red pulp, accounting for the greater part of the splenic volume. The clear spaces represent splenic sinuses, for the most part, but also pulp veins and trabecular veins. The splenic cords constitute the relatively solid tissue lying between the sinuses. ×225. (From L. Weiss. *J. Anat.,* **93:**465, 1959.)

cords. In the red pulp and in the marginal zone, the blood reaches the splenic sinuses which are tributaries of veins of the pulp. These veins enter the trabeculae as *trabecular veins*. At the hilus, the trabecular veins are continuous with the splenic veins which lie outside the organ. The nature of the vascular connections between the arterial terminations and splenic sinuses, the so-called intermediate circulation of the spleen, is difficult to analyze. Further consideration of blood flow will be deferred until a discussion of the structure of the pulp is presented.

LYMPH FLOW

Lymphatic vessels are associated with a fluid flow through the spleen counter to blood flow. The fluid wave originates at the venular end of the red pulp, sweeps across the red pulp, marginal zone, and white pulp and enters lymphatic vessels which lie in white pulp girdling the proximal portions of the central arteries and in trabeculae (Fig. 15-6).

WHITE PULP

The white pulp of the spleen is a lymphatic tissue consisting of lymphocytes, plasma cells, macrophages,

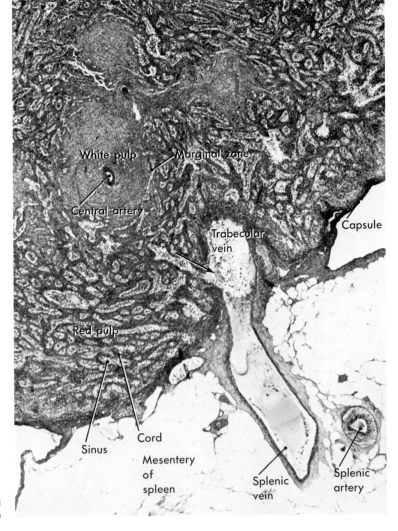

FIGURE 15-3 Spleen of a hedgehog. In this low-power field, the white pulp, red pulp, blood outflow tract, and splenic mesentery are shown. The white pulp, occupying a relatively small volume, surrounds a central artery. The red pulp occupies most of the field. It is made up almost entirely of relatively clear spaces, the splenic sinuses, which form an anastomosing system of venous vessels. The splenic cords, darkly stained tissue lying between the sinuses, consist of a reticular meshwork which contains blood cells and macrophages and receives arterial terminations. Blood is carried out of the spleen through trabecular veins which drain into the splenic vein. Splenic veins leave the spleen at the hilus and enter the splenic mesentery. At the arrow, splenic sinuses empty into a pulp vein which drains into a trabecular vein. The marginal zone lies between white pulp and red pulp. The mesentery contains a branch of the splenic artery which will enter the spleen at the hilus. ×150. (From V. Janout and L. Weiss, *Anat. Rec.*, **172**:197, 1972.)

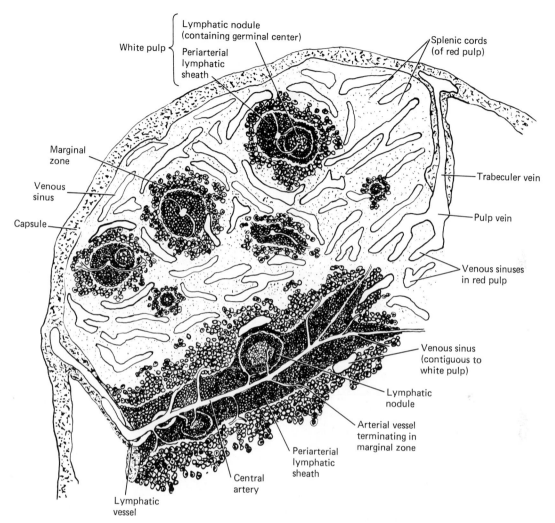

FIGURE 15-4 Schematic view of the organization of the human spleen. The white pulp has two components: periarterial lymphatic sheaths and lymphatic nodules. The latter may be made up of a germinal center and a surrounding mantle zone. The white pulp is surrounded by the marginal zone. The remainder of the tissue depicted is the red pulp, which consists primarily of splenic sinuses separated by splenic cords. The pattern of blood flow is as follows. A trabecular artery enters the white pulp and becomes the central artery. The central artery passes through white pulp and gives rise to many branches. A few end within white pulp; some supply the germinal center and mantle zone of the secondary nodule. Most terminate at the periphery of the white pulp, emptying in or near the marginal zone. A number of arterial vessels emerge from the white pulp, pass into the marginal zone, reach the red pulp, and curve back to empty into the marginal zone. Some arterial branches, in addition to the main stem of the central artery, run into the red pulp. Almost all terminate in the cords. Here, too, variation exists. Some arterial vessels terminate in a cord close against a sinus wall whereas others terminate in the midst of a cord, away from any sinus. Arterial vessels may terminate as capillaries or as somewhat larger vessels. Some arterial vessels may bear sheaths shortly before termination. The sinuses drain into pulp veins which, in turn, drain into trabecular veins. A sinus may abut the white pulp and receive lymphocytes or other free cells which migrate from white pulp across its wall and into its lumen. Efferent lymphatic vessels lie about the proximal portion of the central artery and run out of the spleen through the trabeculae. (From L. Weiss and M. Tavossoli, Sem. in Hemat., **7:**372, 1970). (See text and Figs. 15-26 and 15-27.)

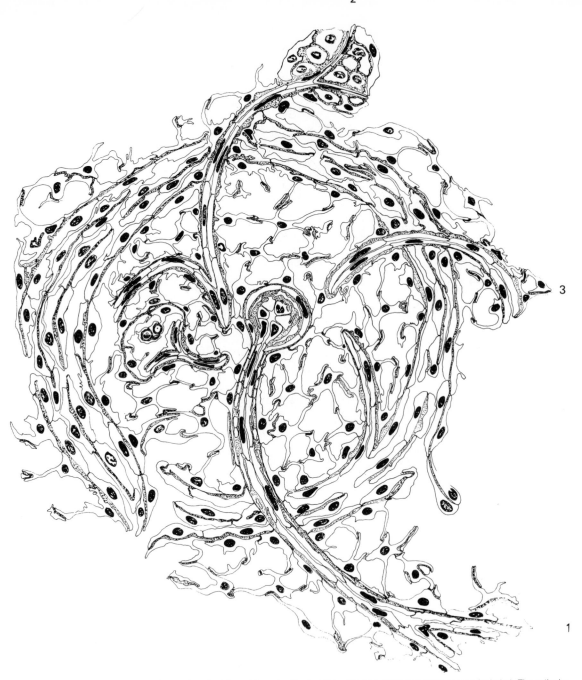

FIGURE 15-5 A sketch of the reticular meshwork of the white pulp. The lymphocytes and other free cells are not included. The reticular cells are indicated as nucleated outlines. The reticular fibers, such as are stained in Fig. 15-2, are stippled. Virtually the entire field is taken by a cross section of the periarterial lymphatic sheath (PALS), in the center of which is the cross section of the central artery. In the vicinity of the central artery the reticular meshwork may not be markedly specialized. Toward its periphery, the reticular meshwork of the PALS is organized in a decidedly circumferential fashion (see Figs. 15-2 and 15-7). To the left of the central artery, the reticular meshwork supports a small lymphatic nodule with several small arterioles playing upon and in it. There are several large branches of the central artery. One branch curves down and to the right, reaching the red pulp where it bifurcates (1). (The relationships of arterial vessels within the red pulp is schematized in Fig. 15-14.) Another large branch travels toward 12 o'clock and terminates in the marginal zones as sheathed capillaries (2). Another vessel arches toward 2 o'clock and opens into the marginal zone by simply terminating (3). Unlike the sheathed capillary, it bears no specialization. (From L. Weiss, "Cells and Tissues of the Immune System," Prentice-Hall, Inc., Englewood Cliffs, N.J., 1972.)

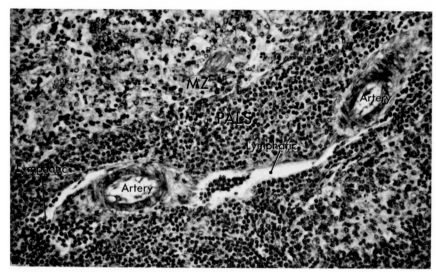

FIGURE 15-6 Spleen of a hedgehog. Lymphatic vessels are shown in this field. They lie within the periarterial lymphatic sheath (PALS) of white pulp in relation to the central artery, two branches of which are shown. The PALS consists of a reticular meshwork obscured by many lymphocytes crowded together. Outside the PALS is the marginal zone (mz) ×950. (From V. Janout and L. Weiss, *Anat. Rec.,* **172:**197, 1972.)

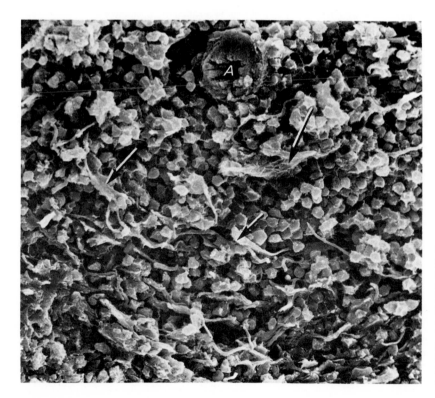

FIGURE 15-7 Periarterial lymphatic sheath; rat spleen; scanning electron micrograph. The central artery (A) is surrounded by reticular cells which tend to follow a circumferential pattern about the central artery (see Figs. 15-2 and 15-5). The small round cells are preponderantly T lymphocytes (see Fig. 15-28). ×2320. (From L. Weiss, *Blood,* **43:**665, 1974.)

and other free cells lying in a reticular meshwork and surrounding the major arterial vessels of the spleen. The white pulp is divisible into *periarterial lymphatic sheaths* and *lymphatic nodules* (Figs. 15-7 to 15-9). The periarterial lymphatic sheaths are of cylindrical form and axially surround the central artery. For this reason the term *central* artery is used. The sheath consists of a reticulum fashioned of reticular cells and fibers. These elements tend to be arranged in circumferential layers about the central artery. The reticulum represents a scaffolding packed with lymphocytes. Lymphocytes are the most numerous of the free cells in these sheaths. They are preponderantly T lymphocytes and most of them are small. Periarterial lymphatic sheaths persist about arterial vessels until the vessels become small arterioles, at which point they are quite attenuated. Lymphatic nodules, spherical or ovoid structures resembling nodules of the cortex of the lymph nodes, lie here and there within the periarterial lymphatic sheath, often at arterial bifurcations. They represent concentrations of B lymphocytes. These nodules, like those of lymph nodes, may contain germinal centers. In a nodule which contains a germinal center, the peripheral zone of small lymphocytes may be termed the *mantle* (Fig. 15-7). The nodules push the central artery aside, forcing it to assume an excentric position in the periarterial lymphatic sheath. The nodules in the human spleen may be several millimeters in diameter and grossly visible on the cut surface of the spleen. They have been termed *malpighian corpuscles*.

There is a marked species variation in the development of the two components of white pulp. In the rabbit and rat, the periarterial lymphatic sheaths are well developed, and the lymphatic nodules, although often present, are not large. In the cat and dog, however, nodules are large and the periarterial lymphatic sheaths are not.

Vascular Supply of White Pulp

The central artery is a medium-sized muscular artery which gives off many branches as it courses through the periarterial lymphatic sheath (Figs. 15-10 and 15-11). The branches tend to run radially, at right angles to the principal stem, toward the periphery of the white pulp. Many go beyond the white pulp and empty into the marginal zone. A moderate number

travel further, reaching the red pulp, and terminate, as described below. For lymph flow see p. 548.

Lymphatic nodules are supplied by two sets of arterioles: one which penetrates to their center; the other which plays on their periphery. Snook has described a distinctive arrangement in human spleen wherein lymphatic nodules of white pulp are supplied by recurrent arteries which curve back from red pulp.

MARGINAL ZONE

The marginal zone consists of an unusually fine meshed spongework made of branched reticular cells associated with reticular fibers. Many arterial vessels open into the reticular meshwork of the marginal zone. They may terminate in a funnel-shaped orifice and often bifurcate just before ending. Venous sinuses regularly come into the marginal zone. Infrequently, a terminating arterial vessel may open directly into such a sinus. The cords of the red pulp are directly continuous with the marginal zone and have a similar structure (see below).

RED PULP

The red pulp is a reticular spongework, or meshwork, supplied by arteries and drained by vascular sinuses (Figs. 15-12 and 15-13). The reticular meshwork is honeycombed by an anastomosing system of sinuses. As a result, the reticular meshwork takes the form of a branching system of cords lying between and complementary to the sinuses. After distributing branches to the white pulp and marginal zone (Figs. 15-2 and 15-4), the attenuated main stem of the central artery, with some branches, runs on into the cords of red pulp, and branches into straight, nonanastomosing slender vessels, about 25 μm in outside diameter, called *penicilli*. The penicilli may terminate as such or may go on to become finer *arterial capillaries*. Some arterial capillaries in human spleen are sheathed (see below). While a few arterial vessels may connect directly with vascular sinuses, virtually all terminate, as observed in histological section, by opening directly into the reticular meshwork of the cords. The interstices of this cordal meshwork are typically crowded with erythrocytes, macrophages, platelets, and plasma cells and some granulocytes. Macrophages are often the predominant cells. They may rapidly differentiate from monocytes sequestered from the circulation. (See the section on Functions of the Spleen below for

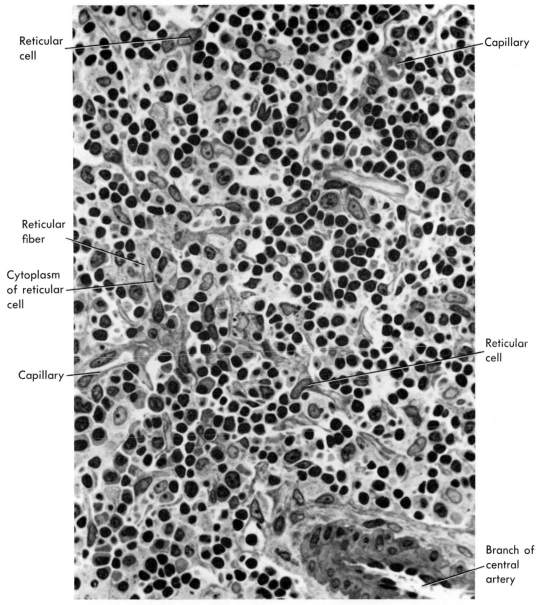

FIGURE 15-8 Spleen of a rabbit, periarterial lymphatic sheath of white pulp. A large branch of the central artery lies in the right lower corner. The larger part of the field consists of a reticular meshwork within which lies the small, densely stained round lymphocytes and related free cells. The meshwork is made of branching reticular cells and reticular fibers. The reticular cells ensheath the more lightly stained reticular fibers. Small blood vessels are present in places in this field. Their adventitial layers are continuous with the reticular meshwork, as are the adventitial layers of the branch of the central artery in the right lower corner. × 600. (From L. Weiss, *Bull. Johns Hopkins Hosp.,* **115:**99, 1964.)

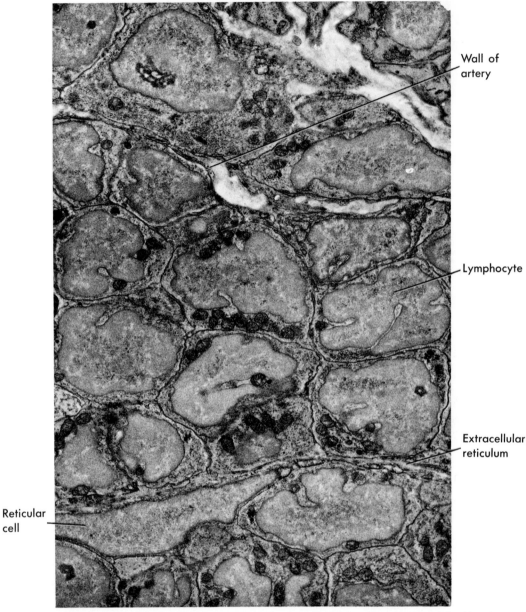

Wall of
artery

Lymphocyte

Extracellular
reticulum

Reticular
cell

FIGURE 15-9 Spleen of a rat, periarterial lymphatic sheath of white pulp. This electron micrograph illustrates the relationships of an arterial vessel, lymphocytes, and the reticular meshwork. The adventitia of a large branch of the central artery is in the upper part of the field. Small lymphocytes are present, tightly packed together. Note that their scanty cytoplasm is rich in ribonucleo-protein and in mitochondria but lacks endoplasmic reticulum. These cells are preponderantly T lymphocytes (see Fig. 15-28). A reticular cell in the lower part of the field is associated with a small segment of extracellular reticulum. ×15,000. (From L. Weiss, *Bull. Johns Hopkins Hosp.,* **115:**99, 1964.)

further discussion.) The T lymphocytes and B lymphocytes are diverted from the cords and are concentrated in the white pulp (see below). The cords are part of the vascular pathway, interposed between arterial terminals and vascular sinuses (see below). They may be regarded as cavernous, vascular spaces inasmuch

as they receive blood from arterial vessels and can convey it to the venous sinuses. The free cells lying in the cordal meshwork may be in rather rapid passage across the cords and into the sinuses or, as is distinctive to the circulation of the spleen, they may be delayed in their passage by remaining in the cords for variable periods (see below). Indeed, the cords may become the site of extramedullary hematopoiesis on the basis of cells sequestered from the blood and prevented from reentering the circulation. The cords are a site where damaged blood cells may be phagocytized and removed from the circulation. The cords, then, are a three-dimensional filter through which blood flows: some elements of the blood may be passed through rather quickly; others may be detained with diverse consequences.

FIGURE 15-10 Human spleen, white pulp. A. Where the cells are stained with Giemsa stain, a central artery (ca) surrounded by the small lymphocyte-rich periarterial lymphatic sheath (PALS) curves into the field from the left. At the left leader it is cut in longitudinal section; at the right leader, in cross section. Hanging from the lower border of the PALS is a large lymphatic nodule, consisting of a large germinal center surrounded by a dense mantle (m) of small lymphocytes. B. In a reticulum preparation, in which the extracellular reticulum is blackened by silver, a similar field is shown. A central artery (ca) curves in from the right. It probably comes from the nearby trabecula. The central artery is surrounded by a PALS. Note the circumferential pattern of the reticulum of the PALS around the central artery. Again, a large lymphatic nodule hangs from the PALS. The periphery of the nodule, constituting the mantle (m) of small lymphocytes, actually represents the PALS which has been carried out by the presence of the large germinal center (gc). × 450. (From the preparation of K. Richardson.)

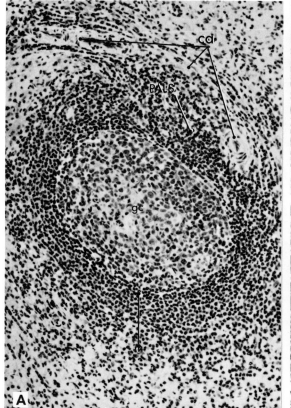

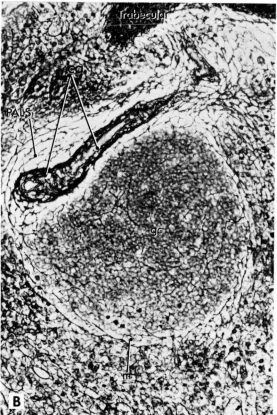

Splenic Sinuses

Splenic sinuses (Figs. 15-14 to 15-25) are long vascular channels 35 to 40 μm in diameter with a unique endothelium and basement membrane. The endothelial cells are elongate with tapered ends and lie parallel to the long axis of the vessel. In cross sections of sinuses, therefore, the endothelial cells are cut in cross section and present a cuboidal shape. They lie side by side with only a slitlike space separating them, free of desmosomes or other membranous attachments. Blood cells cross the wall of the splenic sinus between endothelial cells (Fig. 15-24). Endothelial cells contain bundles of microfilaments in their basal portion. These bundles are disposed in rows running parallel to the long axis of the cells. They may, in some manner, control the width of the interendothelial slit and hence the ease of blood-cell passage across the sinus wall.

The endothelium lies upon a basement membrane, which may be deeply stained in the PAS reaction and impregnated by silver. The arresting feature of the membrane is that it is perforated by large regularly arranged, uniform, polygonal fenestrae so that the little material that remains of the basement membrane is reduced to slender strands separating and outlining the openings. The picture it presents on surface view is that of an almost rectilinear net or of chicken wire. In human beings, the transverse component of the basement membrane is heavy and the longitudinal links relatively slight. The arrangement can be likened to a barrel in which the wooden staves correspond to the endothelium and the hoops to the basement membrane. In section, the membrane appears as a succession of points or short lines of PAS-reactive, or silver-impregnable, substance. By electron microscopy the basement membrane consists of relatively few collagenous and other fibers embedded in a granular matrix. Its composition thus resembles that of

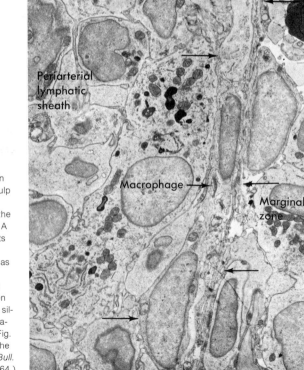

FIGURE 15-11 Spleen of a rat. In this field, the periphery of white pulp (the periarterial lymphatic sheath, PALS) is present. On the left are the closely packed cells of the PALS. A large macrophage may be seen. Its location at the periphery of white pulp is characteristic. The PALS has a well-defined rim of concentric strands of reticulum, running from top to bottom of this field (between arrows). This rim is well shown in silver preparations in which the extracellular reticulum is stained (see Fig. 15-10). The marginal zone is on the right. ×19,000. (From L. Weiss, *Bull. Johns Hopkins Hosp.,* **115:**99, 1964.)

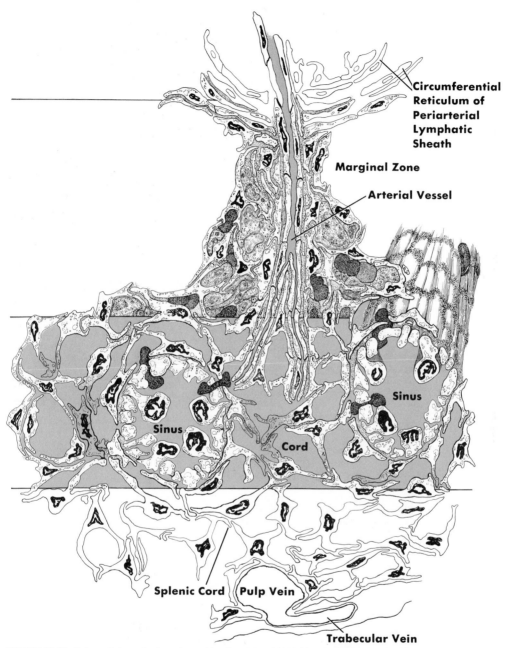

Circumferential Reticulum of Periarterial Lymphatic Sheath

Marginal Zone

Arterial Vessel

Sinus

Sinus

Cord

Splenic Cord   **Pulp Vein**

Trabecular Vein

FIGURE 15-12 Spleen. Schematic view of artery leaving the periarterial lymphatic sheath of white pulp and entering red pulp. It enters a splenic cord and bifurcates between two sinuses. (From L. Weiss, "The Cells and Tissues of the Immune System." Prentice-Hall, Inc., Englewood Cliffs, N.J., 1972.)

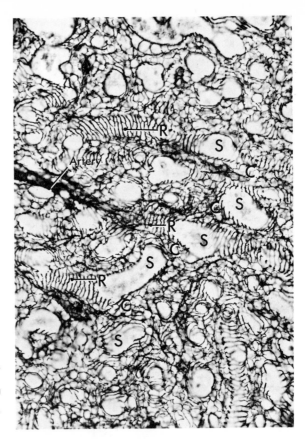

FIGURE 15-13 Red pulp of human spleen, reticulum stain. Sinuses are present as clear spaces (s). Their basement membrane is exposed as consisting primarily of "ring fibers" (R), deeply stained. This membrane is continuous with the reticular fibers of the cords (C). An artery (art) entering from the left appears to open into the cord. ×600. (From the preparation of K. Richardson.)

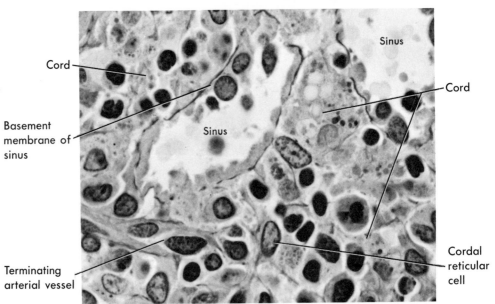

FIGURE 15-14 Rabbit spleen, red pulp. Sections of two sinuses with intervening cords are present in this light micrograph. The basement membrane, stained deeply with the PAS reaction, is interrupted (see Figs. 15-12 and 15-13) in this section because of its fenestrated character. The cords are crowded with macrophages. Reticular cells and PAS-stained reticular fibers are present in the cords. An arterial vessel which opens into a cord is also present. PAS-hematoxylin stain. ×1200. (From L. Weiss, *J. Anat.,* **93**:465, 1959.)

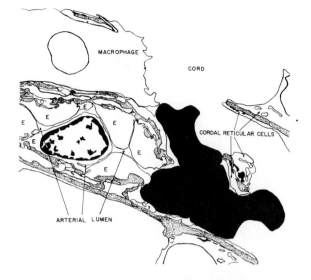

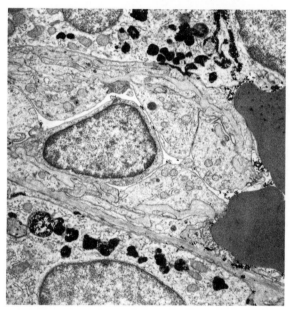

FIGURE 15-15 Spleen of a rabbit, red pulp. An arterial vessel ends in a cord. This vessel is typical of many terminating arterial vessels in red pulp. It is a small arteriole. Its endothelium (E in tracing) is high. Its lumen and the surrounding red pulp contain Thorotrast, which was injected intravenously several minutes before splenectomy. About two layers of extracellular reticulum (stippled in tracing) are present in the vessel wall. The inner one underlies the endothelium and constitutes a basement membrane. Portions of two macrophages lie above and below the vessel. The vessel opens to the right, and several erythrocytes lie just outside the orifice. ×18,000. (From L. Weiss, *Am. J. Anat.*, **113**:51, 1963.)

reticular fibers of the cords, with which the basement membrane is continuous (see below). Reticular cells are applied over the outside surface of the basement membrane of the sinuses. They thus occupy an adventitial position. These reticular cells extend branches into the surrounding cords and are thereby part of the cordal reticular meshwork. They are associated with reticular fibers which, as described above, are continous with the basement membrane of the splenic sinuses. The interendothelial slits of these vascular sinuses constitute a major element in the vascular pathway through the spleen. Blood passes through the cords, through these slits, into the lumen of the sinuses, and then into splenic veins.

Splenic Veins

Sinuses are tributaries of the *veins of the pulp* and these in turn drain into the *trabecular veins* (Figs. 15-3 and 15-4). The transition of splenic sinus into pulp veins is almost insensible, the latter being somewhat larger. Before these veins join the trabecular veins, the lining cells become typical squamous endothelium, the basement membrane becomes an unperforated sheet, and the medial and adventitial tunics become represented by a few strands of muscle and some fibroblasts.

Splenic vein blood is often rich in macrophages and other elements not usually thought of as blood cells. Undoubtedly many of these cells are filtered from the circulation by the liver and, should they pass the liver, by the lung.

Sheathed Capillaries

Terminal arterial capillaries may be modified by a spherical, elliptical, or cylindrical sheath of closely packed macrophages (Figs. 15-23 and 15-24). In the dog and cat these sheaths are very prominent and because of their shape are called *ellipsoids*. Rabbits lack sheathed capillaries. The sheaths in human spleen are relatively small and not every arterial capillary bears one. The endothelium in the sheath is quite rich in microfilaments and may be contractile. The exceptional phagocytic capacity of the sheath may be demonstrated by its efficient concentration of India ink or other particulate matter injected intravascularly.

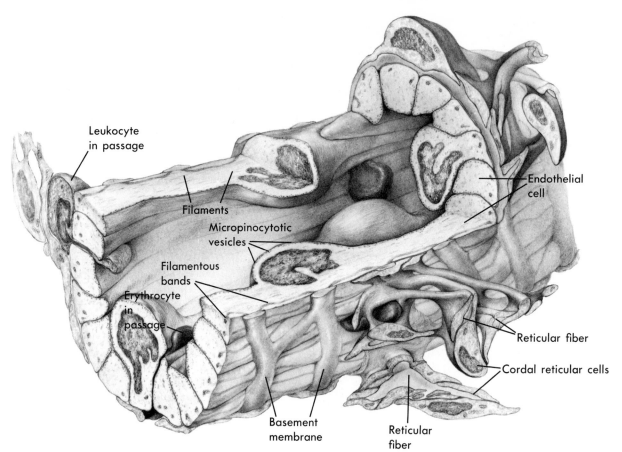

Leukocyte
in passage

Filaments

Micropinocytotic
vesicles

Filamentous
bands

Erythrocyte
in
passage

Endothelial
cell

Reticular fiber

Cordal reticular cells

Basement
membrane

Reticular
fiber

FIGURE 15-16 A schematic drawing of a human splenic sinus in red pulp. The endothelial cells are tapered rods which lie side by side with their long axis parallel to the long axis of the vessel. Virtually all arterial vessels end in the surrounding cords without direct connection to the sinuses. Accordingly, blood entering the vascular sinus must enter from the surrounding cord, squeezing through the slitlike spaces between sinus endothelial cells. Note that several blood cells in passage across the sinus wall are shown. The endothelial cells show several distinctive cytological features. These include a row of pinocytotic vesicles just beneath the plasma membrane on the luminal and lateral surfaces, and two sets of cytoplasmic filaments. One set of filaments, rather loosely organized, runs longitudinally through the cytoplasm. The other set is tightly organized into dense bands in the basal cytoplasm. These bands arch between strands of the basement membrane. They appear to insert into the plasma membrane where it overlies the basement membrane and then continue through the plasma membrane into the substance of the basement membrane. These filaments are likely part of the cytoskeletal system which stiffens the basal cytoplasm and maintains the shape of endothelial cells and the slitlike interendothelial space. They, or the other set of filaments, may be contractile. They play an important role in the spleen's capacity to recognize damaged blood cells and destroy or modify them (see text).

The basement membrane is fenestrated having heavy strandlike transverse "ring" components and lighter longitudinal strands joining the rings. The large fenestrae or apertures in the basement membrane leave ample unimpeded space for blood cell passage through the sinus wall. The cordal surface of the basement membrane is covered by cordal reticular cells which branch into the surrounding cord. (From L-T. Chen and L. Weiss, *Am. J. Anat.,* **134:**425, 1972.)

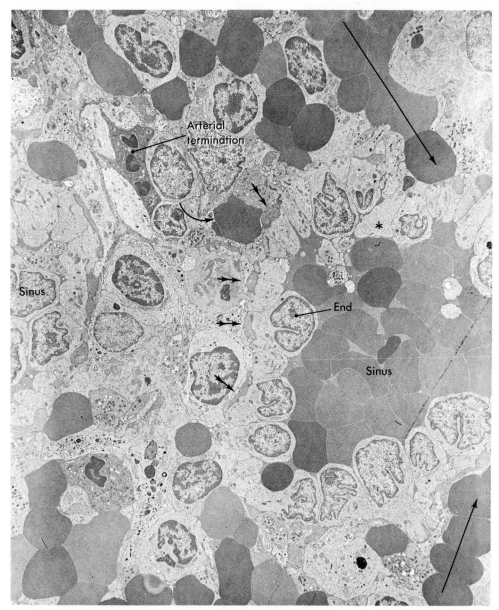

FIGURE 15-17 Human spleen, red pulp. Two sinuses and surrounding cords are present in this low-power electron micrograph. The sinus on the right is filled with erythrocytes. Its wall is cut in cross section. The endothelium consists of tapered rod-shaped cells lying longitudinally and is, therefore, cut in cross section. Nucleated sections of the endothelium protrude into the lumen. Cells are present in passage across the wall (*) between endothelial cells. The basement membrane (double-headed arrows) is present as segments. The sinus on the left is almost collapsed. The cords contain lymphocytes, platelets, erythrocytes, and other free cells. Two columns of erythrocytes are present (arrows) which may represent paths of flow through cords, across the sinus wall, and into the sinus lumen. An arterial capillary is present. It is completely surrounded by a basement membrane except at one point where it opens into a cord. In fact, a cell (arrow) is passing through the aperture of the capillary and into the cord. A granulocyte occupies the capillary lumen. ×2500. (From L-T Chen and L. Weiss, *Am. J. Anat.,* **134:**425, 1972.

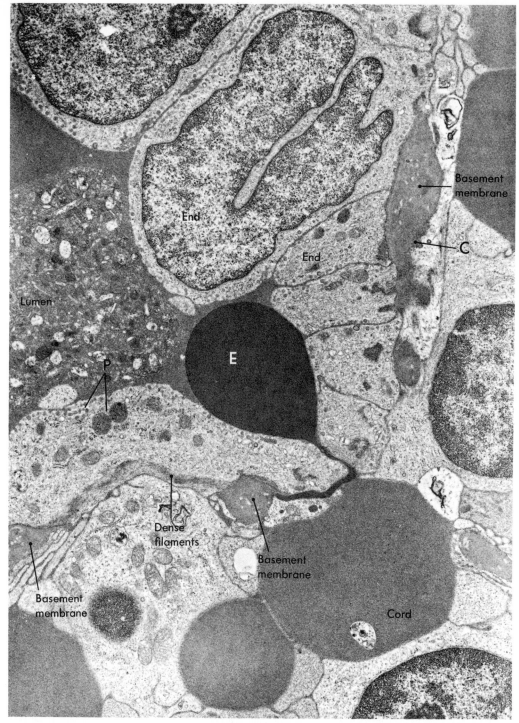

FIGURE 15-18 Human spleen, red pulp. An erythrocyte passes from a cord and through the sinus wall between endothelial cells (end) into the lumen of the sinus. The erythrocyte is drawn into a thin strand as it passes through the mural slit. The endothelial cells contain many pinocytotic vesicles (P) at the luminal surface and dense filaments in the basal cytoplasm which arches across the fenestrae of the basement membrane (BM). Small portions of cordal reticular cells applied to the abluminal surface of the basement membrane are present. The cord is filled with erythrocytes and other free cells. ×10,000. (From L-T. Chen and L. Weiss, *Am. J. Anat.,* **134:**425, 1972.)

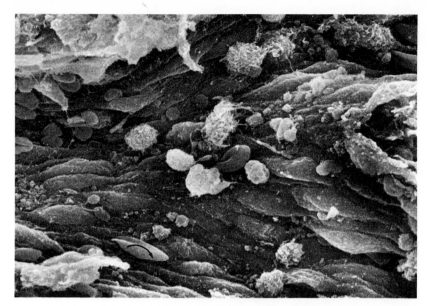

FIGURE 15-19 Rat spleen, red pulp, showing the surface of the endothelium facing the lumen of a vascular sinus. The vessel runs from left to right bifrucating on the right. The endothelial cells lie side by side, their long axis running from left to right. The cells bulge into the lumen in their nuclear zone. There appears to be no interendothelial space. At the curved arrow a red cell appears to be passing through the wall of the vascular sinus by squeezing between endothelial cells. Compare with Fig. 15-18 and see discussion in text. ×1000. (From L. Weiss, *Blood*, **43:**665, 1974.)

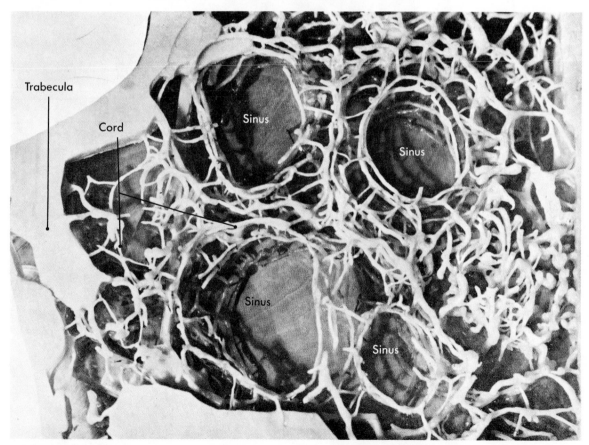

FIGURE 15-20 Human spleen. Reconstruction of extracellular reticulum of red pulp. Four sinuses are present in this field, outlined by the "ring fibers" of the basement mernbrane. The reticular fibers in the cords form a meshwork. In the human spleen the reticular fibers of the cords, as seen well between the upper two sinuses, form a collar or circlet about the sinus. The reader is referred to Koboth's work for additional valuable reconstructions of red pulp. (From E. Koboth, *Beitr. Pathol. Anat.,* **103:**11, 1939.)

THE CIRCULATION OF BLOOD THROUGH THE SPLEEN

Several pathways of blood flow exist in the spleen, since arterial vessels terminate in different places.

Rate studies of erythrocytes tagged with radioactive chromium indicate that normal red cells flow through normal spleens as rapidly as they pass through other organs. But the flow of abnormal red cells or normal red cells in certain abnormal spleens is retarded.

Histologic study of sections of fixed spleen of virtually any species indicates that most of the arterial endings open into the vascular spaces of marginal zone and cords, whereas only a few open into sinuses.

An effort to determine the pathway of blood by direct observation of the living circulation was made by Knisely. The spleen of several animals, among them the mouse and the kitten, was partially exposed in a lightly anesthetized animal and transilluminated by a quartz rod placed beneath the organ and studied through water-immersion lenses. Knisely's conclusions were that blood flow in the spleen is through preformed channels, from arterial vessels directly into

FIGURE 15-21 Rabbit spleen. Low-power scanning electron micrograph of a cut surface of red pulp. Winding furrows or caves with their wall of a latticelike appearance are sinuses cut open (S), among which the cords (C) show a spongy profile. ×360. (From M. Miyoshi, T. Fujita, and J. Tokunaga, *Arch. Histol. Jap.*, **32**:289, 1970.)

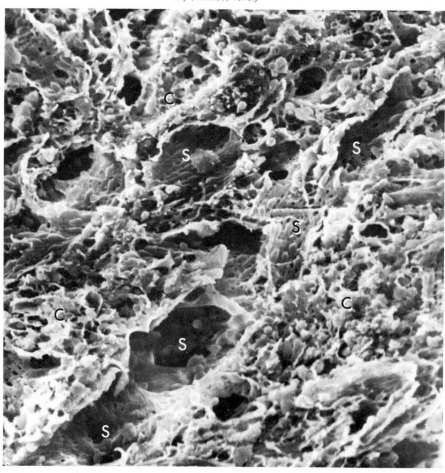

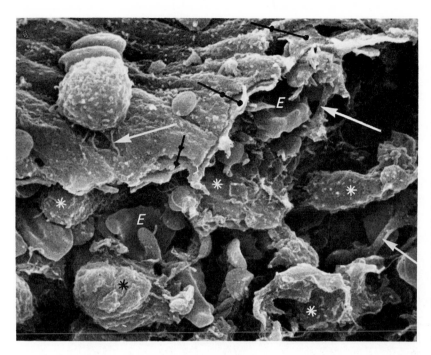

FIGURE 15-22 Rat spleen, red pulp, showing both a vascular sinus and cord. The luminal surface of a vascular sinus is in the upper-left quadrant of this field. The endothelial cells are oriented longitudinally and lie close to one another (see also Figs. 15-19, 15-24, and 15-25). At the cut edge of the sinus the black bars indicate, at the midball, the endothelium and, at the terminal ball, the reticular cells which are adventitial in the sinus wall and branch into the surrounding cord. The blood cell lying on the endothelium sends long microvilli which touch the endothelium (top white arrow). Below the cut edge of the vascular sinus is the cord. It contains a number of reticular cells (asterisks) and strands of reticular fibers (two white arrows on the right). Two erythrocytes (E) in the cord show a crenulated appearance, which may reflect stress imposed by passage through the cords (see text). ×5100. (From L. Weiss, *Blood,* **43:**665, 1974.)

FIGURE 15-23 Spleen of a dog, red pulp. In this light micrograph, an arterial vessel, which is actually a capillary, bifurcates within the sheath. Its endothelium is high, effacing the lumen. The sheath consists of phagocytes with strands of extracellular reticulum running between them. The sheath is about 75 μm in diameter. The surrounding red pulp contains sinuses. The darkly stained free cells in the red pulp are granulocytes. One, in the left upper corner of the field, is crossing the wall of a sinus. Erythrocytes, which abound in red pulp, are unstained in this preparation. PAS-hematoxylin stain. ×650. (From L. Weiss, *Am. J. Anat.,* **111:**131, 1962.)

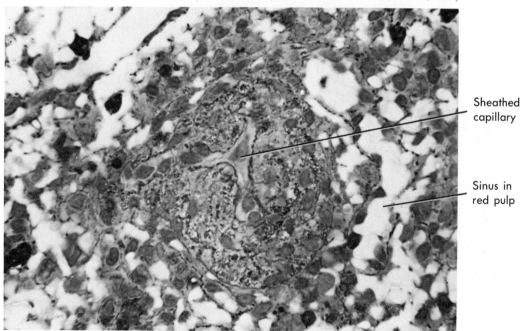

Sheathed capillary

Sinus in red pulp

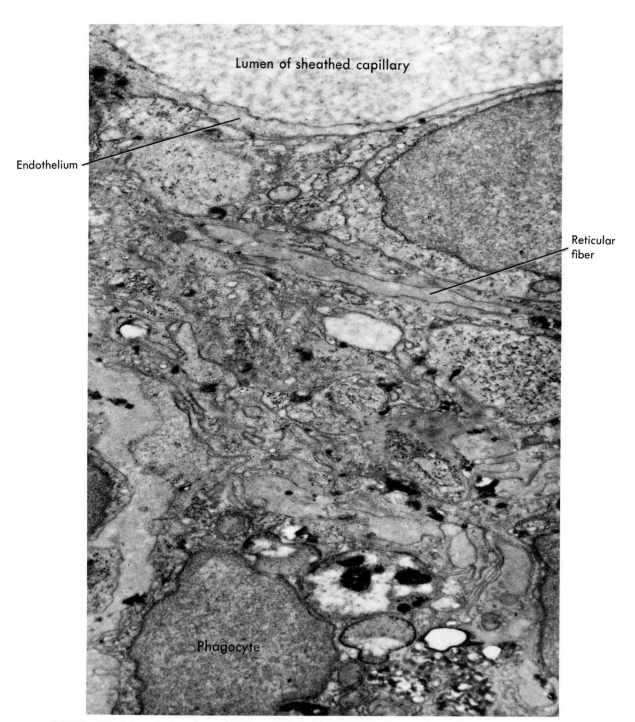

Endothelium

Lumen of sheathed capillary

Reticular
fiber

Phagocyte

FIGURE 15-24 Spleen of a dog, sheathed capillary. In this electron micrograph, the endothelium is quite low. The surrounding cells constituting the sheath are enmeshed in extracellular reticulum. They are phagocytes and contain diverse phagocytic vacuoles. ×22,500. (From L. Weiss, *Am. J. Anat.,* **111:**131, 1962.)

venous sinuses. He observed, moreover, that blood cells could be retained in sinuses, held by sphincter action at the distal end of the vessel, and that the retained plasma left the sinus by seeping through its wall. As a result, the blood cells within the sinus became a pasty mass. Knisely's work has been confirmed by several investigators, including Peck and Hoerr and Bloch; and although there has been some dissent, his findings are generally accepted. It is difficult to relate observations on living spleen with those on fixed histologic sections, but despite the fact that few direct artery-to-sinus connections are found in sections of the spleen, studies of fixed, sectioned spleen and of transilluminated living spleen can be reconciled. The cords and marginal zone are compartmentalized by reticular cells with broad, saillike processes and with an extracellular reticulum associated with these cells. In some cordal areas, the interstices of the reticular

meshwork are plugged with macrophages and other sequestered cells. Such areas would not permit direct and rapid flow of blood. In other places, the reticular meshwork is empty and the processes of reticular cells can adopt a tubular conformation, making possible the same kind of flow that exists in direct vascular connections.

An arterial vessel which terminates in a cord, moreover, may terminate close to the wall of a sinus. Blood passing through this vessel may pass readily through the fenestrated basement membrane of the sinus and between its lining cells, and thus enter the lumen of the sinus. Such flow in the living spleen may appear to be through continuous vessels and be as efficient as through such vessels.

EMBRYOLOGY

The spleen originates in the dorsal mesogastrium at about 5-mm crown-rump length (CRL) in human embryos. At 40-mm CRL the spleen consists of an encapsulated vascular spongework (Figs. 15-25 through 15-27). By 55 mm primitive sinuses are evident and the spongework is much more open. It contains many free blood cells and macrophages (Fig. 15-27). A rich vascular supply quickly develops. By 100-mm CRL, reticular cells tend to lay out the plan of the spleen and assume a circumferential pattern around arteries, defining the periarterial lymphatic sheaths and marginal zone. Soon thereafter, lymphocytes move into the periarterial sheaths. By the end of the first half of gestation, the periarterial lymphatic sheaths are rather clearly developed. In the latter half (by 200 mm), sinuses are present but the full development of their basement membrane and endothelium does not occur until after birth.

In the first trimester of pregnancy, the fetal spleen is erythropoietic and myelopoietic. These functions are preempted successively by the liver and the marrow. In mice, however, they may remain splenic, on a reduced level, through life, supplementing a fully hematopoietic marrow. In human beings, splenic erythropoiesis fades after the fifth prenatal month.

COMPARATIVE ANATOMY

Many differences exist between spleens of different species. The dog's spleen is a large organ, weighing more than 100 g in a small dog. In a big rabbit the spleen may weigh only a few grams. In dogs and humans the spleen is an ovoid structure in the upper left abdominal quadrant. In rabbits, rats, and mice it is a ribbonlike organ lying upon the greater curvature of the stomach. The capsule in the spleen of dogs, oxen, and armadillos is rich in muscle, whereas in human beings and rabbits little muscle is present. Vascular arrangements in the red pulp may be quite different from spleen to spleen. Sinuses are well developed in humans, rabbits, and dogs but not in cats and mice. The spleen of dogs has large and well-developed ellipsoidal sheaths about terminal arterial capillaries. Rabbits have none. Lymphatics are well developed and extensive in hedgehogs and men, but not in rats. Megakaryocytes are normally present in large number

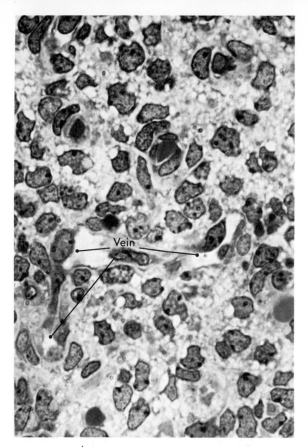

FIGURE 15-25 Spleen of human fetus, 42-mm crown-rump length (approximately 9 weeks' gestational age). The spleen at this stage consists primarily of a spongework of reticular cells containing vessels (a vein crosses this field). See Figs. 15-26 and 15-27. ×1000.

FIGURE 15-26 Spleen of human fetus, 42-mm crown-rump length. The primary reticulum is present as a relatively closed spongework of primitive reticular cells at this fetal stage. Collagen fibrils lie between the reticular cells. Free erythrocytes may be present in the reticular meshwork. ×9500.

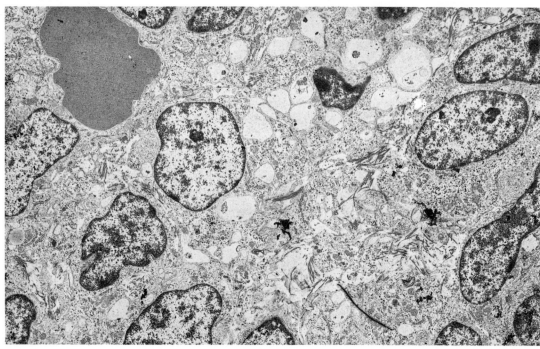

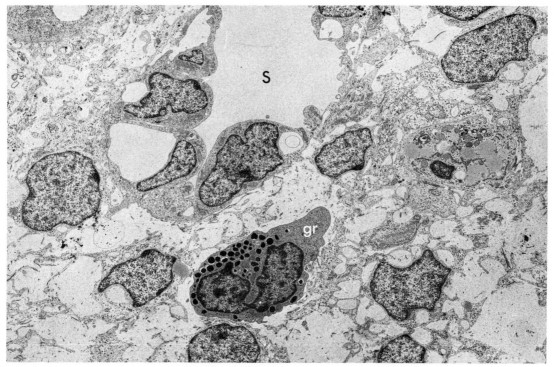

FIGURE 15-27 Spleen of human fetus, 57-mm crown-rump length (approximately 10.5 weeks' gestational age). The primary reticular meshwork has become much more open. A primitive sinus (S) is present. A granulocyte (gr) lies in the meshwork. ×9000.

in the spleen of mice, but are few in humans. The white pulp consists primarily of periarterial lymphatic sheaths in rabbits and rats, whereas lymphatic nodules in cats are the major element of white pulp. Nonetheless, it is common with all these spleens that arterial vessels terminate in a reticular spongework beset with macrophages and that blood is carried out of these spongeworks by venous vessels. Large arterial vessels, moreover, are tightly surrounded by aggregations of lymphocytes, forming white pulp.

FUNCTIONS OF THE SPLEEN

SEPARATION OF BLOOD CELLS AND PLASMA

Plasma is separated from cells in the splenic circulation, so that blood cells are unusually concentrated in the red pulp, as determined both by direct puncture of the spleen and by microscopic study of the living circulation.

The mechanism of separation depends upon muscular constriction of the splenic vein following sympathetic stimulation, so plasma is forced out of sinuses and cords and picked up by the lymphatics. The lymphatics carry the plasma out of the spleen to the thoracic duct. Barcroft and Poole (1927) abolished the spleen's capacity to remove plasma by cutting its nerve supply.

Concentration of blood cells in the spleen enhances its storage function. In animals having a muscular capsule, such as dogs, a reserve mass of blood cells may be rapidly reintroduced into the circulation by adrenergic stimulation, which is followed by massive capsular contraction. The removal of certain elements of the blood and their consequent storage, phagocytosis, or transformation are major functions of the spleen.

The spleen monitors circulating erythrocytes, permitting viable cells passage but detaining and destroying or modifying damaged or aged erythrocytes. This role appears to be carried out in the cords and sinuses of red pulp. The cords pose hazards to erythrocytes. They consist of a reticular meshwork loaded with macrophages. Erythrocytes discharged into this meshwork must travel through it in order to get to the vascular sinuses and exit. The interstices of the meshwork are rather fine, but when filled with bulky macrophages, erythrocytes must be pliant in order to squeeze through. As an erythrocyte ages, it becomes mechanically more fragile and less apt to survive this cordal pathway. Indeed, the oxygen tension and cholesterol and glucose concentration of the cords are likely low. These tend to make erythrocytes more rigid by effects on hemoglobin, plasma membrane, and energy-producing capacity, respectively, and may throw a marginally viable erythrocyte toward phagocytosis. The unshielded presence of macrophages in this cordal pathway, moreover, not only places erythrocytes in passage within direct range of these phagocytes but causes the extracellular fluids of the cords to have a high concentration of hydrolytic enzymes which bathe the erythrocytes in passage. An aged erythrocyte appears to readily lose sialic acid on its surface, exposing galactose residues. By mechanisms unknown, the spleen may "recognize" these galactose moieties and cause such erythrocytes to pool in the reticular meshwork of the cords and be phagocytized. Passage through the wall of vascular sinuses also constitutes a trial for erythrocytes. They must be pliant enough to slip through the interendothelial slits which are likely no wider than 0.5 μm. Rigid erythrocytes, as those in sickle-cell disease and congenital spherocytic anemia, fail to gain the lumen of the vascular sinuses and are "hung up" in the interendothelial slits or pool in the cords. Pliant erythrocytes, which contain rigid particles, as parasitic malarial organisms may have the rigid inclusion "pitted out" at the sinus wall. The pliant portion of the erythrocyte passes through the interendothelial slit of the vascular sinus while the rigid portion is held back. The pliant portion snaps off and enters the lumen of the sinus and thence the circulation as a minierythrocyte. The rigid part remains behind and contributes to the high concentration of

parasites in the spleen in the course of malarial infection.

Lymphocytes released from the marrow (B cells) and from the thymus (T cells) are received in the spleen and with antigen that is also held in the spleen interact to mount an immune response. Recirculating small lymphocytes take a distinctive pathway through the spleen. They enter the white pulp from the marginal zone where they are selectively released from the circulation. If not involved in an immune response, they pass through the white pulp and leave the spleen through deep lymphatics. The route is quite analogous with that of lymphocytes through lymph nodes. Within the white pulp, T and B cells are sorted, presumably by the reticular meshwork; T cells go to the periarterial lymphatic sheath and B cells to the nodules (Fig. 28A and B). Blood-borne antigen is taken up by the spleen. The arrangement favors the interaction of cells with antigen that underlies an immune response (see below).

Monocytes are sequestered in the white pulp, the marginal zone, or the cords. They rapidly undergo conversion into macrophages. In traumatic shock, the circulating leukocytes may fall from a concentration of 10,000 per ml^3 of blood to 700 or fewer per ml^3. Many of these cells lost to the circulation are taken up by the spleen. Approximately one-third of the platelets of the body is normally stored in the spleen in ready reserve. Under certain conditions, however, platelets may be trapped in the spleen with such avidity that there are too few in the circulation and bleeding results. Similarly, the spleen may remove slightly damaged but functionally competent erythrocytes with such zeal that an anemic crisis is precipitated. These conditions are cured by splenectomy.

In addition to the entrapment and subsequent processing of blood cells, the spleen removes particulate material from the blood. Thus, if carbon is injected intravenously, it is rapidly removed from the circulation by the spleen. The material is phagocytized in marginal zone, cords, or sheathed capillaries.

The capacity of the spleen to clear materials from the blood may be estimated by tagging such materials with radioactive isotopes, injecting them intravascularly, and determining the rate of accumulation of the isotope in the left upper quadrant of the abdomen by linear counters moved slowly over the surface of the body.

While the lungs, liver, bone marrow, and other reticuloendothelial tissues also clear the blood, it is likely that the spleen's clearance capacity per gram of tissue is greatest.

The spleen is specialized for trapping blood-borne antigen, immunologically competent cells, and, mounting a large-scale antibody production. It will, however, respond to antigen introduced by routes other than the blood, since such antigen usually finds its way rapidly into the circulation.

Antigen is first trapped and then phagocytized by macrophages in the marginal zone. It subsequently moves into the white pulp and surrounds lymphatic nodules. It thus comes to lie at the junction of T- and B-cell zones. Within the nodules, the antigen is trapped on the surface of macrophages or branched cells, which may be reticular cells.

In a primary immune response, antibody-producing cells appear first within the periarterial lymphatic sheath as part of lymphoid clusters of 20 to 100 or more cells. They move to the periphery of the sheath and then either through blood or lymph are probably carried out of the spleen into the circulation. They

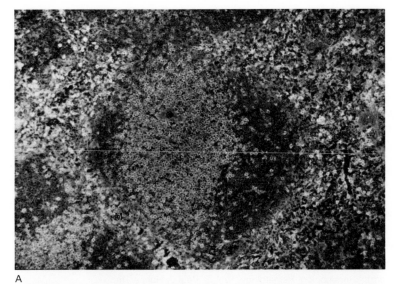

A

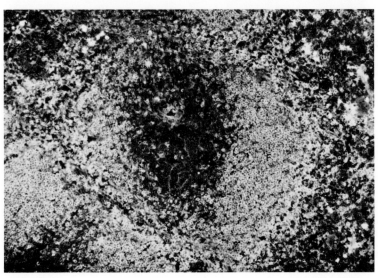

B

FIGURE 15-28 Spleen, mouse. Distribution of T and B lymphocytes as revealed by fluorescence immunocytochemistry. T and B cells are specifically stained in these frozen sections by a technique dependent on antibodies to the surface of T and B cells, respectively. The antibody is conjugated to a fluorescent marker, visible by fluorescence microscopy. In A, the central artery (C) is surrounded by the periarterial lymphatic sheath (P), which is stained by the anti-T-cell reagent, whereas the lymphatic nodule in the field (F) is largely unstained. The marginal zone (M) is stained. R = red pulp. Thus T lymphocytes are concentrated in the periarterial lymphatic sheath and marginal zone. In B, B lymphocytes are stained. Here the lymphatic nodule (F) and the marginal zone (M) are stained. Thus B lymphocytes are concentrated in lymphatic nodules and are largely absent from the periarterial lymphatic sheath. Both T and B cells are present in the marginal zone. See text and see Fig. 14-23 for distribution of T and B lymphocytes in lymph nodes. (From I. L. Weissman, *Trans. Rev.*, **24**:159, 1975.)

rapidly find their way back into the spleen, however, and accumulate in marginal zone and red pulp cords. Alternatively, it is possible that as B cells differentiate into plasma cells, they may migrate directly from white pulp to red pulp. Thus, although red pulp is not the primary site of antibody formation, it may accumulate large numbers of plasma cells.

Somewhat after the periarterial response, the tempo varying with species, antigen, dose, and route of administration, large-scale antibody production by germinal centers begins and may dominate the picture. In secondary responses, as in lymph nodes, the germinal center response is almost immediate and large-scale. [The general discussion of cellular immunology is presented under Lymphocytes in Chap. 10. See also discussions relative to bone marrow (Chap. 11), thymus (Chap. 21), and lymph nodes (Chap. 14).]

REFERENCES

BARCROFT, J., and H. W. FLOREY: Some Factors Involved in the Concentration of Blood by the Spleen, *J. Physiol. (Lond.)*, **66:**231 (1928).

BARCROFT, J., and L. T. POOLE: The Blood in the Spleen Pulp, *J. Physiol. (Lond.)*, **64:**23 (1927).

BJÖRKMAN, S. E.: The Splenic Circulation. With Special Reference to the Function of the Spleen Sinus Wall, *Acta Med. Scand.,* [Suppl. 191] **128:**1 (1947).

CHEN, L. T., and L. WEISS: Electron Microscopic Study of the Red Pulp of Human Spleen, *Am. J. Anat.,* **134:**425 (1972).

CHEN, L. T., and L. WEISS: The Role of the Sinus Wall in the Passage of Erythrocytes through the Spleen, *Blood,* **41:**529 (1973).

GALINDO, B., and T. IMAEDA: Electron Microscope Study of the White Pulp of the Mouse Spleen, *Anat. Rec.,* **143:**399 (1962).

JANOUT, V., and L. WEISS: Deep Splenic Lymphatics in the Marmot: An Electron Microscopic Study, *Anat. Rec.,* **172:**197 (1972).

KLEMPERER, P.: The Spleen, in H. Downey (ed.), "Handbook of Hematology," vol. 3, Paul B. Hoeber, Inc., New York, 1938.

KNISELY, M. H.: Spleen Studies. I. Microscopic Observations of the Circulatory System of Living Unstimulated Mammalian Spleens, *Anat. Rec.,* **65:**23 (1936).

KOBOTH, I.: Über das Gitterfasergeriist der roten Milzpulpa mit einem Bertrag Zu ihrer Gefässtruktur und Blutdurchströmung, *Beitr. Pathol. Anat.,* **103:**11 (1939).

MALL, F. P.: On the Circulation through the Pulp of the Dog's Spleen, *Am. J. Anat.,* **2:**315 (1902).

MILLS, E. S.: The Vascular Arrangements of the Mammalian Spleen, *Qt. J. Exp. Physiol.,* **16:**301 (1926).

SNOOK, T.: The Histology of Vascular Terminations in the Rabbit's Spleen, *Anat. Rec.,* **130:**711 (1958).

SNOOK, T.: A Comprehensive Study of the Vascular Arrangements in Mammalian Spleens, *Am. J. Anat.* **87:**31 (1950).

WEISS, L.: "The Cells and Tissues of the Immune System," Prentice-Hall, Inc., Englewood Cliffs, N.J., (1972).

WEISS, L.: The White Pulp of the Spleen: The Relationships of Arterial Vessels, Reticulum and Free Cells in the Periarterial Lymphatic Sheath, *Bull. Johns Hopkins Hosp.,* **115:**99 (1964).

WEISS, L.: The Structure of Intermediate Vascular Pathways in the Spleen of Rabbits, *Am. J. Anat.,* **113:**51 (1963).

WEISS, L.: The Structure of Fine Splenic Arterial Vessels in Relation to Hemoconcentration and Red Cell Destruction, *Am. J. Anat.,* **111:**131 (1962).

WEISS, L.: A Scanning Electron Microscopic Study of the Spleen, *Blood,* **43:**665, 1974.

WEISS, L., and L. T. CHEN: The Differentiation of White Pulp and Red Pulp in the Spleen of Human Fetuses. (72–145 mm Crown Rump Length), *Am. J. Anat.,* **141:**393, 1974.

WEISS, L.: The Development of the Primary Vascular Reticulum in the Spleen of Human Fetuses (38–57 mm Crown Rump Length), *Am. J. Anat.,* **136:**315, 1973.

Skin

JOHN S. STRAUSS AND A. GEDEON MATOLTSY

The skin is an organ consisting of an epidermis and a dermis (Fig. 16-1). The former is of ectodermal and the latter is of mesodermal origin. The cutaneous appendages such as hair, nails, and sebaceous and sweat glands develop from germinative cells of the epidermis. The dermis primarily consists of collagen and elastic fibers, along with fibroblasts and other mesenchymal cells, blood vessels, lymphatics, and nerves. The pigment cells, which come from the neural crest, are primarily found in the epidermis and the hair. The primary function of the skin is to separate and protect the body from the environment. Most important is the protection that the skin provides against the loss of body fluids and the penetration of noxious agents into the body.

EPIDERMIS

The epidermis is a protective tissue noted for its high structural stability and chemical resistance. It extends over the body as a continuous sheet about 0.1 mm thick. On the surface, horny ridges and valleys form characteristic patterns which are best seen on the palms and soles. At the base, numerous ridges interdigitate with dermal papillae. The epidermis consists of epithelial cells arranged in tightly bound layers (Figs. 16-2 and 16-3) along with scattered pigment cells and nerve endings, but no capillaries; the epidermis receives its nutrients by diffusion from the dermis.

    With light microscopy, the epidermis can be divided into four cell layers, called (proceeding from the deepest layer to the surface) the strata basale, spinosum, granulosum, and corneum (Fig. 16-3). The stratum basale consists of a single row of basal cells which rest on the underlying dermis and have large nuclei and relatively scant cytoplasm containing many tonofibrils. The stratum spinosum is several layers of polyhedral spinous cells that become flattened as they approach the surface. The spinous cells appear to be connected to one another by numerous intercellular bridges, the "prickles." The thickness of the stratum granulosum varies. The cells are flattened but larger than the spinous cells. They contain the irregular granular material keratohyalin in their cytoplasm. The stratum corneum is made up of a series of tightly packed, flat, amorphous-appearing cells. On examination with a polarizing microscope, the stratum corneum shows positive double refraction with reference to the surface plane, indicating the presence of an ordered molecular structure in the horny material. The tonofibrils also show double refraction, but keratohyalin granules are not birefringent.

575

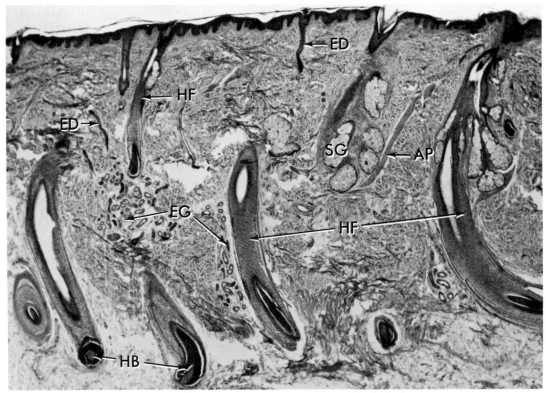

FIGURE 16-1 Photomicrograph of skin from the human scalp. The dense cellular layer at the top is the epidermis. Below this is the thick and compact connective tissue layer, the dermis. At the bottom of the section some of the subcutaneous tissue is shown. Several hair follicles (HF) are present. In the larger follicles, the hair bulb (HB) with its dermal papilla is in the subcutaneous tissue. An arrector pili (AP) muscle is present. There are several sebaceous glands (SG). Eccrine sweat glands (EG) and their ducts (ED) are also present. ×30.

FIGURE 16-2 Photomicrograph of human skin from the interdigital space of the foot. The epidermis (E) is relatively thick. The portion of the dermis (D) that is shown is not compact and represents the pars papillaris. Dermal papillae (DP) and their capillary loops (CL) are well developed. ×220.

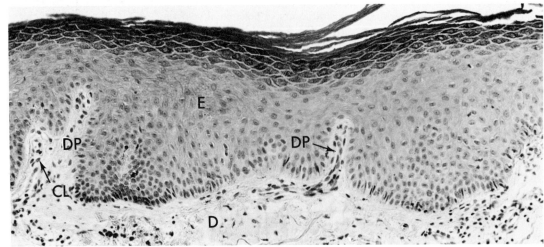

In the electron microscope, the epidermis is seen separated from the dermis by a 50- to 70-nm-thick basal lamina bound to the dermis by relatively short anchoring fibrils having a repeating band pattern of 70 to 120 nm (Fig. 16-4). All the cells of the epidermis, except those of the stratum corneum, are limited by an ordinary trilaminar plasma membrane, which is usually straight and forms specialized structures, the desmosomes, at the attachment sites between adjacent epidermal cells (Fig. 16-5). Each desmosome is composed of two dense plaques on opposing plasma membranes, intersected by a thin intracellular lamella. Filaments converge upon the dense plaques of desmosomes, but they do not cross between cells, as was once assumed from light microscopy. The desmosomes are numerous between adjacent epidermal cells and play an important role in the cohesiveness of the

epidermis. Basal cells have many hemidesmosomes at their base, which provide a firm attachment to the basal lamina (Fig. 16-4).

The cytoplasmic matrix of the basal cells is relatively dense and contains many 60- to 80-Å filaments, either singly or in bundles scattered throughout the cytoplasm. Ribosomes are numerous and clustered; mitochondria are present in moderate numbers; and there are few Golgi vesicles and rough ER membranes. Pinocytotic vesicles are occasionally seen at the base of these cells (Fig. 16-4).

The spinous cells contain the same complement of organelles and inclusions as basal cells, along with new cytoplasmic components called lamellated granules or membrane-coating granules (Fig. 16-6). These ovoid granules vary in size from 0.1 to 0.5 μm. They are covered by a double-layered membrane and are filled with parallel lamellae about 20 Å thick oriented

FIGURE 16-3 Higher magnification of Fig. 16-2, showing the basal (B), spinous (SP), granular (G), and horny (H) layers of the epidermis. Note "prickles" between spinous cells. Tonofibrils can be seen in both basal and spinous cells. ×750.

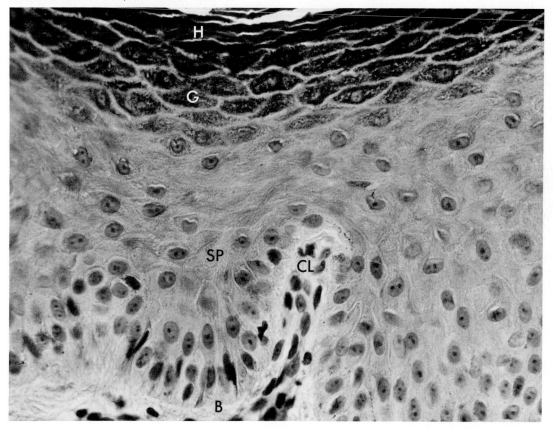

along the short axis of the granule (Fig. 16-7). Lamellated granules usually appear first in the vicinity of Golgi vesicles but later are seen throughout the cytoplasm.

Granular cells contain synthetic organelles and numerous filament bundles, lamellated and keratohyalin granules (Fig. 16-6), and occasional lysosomes. In these cells, the lamellated granules have migrated to the cell periphery or are discharged into the intercellular space with their lamellae spreading between the cells (Fig. 16-8). The keratohyalin granules, which are the distinguishing characteristic of the granular cells,

FIGURE 16-4 Electron micrograph of a portion of the basal epidermis cell from human foreskin. The cytoplasm contains ribosomes (R), endoplasmic reticulum (ER), mitochondria (MI), melanin granules (ME), abundant filaments (F), and pinocytotic vesicles (PV). The basal cell is attached to the basal lamina (BL) by half-desmosomes (HD). The basal lamina is bound to the dermis by anchor filaments (AF). Collagen fibrils (C) appear scattered in the dermis. On the left, a small portion of a melanocyte (MC) is shown with melanosomes, revealing different stages of maturation. ×37,000. (Courtesy of Dr. T. Huszar, Boston University School of Medicine.)

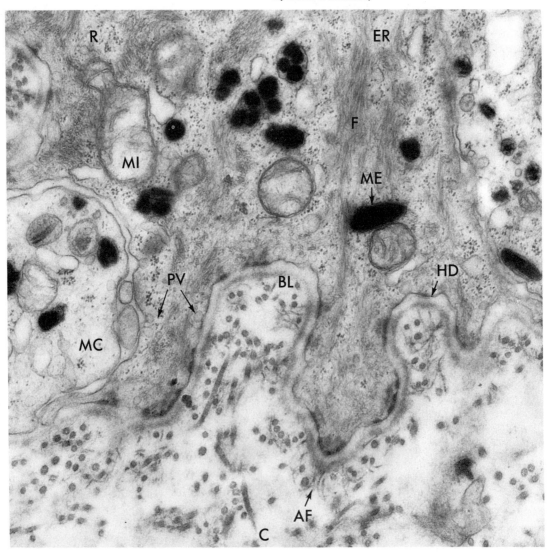

may be round or irregularly shaped, and vary in size from submicroscopic to microscopic dimensions (Fig. 16-6). They are not membrane-bound, and their bulk consists of closely packed, amorphous, 20-Å particles. Filament bundles may pass across the entire length of the keratohyalin granules or be blended into their peripheral parts (Fig. 16-9).

There are relatively few remnants of cell organelles in the stratum corneum; the cells are mainly filled by 60- to 80-Å filaments embedded in an amorphous matrix (Figs. 16-10 and 16-11). The horny cells are enveloped by a modified plasma membrane 150 to 200 Å thick. The plasma membrane thickens from the inside of the cell by deposition of an amorphous material. This fuses with the 20-Å inner leaflet and ultimately forms a single 100- to 150-Å electron-dense layer. The 20-Å outer and mid leaflets reveal comparatively minor changes; their thickening is in the range of 10 Å, respectively (Fig. 16-12). This modified membrane is highly convoluted and interdigitates with adjacent cell membranes. Desmosomes are present in a more or less preserved form (Fig. 16-10). The intercellular spaces are filled and the surface of horny cells covered by material partially derived from lamellated granules; it is occasionally seen as broad sheaths composed of bileaflets (Fig. 16-12).

Functionally, basal cells correspond to reproductive cells, spinous and granular cells to differentiating cells, and horny cells to differentiated cells—that is, to the terminal products of the epidermis. The basal cells maintain the epidermis by mitosis, and for each division, a basal cell enters the course of differentiation. The differentiating cells abandon mitotic activity and form new products. They are constrained to a specific pathway, and subsequent events run their courses irreversibly. The differentiated cells are retained in the horny layer until they are lost into the environment by shedding. Thus, the life history of the cells shows that the epidermis is continuously self-renewing; mitotic reproduction below and desquamation at the surface are balanced to achieve a steady state. Renewal time varies among different species and within various body regions. In general, epidermal renewal takes 3 to 4 weeks in human beings.

Keratinization may be regarded as a form of epithelial cell differentiation consisting of both a synthetic phase and a degradative stage. After mitosis, epidermal cells pass through these stages more or less independently (Fig. 16-13). During the synthetic stage, differentiation products such as filaments, keratohyalin granules, and lamellated granules are formed in large numbers. The filaments and keratohyalin granules are largely composed of protein synthesized by ribosomes. The lamellated granules store large amounts of bipolar lipids and some hydrolytic enzymes such as are present in most secretory granules. The enzymes are presumably involved in exocytosis of the granules. After the epidermal cells become filled

FIGURE 16-5 Electron micrograph of the interface between two adjacent human epidermal cells showing details of desmosomes. ×52,000.

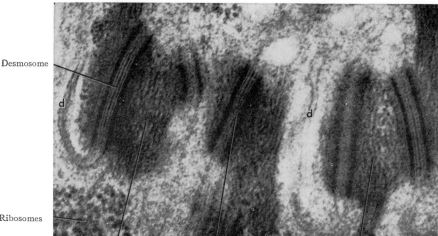

Desmosome

Ribosomes

Tonofilaments　　　Desmosome　　　Tonofilaments

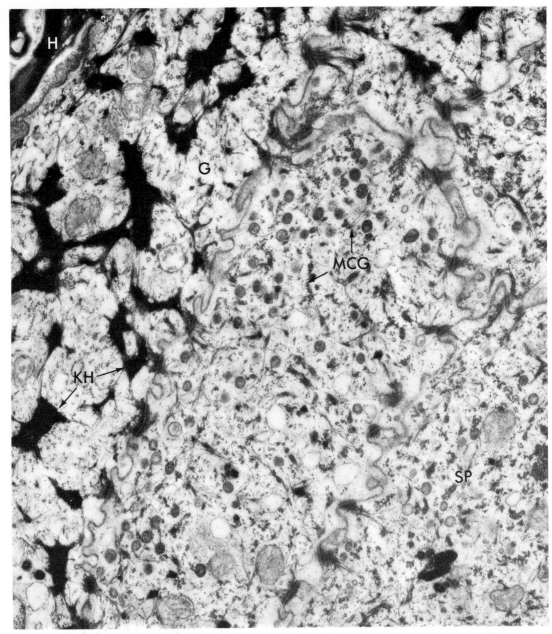

FIGURE 16-6 Electron micrograph of the midportion of the epidermis from human foreskin showing portions of spinous (SP), granular (G), and horny (H) cells. The rounded granules in the spinous cell are membrane-coating granules (MCG). The irregular bodies in the granular cell are keratohyalin granules (KH). ×23,000. (Courtesy of Dr. T. Huszar, Department of Dermatology, Boston University School of Medicine.)

with the synthetic products, the membrane of the lamellated granules fuses with the plasma membrane and the lamellae are discharged into the intercellular spaces and their remnants fill the spaces and coat the surface of the cells. Subsequently, the remaining synthetic organelles are degraded by activation of specific enzymes. However, the filaments and keratohyalin remain unaffected. Concomitant changes in the plasma membrane result in the loss of degraded materials into the intercellular space. Ultimately, the remaining cell content, composed mainly of filaments and keratohyalin masses, consolidates into a fibrous-amorphous material and becomes encased by a thickened cell envelope. Thus, keratinization is a complex process, and the protective material formed may be regarded as being composed of three basic structural units: (1) 60- to 80-Å filaments (2) an amorphous horny matrix, and (3) a thickened cell envelope.

The structural stability and chemical resistance of the protective layer is primarily assured by large amounts of sulfur-containing proteins. These proteins are relatively insoluble owing to the presence of covalent bonds such as disulfide cross-linkages between the

polypeptide chains. These proteins, referred to as keratin, belong to the KMF class of α-proteins (keratin-myosin-fibrin) since they have a characteristic α-keratin x-ray diffraction diagram. Detailed studies have shown that the fibrous proteins in the filaments contain a comparatively small amount of sulfur. The basic unit is a three-stranded dimer having segments about 200 Å long with an α-helical structure. These segments are responsible for the α-type x-ray diffraction pattern given by the filaments. The α-protein is insoluble in buffers pH 3 to 11, but it passes into solution in acid buffer pH 2.6. After solubilization, it retains its ability to reaggregate into filaments comparable to those seen in situ.

The horny matrix consists largely of an amorphous protein which originally was part of the keratohyalin granules. This amorphous protein is stabilized by abundant disulfide bonds and is insoluble in buffers pH 2 to 11. However, if the disulfide bonds are reduced, it dissociates into macromolecules and readily reaggregates into an amorphous particulate material upon reoxidation of the sulfhydryl groups. The association of fibrous α-protein with amorphous protein

FIGURE 16-7 Electron micrograph of a membrane-coating granule showing the lamellar structure. ×236,000. (Courtesy of A. G. Matoltsy and P. F. Parakkal, in A. G. Zelickson (ed.), "Ultrastructure of Normal and Abnormal Skin," Lea & Febiger, Philadelphia, 1967.)

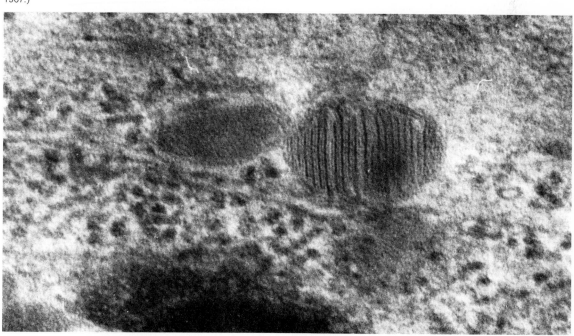

(filament-matrix complex) affords flexibility, elastic recovery, and structural stability for the horny cell.

This fibrous-amorphous complex is encased by a modified plasma membrane with an 100- to 150-Å inner layer; this is the most chemically resistant component of the horny cell. The inner layer contains an amorphous protein which cannot be dissociated into macromolecules by conventional techniques because it is stabilized by an unidentified resistant bond, in addition to ample disulfide bonds. The membrane

protein protects the horny cell and is responsible for the integrity of the stratum corneum.

Whereas the protection offered by the epidermis is provided by the highly resistant horny cells, the stratum corneum as a whole acts as a barrier to the

FIGURE 16-8 Electron micrograph of mouse oral epithelium showing attachment of a membrane-coating granule to the plasma membrane prior to discharge (D) of its content into the intercellular space. Discharged lamellae (L) appear in the intercellular space between adjacent granular and horny cells. Note that the plasma membrane of the horny cell (TPM) is thickened, whereas that of the granular cell (PM) is normal. ×18,000. (Courtesy of A. G. Matoltsy and P. F. Parakkal, *J. Cell Biol.,* **301**:24, 1965.)

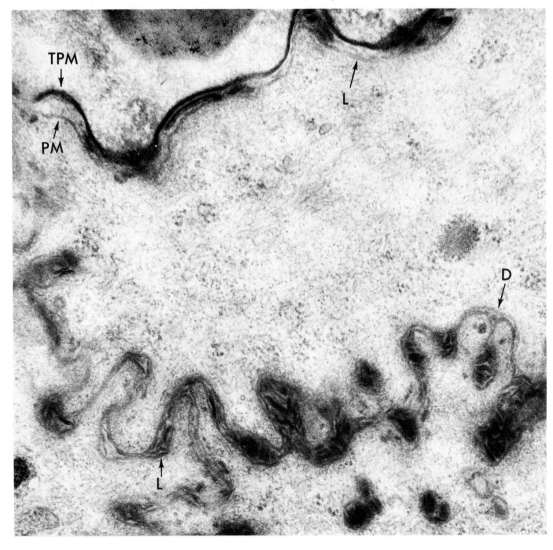

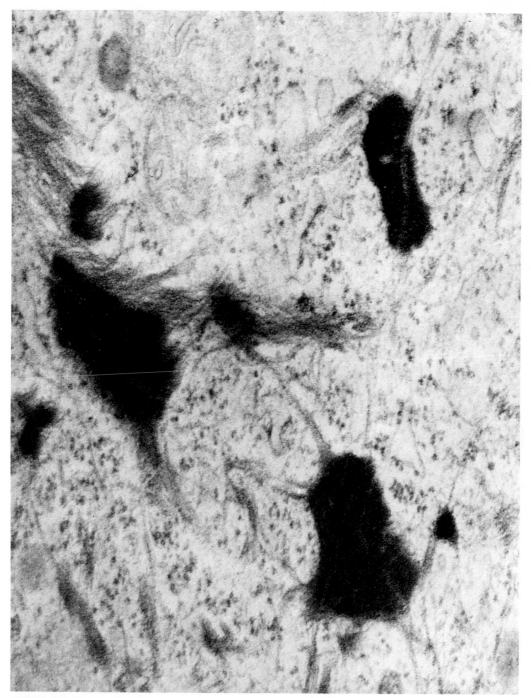

FIGURE 16-9 Electron micrograph of keratohyalin granules of human epidermis. Note filaments passing across the granules and attached to their surfaces. ×83,600. (Courtesy of R. M. Lavker and A. G. Matoltsy, *J. Ultrastruct Res.,* **35:**575, 1971.)

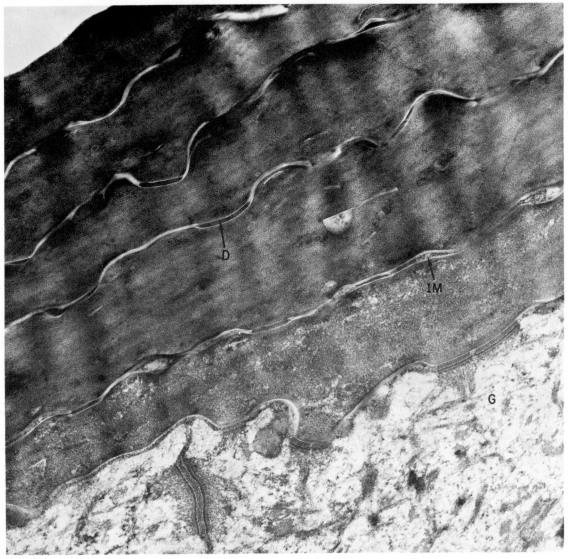

FIGURE 16-10 Portions of a granular (G) and five horny cells of the stratum corneum of human epidermis. The horny cells are filled by a filament-amorphous matrix complex. Desmosomes (D) and intercellular material (IM) are relatively well preserved. ×48,000. (Courtesy of J. A. Bednarz and A. G. Matoltsy.)

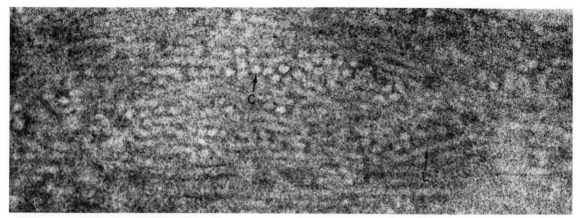

FIGURE 16-11 High-resolution electron micrograph of a portion of a horny cell. The lightly stained filaments are shown in both longitudinal (L) and cross (C) sections. The matrix is darkly stained. ×280,000. (Courtesy of J. A. Bednarz and A. G. Matoltsy.)

FIGURE 16-12 Portion of the stratum corneum showing the modified plasma membrane of the horny cells with a thick layer (TIL) and a thin outer layer (TOL). Membranes with bileaflets originating from lamellated granules are present in the intercellular spaces (MBL). ×74,000 (Courtesy of R. M. Lavker)

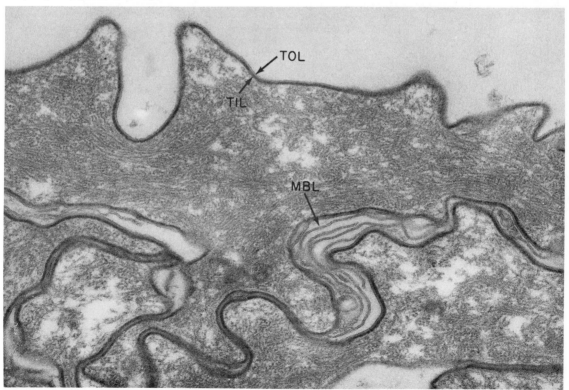

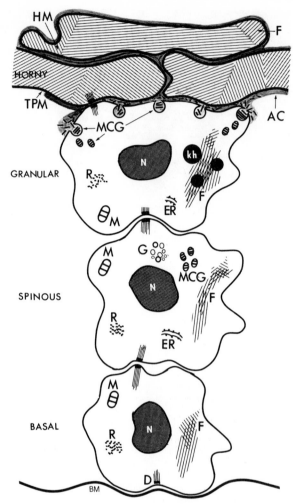

FIGURE 16-13 Schematic illustration of ultrastructural changes of a keratinizing epithelial cell: basement membrane (BM); desmosome (D); filament (F); ribosome (R); nucleus (N); mitochondrion (M); endoplasmic reticulum (ER); membrane-coating granule (MCG); Golgi complex (G); keratohyalin granule (KH); thickened plasma membrane (TPM); amorphous coat (AC); horny matrix (HM). (Courtesy of A. G. Matoltsy and P. F. Parakkal, in A. S. Zelickson (ed.), "Ultrastructure of Normal and Abnormal Skin," Lea & Febiger, Philadelphia, 1967.)

movement of material across the skin. Loss of body fluids into the environment or passage of water into the skin via intercellular spaces is primarily prevented by large deposits of bipolar lipids between horny cells originating from the contents of lamellated granules.

NAIL

The nail is a rather rectangular horny plate which is attached to the nail bed, with its proximal end continuous with the nail matrix. Proximally and laterally, cutaneous folds cover the edges of the nail, with the underlying soft epithelial mass merging with the living part of the epidermis. The distal end of the nail plate extends over the dorsum of the distal phalanx of the fingers and toes. Between the epidermis and the distal end of the nail bed, a boundary called the *hyponychium* is formed. The nail is semitransparent and shows the color of the underlying blood-vessel-rich tissues. Near the proximal cutaneous fold is the whitish, semicircular portion of the nail called the lunula, which is the matrix of tightly packed epithelial cells from which the nail grows (Fig. 16-14). At the base of the matrix, deep ridges interdigitate with the dermal papillae. The cells of the deepest layer of the matrix are cylindrical; above them are several layers of polyhedral cells. Both cell types have a relatively large nucleus, and the cytoplasm contains tonofibrils. As the cells approach the surface, they become somewhat larger and flattened and contain more tonofibrils. A distinguishing characteristic of cellular differentiation in the nail is the absence of keratohyalin. The horny cells are flat and filled with a homogeneous-appearing material. The tonofibrils are birefringent, and the nail plate shows double refraction perpendicular to the direction of growth.

In the electron microscope, the nail matrix is seen separated from the dermis by a basal lamina similar to that separating the epidermis from the dermis. The fine structure of cylindrical and polyhedral matrix cells is comparable to that of basal cells of the epidermis. The cells of the higher layers do not contain lamellated granules or keratohyalin granules; instead, they possess abundant 60- to 80-Å filaments assembled into heavy bundles. The horny cells are enveloped by a thickened plasma membrane and filled with filaments embedded in an amorphous matrix. Desmosomes appear between all the cells of the matrix and horny cells of the nail plate.

The cylindrical matrix cells are reproductive cells which divide frequently and are responsible for continuous growth of the nail. The polyhedral and flattened matrix cells are differentiating cells which be-

FIGURE 16-14 Longitudinal section through distal digit of squirrel monkey showing characteristic nail structures: matrix (M); nail bed (NB); nail plate (NP); and, hyponychium (HN). (Courtesy of Dr. N. Zaias, School of Medicine, University of Miami.)

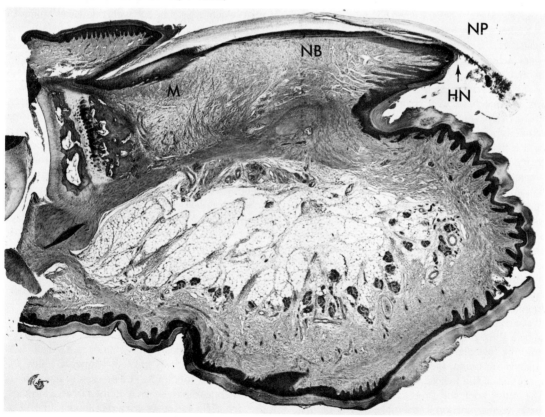

come filled with the fibrous-amorphous mass of insoluble proteins known as *nail keratin*. Nail keratin has a higher sulfur content than does epidermal keratin, which probably explains its higher structural stability and chemical resistance.

The nail bed is continuous with the lower part of the matrix and is formed by layers containing cylindrical and polyhedral cells. Ridges of the nail bed penetrate deeply into the dermis and interdigitate with dermal papillae rich in blood vessels. The polyhedral cells do not reveal structural manifestations of differentiation; they appear as "resting" cells providing attachment and support for the growing nail plate.

HAIR

In humans there are two types of hairs. The very short, soft, usually colorless hairs which cover much of the body are the *vellus hairs*. When small, these hairs cannot be seen with the naked eye. In contrast, the *terminal hairs* are longer and coarser and usually intensely pigmented. The fine hairs found on the forehead or the bald scalp are typical of vellus hairs. The pigmented scalp, eyelid, beard, axillary, pubic, arm, and leg hairs are examples of terminal hairs. Unfortunately, no absolute classification can be made, because there are hairs that are intermediate between these two hair types.

Hairs are hardened epithelial fibers of various lengths and thicknesses emerging from a soft, bulb-shaped *follicle* residing in the dermis, although the bottoms of large hairs may be in the subcutaneous tissue. The neck of the follicle joins the epidermis, and its bottom is invaginated and filled with a dermal papilla rich in blood vessels (Fig. 16-15). The lower bulb-shaped portion, called the *matrix*, is the germinative center of the hair. Above the matrix, the emerging hair and concentric epithelial sheaths, such as the outer and inner root sheaths, appear (Fig. 16-16). The hair itself is composed of a cuticle, cortex, and medulla. The entire follicle is encased by a connective tissue sheath attached by one end to the papillary layer of the dermis by a band of smooth muscle fibers known as the *arrector pili muscle,* which can move the hair into a more vertical position (Fig. 16-1). The development of this muscle varies greatly. The sebaceous gland is connected to the upper part of the follicle by a short duct through which sebum is delivered into the follicular canal. In areas in which apocrine glands are found, they are also attached to the upper portion of the follicle.

The outer root sheath is continuous with the epidermis. At the junction it resembles the epidermis in structure but is distinguished from it by formation of glycogen, as glycogen normally is not seen in epidermal cells. Deeper in the follicle, the outer root sheath thins out and terminates as a single layer when it reaches the matrix area of the follicle. A horny layer is not normally formed by the outer root sheath; it consists only of layers comparable to the basal and spinous cell layers of the epidermis. In the electron microscope, the entire hair follicle is seen separated from the surrounding connective tissue sheath by a basal lamina which is continuous with the basal lamina of the epidermis. Matrix cells and outer root sheath cells are attached to this lamina by hemidesmosomes.

The matrix cells have a comparatively large nucleus which occupies most of the cell. The cytoplasm contains numerous ribosomes and a moderate number of mitochondria. Rough-surfaced ER is scanty, and there are relatively few Golgi vesicles. The plasma membranes of adjacent cells lie close and, at scattered points, are attached by desmosomes. There are only a few short filaments; they occur mainly near the desmosomes. The matrix cells divide more frequently than basal epidermal cells and produce four types of differentiating cells (Fig. 16-17). Those appearing in the periphery of the matrix form a circular multilayered *inner root sheath*, which desquamates as it reaches the skin surface. The more centrally located differentiating cells produce the cuticular, cortical, and medullary layers of the emerging hair. The medulla is poorly developed in humans; human hairs essentially consist of a thin cuticle and a thick cortex.

Within the cytoplasm of various types of differentiating cells emerging from the matrix, various products are formed. The columnar inner root sheath cells first develop many 60- to 80-Å filaments which are packaged into tonofibrils. Later, small amorphous particles appear in the vicinity of the filament bundles; these are early forms of trichohyalin granules (Fig. 16-18). The fully formed trichohyalin granules are comparable to keratohyalin granules of epidermal cells. After inner root sheath cells become filled with filaments and trichohyalin granules, the synthetic organelles disintegrate and the trichohyalin granules disperse. The remaining cell contents become condensed, and a filament-matrix complex is formed. The cell envelope thickens, and the widened intercellular spaces are filled with an amorphous substance.

The cuticular cells contain only a few filaments;

their cytoplasm is filled with 300- to 400-Å granules which are not observable in the light microscope (Fig. 16-18). The granules are not limited by a membrane, and they grow both by continuous deposition of an amorphous material and by coalescence. Cuticular cells are mainly filled with this amorphous material

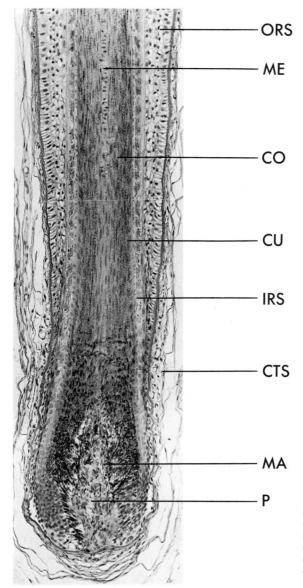

ORS

ME

CO

CU

IRS

CTS

MA

P

FIGURE 16-15 Photomicrograph of a hair follicle from human scalp: papilla (P); matrix (MA); connective tissue sheath (CTS); inner root sheath (IRS); cuticle (CU); cortex (CO); medulla (ME); outer root sheath (ORS). ×160.

when they elongate, overlap, and form the outer layer of the hardening hair fiber (Fig. 16-19).

The differentiating cortical cells, which are the structural cells of the hair, develop many 60- to 80-Å filaments which are assembled into heavy bundles (Fig. 16-18). As these cells assume a spindle shape and form the cortex of the emerging hair fiber, they become filled with filaments between which an amorphous matrix is deposited.

The medullary cells, which are few in number, develop spherical granules 300 to 500 Å in diameter. These granules grow extensively and may reach dimensions of several micrometers. The granules eventually coalesce, and an amorphous mass fills the cell in the medulla of the hair.

As in the epidermis, the keratinization process may be divided into a synthetic phase and a degrada-

tive stage. Keratinization of the hair, however, is more complicated than in the epidermis, since the matrix forms four different cell types, each of which ultimately changes into a structurally and chemically different horny cell. The factors which induce and direct the various differentiative pathways are not understood. Chemical studies indicate that the keratinized inner root sheath cells and cortical cells are filled with a sulfur-poor fibrous protein and a sulfur-rich amorphous protein. The fibrous protein makes these cells birefringent and produces the α-keratin x-ray diffraction pattern given by the hair fiber. Cornified cuticular cells contain a sulfur-rich amorphous protein, and medullary cells an amorphous protein with little or no sulfur.

The hair does not grow continuously as the nail does; it is lost and renewed periodically. Hair loss

FIGURE 16-16 Photomicrograph of midportion of the hair follicle from human scalp: medulla (ME); cortex with melanin granules (CO); cuticle (CU); inner root sheath (IRS); outer root sheath (ORS). ×750.

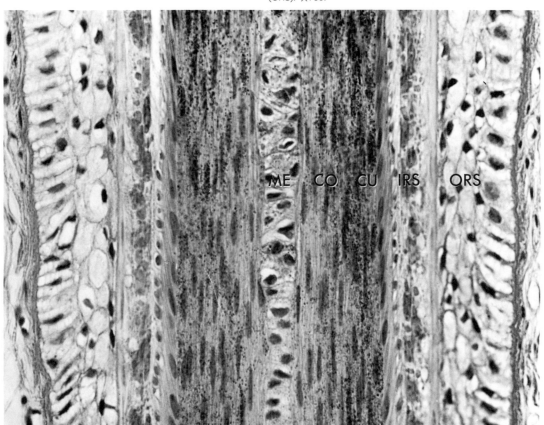

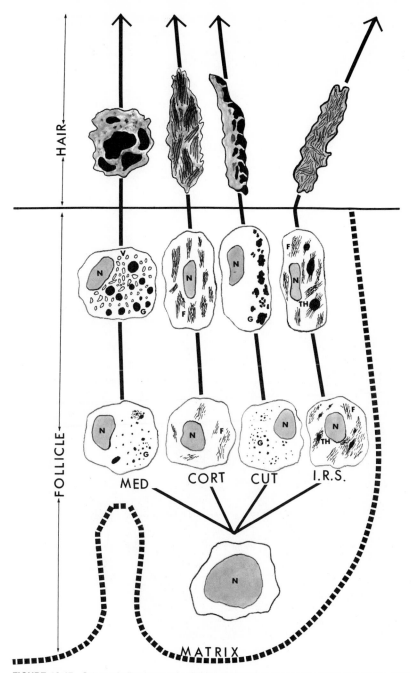

FIGURE 16-17 Schematic illustration of cell lines arising from the matrix of the hair follicle. Differentiation products, observable in the electron microscope, are shown. Medulla cells (MED) form abundant amorphous granules (G) and vesicles (V), which are ultimately filled with large masses of amorphous material. Cortical cells (CORT) develop many filaments (F) and terminally contain a filament-amorphous matrix complex. Cuticular cells (CUT) contain small amorphous granules (G) which coalesce and accumulate at the cell periphery facing the hair surface. Inner root sheath cells (IRS) form both filaments (F) and trichohyalin granules (TH). Terminally, the horny cells are filled with a filament-amorphous matrix complex.

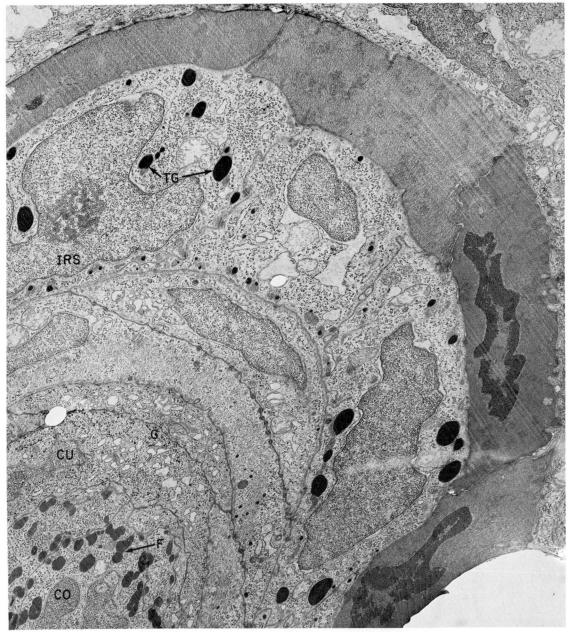

FIGURE 16-18 Electron micrograph of part of a cross section of a hair follicle. Note the heavy filament bundles (F) in the cortical cells (CO), the small amorphous granules (G) in the cuticular cells (CU), and the trichohyalin granules (TG) in the inner root sheath cells (IRS). The outer layer of the inner root sheath consists of keratinized cells containing nuclear remnants (NR). ×10,000. (Courtesy of Dr. A. G. Matoltsy.)

begins when matrix cells cease dividing, so that new cells no longer start to differentiate, and the differentiation process runs its course within cells which have already started. Soon all cells which have left the matrix undergo keratinization in situ and form a clublike mass attached to the hair. Such *club*, or

telogen, hairs (Fig. 16-20) lack firm anchorage to the scalp and can be easily plucked from the follicle. These are the hairs that form the normal defluvium of the scalp. Normally about 5 percent of the scalp hairs are in telogen. During the rest period, many matrix cells become atrophic, and the follicle is rebuilt by a relatively small number of matrix cells. The growing hair, known as an *anagen hair* (Figs. 16-1 and 16-15), is firmly attached to the follicle by the root sheaths and

FIGURE 16-19 Electron micrograph showing part of a cross section of a hair follicle close to the skin surface. The emerging hair fiber (HF) is composed of consolidated cortical cells and a thin cuticle. The hair fiber is surrounded by a layer of keratinized inner root sheath cells. Next to these cells differentiated inner root sheath cells appear filled by trichohyalin granules (TG) and keratinized inner root sheath cells are present around these cells. ×6,600. (Courtesy of J. A. Bednarz and A. G. Matoltsy.)

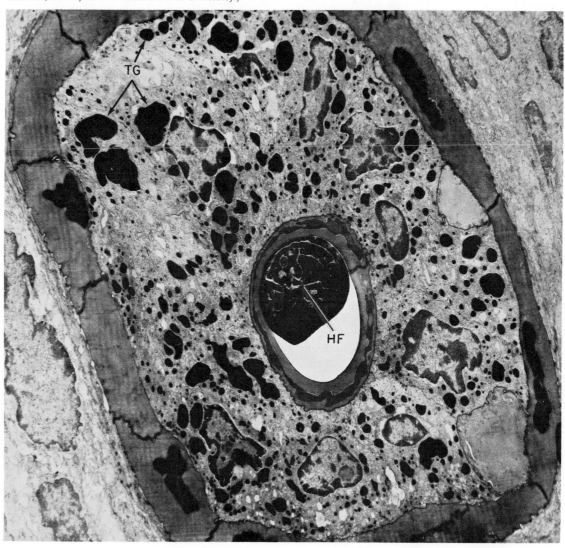

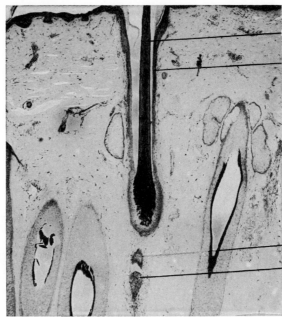

——— Club hair

——— Resting hair follicle

——— Tangential section of active follicle

——— Hair germ and its potential hair papilla

FIGURE 16-20 Club hair in resting follicle in human scalp. Compare this with active growing follicles shown in Figs. 16-1 and 16-15. ×40.

is not easily dislodged. The thickness at the bulb determines hair thickness—the larger the bulb, the more mitotic activity there is and the thicker the hair produced. The length of the growth period determines the ultimate length of the hair. Thus, scalp hairs have a very long anagen phase, whereas the vellus hairs have a short anagen phase. Growth and rest progress in cycles, and in humans each hair follicle has a different growth and rest period, so the follicles are independent of each other. In rodents, hair grows in successive waves over the body, and the duration of growth and rest is remarkably constant.

MELANOCYTES

Normally, the number of melanocytes found in the skin of Caucasoids, Negroids, and Mongoloids are relatively constant. On the head and forearm there are approximately 2000 melanocytes per square millimeter; on the rest of the body, there are approximately 1000 melanocytes per square millimeter. It is thus easy to see that pigmentation is not entirely dependent on the number of melanocytes. As will be discussed, skin color is based upon complex relationships between pigment-producing cells and the cells of the epidermis. Skin color itself is of two types. The basic *constitutive skin color* is the natural color that is not related to the influence of exogenous agents. It is usually considered to be that color which is seen in the unexposed skin; but in its purest form it is that seen in the newborn child. Any increase over this skin color is considered to be the second type of skin color, known as an *inducible or faculatative skin color*. Such changes can be caused by various circumstances such as exposure to ultraviolet light, pregnancy, or the influence of hormones.

The melanocytes are comparable to unicellular exocrine glands. Their excretory product, the melanomes, contain melanin, a brown biochrome which is not found free but is complexed with the structural proteins or melanomes (melanoprotein). Melanin itself is a dense, insoluble, high-molecular-weight polymer. Tyrosinase, a copper-containing aerobic oxidase, is the enzyme responsible for the conversion of both the naturally occurring amino acid tyrosine to dihydroxyphenylalanine (dopa) and dopa to dopa quinone. These are the initial steps in melanin formation. The presence of tyrosinase is used to identify melanocytes. In ordinary histologic sections, the melanocytes appear as small, clear cells intermixed with the basal cells. The melanocytes are best identified by incubating skin sections in a solution of dopa (Fig. 16-21). Owing to the presence of tyrosinase, melanin is formed and the melanocytes become brown-black. The morphologic characteristics of the melanocytes are best seen in whole mounts of the epidermis stripped from the underlying dermis. Under these circumstances, melanocytes appear as a discontinuous network of dendritic cells whose processes fan out in all directions (Fig. 16-22).

On electron-microscopic examination, the melanocytes are easily distinguished from epidermal cells by the absence of desmosomes and by the presence of their unique cytoplasmic components, melanosomes, wherein melanin is synthesized. Melanocytes have an abundance of ribosomes and rough ER and a prominent Golgi zone, all of which are in keeping with the synthetic role of the cell. Tyrosinase is believed to be synthesized in the ribosomes and then transferred via the rough ER to the Golgi complex where it is packaged within a smooth membrane to form a spherical vacuole. The vacuoles can be identified as early melanosomes (stage I) by the electron-microscopic demonstration of either tyrosinase or filaments or both with a distinctive periodicity of approximately 100 Å. The melanosomes then undergo a series of changes as melanin accumulates (Fig. 16-23). Stage II melanosomes are elliptical organelles measuring, on average, $0.5 \times 0.3 \ \mu m$ (in Caucasian skin). They contain a

distinct internal lamellar organization with a periodicity of approximately 100 Å, but they are not yet melanized. There may or may not be cross-linking of the lamellae of filaments which are oriented along the long axis of the organelle. As electron-dense melanin begins to accumulate in stage III melanosomes, the internal structure is partially obscured. Stage IV melanosomes are electron-opaque; the internal structure is completely obliterated by melanin deposition.

The melanosomes and their contained melanin is excreted through the dendritic processes to the adjacent epidermal cells. The individual melanocyte and its adjacent epidermal cell population, the "epidermal melanin unit," has a ratio of approximately 36 epidermal cells for each melanocyte. Even though the epidermal melanin unit as a whole is responsible for skin color and plays a major role in the protection of the body from ultraviolet radiation, it is the number, size, degree of melanization, and distribution pattern of the melanosomes within the epidermal cells which are of ultimate importance. Melanosomes function by scattering light, absorbing ultraviolet light, and serving as a repository for free radicals formed by the interaction of radiant energy with the cellular components. Four basic biologic processes are distinguished in the normal pigmentation process, and each may be altered in specific diseases (Fig. 16-24). These four factors are

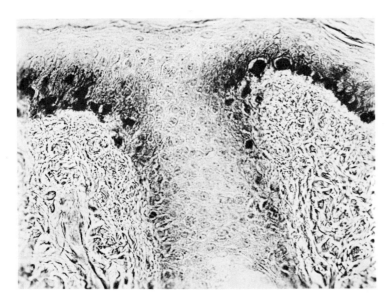

FIGURE 16-21 Thick section of human retroauricular skin. The darkly stained, dendritic melanocytes in the basal layer are demonstrated in this dopa-treated section. The melanocytes are somewhat shrunken and surrounded by a clear halo. ×330. (Courtesy of Dr. G. Szabó, Harvard University.)

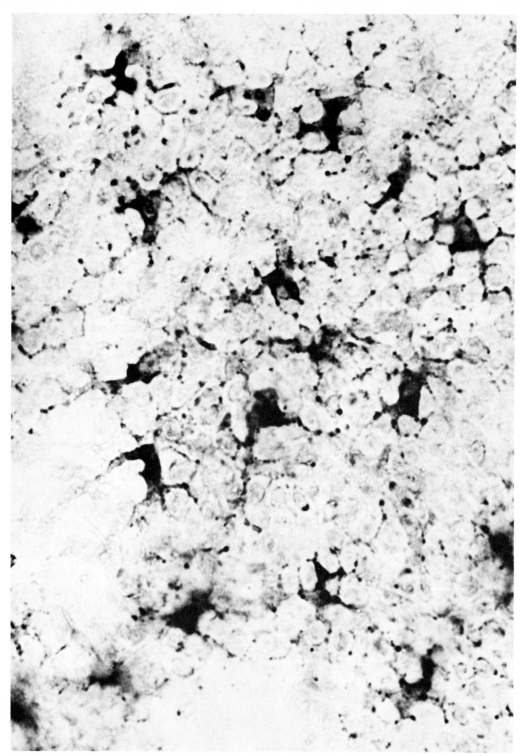

FIGURE 16-22 Epidermal sheet from human thigh skin, prepared by treating the excised skin with trypsin. The epidermal sheet was incubated in dopa. The melanocytes, with many dendritic processes which project between the basal cells of the epidermis, are easily seen. The melanocyte in this location is $720 \pm 45/mm^2$. ×1,000. (Courtesy of Dr. G. Szabó, Harvard University.)

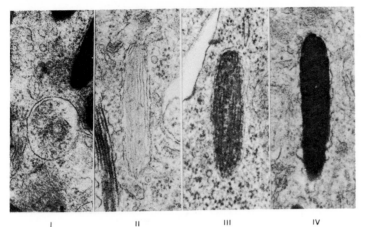

I   II   III   IV

FIGURE 16-23 Stages in melanosome development in melanocytes. The membrane-delineated vesicle can be identified as a melanosome (stage I) if it can be shown to contain tyrosinase or filaments with a distinct periodicity. The stage II melanosome is oval and contains numerous membranous filaments, with or without cross-linking, and with a 100-Å periodicity. In stages III and IV melanosomes, there is progressive accumulation of electron-opaque melanin until all internal structure is obliterated. (From Dermatology in General Medicine, edited by T. B. Fitzpatrick, K. A. Arndt, W. H. Clark, Jr., A. Z. Eisen, E. J. Van Scott, and J. H. Vaughn, copyrighted by McGraw-Hill, Inc., 1971. Published with permission of the publisher and editors.)

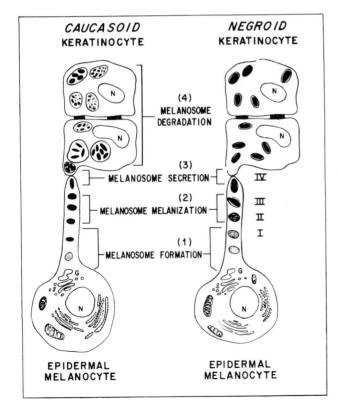

FIGURE 16-24 Four biologic processes underlying melanin pigmentation. These are melanosome formation, melanosome melanization, melanosome secretion, and melanin degradation. In the Caucasoid epidermal cell (keratinocyte), groups of melanosomes are aggregated within membrane-limited lysosome-like organelles and the melanosomes often appear fragmented. In the Negroid epidermal cells, the melanosomes remain discrete (G, Golgi apparatus; N, nucleus). (From Dermatology in General Medicine, edited by T. B. Fitzpatrick, K. A. Arndt, W. H. Clark, Jr., A. Z. Eisen, E. J. Van Scott, and J. H. Vaughn, copyrighted by McGraw-Hill, Inc., 1971. Published with permission of the publisher and editors.)

(1) melanosome formation within the melanocyte; (2) melanization of the melanosomes within the melanocyte; (3) secretion or transfer of the melanosomes within the epidermal cells; and (4) melanin packaging, dispersement, and degradation within the epidermal cells. The first two points have already been discussed. The melanosomes of Caucasoids in general are smaller (0.5 to 0.7 μm $\times$ 0.3 to 0.4 μm) than those with darkly pigmented skin such as African and American blacks and Australian aborigines in whom the melanosomes average 0.8 to 1.0 μm $\times$ 0.4 to 0.5 μm in dimensions (Fig. 16-25). In the melanocytes of Caucasoids, tyrosinase activity is less than in Negroids, and the melanocytes themselves are less pigmented and not as well developed (more stage III melanosomes are present).

The exact mechanism of transfer of the melanosomes to the epidermal cells is not known, but it is believed that under normal circumstances, most of the melanosomes are transferred to basal and suprabasal cells. Ultraviolet exposure will induce epidermal cell proliferation, and it is believed that this proliferation produces the stimulus for increased transfer of melanosomes to the epidermal cells. There may thus be a feedback mechanism controlling pigment transfer.

Within the epidermal cells there are marked differences in the distribution patterns of the melanosomes (Fig. 16-25). In the Negroid, the melanosomes, which as already indicated are larger and more melanized, characteristically remain as single, nonaggregated units throughout the maturation and upward progression of the epidermal cells. In contrast, in Caucasoids, the melanosomes which are smaller and less melanized are aggregated within membrane-limited vesicles (the melanosome complex). These vesicles resemble lysosomal vesicles and as the epidermal cells progress toward the surface, degradation of the melanosomes is likely to occur with the formation of small amorphous grains within the membrane-bound organelles. Melanosome aggregation appears to be a size-dependent phenomenon.

The melanocytes are derivatives of the neural crest and migrate to the skin during embryogenesis by 3 to 4 months of age. Pigmented cells are found in the central nervous system and more importantly in the eye. The melanocytes in these areas produce melanin only during embryonic and possibly early life. On the other hand, the melanocytes in the hair follicles are secretory, although their activity varies with the hair

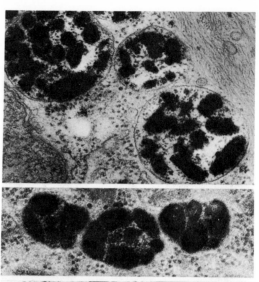

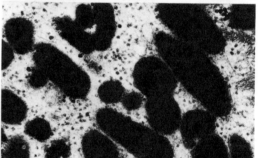

FIGURE 16-25 Melanosome complexes in spinous cells of a Caucasoid, Mongoloid, and Negroid. (a) In the Caucasoid, the melanosomes are grouped in membrane-limited organelles. In addition to stage IV melanosomes, small fragments of melanosomes are present. (b) In the Mongoloid (Chinese), the melanosomes are more densely packed than in the Caucasoid. (c) In the Negroid, almost all the melanosomes are individually dispersed and are larger than those of the Caucasoid or Mongoloid (all $\times$75,000 reduced by 39 percent). (From G. Szabó, A. B. Gerald, M. A. Pathak, and T. B. Fitzpatrick, *Nature,* **222:**1081, 1969, with permission.)

cycle. During telogen, the melanocytes are hard to recognize because they are present as tryosinase-negative "clear cells." Soon after anagen starts, the melanocytes divide and become positive, being filled with melanized melanosomes. As in the epidermis, the melanosomes are transferred to the epithelial cortical cells. Hair color is determined by both the number of melanosomes present in the cells of the hair shaft (black or blond hair) and by chemical alterations of the black melanin pigment eumelanin to cysteine-containing, reddish pheomelanin.

LANGERHANS' CELLS

In the past, Langerhans' cells of the skin have been generally discussed in the section on melanocytes. The basis for this was that these dendritic clear cells, found high in the epidermis, were considered to be related to the melanocytes because of their similarities on a light microscopic level. They were considered to be "effete," or worn-out, melanocytes in the process of being shed during the process of keratinization. This concept is no longer acceptable; the Langerhans cells are now considered to be of mesodermal rather than of ectodermal neural-crest origin. Strong support for a difference of origin of these two types of cells is the finding that Langerhans' cells are found in limbs that have no neural-crest components, whereas melanocytes are not present in such limbs.

On electron-microscopic examination the nuclei of Langerhans' cells are highly convoluted (Fig. 16-26). Their most distinctive characteristic is Langerhans' granules or bodies which are rod or racquet-shaped cytoplasmic organelles (Fig. 16-27). Granules identical in appearance have been found in the infiltrative cells of histiocytosis X. The Langerhans cells, far from being effete, incorporate thymidine and contain abundant active cell organelles (ribosomes, mitochondria, well-defined Golgi zone). Occasionally the Langerhans cells contain materials of lysosomal nature reflecting their mesodermal functions as a macrophage or phagocyte.

DERMIS

The dermis, or corium, is the thick, dense connective tissue layer which extends from the epidermis to the fatty, areolar subcutaneous tissue (Fig. 16-1). It is in this connective tissue stroma that the cutaneous appendages as well as the blood vessels, lymphatics, and nerves are embedded. The dermis can be subdivided into the upper part which is in contact with the epidermis (the *pars papillaris*) and the thicker, denser *pars reticularis*. The papillary layer extends up into the spaces between the epidermal rete ridges (Fig. 16-2). These are the dermal papillae, which are best developed on the palms and soles. Along the border between the epidermis and the dermis there is a PAS-positive layer generally referred to as the *basement membrane*. The collagen fibers of the papillary dermis are arranged in thin bundles in a loose network. In contrast, the collagen of the reticular dermis is arranged in much thicker bundles. Below, the reticular dermis merges along a rather indistinct border with the subcutaneous tissue, an areolar area containing considerable fatty tissue. The connective tissue of the subcutaneous area merges with, and is continuous with, that of underlying tissues.

In addition to collagen fibers the dermis contains a dense network of elastic fibers (Figs. 16-28 and 16-29) that are thinner in the region of the PAS-positive basement membrane (Fig. 16-29). Interspersed between the fibrous components of dermis is the ground substance which contains acidic glycosamino-glycans (hyaluronic acid and chondroitin sulfate). The metachomasia of the glycosaminoglycans is most prominent in the papillary layer near the basement membrane. There are numerous mast cells in the dermis, as well as connective tissue cells such as macrophages and fibroblasts. These cellular components are also more numerous in the papillary dermis.

The blood vessels of the skin are restricted to the dermis. The larger vessels lead to a deep anastomosing network, the cutaneous plexus, from which vessels ascend to the upper dermis where there is another anastomosing network, the subpapillary plexus (Fig. 16-30). Vessels from the deep network supply the fat lobules, the sweat glands, some of the deep sebaceous glands, and the hair bulbs, which are surrounded by a rich network of capillaries. A capillary loop ascends into the dermal papilla of the hair. The capillary bed around the sweat glands is also very well developed. Vessels from the superficial plexus supply vessels for the more superficial portion of the cutaneous appendages. From this same plexus, numerous small vessels ascend into each of the dermal papillae to provide the blood supply for the epidermis (Fig. 16-3), although no vessels actually enter the epidermis.

The venous side of the cutaneous vascular tree is like the arterial supply, with two anastomosing arcades in the superficial and deep dermis. Furthermore, in certain areas such as the tips of the fingers and toes,

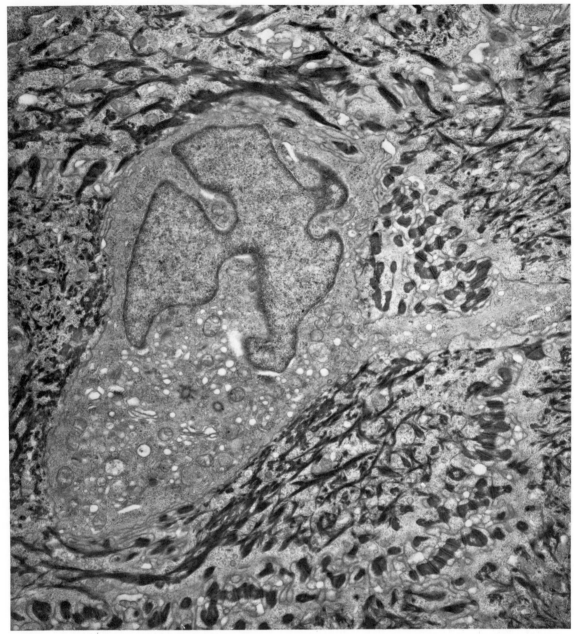

FIGURE 16-26 Electron micrograph of a Langerhans cell. In contrast to the surrounding epidermal cells, there are no desmosomes or tonofilaments. Many mitochondria and Langerhans' bodies are present in the cytoplasm; the nucleus is convoluted. (Courtesy of G. F. Odland; from Clinical Dermatology, edited by D. J. Demis, R. G. Crounse, R. L. Dobson and Joseph S. McGuire, Jr., Harper & Row, Publishers, with permission.)

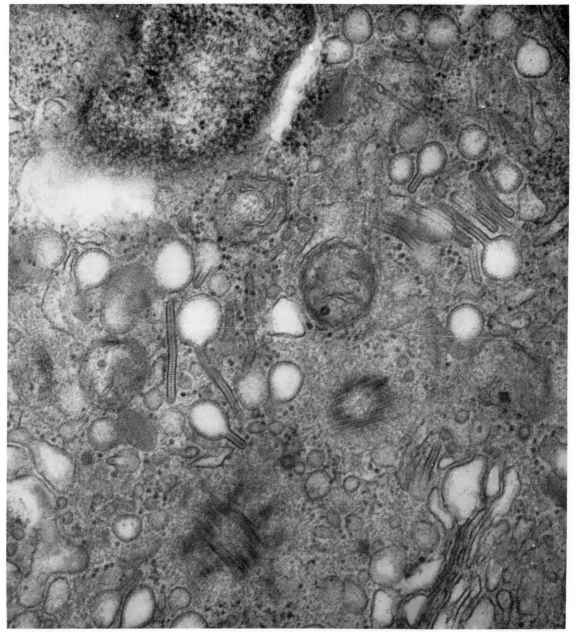

FIGURE 16-27 Higher power electron micrograph of the Langerhans cell in Fig. 16-26. There are many Langerhans' bodies, some of which are indicated by arrows. (Courtesy of G. F. Odland; from Clinical Dermatology, edited by D. J. Demis, R. G. Crounse, R. L. Dobson and Joseph S. McGuire, Jr., Harper & Row, Publishers, with permission.)

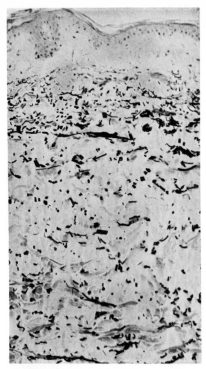

FIGURE 16-28 Verhoeff stain of human abdominal skin. The elastic fibers are darkly stained. The elastic fibers in the pars papillaris are thinner. ×120.

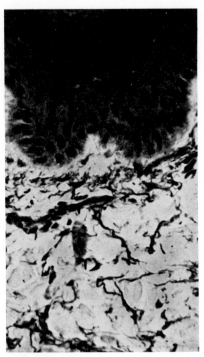

FIGURE 16-29 Verhoeff stain of human skin of the sole. The thin elastic fibers of the pars papillaris are well illustrated. ×350.

there are direct arterial-venous shunts which help to regulate temperature by shunting blood away from the peripheral capillary bed where heat loss occurs through radiation and convection. The condition of the vascular bed, as well as the oxygenation of its contained hemoglobin, is an important determinant of skin color.

The dermis also contains a lymphatic collection system which drains to the regional lymph nodes. It, too, is arranged in a superficial and a deep plexus, corresponding with those of the vascular tree.

The skin, which, is richly provided with nerve fibers, is an important sensory organ. Studies based upon comparative anatomy would indicate that there are specialized nerve endings for touch, pain, and pressure, but the function of such specialized organs in the human being is open to question, and all sensation may depend upon the distribution of free nerve endings, some of which penetrate into the epidermis. Nerve networks are also found around the various cutaneous appendages and the blood vessels. The capillary loops do not contain any nerves, but the nerves of the arteriovenous anastomosis are well developed and obviously extremely important.

THE GLANDS OF THE SKIN

The human skin contains three glandular structures. The *sebaceous glands* produce a lipid end product through a process of holocrine secretion in which the entire differentiated cell, after undergoing lipid differentiation, is discharged into the excretory stream. These glands, as well as the apocrine sweat glands, are an integral part of the pilosebaceous apparatus. *Apocrine sweat glands,* found in specialized areas, secrete a milky material. Although the development of these glands is restricted in humans, phylogenetically they are extremely important glands which produce territorial marking substances and sexual attractants. In contrast, the third type of gland, the *eccrine sweat gland,* is found in only limited areas in lower animals but is distributed over almost the entire body in humans. As humans have lost their hair overcoat, the eccrine sweat glands have assumed an important thermoregulatory role. They develop independently of the other epidermal appendages, all of which are grouped together in the *pilosebaceous unit.*

THE SEBACEOUS GLANDS

In humans, sebaceous glands are found over the entire body surface, except for the palms, soles, and dorsum

FIGURE 16-30 Oblique section of the dorsum of the human toe prepared after India ink injection, demonstrating the subpapillary venous plexus together with some of its tributory capillaries. ×110. (Courtesy of R. K. Winkelmann, S. R. Scheen, R. A. Pyka, and M. B. Coventry, in W. Montagna and R. A. Ellis (eds.), "Blood Vessels and Circulation," Advances in Biology of Skin, vol. 2, Pergamon Press, New York, 1961.)

of the feet. The sebaceous glands are an integral part of the pilosebaceous apparatus and empty into the follicular canal through a short duct. However, in the mucous membranes, they open directly to the surface. Sebaceous glands not associated with hairs may also be found at the mucocutaneous junction. In the eyelids, large sebaceous glands, the *meibomian glands,* are found.

The sebaceous glands are relatively small over most of the body and are usually found in a density of less than 100 per square centimeter of body surface. The glands of certain areas such as the face and scalp are much larger and more numerous, with a density of up to 800 glands per square centimeter. These large

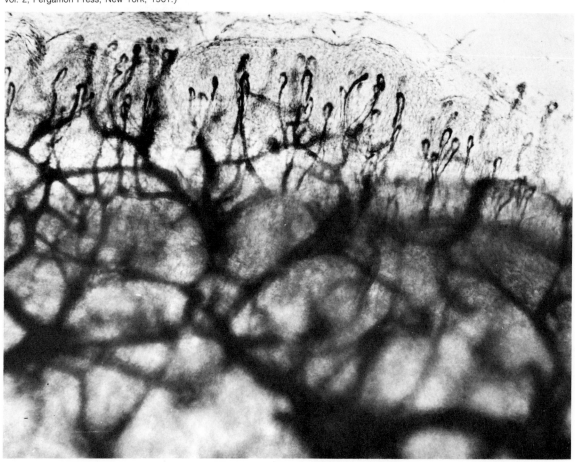

glands are hormone-dependent, being stimulated by androgens, so they make their appearance at the time of puberty, and in elderly individuals they may atrophy. There is no relationship between sebaceous gland size and hair size. The largest glands occur in specialized pilosebaceous units called *sebaceous follicles* which have a small vellus hair and a widely dilated follicular canal. The orifice of such follicles is visible as the "pore" seen on the face.

Regardless of size, all sebaceous glands have the same structure (Fig. 16-31). The duct is a transitional zone between the follicular canal and the lipid-producing cells of the individual sebaceous acinus.

FIGURE 16-31 Sebaceous acinus from the human face. The basal cells (BC) appear as small, dark-staining peripheral cells. As lipid differentiation occurs, the cells enlarge and become foamy. Ruptured cellular remnants appear in the secretory stream (SS) in the region of the sebaceous duct (SD). Dark-staining areas in the center of the acinus are fibrous tissue trabelculae (FT). ×180. (Courtesy of J. S. Strauss and P. E. Pochi, in O. Gans and G. K. Steigleder (eds.), "Normale und Pathologische Anatomie der Haut I," Springer-Verlag, Berlin, 1967.)

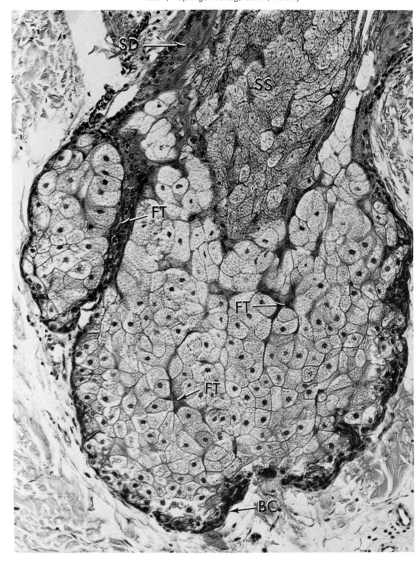

Therefore, although a granular layer is present at the junction with the follicular canal, it disappears below, and there is an abrupt transformation to lipid-producing cells. The outermost cells of the acinus, the basal cells, rest on a basal lamina comparable to that of the epidermis. The basal cells are the germinative cells of the gland. They are small, flattened or cuboidal, and densely basophilic. Usually there is only one layer of basal cells. It may be thrown into folds so that there are invaginations into the center of the acinus. As the cells proceed toward the center of the acinus, there is a progressive accumulation of lipid. The cells become ladened with lipid droplets so their basophilic cytoplasm becomes compressed into a fine reticulated pattern. The cells enlarge greatly, their nuclei become distorted and disintegrate, and eventually the cells rupture, thus forming sebum, the lipid product of the glands.

In the electron microscope three types of cells are demonstrated. The peripheral (basal) cells contain abundant smooth and rough ER, free ribosomes, glycogen particles, mitochondria, and 60- to 80-Å filaments (Fig. 16-32). Filaments are most prominent in the desmosomal regions. A Golgi zone is present, but there are very few lipid droplets in the basal cells. The partially differentiated cell may have a highly convoluted plasma membrane. Its cytoplasm contains more smooth endoplasmic reticulum, and there are membrane-limited lipid droplets of various sizes (Fig. 16-32). It is believed that both the Golgi apparatus and the smooth ER contribute to the formation of lipid droplets.

In the fully differentiated cell the nucleus is irregular in shape, with clumped chromatin, and the nucleolus becomes dispersed (Fig. 16-33). The entire cell is occupied by large lipid droplets which compress the cellular remnants into thin strands that seem to surround the droplets.

Sebum is a complex mixture of lipids, including a large proportion of triglycerides which undergo lipolysis in the follicular canal and liberate free fatty acids. Wax esters and squalene are also prominent in sebum, but there is very little, if any, sterol. However, the lipid recovered from the surface of the skin consists of sebum plus lipids formed by the epidermal cells. Sterols are present in the surface film and they are believed to be of epidermal origin. Lipid collected from the surface of the face, where the glands are large, is predominantly from sebaceous glands, whereas that derived from other areas has a greater percentage of epidermal lipid.

The functions of sebum are not well understood. It has not been shown to be a part of the skin barrier, nor to have any significant role in keeping the skin soft and supple. Although it has some antibacterial and antifungal activity, these effects do not appear to be very significant.

APOCRINE SWEAT GLANDS

Apocrine sweat glands are found over the entire skin surface of many lower animals, but in humans they are restricted to certain areas such as the axilla, the anogenital region, the mammary areola, the ear canal (ceruminous glands), and the eyelid (glands of Moll), with scattered single glands found elsewhere on the body. Apocrine sweat glands are simulated by sexual hormones, and therefore appear at puberty, as do the sebaceous glands.

The apocrine glands are large, branched, tubular structures which open into the upper portion of the follicular canal by a relatively straight duct (Fig. 16-34). In sections containing both eccrine and apocrine glands, the differences are easily recognized. The apocrine glands are large enough to be seen without magnification in excised specimens from gland-rich areas such as the axilla. Their tubules have a single type of eosinophilic secretory cell which may be either cuboidal or columnar and whose nucleus, which is round and contains a prominent nucleolus, is located in the basilar portion of the cell. Secretory droplets accumulate in the more columnar cells and are probably discharged directly into the widely dilated canal. These secretory droplets have been seen by electron microscopy. In the past it has been assumed that the luminal portion of the cell was actually pinched off and discharged ("apocrine secretion"), but this is probably an erroneous concept resulting from a fixation artifact. Myoepithelial cells surround the secretory cells. The duct of these glands is straight and empties into the follicular canal. The ductal portion of the apocrine sweat gland is difficult to distinguish from the eccrine sweat gland duct.

The secretory product of the apocrine sweat gland is a milky product which may contain chromogens. In contrast to eccrine sweat, the secretory product contains protein. The apocrine glands respond to stimuli such as fright and pain but not to heat. Apocrine sweating is a two-phase process. The secretory

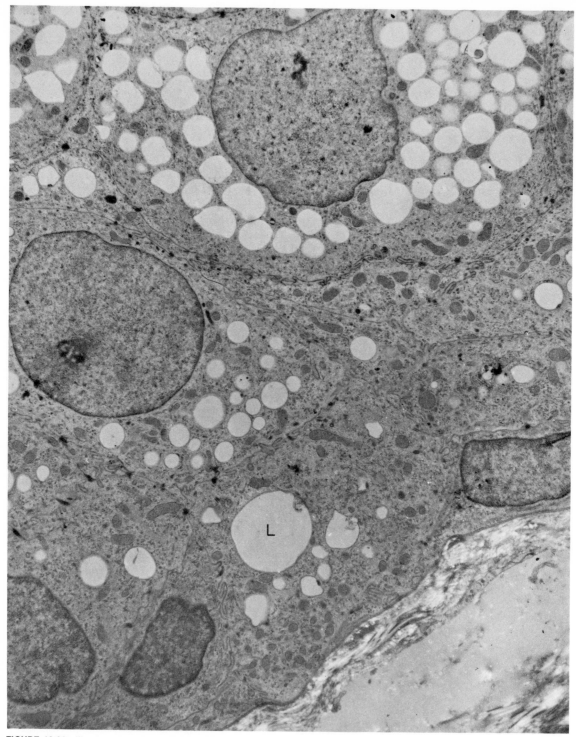

FIGURE 16-32 Electron micrograph showing peripheral and differentiating cells of the sebaceous gland. A portion of the dermis is present in the lower part of the picture. The peripheral cells contain ER, ribosomes, mitochondria, filaments, and a few lipid droplets (L). Lipid droplets are larger and more numerous in the innermost cells. ×7,300. (Courtesy of Dr. R. M. Lavker.)

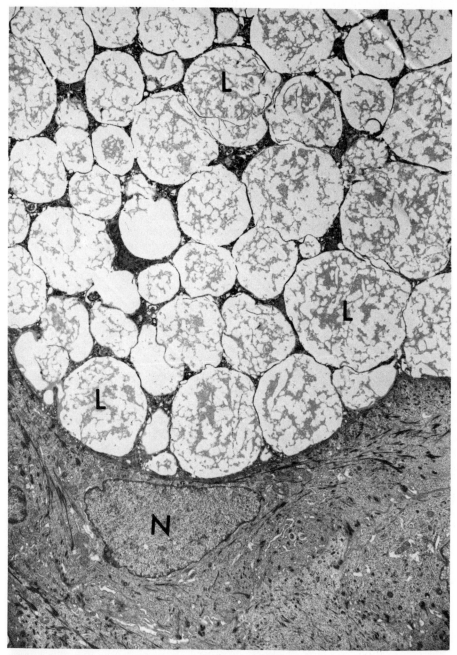

FIGURE 16-33 Electron micrograph of a fully differentiated sebaceous cell in the region of the sebaceous duct. The duct cell is darkly stained with a prominent nucleus (N). Lipid droplets (L) completely fill the differentiated cell. ×3,400. (Courtesy of J. S. Strauss and P. E. Pochi, in O. Gans G. K. Steigleder (eds.), ''Normale und Pathologische Anatomie der Hautasl,'' Springer-Verlag, Berlin, 1967.)

cells secrete their product into the tubular canal, which has a relatively large storage capacity. Then upon adrenergic stimulation, the myoepithelium contracts and forces the contents of the tubule to the surface. There then follows a refractory period of up to 48 h until enough sweat can accumulate for the myoepithelium to force to the surface. Apocrine sweat is odorless on secretion but becomes odoriferous when acted upon by cutaneous bacteria. Although modern society has attached an undesirable quality to this odor, apocrine sweat was extremely important in lower animals as a sex attractor and territorial marker.

ECCRINE SWEAT GLANDS

The eccrine sweat glands are the most important cutaneous glands and the only ones with a known function in humans. They are not connected with the pilosebaceous apparatus; they open directly onto the skin surface by a corkscrewlike duct. The eccrine sweat glands are distributed over the entire body surface except for the lips, the glans penis, the inner surface of the prepuce, the clitoris, and the labia minora. They are most dense on the palms and soles, where their tiny ducts are visible under low magnification on the peaks of the dermatoglyphic ridges. The sweat ducts enter the epidermis at the base of the rete ridges. Sweat gland density is less in the adult than in the

child because there is no neogenesis after birth; and as the skin expands, the glands are spread farther apart. Estimates of the number of sweat glands range from 2 to 5 million per person.

The secretory tubule of the eccrine sweat gland is usually unbranched and has a relatively narrow lumen (Fig. 16-35). There are three types of cells in the sweat gland tubule. Around the periphery of the secretory tubule is a layer of myoepithelial cells which rests on the basement lamella. These are spindle-shaped cells which are arranged parallel to the tubule and do not form a complete envelope for the sweat coil. The secretory cells of the eccrine glands are of two types. Most obvious are the large *clear cells* which appear to rest both on the myoepithelial cells and directly on the basement lamella between these cells. The broad base of the clear cells is on the outside of the tubule and their luminal border is narrow. These cells have an acidophilic cytoplasm. Interspersed between these clear cells are the smaller *dark cells* which have basophilic cytoplasm and an inverted pyramidal shape with the broad base on the luminal surface.

Electron microscopy has clarified the functional properties of these two cell types. The clear cells contain abundant mitochondria, glycogen particles, and considerable smooth ER (Fig. 16-36). Between adjacent clear cells there are well-developed canaliculi which open into the lumen of the tubule. These cells resemble other types of serous secretory cells, such as those found in lacrimal or salivary glands, and are therefore probably responsible for the watery sweat.

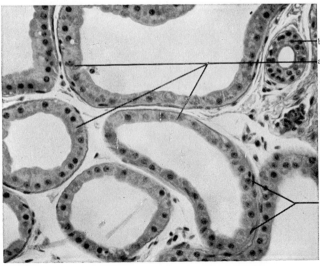

FIGURE 16-34 Apocrine glands from the axilla of adult human being. In addition to the large secretory acini (a) containing cells of varying height, a portion of the small duct (b) is included. The elongated nuclei (c) of the myoepithelial cells can be visualized along the periphery of the secretory cells. ×200.

Indirect evidence for such a function is provided by the depletion of glycogen particles in the clear cells on prolonged sweating, as well as by the observation of eccrine sweating in species that contain no dark cells.

Electron microscopy of the dark cells shows that they are filled with electron-dense vacuoles which are believed to be made up of mucin, and these cells are assumed to secrete mucopolysaccharide. They have fewer mitochondria than the clear cells, whereas the rough ER is comparable. Their luminal surface is made up of a large number of microvilli. The secretory tubule forms approximately half of the sweat gland unit. The duct forms approximately half of the sweat gland unit. The duct is easily distinguished from the secretory portion of the ductal coil by its double row of cells, the lack of a myoepithelium, and the acidophilic luminal coating material, which may be the mucopolysaccharide produced by the dark cells.

Eccrine sweat glands are innervated by postganglionic sympathetic nerve fibers, but under physiologic conditions the glands primarily respond to cholinergic stimuli. Eccrine sweating can also be stimulated by

adrenergic drugs, but this sweat has a different composition from sweat resulting from thermal stimulation. The sweat glands play a significant role in thermal regulation. Heat prostration or heat stroke is prone to occur in an individual with a congenital lack of sweat glands or blockage of the sweat glands through disease. Whenever convection and radiation heat loss from vascular changes are inadequate to maintain thermal homeostasis, the sweat glands are recruited to produce sweat for evaporative heat loss.

There are many factors that influence the composition of sweat, so no absolute composition can be easily defined. Sweat is a hypotonic solution derived from plasma. Its major cation, sodium, is transported into the canaliculi between the clear cells by an active sodium pump, and water is then passively transferred to restore the isotonicity of sweat. Sweat becomes hypotonic due to the reabsorption of sodium in the sweat duct. Sweat also contains chloride, potassium, urea, and lactate. Its composition may change profoundly in disease states. For instance, the increase in sodium concentration in cystic fibrosis is a reliable test for the disease, and sweat-sodium studies have been

FIGURE 16-35 Human sweat gland from the abdominal skin. Both the coiled portion of the sweat duct (a) and the secretory portion (b) are present. The secretory portion is much smaller than that of the apocrine sweat gland shown in the same magnification in Fig. 16-34. ×200.

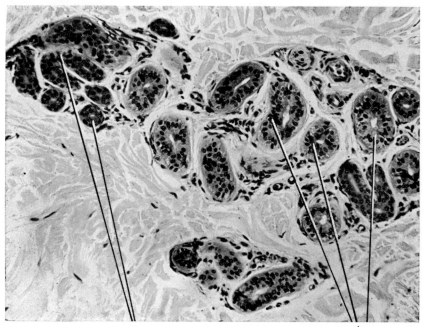

a   b

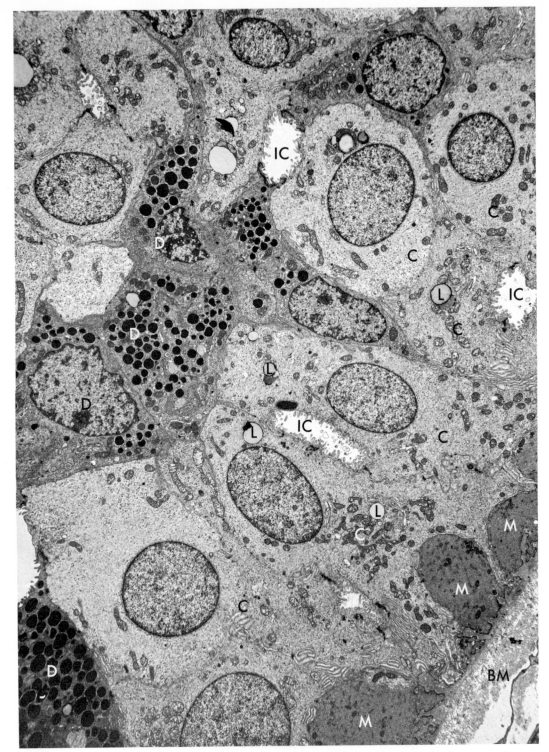

FIGURE 16-36 Electron micrograph of a portion of the secretory coil of an eccrine sweat gland. Three types of cells are present: myoepithelial (M), clear (C), and dark (D). The myoepithelial cells rest on the basement membrane (BM). Intercellular canaliculi (IC) are prominent between clear cells, and several of the clear cells have lipid inclusions (L). The dark cells contain dense secretory granules. ×48,000. (Courtesy of R. E. Ellis, in A. S. Zelickson (ed.), "Ultrastructure of Normal and Abnormal Skin," Lea & Febiger, Philadelphia, 1967.)

an important tool in family studies. Drugs such as desoxycorticosterone or corticotropin will influence sweat composition, and as an adaptive measure, the sweat sodium decreases during protracted heat exposure, a phenomenon called *acclimatization*. It is thus obvious that the sweat gland is well adapted for its role in maintaining the body temperature within normal limits on heat exposure. Humans, with their large number of eccrine glands, make use of the evaporative water loss from a large area of nonhairy skin. In contrast, animals such as dogs have eccrine sweat glands restricted to the paw pads. Since their skin is well insulated by fur, and eccrine glands are restricted to an area from which evaporative water loss is difficult, their thermal regulation depends upon respiratory heat loss, and they pant when they are hot.

REFERENCES

General

BUTCHER, E. O., and R. F. SOGNNAES (eds.): "Fundamentals of Keratinization," American Association for Advancement of Science, Washington, D.C., Publ. 70, 1962.

GANS, O., and G. K. STEIGLEDER (eds.): "Normale und Pathologische Anatomie der Haut I," Springer-Verlag, Berlin, 1969.

LYNE, A. G., and B. F. SHORT (eds.): "Biology of the Skin and Hair Growth," Angus and Robertson, Sydney, 1965.

MONTAGNA, W., and P. F. PARAKKAL: "The Structure and Function of Skin," 3d ed., Academic Press, Inc., New York, 1974.

MONTAGNA, W., and W. C. LOBITZ, JR. (eds.): "The Epidermis," Academic Press, Inc., New York, 1964.

ZELICKSON, A. S. (ed.): "Ultrastructure of Normal and Abnormal Skin," Lea & Febiger, Philadelphia, 1967.

Epidermis

ELIAS, M. E., and D. S. FRIEND: The Permeability Barrier in Mammalian Epidermis, *J. Cell Biol.*, **65:**180 (1975).

LAVKER, R. M., and A. G. MATOLTSY: Formation of Horny Cells, *J. Cell Biol.*, **44:**501 (1970).

MATOLTSY, A. G.: Desmosomes, Filaments and Keratohyalin Granules; Their Role in the Stabilization and Keratinization of the Epidermis, *J. Invest. Dermatol.*, **65:**127 (1975).

MATOLTSY, A. G., and M. N. MATOLTSY: The Chemical Nature of Keratohyalin Granules of the Epidermis, *J. Cell Biol.*, **47:**593 (1970).

MATOLTSY, A. G., and P. F. PARAKKAL: Keratinization, in A. S. Zelickson (ed.), "Ultrastructure of Normal and Abnormal Skin," Lea & Febiger, Philadelphia, 1967.

ODLAND, G. F., and T. H. REED: Epidermis, in A. S. Zelickson (ed.), "Ultrastructure of Normal and Abnormal Skin," Lea & Febiger, Philadelphia, 1967.

Nail

ZAIAS, N., and J. ALVAREZ: The Formation of the Primate Nail Plate, *J. Invest. Derm.*, **51:**120 (1968).

Hair

PARAKKAL, P. F.: The Fine Structure of Anagen Hair Follicle of the Mouse, in W. Montagna and R. L. Dobson (eds.), "Advances in Biology of Skin," vol. 9, Pergamon Press, Oxford, 1969.

RHODIN, J. A. G., and E. J. REITH: Ultrastructure of Keratin in Oral Mucosa, Skin, Esophagus, Claw and Hair, in E. O. Butcher and R. F. Sognnaes (eds.), "Fundamentals of Keratinization," American Association for the Advancement of Science, Washington, D.C., Publ. 70, 1962.

Melanocytes

JIMBOW, K., and A. KUKITA: Fine Structure of Pigment Granules in the Human Hair Bulb, in T. Kawamura, T. B. Fitzpatrick, and M. Seiji (eds.), "Biology of Normal and Abnormal Melanocytes," University Park Press, Baltimore, 1971.

MONTAGNA, W., and F. HU (eds.): "The Pigmentary System," Advances in Biology of Skin, vol. 8, Pergamon Press, Oxford, 1967.

SEIJI, M.: Melanogenesis, in A. S. Zelickson (ed.), "Ultrastructure of Normal and Abnormal Skin," Lea & Febiger, Philadelphia, 1967.

SEIJI, M. K., K. SHIMAO, M. S. C. BIRBECK, and T. B. FITZPATRICK: Subcellular Localization of Melanin Biosynthesis, *Ann. N.Y. Acad. Sci.,* **100:**497 (1963).

SZABÓ, G.: The Biology of the Pigment Cell, in E. B. Bittar and N. Bittar (eds.), "The Biological Basis of Medicine," vol. 6, Academic Press, Inc., New York, 1969.

ZELICKSON, A. S.: Melanocyte, Melanin Granule, and Langerhans Cell, in A. S. Zelickson (ed.), "Ultrastructure of Normal and Abnormal Skin," Lea & Febiger, Philadelphia, 1967.

Dermis

MONTAGNA, W., J. P. BENTLEY, and R. L. DOBSON (eds.): "The Dermis," Advances in Biology of Skin, vol. 10. Appleton Century Crofts, New York, 1970.

Blood Vessels

MONTAGNA, W., and R. A. ELLIS (eds.): "Blood Vessels and Circulation," Advances in Biology of Skin, vol. 2, Pergamon Press, New York, 1961.

MORETTI, G.: The Blood Vessels of the Skin, in O. Gans and G. K. Steigleder (eds.), "Normale und Pathologische Anatomie der Haut I," Springer-Verlag, Berlin, 1969.

Nerves

MONTAGNA, W. (ed.): "Cutaneous Innervation," Advances in Biology of Skin, vol. 1, Pergamon Press, New York, 1960.

Sebaceous Glands

ELLIS, R. A.: Eccrine, Sebaceous and Apocrine Glands, in A. S. Zelickson (ed.), "Ultrastructure of Normal and Abnormal Skin," Lea & Febiger, Philadelphia, 1967.

MONTAGNA, W., R. A. ELLIS, and A. F. SILVER (eds.): "The Sebaceous Glands," Advances in Biology of Skin, vol. 4, Pergamon Press, Oxford, 1963.

STRAUSS, J. S., and P. E. POCHI: Histology, Histochemistry, and Electron Microscopy of Sebaceous Glands in Man, in O. Gans and G. K. Steigleder (eds.), "Normale und Pathologische Anatomie der Haut I," Springer-Verlag, Berlin, 1969.

Apocrine Sweat Glands

ELLIS, R. A.: Eccrine, Sebaceous and Apocrine Glands, in A. S. Zelickson (ed.), "Ultrastructure of Normal and Abnormal Skin," Lea & Febiger, Philadelphia, 1967.

HURLEY, H. J., and W. B. SHELLEY: "The Human Apocrine Sweat Gland in Health and Disease," Charles C Thomas, Springfield, Ill., 1960.

Eccrine Sweat Glands

ELLIS, R. A.: Eccrine, Sebaceous and Apocrine Glands, in A. S. Zelickson (ed.), "Ultrastructure of Normal and Abnormal Skin," Lea & Febiger, Philadelphia, 1967.

ELLIS, R. A.: Eccrine Sweat Glands: Electron Microscopy, Cytochemistry and Anatomy in O. Gans and G. K. Steigleder (eds.), "Normale und Pathologische Anatomie der Haut I," Springer-Verlag, Berlin, 1969.

KUNO, Y.: "Human Perspiration," Charles C Thomas, Springfield, Ill., 1956.

MONTAGNA, W., R. A. ELLIS, and A. F. SILVER (eds.): "Eccrine Sweat Glands and Eccrine Sweating," Advances in Biology of Skin, vol. 3, Pergamon Press, New York, 1962.

WEINER, J. S., and K. HELLMAN: The Sweat Glands, *Biol. Rev.,* **35:**141 (1960).

Teeth

ROBERT M. FRANK AND REIDAR F. SOGNNAES

THE WHOLE TOOTH

A tooth consists of three parts: crown, neck, and root, seated in bone (Fig. 17-1). The clinical *crown* is the portion that projects above the *gingiva* (or gum); the *root* is the part inserted in the alveolus or socket in the bone of the jaw; and the *neck* is the point of junction between the root and the crown. These hard portions surround a dental chamber which contains the *pulp,* a jellylike type of connective tissue. The chamber extends through the root canal to the root apex, where it opens to the exterior of the tooth at the apical foramen. The solid portion of the tooth consists of three calcified substances: the *dentin* (or ivory), the *enamel,* and the *cementum.* Of these, the dentin is the most abundant. It forms a broad layer around the pulp chamber and root canal and it is interrupted only at the apical foramen. Nowhere does the dentin reach the outer surface. In the crown it is covered with enamel; in the root it is enclosed by cementum. The enamel is thickest at the cusp tips, whereas the cementum is thickest at the root apex. Both tissues thin toward the neck where they join in a variable manner. The cementum, and with it the tooth, is attached to the bony socket by the *periodontal ligament,* a connective tissue membrane, which is continuous with the connective tissue of the gingiva. Together these three structures—the cementum, periodontal ligament, and gingiva—serve as the supporting tissues of the tooth. The dental hard tissues, like bone, consist of a densely mineralized organic matrix. Embryologically, the dentin, cementum, pulp, and periodontal ligament of the teeth come from the mesoderm, like bone and other connective tissues, whereas the enamel is a highly specialized ectodermal structure.

BEGINNING TOOTH DEVELOPMENT

Tooth development involves a long process of growth and calcification before the teeth erupt to function in the mouth. The first indication of tooth development is a thickening of the oral epithelium, which has been observed in 6- to 7-week-old human embryos. At this stage the tongue is well developed, but the upper and lower lips are not yet separated by depressions from the structures within the mouth. Although the oral plate, which marks the boundary between oral ectoderm and pharyngeal entoderm, has wholly disappeared, it is evident that this thickening takes place in the oral ectoderm. Soon after its formation, this epithelially derived plate grows into the subjacent mesenchymal tissues following the parabolic curvature of each jaw. The invaginated epithelium undergoes the same type of transformation in both the maxilla and mandible, and the following description of the conditions in the mandible is therefore applicable to both. As the plate descends into the mesenchyme, it divides into two parts. In front, the *labial lamina separates* the lip from the gum. Behind, the *dental lamina* (Fig. 17-2) produces the teeth. Taken as a whole, the dental lamina is a crescentic plate of cells following the line of the gingiva, along which the teeth will later appear. In Fig.

17-2A to D each drawing represents diagrammatically a part of the oral epithelium above and dental lamina below, free from the surrounding mesenchyme. The labial side is toward the left and the lingual side toward the right. Almost as soon as the dental lamina has formed, it produces a series of inverted cup-shaped enlargements along the labial surface (Fig. 17-2B). These become the *enamel organs* (Fig. 17-3).

ENAMEL ORGANS OF DECIDUOUS AND PERMANENT TEETH

There is a separate enamel organ for each of the 10 *deciduous*, or *milk*, *teeth* in each jaw, and they are all present in embryos of $2\frac{1}{2}$ months. The enamel organs not only produce the enamel but subsequently extend over the roots as an epithelial sheath (Hertwig's sheath). The tissue enclosed by the enamel organ is a denser mesenchyme, constituting the dental papilla (Fig. 17-3). This is the primordium of the pulp of the tooth, and it produces at its periphery the bulk of the tooth substance, the layer of *dentin*. An epithelial-mesenchymal tissue interaction is evidently very important in *odontogenesis*. Experiments with mouse embryos have been conducted by recombining isolated dental papilla mesenchyme from incisors and molars with epithelium isolated from nonoral sites within the embryo. As reviewed by Slavkin, such investigations clearly demonstrate the inductive instructive role of the dental papilla mesenchyme.

FIGURE 17-1 Section of a tooth with its supporting tissues in position in the jaw bone.

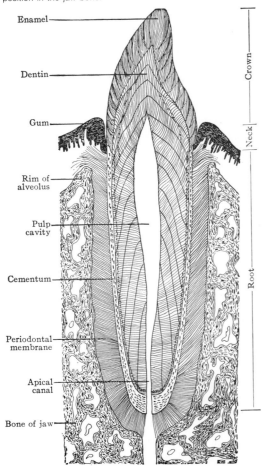

FIGURE 17-2 The dental lamina (A) and the early development of three teeth (B–D). The anterior tooth is shown in vertical section.

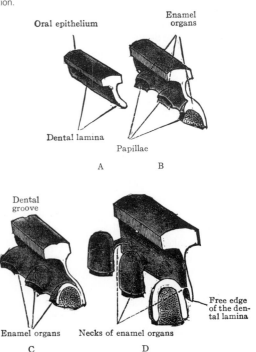

As the tooth develops, the connection between its enamel organ and the dental lamina becomes reduced to a flattened strand of epithelial tissue, which subsequently disintegrates.

The *permanent teeth,* 16 in each jaw, develop similarly. The dental lamina grows backward to produce enamel organs for the three permanent molars, which develop behind the deciduous teeth on each side of the jaws. The enamel organ for the first permanent molar forms at about the seventeeth week of fetal life; the enamel organ for the second molar forms about half a year after birth, and that for the third molar (wisdom tooth) at 5 years.

The permanent teeth anterior to the permanent molars (that is, *incisors, canines,* and *premolars*) develop from enamel organs of the deep portion of the dental lamina. Owing to the obliquity of the lamina, the permanent teeth are on the lingual side of the deciduous teeth. The enamel organs for the incisors

develop slightly before those for the canines, but all these are discernible in a 24-week fetus. Between the canines and molars there are two premolars in each quadrant of the jaw. The enamel organs for the first premolars develop in the eighth month. Each permanent tooth anterior to the molars undergoes a complicated series of spatial changes during its development. Between 6 and 12 years, when the deciduous teeth are being shed one after another, the bony partitions are resorbed together with the roots of the deciduous teeth (Fig. 17-4). It is interesting that the resorption of all the dental hard tissues is accompanied, as in bone, by the appearance of osteoclastlike cells in Howship's lacunas. After the deciduous teeth are shed, entirely new alveolar bone and other investing tissues are produced for the support of the permanent teeth (Fig. 17-4).

The portion of the dental lamina not used in producing enamel organs normally disintegrates, but epithelial remnants may occasionally develop abnormally, forming cysts and tumors (ameloblastomas).

FIGURE 17-3 The enamel organ. This projection drawing (×50) of parasagittal section passes through the primordium of a lower incisor of a fourteenth-week human embryo. On the lower left the small sketch indicates the jaw relations of the area represented. (From B. M. Pattern, ''Human Embryology''; embryo of 104-mm C-R length, University of Michigan Collection.)

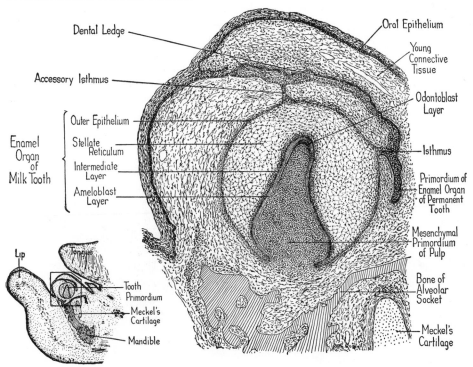

FORMATION AND STRUCTURE OF DENTAL TISSUES

Tooth formation is initiated by the inner development of a thin layer of coronal dentin, followed by outer deposition of enamel. The extracellular formation of the organic matrices of both tissues is under the control of cellular secretion. The odontoblasts, of mesenchymal origin, will secrete a collageneous matrix, called the *predentin,* which undergoes calcification secondarily. Dentin formation is the result of rhythmic incremental development. The epithelial ameloblasts secrete an organic matrix with special biochemical properties which begins to calcify as soon as it is deposited extracellularly.

However, odontogenesis is not a simultaneous event throughout the tooth. The first dentin and enamel formation begins at the tips of cusps of multicusped teeth or the uppermost portions of unicusped teeth. Following completion of the crown, root formation begins. Here the epithelial root sheath induces radicular pulpal cells to become odontoblasts: following root dentin formation, the adjacent mesodermal connective tissue cells are induced to become cementoblasts and to form cementum.

ENAMEL

The internal cells of the enamel organ (see Fig. 17-3) are at first in close contact, like those of ordinary epithelium; after further differentiation and through an accumulation of viscous intercellular substance, they constitute a reticulum which resembles mesenchyme and is known as the *stellate reticulum* (Figs. 17-3 and 17-5A, see color insert). Toward the oral cavity the stellate reticulum is bounded by the outer enamel epithelium, a single layer of cuboidal cells; toward the dental papilla it is bounded by the inner enamel epithelium, the cells of which elongate and become the enamel-producing ameloblasts. These tall cells are separated from the stellate cells by a layer of flattened cells, the *stratum intermedium* (Fig. 17-6). A basement membrane limits the outer and inner enamel epithelium from the surrounding mesenchymal tissues.

Histochemical reactions reveal that the enamel epithelium first secretes a mucopolysaccharide, forming the ground substance of the stellate reticulum (Fig. 17-5A, see color insert); later, after reversing the polarity of its cells, the inner enamel epithelium, transformed into ameloblasts, will secrete the organic matrix of enamel which gives reaction for sulfhydryl groups (Fig. 17-5D, see color insert). The cells of the stellate reticulum are rich in glycogen and alkaline phosphatase, and the ground substance between them is markedly metachromatic, but is not stained by the periodic acid—Schiff procedure. It is destroyed by

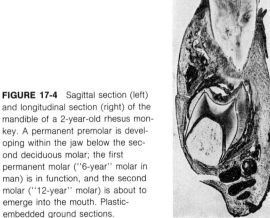
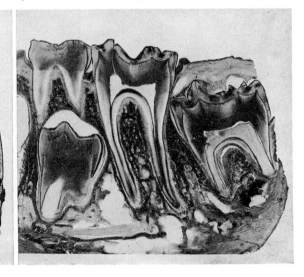

FIGURE 17-4 Sagittal section (left) and longitudinal section (right) of the mandible of a 2-year-old rhesus monkey. A permanent premolar is developing within the jaw below the second deciduous molar; the first permanent molar ("6-year" molar in man) is in function, and the second molar ("12-year" molar) is about to emerge into the mouth. Plastic-embedded ground sections.

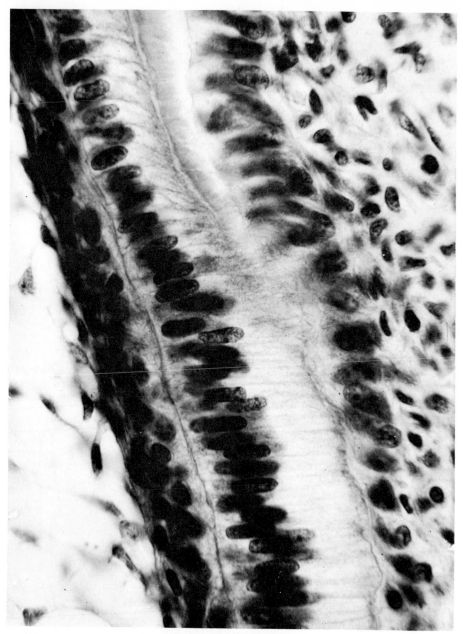

FIGURE 17-6 Enamel- and dentin-forming cells of the enamel organ. Left to right there are the stellate reticulum, stratum intermedium, inner enamel epithelium, odontoblasts, and pulpal cells. Note the cytomorphologic changes in functionally maturing ameloblasts (left) and odontoblasts (right): The ameloblasts decrease in height, while the odontoblasts become columnar as dentin and enamel formation begins at the upper half of the figure.

hyaluronidase and has no metachromatic antecedent visible in its constituent cells. An intense alkaline phosphatase reaction has been demonstrated in the stratum intermedium as well as in the ameloblasts.

The ameloblasts produce enamel along their distal surfaces (Figs. 17-7 and 17-8). These tall cells, which are directed toward the dental papilla, have

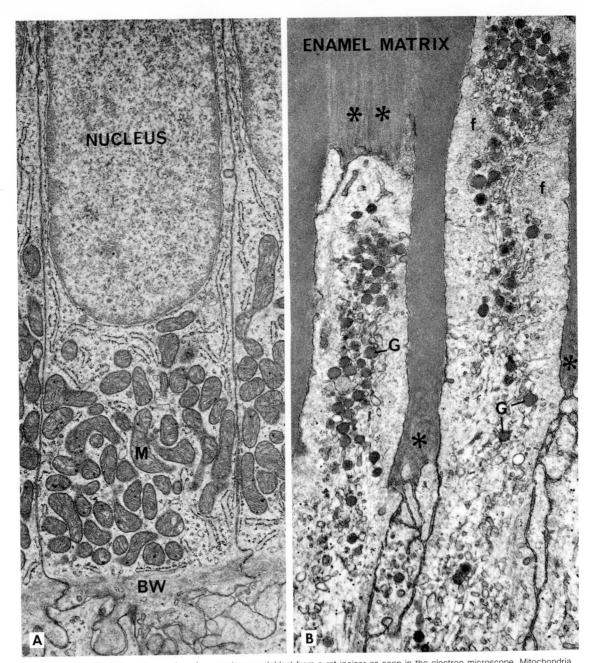

FIGURE 17-7 A. The infranuclear region of a secretory ameloblast from a rat incisor as seen in the electron microscope. Mitochondria (M) with dense matrices, characteristic of this cell type, abound within the infranuclear cytoplasm. Also present are scattered elements of rough endoplasmic reticulum, the flattened profiles of which may be seen distributed between the mitochondria and adjacent to the lateral cell membrane. A prominent basal web (BW) composed of densely packed microfilaments is located at the base of the cell. ×15,000. (Courtesy of Alfred Weinstock, University of California, Los Angeles). B. An electron micrograph of the apical (Tomes's) processes of two ameloblasts from a rat incisor showing their architecture and relationship to the enamel matrix. Each process is limited by a plasma membrane which is closely applied to the matrix. The *distal* portion (upper two-thirds of micrograph) is embedded within the matrix. Secretory granules (G), each delimited by a unit membrane, abound within the central core of cytoplasm in association with microtubules and smooth vesicular or tubular elements. This core is usually ensheathed by a feltwork of fine filaments (f) which extends to the plasma membrane. The *proximal* portion of each process (lower one-third of micrograph) is not embedded in matrix and contains scattered secretory granules. Although the enamel matrix appears relatively homogeneous at this magnification, it shows an arrangement of parallel lines in two regions; (1) the matrix abutting the distal end of each process (**, upper left), and (2) at the proximal ends of the prongs of matrix (*) projecting between the processes. This striated matrix, lying opposite the secretory zones, represents the most recently deposited matrix and corresponds to the so-called growth regions of enamel. ×21,000. (From A. Weinstock, and C. P. Leblond, *J. Cell Biol.,* **51:**26, 1971.)

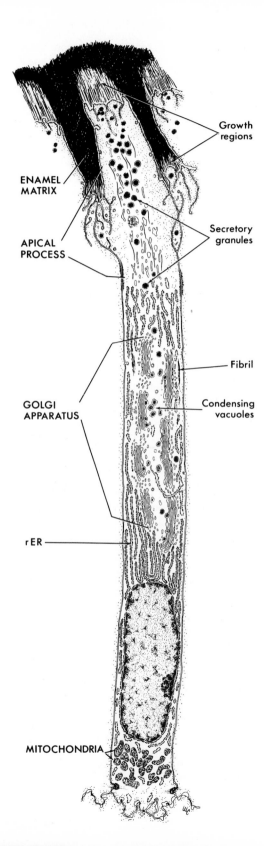

ENAMEL
MATRIX

APICAL
PROCESS

GOLGI
APPARATUS

r ER

MITOCHONDRIA

Growth
regions

Secretory
granules

Fibril

Condensing
vacuoles

their nuclei nearer the stellate reticulum. The Golgi apparatus, which was originally on the side of the nucleus toward the stellate reticulum, shifts to the opposite position. At the stage of active matrix formation, the Golgi apparatus becomes highly developed, as does the rough endoplasmic reticulum. The cytoplasm is rich in ribosomes, microfilaments, and microtubules. The ameloblasts are initially separated from the odontoblasts by a basement membrane, but as soon as the first layer of dentin has calcified, this membrane disappears.

At the apical surface of each ameloblast, a tapering projection known as the *Tomes process* develops. A great concentration of round secretory granules accumulate within the Tomes process. These secretory granules are elaborated in the Golgi apparatus and migrate to the distal end of the cell. Electron-microscopic autoradiography suggests that the material in the secretory granules is released in the extracellular space without any discontinuity of the cell membrane and that an important part of the enamel matrix precursors are secreted through these granules. The precursors contain proteins and glycoproteins.

Autoradiography involving both light and electron microscopy have shown that ^{45}Ca can be directly transferred to enamel through the extracellular spaces. Though a transcellular pathway through the ameloblast is also possible, this intracellular transfer does not appear to be associated with the secretory ameloblastic bodies. The mitochondria, the endoplasmic reticulum, and the Golgi apparatus are the organelles most highly labeled with ^{45}Ca.

During the different phases of enamel development, the ameloblasts assume multiple functions of

FIGURE 17-8 Diagrammatic representation of the structure of a whole secretory ameloblast (combining Fig. 17-7A and B), from the region of enamel matrix secretion in a rat maxillary incisor. Mitochondria are grouped in the infranuclear region between the basal web and the nucleus. The supranuclear region contains the elongated, tubular-shaped Golgi apparatus which is surrounded on all sides by the rough endoplasmic reticulum (rER). Within the central core of cytoplasm demarcated by the Golgi saccules are condensing vacuoles and a few secretory granules. The apical (Tomes) process extends apically from the terminal web, and its distal portion is embedded in the enamel matrix. Secretory granules abound within its central core. The growth regions represent the most recently deposited matrix. (From A. Weinstock and C. P. Leblond, *J. Cell Biol.*, **51:**26, 1971).

secretion, absorption, and transfer. Biochemically the organic matrix of developing enamel undergoes marked changes, notably a loss in proteins and a change in the amino acid composition. Histochemical studies have indicated the presence in the ameloblast of several lysosomal enzymes and have suggested the presence of an acid phosphatase activity in the highly developed Golgi complex and perhaps in the secretory granules.

The enamel is built up layer by layer. Its formation begins at the top of the crown of each tooth and spreads downward over its sides. If the tooth has several cusps, a cap of enamel forms over each, and these caps coalesce. As soon as the enamel matrix is deposited extracellularly, it starts to calcify, forming enamel rods or prisms approximately 5 μm thick, bounded by zones classically described as rod or prism sheaths (Fig. 17-5E, see color insert) and interrod or interprismatic substance (Figs. 17-9 and 17-10A). Ini-

tially, the prism sheath appears as a thin, noncalcified area filled with organic material and limited by apatite crystals of the prism and the interprismatic substance. With advancing calcification, the prism sheath shrinks, and in the adult enamel, it is practically reduced to a submicroscopic space recognizable by the fact that the limiting apatite crystals on both sides have a different orientation. As enamel increases in thickness, the ameloblasts migrate outward. To accommodate themselves to the greater area of the outer surface of the enamel, the prisms become slightly broader as they develop radially. By the time the tooth is ready to erupt, the enamel organ has ceased to function and is a much reduced structure. When the tooth is functioning, the worn surfaces of enamel become covered by a thin organic layer called the *acquired pellicle*, which comes from saliva.

The fully calcified enamel is the hardest substance

FIGURE 17-9 Transverse section through human fetal enamel rods (R). Note the arcade-shaped form of the peripheral rod sheath areas (S). The rods are continuous with the interrod substance (IP) on one side. ×14,000.

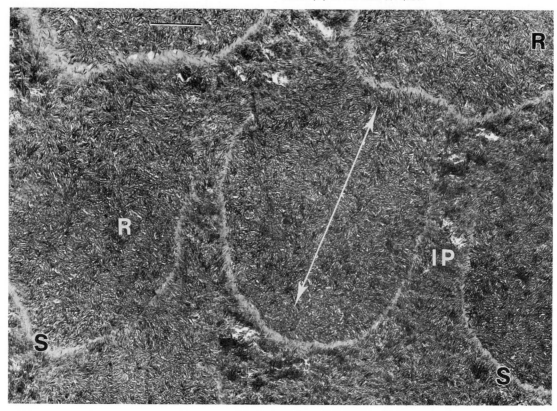

in the body. Both the prisms and the interprismatic substance are calcified and contain from 96 to 98 percent inorganic material, 90 percent of which is hydroxyapatite. Amorphous calcium phosphates have also been observed. Traces of calcium carbonate, acid magnesium phosphate, calcium fluoride, and other salts form the remainder. Enamel contains no cells or other cytoplasmic structures (see Table 17-1).

The enamel apatite crystals, the largest of all found in human calcified tissues, are elongated cylinders which, in transverse section, are sometimes flat-

tened hexagons but more frequently are irregular and more or less circular. Their dimensions in human enamel vary from 400 to 1200 Å in width and from 2000 to 10,000 Å in length in bright-field and dark-field electron microscopy. Through high-resolution transmission electron microscopy, periodic lattice fringes corresponding to different crystallographic planes have been demonstrated in apatite crystals of normal human enamel (Fig. 17-10B and C). In the prisms and the interprismatic substance, the crystals are closely packed and the intercrystalline spaces are about 20 to 30 Å in width. The organic fraction of enamel has a characteristic amino acid composition that is different from both collagen and keratin and contains small amounts of glycoprotein and lipid.

In the prisms, the apatite crystals have their long axis (c axis) approximately parallel to the longitudinal

FIGURE 17-10A Longitudinal section through arcade-formed human fetal enamel rods in a plane indicated by the white arrow on Fig. 17-9. The divergent orientation of the apatite crystals in the rods (R) versus the interrod substance (IP) is apparent. The central rod is separated on the right from the interrod substance by a sheath (S), whereas on its left side, it is continuous with the interrod substance. This configuration is accounted for by examining the longitudinal plane of the section indicated by the arrow on Fig. 17-9. (The upper right part on Fig. 17-9 corresponds to the left part of Fig. 17-10A.) ×17,000.

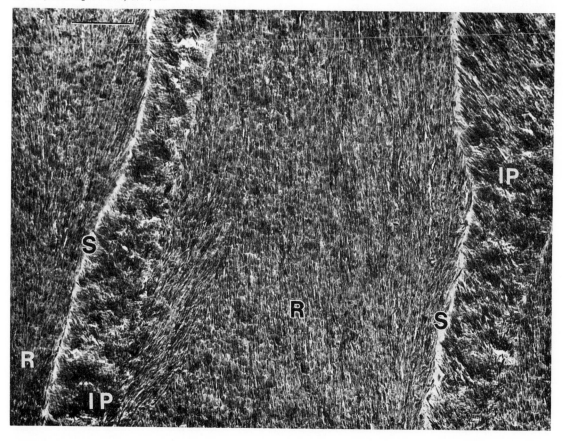

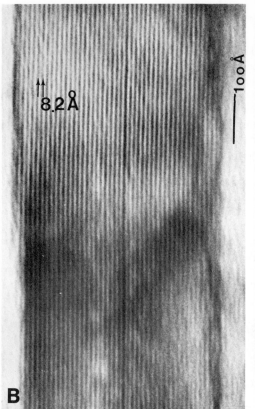

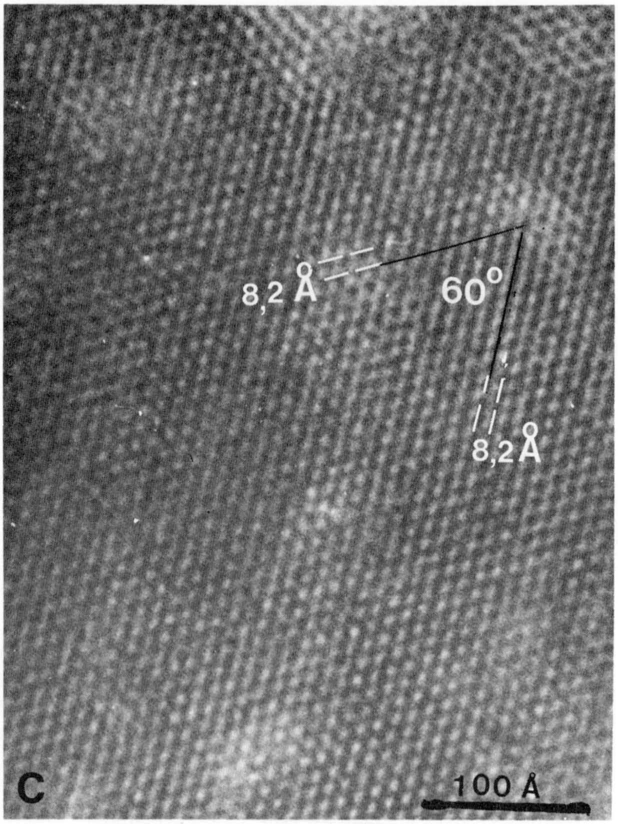

FIGURE 17-10B Transmission electron micrograph of apatite crystal in human dental enamel with the c axis near the longitudinal axis. The a axis is perpendicular to the sectioning plane and the b axis forms an angle of +120° with the plane formed by the two first axes. The periodic lattice fringes are in the order of 8.2 Å. ×1.530.000.

FIGURE 17-10C Demonstration of three series of equidistant 8.2-Å lattice fringes, corresponding to the (100) lattice planes in an apatite crystal of normal adult human enamel. The angle formed between the different striations is 60°. The axis of the electron beam and the crystal c axis can be considered as parallel. ×2.620.000.

TABLE 17-1 COMPARISON OF HARD TISSUES

MAIN COMPONENTS	BONE	CEMENTUM	DENTIN	ENAMEL
Inorganic crystals	Calcium phosphate	Calcium phosphate	Calcium phosphate	Calcium phosphate
Amorphous ground substance	Glycoprotein	Glycoprotein	Glycoprotein	Glycoprotein and
Principal organic component	Collagen	Collagen	Collagen	special protein
Internal cells	Osteocytes	Cementocytes	Cell processes	Absent
Adjacent cells	Osteoblasts osteoclasts	Cementoblasts	Odontoblasts	Absent
Blood vessels	Present	Absent	Absent	Absent
Adjacent fluid	Connective tissue fluid	Connective tissue fluid	Connective tissue fluid	Saliva

axis of the prism, whereas in the interprismatic substance the long axis of the crystals forms an angle of more than 40° with that of the prisms. On cross sections of human enamel, it has been shown that the relationships between prism, interprismatic substance, and prism sheath can be variable. Traditionally, the most frequent type has been described as "arcade-formed" enamel, because the prism profile has an arcade shape (Fig. 17-9). Other studies suggest a keyhole configuration in which the cross-cut prisms have a head and a tail. In the head, the long axis of the apatite crystals is approximately parallel to that of the prism, whereas toward the tail, the crystal axis diverges progressively from that of the prism.

Various markings can be seen on the enamel surface or in ground sections. The outer surface of the enamel, especially of young permanent teeth, presents a succession of circular ridges and grooves which may be seen with a hand lens (Fig. 17-11). These ripple marks, or *perikymata* as they are now called, were discovered by Leeuwenhoek in 1687. When a tooth is split in two and the exposed enamel is examined with a hand lens, a set of lines or bands can be seen to cross the enamel radially, taking the shortest course from the dentin toward the free surface. These radial lines are said to be owing to the arrangement of the enamel prisms, and fractures of the enamel tend to follow

them. It is also suggested that they may reflect differences in composition. Seen in reflected light under low magnification, they appear as alternating light and dark zones called *lines of Hunter-Schreger* (Fig. 17-12). The bundles of prisms, in crossing the enamel, are bent so that in a radial section they appear as alternating zones of oblique and longitudinal sections. These zones also differ in degree of calcification, as evidenced by the affinity for stain in alternating areas (see also Fig. 17-5F, color insert).

The enamel shows other striations, which are broadest and most distinct toward the free surface. Apparently these striations indicate the shape of the entire enamel at successive stages in its development (see Fig. 17-1), and for this reason they are called *growth lines* or *lines of Retzius*. These lines may also represent differences in structure and composition of the enamel. They tend to obstruct transmitted light when viewed in both decalcified and ground sections (Fig. 17-13). Metabolic disturbances occurring during the development of the teeth often accentuate these lines and are permanently recorded. Similarly, the physiologic change in metabolism at birth stamps an imprint on the teeth known as the *neonatal line*.

In the internal enamel, near the dentin-enamel

FIGURE 17-11 Intact enamel surface. The appositional growth pattern of the enamel is reflected in the circular ridges and depressions.

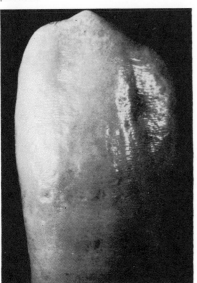

FIGURE 17-12 Ground section of a tooth photographed in reflected light. The light enamel layer with the alternating dark and light bands of Hunter-Schreger is clearly distinguishable from the dentin. (Meyer-Churchill.)

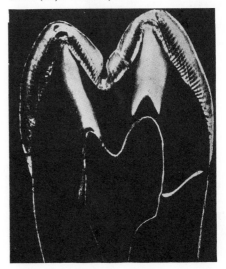

border, structures called *enamel tufts* often appear and extend various distances between the enamel prisms (Fig. 17-13A). Heavy organic bands derived from saliva and elsewhere, known as *enamel lamellae,* are frequently found along cracks between the enamel prisms (Fig. 17-14). Other structures extend for short distances into the enamel at an angle to the prisms; these are called *enamel spindles* (Fig. 17-15) and are thought to represent extensions of dentinal tubules.

Individual enamel prisms, when seen lengthwise, exhibit transverse markings usually, but not always, aligned to form continuous striations across many

FIGURE 17-13 A. Paraffin section of decalcified enamel of deciduous molar. The several incremental (Retzius) lines and one accentuated birth line correspond to areas with relatively thicker interprismatic organic matter. B. Undecalcified ground section of enamel and dentin of permanent molar. The enamel shows several incremental lines running parallel and a few tufts extending into enamel from underlying dentin.

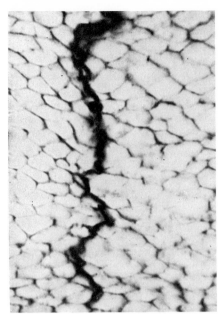

FIGURE 17-14 Enamel lamella ending blindly between enamel prisms. Paraffin section of decalcified enamel.

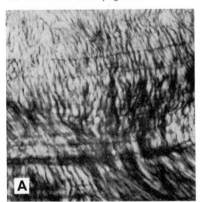

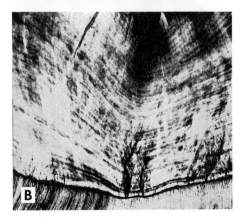

FIGURE 17-15 Enamel spindle running from dentin surface at an angle to the enamel prisms and ending blindly in the enamel. Ground section.

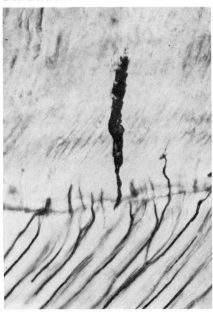

prisms (Fig. 17-5E, see color insert). It is apparent that the prismatic striations reflect a periodic rhythm of incremental activity.

For a summary of the characteristic differences between enamel and other hard tissues, refer to Table 17-1.

DENTIN

Following the differentiation of the ameloblasts of the enamel organ, the outermost cells of the dental papilla become elongated and arranged in an epithelioid layer and are called *odontoblasts* (Fig. 17-6). They are tall columnar cells, with one or more thin processes directed toward the enamel. As dentin matrix is formed, the odontoblasts recede centripetally, narrowing the

pulpal chamber. The cells leave behind an apical extension, the odontoblastic process (*Tomes's fiber*), surrounded by a canalicular structure termed the *dentinal tubule* (Fig. 17-16). The odontoblastic processes should not be confused with the previously described Tomes's processes of the ameloblasts. The thin outermost layer of dentin is the mantle dentin, characterized by an arborescent pattern of dentinal tubules. The bulk of the dentin, the circumpulpal dentin, contains essentially straight tubules that branch dichotomously at the tips and bear smaller side branches. Each process occupies a canaliculus in the dentinal matrix; but the odontoblasts remain always at the inner border of the dentin, receding centripetally, and unlike osteoblasts, do not become buried. They are in contact with adjacent cells and with cells more central in the pulp.

FIGURE 17-16 The odontoblastic process (O) of cat dentin (D) is separated from the wall of the tubule by a periodontoblastic organic space (S), containing some collagen fibrils and ground substance. P = predentin. ×32,000.

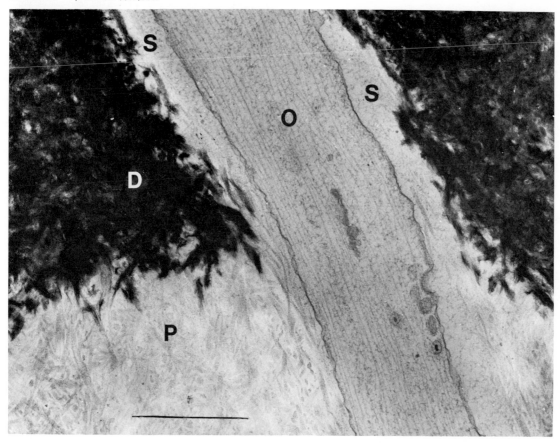

The odontoblast, with an oval-shaped nucleus, contains a well-developed Golgi zone located near the nucleus, on the side facing the enamel, as well as endoplasmic reticulum, mitochondria, ribosomes, microtubules, and microfilaments. Laterally the odontoblasts can be attached by tight, intermediary junctions and desmosomes. Along the predentin, a complex junctional attachment can be seen. The odontoblastic process is limited by the cell plasmalemma and contains a cytoplasmic mass rich in microtubules and microfilaments (Fig. 17-16).

It was thought that during the early stages of dentinogenesis, the first fibrils to be formed in mantle dentin originated in mesenchymal pulpal cells and fanned out in the predentin, passing between odontoblasts. With the light microscope these fine argyrophilic fibers, known as Korff's fibers, have been described in the mantle dentin. With the electron microscope, these fibrils show the classical periodic cross-striations typical of collagen, and the main bulk of the dentinal organic matrix, known as *predentin,* is mainly composed of collagen fibrils embedded in a ground substance (Fig. 17-17). Through electron-microscope autoradiography, it has been shown that the secretion of collagen precursors of predentin is mainly under the control of the odontoblast; and it must be noted that only a few collagen bundles could be observed in the lateral extracellular space between odontoblasts. During active dentinogenesis, different types of dense elongated granules and coated vesicles are found in the odontoblast process. An important

FIGURE 17-17 Longitudinal section of an odontoblastic process (O) in the predentin of a newborn cat 1 h after intravenous injection of tritiated proline. Numerous silver grains are visible in the odontoblastic process containing dense elongated granules (G), some of which are labeled. The collagen fibrils surrounding the process are only slightly labeled at this stage. However, 24 h after the intravenous injection of tritiated proline, the collagenous matrix is labeled almost exclusively, whereas the odontoblastic process is free of silver grains. ×28,000.

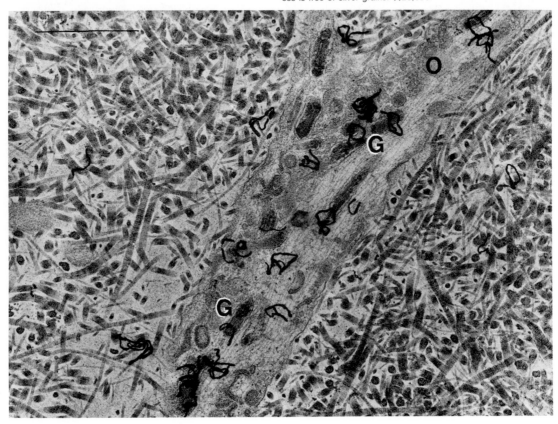

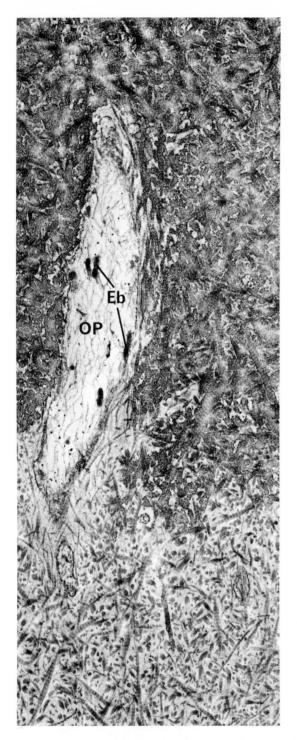

part of the collagen precursors migrate through the odontoblast in the elongated granules (Fig. 17-17), which are formed within the Golgi zone, as can be demonstrated with ultrastructural autoradiography after injection of tritiated proline.

Glycoproteins are evidently elaborated in the Golgi apparatus and transferred through the dense elongated vesicles to the odontoblast process, where secretion into the extracellular space appears to depend upon exocytosis. Calcium transfer in dentinogenesis has been studied by light and electron-microscopic autoradiography. A direct pathway from the capillaries appears to follow the intercellular spaces so as to reach the dentin via the predentin. A second route involves a transcellular transfer through the odontoblast where the mitochondria and the Golgi apparatus show the most intense ^{45}Ca labeling. The calcium diffusion through the cytoplasm of the odontoblastic process occurs without being associated with the dense elongated granules.

Even though the odontoblasts differentiate later than the ameloblasts, the dentin matrix is first laid down as a thin layer of predentin below the row of ameloblasts (Fig. 17-6). Calcification is induced through hydroxyapatite growth in this collageneous matrix. The mature apatite crystal in dentin has been described as a needle- or platelike crystal.

If the inorganic crystals are removed, it is found that the organic matrix of decalcified dentin has a greater electron density than the predentin precursor (Fig. 17-18). Dentin is elaborated through incremental deposition of predentin layers followed by either homogeneous or globular calcified masses. Here, as in the young enamel, one can observe a very marked phosphorus uptake in ^{32}P-injected animals accompanied by an intensive alkaline phosphatase activity in

FIGURE 17-18 An electron micrograph demonstrating the dentin (upper two-thirds of micrograph) and the predentin (lower one-third of micrograph) from an EDTA-demineralized rat incisor. The dentin. This process contains elongated granules (Eb); microwhich, after demineralization, appear to be associated with an electron-dense material. In contrast, the collagen bundles in the predentin lack this dense material. A portion of an odontoblastic process (OP) may be seen penetrating the dentin from the predentin. This process contains elongated granules (Eb), microtubules, and microfilaments. ×15,000. [From A. Weinstock, in G. H. Bourne (ed.), ''Elaboration of Enamel and Dentin Matrix Glycoproteins,'' p. 121, Academic Press, Inc., New York, 1972.]

the adjacent tooth-forming cells of the dental papilla and enamel organ (Figs. 17-19 and 17-20).

When fully calcified, dentin is not so hard as enamel, since it contains much more organic matter (approximately 30 percent, roughly similar to bone). When the inorganic substances are removed from enamel, the remaining organic framework scarcely holds together, whereas the demineralization of dentin and bone leaves a coherent matrix which preserves the form of the original object.

The dentinal tubules pass radially through the dentin, often following a somewhat S-shaped course (Fig. 17-21), sometimes with spiral twists and secondary curves. As the tubules penetrate the dentin, they give off many slender lateral branches, some of which seem to anastomose with those from adjacent tubules. They finally become very slender and end blindly.

The tubules of the inner third of calcified dentin are permeated by portions of odontoblastic process (Fig. 17-5G and H, see color insert) that do not completely fill the tubule but leave an organic periodontoblastic space, containing some uncalcified collagen fibrils and ground substance, between the process and the calcified tubule wall (Fig. 17-16). In the peripheral parts of the odontoblastic process, an accumulation of large vacuoles has been observed. On cross sections, the process appears as an annular condensation of hyaline cytoplasm with a central vacuole (Fig. 17-22).

In the inner layer of dentin, near the predentin,

FIGURE 17-19 Radioautograph of the jaw of ^{32}P-injected rhesus monkey. Note intense activity in the internal dentin.

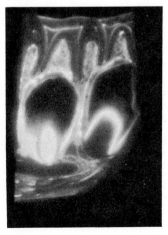

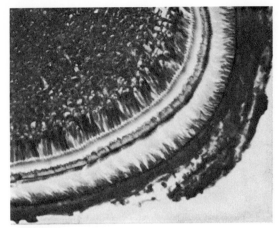

FIGURE 17-20 Alkaline phosphatase activity in the cells of the enamel organ and dental papilla of developing rat incisor. Paraffin section of the uncalcified growing part of tooth.

the dentinal tubules are directly bordered by intertubular dentin consisting of a calcified collageneous matrix (Fig. 17-16). In more peripheral layers are found hypercalcified tubular walls known as peritubular dentin (Fig. 17-22). The peritubular dentin, which is continuous with intertubular dentin, is rich in closely packed inorganic crystals. The exact nature of the scarce organic matrix of the peritubular dentin is still a matter of debate.

Histochemical techniques have revealed basophilic and metachromatic reactions in the areas surrounding the processes of the odontoblasts (Fig. 17-5I and J, see color insert). Besides the collagenous framework (Fig. 17-5G, color insert), a PAS-positive component is interspersed in the ground substance of the dentin (Fig. 17-5H, color insert).

Investigations with the light microscope have alternatively confirmed and denied the presence of nerve fibrils in adult predentin and dentin stained by silver impregnations. A few unmyelinated nerve fibrils in close contact with the odontoblastic processes have been identified with the electron microscope, in predentin as well as in some tubules of the inner dentin (Fig. 17-23). In contrast to the odontoblastic process, they contain many mitochondria, as well as some vesicles and neurotubules.

The juncture between dentin and enamel is slightly scalloped. Toward the root of the tooth, where the dentin is in contact with the cementum, it exhibits a more or less continuous layer of especially small interglobular spaces known as Tomes's granular layer. According to its appositional pattern, dentin shows parallel incremental lines (of Ebner), and sometimes even broader contour lines of Owen (see Fig. 17-21) corresponding to accentuated lines of Retzius in the enamel (compare with Fig. 17-13).

In human teeth, the dentin matrix is often incompletely calcified, leaving interglobular dentin spaces which appear black in ground sections (Fig. 17-22). They are usually located in the peripheral coronal dentin and are parallel to the dentin-enamel junction.

Dentin continues to be formed slowly throughout life, so that the pulp cavity becomes reduced in size with age. Injury causes an increased deposit of new or secondary dentin. In response to wear and tear, the lumen of the dentinal tubules can be totally occluded by calcification, and this age change produces what is referred to as transparent, or sclerotic, dentin.

PULP

The pulp originates from the dental papilla (see Fig. 17-3), which is composed of condensed mesenchyme. It is enclosed and probably molded by the enamel

organ. The young papilla is very cellular. The cells are round or polyhedral and moderately large, with pale, almost unstained cytoplasm and large nuclei. In humans and monkeys, these round cells have been encountered only in the pulp of fetal teeth. They appear to have no counterpart in other connective tissues, unless it be some resemblance to cartilage cells. The round cells are surrounded by the ground substance of the dental papilla, which in fetal teeth and in the growing incisors of rodents exhibits marked metachromasia (Fig. 17-5B, color insert). As the pulp matures, the round cells of the dental papilla become spindle-shaped and their metachromasia diminishes, whereas an intense alkaline phosphatase reaction persists. Glycogen is plentiful in the pulp cells of growing teeth, and a multitude of sudanophilic particles which are presumably mitochondria has been observed in their cytoplasm.

Besides the odontoblastic layer already described, it appears that the predominant cells of the adult pulp are fibrocytes and fibroblasts (Figs. 17-24 and 17-25). The intercellular spaces are filled with ground sub-

FIGURE 17-21 Ground section of human molar. Several accentuated growth lines in concurrently developed dentin and enamel form V-shaped patterns with the apex at the dentin-enamel junction.

Contour lines of Owen   Dentin-enamel junction   Contour lines of Retzius

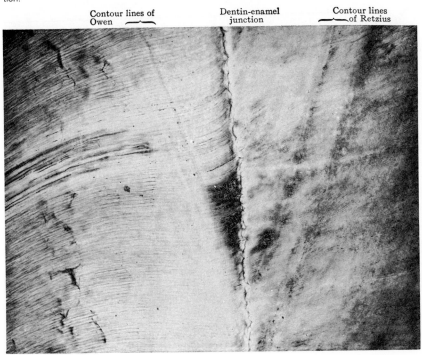

stance and a few bundles of collagen fibrils. With the electron microscope it is possible to identify some scarce bundles of small unstriated filaments about 150 Å in diameter. These bundles are ultrastructurally close to elastic fibers and similar to other microfilaments observed in the supporting tissues of the teeth.

The pulp is very vascular. Small arteries enter the apical foramina, then branch and divide into numerous capillaries which may pass between the odontoblasts but normally do not enter the predentin. The pulpal capillaries can have continuous walls with endothelial cells lined by pericytes and a basement membrane, but fenestrated capillaries with pores in their walls have been observed with the electron microscope (Fig. 17-25). Similar structures are found elsewhere, such as in endocrine glands and kidneys, where fast and important liquid exchanges occur. The pulpal blood capillaries empty into very thin-walled

veins which are larger in diameter than the arteries. These vessels become smaller and leave the pulp in company with the entering arteries. Whether or not lymphatic vessels are present in the pulp has not been proved. Attempts to inject lymphatics either directly or indirectly sometimes show the injected mass within the pulp, but no conclusive evidence for the presence of such vessels has been presented to date.

The nerves of the pulp are either myelinated or unmyelinated and often twist spirally around the vessels. Myelinated nerve fibrils consist of a central axon, surrounded by a lamellated myelin sheath and a Schwann cell, limited by a basement membrane. The unmyelinated nerve fibrils are covered by a Schwann cell with typical mesaxons. They are also circumscribed by a basement membrane. These unmyeli-

FIGURE 17-22 Transverse section through a dentinal tubule located in the middle third of adult human coronal dentin. The odontoblastic process contains a centrally located vacuole (v) with peripheral condensation of hyaline cytoplasm (c). Highly calcified peritubular dentin (Pd) surrounds the tubular lumen. Id = Intertubular dentin. ×35,000.

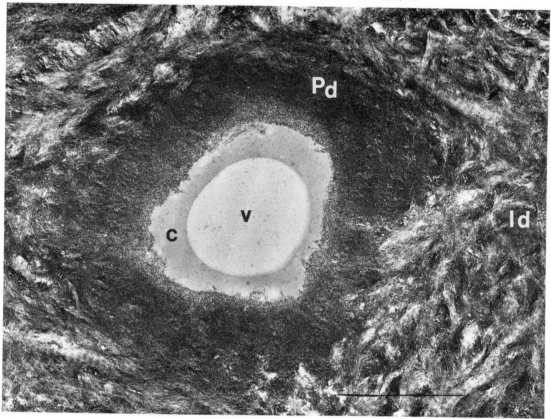

nated nerve fibrils are prominent in the subodonto-blastic layer. Some of the unmyelinated nerve fibrils can be followed with the electron microscope in the predentin (Fig. 17-23) and the inner third of dentin, where they end along the odontoblastic process.

DENTAL SUPPORTING TISSUES

The cells of the inner and outer enamel epithelium together form the *epithelial sheath* of the root, generally referred to as *Hertwig's sheath.* This sheath determines the extent and shape of the downward growth of the root. Each tooth germ, consisting of its enamel organ and papilla (see Fig. 17-3), is completely surrounded by mesenchyme, forming the *dental sac.* After the dentin of the root is formed, the ectodermal

layers degenerate, at first in the region of the neck, leaving the outer surface of the dentin exposed to the surrounding mesenchyme. The mesenchymal cells become similar to osteoblasts. These cells, the cementoblasts, form a modified appositional bone on the dentinal surface, the so-called cementum.

Cementum

A thin layer of cementum is deposited before the tooth erupts. This is noncellular, since none of the cementoblasts becomes embedded, and is designated *primary cementum.* After eruption a new layer of cementum forms against the external root surface, and this time the *secondary cementum* becomes much thicker and contains several layers of cells (Fig. 17-26A). These cells, the *cementocytes,* seem to have their largest and most numerous processes directed away from the dentin, a condition that is reflected in the shape of the lacunas and canaliculi (Fig. 17-26B).

FIGURES 17-23 Transverse section through an odontoblastic process (Op) in predentin layer of adult human premolar. An unmyelinated nerve fiber (N) can be seen in close association with the process. The axoplasm contains numerous mitochondria and some vesicles. Pd = noncalcified predentinal collagenous matrix. ×61,000.

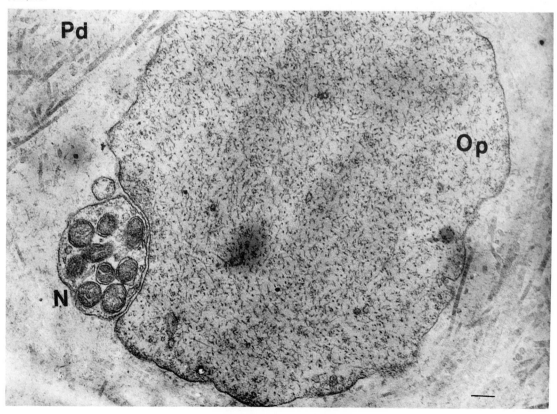

Besides supplying cementoblasts to form the secondary cementum, the mesenchyme of the dental sac also produces the thick collagenous fibers of the periodontal ligament which become embedded in the bonelike cementum matrix. These are called *Sharpey's fibers,* as are comparable structures in bone.

Periodontal Ligament

The connective tissue lying in the narrow space between the cementum and the bony alveolar process is referred to as the *periodontal ligament.* Aside from the ground substance and the cellular elements, among which the fibrocytes and fibroblasts are prominent, the periodontal ligament is essentially a ligament made of bundles of collagen fibrils, with some few bundles of small unstriated microfilaments, ultrastructurally reminiscent of elastic fibers.

Some of the collagen bundles, embedded at one end in cementum (Sharpey's fibers), extend from the cementum across the periodontal space and are inserted into the bone of the alveolar process, which forms the tooth socket. They support the tooth while allowing a certain amount of motion in order to withstand the shock of biting and chewing. The fiber direction varies at different regions of the tooth (see the diagram in Fig. 17-1). From the root end to the rim of the alveolar process the fiber bundles may be grouped into apical, oblique, horizontal, and alveolar crest fibers, according to their directions and attachments. Above the alveolar processes, the transseptal fibers run between adjacent teeth, and the gingival fibers are attached to the dense connective tissue of the gum.

In addition to the cementoblasts and Sharpey's fibers, the periodontal structures include not only the usual constituents of dense collagenous connective tissue but also, importantly, occasional epithelial nests or cords. These are remnants of Hertwig's epithelial sheath, and proliferation of this epithelium is significant in certain diseases.

The blood vessels in the periodontal ligament pass parallel to the tooth, communicating with intra-alveolar and gingival vessels. They form fine capillary loops toward the tooth. The lymphatic vessels also form loops toward the tooth but are more tortuous. The periodontal ligament is richly innervated, having an extremely wide range of sensitivity.

FIGURE 17-24 Normal pulp of adult human tooth. Dentin and a light zone of predentin are seen at left adjacent to the row of odontoblasts along the periphery of the pulp. Centrally, note the delicate walls of the blood vessels of the pulp. Decalcified section; H&E. ×100.

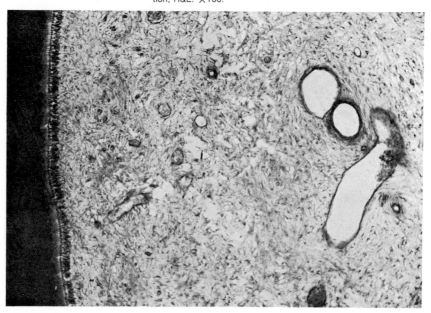

Gingiva

The gum, or gingiva, forms a collar of soft tissue around the neck of each tooth (see diagram in Fig. 17-1). The gum tissue that separates adjacent teeth is called the interdental papilla. A narrow sulcus, normally less than 2 mm deep, separates the gingival margin from the tooth surface (Fig. 17-27). At the base of this sulcus, the gingiva is in contact with the tooth surfaces by a region known as the *epithelial attachment*. Two different situations have been described between the superficial epithelial cells and the enamel surface. In unerupted and in functioning erupted teeth, the plasmalemmas of the epithelial cells exhibit numerous hemidesmosomes and are separated from the enamel apatite crystals by an extracellular space containing an amorphous and granular material (Fig. 17-28, left). Histochemical methods revealed

polysaccharides and proteins in this space. The space situation has been observed exclusively in erupted teeth and consists of a cuticular structure, directly in contact with the enamel apatite crystals, being separated by a small extracellular space from the epithelial cell membranes which contain hemidesmosomes (Fig. 17-28, right). This cuticle is elaborated after eruption by either epithelial or connective tissue.

In normal conditions, a certain number of lymphocytes and polymorphonuclear leukocytes cross the epithelial attachment and the sulcular epithelium and penetrate into the oral cavity.

Histologically the gingival tissue resembles the epidermis of the skin in many respects, even to the point of cornification. It is capped by a thick layer of stratified squamous epithelium, but unlike skin, this is indented by many long, basal, connective tissue papil-

FIGURE 17-25 Human dental pulp with numerous elongated fibrocytes separated by intercellular spaces filled with some collagen bundles. A blood capillary, with fenestrated walls (see arrows), contains an erythrocyte. ×11,000.

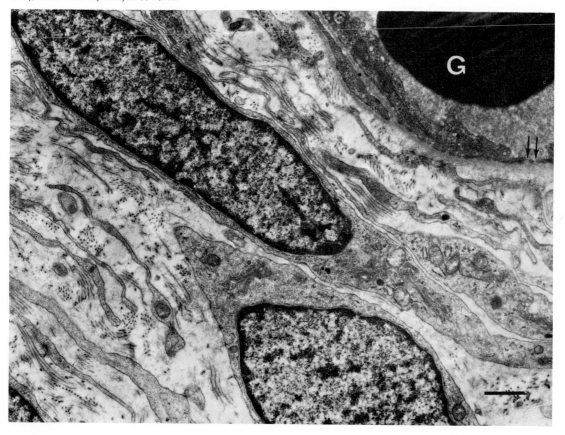

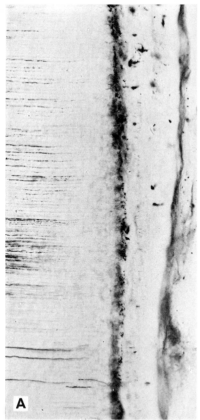

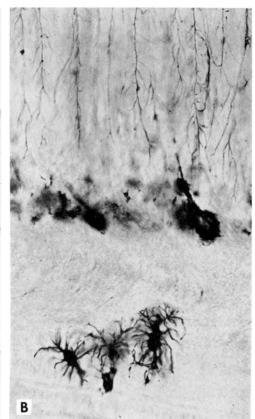

FIGURE 17-26 Longitudinal ground
section of root of human tooth. A. Left to
right: Dentin, Tomes's granular layer, and
cementum, largely acellular. B. A higher
magnification of A, showing three cementocytes, granular layer, and dentin
with ramifying dentinal tubules.

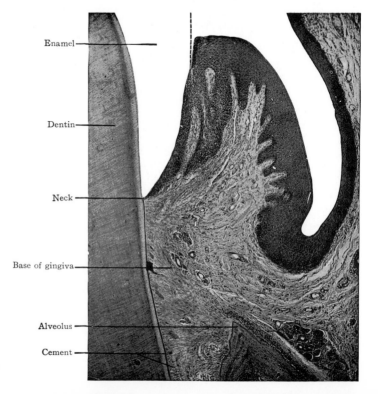

FIGURE 17-27 Tooth, periodontal
ligament, and gingiva. Decalcified
section. The enamel has been dissolved, but it once occupied the
wedge-shaped space between dentin,
gingiva, and the dotted line.

Enamel

Dentin

Neck

Base of gingiva

Alveolus

Cement

lae. The cell layers and the papillae become fewer as the gum dips to enclose the enamel. The degree of cornification varies a good deal from person to person and in time, but cornification is absent within the gingival sulcus. The gingiva contains bundles of collagen in the form of transseptal and gingival fibers. These are so firmly attached to the neck and root surface of the tooth that they have been referred to as a circular ligament. In the gingival lamina propria, special bundles of small unstriated filaments can be observed among the collagen fibrils (Fig. 17-29). Elongated loops of blood and lymphatic capillaries are

found in the tall connective tissue papillae under the epithelium. The gingiva is richly innervated and has several different types of encapsulated and nonencapsulated terminal bulbs and coils in addition to free endings, some of which pass into the epithelium between the cells.

Delicate sudanophilic staining is visible in the intercellular bridges of the cells of the stratum spinosum of the Malpighian layer of the gingival epithelium. The ground substance of the gingival connective tissue and periodontal ligament is quite perceptibly metachromatic. The stroma of the gingival tissue varies considerably in this regard, but in places it is deeply metachromatic and contains exceptionally large numbers of mast cells (see Fig. 17-5C, color insert), surpassing in this respect most other normal connective tissues. Glycogen is present in the stratified epithelium of the gingival mucous membrane, especially in the

FIGURE 17-28 Junctions between the superficial cells of the epithelial attachment and the enamel surface (e) of adult human erupted tooth. On the left, an intercellular space (i), filled with granular and amorphous material, separates the cell membrane, which is coated with hemidesmosomes (see arrows), from the enamel apatite crystals (e). On the right, a cuticle (C), the so-called acquired endogenous pellicle, is interposed between the enamel apatite crystals (e) and the intercellular space (i). The epithelial cell membrane is also coated by hemidesmosomes (see arrows). ×44,000.

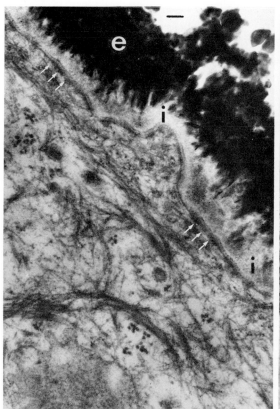
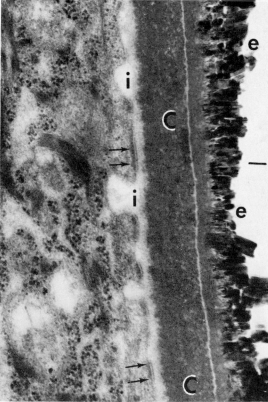

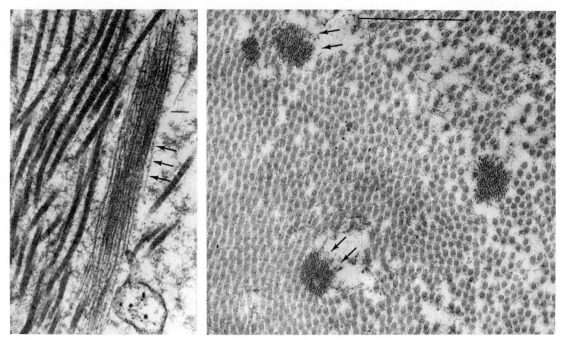

FIGURE 17-29 Intercellular spaces of the lamina propria of the human gingiva contain typical collagen fibrils as well as bundles of small nonstriated filaments (arrows), seen in a longitudinal section on the left (×38,000) and in a transverse section on the right. (×29,000).

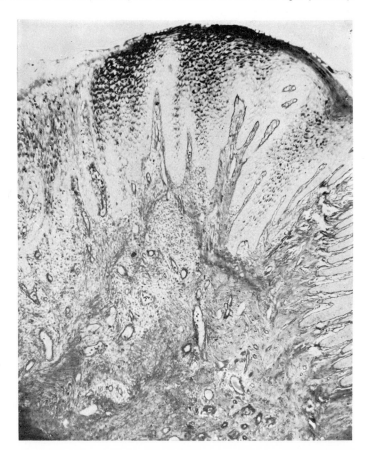

FIGURE 17-30 Gingival tissue from adult man. Note the tall, slender connective tissue papilla. Stained with the periodic acid–Schiff method, the darkest areas indicate that glycogen is especially abundant in the stratum spinosum of the squamous epithelium. ×90.

prickle cell layer (Fig. 17-30). The supporting structures of growing and adult teeth also give a marked reaction for alkaline phosphatase. The lamina propria of the gingiva contains variable quantities of this enzyme, the reaction involving, to various degrees, the cells, fibers, ground substance, and walls of the arterioles.

The continuing persistence of metachromatic ground substance (acid mucopholysaccharide) and alkaline phosphatase in the periodontal membrane and especially in the tunica propria of the gingiva may suggest that the tissues involved are permanently in a state of elevated metabolic activity. The excess of these substances in the gingival tissue may be a response to constant friction, irritation, and abrasion to which the supporting structures of the teeth are continuously subjected.

Alveolar Bone

The alveolar bone is part of the tooth-supporting tissues, closely associated to the periodontal ligament

and the gingiva. Anatomically the alveolar bone can be defined as the part of the mandible or the maxilla surrounding the dental roots. The alveolar bone is continuous with the body of the upper or lower jaw without distinct boundary.

Alveolar bone consists of a thin layer of lamellar bone, the lamina dura or cribriform plate, limiting the socket, and a cortical plate of compact lamellar bone. A small amount of spongy bone, with medullary spaces, is found between the two plates of lamellar bone. The principal fibers of the periodontal ligament penetrate the alveolar bone as Sharpey's fibers. Along the lamina dura, osteoblasts and some osteoclasts can be found in the periodontal ligament. Communicating with the marrow spaces, the lamina dura is perforated by many openings, through which nerves and blood vessels can pass into the periodontal ligament.

REFERENCES

ANDERSON, D. J., A. G. HANNAM, and B. MATTHEWS: Sensory Mechanisms in Mammalian Teeth and Their Supporting Structures, *Physiol. Rev.,* **50:**171 (1970).

ARWILL, T., L. EDWALL, J., LILJA, L. OLGART, and S. E. SVENSON: Ultrastructure of Nerves in Dentinal Pulpal Border Zone after Sensory and Autonomic Nerve Transection in the Cat, *Acta Odontol. Scand.,* **31:**273 (1973).

BRODIE, A. G.: On the Growth Pattern of the Human Head from the Third Month to the Eighth Year of Life, *Am. J. Anat.,* **68:**209 (1941).

CARMICHAEL, G. G., and H. M. FULLMER: The Fine Structure of the Oxytalan Fiber, *J. Cell Biol.,* **28:**33 (1966).

CRABB, H. S. M., and A. I. DARLING: The Pattern of Progressive Mineralization in Human Dental Enamel, in "International Series of Monographs on Oral Biology," vol. 2, Pergamon Press, New York, 1962.

EASTOE, J. E.: The Amino-acid Composition of Proteins from the Oral Tissues: II. The Matrix Proteins in Dentine and Enamel from Developing Human Deciduous Teeth, *Arch. Oral Biol.,* **8:**633 (1963).

FINN, S. B.: "Biology of the Dental Pulp Organ: A Symposium," University of Alabama Press, University, Ala., 1968.

FRANK, R. M.: Autoradiographie Quantitative de l'Amélogenèse en Microscopie Electronique à l'Aide de la Proline Tritiée Chez le Chat, *Arch. Oral Biol.,* **15:**569 (1970).

FRANK, R. M.: Étude Autoradiographique de la Dentinogenèse en Microscopie Électronique à l'Aide de la Proline Tritiée Chez le Chat, *Arch. Oral Biol.,* **15:**583 (1970).

FRANK, R. M., and G. CIMASONI: Ultrastructure de l'Epithélium Cliniquement Normal du Sillon et de la Jonction Gingivo-dentaire, *Z. Zellforsch.,* **103:**356 (1970).

FRANK, R. M., and P. FRANK: Autoradiographie Quantitative de l'Ostéogenèse en Microscopie Electronique à l'Aide de la Proline Tritiée, *Z. Zellforsch.,* **99:**121 (1969).

GARANT, P. R., G. SZABÓ, and J. NALBANDIAN: The Fine Structure of the Mouse Odontoblast, *Arch. Oral Biol.,* **13:**857 (1968).

GLIMCHER, J. M., E. J. DANIEL, D. F. TRAVIS, and S. KAMHI: Electron Optical and X-ray Diffraction Studies of the Organization of the Inorganic Crystals in Embryonic Bovine Enamel, *J. Ultrastruct. Res.* (suppl. 1), **7:**77 (1965).

GREEP, R. O. (ed.): Recent Advances in the Study of the Structure, Composition and Growth of Mineralized Tissues, *Ann. N.Y. Acad. Sci.,* **60:**541 (1955).

GREEP, R. O., C. J. FISCHER, and A. MORSE: Alkaline Phosphatase in Odontogenesis and Osteogenesis and Its Histochemical Demonstration after Demineralization, *J. Am. Dent. Ass.,* **36:**427 (1948).

KALLENBACH, E.: Fine Structure of Rat Incisor Ameloblasts during Enamel Maturation, *J. Ultrastruct. Res.,* **22:**90 (1968).

KATCHBURIAN, E., and S. J. HOLT: Role of Lysosomes in Amelogenesis, *Nature,* **223:**1367 (1969).

LEHNER, J., and H. PLENK: Die Zähne, in W. von Möllendrof (ed.), "Handbuch mikroskop. Anat. Menschen," vol. 5, pt. 3, Springer-Verlag, Berlin, 1936.

LISTGARTEN, M. A.: Electron Microscopic Study of the Gingivodental Junction of Man, *Am. J. Anat.,* **119:**147 (1966).

LORBER, M.: A Study of the Histochemical Reactions of the Dental Cementum and Alveolar Bone, *Anat. Rec.,* **111:**129 (1951).

MECKEL, A. H., W. J. GRIEBSTEIN, and R. J. NEAL: Structure of Mature Dental Enamel as Observed by Electron Microscopy, *Arch. Oral Biol.,* **10:**775 (1965).

MILES, A. E. W.: "Structural and Chemical Organization of Teeth," vol. II, Academic Press, New York, 1967.

MUNHOZ, C. O. G., and C. P. LEBLOND: Deposition of Calcium Phosphate into Dentin and Enamel as Shown by Radioautography of Sections of Incisor Teeth Following Injection of ^{45}Ca into Rats, *Calcif. Tissue Res.,* **15:**221 (1974).

NAGAI, N., and R. M. FRANK: Electron Microscopic Autoradiography of Ca^{45} during Dentinogenesis, *Cell Tissue Res.* **155:**513 (1974).

NAGAI, N., and R. M. FRANK: Transfert du Ca^{45} par Autoradiographie en Microscopie Électronique au Cours de l'Amélogenèse, *Calcif. Tissue Res.* (1975).

NYLEN, M. U. and D. B. SCOTT: An Electron Microscopic Study of the Early Stages of Dentinogenesis, *U.S. Public Health Service Publ.* 613, 1958.

REITAN, K.: Tissue Behavior during Orthodontic Tooth Movement, *Am. J. Orthod.,* **46:**881 (1960).

REITH, E. J.: The Ultrastructure of Ameloblasts during Early Stages of Maturation of Enamel, *J. Cell Biol.,* **18:**691 (1963).

REITH, E. J.: The Ultrastructure of Ameloblasts from the Growing End of Rat Incisors, *Arch. Oral Biol.,* **2:**253 (1960).

RÖNNHOLM, E.: The Structure of the Organic Stroma of Human Enamel during Amelogenesis, *J. Ultrastruct. Res.,* **3:**368 (1962).

SCHROEDER, H. E., and J. THEILADE: Electron Microscopy of Normal Human Gingival Epithelium, *J. Periodont. Res.,* **1:**95 (1966).

SELVIG, K. A.: The Crystal Structure of Hydroxyapatite in Dental Enamel as Seen with the Electron Microscope, *J. Ultrastr. Res.,* **41:**369 (1972).

SELVIG, K. E.: Electron Microscopy of Dental Enamel: Analysis of Crystal Lattice Images, *Z. Zellforsch.,* **137:**271 (1973).

SLAVKIN, H.: Embryonic Tooth Formation. A Tool for Development Biology, *Oral Sci. Rev.,* **4:**3 (1974).

SOGNNAES, R. F.: Dental Aspects of the Structure and Metabolism of Mineralized Tissues, in Comar and Bronner (eds.), ''Mineral Metabolism—An Advanced Treatise,'' vol. 1, part B, p. 677, Academic Press, New York, 1961.

SOGNNAES, R. F. (ed.): Calcification in Biological Systems, Publ. 64, American Association for the Advancement of Science, Washington, D.C., 1960.

SOGNNAES, R. F.: Microstructure and Histochemical Characteristics of the Mineralized Tissues, in ''Recent Advances in the Study of the Structure, Composition, and Growth of Mineralized Tissues,'' *Ann. N.Y. Acad. Sci.,* **60:**541 (1955).

SQUIER, C. A., and J. P. WATERHOUSE: Lysosomes in Oral Epithelium: The Ultrastructural Localization of Acid Phosphatase and Non-specific Esterase in Keratinized Oral Epithelium in Man and Rat, *Arch. Oral Biol.,* **15:**153 (1970).

STACK, M. V., and R. W. FEARNHEAD: ''Tooth Enamel: Its Composition, Properties and Fundamental Structure,'' John Wright & Sons, Bristol, England, 1965.

SYMONS, N. B. B. (ed.): ''Dentine and Pulp: Their Structure and Reactions,'' E. & S. Livingstone, Edinburgh, 1968.

TRAVIS, D. F.: Comparative Ultrastructure and Organization of Inorganic Crystals and Organic Matrices of Mineralized Tissues, in P. Person (ed.), ''Biology of the Mouth,'' Pub. 89, p. 236, American Association for the Advancement of Science, Washington, D.C., 1968.

VOEGEL, J. C., and R. M. FRANK: Microscopie Électronique de Haute Resolution du Cristal d'Apatite d'Émail Humain et de sa Dissolution Carieuse. *J. Biol. Buccale,* **2:**39 (1974).

WARSHAWSKY, H.: The Fine Structure of Secretory Ameloblasts in Rat Incisors, *Anat. Rec.,* **161:**211 (1968).

WATSON, M. L.: The Extracellular Nature of Enamel in the Rat, *J. Biophys. Biochem. Cytol.,* **7:**489 (1960).

WEINSTOCK, A.: Elaboration of Enamel and Dentin Matrix Glycoproteins, in G. H. Bourne (ed.), ''The Biochemistry and Physiology of Bone,'' 2d ed., vol. II, Academic Press, New York, 1972, p. 121.

WEINSTOCK, A., and J. T. ALBRIGHT: The Fine Structure of Mast Cells in Normal Human Gingiva, *J. Ultrastruct. Res.,* **17:**245 (1967).

WEINSTOCK, A., and C. P. LEBLOND: Elaboration of the Matrix Glycoprotein of Enamel by the Secretory Ameloblasts of the Rat Incisor as Revealed by Radioautography after ^{3}H-Galactose Injection, *J. Cell Biol.,* **51:**26 (1971).

WEINSTOCK, A., M. WEINSTOCK, and C. P. LEBLOND: Autoradiographic Detection of ^{3}H-Fucose Incorporation into Glycoprotein by Odontoblasts and Its Deposition at the Site of the Calcification Front in Dentin, *Calcif. Tissue Res.,* **8:**181 (1972).

WISLOCKI, G. B., and R. F. SOGNNAES: Histochemical Reactions of Normal Teeth, *Am. J. Anat.,* **87:**239 (1950).

YOUNG, R. W., and R. C. GREULICH: Distinctive Autoradiographic Patterns of Glycine Incorporation in Rat Enamel and Dentine Matrices, *Arch. Oral Biol.,* **8:**509 (1963).

The Digestive Tract

HELEN A. PADYKULA

The microscopic structure of the digestive tract will be approached in relation to the sequential functional changes that occur as food is propelled from the mouth toward the anus. The propulsion is effected primarily by waves of involuntary muscular contraction (peristalsis). The food is digested en route by enzymes secreted by the mucosae in fluids of appropriate pH and ionic composition. Current research has provided better definition of the local endocrine control mechanisms that influence this secretory and peristaltic activity; a diffusely distributed system of endocrine cells occurs throughout the gastrointestinal epithelia. Thus, locally produced hormones, such as gastrin, secretin, glucagon, affect the physiologic activity of the digestive tract and of the pancreas and liver as well. Certain components of the food are digested and absorbed. An important final physiologic action is the reabsorption of fluid that was poured into the digestive cavity as part of the salivary and gastrointestinal secretions. Undigested material is eliminated by a combined involuntary and voluntary muscular activity. These functions occur in a well-defined progression and are reflected by distinctive gross, histologic, and cellular variations along the length of the digestive tube. After the *oral cavity*, the hollow digestive tube is differentiated into four major organs: *esophagus, stomach, small intestine,* and *large intestine.* Grossly the organs are separated by muscular valves or *sphincters* (G. *sphinkter,* that which binds tight); these control the passage of contents from one organ to the next.

At the junctions between organs of the digestive tube, the nature of the lining layer, the *mucous membrane* or *mucosa,* also changes abruptly. The digestion of carbohydrates is initiated in the oral cavity, but most of the digestion and absorption is accomplished by the mucosae of the stomach and small intestine in coordination with the secretions of the pancreas and liver. Although it has long been known that lymphatic tissue occurs in abundance in the digestive tube, its participation as a *local immune system* in the body's defense mechanisms has only recently begun to be appreciated. We now know that, in response to the presence of living microorganisms in the lumen, the mucosae produce antibodies, especially immunoglobulin A. The alimentary tract also serves as an avenue of *excretion,* eliminating certain waste products, some of which are secreted by the liver and carried in the bile to the duodenum, and some of which are secreted by the large intestine.

Except for the oral cavity, the histologic organization of the digestive tube has a common plan which is evident throughout its length. This plan will be presented after the description of the principal features of the human oral cavity and of the major salivary glands.

ORAL CAVITY

The initial processing of food occurs in the mouth by chewing. This is assisted by the movements of the tongue which also "tastes" the ingested food through specialized receptors. The digestion of carbohydrates commences through the action of salivary amylase. In addition, defense mechanisms, represented by salivary immunoglobulins and lactoperoxidase, control microbial growth.

In the oral cavity, stratified squamous epithelium covers the red border of the *lip,* the *oral mucosa,* the *tongue,* and the *tonsils* (Figs. 18-1 to 18-3). Embryologically, the oral epithelium gives rise to a variety of *oral glands.* The densely calcified outer enamel layer of the *teeth* also originates from the oral epithelium, through a complex process of invagination, growth, differentiation, and calcification.

The mouth is lined by a mucous membrane (*mucosa*) which has two components, a *stratified squamous epithelium* that is smooth-surfaced and an underlying layer of reticular connective tissue called the *lamina propria* which often has accumulations of lymphoid cells. The epitheliostromal interface is usually distinctly scalloped to varying degrees by stromal *papillae* ("pegs") that carry blood, lymphatic, and neural systems into close association with the thick epithelium (Fig. 18-2). In some regions, such as the soft palate and cheeks, a deeper layer of connective

tissue called the *submucosa* occurs. No smooth muscle intervenes, however, between these two layers of connective tissue. The submucosa in the oral cavity contains adipose cells and the secretory portions of glands. Wherever the submucosa is well developed, the mucosa can be moved, as, for example, in the cheeks.

KERATINIZED SURFACES

In regions subject to the mechanical forces related to mastication, the stratified squamous epithelium is keratinized and closely resembles the epidermis, even at the ultrastructural level (Schroeder and Theilade, 1966) It has the strata, the basalis, spinosum, granulosum, and corneum (Figs. 18-1 and 18-3). Such cornified epithelia occur in the *gingiva* (oral mucosa that surrounds the teeth and the external surfaces of the alveolar processes, that is, the gums), *hard palate,* and *dorsal surface* of the *tongue.* As in the epidermis, there is a labyrinthine intercellular space in the epithelium which is sealed at the free surface by tight junc-

FIGURE 18-1 Vertical section through the lower lip of a man 19 years of age. At the right, the skin is represented by epidermis and dermis (corium); at the left, the oral mucosa is shown with its thicker epithelium and accompanying lamina propria and submucosa. x10.

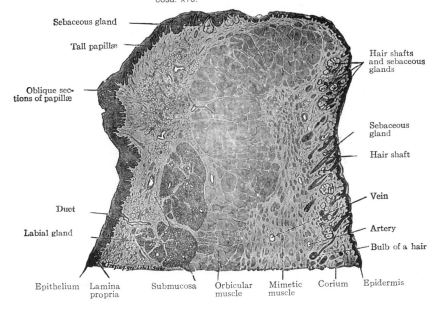

Sebaceous gland

Tall papillæ

Oblique sections of papillæ

Duct

Labial gland

Hair shafts and sebaceous glands

Sebaceous gland

Hair shaft

Vein

Artery

Bulb of a hair

Epithelium Lamina propria Submucosa Orbicular muscle Mimetic muscle Corium Epidermis

tions and is open toward the basal lamina. A dense material is present in the intercellular spaces associated with the upper layers of the stratum granulosum. Hemidesmosomes occur along the surface of the basal cells associated with the basal lamina. This keratinized mucosa differs from the epidermis in that glycogen

may be stored in the cells of the upper spinosum and stratum granulosum. The keratinized epithelia of the gingiva and hard palate are associated with a dense fibrous lamina propria that is firmly attached to cementum of the tooth or to bone.

The gingiva is being intensively studied now because of its involvement in dental disease. Investiga-

FIGURE 18-2 A. Keratinized stratified squamous epithelium of the adult human gingiva. Note the deep papillae (P) in the lamina propria. SC, stratum corneum. Toluidine blue. B. Desquamated cells in the normal human oral cavity. (Courtesy of Dr. G. Shklar.)

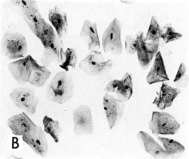

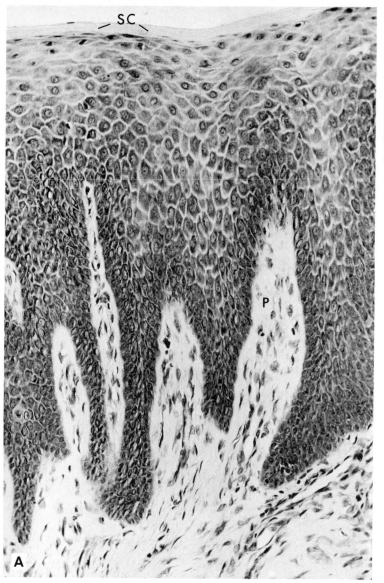

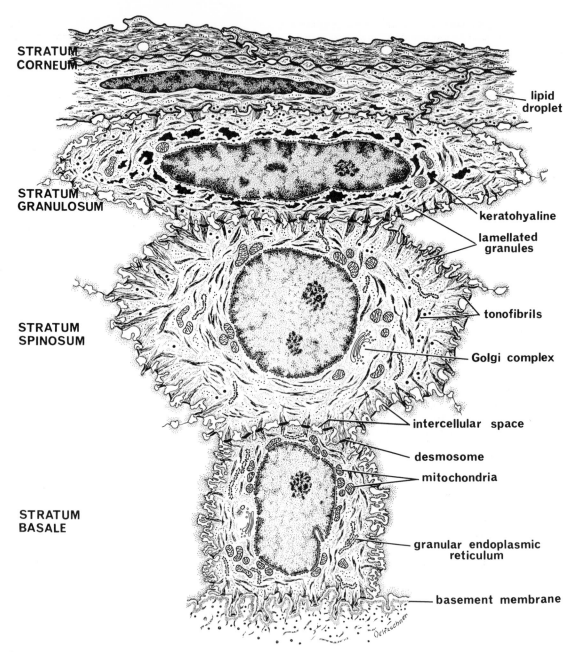

STRATUM CORNEUM

STRATUM GRANULOSUM

STRATUM SPINOSUM

STRATUM BASALE

lipid droplet

keratohyaline

lamellated granules

tonofibrils

Golgi complex

intercellular space

desmosome

mitochondria

granular endoplasmic reticulum

basement membrane

FIGURE 18-3 An ultrastructural diagram of keratinized stratified squamous epithelium obtained from biopsies of the human hard palate. Each cell is representative of those usually found in the four successive cell layers indicated on the left. Overall the cellular layering as well as the ultrastructural features are comparable to those of epidermis. (Courtesy of Dr. Alfred Weinstock.)

tors have long tried to determine the mode of attachment of the gingival stratified squamous epithelium to the tooth. Ultrastructural evidence indicates that this epithelium is attached directly to the enamel and "cuticles" of the teeth by an apparatus consisting of a basal lamina and hemidesmosomes (Listgarten, 1966). This adhesion is similar to that occurring between any epithelium and its underlying connective tissue, however, it should be pointed out that enamel is not of connective tissue origin. The gingival epithelium, like the epidermis, contains melanocytes. It is renewed every 1 to 2 weeks (monkey); this renewal here and elsewhere in the oral mucosa is subject to diurnal variations.

NONKERATINIZED SURFACES

Nonkeratinized surfaces occur in regions of lower mechanical stress, such as the vestibule, floor of the mouth, cheeks, soft palate, and ventral surface of the tongue. This stratified squamous epithelium differs from that of the gingiva and hard palate in that it lacks a stratum granulosum and stratum corneum. Above the strata germinativum and spinosum, there are desquamating layers of flattened, nucleated cells (stratum disjunctum) that are held together loosely and are easily scraped off. High glycogen content is a characteristic of the nonkeratinized epithelium; during epithelial migration, glycogen accumulates gradually, and peak storage occurs in the upper squamous layers. The shed cells occur in large numbers in the saliva (Fig. 18-2B).

An ultrastructural investigation of the human posterior buccal mucosa has revealed that it is remarkably similar to embryonic skin (Hashimoto et al, 1966). Progressive thickening of the plasma membranes occurs during cytomorphosis in the absence of obvious keratinization, and tonofilaments are relatively few in number. Active melanocytes occur here also. In addition, lymphocytes have been observed in migration through the epithelium.

Lips

The red border occurs only in humans and is a transitional zone between the external skin and the internal oral mucosa (Fig. 18-1). Here the stratified squamous epithelium has a well-developed stratum lucidum and a thin corneum. This transparent epithelium is associated with deep stromal papillae that are richly vascularized, creating the red appearance. The lips and oral mucosa are the most accessible parts of the digestive

canal and hence are usually examined as an index of health or disease.

MINOR SALIVARY GLANDS

Minor salivary glands occur throughout the oral mucosa, except in the gingiva and portions of the hard palate. They are either pure mucous glands or mixed glands that have more mucous than serous cells (see the section on major salivary glands for definitions). They serve to moisten the lips (*labial,* mixed type), cheeks (*buccal,* mixed type), palate (*palatine,* pure mucous type), and the floor of the mouth (*minor sublinguals,* mixed type).

TONGUE

The anterior and posterior regions of the adult human tongue have different embryonic origin; the boundary between the two regions is V-shaped and is the location of the principal gustatory receptors, the circumvallate (vallate) papillae (Fig. 18-4). In the adult the dorsal surface of the anterior region of the tongue is rough because of several types of elevations or *papillae,* whereas the ventral surface is smooth. The *lingual tonsils* are located on the posterior part behind the circumvallate papillae.

The core of this highly muscular organ consists of interwoven bundles of skeletal muscle fibers that constitute the various intrinsic and extrinsic *lingual muscles.* Some of the muscle bundles are oblique in orientation, whereas others cross at right angles in either horizontal or vertical planes. These muscles are innervated by lingual branches of the hypoglossal nerve which supply all the lingual muscles except the palatoglossus; the latter is supplied by fibers from the vagus nerve. The intricate arrangement of the muscle bundles forms the mechanical basis for the highly varied and delicate voluntary movements that are possible with the tongue.

This muscular mass is covered by a highly specialized mucous membrane that consists of a keratinized stratified squamous epithelium and a dense lamina propria that is continuous with the connective tissue partitions among the lingual muscles. A submucosa occurs only on the ventral surface beneath a typical nonkeratinized oral mucosa. Lingual glands occur in the connective tissue layers, including the

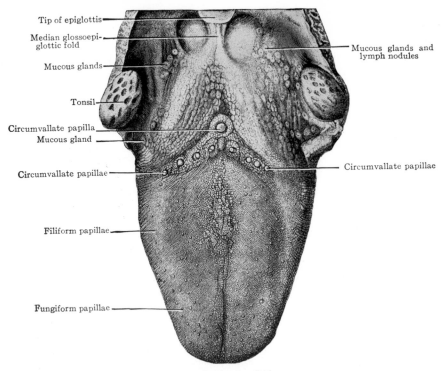

FIGURE 18-4 Dorsum of the human tongue, showing the distribution of papillae and the palatine tonsils. (Sappey.)

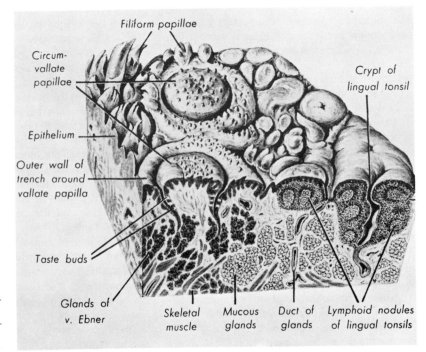

FIGURE 18-5 Reconstruction of the dorsum of the tongue at its junction with the root. (Original drawing by Braus. This modified drawing taken from W. M. Copenhaver, R. P. Bunge, and M. B. Bunge, ''Bailey's Textbook of Histology,'' The Williams & Wilkins Company. Baltimore, 1971.)

stromal partitions among the muscle bundles. The *anterior lingual gland* contains mixed secretory tubules with demilunes and, in some portions, tubules with only seromucous cells (*see* below). The circumvallate papillae are surrounded by a deep trench which is a circular invagination of the mucosa (Figs. 18-5 and 18-7). This trench is irrigated by pure serous secretion from the *glands of von Ebner.* The *posterior lingual glands* are the pure mucous type.

The velvety appearance of most of the dorsal surface of the tongue is created by mucosal projections called *lingual papillae* (Figs. 18-5 to 18-7), all of which have a stratified squamous epithelial cover. The

most numerous, slender, and smallest are the *filiform papillae* that are arranged approximately in rows aligned in relation to the V-shaped gustatory region. The cornified squamous cells are oriented toward the tip of the papilla and are stacked like superimposed hollow cones. The underlying connective tissue core (the *primary papilla*) is thrown into *secondary papillae,* a device for increasing epitheliostromal interaction. Scattered among the filiform projections are the fungiform papillae which are conspicuous elevations that have flattened domelike surfaces (Fig. 18-6). Their epithelium is thinner because of less cornification and thus the underlying high vascularity of the

FIGURE 18-6 Fungiform and filiform papillae on the human tongue. Note the primary and secondary papillae. Zenker fixation; H&E.

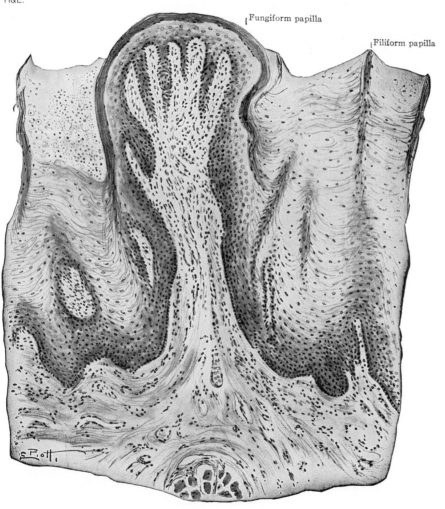

Fungiform papilla

Filiform papilla

secondary papillae is manifested as redness. The *circumvallate papillae,* generally 6 to 12 in number, occur along the V-shaped boundary of the anterior and posterior parts of the tongue. These broad papillae (1 to 3 mm wide and 1 to 1.5 mm tall) do not protrude beyond the lingual surface but rather each is surrounded by circular invagination of the surface (*papillary crypt*) that forms a moat around it (Figs. 18-5, 18-7, 18-9, and 18-10). Taste buds are located within the epithelial cover along the lateral walls of the papillae. The upper surface is covered by a smooth thin epithelium that is ridged by the underlying secondary papillae. A fourth type, the *foliate papilla,* is a leaflike mucosal fold that occurs on the lateral surface of the tongue (Fig. 18-8). These papillae are less pronounced in humans than in other mammals, such as the rabbit, where they constitute the principal organ of taste. Although taste buds in humans occur primarily on the circumvallate and foliate papillae, they occur also to some extent on the fungiform papillae, soft palate, and laryngeal surface of the epiglottis. The gustatory nerves are the chorda tympani, glossopharyngeal, and vagus.

Taste buds are oval groups of elongate epithelial cells that extend from the basal lamina toward the *taste pore,* which is a small opening in the surrounding epithelium (Fig. 18-9). The gustatory receptors are thus protected by their enclosure within the stratified squamous epithelium from any injury by friction. Taste buds are conspicuous in histochemical preparations that demonstrate membrane ATPase activity (Fig. 18-10A). Light microscopists have generally identified two types of cells in the taste bud: (1) sensory *taste cells* (neuroepithelial taste cells) which have a *taste hair* on their free surface and occupy a central location in the taste bud and (2) *supporting cells* that occur mainly on the periphery. Autoradiographic study of the renewal of cells in the rat taste bud indicates that germinal cells occur in the periphery of the taste bud and that certain daughter cells move in and migrate toward the center (Beidler and Smallman, 1965). It was determined that about one cell enters the taste bud every 10 h and that the life-span of an average cell is about 250 h. There is evidence also of cell death within the taste bud. It is thus a differentiating system

FIGURE 18-7 Vertical section of a human circumvallate papilla. ×25.

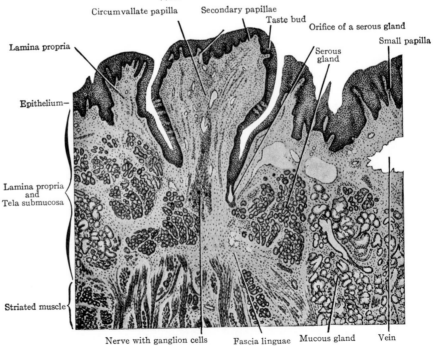

Circumvallate papilla
Secondary papillae
Taste bud
Orifice of a serous gland
Small papilla
Lamina propria
Serous gland
Epithelium
Lamina propria and Tela submucosa
Striated muscle
Nerve with ganglion cells   Fascia linguae   Mucous gland   Vein

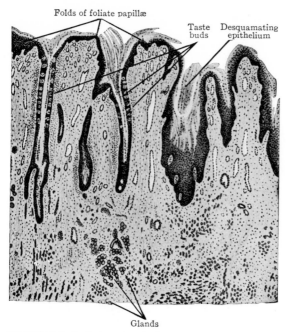

Folds of foliate papillæ   Taste buds   Desquamating epithelium

Glands

FIGURE 18-8 Vertical section of a human foliate papilla. Zenker fixation; H&E. (Sobotta.)

of sensory receptor cells that establish contact with intraepithelial gustatory nerve endings. The existence of taste buds is dependent on intact innervation (Fig. 18-10B). Ultrastructural studies of rabbit taste buds have identified three types of cells, only one of which is extensively associated with nerve endings in a synaptic association and thus may be the gustatory receptor (Murray et al., 1969). Naked nerve terminals occur in an intraepithelial position and are closely apposed to the surface of the neuroepithelial taste cells; vesicles, some with dense cores, are numerous on the "presynaptic side." Ultrastructural interpretation is complicated by the fact that the cells of the taste bud constitute a dynamic differentiating system in which the cells have a relatively short life-span. Interesting functional speculations have been made about the possibility that sensitivity to different taste stimuli may change during the life-span of a gustatory receptor (Beidler and Smallman, 1965).

Ciliated cells have been identified near the floor of the papillary crypt of human circumvallate papillae (Mattern et al., 1970). These mitochondria-rich cells are located 0.25 to 0.5 mm below the taste buds and somewhat above the openings of the ducts of von Ebner's glands. Thus, the ciliated cells are equipped, by their cellular machinery and their position, to be a microcirculatory system in the crypt for the movement of gustatory stimuli.

FIGURE 18-9 Section on the side (left) and through the center (right) of taste buds of a camel's tongue. Methylene blue and eosin stain.

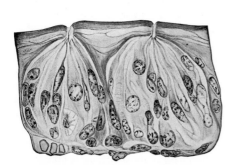

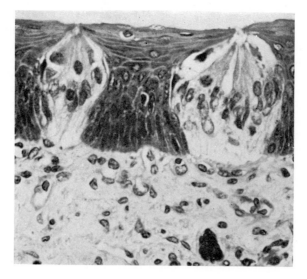

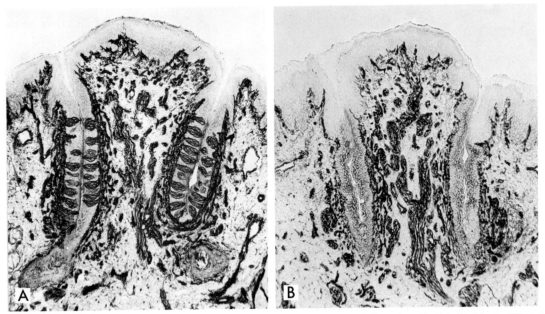

FIGURE 18-10 ATPase activity in the taste buds of circumvallate papillae (rat). ×70. A. Normal papilla. Note the intense ATPase activity in the numerous taste buds in the epithelium that lines the trench. B. Papilla 2 weeks after denervation. The taste buds have disappeared. (From A. A. Zalewski, *Exp. Neurol.*, **30:**510, 1971.)

MAJOR SALIVARY GLANDS

The parotid, submandibular (formerly submaxillary), and sublingual glands elaborate a major portion of the saliva. These compound tubuloacinar glands secrete proteins, glycoproteins, electrolytes, and water into the oral cavity. This secretory activity is controlled almost entirely by the autonomic nervous system. The best-known protein of saliva is the enzyme salivary amylase, which initiates the digestion of carbohydrate. The average daily output of saliva in humans is about 750 to 1,000 ml; saliva is a dilute aqueous fluid which is not an ultrafiltrate of the blood since it differs in the concentration of hydrogen ions, chloride ions, glucose, proteins, and in other constituents as well. Within minutes after an intravenous injection of iodide, the concentration of this ion in the saliva is at least 20 times greater than in the serum. This distinctive composition indicates that the secretion of saliva is an energy-requiring process. Furthermore, it has recently become known that saliva contains gamma globulins, the predominant one being immunoglobulin A (IgA). Lactoperoxidase has also been recently iden-

tified as a component of saliva; this enzyme, along with IgA, are part of a salivary antibacterial system.

From this brief physiologic introduction, it should be evident that the histologic-cytologic organization of these exocrine glands reflect mechanisms for protein and glycoprotein synthesis and transport, as well as mechanisms related to the transport of water and electrolytes. It should be noted that among different mammals there is considerable morphologic variation in these glands, which is probably related primarily to dietary differences (carnivores as against herbivores).

These exocrine glands are organized around a branching duct system that carries the secretion to the oral cavity. The secretory cells are arranged as *acini* or secretory end pieces around the smallest branches of the duct system to form many individual lobules which may be viewed as secretory units (Figs. 18-11 and 18-12). Each acinus is limited by a distinct basement membrane, and two types of secretory cells occur in the acinar epithelium, the *serous cells* and the *mucous cells*. The parotid gland of most species is composed entirely of serous acini (Fig. 18-13), whereas the submandibular and sublingual glands contain both (Figs. 18-14 and 18-15, see color insert). In the submandibular gland of humans, serous cells outnumber the mucous cells, whereas the opposite is true for the sublingual gland.

The cytology of the *serous cells* of the salivary glands is most easily comprehended by viewing them as variations of the pancreatic acinar cell. Radioautographic and other evidence demonstrates that the parotid acinar cell (rabbit) synthesizes, transports, and stores secretory enzymes in a manner comparable to the pancreatic acinar cell (Castle et al., 1972). The parotid gland is favored in experimental studies because its secretory cells are entirely of the serous type.

At the light-microscopic level, the serous cells are pyramidal in shape, their nuclei are basal, cell boundaries are indistinct, the basal and perinuclear cytoplasm are basophilic (Fig. 18-13), and the apical cyto-

plasm contains secretory granules that vary in number according to functional state. There are two major variants which can be distinguished by the presence or absence of histochemically demonstrable carbohydrate polymer in the cytoplasmic granules. According to this classification (Munger, 1964), the pancreatic acinar cells and the gastric chief cells are termed *serous cells* on the basis of the relative absence of such carbohydrate, whereas in the human submandibular gland, where the granules contain sialomucin and sulfomucin, the cells are called *seromucous* cells (Leblond).

At the ultrastructural level, the cytoplasmic basophilia of the serous cells corresponds to an abundant rough endoplasmic reticulum (ER); and the secretory granules occur within the membranes of the supranuclear Golgi complex (Fig. 18-16). These features are typical of cells that produce protein for export. In addition, ultrastructural variations occur that may be related to the secretion of saliva in partic-

FIGURE 18-11 Diagram of the histological organization of the salivary glands. Parotid gland is at the left, submandibular gland in the middle, and sublingual gland at the right. (From E. V. Cowdry, "A Textbook of Histology," Lea & Febiger, Philadelphia, 1950.)

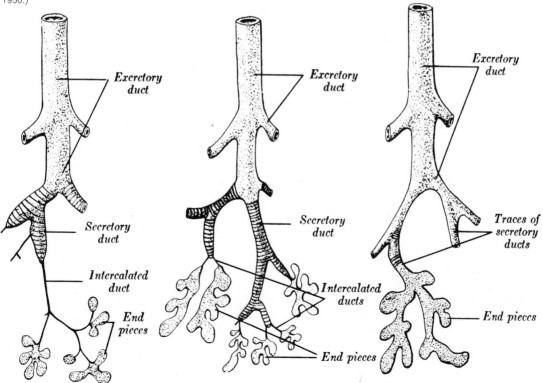

ular. For example, the serous cells of the human submandibular gland possess numerous slender basal projections that extend beyond the lateral margins as radiating foot processes that interdigitate with adjacent cells. This device increases surface area directed toward the vascular pole by at least sixtyfold and may be a specialization for transport of electrolytes and water into the primary secretion that enters the acinar lumen. Amylase is produced by the serous cells of the parotid gland. Peroxidase has been localized in the secretory granules of serous cells in the salivary glands of several species.

The *mucous cells* of the salivary glands may be viewed as variations of the intestinal goblet cell which has been the subject of considerable ultrastructural and analytic interpretation (see below). In the fresh condition, the cytoplasm may be filled with numerous droplets of mucigen; in routine preparations these droplets are usually dissolved out and the cytoplasm assumes an empty or vacuolated appearance (Figs. 18-14 and 18-15, see color insert). The mucous droplets are intensely reactive in the periodic acid Schiff (PAS) procedure, since they contain neutral glycoproteins and acid mucosubstances, such as sulfomucins or sialomucins (containing hexosamine and sialic acid in combination with protein) (see Leppi and Spicer, 1966). Some mucous cells produce sulfomucin (for example, most acini of the human sublingual) whereas others produce sialomucin or mixtures

FIGURE 18-12 Reconstruction of the secretory end piece and intralobular ducts of the submandibular gland. D, demilune composed of serous cells; M, mucous cells; My, myoepithelial cells; SC, secretory capillaries in a serous acinus; ID, intercalated duct; SD, striated duct. A. Cross section through the striated duct. B. Cross section through the intercalated duct. C. Cross section through a mucous acinus. D. Cross section through a serous acinus. (From H. Braus, ''Anatomie der Menschen,'' Springer-Verlag OHG, Berlin, 1924.)

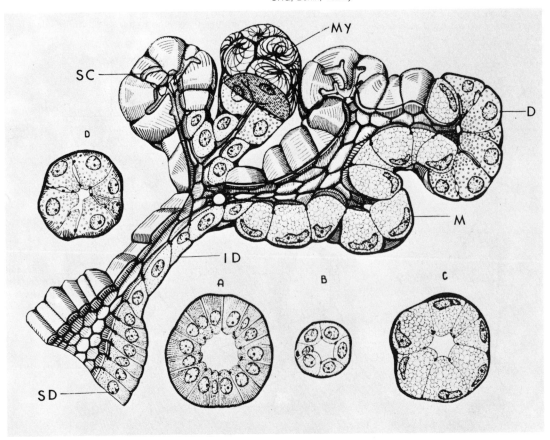

of the two (human submandibular). When the acid mucosubstances are preserved in a tissue section, the droplets are strongly basophilic. In a fully laden cell, the nucleus is basal and appears to be compressed by the accumulated secretion. The ultrastructure of the mucous cell is essentially similar to that of the goblet cell; that is, most of the supranuclear cytoplasm is filled with secretory droplets that have been derived from the large central supranuclear Golgi complex. As secretion accumulates, the mitochondria and rough ER are relegated to the lateral and basal cytoplasm.

A secretory end piece or acinus may be composed entirely of serous cells or mucous cells or may contain both cell types. In the latter situation, the serous cells occupy the fundus of the acinar sac, and the mucous cells are located closer to the opening to the initial duct segment (intercalated duct). Thus the serous cells form basophilic crescent-shaped groups that are called *demilunes* (Figs. 18-12 and 18-14). The cells of the demilune seem to be separated from

the acinar lumen by the mucous cells, but actually they are directly connected by the *secretory capillaries* which are extensions of the acinar lumen that may penetrate deeply between serous cells (Fig. 18-12). Microvilli occur along these secretory capillaries and thereby increase free-surface area.

Another component of the acinus is the *myo-epithelial cell* which, as the name suggests, has generally been regarded as a contractile element. Myo-epithelial cells have a distinctive form and occupy a unique position; they are flat cells with long cytoplasmic processes which extend over the outer surface of the acinus in a basketlike configuration (Fig. 18-12). They are located between the secretory cells and the basal lamina (Fig. 18-16). Their stellate form is difficult to discern in routine light-microscopic preparations because usually only their nuclear regions are recognizable in a given section. Since these cells possess relatively strong alkaline phosphatase activity, their form is better observed in histochemical preparations

FIGURE 18-13 Section of a human parotid gland. A. Section of a striated duct. B. Serous cell. C. Basal striations of serous cells. Zenker fixation; methylene blue and eosin.

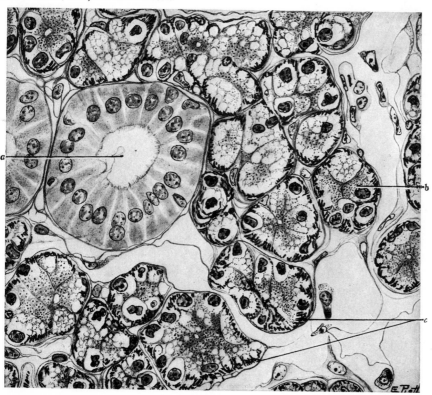

that demonstrate this enzymatic activity. The ultrastructure of the myoepithelial cells resembles that of smooth muscle cells; in particular, there are numerous parallel fine filaments that occupy large areas of the cytoplasm. The surface of the myoepithelial cell is smooth and is closely apposed to the secretory cell surface, with occasional desmosomal associations. The geometry and arrangement of the myoepithelial cells, as well as their ultrastructural features, suggest a role in moving the primary secretion.

The primary secretion is most likely modified during its passage through the branching duct system, since certain cytologic features, especially those of the

FIGURE 18-14 Human submandibular gland showing demilunes (arrows) of the mixed acini. M, mucous cells; S, serous cells.

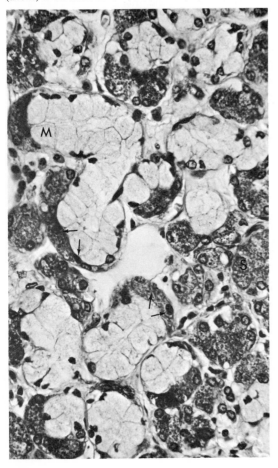

striated ducts, suggest participation in transport activities. The first two segments, the *intercalated duct* and the *striated duct*, also called *secretory* or *salivary duct*, are intralobular (Fig. 18-12). The secretion first enters the intercalated ducts which have a low cuboidal epithelium (Fig. 18-19A) and also have associated myoepithelial cells. Then it moves into the larger striated ducts which are lined by a tall columnar epithelium that is distinctly acidophilic. This segment derives its name from the light-microscopic appearance of the basal cytoplasm of the columnar cells; parallel striations are created by the vertical orientation of mitochondria within numerous slender cytoplasmic compartments that are outlined by deep infoldings of the basal plasma membrane (Fig. 18-17). These basal cytoplasmic compartments represent interdigitating foot processes of adjacent cells, similar to those which occur in the distal tubule of the nephron. This specialization, which creates a vast basal surface area and associates it closely with energy-producing mitochondria (Fig. 18-18), is characteristic of other epithelia known to be involved in rapid transport of ions and water. Myoepithelial cells are absent from the striated ducts. Larger ducts, known as *interlobular ducts*, course through the stroma, become progressively larger, and finally join the primary duct that leads into the oral cavity. The interlobular ducts are initially simple columnar and then pseudostratified columnar with occasional goblet cells. The largest ducts are lined by stratified epithelia, which may be stratified columnar (Fig. 18-19B), and those near the orifice are usually stratified squamous in form.

The salivary glands differ in the extent to which the intralobular ducts are developed (Fig. 18-11). The intercalated ducts are longest in the parotid, and the striated ducts are best developed in the submandibular gland. Both types of intralobular ducts are quite inconspicuous in the sublingual gland. The varying proportions of striated ducts among the glands should have considerable functional significance.

It has long been known that the connective tissue among the acini of the salivary glands is a reticular connective tissue that contains many plasma cells and some small lymphocytes, as well as the usual stromal cells and fibers. In 1965, in an important discovery, Tomasi and his associates demonstrated the presence of IgA in most of the plasma cells in the interstitium of the human parotid gland (via the fluorescent antibody technique). Also, plasma cells containing IgG and IgM occur in the periacinar stroma but in fewer numbers. Further work led to the following hypothesis: IgA is

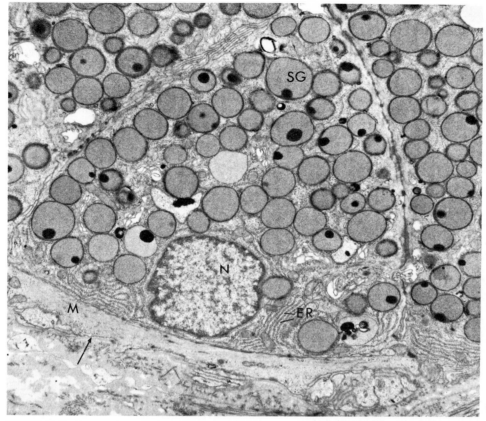

FIGURE 18-16 Human submandibular gland, serous cell, electron micrograph. Rough endoplasmic reticulum (ER) occurs in the basal cytoplasm. Secretory granules (SG) occupy most of the cell. A process of a myoepithelial cell (M) occurs between the serous cell and the basal lamina (arrow). ×9000. (Courtesy of Dr. Bernard Tandler.)

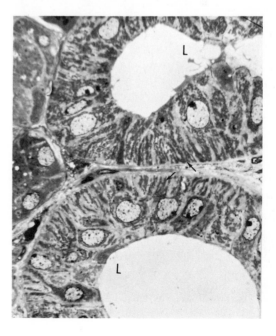

FIGURE 18-17 Human submandibular gland. Portions of two striated ducts are shown. The basal striations (arrows) created by parallel alignment of mitochondria are evident. L, lumen. Toluidine blue; 1-μm section. ×1300. (Courtesy of Dr. Bernard Tandler.)

produced in local plasma cells, it combines with a unique protein called the *secretory piece* which is believed to be produced by the acinar epithelial cells, and then it is released into the secretion as *secretory IgA,* which is resistant to proteolysis. It is likely that secretory IgA plays an important role in the oral cavity in defense against pathogens.

The major blood vessels course through the connective tissue, following the route of the large branch-

FIGURE 18-18 Human submandibular gland. A horizontal section through the base of the striated duct reveals the close association of mitochondria (M) with infoldings of basal plasma membrane (arrows). Electron micrograph. ×17,000. (Courtesy of Dr. Bernard Tandler.)

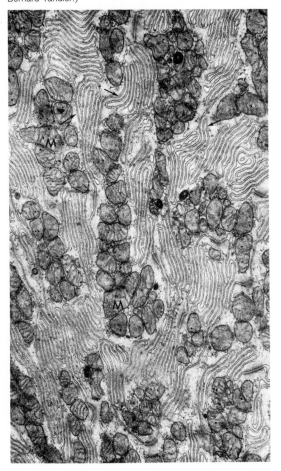

ing ducts. Within the lobules, some arteries form rich capillary networks around the intralobular ducts, whereas other arterial branches continue to create capillary plexuses around the acini. The periductal capillaries are denser than the periacinar ones (Leeson). The venous drainage retraces the arterial pathway. Arteriovenous anastomoses have been reported to occur. An extensive system of lymphatic drainage follows the course of the duct system.

Each major salivary gland is innervated by both the parasympathetic and sympathetic divisions of the autonomic nervous system, and it is generally agreed that secretory activity is mainly under neural control. Stimulation of either the sympathetic or parasympathetic innervation produces qualitatively different salivas. Parasympathetic stimulation produces a more voluminous saliva than does sympathetic activation. The manner in which this dual innervation influences the functional activity of the acinar and ductal cells remains a problem for investigators. Species variation among salivary glands is great, and this complicates interpretation. Ultrastructural observations on the cat submandibular gland indicate that terminations of both sympathetic and parasympathetic fibers are associated with the surface of one acinar cell (Hand, 1970). An important anatomic feature of this innervation is illustrated in Fig. 18-20, which demonstrates that autonomic nerve fibers penetrate the acinar basal lamina and acquire an intraepithelial position. Within the acinar epithelium, the axons are naked and come into close association with both the secretory and myoepithelial cells. The axons may penetrate deeply between acinar cells or within invaginations of the acinar cell surface. A 20-nm space separates the surfaces of the neuronal and epithelial cells. The nerve fibers have small enlargements that contain many axoplasmic vesicles and mitochondria, ultrasturctural features that typify nerve terminals. Acetylcholinesterase activity has been demonstrated in these regions of close apposition. Another significant anatomic feature is the occurrence of autonomic networks around intralobular ducts which in some glands may be denser than around the acini.

SUMMARY OF THE MAJOR FEATURES OF HUMAN SALIVARY GLANDS (Fig. 18-11)

The *parotid gland* is an almost purely seromucous gland (Figs. 18-13 and 18-19A). The secretory granules are PAS-positive, indicating that they contain a carbohydrate-protein polymer. The intercalated ducts are long and abundant, whereas the striated ducts are less elaborate.

The *submandibular*[1] (formerly called submaxillary) gland (Fig. 18-14) is a mixed gland with seromucous acini and demilunes predominating over the purely mucous acini. However, lobules vary somewhat in this proportion, with some having a predominance of mucous acini (Leppi and Spicer, 1966). The secretory granules of the seromucous cells are PAS-posi-

---

[1] Portions of the human submandibular and sublingual glands intermingle in a manner that constitutes a gross submandibular sublingual complex (Leppi, 1967). This intermingling can create a sampling problem in microscopic study.

FIGURE 18-19 Portions of the duct system of salivary glands. A. The intercalated duct of the human parotid with a flattened simple epithelium. The arrows are within the lumen of the duct. B. A large excretory duct of the human sublingual lined with a two-layered stratified columnar epithelium.

tive; they are rich in sialomucin although some cells contain sulfomucin. The mucous cells contain either sialomucin or sulfomucin or a mixture of both. The striated ducts are best developed in the submandibular gland; the intercalated ducts are present but less conspicuous.

The sublingual gland[1] is a mixed gland composed mainly of mucous acini although there may be considerable variation in the proportion of mucous to seromucous acini and demilunes in different regions of the gland (Fig. 18-15, see color insert). Sulfomucin is the major component of the abundant mucous secretion. The seromucous cells are rich in sialomucin. Both segments (intercalated and striated ducts) of the intralobular duct system are poorly developed.

The *pharynx* is a component of both the digestive

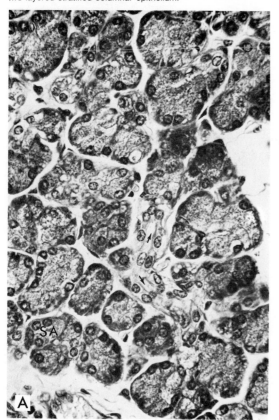

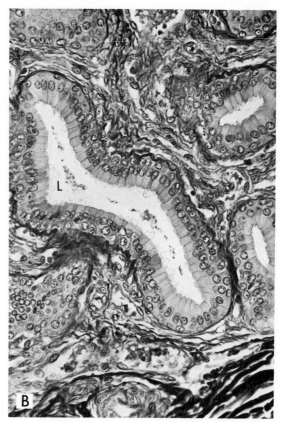

and respiratory systems; it is here that the pathways for the passage of gases and food merge and cross. In its upper regions, the histologic organization follows that of the respiratory system whereas the lower part resembles that of the oral cavity.

The remainder of the digestive tract is organized around a common histologic plan. The following de-scription of the general structural plan pertains to the remainder of the digestive tube. Also, essential termi-nology that is needed to analyze the microscopic anat-omy of these organs is presented.

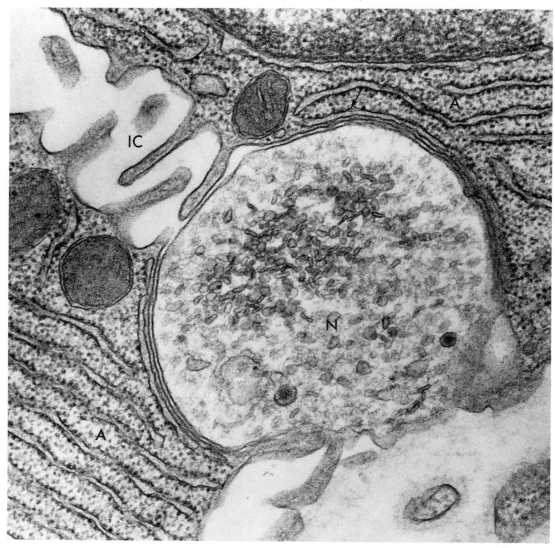

FIGURE 18-20 Intraepithelial autonomic nerve terminal (N) be-tween two acinar cells (A) of the rat parotid gland. Note regions of close apposition between the surfaces of the nerve fiber and the secretory cells. A. cisterna of endoplasmic reticulum (arrows) parallels the apposed surfaces. IC, intercellular space. ×57,000. (From Hand, 1970.)

GENERAL STRUCTURAL PLAN FOR THE ESOPHAGUS, STOMACH, AND INTESTINES

LAYERS

The digestive tube from the esophagus through the large intestine is made up of four concentric layers which exhibit considerable regularity. Named in order from the lumen outward, these are the *mucosa,* the *submucosa,* the *muscularis,* and the *adventitia* or *serosa* (Fig. 18-21). The *mucosa,* or mucous membrane, has three components: (1) a superficial *epithelium;* (2) an underlying stroma composed of a vascularized, highly cellular, reticular connective tissue (*lamina propria*); and (3) a relatively thin layer of smooth muscle (*muscularis mucosae*). Typically, the fibers in the muscularis mucosae are subdivided into an inner circular and an outer longitudinal layer. Large accumulations of typical lymphatic tissue are often present in the stroma. Furthermore, because of the abundance of plasma cells and lymphocytes, the entire lamina propria of much of the gut is a major site of immunologic response.

The lining epithelium may form glands that extend into the lamina propria (*mucosal glands*) or submucosa (*submucosal glands*), or ducts that lead from the wall of the tract to glands situated outside the tube proper (*liver, pancreas*). In other instances the entire mucosa projects into the lumen as folds (*plicae and rugae*) or fingers (*villi*). These invaginations and evaginations of the lining of the gut enlarge its effective surface tremendously.

The *mucosa* differs considerably from segment to segment of the alimentary tract in relation to the changing functional activity. Considerable emphasis will be placed in the following descriptions on the specialized mucosal cells involved in secretion and absorption. On the other hand, the surrounding, supportive and muscular layers change relatively little, and thus only their distinctive features will be noted.

The *submucosa* is a fibrous, rather than a highly cellular, connective tissue layer, often containing accumulations of lymphatic tissue as well as glands that

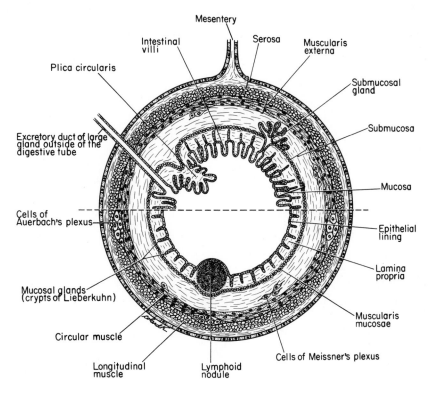

Mesentery

Intestinal villi

Serosa

Muscularis externa

Plica circularis

Submucosal gland

Submucosa

Excretory duct of large gland outside of the digestive tube

Mucosa

Cells of Auerbach's plexus

Epithelial lining

Lamina propria

Mucosal glands (crypts of Lieberkuhn)

Circular muscle

Muscularis mucosae

Longitudinal muscle

Lymphoid nodule

Cells of Meissner's plexus

FIGURE 18-21 Diagrammatic representation of the overall histological organization of the digestive tract from the esophagus through the large intestine. (From W. Bloom and D. W. Fawcett, "A Textbook of Histology," 10th ed., W. B. Saunders Company, Philadelphia, 1975.)

extend from the mucosa. The submucosa is also a vascular service area containing large blood vessels that send finer vessels into the layers that embody the specific functions, the mucosa and muscularis.

The *muscularis* contains at least two layers of muscle. The muscle is smooth in all parts except the upper esophagus and the anal sphincter, where it is composed of skeletal muscle fibers. The fibers of the inner layers are disposed in a roughly circular fashion around the tube (*circular layer*), and those of the outer layer are disposed lengthwise along the tube (*longitudinal layer*). Contractions of the circular layer constrict the lumen, contractions of the longitudinal layer shorten the tube. At the various sphincters and valves along the tube (pharyngoesophageal, esophagogastric, pyloric, ileocecal, and anal), the layer of circular muscle is greatly thickened. Careful dissection of the muscle layers has shown that the fibers are actually disposed in a helical fashion, those in the circular layer forming a tight helix and those in the longitudinal layer an elongated one. The connective tissue fibers in the submucosa and adventitia are likewise oriented helically.

The *adventitia* of the tract is composed of several layers of loose connective tissue, alternately collagenous and elastic. Where the tract is suspended by a peritoneal fold, it is covered by a mesothelium continuous with that of the peritoneum (see later section). Wherever a mesothelial covering occurs, the adventitial layer is customarily termed a *serosa*.

BLOOD VESSELS

At intervals, blood and lymphatic vessels and nerves enter the tract from the surrounding tissues or via the supporting peritoneal fold. The largest arteries are disposed longitudinally in the submucosa, and smaller branches also run in the serosa (Fig. 18-22A). From these two sets of vessels, branches ramify perpendicularly to both the mucosa and the muscularis. In the latter, the capillaries run parallel with the muscle fibers. In the mucosa, the arteries supply an irregular capillary plexus around the glands and, in the small intestine, send terminal branches into the villi. The small capillaries associated with the intestinal epithelium typically have fenestrated endothelial cells.

The veins arising in the mucosa anastomose in the submucosa and pass out of the intestine beside the arteries. The muscularis mucosae has been described as forming a sphincter for the veins penetrating it. Valves are found in the larger veins only in the adventitia or serosa; they disappear again in the mesentery where these veins form the branches of the portal vein leading to the liver.

FIGURE 18-22 Diagrams of blood vessels (A), lymphatic vessels (B), and nerves (C) of the alimentary tract, as occur in the small intestine. The layers of the tract are m, mucosa; mm, muscularis mucosae; sm, submucosa; cm, circular muscle layer; ic, intermuscular connective tissue; lm, longitudinal muscle; s, serosa. In A, arteries are shown as coarse black lines, capillaries as fine black lines, and veins shaded. In B, lymphatic vessels are shown as open channels. In C, neurons and nerve fibers are shown. Additional abbreviations: n, lymphatic nodule; s pl, submucosal plexus; m pl, myenteric plexus.

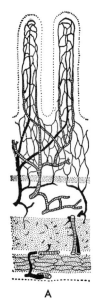

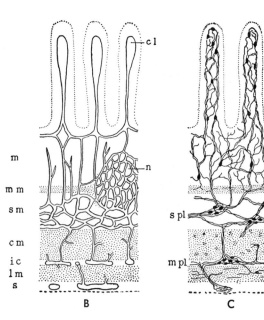

A   B   C

The alimentary tract is richly supplied with lymphatic vessels, which arise as blind tubes in the mucosa. In the small intestine, each villus usually contains a single central lymphatic vessel known as a *lacteal* (Fig. 18-22B). In some stages of digestion, the distention of these lymphatics is great and they are easily recognized in sections. When the vessels are collapsed, their walls are difficult to distinguish from the surrounding reticular connective tissue. Viewed at the ultrastructural level, these lymphatic capillaires lack endothelial pores—thus differing from the local blood capillaries—and have little or no basal lamina.

In the submucosa, the larger lymphatic vessels branch freely and have numerous valves. They cross the muscle layers, spreading in the intermuscular tissue and serosa, and pass through the mesentery. Unlike lymphatic vessels in many other parts of the body, those in the mesentery possess muscular walls and are thus able to propel their contents.

LYMPHATIC TISSUE

The lymphatic tissue of the alimentary tract occurs primarily in the lamina propria and assumes three forms: diffuse lymphatic tissue, solitary lymphatic nodules (Figs. 18-40 and 18-58), and aggregate nodules (Figs. 18-54A, B, C and 18-60). Large lymphatic masses may break through the muscularis mucosae and spread into the submucosa, as shown in Figs. 18-54A, B, C and 18-58. The superficial lymphatic vessels form a plexus as they pass through the nodule (Fig. 18-22B). Blood vessels also form a net in the lymphatic tissue.

Diffuse lymphatic tissue occurs under the simple epithelia of the intestines. The degree of cellularity has been related to the bacterial count in the lumen. This local lymphatic tissue produces IgA in association with the lining epithelium. This antibody occurs along the luminal surface like an "antiseptic paint" (Walker and Hong, 1973). Antigens that pass through the lining epithelium effect an immune response in this local lymphatic tissue. The cells found most abundantly are lymphocytes, macrophages, plasma cells, and eosinophils.

Solitary nodules occur in the esophagus, in the pylorus of the stomach, and along the entire length of the small and large intestines.

Aggregate nodules (Peyer's patches) occur in the small intestine and in the appendix (Figs. 18-54 and 18-60). They are oval bodies, usually from 1 to 4 cm long but occasionally much larger, composed of 10 to 60 nodules in close contact. These patches distort and push aside the nearby glands, and immediately above the nodules villi are largely effaced. There are 15 to 30 such patches in the human intestine, principally in the lower part of the ileum on the side opposite the mesenteric attachment. A few occur in the jejunum and lower duodenum. Aggregate nodules are always present in the vermiform appendix (Fig. 18-60) but do not occur elsewhere in the large intestine.

This widely distributed tissue is part of the local immune system that responds to antigenic stimuli by producing primarily secretory immunoglobulin and other antibodies.

NERVES

The nerves consist of both autonomic motor and sensory fibers. (At the two extremes of the tract there is, of course, voluntary innervation of the skeletal muscle fibers.) The motor fibers are both parasympathetic and sympathetic. The fibers of both ramify in the wall of the tract as shown in Fig. 18-22C, forming plexuses in each of the layers. The ganglia of the sympathetic nerves are external to the gut wall, lying in the celiac plexus and in the superior and inferior mesenteric plexuses. The parasympathetic nerves are derived from the vagus and the sacral outflow.

The neurons of the intramural parasympathetic ganglia occur in two locations: (1) in nodes of the *submucosal plexus* (of Meissner) and (2) between the two layers of the muscularis, in the *myenteric plexus* (of Auerbach). The ganglia and the associated fibers form an irregular rectilinear pattern when viewed from the surface. The autonomic ganglion cells, surrounded by the usual satellite cells, possess many dendrites and have eccentrically located nuclei (Fig. 18-23). Sympathetic fibers ramify through the wall of the tube along with the parasympathetic fibers to innervate the muscularis and the blood vessels.

Stimulation of the parasympathetic nerves to the intestinal tract, generally speaking, increases muscular activity, circulation, and secretion, whereas these activities are decreased by stimulation of the sympathetic nerves. Since the postganglionic parasympathetic fibers arise locally, their influence may be limited to a fairly short length of the tube. Postganglionic fibers of

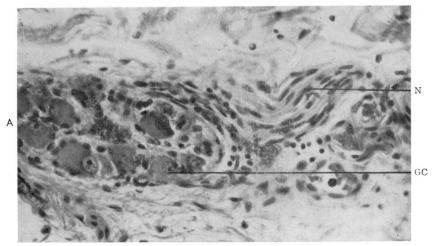

A   N

GC

FIGURE 18-23 Parasympathetic ganglion in the submucosa of the human stomach wall. N, nerve fibers; GC, large ganglion cell, surrounded by satellite cells. H&E. ×300.

the sympathetics, however, arise from ganglia external to the gut and possess much wider distribution. Sympathetic activity is reinforced, moreover, by the concomitant release of catecholamines from the adrenal medulla.

SUSPENSORY FOLDS

The esophagus runs through the thorax within the superior and posterior mediastina and lacks any special support. The stomach and intestines are mostly supported by suspensory folds from the peritoneal wall known as the *omenta* and *mesenteries,* respectively. However, the duodenum and the ascending and descending limbs of the colon adhere to the posterior wall of the abdominal cavity and are thus considered *secondarily retroperitoneal.*

Suspensory folds are composed of a serous membrane covering the "ventral" surface and sides of the tube and a double-layered suspending membrane, continuous on each side with the peritoneal lining of the cavity. The *peritoneum* thus forms a closed sac and is divisible into the *visceral peritoneum,* covering the viscera, and the *parietal peritoneum,* which lines the body walls. In all cases, its free surface is covered with a single layer of closely packed, polygonal cells, the *mesothelium.* Although very flat, these cells have scattered microvilli on the free surface and may be somewhat phagocytic.

ESOPHAGUS

The esophagus is a tubular passageway for the chewed, partly digested food received from the oral cavity. In the adult human it is about 25 cm long. There is considerable regularity in the arrangements of the component tissue layers (Fig. 18-24) which are continuous superiorly with those of the pharynx and inferiorly with those of the stomach. Because of the tonus of the circular layer, its mucous membrane is thrown into many temporary longitudinal folds (Fig.

18-24) that flatten out during passage of a bolus of food.

A thin layer of connective tissue, with cells, elastic networks, and interwoven bundles of collagenous fibers, occupies the interval between the two epithelial layers. It is here that the lymphatic vessels, blood vessels, and nerves that supply the various alimentary organs are to be found running together. Mast cells are common, and eosinophils, monocytes, lymphocytes, macrophages, and adipose tissue also occur. Mesothelial cells and the various wandering cells are frequently found free in the peritoneal fluid.

The stomach is peculiar in that it retains a ventral suspensory fold and thus possesses both a *dorsal* (greater) *omentum* and a *ventral* (lesser) *omentum*. The omenta differ from the mesenteries proper in that they are perforated. Especially numerous in these sheets, and also in the peritoneum covering the diaphragm, are "milky spots," which consist of aggregations of blast cells, monocytes, and macrophages. These aggregations apparently play an important role in combating infection in the peritoneal cavity.

The epithelium of the mucosa is stratified squamous (Fig. 18-26) and extremely thick (about 300 μm). In humans, complete keratinization of the epithelium is rare unless the esophagus is subject to an unusual degree of trauma. Such keratinization occurs normally in some mammalian species, especially in herbivores.

The lamina propria of the esophagus is less cellular than that of lower parts of the digestive tube. Lymphatic nodules occur occasionally, especially around the ducts of glands. The muscularis mucosae is broad,

being 200 to 400 μm thick. It is unusual in that it consists of longitudinally directed fibers. It replaces the elastic layer of the pharynx at the level of the cricoid cartilage.

The submucosa is thick (300 to 700 μm) and is characterized by abundant, coarse elastic fibers, which permit distention.

The muscularis (0.5 to 2 mm) comprises an inner circular layer and outer bundles of longitudinal fibers, arising at the level of the cricoid cartilage. At its upper extremity, there is the *superior esophageal* (pharyngoesophageal) *sphincter,* consisting of a thickened layer of circular (oblique) muscles. In the upper quarter of the tube the fibers are skeletal rather than smooth. Striated and smooth muscle fibers intermingle in the second quarter of the tube (Fig. 18-25). Only smooth muscle fibers occur in the lower half and mark the beginning of a continuous muscularis of smooth muscle that extends throughout the stomach and intestines to the anus.

The adventitia is loose connective tissue contain-

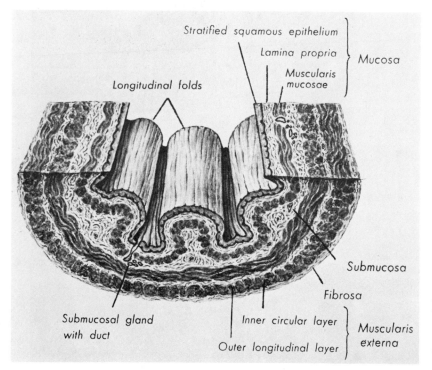

FIGURE 18-24 Reconstruction of a segment of the dorsal half of the human esophagus. (From W. M. Copenhaver, R. P. Bunge, and M. B. Bunge, "Bailey's Textbook of Histology," The Williams & Wilkins Company, Baltimore, 1971.)

666

ing many longitudinally directed blood vessels, lymphatic vessels, and nerves. For 2 to 3 cm above the stomach, elastic fibers are numerous and attach the esophagus to the diaphragm.

The orifice between the esophagus and stomach is bounded by a broad band of circular muscles, the *inferior esophageal* (esophagogastric) *sphincter.* There is generally an abrupt change at the esophageal-cardiac junction from stratified epithelium to the simple columnar epithelium that characterizes the stomach (Fig. 18-29).

Glands are isolated in the esophagus and are only of the mucous type. By position, they are classified as superficial (mucosal) and deep (submucosal). The *mucosal glands* are limited to narrow zones near the two ends of the esophagus, between the level of the cricoid cartilage and the fifth tracheal ring and again near the entrance of the stomach (Fig. 18-29). The mucus formed by these superficial glands does not stain metachromatically, as does that of the deep glands. Because of the resemblance of the mucosal glands to those occurring at the cardiac end of the stomach, an alternative name is *cardiac glands.*

The submucosal glands are scattered, tubular downgrowths that pass through the lamina propria and muscularis mucosae into the submucosa (Figs. 18-26, 18-27, and 18-29). The cells have the typical cytologic characteristics of mucous cells. The smallest ducts are lined with simple columnar epithelium; the main ducts that enter the mucosa are lined with stratified epithelium. The number of deep glands varies greatly in different individuals. They usually predominate in the upper half of the esophagus.

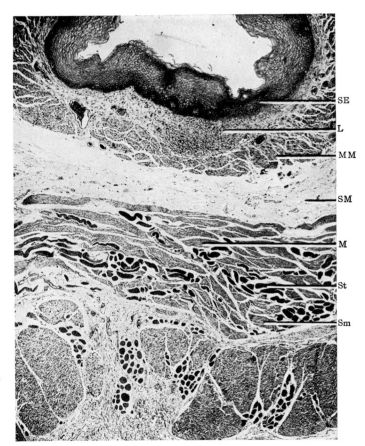

FIGURE 18-25 Midregion of the human esophagus, cross section. At this level, the muscularis contains skeletal muscle fibers in addition to smooth muscle fibers. SE, stratified squamous epithelium; L, lymphatic tissue in lamina propria; MM, muscularis mucosae; SM, submucosa; M, muscularis; St, striated (skeletal) muscle fiber; Sm, smooth muscle fibers. Eosin and methylene blue. ×45.

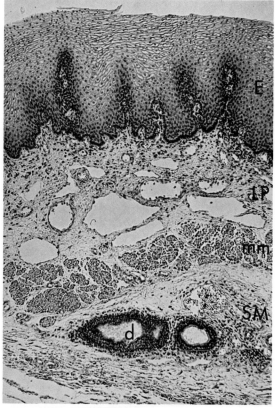

FIGURE 18-26 Monkey esophagus, mucosa with a portion of submucosa. The nonkeratinized stratified squamous epithelium (E) rests on a relatively acellular lamina propria (LP). The muscularis mucosa (mm) is thick. Ducts (d) of esophageal glands occur in the submucosa (SM). H&E.

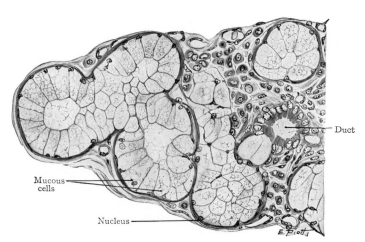

FIGURE 18-27 The end of a submucosal gland, esophagus of a child. The secretory end pieces produce mucus. H&E.

STOMACH

The stomach is a remarkable exocrine secretory organ in that it produces after each meal a large volume of acidic (pH2) secretion that contains the protease pepsin. This enzyme initiates protein digestion which is continued in the intestinal lumen by pancreatic enzymes. The gastric surface is protected from the highly acidic secretion by a thin film of mucus which is being constantly produced by the surface epithelial cells. Another exocrine gastric product is an intrinsic factor, a glycoprotein, that combines with vitamin B_{12} to produce a complex necessary for the maturation of red blood cells. The stomach is also, in part, an endocrine gland that produces the hormone gastrin, which influences the activity not only of the gastric exocrine and muscular cells but also the physiologic activity of the pancreas and small intestines. Gastric digestion is facilitated by contractions of the heavy muscularis which churn the food.

The opening through which the esophagus connects with the stomach is the *cardiac orifice,* and the opening from the stomach to the intestine is the *pyloric orifice* (G, *pyloros,* gatekeeper). The lining of the stomach is thrown into major longitudinal folds, or *rugae,* when the organ is not distended with food (Fig. 18-28).

HISTOLOGIC ORGANIZATION

In humans, the *gastric epithelium* is simple columnar throughout. At the cardiac opening, the cells are continuous with the basal layer of the stratified epithelium of the esophagus (Fig. 18-29). The lining of the organ is indented by multitudinous pits (foveolae), leading from *branched, tubular glands.* There are about 3.5 million foveolae on the stomach wall, serving some 15 million glands. All the glands occur in the mucosa.

The glands of the stomach are divided into three categories: The *cardiac glands* are in the first 5 to 40 mm from the cardiac orifice; the *pyloric glands* are along the 4 cm from the pyloric vestibule to the pyloric sphincter; between these two extremities lie the *gastric* (or, erroneously, fundic) *glands.* The cells of the cardiac and pyloric glands are primarily mucous. The epithelium of the gastric glands is more diversified, containing enzyme- and acid-secreting cells as well as mucous cells. The cardiac and pyloric glands are conspicuously coiled (Fig. 18-29 and 18-30B), whereas the gastric glands are relatively straight (Fig. 18-30A). The pyloric region is distinguished by foveolae that occupy nearly one-half the depth of the mucosa; in the cardia and body of the organ, the pits occupy only one-fourth the thickness of the mucosa.

The *mucous membrane* of the stomach measures 0.3 to 1.5 mm in width, being thinnest in the cardiac region. Underlying the epithelium is a richly vascularized lamina propria, which is often quite cellular, especially in the pylorus (Fig. 18-30B). Occasionally lymphatic nodules occur. As in the intestines, the gastric lamina propria is the site of immunologic response. Smooth muscle fibers extend upward from the muscularis mucosae around the glands, and their shortening may aid in the expulsion of secretory products.

The *submucosa* consists of coarse collagenous bundles and many elastic fibers, plus blood and lymphatic vessels and the submucosal nerve plexus. Clusters of fat cells are common in older people.

The *muscularis* is composed of three primary layers—an inner oblique, a middle circular, and an outer longitudinal layer. The oblique layer is best developed at the cardiac end and in the body of the organ. The circular bundles are thickened at both ends in the regions of the sphincters. The myenteric nerve plexus occurs in the connective tissue lamina separating the circular from the longitudinal muscle layer. The extensive muscle coat produces the churning and homogenization of ingested food as gastric juices are added to it.

The *serosa,* consisting of connective tissue plus mesothelium, is continuous, via the omenta, with the peritoneum.

FIGURE 18-28 Interior of the human stomach showing regional differences and the internal folds or rugae. (From H. Gray and C. M. Goss, "Gray's Anatomy," 28th ed., Lea & Febiger, Philadelphia, 1966.)

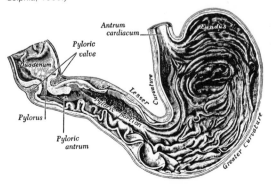

The entire gastric surface and the glands are lined by simple columnar epithelium. Cells of four major types occur: (1) *surface mucous cells,* (2) *neck* mucous cells, (3) parietal, or oxyntic, cells, and (4) chief, or peptic, cells (Fig. 18-31, see color insert). In addition to these, there are *enterochromaffin cells,* which contain granules that may be blackened by silver methods or oxidized by chromates or osmium tetroxide. These cells have recently been identified as endocrine cells by immunocytochemistry.

The surface of the stomach is lined entirely by *surface mucous cells* which form a uniform simple columnar epithelium that extends into the pits (foveolae) (Figs. 18-32 and 18-34A). They secrete a neutral polysaccharide-protein continuously which forms a mucous film that protects the mucosa from the high acidity of the gastric fluid. These luminal cells are constantly being shed into the lumen and replaced

from below. In routine preparations (Fig. 18-32) the mucus is usually not preserved and thus the apical cytoplasm appears empty or foamy. This mucus is demonstrable by the PAS procedure (Fig. 18-34A). At the ultrastructural level, the mucous droplets are ovoid, spherical, or discoid dense granules located within the membranes of the well-developed Golgi complex. The endoplasmic reticulum is relatively sparse.

The *neck mucous cells* are located in the upper ends of the gastric gland (that is, immediately below the base of the pit), where they are interspersed among parietal cells (Figs. 18-31 and 18-33). These cells which produce an acidic mucus (glycosaminoglycan) (Fig. 18-34B) differ structurally and functionally from the surface mucous cells which produce a neutral mucus. Neck mucous cells exhibit more cytoplasmic basophilia in light microscopic preparations and more rough ER in electron-microscopic preparations than do the surface mucous cells. The Golgi complex is exceptionally well developed. The droplets are larger and more spherical than those of the surface cells; mucous droplets often lie deep in the cell as well as near the apex.

The *parietal,* or *oxyntic, cells* secrete 0.1 *N* hy-

FIGURE 18-29 Longitudinal section through the junction of the human esophagus and stomach. Note the sharp transition from stratified epithelium of the esophagus (left) to the simple columnar epithelium of the stomach (right). The simple epithelium is continuous with the basal layer of the stratified epithelium. a. Duct of a mucosal esophageal gland. b. Esophageal epithelium. c. Gastric epithelium. d. Tubule of mucosal gland. e. Lymphatic nodule. f. Lymphatic vessel. g. Muscularis mucosae.

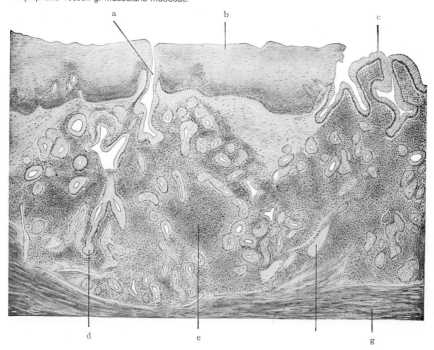

670

drochloric acid. Since this concentration of acid can destroy living cells, this remarkable secretory feat has attracted much interest. Parietal cells are located principally in the upper half of the gastric gland proper, but they also occur in the lower half among the pepsin-producing chief cells (Figs. 18-31 and 18-33). They are also present in fewer numbers in the pyloric glands. At the light microscopic level, these cells are easily identified by their large size (Fig. 18-32) and intensely acidophilic cytoplasm (Fig. 18-31). They usually contain one nucleus but may also be binucleate.

A distinctive morphologic feature of these acid-secreting cells is the presence of *intracellular (or secretory) canaliculi* which are trenchlike invaginations of the apical cell surface (Figs. 18-34 and 18-35). (These deep invaginations may also be interpreted as extensions of the glandular lumen.) The canaliculi are

lined by numerous microvilli, and thus the surface area of the apical plasma membrane is greatly increased. The secretion of HCl is believed to occur along this vast internalized surface.

The intense cytoplasmic acidophilia of the parietal cells reflects the abundance of smooth membranes and mitochondria and a relatively small representation of rough endoplasmic reticulum (Fig. 18-35). The Golgi complex is small and basal in location. The smooth membranes have been described as the *tubulovesicular system*, which is continuous with the plasma membrane lining the canaliculi. During acid secretion, microvilli become more abundant, whereas the tubulovesicular system diminishes (Fig. 18-36). When acid secretion is inhibited experimentally, the

FIGURE 18-30 Mucosal surfaces of the human stomach. Arrows indicate the bottoms of the gastric pits. Muscularis mucosae (mm). A. Gastric glands from the body of the stomach. B. Pyloric glands. Note the deeper pits in the pyloric glands in comparison with those of the gastric glands. Contrast the relative straightness of the gastric glands with the coiled nature of the pyloric glands. H&E.

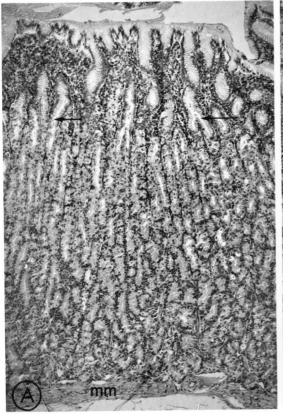
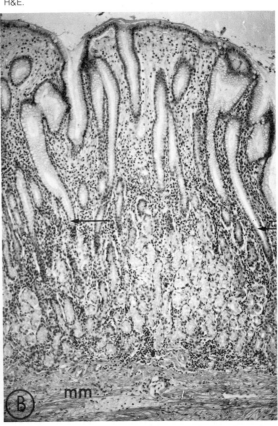

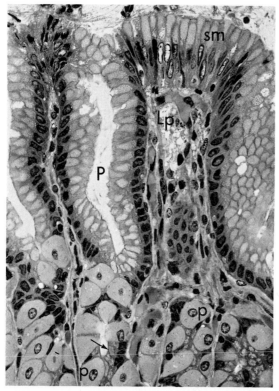

FIGURE 18-32 Gastric glands, monkey, H&E. The luminal epithelium is composed of surface mucous cells (sm) which also form the lining of the gastric pit (P). The upper portions of the gland are visible where parietal cells (p) and neck mucous cells (arrow) are evident. Lp, lamina propria.

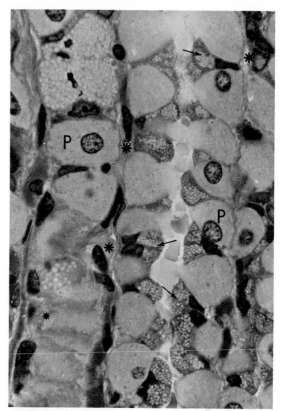

FIGURE 18-33 Human gastric glands, upper half. The epithelium is composed primarily of large, clear, parietal cells (P) and smaller neck mucous cells (arrows) with vacuolated cytoplasm and basal nuclei. The asterisks identify the narrow lamina propria. (Courtesy of Dr. Marion Neutra.)

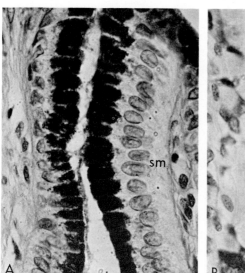

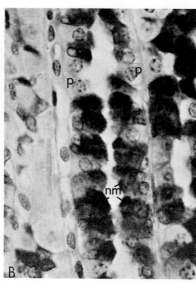

FIGURE 18-34 Gastric gland, grasshopper mouse. PAS&H. Note the differences in the size, shape, and distribution of mucous droplets in the surface mucous cells (panel A, sm) and neck mucous cells (panel B, nm). p, parietal cells.

reverse morphologic relationship is observed. The tubulovesicular system may thus represent a membrane reserve that is translocated to the surface during acid secretion. Overall, it is evident that active acid secretion requires a large area of free surface. Also physiological evidence indicates that acid secretion has a high energy requirement (oxidative metabolism); this is reflected morphologically by an abundance of mitochondria that have many cristae and matrix granules (Fig. 18-35).

The pepsin-producing cells are located primarily in the basal half of the gastric glands; they have been called *chief (or peptic or zymogenic) cells* (Fig. 18-31, see color insert). They are typical serous zymogenic cells, resembling the pancreatic acinar cell. The basal cytoplasm contains an extensive rough ER (Fig. 18-37), which is reflected light microscopically as a striated basophilic region. The supranuclear region is filled with basophilic *zymogen granules* which are often not preserved in routine preparations. These secretory granules form in the Golgi complex and are believed to be released in the same manner as the zymogen granules of pancreatic acinar cells.

The chief cells contain *pepsinogen*, the precursor of the active enzyme pepsin which hydrolyzes proteins

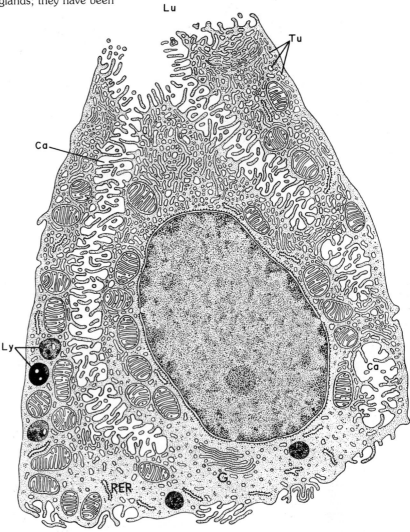

FIGURE 18-35 Drawing representing the ultrastructural features of the gastric parietal cell. The secretory canaliculus (Ca), a deep, troughlike invagination of the apical surface, is a principal distinctive feature. It has numerous microvilli along its surface that additionally increases surface area. The cytoplasmic membrane system consists primarily of the smooth tubulovesicular system (Tu) which is concentrated beneath the surface of the canaliculus. Mitochondria are abundant. Note the relative sparcity of the rough ER (RER) and Golgi membranes (G). The dense bodies (Ly) may be derivatives of the lysosomal system. (From T. L. Lentz, "Cell Fine Structure," W. B. Saunders Company, Philadelphia, 1971.)

into smaller molecules. The acid milieu of the stomach is required to convert pepsinogen to pepsin. Another proteolytic enzyme, *rennin,* which digests milk proteins, is also secreted by the stomach.

Considerable current interest centers around ul-

trastructural and immunocytochemical studies of a group of endocrine cells which are widely distributed throughout the gastrointestinal mucosae. It has long been known that small cells with minute acidophilic granules (Fig. 18-38, see color insert) occur in the epithelia of the stomach, small and large intestine, appendix, and even in the ducts of the pancreas and liver. Typically the granules are concentrated in the

FIGURE 18-36 Gastric gland of a bat, cross section; electron micrograph. Portions of parietal (oxyntic) cells are shown. This stomach has been stimulated in vitro to produce hydrochloric acid. The secretory canaliculi (C) are occluded, and their lumens are filled with numerous microvilli (MV). Mitochondria (M) are numerous. L, Lumen of gland. (From Ito, 1967.)

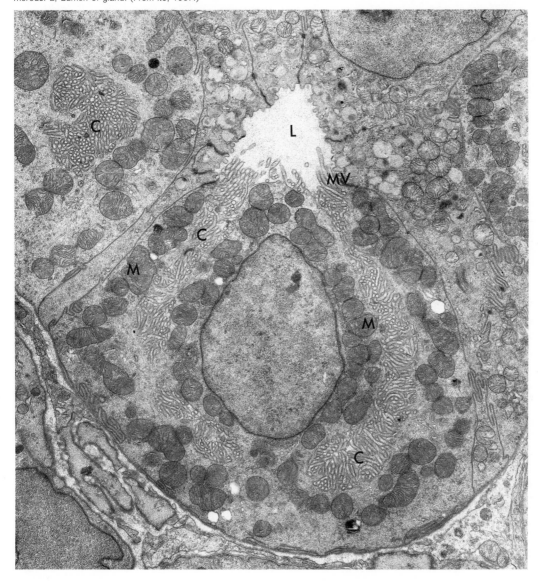

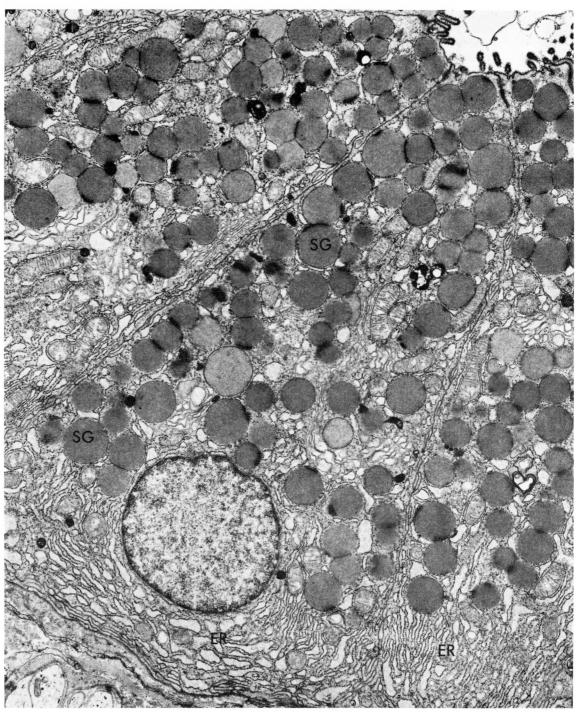

FIGURE 18-37 Chief (peptic) cells of the human gastric glands. Electron micrograph. The characteristics of zymogenic cells are evident in the abundant basal rough cisternal endoplasmic reticulum (ER) and the numerous secretory granules (SG). ×11,000. (From Rubin et al., 1968).

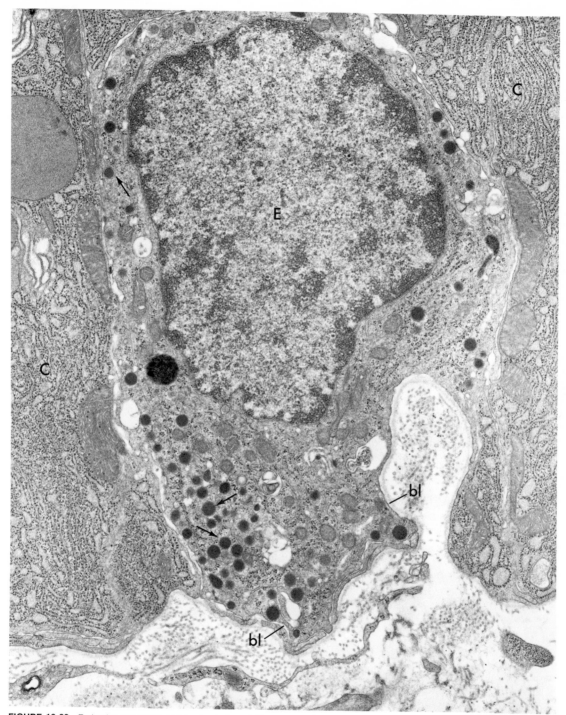

FIGURE 18-39 Endocrine cell of the gastric gland of a rat. The enterochromaffin cell (E) occurs between two chief cells (C). Its basal surface rests against the basal lamina (bl), and its cytoplasm contains small round dense granules (arrows) that are membrane-limited. ×18,000. (Courtesy of Dr. Susumo Ito.)

basal cytoplasm. At the light microscopic level, several reactions identify the granules of these cells. They are colored by osmic acid or with potassium dichromate, for which reason they were called *enterochromaffin cells*. The granules of most of these cells precipitate silver when treated with ammoniacal silver nitrate (Fig. 18-38)—thus the name *argentaffin cells*. A minority of the enterochromaffin cells are impregnated by silver only when a reducer is employed.

These various reactions suggested heterogeneity among the granular epithelial cells, but with the light microscope it could not be ascertained whether one or more cell types were responsible for these reactions. This system of cells was first associated with the secretion of 5-hydroxytryptamine (serotonin) by the gastrointestinal mucosa. The cells were identified by their uptake of radioactive precursors, such as 5-hydroxytryptophan. The serotonin producers are numerous and widely distributed in the gastrointestinal tract. The *gastrin cell (G cell)* has been identified through immunocytochemical identification of intracellular gastrin (peptide) by its antibody. G cells occur in the pyloric glands (distally in the pyloric antrum) and also in the proximal duodenum; they are cells with a broad base and a narrow apical end covered with microvilli. The gastrin-containing granules (150 to 200 nm) occur within smooth membranes in the basal cytoplasm. The stomach also contains glucagon-producing cells which resemble the A cells of the endocrine pancreas.

In their ultrastructure, the enterochromaffin cells as a group resemble peptide-synthesizing endocrine cells. The granules are enclosed in smooth membranes, and the rough ER and Golgi membranes are well developed (Fig. 18-39). Free ribosomes and lysosomal derivatives occur quite regularly. The general polarization of most of these cells suggests that they secrete into the surrounding tissues and bloodstream rather than into the gastric lumen. It seems likely that these cells may be involved in the synthesis of catecholamines, gastrin, secretin, glucagon, and other hormones. The secretory and muscular activities of the gastrointestinal tract itself, and of the pancreas and gallbladder, are controlled to a considerable degree by hormones secreted by the gut wall in response to changing properties of the substances in the lumen.

REPLACEMENT OF GASTRIC EPITHELIAL CELLS

In the gastric glands proper, mitotic activity occurs principally at the base of the pits and the uppermost portions (neck) of the glands. Undifferentiated epithelial cells with prominent nucleoli and numerous free polysomes occur in this region. Labeling this dividing population with [3H]thymidine has established that most of these cells migrate upward along the pit to replace the surface epithelium. Thus the surface mucous cells are continually replaced, and in human beings the gastric surface epithelium is replaced every 4 to 5 days. At the base of the foveolae, precursors of the neck mucous, peptic, and oxyntic cells occur in a region known as the *isthmus*. From here the differentiating cells migrate deeper into the gland. Evidence indicates that the chief and oxyntic cells are renewed at a slow rate.

Studies made on the regeneration of the epithelium in the body of the stomach over areas denuded either by mechanical means or by treatment with alcohol have revealed that cells in the pit and neck divide and migrate out from the edges of the wound to cover the lesion. Then new pits and glands form, and in them the specialized cells of the glands differentiate.

SMALL INTESTINE

Macromolecular nutrients in food are digested extracellularly in the small intestine largely by the action of pancreatic enzymes. The terminal digestion of proteins and carbohydrates occurs at the mucosal surface by enzymes of intestinal origin. The resultant amino acids, monosaccharides, fatty acids, and monoglycerides are absorbed along a vast internal absorptive surface created by various gross and microscopic devices for increasing surface area. Water and electrolytes from salivary, gastric, and pancreatic secretions are also reabsorbed.

The human small intestine is a thin-walled tube

about 4 m in length, extending from the pylorus of the stomach to the colon. At the pylorus, the smooth-surfaced gastric mucosa changes abruptly to a rough-surfaced intestinal mucosa composed of numerous projections (villi) (Fig. 18-40). The intestine consists of three portions: the duodenum, jejunum, and ileum. The duodenal-jejunal junction is marked externally by the suspensory ligament of Treitz; a thickening of the mesentery. Otherwise, no definite structural land-marks distinguish the three segments, although certain distinctive histologic features characterize their muco-sae (see below). In addition, functional differences in absorptive activities have been demonstrated along the length of the small intestine.

HISTOLOGIC ORGANIZATION

The lining of the small intestine possesses gross and microscopic devices for increasing the surface area available for digestive and absorptive activities. The

lining is thrown into large elevations that include the submucosa as well as the mucosa. These are the circularly arranged folds (*plicae circulares,* or *valves of Kerckring*), which are relatively permanent struc-tures. The plicae are highly developed in the jejunum, forming its most conspicuous feature (Fig. 18-41). In the duodenum and ileum they are less conspicuous, and they generally end 2 ft above the entrance to the colon.

The surface of the small intestine is studded with innumerable *villi,* or mucosal projections, that give it a velvety appearance grossly. They are the absorptive units, which are unique to this segment of the adult digestive tract. At their bases are simple tubular invag-inations or pits that extend to the muscularis mucosae but do not penetrate it; these are the *intestinal glands,* or crypts of Lieberkühn (Fig. 18-42). The crypts have

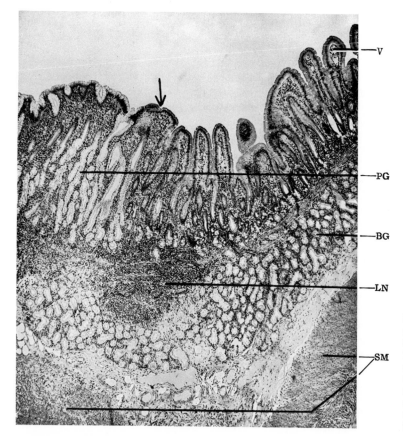

FIGURE 18-40 Longitudinal section of the junction between the pylorus and the duodenum of a monkey. In the epithelium, the junction occurs approximately at the arrow. V, villus; PG, pyloric gland; BG, Brunner's (du-odenal) gland in the submucosa; LN, diffuse lymphatic nodule; SM, sphinc-teric (circular) muscles. Bouin fixa-tion; H&E. ×50.

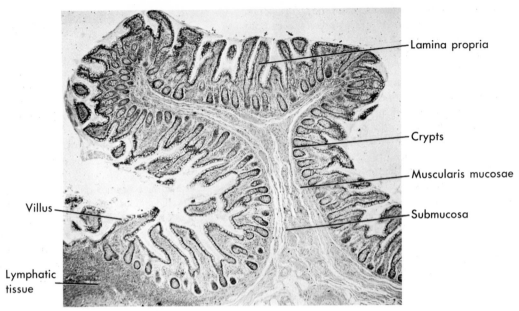

FIGURE 18-41   Plica circularis of the human jejunum. The isolated bodies lying near the villi are sections of villi that were bent so that their ends appear in the plane of the section. H&E. ×40.

generative and secretory functions, as will be described later.

The villi are essentially evaginations or folds of the mucosa; they have a simple columnar epithelial cover and a core of highly cellular reticular connective tissue (lamina propria) capable of immunologic response. Villi vary in height and form in different regions of the human small intestine. Each villus contains an artery, a capillary network, a vein, and a central lymphatic or lacteal (Fig. 18-22). A rich network of blood capillaries ramifies through the lamina propria and is closely apposed to the basement membrane of the absorptive epithelium (Figs. 18-43 and 18-45). The vascularity of the villi is considerably greater than that of the tissue around the crypts.

The villi change in length and produce wavelike motions. This contractility arises from narrow strands of smooth muscle cells that extend from the muscularis mucosae into the villi. These muscle fibers, arranged lengthwise in the villus, may also aid circulation through the lymphatic vessels. With the electron microscope, small bundles of unmyelinated nerves have been observed in the lamina propria in association with blood vessels and smooth muscle fibers.

The intestinal mucosa is divided into two histologically distinct regions, the germinative crypts and the absorptive villi (Fig. 18-42). The simple columnar epithelium that lines the crypts and covers the villi is a continuous sheet, which is constantly being renewed.

It is composed of at least five distinct types of epithelial cells. In the crypt, the principal cell type is the relatively *undifferentiated columnar cell;* this cell has a basophilic cytoplasm and divides frequently. On the villus, the *absorptive cell* is the principal cell type (Figs.

FIGURE 18-42   Spatial scheme of the intestinal epithelium. The epithelium of the crypts is continuous with that covering the villi. Epithelial cells originate in the crypt of Lieberkühn; they differentiate and migrate along the villus to its apex, where they are shed at the extrusion zone. (From Quastler and Sherman.)

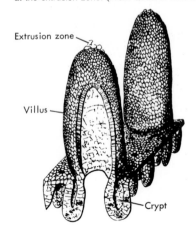

18-44, 18-45 and 18-46). It has a moderately baso-philic cytoplasm and a conspicuous microvillous sur-face, the *striated border*. Interspersed among these major cell types, both in the crypts and on the villi, are mucus-secreting *goblet cells* and *argentaffin cells*. (See enterochromaffin cells under Stomach.) The bottom of the crypt is lined with a cluster of *Paneth cells*, which have the cytologic characteristics of zymogenic cells (Figs. 18-47 and 18-48). These different cell types will be described in greater detail below. Lymphoctyes occur frequently between the epithelial cells (Figs. 18-44 and 18-45).

The epithelial cells rest on a well-defined but delicate basement membrane. The connective tissue that forms the core of the villi and surrounds the glands is highly cellular reticular connective tissue typical of the alimentary tract. Lymphatic nodules and aggregates are common. The submucosa and muscu-laris follow the common pattern described earlier in this chapter.

The distribution of blood and lymphatic vessels and nerves in the small intestine has been described earlier (Fig. 18-22).

CYTOLOGY OF THE INTESTINAL EPITHELIUM

The *absorptive cells* of the villi are tall columnar,

approximately 25 μm high and 8 μm wide, with oval nuclei located in the lower half of the cell. The ab-sorptive cells of mammals have a common design, and the following description refers to the well-described cells in the intestinal villi of the (fasted) rat.

Light microscopy shows that the free surface of these cells is a specialized *striated border* (Fig. 18-46) which consists of minute rodlike projections or *micro-villi* in a uniform, parallel array (Fig. 18-50). These numerous surface projections tremendously increase the cellular surface area presented to the intestinal contents. (They are about 1.4 μm long and 0.08 μm in diameter in human jejunal cells.) The border is highly PAS-positive (Fig. 18-45) due to a *cell coat* over the microvilli of fine filaments (Fig. 3-23) made of glyco-protein that is rich in acid residues. The surface coat is prominent in humans but is developed in varying degrees among other species. Recent radioauto-graphic evidence indicates that the carbohydrate por-tion of this glycoprotein is synthesized in the Golgi complex and linked to the protein moiety; this secre-tion migrates through the cytoplasm and is added to the cell coat (Bennett, 1970).

Intestinal microvilli are also contractile. Each mi-crovillus contains a core of longitudinal filaments

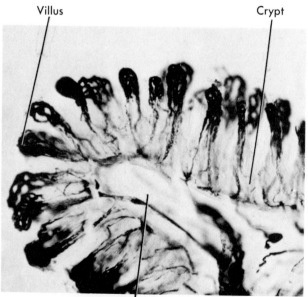

Villus   Crypt

Submucosa

FIGURE 18-43 Human jejunal mu-cosa. India-ink injection of a branch of the mesenteric artery within 1 to 2 hr postmortem. A profuse capillary network exists at the tip of the villus. Note the lower vascularity in the re-mainder of the mucosa. (Courtesy of W. T. Cooke, G. I. Nicholson, and A. Ayres.)

FIGURE 18-44 Longitudinal section of an intestinal villus of a monkey duodenum. SB, striated border on absorptive cell; L, lymphocyte migrating through epithelium; BM, basement membrane; GC, globet cell. Bouin's fixation; H&E. ×500.

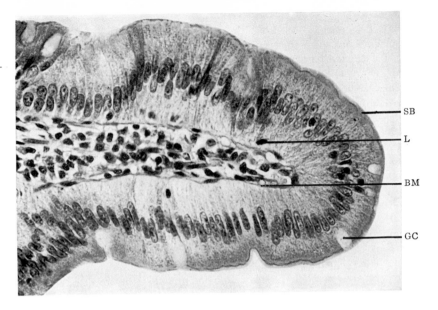

— SB

— L

— BM

— GC

FIGURE 18-45 Normal human absorptive epithelium. This specimen was obtained with an intraluminal biopsy capsule. The striated border of this simple columnar epithelium is strongly PAS-positive, indicating the presence of a carbohydrate-protein polymer. Note also the fine PAS-positive droplets in the apical cytoplasm of the absorptive cells. Lymphocytes are migrating into the epithelium. Note venules in the lamina propria. Plastic section; osmium tetroxide fixation; periodic acid Schiff procedure. ×1000. (Courtesy of H. A. Padykula, E. W. Strauss, A. J. Ladman, and F. H. Gardner.)

Lymphocytes   Venule

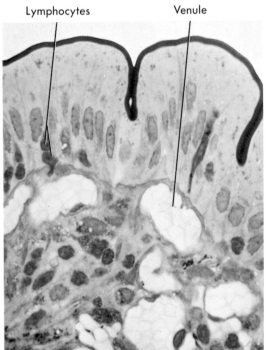

FIGURE 18-46 Portion of an intestinal villus, monkey. H&E. The microvillous (striated) border of the absorptive cells is distinct. Goblet cells are interspersed among the absorptive cells. Note the richly cellular lamina propria.

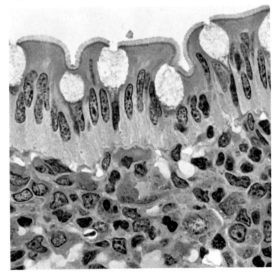

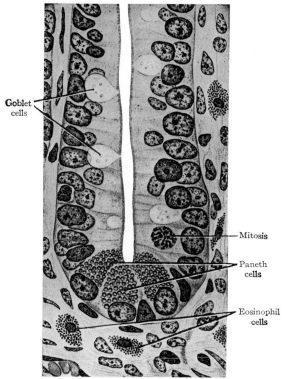

Goblet
cells

Mitosis

Paneth
cells

Eosinophil
cells

FIGURE 18-47 Cell types at the base of an intestinal gland of human jejunum. In addition to Paneth cells and goblet cells, there are the relatively undifferentiated cells destined to become various epithelial cells. Mitoses occur characteristically in these cells. Zenker fixation; H&E. ×1000. (Von Möllendorff.)

which merge just beneath the microvillous border with the *terminal web,* a dense meshwork of filaments that lie mostly in a plane parallel to the free surface of the cell and insert into the lateral surfaces of the cell at junctional complexes (Figs. 18-50, 18-51, and 18-52). The longitudinal filaments in the microvilli are actin filaments that are connected with the plasma membrane at the top of the microvillus as well as along its length. A current model (Fig. 18-51) suggests that the microvillar actin filaments are anchored at the tip in a dense matrix that contains α-actinin, which provides anchorage comparable to that of the Z line of muscle. With evidence that myosinlike filaments occur in the terminal web, a macromolecular framework for microvillar contractility has recently been provided (Mooseker and Tilney, 1975).

The rigid apical ectoplasm composed of the striated border and the terminal web can be readily isolated from homogenates of intestinal mucosa as a

morphologically distinct entity. The surface plasma membrane invaginates into the cytoplasm between the bases of the microvilli.

The apical cytoplasm immediately beneath the terminal web contains vesicles and tubules of the labyrinthine smooth ER (Figs. 18-51 and 18-52). This dense, tubular network is continuous below, nearer the nucleus, with the rough ER whose anastomosing membranes are oriented in the long axis of the cell. Immediately above the nucleus, the Golgi complex can be selectively demonstrated by metallic impregnation methods or by the cytochemical localization of nucleoside diphosphatase activity. It has the typical configuration of stacked cisternae and associated small and large vesicles. Absorptive cells are characterized by numerous typical mitochondria, generally filamentous, although they may also be branched or spherical. They occur mainly in the apical cytoplasm

FIGURE 18-48 Longitudinal section through a crypt in the small intestine (mouse). Several mitotic figures are shown. M^1 and M^2 occur among the Paneth cells at the bottom of the crypt. Undifferentiated columnar cells are evident in the upper crypt. (From Hampton.)

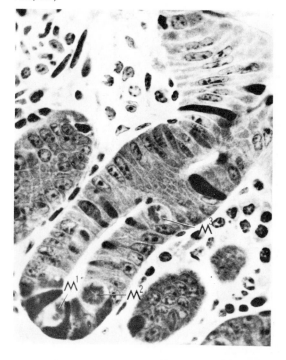

where they are oriented parallel to the long axis of the cell; the infranuclear mitochondria are oriented more randomly. Thus the absorptive cell is highly polarized, with a characteristic arrangement of membrane systems and mitochondria.

FIGURE 18-49 Human small intestinal mucosa, immunocytochemical localization of lysozyme, an antibacterial enzyme. Lysozyme is concentrated in the Paneth cells at the bottom of the crypts (arrows). The remainder of the mucosa is unreactive. Ultrastructural study of this material reveals that lysozyme is localized in the secretory granules. V, villus, C, crypt. (Courtesy Dr. S. Erlandsen.)

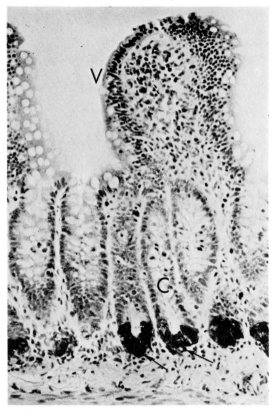

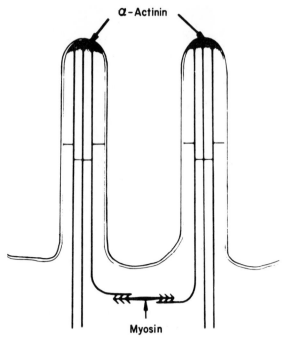

FIGURE 18-50 Mooseker-Tilney model for functional interaction of microvillar contractile proteins. (*J. Cell Biol.,* **67:**725, 1975.)

The lateral surfaces of absorptive cells form a well-developed junctional complex, as described and illustrated in Chap. 3, that binds the various cells to each other throughout the intestinal epithelium and prevents passage of substances from the lumen into the intercellular epithelial compartments. Below the junctional complex, the lateral cell surfaces are plicated; near the base of the cell, small footlike processes abut against adjacent cells. The intercellular space is approximately 10 nm wide, although intercellular dilations as great as 200 nm occur in the basal regions of the epithelium (Figs. 18-51 and 18-57). The basal surface of the cell is flattened on a thin basal lamina.

The villous epithelium is coated by a protective layer of mucus produced by goblet cells located in the

FIGURE 18-51 Intestinal epithelium of the villus of a fasted rat. Several absorptive cells and a portion of a goblet cell are shown. The polarity of the absorptive cells is evident in structural differences between the free and attached surfaces and also in the distribution of the organelles. The luminal surface is composed of closely packed, regularly arranged microvilli (MV); the subjacent cytoplasm, which is relatively free of organelles, is the region of the terminal web (TW). Below the terminal web the cytoplasm contains smooth endoplasmic reticulum (SER), whereas somewhat deeper the rough form (RER) occurs. The Golgi complex (G) occurs immediately above the nucleus. Mitochondria are widely distributed and here are heavily concentrated in the infranuclear cytoplasm. The lateral cell surfaces on the supranuclear region are closely apposed and sometimes folded (arrows), whereas below the nucleus (N) the lateral surfaces form interdigitating processes (P) and the intercellular space is wider (*). BL, basal lamina; LP, lamina propria. ×6000. (R. R. Cardell, S. Badenhausen, and K. R. Porter, *J. Cell Biol.,* **34:**123, 1967.)

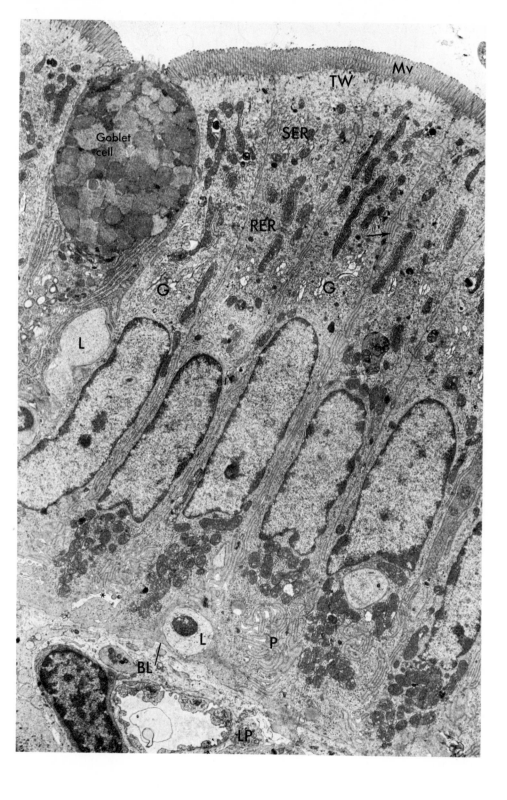

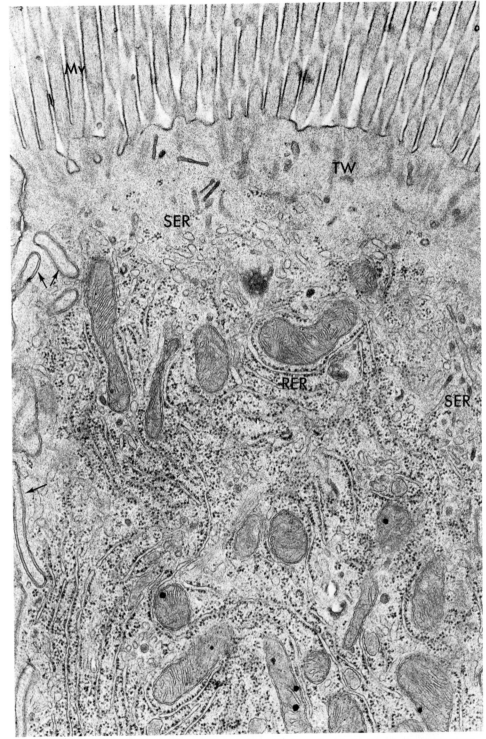

FIGURE 18-52 Supranuclear cytoplasm of an intestinal absorptive cell in a fasted rat. The smooth endoplasmic reticulum (SER) occurs beneath the terminal web (TW), while the rough endoplasmic reticulum (RER) occupies a deeper location. The interdigitating lateral cell surfaces are indicated by arrows. Mv, microvilli. ×37,800. (H. I. Friedman and R. D. Cardell, Jr., *J. Cell Biol.,* **52:**15, 1972.)

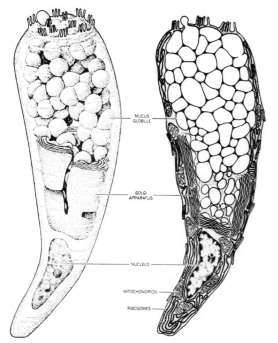

FIGURE 18-53 Diagrammatic representations of the intestinal goblet cell. (Neutra and Leblond.)

expands and increases in complexity, and secretory material accumulates in its vesicles.

Radioautographic studies have demonstrated that the protein moiety of mucus glycoprotein is synthesized in the rough ER whereas the carbohydrate moiety is produced and linked to protein in the Golgi membranes (Neutra and Leblond, 1966). The final product is collected and segregated in the Golgi membranes. As secretory material begins to crowd the supranuclear cytoplasm, the mitochondria and the ER sacs are displaced to the peripheral cytoplasm, the lateral folds of the cell surface become ironed out, and the microvilli are flattened. The droplets of mucus coalesce, to some extent, and begin to lose their surrounding membranes. Finally, the secretion is released in an apocrine manner by the bursting of the plasma membrane at the apex of the cell, and the contents of the Golgi membranes flow into the intestinal lumen. Radioautographic evidence indicates that synthesis and release of mucus occur continually during the 2 to 3 days of the goblet cell's life.

Protein-producing *Paneth cells* line the bottoms of the intestinal crypts (Figs. 18-47 to 18-49). They are pyramidal in shape and have cytologic characteristics typical of serozymogenic cells. The basal cytoplasm is strongly basophilic, being rich in ribonucleoprotein; in the supranuclear Golgi region there are conspicuous, large refractile granules. These brightly acidophilic secretory granules contain an argenine-rich basic protein as well as mucopolysaccharide (PAS-positive). Overall the ultrastructural features resemble that of a pancreatic acinar cell. Since it was observed that the granules accumulate during fasting, and are released after ingestion of food, it was generally assumed that these cells were enzyme producers.

Their secretory function has only recently been specifically characterized through the immunocytochemical localization of the enzyme lysozyme, in the granules (Erlandsen, Parsons, and Taylor, 1974). Lysozyme is a highly cationic protein which is bacteriolytic. The strong positive charge on this protein explains the intense acidophilia of the granules (overall isoelectric point exceeds pH 10). Although the precise in vivo role of intestinal lysozyme remains to be defined, recent evidence (Erlandsen et al., 1976) suggests that the Paneth cells may play a role in the regulation of intestinal flora.

crypts and on the villi (Fig. 18-51). This mucus lies outside the surface coat of the microvilli (Fig. 3-13). Active goblet cells can easily be recognized by their secretory product, which is strongly basophilic, metachromatic, and PAS-positive. This sulfated mucoprotein material appears as small droplets in the immediately supranuclear region of the goblet cell where the Golgi apparatus is located. As the mucoid store increases, it begins to fill the entire supranuclear cytoplasm; the cell acquires the rounded contours of the goblet, and the basal nucleus becomes somewhat flattened. The cytoplasm of goblet cells is basophilic, being rich in ribonucleoprotein.

With the electron microscope, many additional cytologic features of the production and release of the secretory product are revealed. The ultrastructural changes that occur during the secretory cycle of the goblet cell have been described in detail for the rat jejunum (Fig. 18-53). At the onset of secretion the membrane systems begin to proliferate. The cytoplasm becomes filled with large, branching rough ER cisternae that are longitudinally oriented and contain a dense material. The supranuclear Golgi apparatus

REGIONAL DIFFERENCES

The three regions of the small intestine, the duodenum, jejunum, and ileum, can be distinguished to some extent by histologic criteria. The upper duodenum is characterized by *Brunner's glands,* which are submucosal in position (Fig. 18-40). These mucus-producing glands are branched and tubuloalveolar in form; they empty into the intestinal crypts. The secretory cells possess tiny supranuclear droplets, rather than the large masses found in goblet cells. This mucus does not stain metachromatically. It probably lubricates the entering gastric contents and possibly separates and suspends solid food particles.

Plicae circulares occur in all three regions but are best developed in the jejunum (Fig. 18-41). Form differences in the villi occur in the three regions of the human small intestine. In the duodenum they are short, leaflike folds (0.2 to 0.5 mm high) that may be branched; in the jejunum they are rounded, fingerlike projections; whereas in the ileum, they tend to have a clublike form. These differences are not easily recognized in sections. In the jejunum and ileum, the villi are 0.2 to 1.0 mm in height, standing 10 to 40 to the square millimeter; they are taller and more numerous in the jejunum than in the ileum. They disappear in the region of the ileocecal valve. The number of goblet cells in the villous epithelium increases progressively from the duodenum to the ileocecal valve, and the basophilia of the mucus likewise increases steadily. Thus the villous epithelium of the ileum has a high percentage of goblet cells.

Functional differences in absorptive activity have been described along the length of the small intestine. For example, maximal absorption of triglycerides occurs in the proximal small intestine, whereas bile salts and vitamin B_{12} are absorbed by the distal segment. A gradient in the alkaline phosphatase activity along the length of the small intestine of the mature mouse has been demonstrated biochemically; the activity of homogenates is highest in the duodenum, falls sharply to a lower level in the jejunum, and remains low in the ileum. This enzyme is heavily concentrated in the microvilli.

Solitary lymphoid nodules may occur along the entire intestine, but they tend to be more numerous in the ileum, where they are grossly recognizable aggregates called *Peyer's patches* (Fig. 18-54A). The patches are generally oval and usually located in the antimesometrial wall of the intestine. Their number changes with age, being maximal (300) at puberty. Considerable interest centers on Peyer's patches now because experimental immunologic evidence indicates that these patches provide the precursors of intestinal plasma cells that produce immunoglobulin A (IgA). The precursors (plasmoblasts) enter the lymphatic circulation, and then the blood vascular system, from whence they become localized and widely distributed in the lamina propria of the small intestine. This migration suggests a selective homing by these lymphoid cells. The resulting intestinal plasma cells are part of the local antibody system that produces primarily IgA. The several components of secretory IgA are produced by plasma cells and the intestinal epithelium (Fig. 18-54D). The nodules may form bulges along the luminal surface; at such loci the villous form of the mucosa flattens into a smooth cover (Figs. 18-54B and 18-54C). The nodules may occupy the lamina propria and submucosa (Fig. 18-54C).

FIGURE 18-54 A. Low-power diagrammatic representation of a portion of one Peyer's patch. (From W. M. Copenhaver, R. P. Bunge, and M. B. Bunge, "Bailey's Textbook of Histology," The Williams & Wilkins Company, Baltimore, 1971.) B. Scanning electron micrograph of the human ileum. The rounded surfaces represent loci of bulging lymphoid follicles. Note the surrounding villi, some of which overhang the follicular surfaces. Compare with Fig. 18-54C. (From R. L. Owen, and A. L. Jones, *Gastroenterology,* **66:**189, 1974.) C. Lymphoid follicles in the monkey ileum. Note the occurrence of lymphoid follicles (asterisks) in the lamina propria and submucosa. Nearby villi overhang the rounded surface of the follicular areas. Compare with Fig. 18-54B. D. Diagrammatic representation of the local antibody system illustrating the cellular mechanisms involved in the synthesis of secretory immunoglobulin (SIgA). Secretory IgA is the predominant immunoglobulin in various exocrine secretions where it exists as a dimer of serum IgA linked by a polypeptide J chain. It coats the mucous epithelial surfaces that are regularly exposed to bacteria. Here it functions as an "antiseptic paint." The plasma cells of the lamina propria synthesize the dimer with its J chain. This SIgA is transported through the epithelial cells, which add a glycoprotein called secretory component (SC) to the immunoglobulin dimer. The secretory component makes the antibody more resistant to proteolytic enzymes, such as trypsin and chymotrypsin, and may also play a role in its transepithelial transport. The local antibody system may control bacterial growth as well as prevent attachment of antigens to the epithelial surfaces. With stronger antigenic stimulus, both SIgA and serum IgA (7 SIgA) are produced, and the latter enters the lymphatic capillaries. Note also that the lamina propria of the gastrointestinal tract is able to produce other immunoglobulins. (From T. B. Tomasi, Jr., *N. Engl. J. Med.,* **287:**500. 1972.)

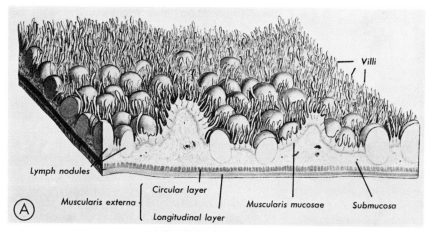

Villi

Lymph nodules

Muscularis externa { Circular layer / Longitudinal layer

Muscularis mucosae

Submucosa

(A)

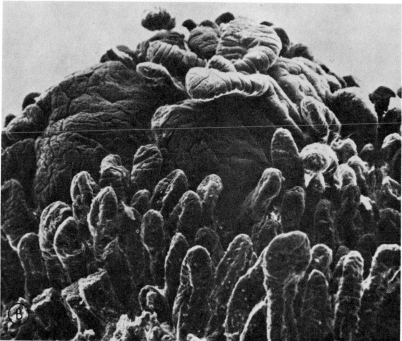

(B)

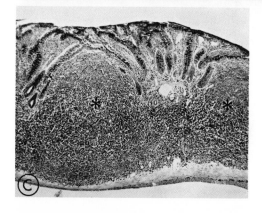

(C)

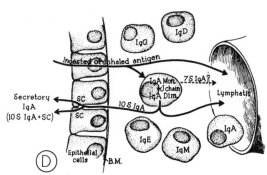

(D)

Ingested or inhaled antigen

IgG

IgD

IgA Mon.
J chain
IgA Dim

7S IgA?

Secretory
IgA
(10 S IgA + SC)

SC

SC

10 S IgA

Lymphatic

IgA

Epithelial
cells

B.M.

IgE

IgM

EPITHELIAL REPLACEMENT

The histologic concept of the continuous replacement of the intestinal epithelium in the adult has been developed since 1948, largely through radioautographic studies of Leblond and his associates. It has long been known that there is intensive mitotic activity in the undifferentiated cells in the crypts of Lieberkühn and that mitosis occurs rarely in the normal villous epithelium. It has been established that the absorptive cells and goblet cells originate in the crypts, migrate onto the villus, and move toward its apex, where they are extruded at a specific site called the *extrusion zone* (Fig. 18-42).

The most convincing evidence for this epithelial migration is derived from the tagging of dividing cells with tritiated thymidine. This precursor of DNA is incorporated into the dividing cells in the crypt (Fig. 18-55), and then the radioactive tag is carried by the daughter cells during their migration. The radioactive label is picked up by undifferentiated columnar cells (Fig. 18-48) that become absorptive cells and also by *oligomucous cells* that are precursors of goblet cells. The dividing oligomucous cell has been most likely derived from an undifferentiated columnar cell. Such isotopic labeling reveals that the life-span of the cells of the villous epithelium is very short; in experimental animals there is a complete replacement within 2 or 3 days. In humans there is likewise evidence that the whole epithelial lining of the gastrointestinal tract, from stomach to rectum, is completely renewed every 2 to 4 days.

Mitosis in Paneth cells has not been observed. However, these cells are slowly replaced by progenitors that proliferate at the bottom of the crypt (Fig. 18-48). In the mouse the turnover time for the Paneth

FIGURE 18-55 Radioautographs of mouse jejunum 8 h (A) and 72 h (B) after injection of tritiated thymidine. The horizontal marker indicates the approximate junction of the crypt and villus. At 8 h, radioactivity is limited to the upper crypts whereas by 72 h it is located in the surface epithelium of the upper third of the villus. (From Leblond and Messier.)

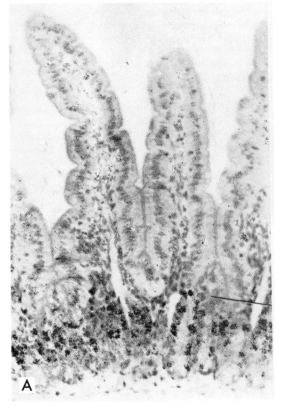

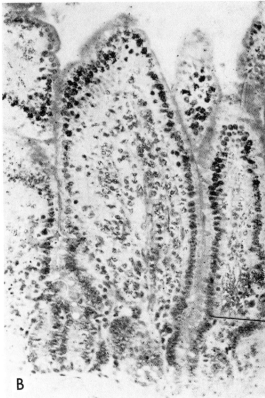

cells is about 3 weeks. The argentaffin and other endocrine cells of the mouse intestine originate from precursors in the lower half of the crypt and migrate to the villus. Their turnover time is about 4 days.

The extrusion zone at the apex of the villus is marked by a distinct cleft in the epithelium, and the emerging cells round off somewhat as they are shed into the intestinal lumen. Leblond and Walker have presented the interesting concept that the normal histologic appearance of the intestinal mucosa is a result of the balance between cell proliferation in the crypts and cell loss at the extrusion zones. Irradiation upsets this balance by interfering with cell division in the crypts, cell loss at the extrusion zones continues, and the result is atrophy of the villi.

A variety of evidence suggests that during the migration of the absorptive cells toward the apex of the villus they differentiate progressively. For example, the microvilli of the absorptive cells become longer, narrower, and more numerous. This progressive differentiation results in a great increase in the surface area of the plasma membrane at the crest of the villus. There is evidence that in the human jejunum the absorptive cells at the tip of the villus may have a lower RNA content than those at the base. Histophysiologic experiments have demonstrated that the absorptive cells at the villous crest can concentrate lipids, sugars, and amino acids to a greater degree than the younger, more basal absorptive cells. The evidence supports the hypothesis that the differentiation of the intestinal epithelium culminates in the formation of a highly specialized digestive and absorptive surface at the apex of the villus (Fig. 18-56).

MORPHOLOGIC ASPECTS OF DIGESTIVE AND ABSORPTIVE FUNCTIONS

Locus of Digestive Activity

Extracellular digestion is characteristic of the intestines of higher animals, including mammals. Complex molecules are degraded by enzymes secreted into the lumen by glands associated with the digestive tract. The resulting smaller molecules are taken in by the absorptive cells of the small intestine. In addition, recent evidence indicates that certain large molecules can be absorbed directly.

The intestinal juice has a low enzymic content that increases with increasing cellular content. When the shed epithelial cells in the intestinal juice are broken up by homogenization, the enzymatic activity increases. Furthermore, digestive activity of the human

small intestine toward disaccharides is greater than can be accounted for by the enzymic content of the juice. This evidence led to the suggestion that the terminal hydrolytic digestion in the small intestine may occur on or in absorptive cells rather than in the intestinal lumen.

Although there is virtually no phosphatase in the lumen, phosphate esters are rapidly hydrolyzed by the small intestine. Histochemists have long been aware that the striated border is rich in phosphatases active in the neutral and alkaline range of pH, including ATPase. Recent ultrastructural identification of phosphatase activity localizes it in (or near) the plasma membrane. The isolated microvillous border contains practically all the sucrase and maltase activities of the total mucosal homogenate. Furthermore, 75 percent of all the aminopeptidase and alkaline phosphatase activities of whole intestinal homogenates is recovered in the isolated microvillous border. From in vitro experiments it has been suggested that the hydrolysis of disaccharides, peptides, and sugar phosphates occurs within the microvillous border at an intracellular locus. Recently the synthetic enzymes glycosyltransferase and glyceride synthetase have been localized in the intestinal microvillous border. From this evidence it seems highly probable that the striated border, in addition to providing abundant surface area for absorption, is a locus of hydrolysis and active transport.

Morphologic Aspects of Absorption

In a morphologic study of absorption, it is necessary that the substance being transported be identifiable by some visible tag in tissue sections. The absorption of fats has lent itself to such study because the lipid droplets are sudanophilic and osmiophilic. This process has been analyzed in considerable detail by histochemical identification of lipids with Sudan dyes and with the electron microscope. Some information concerning the absorption of proteins, such as antibodies, has been derived from the use of proteins carrying flourescent or other labels. Only fragmentary information exists concerning morphologic aspects of the absorption of carbohydrates.

Although the morphologic aspects of lipid absorption have long been studied in laboratory animals, it is only in recent years that it has been possible to study this problem in the normal human being. Intraluminal biopsy procedures have permitted study of the normal and abnormal intestinal mucosa. Within 20 min after a fasted normal human being (or other mammal) ingests fat, such as corn oil, lipid droplets appear within the absorptive epithelium of the proximal small intestine. The absorbed lipid is restricted to the villus, and a conspicuous gradient in the amount of intraepithelial lipid is evident (Fig. 18-56). Most of the droplets are concentrated at the upper half of the villus, and the amount of lipid diminishes progressively from the tip of the villus to its base. Cytologic study with the light microscope reveals that in the absorptive cells nearest the tip of the villus the droplets occur throughout the apical endoplasm; the droplets in the supranuclear Golgi region are generally larger.

Observations with the electron microscope have added greatly to our knowledge of the pathway followed by lipid in the intestinal absorptive cell. Several physiological facts should be considered before the ultrastructural descriptions of the intracellular pathway of lipid absorption are given. In the intestinal lumen, pancreatic lipase hydrolyzes triglyceride principally to fatty acid and 2-monoglyceride. The absorption of long-chain fatty acids is known to be a passive process. Resynthesis of triglyceride occurs in the endoplasmic reticulum of the absorptive cell. After intracellular resynthesis of triglyceride, phospholipid, and cholesterol ester, these lipids are assembled into lipoprotein particles, called chylomicrons. The chylomicrons leave the cells and enter the lymphatic circulation.

The following ultrastructural changes occur in the absorptive cells soon after instillation of an oil into the stomach of a fasted animal. Small lipid droplets (65 nm in maximal diameter) are lodged in the spaces among the microvilli of the jejunal absorptive cells; no droplets are observed within the microvilli (Fig. 18-57). Droplets are then seen within small vesicles which, beneath the terminal web, join the smooth ER. Here the lipid droplets are generally larger (50 to 240 nm). The labyrinthine network of smooth-surfaced tubules is continuous with the rough ER. Lipid droplets occur also within membranes studded with ribosomes. Lipid accumulates in the Golgi cisternae as droplets of varying sizes (40 to 150 nm). Droplets have been observed also in the nuclear envelope. Since they occur therefore in all parts of the cytoplasmic membrane systems (Fig. 18-57), they have been interpreted as markers of a physiologic continuity of the cell surface with all parts of the membranes of the apical cytoplasm.

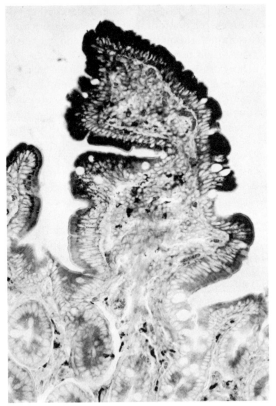

FIGURE 18-56 Normal human jejunal mucosa biopsied 20 min after ingestion of corn oil. Lipid droplets have accumulated principally in the absorptive epithelium of the upper half of the villus. Epithelial cells at the base of the villus and in the crypt are free of lipid droplets. Heavily sudanophilic cells in the lamina propria are tissue eosinophils. Formalin-fixed; frozen section stained with Sudan black. ×200. (Courtesy of A. J. Ladman, H. A. Padykula, and E. W. Strauss.)

After coursing through the membranous system, the droplets (chylomicrons) are discharged from the lateral surfaces of the absorptive cells at the nuclear level into the intercellular spaces, and so the basal part of the cell is bypassed. Lipoprotein droplets, devoid of membranes, travel through the extracellular space toward the basal lamina, above which they accumulate in large clusters; they then pass through this into the connective tissue spaces. From here they gain entrance to the lacteals by passing between endothelial cells. Although numerous lipid droplets can be seen entering the lacteals, only rarely do they occur in the blood capillaries. Physiologic experiments have indicated that triglycerides are selectively absorbed by the lymphatic vessels, whereas water-soluble, short-chain fatty acids enter the blood capillaries.

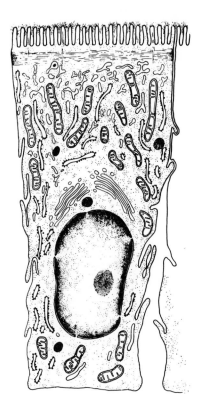
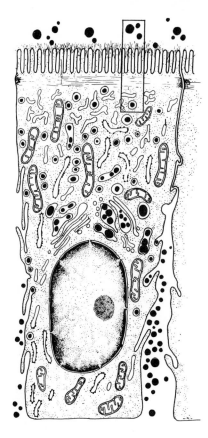

FIGURE 18-57 Diagrammatic representations of the ultrastructure of the intestinal absorptive cells in the fasted condition (left) and during lipid absorption (right). (From W. Bloom and D. W. Fawcett, "A Textbook of Histology," W. B. Saunders Company, Philadelphia, 1975. Derived from an original plate by Cardell, Badenhausen, and Porter, 1967.)

The observation that absorbed lipid droplets are closely invested by membranes in the apical cytoplasm suggests that the triglyceride droplets have entered the cell by pinocytosis and that the membranes are derived from the cell surface (Fig. 18-57). It is known, however, that lipid is hydrolyzed in the intestinal lumen, and that the products of hydrolysis are absorbed by diffusion. Compelling evidence is presented in studies which demonstrate that the initial phase of absorption is not temperature-dependent and thus most likely does not represent pinocytosis, which is an active process. In addition, observations following the exposure of the intestinal mucosa to lipid containing electron-opaque markers further suggest that pinocytosis is not a primary mechanism because the membrane-enclosed droplets are free of the accompanying markers. Since it is known that triglyceride can be resynthesized by the microsomal fraction of these cells, the droplets accumulated within the endoplasmic reticulum may reflect newly synthesized triglyceride.

LARGE INTESTINE

The histologic organization of the large intestine reflects its principal function of elimination of the undigested material, the feces. Water is reabsorbed and mucus is secreted in large amounts to facilitate elimination of the dehydrated feces by lubrication of the mucosal surface. The thick muscularis has a distinctive arrangement into three longitudinal bands in the colon. Lymphatic tissue is abundant.

The large intestine, or colon, begins at the ileocecal valve and consists of a *cecum* and *appendix;* the *ascending, transverse,* and *descending segments;* the *sigmoid colon;* and a terminal portion, the *rectum,* ending at the external orifice or *anus.* Its total length is roughly 150 cm in human beings.

COLON

The mucosa of the large intestine everywhere lacks villi; it has deep straight glands (about 0.5 mm). The lamina propria contains frequent solitary lymphatic nodules, often so large as to extend into the submucosa (Fig. 18-58). The submucosa contains the usual constituents plus large accumulations of fat cells.

The surface epithelium consists of a mixture of

FIGURE 18-58 A. Longitudinal section of mucosa and submucosa of the human colon. IG, intestinal gland; LN, lymphatic nodule, which has perforated through the muscularis mucosae into the submucosa; LV, lymphatic vessel filled with lymphocytes; V, vein; A, artery. ×50. B. Section through the base of a gland of the large intestine of a monkey. M, mitotic figure in an epithelial cell; PC, plasma cells in the periglandular stroma; L, lymphatic vessel; MM, muscularis mucosae. Bouin fixation. ×600.

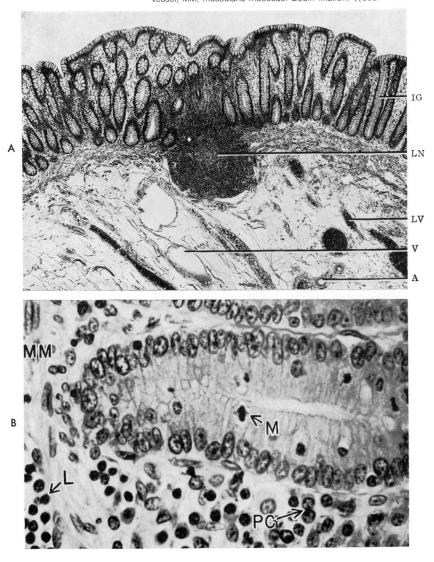

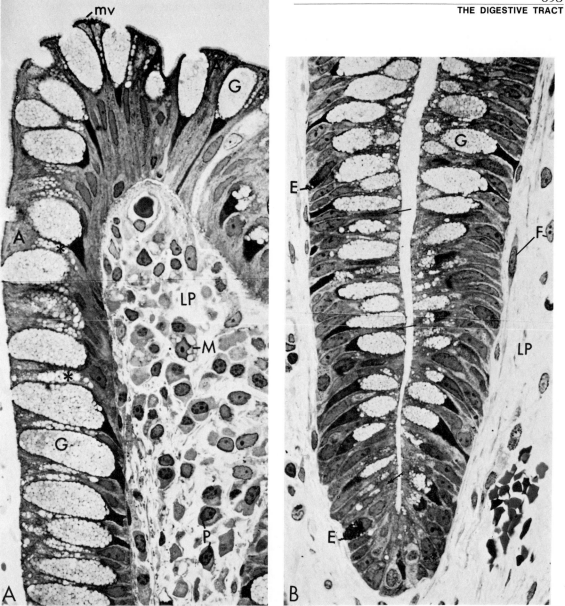

FIGURE 18-59 Mucosa of the human large intestine. A. Luminal surface, including a portion of a mucosal gland (left margin) and the lamina propria (LP). The luminal epithelium consists of absorptive cells (A) with microvilli (mv) and interspersed goblet cells (G). These same cell types are evident in the glandular epithelium (left margin) where vacuolization (*) is conspicuous in the absorptive cells. In the lamina propria (LP), macrophages (M) and plasma cells (P) are evident but lymphocytes are less easily identified in this micrograph. B. Mucosal gland and surrounding lamina propria (LP). Goblet cells (G) are numerous and are interspersed with tall columnar cells (arrows) which in the upper part of the gland are absorptive cells but in the lower region are undifferentiated precursor cells. Endocrine cells (E) with aggregates of infranuclear granules are less numerous. (Courtesy of Dr. Marion Neutra.)

columnar absorptive cells, with striated borders, and mucous goblet cells (Fig. 18-59). The crypts consist principally of tall mucous cells. In the human rectum, enterochromaffin cells occur at the bottom of the crypt. Epithelial proliferation occurs in the lower half to two-thirds of human rectal crypts to provide cells needed for the constant replacement. Replacement time in the human rectum has been estimated as 5 to 6 days.

The lamina propria, as in the small intestine, contains macrophages, lymphocytes, and plasma cells (Fig. 18-59), which reflect local production of IgA.

The muscularis of the colon and cecum has a characteristic arrangement not found in the vermiform appendix or the more proximal portions of the alimentary tract. The longitudinal smooth muscle fibers of the outer layer gather into three equidistant longitudinal strands known as *taeniae* (G., bands). Between them, the longitudinal fibers form a thin, sometimes interrupted layer. Because of the tonus of the taeniae, the wall of the colon bulges outward as sacculations or *haustra* (L., buckets). Between these sacculations, the wall is thrown into crescentic *plicae semilunares* that project into the lumen. The ileocecal valve consists of two folds resembling such plicae. A peculiarity of the colon is that fascicles of longitudinal fibers from the taeniae frequently join the circular layer. This arrangement interrupts the continuity of the circular layer, and different intertaenial areas may contract independently.

The serosa is incomplete, since the ascending and descending limbs of the colon are retroperitoneal. It may contain lobules of fat that form pendulous projections (*appendices epiploicae*).

CECUM AND VERMIFORM APPENDIX

The *cecum* is a blind pouch at the proximal end of the colon, and its terminal thin tip is known as the *vermiform appendix*. The structure of the cecum resembles that of the rest of the colon, and the vermiform appendix has a similar structure in miniature (Fig. 18-60), except that taeniae are absent. The glands are simple tubes, sometimes forked; the epithelium consists mainly of mucous cells. Lymphatic nodules are abundant and more or less confluent. The wealth of lymphatic vessels and lymphatic tissue is the most conspicuous histologic feature of the appendix.

The lumen of the normal appendix in the adult, when empty, is thrown into folds separated by deep pockets. But this normal condition is found in scarcely 50 percent of individuals over 40 years of age because of a history of subclinical appendicitis. Often the lumen

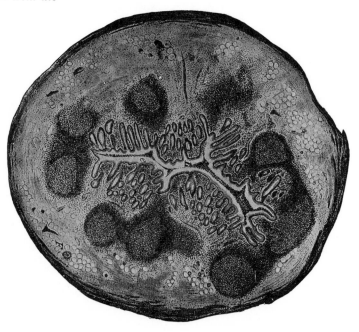

FIGURE 18-60 Cross section of the human appendix. Note abundance of lymphatic nodules. Only a part of the circular layer of the muscularis is included. ×20. (Sobotta.)

is narrowed or even obliterated. The epithelium and the underlying lymphatic tissue then disappear and are replaced by an axial mass of fibrous tissue.

RECTUM

The rectum is divided into two parts, an upper part that extends from the third sacral vertebra to the pelvic diaphragm, and a lower part, or anal canal, that continues down to the anus. The lining of the first part is thrown into several large, semilunar, circular folds, the *plicae transversales recti.* For most of its length the anal canal presents on its inner wall a number of longitudinal folds, the *anal columns.*

The mucous membrane of the first part of the rectum is similar to that of the colon, but its glands are somewhat longer (0.7 mm) and are composed almost completely of mucous cells. Solitary lymphatic nodules are present. A continuous layer of longitudinal muscle is present. The rectum has no mesentery, and the serosa is replaced by adventitial connective tissue.

The lower portion of the rectum, or anal canal, is 2 to 3 cm in length and roughly elliptical in cross section. It ends at the anus, where its lining becomes continuous with the external skin. In the anal canal, the epithelium changes abruptly from simple columnar to stratified cuboidal at the *pectinate line* (Fig. 18-61). The anal columns join one another somewhat below

this line, creating pocketlike anal valves. Above each valve is a recess termed an *anal sinus.* At this level the muscularis mucosae disappears. The uncornified epithelium of the canal changes into typical keratinized stratified squamous epithelium at the anus proper. In the lower part of the anal canal a few isolated sebaceous glands make their appearance.

The skin immediately around the anus forms the *zona cutanea.* Sweat glands are absent from the region immediately bordering the anus, but at a distance of 1.0 to 1.5 cm there is an elliptical zone, 1.5 cm wide, containing simple tubular glands, the *circumanal glands.* These are apocrine sweat glands, being the terminal representatives of the milk line (see Chap. 24). They secrete an oily fluid that is related, in lower mammals, to sexual activity.

The outer layers of the anal canal include a very vascular submucosa, which contains blood vessels, numerous nerves, and Pacinian corpuscles. The veins form the large hemorrhoid plexus (Fig. 18-61) and are especially susceptible to varicosities. The circular layer of the muscularis becomes thickened at its termination, forming the internal anal sphincter. Beyond this, striated muscle fibers surround the orifice, forming the external anal sphincter.

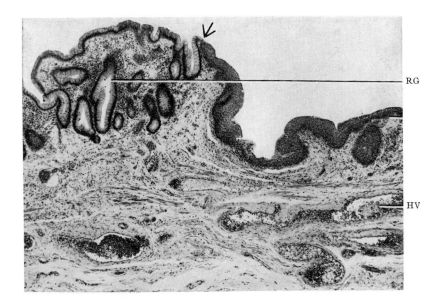

RG

HV

FIGURE 18-61 Longitudinal section through the junction of the human rectum and anal canal. Arrow marks pectinate line. RG, rectal gland; HV, hemorrhoidal vein in the submucosa. ×35.

REFERENCES

ORAL CAVITY

BEIDLER, L. N., and R. L. S. SMALLMAN: Renewal of Cells within Taste Buds. *J. Cell Biol.,* **27:**263 (1965).

HASHIMOTO, K., R. J. DIBELLA, and G. SHKLAR: Electron Microscopic Studies of the Normal Human Buccal Mucosa, *J. Invest. Dermatol,* **47:**512 (1966)

LISTGARTEN, M. A.: Electron-microscopic Study of the Gingivo-dental Junction of Man, *Am. J. Anat.,* **119:**147 (1966).

MATTERN, C. F. T., W. A. DANIEL, and R. I. HENKIN: The Ultrastructure of the Human Circumvallate Papilla. I. Cilia of the Papillary Crypt, *Anat. Rec.,* **167:**175 (1970).

MURRAY, R. G., A. MURRAY, and S. FUJIMOTO: Fine Structure of Gustatory Cells in Rabbit Taste Buds, *J. Ultrastruct. Res.,* **27:**444 (1969).

PROVENZA, D. V.: "Oral Histology," J. B. Lippincott Company, Philadelphia, 1964.

SCHROEDER, H. E., and M. A. LISTGARTEN: Fine Structure of the Developing Epithelial Attachment of Human Teeth, "Monographs in Developmental Biology," vol. 2, S. Karger AG, Basel, 1971.

SCHROEDER, H. E., and J. THEILADE: Electron Microscopy of Normal Human Gingival Epithelium, *J. Periodont. Res.,* **1:**95 (1966).

SCHUMACHER, S.: Die Mundhohle, Die Zunge, Der Schlundkopf, in W. von Möllendorff and W. Bargmann (eds.), "Handbuch der mikroskopischen Anatomie der Menschen," vol. 5, pt. 1, Springer-Verlag OHG, Berlin, 1927.

SKOUGAARD, M. R.: Cell Renewal, with Special Reference to the Gingival Epithelium, *Adv. Oral Biol.,* **4:**261 (1970).

ZALEWSKI, A. A.: Combined Effects of Testosterone and Motor, Sensory, or Gustatory Nerve Reinnervation on the Regeneration of Taste Buds, *Exp. Neurol.,* **24:**285 (1969).

Salivary Glands

AMSTERDAM, A., I. OHAD, and M. SCHRAMM: Dynamic Changes in the Ultrastructure of the Acinar Cell of the Rat Parotid Gland During the Secretory Cycle. *J. Cell Biol.,* **41:**753 (1969).

CASTLE, J. D., J. D. JAMIESON, and G. E. PALADE: Radioautographic Analysis of the Secretory Process in the Parotid Acinar Cell of the Rabbit. *J. Cell Biol.,* **53:**290 (1972).

HAND, A. R.: Nerve-acinar Cell Relationships in the Rat Parotid Gland, *J. Cell Biol.,* **47:**540 (1970).

LEESON, C. R.: Structure of Salivary Glands, in C. F. Code and W. Heidel (eds.), "Handbook of Physiology," vol. 2, sec. 6, chap. 1, American Physiological Society, Washington, 1967.

LEPPI, T. J.: Gross Anatomical Relationships between Primate Submandibular and Sublingual Salivary Glands, *J. Dent. Res.,* **46:**359 (1967).

LEPPI, T. J., and S. S. SPICER: The Histochemistry of Mucins in Certain Primate Salivary Glands, *Am. J. Anat.,* **118:**833 (1966).

MUNGER, B. L.: Histochemical Studies on Seromucous- and Mucous-secreting Cells of Human Salivary Glands, *Am. J. Anat.,* **115:**411 (1964).

STRUM, J. M., and M. J. KARNOVSKY: Ultrastructural Localization of Peroxidase in Submaxillary Acinar Cells, *J. Ultrastruct. Res.,* **31:**323 (1970).

TAMARIN, A.: Myoepithelium of the Rat Submaxillary Gland, *J. Ultrastruct. Res.,* **16:**320 (1966).

TANDLER, B.: Ultrastructure of the Human Submaxillary Gland. I. Architecture and Histological Relationships of the Secretory Cell, *Am. J. Anat.,* **111:**287 (1962).

TANDLER, B., C. R. DENNING, I. D. MANDEL, and A. H. KITSCHER: Ultrastructure of Human Labial Salivary Glands. I. Acinar Secretory Cells, *J. Morphol.,* **127:**383 (1969).

TANDLER, B., and L. L. ROSS: Observations of Nerve Terminals in Human Labial Salivary Glands, *J. Cell Biol.,* **42:**339 (1969).

THORN, N. A., and O. H. PETERSEN (eds.): "Secretory Mechanisms of Exocrine Glands," Academic Press, New York, 1975.

TOMASI, T. B., and J. BIENENSTOCK: Secretory Immunoglobulins, *Adv. Immunol.,* **9:**11 (1968).

ZIMMERMAN, K. W.: Die Speicheldrusen der Mundhohle und die Bauchspeicheldruse, in W. von Möllendorff and W. Bargmann (eds.), "Handbuch der mikroskopischen Anatomie der Menschen," vol. 5, pt. 1, Springer-Verlag OHG, Berlin, 1927.

Esophagus

PARAKKAL, P.: An Electron Microscopic Study of the Esophageal Epithelium in the Newborn and Adult Mouse, *Am. J. Anat.,* **121:**175 (1967).

Stomach

BENSLEY, R. R.: The Gastric Glands, in E. V. Cowdry (ed.), "Special Cytology," 2nd ed., vol. 1, Paul B. Hoeber, Inc., New York, 1932.

FORSSMAN, W. G., L. ORCI, R. PICTET, A. E. RENOLD, and C. ROUILLER: The Endocrine Cells in the Epithelium of the Gastrointestinal Mucosa of the Rat. An Electron Microscope Study, *J. Cell Biol.,* **40:**692 (1969).

GROSSMAN, M. I., and I. N. MARKS: Secretion of Pepsinogen by the Pyloric Glands of the Dog, with Some Observations on the Histology of the Gastric Mucosa, *Gastroenterology,* **38:**343 (1960).

ITO, S.: Anatomic Structure of the Gastric Mucosa, in C. F. Code and W. Heidel (eds.), "Handbook of Physiology." vol. 2, sec. 6, chap. 41, American Physiological Society, Washington, 1967.

ITO, S., and G. C. SCHOFIELD: Studies on the Depletion and Accumulation of Microvilli and Changes in the Tubulovesicular Compartment of Mouse Parietal Cells in Relation to Gastric Acid Secretion, *J. Cell Biol.,* **63:**364 (1974).

MACDONALD, W. C., J. S. TRIER, and N. B. EVERETT: Cell Proliferation and Migration in the Stomach, Duodenum, and Rectum of Man: Radioautographic Studies, *Gastroenterology,* **46:**405 (1964).

PLENK, H.: Der Magen, in W. von Möllendorff and W. Bargmann (eds.), "Handbuch der mikroskopischen Anatomie der Menschen," vol. 5, pt. 2, Springer-Verlag OHG, Berlin, 1932.

RUBIN, W., M. D. GERSHON, and L. L. ROSS: Electron Microscope Radioautographic Identification of Serotinin-synthesizing Cells in the Mouse Gastric Mucosa, *J. Cell Biol.,* **50:**399 (1971).

RUBIN, W., L. L. ROSS, M. H. SLEISENGER, and F. H. JEFFRIES: The Normal Human Gastric Epithelia. A Fine Structural Study, *Lab. Invest.,* **19:**598 (1968).

SEDAR, W. W.: Uptake of Peroxidase into the Smooth-surfaced Tubular System of the Gastric Acid-secreting Cell, *J. Cell Biol.,* **43:**179 (1969).

STEVENS, C. E., and C. P. LEBLOND: Renewal of the Mucous Cells in the Gastric Mucosa of the Rat, *Anat. Rec.,* **115:**231 (1953).

Small Intestine

BENNETT, G.: Migration of Glycoprotein from Golgi Apparatus to Cell Coat in the Columnar Cells of the Duodenal Epithelium, *J. Cell Biol.,* **45:**668 (1970).

BROWN, A. L.: Microvilli of the Human Jejunal Epithelial Cell, *J. Cell Biol.,* **12:**623 (1962).

CARDELL, R. R., S. BADENHAUSEN, and K. R. PORTER: Intestinal Absorption in the Rat. An Electron Microscopical Study, *J. Cell Biol.,* **34:**123 (1967).

CHENG, H., J. MERZEL, and C. P. LEBLOND: Renewal of Paneth Cells in the Small Intestine of the Mouse, *Am. J. Anat.*, **126:**507 (1969).

CLEMENTI, F., and G. E. PALADE: Intestinal Capillaries. I. Permeability to Peroxidase and Ferritin, *J. Cell Biol.*, **41:**33 (1969).

CRAIG, S. W., and J. J. CEBRA: Peyer's Patches: An Enriched Source of Precursors for IgA-Producing Immunocytes in the Rabbit, *J. Exp. Med.*, **134:**188 (1971).

ERLANDSEN, S. L., J. A. PARSONS, and T. D. TAYLOR: Ultrastructural Immunocytochemical Localization of Lysozyme in the Paneth Cells of Man, *J. Histochem. Cytochem.*, **22:**401 (1974).

ERLANDSEN, S. L., C. B. RODNING, C. MONTERO, J. A. PARSONS, C. A. LEWIS, and I. D. WILSON: Immunocytochemical Identification and Localization of Immunoglobulin A within Paneth Cells of the Rat Small Intestine, *J. Histochem. Cytochem.*, **24:**1085 (1976).

FERREIRA, M. H., and C. P. LEBLOND: Argentaffin and Other "Endocrine" Cells of the Small Intestine in the Adult Mouse. II. Renewal, *Am. J. Anat.* **131:**331 (1971).

FLOREY, H. W.: The Secretion and Function of Intestinal Mucus, *Gastroenterology*, **43:**326 (1962).

GAGE, S. H., and P. A. FISH: Fat Digestion, Absorption, and Assimilation in Man and Animals as Determined by the Dark-field Microscope, and a Fat-soluble Dye, *Am. J. Anat.*, **34:**1 (1924).

ISSELBACHER, K. J.: The Intestinal Cell Surface: Properties of Normal, Undifferentiated, and Malignant Cells, *Harvey Lec.* **69:**197, (1973–1974).

ITO, S.: The Enteric Surface Coat on Cat Intestinal Microvilli, *J. Cell Biol.*, **27:**475 (1965).

LADMAN, A. J., H. A. PADYKULA, and E. W. STRAUSS: A Morphological Study of Fat Transport in the Normal Human Jejunum, *Am. J. Anat.*, **112:**389 (1963).

LEBLOND, C. P., and B. MESSIER: Renewal of Chief Cells and Goblet Cells in the Small Intestine as Shown by Radioautography after Injection of Thymidine-H^3 into Mice, *Anat. Rec.*, **132:**247 (1958).

MERZEL, J., and C. P. LEBLOND: Origin and Renewal of Goblet Cells in the Epithelium of the Mouse Small Intestine, *Am. J. Anat.*, **124:**281 (1969).

MILLER, D., and R. K. CRANE: The Digestive Function of the Epithelium of the Small Intestine. II. Localization of Disaccharide Hydrolysis in the Isolated Brush Border Portion of Intestinal Epithelial Cells, *Biochim. Biophys. Acta,* **52:**293 (1961).

MOOG, F.: The Functional Differentiation of the Small Intestine. VIII. Regional Differences in the Alkaline Phosphatases of the Small Intestine of the Mouse from Birth to One Year, *Dev. Biol.*, **3:**153 (1961).

MOOSEKER, M. S. and L. G. TILNEY: Organization of an Actin Filament-Membrane Complex. Filament Polarity and Membrane Attachment in the Microvilli of Intestinal Epithelial Cells, *J. Cell Biol.*, **67:**725 (1975).

NEUTRA, M., and C. P. LEBLOND: Synthesis of the Carbohydrate of Mucus in the Golgi Complex as Shown by Electron Microscope Radioautography of Goblet Cells from Rats Injected with Glucose-H^3, *J. Cell Biol.*, **30:**119 (1966).

OCKNER, R. K., and K. J. ISSELBACHER: Recent Concepts of Intestinal Fat Absorption, *Rev. Physiol. Biochem. Pharmacol.*, **71:**107 (1974).

OWEN, R. L., and A. L. JONES: Epithelial Cell Specialization within Human Peyer's Patches: An Ultrastructural Study of Intestinal Lymphoid Follicles, *Gastroenterology,* **66:**189 (1974).

PADYKULA, H. A., E. W. STRAUSS, A. J. LADMAN, and F. H. GARDNER: A Morphologic and Histochemical Analysis of the Human Jejunal Epithelium in Nontropical Sprue, *Gastroenterology,* **40:**735 (1961).

PALAY, S. L., and L. J. KARLIN: An Electron Microscopic Study of the Intestinal Villus, I and II, *J. Biophys. Biochem. Cytol.,* **5:**363, 373 (1959).

PATZELT, V.: Der Darm, in W. von Möllendorff and W. Bargmann (eds.), "Handbuch der mikroskopischen Anatomie der Menschen," vol. 5, Springer-Verlag OHG, Berlin 1936.

STRAUSS, E. W.: Morphological Aspects of Triglyceride Absorption, in C. F. Code and W. Heidel (eds.), "Handbook of Physiology," vol. 3, sec. 6, chap. 71, American Physiological Society, Washington, 1968.

TRIER, J. S.: Morphology of the Epithelium of the Small Intestine, in C. F. Code and W. Heidel (eds.), "Handbook of Physiology," vol. 3, sec. 6, chap. 63, American Physiological Society, Washington, 1968.

WALKER, W. A., and R. HONG: Immunology of the Gastrointestinal Tract. Part I. *J. Pediatr.,* **83:**517 (1973).

WRIGHT, R. D., M. A. JENNINGS, H. W. FLOREY, and R. LIUM: The Influence of Nerves and Drugs on Secretion by the Small Intestine and an Investigation of the Enzymes in the Intestinal Juice, *Quart J. Exp. Physiol.,* **30:**73 (1940).

Large Intestine

CHANG, W. W. L., and C. P. LEBLOND: Renewal of the Epithelium in the Descending Colon of the Mouse, Parts I, II, and III, *Am. J. Anat.,* **131:**73, 101, and 111 (1971).

FLOREY, H. W.: Electron Microscopic Observations on Goblet Cells of the Rat's Colon, *Quart J. Exp. Physiol.,* **45:**329 (1960).

LINEBACK, P. E.: Studies on the Musculature of the Human Colon, with Special Reference to the Taeniae, *Am. J. Anat.,* **36:**357 (1925).

LORENZONN, V., and J. S. TRIER: The Fine Structure of Human Rectal Mucosa. The Epithelial Lining at the Base of the Crypt, *Gastroenterology,* **55:**88 (1968).

MARTIN, B. F.: The Goblet Cell Pattern of the Large Intestine, *Anat. Rec.,* **140:**1 (1961).

VENKATACHALAM, M. A., M. H. SOLTANI, and H. D. FAHIMI: Fine Structural Localization of Peroxidase Activity in the Epithelium of Large Intestine of Rat, *J. Cell Biol.,* **46:**168 (1970).

The Liver and Gallbladder

ALBERT L. JONES AND ELINOR SPRING-MILLS

GENERAL MORPHOLOGY AND FUNCTION

The liver is the largest *gland* in the human body, constituting approximately one-twentieth of the body weight in the neonate and one-fiftieth in the adult. It lies in the right upper quadrant of the abdominal cavity, beneath the diaphragm and attached to it. It is made up of four incompletely separated *lobes*. A thin connective tissue *capsule* (Glisson's capsule), usually covered by reflected peritoneum, lines the external surface of the liver. A definite hilus, the *porta hepatis,* is present where vessels enter and ducts leave the liver, and the surface capsule becomes continuous with the internal stroma. Right and left *hepatic bile* ducts emerging from the gland unite in the porta hepatis to form the *hepatic duct* proper. A short distance outside the liver, the hepatic duct joins the *cystic duct,* or *ductus choledochus,* which enters the duodenum about 10 cm below the pyrloric-duodenal junction.

The liver has a dual blood supply. The *portal vein,* carrying blood which has already passed through the capillary beds of the alimentary tract, spleen, and pancreas, brings approximately 75 percent of the afferent blood volume to the liver. This blood is rich in nutrients and other absorbed substances but relatively poor in oxygen. The *hepatic artery,* a branch of the celiac trunk, carrying well-oxygenated blood, supplies the remaining blood to the liver. Blood from branches of these two vessels mixes in passing to and through the liver lobules (see Figs. 19-1 and 19-2). Sinusoidal blood flows toward the center of each lobule and is collected by the *central vein.* After leaving the lobules, the central veins unite to form the larger *sublobular* or *intercalated* veins which finally join the large *hepatic veins.* Blood returns to the heart via the *inferior vena cava.*

The classic structural unit of the organ is the *hepatic lobule,* a polyhedral prism of tissue, approximately 2 mm long and 0.7 mm wide, containing anastomosing plates of parenchymal cells and a labyrinthine system of blood sinusoids. Branches of the afferent blood vessels and bile ducts run along the edges of the polyhedron, and the central vein runs throughout its center. *Bile,* produced by the parenchymal cells, is secreted into minute *bile capillaries* or *canaliculi* between the glandular epithelial cells. At the periphery of the lobule, bile flows into small *bile ductules,* or canals of Hering, and eventually into the larger *bile ducts.* The liver is composed of approximately 1 million lobular units.

701

The liver is essential for life; mammals survive subtotal hepatectomy mainly because the cells have extraordinary regenerative powers and the capacity to tolerate the increased metabolic demands. The functional diversity and complexity of the liver are rivaled only by the central nervous system. The liver functions both as an *exocrine* and *endocrine gland*. It secretes bile, which flows into the duodenum and contains, among other constituents, *bile salts* which emulsify dietary fats prior to digestion. The liver takes up digested foodstuffs from the afferent blood and stores carbohydrate (glycogen), proteins, vitamins, and some lipids. Stored substances not used by the hepatocyte can be released into the blood unbound (for example,

glucose) or in association with a carrier (for example, triglyceride molecules complexed in a lipoprotein). The liver also synthesizes many substances in response to the body's demands: albumin and other plasma proteins, glucose, fatty acids for triglyceride synthesis, cholesterol, and phospholipids. The liver metabolizes, detoxifies, and inactivates exogenous compounds, such as drugs and insecticides, endogenous compounds, such as steroids, and probably most other hormones. In additon, it has the ability to convert substances into more active forms, for example,

FIGURE 19-1 Liver lobule. Schematic view. The central vein lies in the center of the figure, surrounded by anastomosing cords of blocklike hepatocytes. About the periphery of the schema are six "triads," evenly spaced from one another, lying at an angle in the polyhedron lobule. Each "triad" consists of branches of the portal vein, hepatic artery, and bile duct. See text.

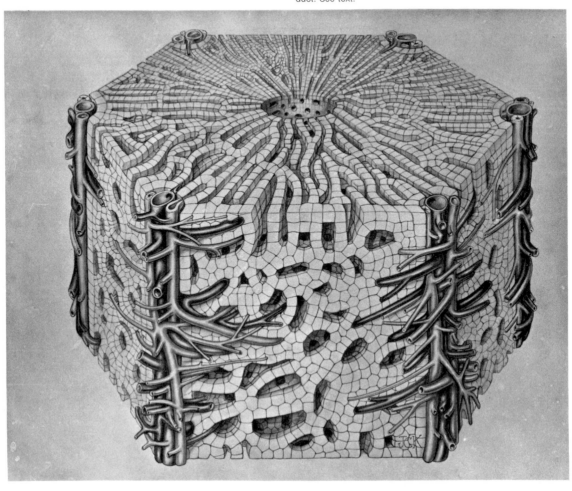

T_4 to T_3. By virtue of its large vascular capacity, it serves as a major storehouse for blood. During embryogenesis and certain diseases of the adult, it is a site of hematopoiesis. Finally, its abundance of phagocytes makes the liver one of the principal filters for foreign

particulate matter, especially for bacteria coming from the gut.

HISTOLOGIC ORGANIZATION OF THE HUMAN LIVER

STROMA

Most of the liver's free surface, except for a small area within its diaphragmatic attachment, is covered by a

single layer of flattened *peritoneal mesothelial cells.* Beneath the mesothelium lies a thin yet distinct *surface capsule* (Glisson's capsule) composed of regularly arranged collagen fibers, scattered fibroblasts, and a few small blood vessels. The capsule surrounds the four incompletely separated lobes and is thickest around the inferior vena cava and the hilus or porta

FIGURE 19-2 Liver lobule—schematic view, higher power of Fig. 19-1. The relationships of branches of the portal vein, hepatic artery, bile duct, vascularsinusoids and hepatocytes are shown. See text.

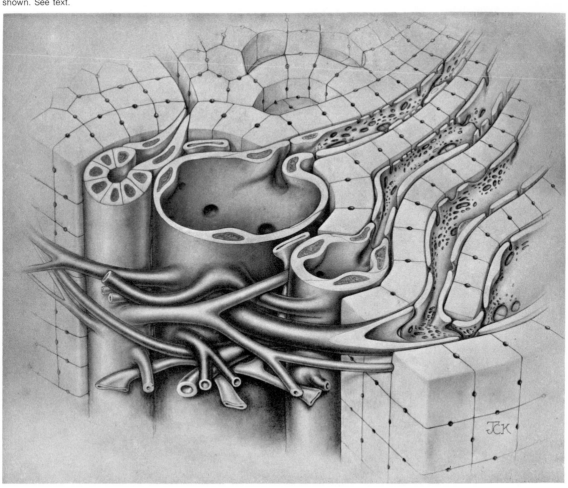

hepatis. The capsule is reflected inwardly at the porta, where its fibers merge with the denser connective tissue surrounding the vascular and biliary branches. Most of the fibrous hepatic stroma is derived from the connective tissue that passes into the liver through the porta. Within the interior of the organ, the connective tissue arborizes to such an extent that no segment of the parenchyma is more than a few millimeters away from one of its branches. It should be kept in mind, however, that examination of liver sections following selective connective tissue staining procedures (for example, Mallory-Azan, silver impregnation, elastic fiber staining) and preparations of isolated hepatic stroma (that is, obtained by macerating away the parenchyma in water) reveal that despite its size, the large, bulky human liver under normal conditions contains relatively little connective tissue.

Nevertheless, this connective tissue (1) provides an internal supporting framework for the hepatic parenchyma, (2) ensheaths most of the vessels and nerves, and (3) subdivides the parenchyma into *lobules*. The only connective tissue within the lobule is the *reticular network* between the sinusoidal endothelium and plates of parenchymal cells. The reticular fibers presumably support the liver parenchyma and also may keep the sinusoids open (see Fig. 19-3 for size and arrangement of reticular fibers). In addition, there is some evidence that when this reticular framework survives hepatic injury, the parenchyma regenerates more rapidly and in a more orderly fashion (Rappaport, 1969). The failure to demonstrate fibroblasts in the sinusoidal areas with conventional light and early electron-microscopic techniques fostered the wide-

FIGURE 19-3 Photomicrograph of the human liver showing the close meshwork of reticular fibers in the perisinusoidal space between the parenchymal cells and the sinusoidal lining. A few perisinusoidal cell nuclei can be seen within the meshes of the reticulum. Silver, gold, hematoxylin, and Van Gieson's.

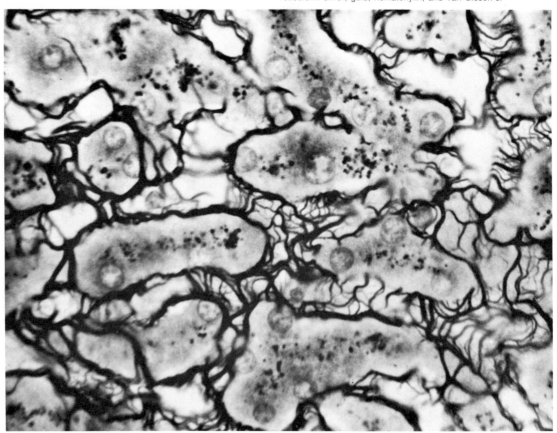

spread speculation that the reticular fibers in these regions are produced by cells other than fibroblasts. The endothelial cells lining the sinusoids were credited with fiber production, even though their ultrastructure revealed none of the usual features associated with the manufacture of extracellular proteins. However, recent electron-microscopic observations and autoradiographic studies have shown that normal livers do contain a few true fibroblasts within the perisinusoidal space of Disse. In addition, it has been suggested that a fat-containing perisinusoidal cell (that is, the so-called Ito cell, or lipocyte) may be the progenitor of the perisinusoidal fibroblast, since fat cells in other tissues can be transformed into fibroblasts (Popper and Udenfriend, 1970).

At the periphery of the lobule, the recticular meshwork of the sinusoids becomes continuous with the *interlobular connective tissue,* which usually contains bundles of collagen, elastic fibers, and occasional fibroblasts. The term *Glisson's capsule* is sometimes applied to both the surface capsule and the internal connective tissue. However, because the interlobular tissue is not composed exclusively of fibrous tissue and in any one site usually serves two or more contiguous

lobules, the broader terms *portal canal, area, space, radicle,* and *tract,* are more commonly used to designate the tissue in these regions. The fibrous stroma forms the bed of a portal canal. It ensheaths and carries the so-called portal triad (that is, branches of the hepatic artery, portal vein, and bile duct), the lymphatic vessels, and the nerves throughout the interior of the liver (see Fig. 19-4). The size of a portal canal depends upon its position in the branching connective tissue stroma. Large portal canals in the thicker branches of connective tissue may contain both large and small vessels derived from the portal vein and hepatic artery. The larger vessels carry blood to more distant sites, whereas the small vessels are usually terminal branches of the vein and artery carrying blood into the adjacent lobules. The smallest portal canals contain only terminal branches of the blood and biliary vessels. Sections through these regions usually reveal no more than four tubular structures (for example, venule from the portal vein, arteriole from the hepatic artery, lymphatic, and bile duct) embedded in a tiny isolated patch of loose connective tissue.

ALTERATIONS IN THE STROMA

Hepatic fibrosis, or excess connective tissue, is an early histologic sign of chronic liver disease; it is im-

FIGURE 19-4 Photomicrograph of a portal canal from human liver. Branches of the portal vein, hepatic artery, bile duct (B), and lymphatic vessel can be found within the connective tissue. Note the large lumen in the portal vein and the cuboidal epithelium which lines the bile duct. Mallory-Azan. ×200.

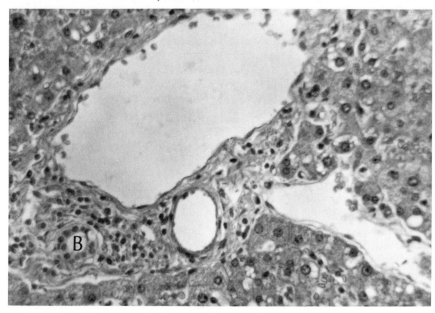

portant to be able to recognize this phenomenon in liver sections. Fibrosis occurs primarily at four sites: (1) in the portal canals, (2) around central veins, (3) around hepatocytes, and (4) around proliferating bile ductules that extend from the portal canals into the parenchyma. It is currently believed that parenchymal cell injury or degeneration or both is one of the primary stimuli for the formation of excess connective tissue. The connective tissue elaborated under these conditions often forms new, irregular septa around nodules of regenerating parenchymal cells, preventing these cells from making appropriate connections with blood and biliary vessels, while the inelastic septa ultimately compress the nodules and restrict their growth. As a result, blood and bile flow through the liver is impeded, cellular nutrition is impaired, and the organ is often unable to restore its normal architecture. Factors responsible for stimulating fibroblasts, deposition, and catabolism of fibers are being investigated with the hope that the insidious fibrotic and cirrhotic changes associated with many liver diseases can be treated and controlled (see Popper and Udenfriend, 1970).

LOBULATION

The presence of small *histologic units,* or *lobules,* within the mammalian liver has been generally accepted since the pioneering observations of Wepfer (1664) and Malpighi (1666), but the validity and usefulness of the traditional definition of a hepatic lobule, based primarily upon the disposition of structural boundaries such as connective tissue septa and vessels within the liver lobes, have been questioned. As a result, three primary schemata have been developed to describe the histologic and functional units of the liver. The names *classic lobule, portal lobule,* and *liver acinus* have been assigned to the three interpretations. Each concept was formulated under different circumstances, yet they are not mutually conflicting. They represent different ways to interpret particular aspects of liver structure and function and thus facilitate our understanding of this organ (see Table 19-1).

The *classic lobule* was described above; it is a polyhedral prism of hepatic tissue about 0.7×2 mm, the boundaries of which are demarcated by connective tissue septa (portal canals) or the regular distribution of biliary and vascular vessels (portal triad), or both. In

cross section, the lobule is roughly hexagonal, but adjacent lobules are not perfectly aligned nor precisely the same size. In the angles of the hexagon are the portal areas containing connective tissue stroma and the portal triad or terminal braches of the hepatic artery, portal vein, and bile duct. The center of the lobule contains the *central vein* or *terminal hepatic venule* (the smallest subdivision of the hepatic veins) surrounded by a minute amount of connective tissue (see Fig. 19-5). One-cell-thick rows of *parenchymal* or *glandular epithelial cells* (hepatocytes) separated on either side by narrow vascular spaces, the *sinusoids,* radiate from the central vein to the portal areas at the periphery of the lobule. In histologic sections, the cell columns appear to be isolated branches or cords of parenchymal cells suspended in an underlying meshwork of blood sinusoids (see Fig. 19-6). Three-dimensional reconstructions of the lobule (Elias, 1949), however, show that the liver parenchyma has a more complicated arrangement than routine two-dimensional histologic sections indicate (Figs. 19-1 and 19-2). In short, these special preparations reveal that (1) the lobules are composed of a continuous system of communicating parenchymal *cell plates,* or laminae, and not single strands or columns of cells; (2) the parenchymal cells throughout an entire lobule are interconnected and subdivided by spaces or lacunae into anastomosing one-cell-thick plates; (3) the sinusoids run within the center, and the perisinusoidal *space of Disse* occupies the periphery of each lacuna; and (4) the lacunae form a continuous labyrinth within each lobule. In addition, stereograms of a liver lobule show that each lacuna opens directly into a *central space* containing the central vein. At the periphery of the lobule, however, the lacunae do not communicate freely with the portal areas. Instead, a *limiting plate* of hepatic cells, surrounding the circumference of the lobule, forms a nearly continuous wall between the interior of the lobule and the space occupied by the portal canals. Only tiny terminal branches of the hepatic artery, portal vein, and bile duct can penetrate the liver parenchyma via the occasional fenestrations in the limiting plate (see Figs. 19-1 and 19-2).

The *classic lobule* is best seen in species (for example, pig, raccoon, camel, polar bear) in which relatively thick bands of interlobular connective tissue almost completely encapsulate each lobule (Fig. 19-7, see color insert). In man, lobulation is incomplete and poorly defined. The sparse perilobular connective tissue does not form a continuous boundary between contiguous lobules, and the parenchyma often appears to be coextensive between adjacent lobules. Nevertheless the approximate boundaries of a human classic lobule can be visualized by first locating a central vein and then following the successive, regularly placed portal triads which encircle the periphery of each lobule (Fig. 19-8, see color insert).

Blood flows from the portal canals (hepatic artery and portal vein) into the lobule, passes along the

sinusoids, and is removed from the lobule by the central vein. Bile, however, flows in the opposite direction, from the parenchymal cells where it is formed to the interlobular bile ducts in the portal canals.

Although the classic lobule is regarded primarily

TABLE 19-1 IMPORTANT FEATURES OF THREE CONCEPTS OF LIVER LOBULATION

	CLASSIC LOBULE	PORTAL LOBULE	LIVER ACINUS
Cross-sectional appearance of three types of hepatic units. Classic lobules (hexagons) outlined in each diagram. Shaded regions show amount of tissue included in each unit and its relationship to classic lobules.	Central vein — Portal canals	Central vein — Portal canals	Central vein — Portal canals
Shape	Polygonal or hexagonal	Roughly triangular or wedge-shaped	Irregular; sometimes oval or diamond-shaped
Morphologic axis	Central vein	Portal area, especially interlobular bile duct	Terminal branches of portal triad lying along border of two adjacent classic lobules
Peripheral landmarks	Approximately six portal areas	Three (or more) central veins	Two (or more) central veins
Relationship to classic lobule	....	Encompasses those portions of all classic lobules which secrete bile into a common interlobular bile duct	Small sectors of two adjacent classic lobules
Direction of blood flow	From periphery (portal areas) to center (central vein)	From center (portal area) to periphery (central veins)	From center (portal area and edges of two adjacent classic lobules) to periphery
Direction of bile flow	From center toward periphery	From periphery to center	From periphery toward center
Advantages of concept	1. Emphasizes endocrine function of liver 2. Useful in understanding histologic changes associated with centrolobular necrosis (for example, CCl_4 poisoning)	1. Emphasizes exocrine function of liver (that is, bile secretion) 2. Makes histologic organization of a hepatic lobule comparable to those of most exocrine glands	1. Offers best explanation for gradient of metabolic activity or zonation within liver, that is, direct correlation between blood supply and metabolism 2. Helps to explain pattern of regeneration 3. Useful in understanding development of cirrhosis
Principal developers of concept	Wepfer; Malpighi; Mascagni; Kiernan; Müeller	Theile; Brissaud and Sabourin; Mall; Arey	Rappaport and coworkers; Novikoff and Essner

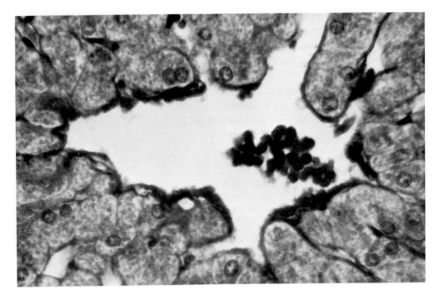

FIGURE 19-5 Several sinusoids empty into the central vein shown in this photomicrograph. Note that the central vein is larger than the sinusoids. It has extremely thin walls and is surrounded by sparse connective tissue. Human liver. Mallory-Azan. ×400.

FIGURE 19-6 Liver parenchymal cells are shown at higher magnification in this photomicrograph. The cells are polyhedral, yet adjacent cells may vary in size and shape. The hepatic cells form branching and anastomosing single-cell-thick plates which are separated by the sinusoids (light areas). Arrows point to binuclear cells. Human liver. Mallory-Azan. ×600.

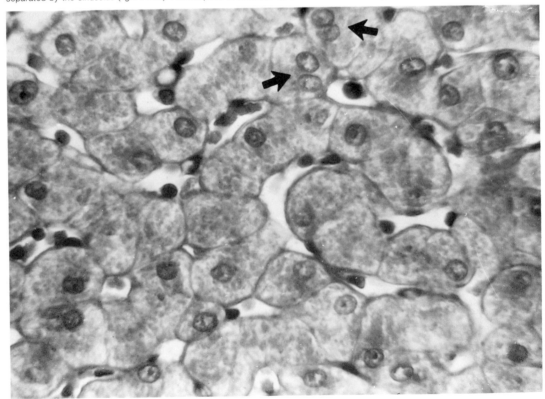

as a structural unit, certain physiologic (for example, fat and glycogen deposition after a meal) and pathologic (for example, necrosis) changes often appear confined to specific areas within the lobule. Such changes may originate and spread through the territory of the classic lobule from either the peripheral (portal areas) or the central areas (central vein), producing an unusual circular gradient in which similar microscopic alterations appear in concentric bands or zones around the central vein (see Table 19-1). Because of this, certain histologists believe that the classic lobule can and should be regarded as both a structural and a functional unit of the liver.

The concept of the *portal lobule* began to emerge during the mid-nineteenth century as histologists discovered that in most mammals liver lobules are *not* well-defined anatomic units and that in many exocrine glands it is more convenient to consider a lobule as a *functional unit* rather than a segment of tissue enclosed by fissures or septa. As a result, in exocrine glands, the term *lobule* became synonymous with a group of secretory cells which release their product(s) into a common duct located in the center of the lobule. Subsequently, three lines of evidence suggested that the classic lobule was not the only logical unit to use in describing the liver parenchyma. Theile observed (1844) that when mammalian livers were crushed and washed in water the resulting specimen resembled a bunch of grapes: The lobules were clustered around branches of the portal vein. Brissaud and Sabourin reported (1844) that lobules in seal liver were formed by epithelial trabeculae radiating from portal canals rather than central veins. And Mall's studies (1906) of corrosion preparations, in which the portal, arterial, or biliary vessels had been injected in situ, demonstrated that arterial and portal vessels, bile ducts, lymphatics, nerves, and connective tissue all radiated from the portal areas. Eventually, these observations culminated in a new concept of hepatic lobulation called the *portal, or functional, lobule.*

The portal lobule is a roughly triangular or wedge-shaped prism of hepatic tissue. Its boundaries, however, are ill defined in most mammals except the seal. It encompasses those segments of three or more contiguous classic lobules which are drained by a common interlobular bile duct situated in a portal canal at their edge (see Table 19-1). The morphologic axis of the portal lobule is the interlobular bile duct in the portal space, and its peripheral limits are formed by three different "central" veins. According to this

schema, bile flows from the periphery to the centrally located bile duct, and blood flows from the center of the lobule to the periphery. Hence, the pathways for bile drainage and blood flow are similar to most exocrine glands. Those who oppose the recognition and use of this concept often argue that it unduly emphasizes the liver's role as an exocrine gland, but since no valid judgment can be made about the relative importance of the exocrine and endocrine activities of the liver, each schema is useful, in its own way, to explain the myriad functions of the liver.

More recently, Rappaport (1969) introduced the concept of the *liver acinus.* In certain respects this unit resembles the portal lobule, but it is much smaller and is usually described as the smallest functional unit within the liver. Observations of hepatic circulation in vivo and preparations of specially injected human liver casts revealed that the tissue around each central vein is derived from different sources, suggesting that this tissue is not one unit but a series of units or liver acini. The *simple liver acinus* is defined as a small, irregular mass of unencapsulated parenchymal tissue lying between two (or more) terminal hepatic venules ("central veins"). Its axis is a small radicle of the main portal canal containing a terminal portal venule, hepatic arteriole, bile ductule, lymph vessel, and nerves. In histologic sections, it includes only small segments of two adjacent classic lobules. The acini extend at right angles from the preterminal branches of the portal veins (at the edges of the classic lobules) to the central veins (see Figs. 19-1 and 19-9 and Table 19-1). The parenchyma is continuous between the classic lobules, and blood flows toward both central veins from the terminal branches of the portal veins. Although there is extensive communication among sinusoids, Rappaport has found that the tissue within each acinus is supplied mainly by its parent vessels. Moreover, the cells within each acinus appear to be grouped into concentric zones around the axis of the acinus. Cells close to the axis and the terminal afferent vessels (for example, zone 1) are the first to receive blood and nutrients, the last to die, and the first to regenerate. Cells in more distant regions receive blood of poorer quality and also appear less resistant to damage. The concept of acinar circulatory zones has been extended by Rappaport to provide an explanation for the histologic appearance of many pathologic changes in the liver.

PARENCHYMAL CELLS

The hepatic plates are composed of large, polyhedral parenchymal cells approximately 30 μm long and 20 μm wide (see Fig. 19-6). These cells make up approximately 80 percent of the cell population within the human liver (Gates et al., 1961). They are different sizes: The smallest ones border perforations in the liver plate, and the largest ones are either polyploid or located in the corners where three cell plates meet. The six or more surfaces on each parenchymal cell are of three different types: (1) those abutting other parencymal cells; (2) those bordering bile canaliculi; and (3) those touching the perisinusoidal space (Disse). In addition, cells bordering the portal zone have a surface in contact with the portal connective tissue. At the light microscopic level the plasmalemma appears fairly uniform and often indistinct, even though fine structural and histochemical studies reveal that the cell membrane undergoes characteristic modifications in each of these three sites. In optimal routine histologic preparations or following special procedures (for example, indigo blue staining, silver impregnation, or staining for adenosine triphosphatase) bile canaliculi are seen on surfaces between contiguous cells. These tiny channels follow an incomplete chicken-wire pattern along contiguous surfaces of parenchymal cells (see Figs. 19-2, 19-10, and 19-11).

The nuclei are large, round, and usually centrally located. They contain one or more nucleoli and scattered clumps of chromatin. Generally the nuclei of parenchymal cells stain less intensely than the smaller nuclei of other cells in the liver. Moreover, in the adult liver, parenchymal cell nuclei can be subdivided into several nuclear-sized groups or classes (Doljanski, 1960). Polyploid nuclei and binucleated and multinucleated cells are easily found. Adult mammalian livers contain 30 to 80 percent polyploid cells, and there appears to be good correlation between nuclear

FIGURE 19-9 Blood supply of the simple liver acinus. The oxygen tension and nutrient level of the blood in sinusoids decrease from zone 1 through zone 3. Zones 1', 2', and 3' indicate corresponding volumes in a portion of an adjacent acinar unit. Circle A encloses the area commonly designated as periportal; B and C represent the areas more peripheral to the portal space (PS). THV, terminal hepatic venules (central veins). (From Fig. 1, A. M. Rappaport, Z. J. Borowy, W. M. Laugheed, and W. N. Lotto, *Anat. Rec.* **119**:11, 1954.)

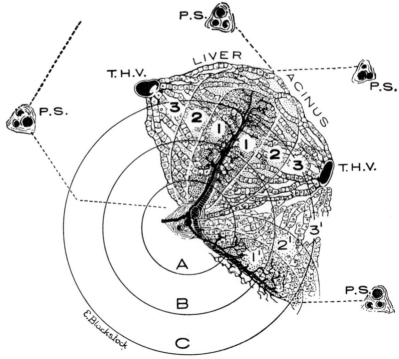

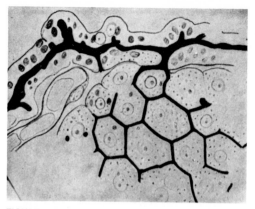

FIGURE 19-10 Drawing of a network of bile canaliculi in dog liver, showing the entrance of canaliculi into a terminal bile ductule at the edge of a lobule. Silver preparation. (Courtesy of H. Elias, *Am. J. Anat.*, **85:**379, 1949.)

size and ploidy, that is, doubling of DNA content being accompanied by an approximate doubling of nuclear volume. The two nuclei of binuclear cells have roughly the same size and staining properties. Both nuclei divide simultaneously and are thought to arise from mononuclear cells through endomitosis. Binuclear cells can account for as much as 25 percent of the parenchymal cell population. The factors influencing the formation of polyploid and binuclear liver cells and the physiologic consequences of these phenomena are not understood. The work of Carriere (1969) and others suggests that certain hormones regulate both the liver's mitotic index and the formation of the polyploid and binuclear cells. Mitotic activity, however, is rare in the intact normal adult liver (1 mitosis per 10,000 to 20,000 cells), and the minimum average life-span of a parenchymal cell is about 150 days. It is hoped that eventually new techniques will reveal more about the submicroscopic organization of these nuclei and their relation to ploidy, cell renewal, regeneration, and nuclear-cytoplasmic interactions.

The cytoplasm of the parenchymal cell is usually

FIGURE 19-11 Scanning electron micrograph of rat-liver parenchymal cells. Hemibile canaliculi connect and form the microvillus lined groove passing between adjacent hepatocytes. ×4774.

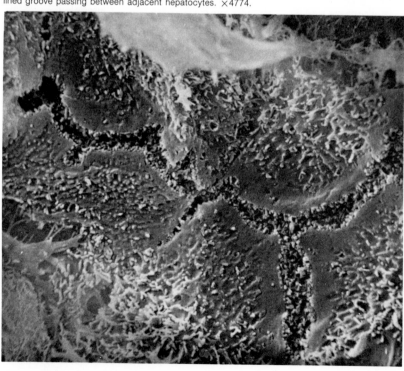

granular; however, it can vary widely in appearance, often reflecting the functional and nutritional state of the cell. Usually large clumps of basophilic *ribonucleoprotein* and abunant mitochondria can be demonstrated throughout the cytoplasm. However, after a prolonged fast, the basophilic bodies decrease and the cytoplasm becomes predominantly eosinophilic. The Golgi complex is ordinarily located near a bile canaliculus, and there is usually more than one Golgi area per section. Stored materials such as glycogen and fat are usually not preserved in conventional histologic sections, but empty round vacuoles in the cytoplasm normally indicate the sites occupied by fat, and irregular empty spaces or flocculent, grainy cytoplasmic regions mark areas that were rich in glycogen.

It is generally assumed that all parenchymal cells can store or secrete any of the substances which are demonstrable histochemically (Fig. 19-12, see color insert). Disparities in the appearance and contents of the cytoplasm are thought to depend upon the position of the cell within the lobule and the nutritional status of the individual. However, in our opinion, these problems have not been resolved and require additional work to determine how uniform liver cells are in metabolic capacity, nutritional requirements, and disease susceptibility (Table 19-2).

BLOOD VESSELS AND SINUSOIDS

The liver is highly vascularized, and its function is intimately related to the distribution and histology of its blood vessels. Blood is brought to the liver via the *portal vein* and *hepatic artery*. The livers of the dog, cat, and human being receive a total blood flow of 100 to 130 ml per min per 100 g tissue; of this 70 to 75 percent is supplied by the portal vein and the remainder by the hepatic artery. Total hepatic blood flow is about one-quarter of the cardiac output. The hepatic arterial resistance is approximately 30 to 40 times greater than the portal resistance (Greenway and Stark, 1971).

The afferent blood vessels enter the organ at the *porta* and promptly form several large branches which initially course between the lobes ensheathed in the largest trabeculae of connective tissue and then follow the successive, graduated branchings of the stroma. The gross intrahepatic vascular anatomy has been studied by combined radiologic and injection-corro-

sion techniques. Specially injected plastic casts of adult human livers reveal that the liver can be divided into segments on the basis of its internal vasculature. Each branch of the afferent vessels entering the liver is essential for proper function, since each one supplies blood to a specific area. Usually there are no anastomoses between the major branches and no accessory or additional portal veins or hepatic arteries which could provide the segment with an adequate blood supply should the major branches be impaired (Healey, 1970).

The incoming portal vein contains no valves, and its lumen is much larger than the lumen of the accompanying hepatic artery. It bifurcates into two trunks in the porta that, in turn, divides into large branches or *rami venae portae*, which are usually *interlobar* vessels. In humans, branches of the portal vein with a diameter of 400 μm or more are called *conducting veins*. They are visible to the unaided eye and include the rami venae portae, their largest branches, and subbranches. These vessels are *large-* and *medium-sized branches* of the portal vein. The histologic organization of the large conducting veins is like that of other large veins, with the exception that the portal vein contains no valves. The smaller branches of the conducting veins often lack a longitudinal layer of smooth muscle and are usually *interlobular*.

In humans, the smallest branches of the portal vein (terminal portal venules or *distributing veins*) have a diameter of 280 μm or less and are essentially endothelial tubes surrounded by a thin layer of smooth muscle fibers. They are found in the smallest portal canals and form the axis of the simple liver acinus. At intervals, they produce short branches (*inlet venules*) which pass through the limiting plate at the periphery of the lobule. Inlet venules arise perpendicularly from the axial distributing vein (see Table 19-3). The extreme ends of the inlet venules (terminal twigs) lead directly into the sinusoids; these terminal segments lack a muscle coat. In certain species, inlet venules may contain contractile endothelial cells, showing sphincter activity that regulates the portal blood flow into the sinusoids.

The largest intrahepatic branches of the hepatic artery are thick-walled. As the arteries branch and form smaller vessels, the muscle coat is reduced. Terminal branches contain only endothelium surrounded by a thin adventitia. Most of the blood within the hepatic arteries is distributed to the stroma, extrahepatic bile ducts, and gallbladder, so that only a very small volume enters the sinusoids directly. Blood from

TABLE 19-2 CYTOCHEMICAL AND ULTRASTRUCTURAL EVIDENCE OF METABOLIC HETEROGENEITY IN LIVER PARENCHYMAL CELLS

SUBSTANCE OR ORGANELLES	EXPERIMENTAL CONDITIONS		DISTRIBUTION		REFERENCES
	ANIMAL	METHOD*	CYTOPLASM	LOBULE	
Glycogen deposits	Fed	LM: PAS or Best's carmine EM: Lead stain	Throughout; often in close association with SER	Appears first in periphery of classic lobule or zone 1 of liver acinus	Deane, 1944; Novikoff and Essner, 1960
	Fasted 21 + h	LM: PAS or Best's carmine EM: Lead stain	Low or absent	Depends upon maximal hepatic glycogen level	Babcock and Cardell, 1974; Deane, 1944
Fat droplets	Fed	LM: Sudan stains; oil red O; osmium impregnation	Random, throughout	Appear transiently after meal in central cells (zone 3)	Deane, 1944
	Ethanol-treated	LM: Sudan stains; oil red O; osmium impregnation	Increased number of droplets; random, throughout	Most numerous in central (zone 3)	Elias and Sherrick, 1969
	Starved	LM: Sudan stains; oil red O; osmium impregnation	Increased after 24 h; random, throughout	Depot fat appears as droplets in peripheral cells (zone 1)	Rappaport, 1969
	Choline deficient	LM: Sudan stains; oil red O; osmium impregnation	Increased; random, throughout	Accumulate first in central cells (zone 3)	Rappaport, 1969
Bile acids	Fed	LM: barium chloride precipitation and acid fuchsin	Random, throughout	Most concentrated in peripheral cells zone 1)	Deane, 1944
Acid phosphatase	Fed	LM, EM: modified Gomori lead salt technique	In lysosomes, especially peribiliary dense bodies	Activity highest in peripheral cells (zone 1)	Novikoff and Essner, 1960
Lysosomes (all categories)	Fed	EM: quantitative stereology	Peribiliary	Most in central cells (zone 3)	Loud, 1968
Krebs' cycle enzymes	Fed	LM, EM: tetrazolium salt techniques	In mitochondria	Activity highest in peripheral cells (zone 1)	Novikoff and Essner, 1960
Mitochondria	Fed	EM: quantitative stereology	Random, throughout	Smaller and more numerous in central cells (zone 3), approximately 800 per cell	Loud, 1968
Pentose shunt enzymes	Fed	LM, EM: tretrazolium salt techniques	Random, throughout	Activity highest in central cells (zone 3)	Isselbacher and Jones, 1964; Wachstein, 1959
Peroxisomes	Fed	EM: quantitative stereology	Random, throughout	Most numerous in central cells (zone 3), approximately 200 per cell	Loud, 1968
Albumin	Fed	Fluorescent antibody techniques	Variable	No evidence of zonation; pronounced variation among adjacent cells	Hamashima et al., 1964
Rough endoplasmic reticulum	Fed	EM: quantitative stereology	Random, throughout	No zonation; about 25,000 μm^2 membrane area per cell	Loud, 1968
Smooth endoplasmic reticulum	Fed	EM: quantitative stereology	Throughout; often in association with glycogen	Membrane area in square micrometers per cell: periphery 15,700 midzonal: 16,900 central: 21,600	Loud, 1968
Golgi complex	Fed	EM: quantitative stereology	Peribiliary	Largest in peripheral cells (zone 1)	Jones et al., 1975

* LM, light microscope; EM, microscope.

terminal branches of the hepatic artery usually enters the peribiliary or periductual capillary plexus within the portal canals. Small bile ducts are surrounded by one subepithelial capillary plexus, whereas larger bile ducts have a subepithelial and a submucosal plexus. These plexi, in turn, are usually drained by small branches of the portal vein. As a result, most arterial blood reaches the hepatic sinusoids via an indirect route (see Figs. 19-2, 19-13, and 19-14 for additional details).

The sinusoids, forming the rich intralobular vascular network, anastomose and converge toward the central vein. They differ from conventional capillaries in several aspects: they are larger and more variable in caliber (9 to 12 μm wide), their cell boundaries do not blacken with silver nitrate, and many of the cells are phagocytic. The sinusoid wall contains two types of

cells: typical, flattened endothelial cells; and large, fixed macrophages, or *Kupffer cells*. The endothelial cell contains a small, compact nucleus, many micropinocytotic vesicles, small mitochondria, and only short profiles of rough ER scattered throughout the cytoplasm. The stellate-shaped Kupffer cells occur at various points along the sinusoidal lining (see Figs. 19-15, 19-16, and 19-17). These cells contain larger, oval nuclei, more mitochondria, and more rough ER than the endothelial cells. They are active phagocytes, and their cytoplasm usually contains phagocytic vacuoles with amorphous debris, engulfed blood cells, or iron, or all three.

The perisinusoidal space of Disse, surrounding the sinusoid wall, lies between the sinusoids and the parenchymal cells. Electron micrographs show that numerous parenchymal cell microvilli project into this space. In addition, bundles of collagen can be seen in this region, but never in the abundance suggested by reticular fiber stains at the light-microscopic level (see

TABLE 19-3 OVERVIEW OF HEPATIC CIRCULATION

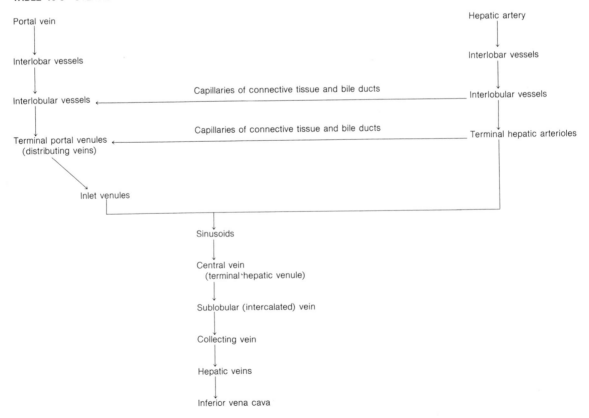

Fig. 19-18). Fat-laden lipocytes are found occasionally. Their function is not understood, although they have been implicated in vitamin A storage and the production of fibroblasts. On rare occasions, cells resembling the pericytes of the capillaries are observed. Although hematopoietic cells are numerous in this region during fetal life, they are seldom seen in the adult except during chronic anemia.

The sinusoid lining in most mammals, except certain ruminants, appears discontinuous (Grubb and Jones, 1971; Wood, 1963). Although some investigators (Wisse, 1970) believe that this appearance is artifactual, this opinion is not widespread at present. The structure of the sinusoids is important for understanding how materials are exchanged between the blood and hepatic cells. It is thought that in most mammals the sinusoid wall and the cells and fibers within the perisinusoidal space of Disse pose no significant morphologic barrier between the fluid phase of blood and the parenchymal cells. This assumption is based on the following observations. (1) Gaps are often present between the attenuated processes of adjacent endothelial cells; (2) the large and small fenestrae in the endothelial cells of most mammals

contain no diaphragm (see Figs. 19-16 and 19-19); (3) the sinusoid endothelium of most mammals, except the ruminants (see Fig. 19-20), does not have a continuous basal lamina; and (4) the cells and reticular fibers in the perisinusoidal space do not form a continuous boundary. Since the fluid phase bathes the microvilli projecting into the space of Disse, it is suspected that this region may be a site for exchange of materials between the fluid and the parenchymal cells (see Figs. 19-16, 19-18, 19-19 and 19-20).

Blood leaves the lobule via the central vein, or *terminal hepatic venule* that runs longitudinally through the middle of the lobule in the so-called central space. Central veins are lined by a simple endothelium covered by an external adventitia composed of a few spirally arranged connective tissue fibers. They are larger than sinusoids (45 μm in diameter), they travel alone, and their extremely thin walls contain numerous pores which communicate directly with the sinusoids. Several sinusoids can be seen opening into the central vein in Fig. 19-5. Note that there is no

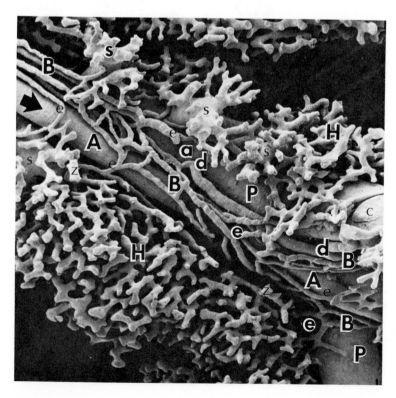

FIGURE 19-13 Methyl methacrylate casts of a small peribiliary plexus and its connecting vessels from a crab-eating monkey are shown after dissection in the scanning electron micrograph. This and similar preparations clearly demonstrate that the afferent vessels supplying the peribiliary blood vascular plexus come from the hepatic artery. In contrast to human beings and rats, in this species the efferent vessels draining the peribiliary plexus empty directly into the hepatic sinusoids. A, hepatic artery branch; B, peribiliary plexus; H, hepatic sinusoids; P, portal vein branch; a, afferent vessels of the peribiliary plexus; c, cut edges of the portal vein; d, collateral branches of the hepatic artery; e, efferent vessels of the peribiliary plexus; s, side branches of the portal vein; thick arrow is directed distally. Approximately ×121. (From T. Murakami, T. Itoshima, and Y. Shimada, *Arch. Histol. Jap.,* **37:**245–260, 1974.)

limiting plate of parenchymal cells as there is around the portal canal. At the periphery of the lobule, the central vein connects at right angles with a *sublobular* or *intercalated vein*. These vessels are larger than central veins. They are usually 90 to 200 μm in diameter and lined by endothelium and surrounded by a distinct inner circular and outer longitudinal layer of connective tissue fibers. Elastic fibers are numerous and arranged irregularly in nets throughout the walls. These veins course along the base of the lobules and enter the stromal trabeculae where they follow a solitary, isolated course, unaccompanied by other blood vessels or ducts. Several sublobular veins join to form larger collecting veins, which subsequently join to form the *hepatic veins* (see Fig. 19-21).

The hepatic veins lack valves and have numerous anastomoses among their branches. The larger branches have a moderately well-developed tunica media and vasa vasorum. They usually travel alone and are surrounded by considerable amounts of connective tissue. Hepatic veins eventually join the *inferior vena cava*.

LYMPHATICS, TISSUE SPACE OF MALL, AND THE PERISINUSOIDAL SPACE OF DISSE

The liver's capsule and stroma contain numerous lymphatic vessels. Just beneath the capsule, *superficial*

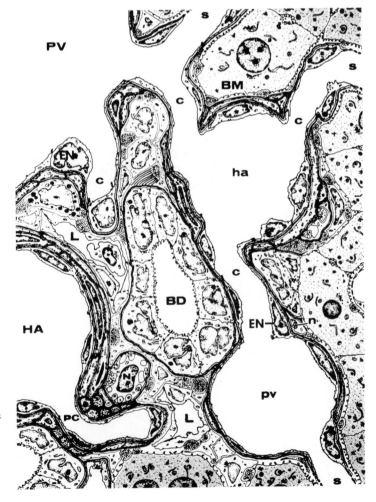

FIGURE 19-14 Terminal branches of the hepatic artery in the rat. Arterioles (HA) and terminal arterioles (ha) give rise to capillaries (c) which surround bile ducts (BD). Capillaries arising from arterioles (PC) have well-developed sphincters. The periductal capillaries terminate by joining portal veins or sinusoids, or both. A few capillaries join larger interlobular veins (PV), and some join terminal distributing veins (pv). Endothelial cell nuclei (EN) are usually located at or near the junctions of capillaries with other vessels. Sinusoids arising from capillaries are identical in structure to those arising from portal veins. At the periphery of the lobule all sinusoids resemble capillaries, having a complete basement membrane (BM) and unfenestrated endothelium. A short distance into the parenchyma they lose their basement membrane, become fenestrated, and are true sinusoids. There are numerous lymphatic vessels (L) and unmyelinated nerves (N, n) in the portal tissue. The nerves supply the smooth muscle of arterioles and precapillary sphincters. Occasionally small nerve fibers (n) are found in close relation to endothelial cells. (Courtesy of W. E. Burkel, *Anat. Rec.,* **167**:333, 1970.)

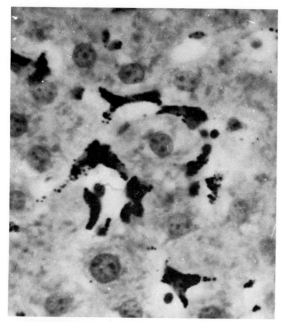

FIGURE 19-15 Kupffer cells within the sinusoid linings are phagocytic and belong to the reticuloendothelial system. They stand out as dark bodies in this photomicrograph because they have ingested carbon particles from the India ink which was injected intravenously before the animal was sacrificed. Rat liver. India ink vascular injection. Formol. H&E. ×700.

lymphatic vessels form loose plexuses which connect at intervals with the *deep lymphatic vessels* within the *portal canals* (see Fig. 19-22). Lymphatic capillary pleuses, coursing within the connective trabeculae, follow and surround branches of the portal vein, hepatic artery, and bile duct to their finest ramifications at the edge of the lobules. Because lymphatic capillaries have not been found between parenchymal cells, the origin and transport of liver lymph have been the subject of extensive investigation and controversy. The most widely accepted theory at present contends that the perisinusoidal space of Disse is the primary site for formation of liver lymph. The connections between the spaces of Disse and the lymphatic vessels in the terminal portal canals have not been demonstrated. This perplexing problem is complicated by the fact that the periphery of the lobule is surrounded by a limiting wall or plate of parenchymal cells. Elias and Sherrick (1969), however, suggest that in human beings, as fluid within the space of Disse reaches the edge of the

lobules, it flows alongside the afferent blood vessels and leaves the lobules via the occasional fenestrations in the limiting plate. From there, the fluid enters the *periportal tissue space of Mall,* which lies between the portal connective tissue and the limiting plate (see Fig. 19-1). Subsequently, the fluid diffuses from the space of Mall through the connective tissue and is collected by the lymphatic capillaries within the portal canal. Lymph is then conveyed by progressively larger lymphatic vessels to the collecting vessels which leave the liver at the hilus. On leaving the hilus, approximately 80 percent of the liver lymph flows into hilar lymph channels and then to the thoracic duct. The remaining lymph presumably originates directly from blood in the large branches of the hepatic veins. These vessels are surrounded by small networks of lymphatics, and their vasa vasorum often contains lymph vessels. Lymph formed in these vessels leaves the liver and enters retrosternal collecting lymphatics which ascend to the neck along the internal thoracic artery.

NERVES

In humans, nerves enter at the hilus. The fibers are mainly unmyelinated and from the autonomic nervous system. A few bundles of unmyelinated fibers and parasympathetic ganglion cells are found in the larger portal canals, gallbladder and capsule. Parasympathetic innervation of the liver is derived from preganglionic fibers in the dorsal efferent nucleus of the vagus. Sympathetic innervation is derived from preganglionic fibers (with cells of origin T_5 to T_9 of the thoracic cord) which synapse in the celiac ganglion. Postganglionic sympathetic fibers from cells in the celiac ganglion are distributed to the hepatic arteries within the liver and the smooth muscle of the gallbladder. The arteries are thought to be innervated by sympathetic fibers only, whereas the bile ducts are innervated by sympathetic and parasympathetic fibers. Some fibers follow the vessels and ducts into the smallest portal canals, but it is questionable whether fibers penetrate the lobules and end on parenchymal cells. Thus, at present, the principal influence of the nervous system is thought to be exerted on the blood and biliary vessels.

ULTRASTRUCTURAL AND FUNCTIONAL ASPECTS OF THE PARENCHYMAL CELLS

ENDOPLASMIC RETICULUM AND GOLGI COMPLEX

Structure

Unlike most cells, both smooth and rough endoplasmic reticulum are well developed in hepatic paren-

chymal cells, although their relative quantities, precise position, and arrangement vary from cell to cell and may be significantly altered during different physio-

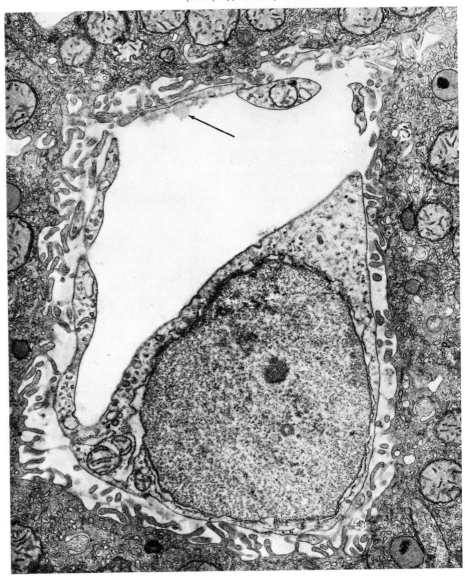

FIGURE 19-16 Rat liver sinusoid. Note the large Kupffer cell filling one-half the lumen and the discontinuity of the sinusoidal lining. A chylomicron is observed within the vascular space (arrow). Approximately ×10,000.

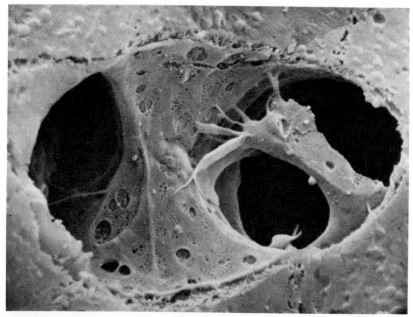

FIGURE 19-17 Scanning electron micrograph of a rat liver sinusoid with a stellate Kupffer cell stretched across the lumen. ×3066.

FIGURE 19-18 Reticular fibers can be seen in this electron micrograph within the perisinusoidal space of Disse between a sinusoid and the vascular surface of a rat hepatocyte. Small bundles of reticular fibers presumably serve as cables which support the liver parenchyma. ×6165.

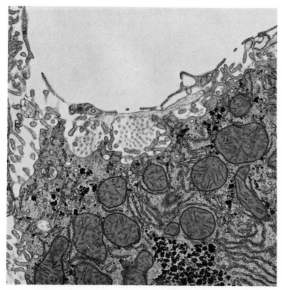

logic and experimental conditions. In addition to the membrane-bound ribosomes of the rough ER, the liver cell contains many free ribosomes and polyribosomes which fluctuate in response to various conditions (see Fig. 19-23).

The rough ER usually forms aggregates of parallel, flattened cisternae scattered randomly throughout the cytoplasm. They correspond to the *basophilic bodies,* or *ergastoplasm,* seen in specially stained histologic sections. In the rat, the surface area of the rough and smooth membranes is equal in cells surrounding the central vein but in the peripheral and midzonal cells, the rough ER has approximately 50 percent more surface area than the smooth (Loud, 1968) (see Table 19-2).

The smooth ER is composed of a complex meshwork of twisting, branching, and anastomosing tubules which frequently communicate with the rough ER and Golgi but never with the nuclear envelope. These tubules follow a highly tortuous course and often exhibit variations in caliber. Smooth ER in the liver often shows local specializations and almost invariably is associated with *glycogen,* although the functional significance of this relationship is unclear. In the rat, the surface area of the smooth ER is significantly higher in central (21,600 μm^2 per cell) and midzonal (16,900 μm^2 per cell) cells than in the pe-

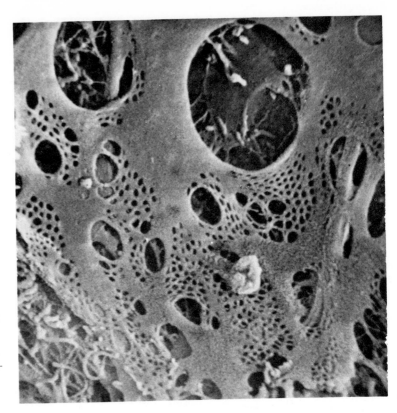

FIGURE 19-19 Scanning electron micrograph of the luminal surface of a rat liver sinusoid. Fenestrations of variable size impart a sievelike appearance to the endothelium. Microvilli and the surface of a hepatic parenchymal cell can be seen through the large fenestrations at the top of the micrograph. ×14,025.

ripheral cells (15,700 μm^2 per cell) of the classic lobule (Loud, 1968).

Golgi profiles are numerous, and each parenchymal cell has been estimated to contain as many as 50 Golgi complexes (Claude, 1970). Early in fetal life, the Golgi complex is paranuclear but migrates into the peribiliary cytoplasm early in the second trimester when bile secretion commences (Koga, 1971). In the rat, Jones et al. have found significantly more Golgi area in the periportal cells. The fine structure of the Golgi complex is similar, but not identical, to those in other cell types. Each complex has three to five closely packed, parallel, smooth-surfaced cisternae and a variable number of vesicles. The bulbous ends of the cisternae and their associated large vesicles are often filled with electron-dense particles, 250 to 800 Å in diameter, which are thought be the triglyceride-rich *very-low-density lipoproteins* (VLDL) which play an important role in the transport of lipids within the plasma (Jones et al., 1967; Hamilton et al., 1967; Mahley et al., 1969).

FIGURE 19-20 Endothelial lining of the sinusoid from sheep liver. Note the diaphragm covering one fenestra (arrow) and basal lamina. S, sinusoidal space; D, space of Disse. (From D. J. Grubb and A. L. Jones, *Anat. Rec.,* **170:**75, 1971.)

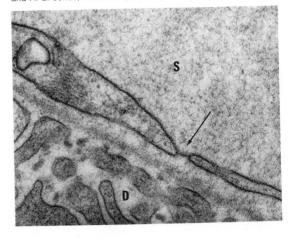

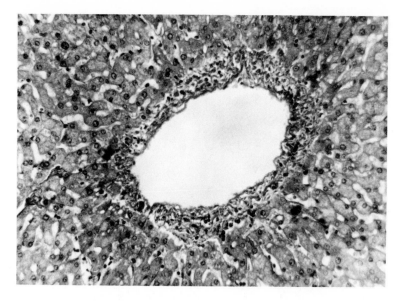

FIGURE 19-21 A branch of the hepatic vein is shown surrounded by a considerable amount of connective tissue. These vessels usually travel alone. Human liver. Zenker formal in H&E.

FIGURE 19-22 Network of lymphatic vessels. The vessels, shown in white, surround branches of the portal vein (to the left), connecting with superficial lymphatics in Glisson's capsule (to the right). ×50. (Teichmann.)

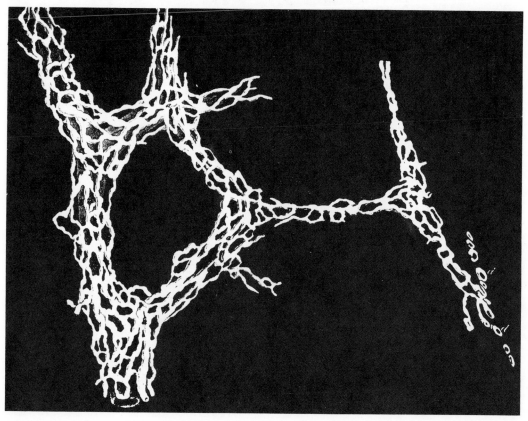

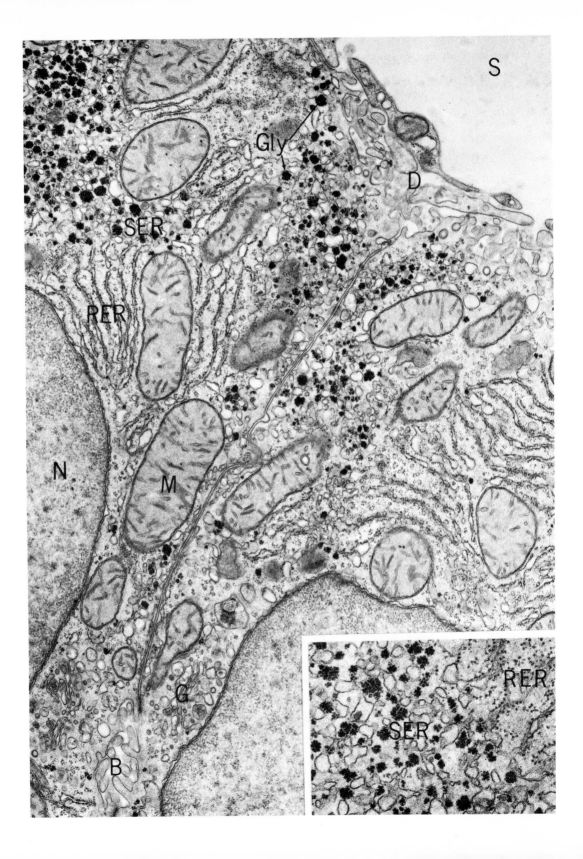

FIGURE 19-23 Electron micrograph of two liver cells from the rat. S, sinusoid; D, space of Disse; Gly, glycogen; M, mitochondria; SER, smooth-surfaced reticulum; RER, rough-surfaced reticulum; B, bile canaliculi; G, Golgi apparatus; N, nucleus. Note the discontinuous endothelial lining, the association of glycogen with the SER (see insert), the flattened lamellar profiles of the RER, the microvilli within the space of Disse and bile canaliculus, and close relationships between the Golgi apparatus and bile canaliculi. ×27,000; insert ×45,000.

Function

The liver microsomal fraction (ER) is known to participate in (1) the synthesis of albumin, fibrinogen, and other plasma proteins; (2) the synthesis of cholesterol for export and bile-salt formation; (3) glucuronide conjugation of bilrubin, drugs, and steroids; (4) metabolism of drugs and steroids; (5) esterification of free fatty acids to triglycerides; (6) the breakdown of glycogen; and (7) deiodination of T_4 to T_3.

Most studies of protein synthesis for export (for example, albumin and other plasma proteins) show that protein synthesis is a function of the rough ER. The product is thought to leave the rough ER and migrate via the smooth ER to the Golgi complex and finally to the cell's vascular surface for release. However, a recent study by Lin and Chang (1975) does not support this theory. Instead, these investigators observed that albumin molecules, synthesized on polysomes bound to the rough ER and nuclear envelope, were discharged into the cytosol, and then into the extracellular spaces.

Cholesterol biosynthesis seems to be a function of the smooth ER. Evidence for this function came from the discovery that liver cells following phenobarbital administration and smooth ER hypertrophy were four times more active in cholesterol biosynthesis than control livers (Jones and Armstrong, 1965) (see Fig. 19-24).

Most lipid-soluble drugs and steroids are metabolized by the liver microsomal fraction. The microsomal *mixed-function oxidase system,* a chain of enzymes such as NADPH cytochrome c reductase and cytochrome P_{450}, is thought to perform these functions. Although there is evidence that this functional chain occurs in both categories of ER, the principal activity of the chain probably resides in the membranes of the smooth ER (Jones and Fawcett, 1966). Most lipid-soluble compounds with diverse chemical structure (for example, phenobarbital as against DDT) are metabolized by the microsomes and also promote a marked hypertrophy of the smooth ER and many of its enzymes. This adaptive response enables the liver to

metabolize more effectively the inducing substances and is obviously valuable in the detoxification of drugs, certain carcinogens, and insecticides. Progesterone and certain anabolic steroids are also inducers of liver smooth ER, its associated cytochrome P_{450}, and the mitochondrial enzyme Δ-aminolevulinic acid synthetase (ALA syn) (Jones and Emans, 1969). Increased ALA syn activity results in increased heme production and stimulates the formation of cytochrome P_{450} (see Fig. 19-25). Interference with the terminal steps of heme synthesis produces an abnormal accumulation of porphyrin and the clinical condition of porphyria (Marver and Schmid, 1972). As a result, it is currently assumed that sex steroids in some way influence the normal quantities of smooth ER and hence certain functional activities within the liver cells. The induction of liver ER and its subsequent effect on porphyrin and drug metabolism should be considered by the physician when administering gonadal hormones for contraceptive purposes.

Deliberate induction of microsomal enzymes, to increase glucuronyl transferase activity, has been found beneficial in certain cases of hyperbilirubinemia. However, liver microsomal enzyme induction is *not* always beneficial. First, the ER induction following the initial exposure to an inducing compound can alter the individual's subsequent response to the same or another therapeutic agent: the additional enzymes may metabolize a drug at a new rate. Second, some compounds metabolized by the ER are more dangerous than the parent compound. One example is 3,4-benzpyrene, a relatively innocuous component of cigarette smoke, which on hydroxylation becomes a potent carcinogen. Another example is carbon tetrachloride: The centrolobular necrosis associated with carbon tetrachloride poisoning is not caused by the parent compound but by a free radical formed during its metabolism.

Fat metabolism is another important liver function associated with the ER. In the parenchymal cell, free fatty acids not utilized for energy or membrane synthesis are reesterified into triglycerides. A small amount of triglyceride is stored in cytoplasmic fat droplets and the remainder is released into the blood as VLDL (see Fig. 19-26). The VLDL particle is a lipid-protein complex. Its triglyceride, or fatty core, is encompassed by a surface apoprotein and a mixture of cholesterol and phospholipid. Presumably the particle

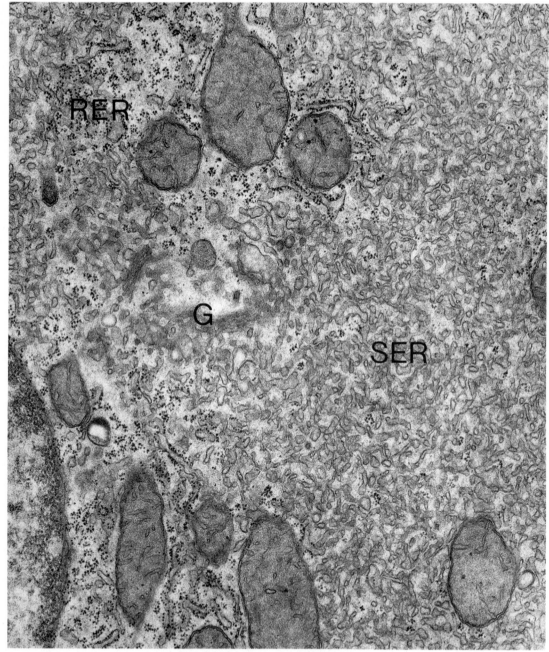

FIGURE 19-24 Liver cell from a phenobarbital-treated animal showing an extraordinary hypertrophy of the smooth-surfaced endoplasmic reticulum (SER). Because of its abundance, the smooth-membraned elements appear to crowd the profiles of rough-surfaced endoplasmic reticulum (RER) into localized areas. The tangential section through the Golgi complex (G) shows several areas of communication between this organelle and the SER. Approximately ×40,000. (From A. L. Jones and D. W. Fawcett, *J. Histochem. Cytochem.*, **14**:215, 1966.)

is synthesized in the ER with the smooth ER forming the lipid and the rough ER synthesizing the protein. The mechanism of complexing the two components is not understood.

Following synthesis, the lipoprotein is transferred through the smooth ER and is released from the cells. This may be accomplished in two ways: (1) smooth vesicles containing lipoproteins may bud off the smooth ER, migrate to the surface, and be released by exocytosis or (2) the lipoproteins within the smooth ER may be sequestered in Golgi vesicles, which in turn are released at the cell surface in a packet (see Figs. 19-26, 19-27, and 19-28). This latter mode of transport is similar to that used by the pancreatic acinar cells for protein secretion. The recent intracellular localization of sugar nucleotide glycoprotein glycosyltransferases in Golgi-rich fractions from liver strongly suggests that the Golgi may be involved generally in glycoprotein production and in the addition of a carbohydrate component to the lipoprotein (see Fig. 19-28).

FIGURE 19-25 A (left) The close association of the rough-surfaced reticulum with mitochondria seen in electron micrographs of intact hepatocytes is diagrammatically represented here. This relationship may be necessary for the production of smooth reticulum and cytochromes. Under the influence of messenger RNA (mRNA), the rough-surfaced endoplasmic reticulum (RER) synthesizes the enzyme Δ-aminolevulinic acid synthetase (ALA syn) which is transferred to the mitochondria. This results in an increased production of heme. Some heme is transferred back to the endoplasmic reticulum for the production of the microsomal heme protein P450. (From A. L. Jones and J. B. Emans, in H. A. Salhanick, D. Kipnes, and R. L. Van de Wiele (eds.), "Metabolic Effects of Gonadal Hormones and Contraceptive Steroids," Plenum Press, Plenum Publishing Corporation, New York, 1969) B (right) Using special techniques, it is now possible to isolate a mitochondrial-RER complex from liver homogenates. Early studies indicate that this may be a functional unit essential for microsomal hemoprotein synthesis. Approximately ×20,000. (Courtesy of U. A. Meyer, P. J. Meier, and M. A. Spycker.)

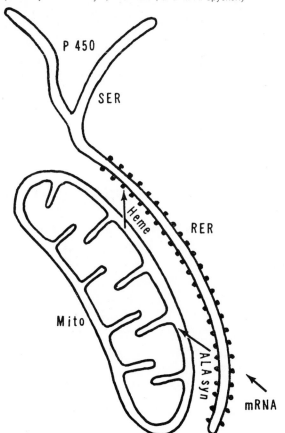

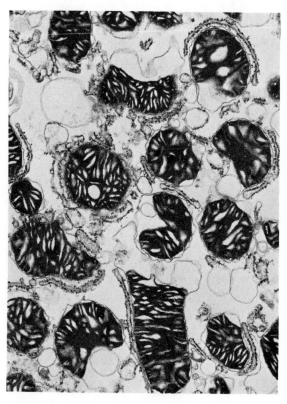

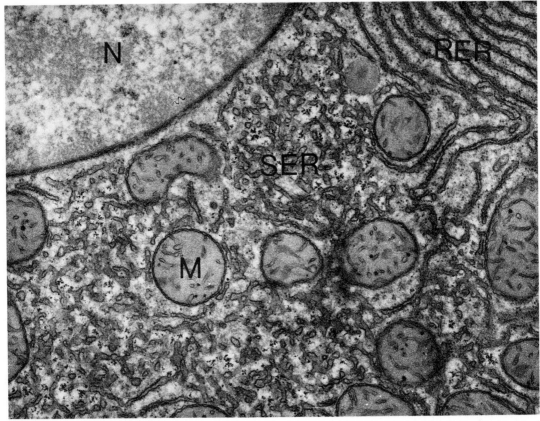

FIGURE 19-26 Certain synthetic and naturally occurring steroids produce a marked hypertrophy of the hepatic smooth-surfaced endoplasmic reticulum (SER). Rough-surfaced endoplasmic reticulum (RER) can be observed partially wrapped around mitochondria during rapid membrane proliferation. N, nucleus; M, mitochondria. ×37,000 (Courtesy of J. A. Hahn.)

FIGURE 19-27 Electron micrographs of very-low-density lipoprotein particles within the Golgi complex of an intact liver cell (A) and within the membranes of the isolated Golgi-rich fraction (B) of rat liver. The lipoprotein particles can be further isolated from the Golgi membranes for analysis. Approximately ×25,000. (Courtesy of R. L. Hamilton.)

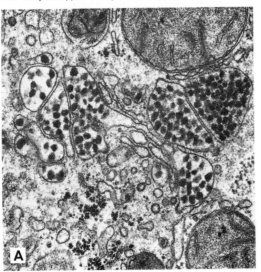

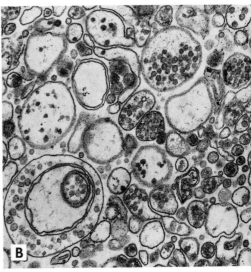

Membrane Synthesis and Turnover

A number of important relationships between the sub-cellular structure and function of hepatic ER have been derived from the elegant studies of fetal and newborn rat livers by Dallner, Siekevitz, and Palade (1966). Three days prior to delivery, there is a marked increase in parenchymal cell glycogen. Although parenchymal cell rough ER is essentially fully developed, the activity of certain microsomal enzymes (for example, mixed-function oxidases and glucose-6-phosphatase) is nearly unmeasurable. Furthermore, there is little or no smooth ER in these cells. After birth, glycogen falls and smooth ER increases within the cells, while the activity of the enzymes mentioned

above begins to rise (although not all enzymes do at the same rate) and the liver acquires the ability to metabolize certain drugs.

Following formation of ER within the hepatocyte, these membranes undergo constant renewal or turnover. The half-life of adult liver ER has been calculated to be 2 to $2\frac{1}{2}$ days (Schimke et al., 1968). It is becoming clear, however, that not all components within these membranes turn over at the same rate. Moreover, recent studies of lipoprotein synthesis show that they can be synthesized and transported out of the liver cell within 5 min. Since each particle or packet of particles is surrounded by a portion of smooth ER or Golgi membrane, or both, which accompanies the particle to the plasmalemma, it appears likely that

FIGURE 19-28 Diagrammatic representation of the possible steps in lipoprotein production and release. (Modified from A. L. Jones, N. B. Ruderman, and M. G. Herrera, *J. Lipid Res.,* **8:**429, 1967.)

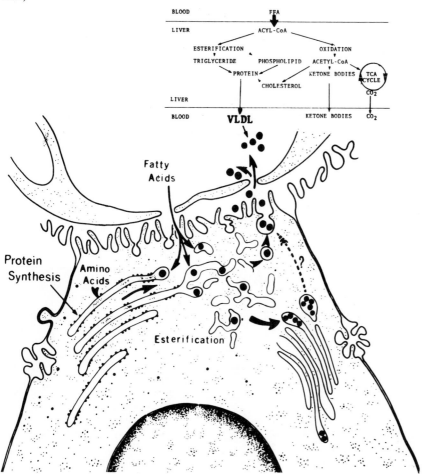

membrane turnover might take minutes rather than days or hours, as previously thought.

LYSOSOMES

Structure

Liver parenchymal cells contain many lysosomes (see Fig. 19-29). They can be found almost invariably within the cytoplasm bordering each bile canaliculus and Golgi complex. Lysosomes in these sites correspond to the so-called peribiliary dense bodies described by early histologists. These highly pleomorphic organelles vary in size, number, and position during different conditions. Since no two lysosomes look alike, their positive identification in electron micrographs requires that the intracellular particle be bounded by a single membrane and exhibit a positive staining reaction for acid phosphatase. Parenchymal cell lysosomes are usually 0.2 to 1 µm in diameter and contain variable amounts of material. Their contents may be homogenous, heterogeneous, dense, or finely granular and may include myelin figures, pigment, intact or partially digested organelles, or inclusions, or all four.

Function

Lysosomes perform a number of digestive and lytic functions for the parenchymal cells. Under normal conditions, they catabolize certain unwanted exogenous substances, effete organelles, and inclusions. The latter two processes are especially important for main-

tenance and rejuvenation of the parenchymal cells, since some products of digestion may be utilized by the cells for energy and repair. Loss of liver mass and the presence of increased numbers of lysosomes in livers of starved animals are associated with the mobilization and release of stored energy-producing substances needed to maintain the entire body. Hepatic lysosomes also appear to participate in the storage of iron. They normally contain ferritinlike substances and accumulate large quantities of these materials in iron-storage diseases, for example, hemochromatosis and hemosiderosis.

There is now considerable evidence that lysosomes have an important role in cellular pathology. Hepatic lysosomes increase in viral hepatitis, cholestasis, and cell injury following anoxia. The livers of children with type 2 glycogenosis (Pompe's disease) lack the enzyme α-glucosidase and contain large glycogen deposits within their lysosomes (see Weissman, 1969, for review).

MICROBODIES (PEROXISOMES)

Structure

The microbody is a single membrane-bounded particle (approximately 0.2 to 1 µm in diameter) with a fine granular matrix. Each parenchymal cell has approximately 200 microbodies or one microbody per four

FIGURE 19-29. (Left) Three hepatic lysosomes near a bile canaliculus. Note the morphologic variation in their matrix and that they are bounded by a single membrane. Approximately ×23,750 **(Right)** This membrane-bounded structure in a human hepatocyte is a lipofuscin pigment granule. These pigment deposits are thought to be undigestible residues of lysosomal activity and are common in livers from older humans and animals. (Micrograph courtesy of H. I. Friedman.)

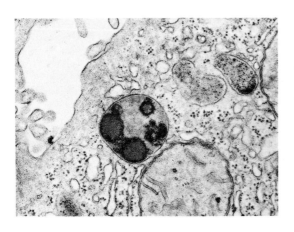
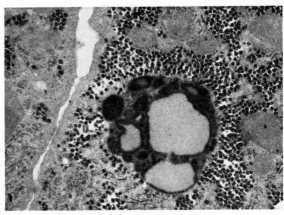

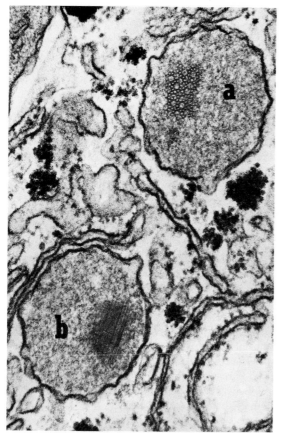

FIGURE 19-30 Microbodies. In the rat, these single-membrane–bounded structures contain a crystalloid enmeshed in a homogenous matrix. Both a cross section (a) and longitudinal section (b) of the crystalloid are observed in this micrograph. (See text). Approximately ×100,000.

mitochondria. They vary greatly in size within the same cell, but there appears to be no difference in enzymatic composition between small and large microbodies having the same structure. Hepatic microbodies in many mammals contain a crystalloid laminated core or nucleoid which distinguishes them from the denser peribiliary bodies, the lysosomes. The structure of the core varies greatly from species to species. In the hamster (Jones and Fawcett, 1966), it appears as a thin flexible sheet; whereas in the rat, it is made up of tubules of two different sizes: small ones, approximately 45 Å in diameter, and large ones, 95 to 115 Å in diameter (see Fig. 19-30). The two types of tubules, in longitudinal section, produce the laminated appearance of the crystalloid. The core is thought to contain urate oxidase whereas catalase and D-amino

acid oxidase presumably are present in the matrix. The livers of uricotelic animals, anthropoid primates, and human beings usually contain anucleoid microbodies deficient in urate oxidase. In some species, the liver contains a mixture of nucleoid and anucleoid microbodies.

Function

The physiologic significance of hepatic microbodies is not known, although it is speculated that they may participate in any one or all of the following: disposal of hydrogen peroxide; metabolism of purines, lipids, and alcohols; oxidation of reduced NAD; and gluconeogenesis (see De Duve and Baudhuin, 1966, for review). Human beings and certain mouse strains with little or no blood and liver catalase activity can survive satisfactorily; hence it appears that this constituent of the microbody is not essential for life.

Proliferation of hepatic microbodies occurs during embryologic development and early postnatal life, during recovery from partial hepatectomy, and following the administration of salicylates and the lipid-lowering agent ethyl-α-p-chlorophenoxyisobutyrate (CPIB, or clofibrate).

MITOCHONDRIA

Parenchymal cells contain numerous well-developed mitochondria (approximately 800 per cell) (see Fig. 19-23). In rat and human livers the mitochondria are usually round or oblong (for example, 0.5 to 1.5 μm in diameter, 1.5 to 4.5 μm in length). These organelles account for approximately 20 percent of the total nitrogen within each cell. The mitochondria appear to be randomly distributed throughout the cytoplasm. However, there is good evidence that the number, size, shape, and enzymatic properties of liver mitochondria are related to the position of the cell within the lobule (Novikoff and Essner, 1960; Loud, 1968).

Mitochondria move about in the cytoplasm and undergo changes in structure and volume. Such morphologic alterations are thought to reflect functional changes. Swelling and contraction of isolated liver mitochondria occur in response to a number of endogenous substances, such as hormones, calcium ions, phosphate ions, and fatty acids, as well as to changes in ion transport and osmotic pressure. Although the precise meaning of these observations is not yet clear, it appears likely that both conformational and chemiosmotic changes are normally involved in energy transduction. The effects of swelling and contraction on the molecular organization and composition of the mitochondrial membranes are not yet completely documented; however, it appears that the flexibility of mitochondrial membranes depends, at least in part, upon the presence of unsaturated fatty acids (Packer, 1970).

Liver mitochondria are thought to be self-replicating bodies with a half-life of about 10.5 days. The presence of mitochondria within lysosomes has fostered the idea that the lysosomes destroy effete mitochondria. And the rapidity with which the mitochondria are thought to turn over, in comparison with the life-span of the cell, presumably accounts for the presence of a few atypical or abnormal mitochondria in otherwise healthy cells. The genesis of the liver mitochondrion, however, is still subject to conjecture. Budding or dividing mitochondria are not readily found in normal liver, but they are commonplace during recovery from simple riboflavin (Tandler et al., 1969) or dietary iron (Dallman and Goodman, 1971) deficiency. The giant mitochondria formed during the course of these diseases are restored to normal di-

mensions by means of division following the onset of replacement therapy.

Intramitochondrial inclusions have been described in hepatic mitochondria in a number of human diseases; however, their significance remains obscure.

AGING

Although very little is known about the structural changes accrued by aging in human liver, several studies indicate that aging leads to significant structural alterations in rat liver. In this species, the number of hepatocytes per unit volume of tissue decreases with age while the cell size and incidence of polyploidy increases (Wheatley, 1972).

Previous investigators have also suggested that the number of mitochondria and microbodies changes with age, but recent quantitative studies do not support this idea (Schmucker, 1975 and 1976). Instead, these investigations show that lysosomes and smooth ER increase with age in rat liver. The additional smooth ER membrane, however, may suffer from age-related changes, since the microsomal drug-metabolizing capabilities of the animal decreases with age. The accumulation of nondigestible materials such as lipofuscin pigment in lysosomes or residual bodies of otherwise healthy liver cells occurs even in young animals, but the number of lysosomes with residua increases as the individual ages.

THE BILIARY SPACE

BILE CANALICULI

The bile canaliculi are the smallest biliary spaces, ranging from 0.5 to 1.5 μm in diameter. They are usually centrally located between adjacent parenchymal cells (see Figs. 19-2, 19-10, 19-11, and 19-31). The bile canaliculi can be isolated from the remainder of the liver by maceration. Misinterpretation of this phenomenon resulted in the erroneous notion that the canaliculi were bounded by a separate cuticular wall. Electron-microscopic evidence has now clearly established that the limiting wall of the bile canaliculus is made up of local surface specializations on adjacent liver cells (Matter et al., 1969). Microvilli of the parenchymal cells protrude into the lumen of the canaliculi (see Fig. 19-23), and fine cytoplasmic

filaments circumscribe the area beneath the canaliculi. They insert into desmosomes and extend into the core of the microvilli. The filament-rich pericanalicular ectoplasm of the liver and the terminal web area of the intestinal absorptive cell have similar staining reactions, indicating that they are composed, at least in part, of the same material (Biava, 1964). Histochemical preparations, such as ATPase and alkaline phosphatase stains, have enabled investigators to clearly observe the biliary network with the light microscope. The finding of ATPase activity in this area suggests that bile secretion is an energy-requiring process.

The biliary space is separated from the other intercellular spaces by junctional complexes between the parenchymal cells (see Figs. 19-32 and 19-33). Immediately adjacent to the canalicular lumen is a

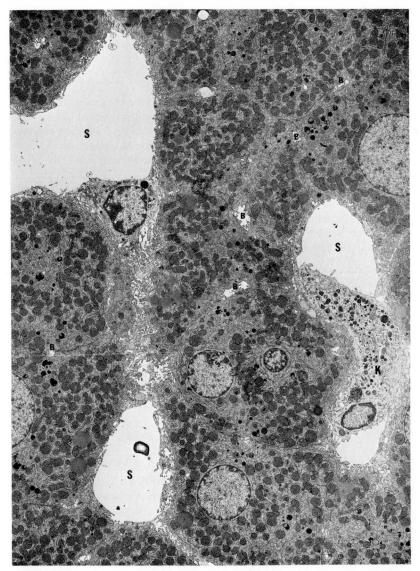

FIGURE 19-31 This low-power electron micrograph of rat liver shows hepatocytes disposed between sinusoids (S), the blood vascular channels within the lobule. Bile canaliculi (B) are centrally located between adjacent parenchymal cells. At this magnification one can appreciate the random distribution of the organelles. Golgi complexes, however, are almost always located between the nucleus and bile canaliculus. A large Kupffer cell (K) extends across part of a sinusoid. Approximately ×2520. (From A. L. Jones and E. Spring-Mills, *Am. J. Drug and Alcohol Abuse,* **1:**111–135, 1974, micrograph courtesy of D. L. Schmucker.)

tight junction (see Fig. 19-32). Lanthanum injected into the portal vein or retrograde up the common bile duct will not normally pass across this junction (Matter et al., 1969). Because of this, it is speculated that certain components of bile, such as conjugated bilirubin, may gain access to the intercellular space by this route during times of chronic biliary obstruction. Another cellular attachment near the canaliculus is the nexus or gap junction. The membranes in this junction are parallel to one another with a 20-Å gap which normally will admit lanthanum. The function of the junction is still not clear, but certain evidence indicates that it provides an electrical communication between cells. The nexus may be observed along any part of the

FIGURE 19-32 Tight junction adjacent to a bile canaliculus (bc) in rat liver. Note the focal merging of the two outer leaflets of the plasma membrane of the parenchymal cells (arrow). Approximately ×100,000. (Courtesy of D. Friend.).

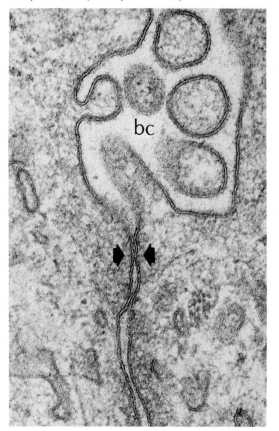

plasmalemma between adjacent liver cells. Desmosomes, when included within the plane of section, appear near the canaliculi.

TERMINAL DUCTULES

Bile flows in the canaliculi to the periphery of the classic lobule and enters small terminal bile ductules or canals of Hering. These canals form short channels that convey bile from the canaliculi through the limiting plate and into the interlobular bile duct of the portal canals.

At first, one or two fusiform-shaped ductular cells share a canalicular lumen with a hepatocyte (see Fig. 19-34). Subsequently, they are lined by two to four cells which become cuboidal as the ductule nears the portal canal. The terminal ductules are smaller than the interlobular ducts, having diameters usually less than 15 μm. Many blunt microvilli project from their lumenal borders. The nuclei are elongated and the mitochondria are smaller than those of neighboring hepatocytes. Endoplasmic reticulum is sparse, but the Golgi complex and pinocytotic vesicles are well developed, suggesting that the ductules are metabolically active. A basal lamina completely encompasses the ductules except at the point of contact between the hepatocytes and ductule cells.

The origin of the terminal ductule cell is a matter of debate. Some feel that it is derived from cells of the larger interlobular ducts, whereas others claim it is of parenchymal origin. During chronic extrahepatic cholestasis, the ductule cells proliferate and almost completely replace the liver cells (Steiner et al., 1962). Wilson believes they are primitive cells capable of differentiating into either parenchymal or bile epithelium. Whatever their source or potentials, the epithelial cells of the terminal ductules are very unusual.

INTRAHEPATIC BILE DUCTS

Bile in the terminal ductules empties into *interlobular bile ducts* (30 to 40 μm in diameter) in the portal canals (see Fig. 19-4). These ducts form a continuous network of passageways whose size increases as they near the porta. They are lined by a single layer of cuboidal or columnar epithelial cells which have microvilli on their lumenal surface (see Fig. 19-35). The epithelium is surrounded by a basal lamina. The basal nuclei are round and contain considerable chromatin often arranged like cartwheel spokes. These cells, like those of the ductules, contain a prominent Golgi complex and vesicles considered to be pinocytotic. Cholesterol crystals have been observed in the cytoplasm. Occasionally, areas of mucus-secreting epithelium surrounded by a vascular plexus have been observed in the larger ducts. The wall of the intrahepatic bile ducts is made up of dense fibrous tissue containing many elastic fibers. Smooth muscle fibers in the walls of the ducts near the hilus of the liver form the morphologic basis for the narrowing of the ducts in this

FIGURE 19-33 Electron micrograph of a replica of a frozen-fractured membrane from an hepatocyte (H) showing the origin of a bile canaliculus. The tight junctions (TJ) appear as anastomosing, thin, linear grooves surrounding the bile canaliculus. The arrow points to a gap junction. The large pits or indentations in the surface are bases of the microvilli (MV). (Courtesy of N. Scott McNutt.)

location often seen in cholangiograms (Rappaport, 1969).

EXTRAHEPATIC BILE DUCTS

The extrahepatic ducts are enclosed by tall columnar cells. Their walls possess the same layers as the intestine, that is, mucosa, submucosa, muscularis, and adventitia. Tubular glands containing cells rich in mucopolysaccharides are occasionally noted at regular intervals in the submucosa. The wall of the extra-

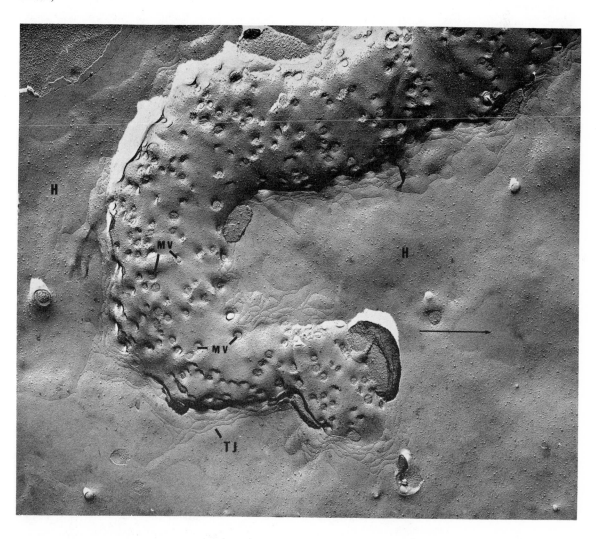

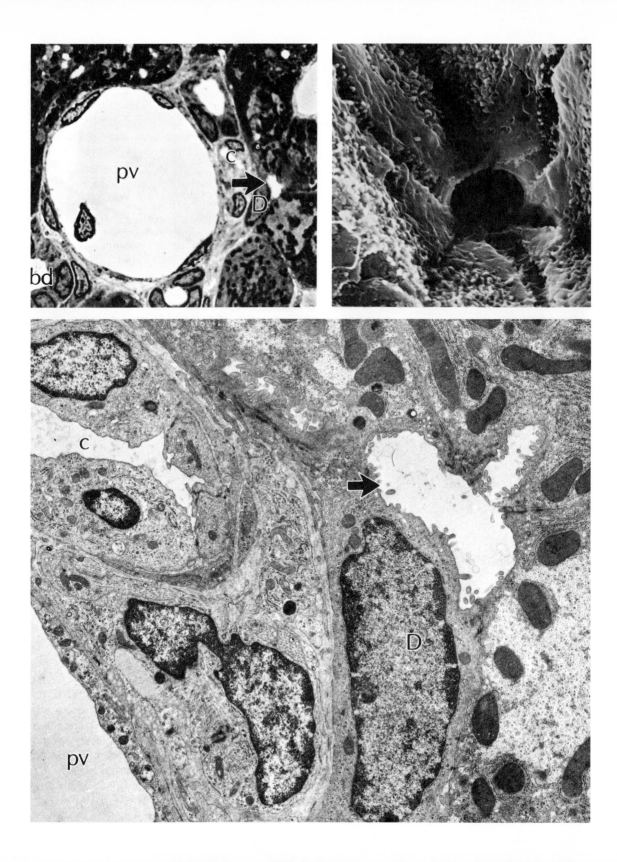

FIGURE 19-34 Adjacent to a portal canal a junction is seen between a terminal ductule cell and three hepatic parenchymal cells (arrow) by both light (upper left figure, ×1,100) and electron microscopy (lower figure, ×8,000). Note the fusiform shape of the ductule cell and its basal lamina. pv, portal vein; c, capillaries; bd, bile duct; D, ductule cell. (Courtesy of R. L. Wood). The scanning electron micrograph (upper right figure, approximately ×5,300) shows three bile canaliculi converging to form a canal of Hering. (From T. J. Layden, J. Schwarz and J. L. Boyer, *Gastroenterology,* **69:**724–738, 1975.)

hepatic ducts receives its blood supply from small branches of the hepatic and gastroduodenal arteries.

The *common hepatic duct* is approximately 3 cm long. It arises at the porta from the confluence of the right and left hepatic lobular ducts. It is joined by the

FIGURE 19-35 Small interlobular bile duct. These ducts are encompassed by a thin basal lamina. The cuboidal cells contain few organelles although pinocytotic vesicles are abundant and the Golgi complex (G), when included in the plane of section, is well developed. Note the microvilli on their luminal surface and the apical zones of adhesion (arrow). Approximately ×12,000.

cystic duct from the gallbladder to form the *common bile duct* (ductus choledochus), which is approximately 7 cm long and empties into the duodenum. Tubular glands containing PAS-positive cells are scattered along the length of the common duct. These glands are more extensive in mammals lacking a gallbladder, such as the rat.

GALLBLADDER

Located on the undersurface of the right liver lobe and connected to the relatively rigid ducts of the biliary tree is a readily distensible bag: the gallbladder. In humans, it is large enough to hold 30 to 50 ml of bile. The surface of the filled gallbladder is stretched evenly, but in the empty, contracted gallbladder it

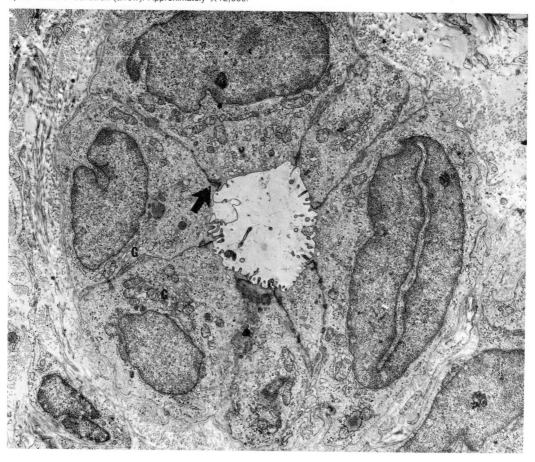

forms numerous elongated, decussating folds or rugae. The wall contains a surface epithelium, lamina propria, muscularis, and a serosa (see Fig. 19-36).

The musosa contains an inner layer of simple columnar epithelium. The apex of each cell contains numerous microvilli (see Fig. 19-37), lateral junctional complexes, and associated tonofilaments. Desmosomes occur at frequent intervals along the entire length of the lateral cell membranes. The Golgi is usually supranuclear and well developed. Rough ER and membrane-bounded granular inclusions are especially prominent in humans. Mitochondria are numerous but relatively small.

The lamina propria is rich in blood vessels and connective tissue fibers. The muscularis consists of a number of layers of smooth muscle separated by a fairly extensive network of elastic fibers. The serosal coat is a broad connective tissue layer containing numerous collagen fibers and the blood vessels and lymphatics which supply the organ. Numerous nerves from the autonomic nervous system can also be noted on the serosal surface. Glands can be found occasionally in the lamina propria of the human gallbladder, especially near the neck. These glands contain goblet cells and a few cells which are identical to the argentaffin cells in the intestine. These so-called mucous glands, sparse in normal tissue, are moderately abundant in persons who have had chronic inflammation of the gallbladder. However, it is difficult to tell whether a common pathologic factor promotes inflammation and stimulates the development of the glands or whether there is a secondary causal relationship between the development of cholecystitis and the presence of these glands.

Rokitansky-Aschoff crypts, or *diverticula,* are invaginations of the surface epithelium. Some of these crypts, or sinuses, extend through the entire width of the muscular layer. They favor bacterial retention and inflammation and are usually regarded as antecedents to pathologic changes.

Luschka's bile ducts are seen occasionally in some gallbladders. Serial sections reveal that these bile ducts, located along the hepatic surface of the gallbladder, open directly into the liver. The epithelium has a variable morphology but is generally similar to normal intrahepatic ducts. They are probably the consequence of some embryologic developmental disturbance.

The arterial supply of the gallbladder is via the *cystic artery,* which usually arises from the right hepatic artery. At the gallbladder it divides into a superficial branch supplying the free or serosal surface and a deep branch which arborizes throughout the deeper, interior layers of the wall. These branches anastomose freely and may send twigs into the adjacent liver substance. Venous drainage from the gallbladder and cystic duct is via the *cytstic vein,* which ends in the right branch of the portal vein. Occasionally, some small venous branches may pass directly into the hepatic parenchyma and join the sinusoids. The lymph vessels of the gallbladder are reportedly intimately connected with lymph vessels of Glisson's capsule.

The neck of the gallbladder is continuous with the *cystic duct.* This duct retains all the layers of the wall of the gallbladder, is about 4 cm long, and joins the common hepatic duct. Its mucous membrane is thrown into a series of folds arranged in a spiral fashion around the tube (spiral valve) (see Fig. 19-38). Many nerve cells are found in the fibromuscular layer of the cystic duct.

CHOLEDOCHODUODENAL JUNCTION

The junction of the common bile duct, pancreatic duct, and the duodenum is an anatomic area of medical and physiologic importance. It regulates the flow of bile and pancreatic enzymes into the duodenum and governs the filling of the gallbladder. Occlusion of the choledochoduodenal junction by small gallstones or tumors results in cholestasis (and various sequelae).

In the human embryo, the ventral pancreatic and common bile duct arise from the hepatic diverticulum of the foregut. In the adult, the associated bile and pancreatic ducts pass obliquely through an opening in the circular musculature of the duodenum. The ducts empty their contents into a duodenal ampulla, the *ampulla of Vater.* The bile and pancreatic enzymes

FIGURE 19-36 Contracted gallbladder. Parts a (×3000) and c (×350) are scanning electron micrographs of the inner surface of guinea pig gallbladder. Part c shows the pronounced folding of the gallbladder mucosa. In a the bulging individual epithelial cells are covered with bristlelike microvilli. Compare with Fig. 19-37. Part b (×90) is a light micrograph of contracted human gallbladder. Note the diverticula (D) into the wall and the mucous gland (MG). The muscularis (M) is present but the serosa has been stripped off. Fixed in Zenker's fluid; H&E. (a and c from J. C. Mueller, A. L. Jones, and J. A. Long, *Gastroenterology,* **62,** 1972.)

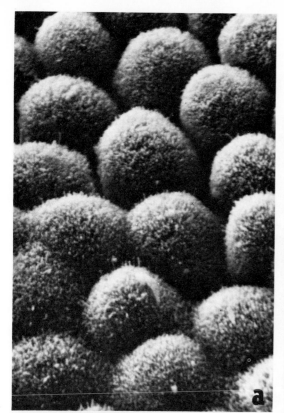

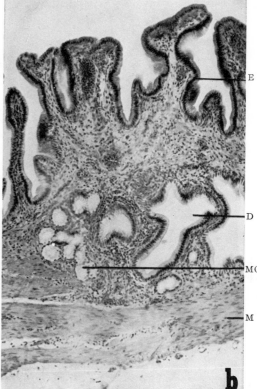

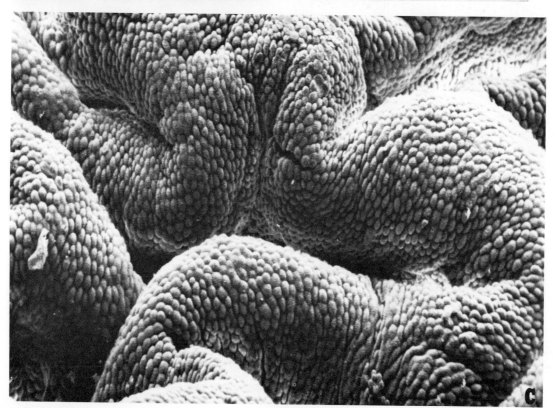

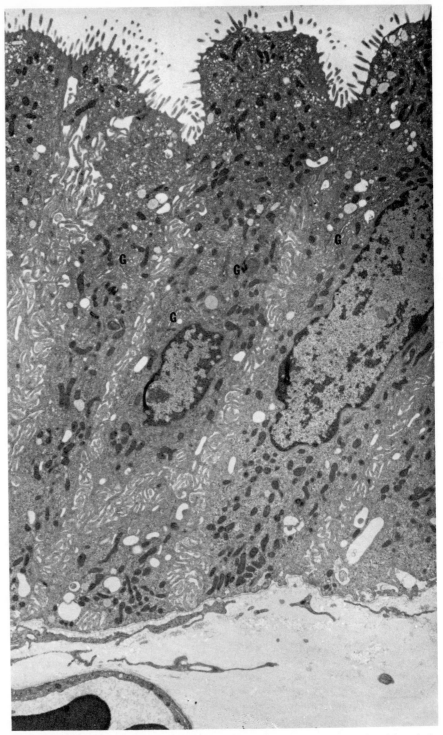

FIGURE 19-37 Epithelial cells from a normal guinea pig gallbladder. Note the long microvilli and the characteristic bulging of the apical region of the cell into the gallbladder lumen. The Golgi (G) apparatus is supranuclear, and the small mitochondria are distributed at random in the cytoplasm. Numerous pinocytotic vesicles and larger PAS-positive granules are in the apical cytoplasm. The lateral cell borders are markedly interdigitated, and a basal lamina encompasses the basal region of the cells. ×7000. (From J. C. Mueller, A. L. Jones, and J. A. Long, *Gastroenterology,* **62:**1972.)

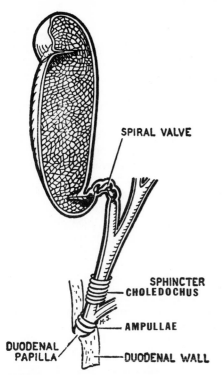

SPIRAL VALVE

SPHINCTER
CHOLEDOCHUS

AMPULLAE

DUODENAL
PAPILLA

DUODENAL WALL

FIGURE 19-38 The mucous membrane of the gallbladder and extrahepatic bile passages. The two sphincters are shown diagrammatically. (From "Grant's Method of Anatomy," The Williams & Wilkins Co., Baltimore, 1965.)

tates the flow of bile into the duodenum. When both the pancreatic and common bile duct end in the ampulla, contraction of the sphincter ampullae may promote reflux of bile into the pancreatic duct, which, in turn, may result in pancreatitis.

BILE PRODUCTION AND TRANSPORT

Although bile is secreted continuously from the hepatic parenchymal cells into the bile canaliculi, the organelles responsible for bile production have not been positively identified. Despite the fact that the Golgi complex is polarized toward the bile canaliculi and hypertrophies during periods of increased bile secretion, components of this complex are seldom observed passing through the ectoplasmic layer (Jones et al., 1975). However, intravascularly administered horseradish peroxidase is picked up at the vascular surface of liver cells and transported by small vesicles to the Golgi cisternae where it is concentrated and later transferred into the bile canaliculus (Matter and Rouiller, 1969). It is possible that the secretory events leading from the Golgi to the canaliculi are so rapid that they are not observed by conventional techniques. Interestingly, retrograde injection of horseradish peroxidase into the biliary tree shows that this substance may return to the space of Disse through the liver cells in vacuoles which appear unassociated with the Golgi complex.

Other organelles, such as lysosomes and multivesicular bodies, are often found near the bile canaliculi, but like the Golgi complex, there is no direct evidence of their participation in bile formation or secretion.

When the flow of bile is impeded (cholestasis), the canaliculi dilate with subsequent flattening of the microvilli. The rough ER partially degranulates and there is a reduction in the amount of Golgi, rough ER, and smooth ER membrane (Jones et al., 1975).

Daily 15 ml of bile per kg body weight is produced by adult human livers. Bile is secreted at a rate of approximately 0.6 ml per min in a 60-kg adult. The rate of synthesis and secretion depends largely on the blood flow to the liver. Bile is produced at a pressure of 200 to 300 mm H_2O. This pressure is regulated by the rate of secretion and viscosity of the bile, the contractility of the gallbladder, and the resistance of the sphincter of Oddi.

pass through the orifice in the ampulla into the lumen of the duodenum (see Fig. 19-38).

During passage through the intestinal wall, the associated bile and pancreatic ducts are invested by a common musculus proprius, termed the *sphincter of Oddi*. The latter structure varies greatly among individuals but usually contains four subdivisions: (1) the *sphincter choledochus*, a strong annular sheath surrounding the common bile duct prior to its junction with the pancreatic duct; (2) the *fasciculi longitudinales*, consisting of longitudinal muscle bundles which span the intervals between the two ducts from the margins of the fenestrae to the ampulla; (3) the *sphincter ampullae*, or terminal musculature surrounding the ampulla of Vater; and (4) the *sphincter pancreaticus*, surrounding the intraduodenal segment of the pancreatic duct, prior to its junction with the ampulla.

Contraction of the sphincter choledochus prevents the flow of bile, whereas contraction of the fasciculi longitudinales shortens the ducts and facili-

The bile is in an aqueous solution containing various organic and inorganic solutes. Bile salts, phospholipids, cholesterol, and bile pigments are the major organic solutes. Lecithin, the chief phospholipid, and cholesterol are insoluble in water but remain in solution even when the bile is concentrated by the gallbladder, presumably because they form mixed micelles with the bile salts. Indeed, Wheeler (1969) states that solubilization of cholesterol is possible only over a narrow range of concentrations of bile salts and lecithin. The protein concentration is very low in human bile, but electrolytes and glucose are found in practically the same concentration as they are in the blood. The latter two compounds probably enter the bile by simple diffusion. Bile salts, pigments, and sulfobromophthalein (BSP), a compound used in liver function tests to measure hepatic clearance, are approximately 100 times more concentrated in bile than in the blood, suggesting that they are actively secreted into the bile against the concentration gradient. Chloride is less concentrated and bicarbonate is more concentrated in the bile than in the plasma. Excess bicarbonate renders the bile alkaline (for example, pH 7.5 to 9.5).

It has been suggested that there is some fluid reabsorption in the intrahepatic bile ducts (see Fig. 19-39). This is a well-established phenomenon in the gallbladder, but direct studies are difficult in intrahepatic bile ducts. Certain gastrointestinal hormones, such as secretin, cholecystokinin (CCK), and gastrin, increase bile flow and bicarbonate concentration. Cholecystokinin reportedly encourages the flow of bile into the intestinal lumen by inducing contraction of the gallbladder and relaxation of the sphincter of Oddi. The parasympathetic vagus nerve is thought to contract the sphincter of Oddi between fatty meals.

The constituents in the bile that reach the intestine are not completely lost. Many are reabsorbed and transported by the portal blood to the liver for reexcretion (enterohepatic circulation). Most bile salts and the fatty acids from the phospholipid and cholesterol in the bile are reabsorbed.

In addition to providing a pool of bile for digestion of fat, the gallbladder also plays a role in concentrating the bile. Absorption in the normal gallbladder is confined largely to water and inorganic ions, especially sodium, calcium, chloride, and bicarbonate. In the dog, water is reabsorbed at a rate of 3 to 6 cm^3 an hour. This concentrates the bile 4 to 10 times (Cameron, 1970). In gallbladders known to be transporting fluid, Kaye et al. (1966) found that the intercellular spaces between the epithelial cells as well as the subepithelial spaces are distended. Studies of sodium localization showed high concentrations in the distended areas. ATPase activity was present along the lateral plasma membrane of the epithelial cells. Hence, it was concluded that solute from the bile is actively transported through the epithelial cell and across the lateral plasma membrane into the intercellular space.

The normal gallbladder secretes a small amount of mucus, but the role of this process in the total economy of the organism is not understood.

THE DEVELOPMENT OF THE LIVER AND GALLBLADDER

ORIGIN OF THE HEPATIC DIVERTICULUM

The liver primordium appears in human embryos (2.5 mm) during the middle of the third week of gestation. It begins as a thickening of the endodermal epithelium lining the cranioventral wall of the foregut near its junction with the yolk sac (that is, the anterior intestinal portal). The thickening rapidly develops into a ventral outgrowth which becomes hollow and lined by columnar epithelium. The cavity of the diverticulum is continuous with the region of the intestine destined to become the duodenum. As the diverticulum enlarges, it grows into the mesenchyme of the *septum transversum* and separates into (1) a cranial, hepatic portion which eventually forms the liver and intrahepatic bile ducts; (2) a smaller caudal, cystic portion which becomes the gallbladder, common bile duct, and cystic duct; and (3) a ventral portion which evolves into a segment of the head of the pancreas.

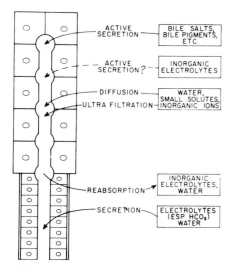

FIGURE 19-39 Diagrammatic summary of some of the mechanisms involved in bile formation. The larger cells represent liver parenchymal cells and the smaller ones the bile duct system. [From H. O. Wheeler, in L. Schiff (ed.), "Diseases of the Liver," 3d ed., J. B. Lippincott Company, Philadelphia, 1969.]

In the diagram, labels read:
- ACTIVE SECRETION → BILE SALTS, BILE PIGMENTS, ETC.
- ACTIVE SECRETION? → INORGANIC ELECTROLYTES
- DIFFUSION → WATER, SMALL SOLUTES, INORGANIC IONS
- ULTRA FILTRATION →
- REABSORPTION → INORGANIC ELECTROLYTES, WATER
- SECRETION → ELECTROLYTES (ESP HCO₃), WATER

THE HEPATIC PARENCHYMA, SINUSOIDS, AND LIGAMENTS

As the hepatic diverticulum invades the septum transversum, the irregularly shaped endodermal cells migrate forward from the original invagination in the form of solid strands or cords. The cords grow between the two *vitelline veins* into the capillary network of the septum transversum that arises from these vessels. In so doing, the hepatic cords subdivide the capillaries in the plexus and become surrounded by them. This process ultimately leads to the development of the complicated adult pattern of the *parenchyma* and *sinusoids,* as the cell cords become hepatic plates and the capillaries become liver sinusoids. The hepatic plates at this stage are three to five cells thick and remain this way until several years after birth. Once the plates are formed, the liver cells become more regular in shape and are usually cuboidal. There are no binucleated cells until after birth, and the cell volume increases as the cells undergo terminal differentiation. In the 10-mm, 6-week embryo, the liver is bilobed. Mesenchymal tissue from the septum transversum forms the *stroma, capsule,* and *mesothelium* of the liver. Reflections of peritoneum off the diaphragm onto the liver's surface will form the triangular and coronary ligaments, whereas the area of original contact with the septum transversum, which is not covered by peritoneum, forms the *bare area* of the liver.

HEMATOPOIESIS

By the tenth week, the liver constitutes approximately 10 percent of the body weight. Hematopoiesis within the liver commences at the 10-mm stage (6 weeks) and contributes much of this weight. For a short time the liver is the primary site for fetal blood formation. The hematopoietic cells are extravascular and in close contact with the parenchymal cells. The ratio of liver to body weight decreases during the last trimester when most hematopoietic sites within the liver disappear.

INTRAHEPATIC BILIARY TREE AND BILE CANALICULI

The first bile canaliculi appear as small vesicles between parenchymal cells of the sixth-week embryo, far in advance of bile secretion. During the sixth to ninth weeks, the remainder of the intrahepatic biliary tree begins to form and apparently is derived from limiting plate hepatocytes abutting the edges of the portal canals. It is thought that certain limiting plate hepatocytes, surrounding lumina or vesicles in the wall, are transformed into ductal epithelium as the mesenchyme penetrates the limiting plate. In later stages, connective tissue separates the transforming cells from the liver parenchyma. Bile production commences at 4 months of gestation. The bile flows into the gallbladder and then to the duodenum, producing the characteristic dark color of the meconium.

EXTRAHEPATIC BILIARY TRACT AND GALLBLADDER

Little is known about the early development of the extrahepatic biliary tract and gallbladder in man. However, as the originally hollow pars cystica elongates, its lumen is obliterated by the migration of cells into the original lumen. Hence, in the 6- to 7-mm embryo, the future gallbladder and common bile duct form a solid epithelial cord in the septum transversum just below the developing liver. Vacuolization of the solid cord produces a lumen in the common bile duct at 7.5 mm, the hepatic duct at 10 mm, the cystic duct at 16 mm, and the gallbladder at 18 mm. However, the gallbladder is not completely hollow until the third month. The mucosa, muscularis, and serosa of the gallbladder are established in the 29-mm embryo, but the mucosal folds are not formed until the very end of gestation.

Congenital atresia of the bile ducts can cause cholestasis and jaundice in the newborn. Untreated infants develop cirrhosis, liver failure, and portal hypertension and usually do not live longer than 2 years.

DEVELOPMENT OF THE HEPATIC VENOUS SYSTEM

The vasculature undergoes drastic changes during fetal life. In the 4.5-mm human embryo (5 weeks), the hepatic diverticulum and its associated capillaries (derived from the vitelline veins) lie between the right and left *umbilical veins* (Fig. 19-40A). During the 5-mm stage, the caudal segments of the vitelline veins begin to form three anastomoses. The anterior anastomosis is formed within the liver, whereas the middle and posterior form outside the liver, dorsal and ventral to the duodenum (Fig. 19-40B). As a result, two venous rings are formed. The right half of the upper ring and the left half of the bottom ring disappear by the 9-mm stage, and a new S-shaped vessel, composed of segments from the cross-connected vitelline veins, is formed. This vessel is the portal vein (Fig. 19-40C).

The efferent hepatic veins which drain the liver are derived from the vitelline veins proximal to the vitelline capillary plexus. In Fig. 19-40A, the vitelline veins are shown entering into the sinus venosus anterior to the liver. The stem of the right vitelline vein enlarges, and by the 9-mm stage it forms the termination of the inferior vena cava.

Except for very early stages, all maternal blood within the placenta flows through the umbilical veins. In the 5-mm embryo, the umbilical veins send ramifications into the liver (Fig. 19-40B). The right umbilical vein and proximal portions of the left umbilical vein disappear during the 6- to 7-mm stage. The remaining distal portion of the left umbilical vein supplies the liver with oxygenated blood from the maternal circulation (Fig. 19-40B).

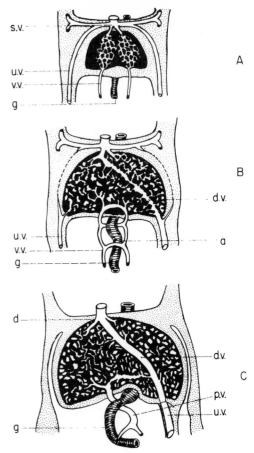

FIGURE 19-40 Diagram showing development of liver veins. sv, sinus venosus; uv, umbilical veins; vv, vitelline veins; g, gut; dv, ductus venosus; a, caudal anastomosis of distal vitelline veins; d, diaphragm. [Courtesy of A. M. DuBois, The Embryonic Liver, in C. Rouiller (ed.), "The Liver" vol. 1, Academic Press, Inc., New York, 1963.]

The ductus venosus, which shunts blood directly from the left umbilical vein to the inferior vena cava, develops within the hepatic diverticulum during the 5- to 6-mm stage (Fig. 19-40B and C). The ductus venosus persists until birth, at which time it collapses and begins to atrophy. Eventually it forms a connective tissue remnant, the *ligamentus venosum*. Concomitantly, the left umbilical vein atrophies, forming the *ligamentum teres*, which extends from the liver to the umbilicus.

REFERENCES

BABCOCK, M. B., and R. R. CARDELL, JR.: Hepatic Glycogen Patterns in Fasted and Fed Rats, Am. J. *Anat.* **140:**299 (1974).

BEAMS, H. W., and R. L. KING: The Origin of Binucleate and Large Monoculeate Cells in the Liver of the White Rat, *Anat. Rec.,* **83:**281 (1942).

BIAVA, C. G.: Studies on Cholestasis: a Re-evaluation of the Fine Structure of Normal Human Bile Canaliculi, *Lab. Invest.,* **13:**840 (1964).

BOYDEN, E. A.: The Anatomy of the Choledochoduodenal Junction in Man, *Surg. Gynec. Obstet.,* **104:**641 (1957).

BRAUER, R. W.: Liver Circulation and Function, *Physiol. Rev.,* **43:**115 (1963).

BRUNI, C., and K. R. PORTER: The Fine Structure of the Parenchymal Cell of the Normal Rat Liver. 1. General Observations, *Am. J. Path.,* **46:**691 (1965).

BUCHER, N. L. R.: Experimental Aspects of Hepatic Regeneration, *New Eng. J. Med.,* **277:**686 (1967).

BURKEL, W. E.: The Fine Structure of the Terminal Branches of the Hepatic Arterial System of the Rat, *Anat. Rec.,* **167:**329 (1970).

BURSTONE, M. S.: New Histochemical Techniques for the Demonstration of Tissue Oxidse (Cytochrome Oxidase), *J. Histochem. Cytochem.,* **7:**112 (1959).

CAMERON, I. L.: Cell Renewal in the Organs and Tissues of the Nongrowing Adult Mouse, Tex. *Rep. Biol. Med.,* **28:**3 (1970).

CAMERON, R. and P. C. HOU: "Biliary Cirrhosis," Charles C Thomas, Publisher, Springfield, Ill., 1962.

CARRIERE, R.: The Growth of the Liver Parenchymal Nuclei and its Endocrine Regulation, *Int. Rev. Cytol.,* **25:**201 (1969).

CARRUTHERS, J. S., and J. W. STEINER: The Fine Structure of Terminal Branches of the Biliary Tree. III. Parenchymal Cell Cohesion and "Intracellular Bile Canaliculi," *Arch. Path.,* **74:**117 (1962).

CHAPMAN, G. B., A. J. CHIARODO, R. J. COFFEY, and K. WIENEKE: The Fine Structure of Mucosal Epithelial Cells of a Pathological Human Gallbladder, *Anat. Rec.,* **154:**579 (1966).

CLAUDE, A.: Growth and Differentiation of Cytoplasmic Membranes in the Course of Lipoprotein Granules Synthesis in the Hepatic Cell. 1. Elaboration of the Elements of the Golgi Complex, *J. Cell Biol.,* **47:**745 (1970).

DALLMAN, P. R., and J. R. GOODMAN: The Effects of Iron Deficiency on the Hepatocyte: a Biochemical and Ultrastructural Study, *J. Cell Biol.,* **48:**79 (1971).

DALLNER, G., P. SIEKEVITZ, and G. E. PALADE: Biogenesis of Endoplasmic Reticulum Membranes. 1. Structural and Chemical Differentiation in Developing Rat Hepatocyte, *J. Cell Biol.,* **30:**73 (1966).

DALLNER, G., P. SIEKEVITZ, and G. E. PALADE: Biogenesis of Endoplasmic Reitculum Membranes. 11. Synthesis of Constitutive Microsomal Enzymes in Developing Rat Hepatocyte, *J. Cell Biol.,* **30:**97 (1966).

DE DUVE, C. and P. BAUDHUIN: Peroxisomes (Microbodies and Related Particles), *Physiol. Rev.,* **46:**323 (1966).

DEANE, H. W.: The Basophilic Bodies in Hepatic Cells, *Am. J. Anat.,* **78:**227 (1946).

DEANE, H. W.: A Cytological Study of the Diurnal Cycle of the Liver of the Mouse in Relation to Storage and Secretion, *Anat. Rec.,* **88:**39 (1944).

DEANE, H. W.: The Cytology of the Mouse Liver in a Controlled Diurnal Cycle, *Anat. Rec.,* **84:**477 (1942).

DOLJANSKI, F.: The Growth of the Liver with Special Reference to Mammals, *Int. Rev. Cytol.,* **10:**217 (1960).

DU BOIS, A. M.: The Embryonic Liver, in C. Rouiller (ed.), "The Liver," vol. 1, p. 1, Academic Press, Inc., New York, 1963.

ELYING, G.: Crypts and Ducts in the Gallbladder Wall, *Acta Pathol. Microbiol. Scand.,* **49** (suppl 135) (1960).

ELIAS, H.: A Re-examination of the Structure of the Mammalian Liver. 1. Parenchymal Architecture; II. The Hepatic Lobule and its Relation to the Vascular and Biliary Systems, *Am. J. Anat.,* **84:**311, **85:**379 (1949).

ELIAS, H., and J. C. SHERRICK: "Morphology of the Liver," Academic Press, Inc., New York, 1969.

ESSNER, E., and A. B. NOVIKOFF: Localization of Acid Phosphatase Activity in Hepatic Lysosomes by Means of Electron Microscopy, *J. Biophys. Biochem. Cytol.,* **9:**773 (1961).

FAWCETT, D. W.: Observations on the Ctyology and Electron Microscopy of Hepatic Cells, *J. Natl. Cancer Inst.,* **15:**1475 (1955).

GATES, G. A., K. S. HENLEY, H. M. POLLARD, E. SCHMIDT, and F. W. SCHMIDT: The Cell Population of Human Liver, *J. Lab. Clin. Med.,* **57:**182 (1961).

GREENWAY, C. V., and R. D. STARK: Hepatic Vascular Bed, *Physiol. Rev.,* **51:**23 (1971).

GRUBB, D. J. and A. L. JONES: Ultrastructure of Hepatic Sinusoids in Sheep, *Anat. Rec.,* **170:**75 (1971).

HAMASHIMA, Y., J. G. HARTER, and A. H. COONS: The Localization of Albumin and Fibrinogen in Human Liver Cells, *J. Cell Biol.,* **20:**271 (1964).

HAMILTON, R. L., D. M. REGEN, M. E. GRAY, and V. S. LEQUIRE: Lipid Transport in Liver. 1. Electron Microscopic Identification of Very Low Density Lipoproteins in Perfused Rat Liver, *Lab. Invest.,* **16:**305 (1967).

HAYWARD, A. F.: The Structure of Gallbladder Epithelium, *Int. Rev. Gen. Exp. Zool.,* **3:**205 (1968).

HEALEY, J. E.: Vascular Anatomy of the Liver, *Ann. N.Y. Acad. Sci.,* **170:**8 (1970).

HERING, E.: The Liver, in S. Stricker (ed.), "Manual of Human and Comparative Histology," vol. 2, The New Sydenham Society, London, 1872.

JONES, A. L., and D. T. ARMSTRONG: Increased Cholesterol Biosynthesis Following Phenobarbital Induced Hypertrophy of Endoplasmic Reticulum in Liver, *Proc. Soc. Exp. Biol. Med.,* **119:**1136 (1965).

JONES, A. L., and J. B. EMANS: The Effects of Progresterone Administration on Hepatic Endoplasmic Reticulum: An Electron Microscopic and Biochemical Study, in H. A. Salhanick, D. Kipnes, and R. L. Van deWiele (eds.), "Metabolic Effects of Gonadal Hormones and Contraceptive Steroids," Plenum Press, Plenum Publishing Corporation, New York, 1969.

JONES, A. L., and D. W. FAWCETT: Hypertrophy of the Agranular Endoplasmic Reticulum in Hamster Liver Induced by Phenobarbital (with a Review of the Functions of This Organelle in Liver), *J. Histochem. Cytochem.,* **14:**215 (1966).

JONES, A. L., N. B. RUDERMAN, and M. G. HERRERA: Electron Microscopic and Biochemical Study of Lipoprotein Synthesis in the Isolated Perfused Rat Liver, *J. Lipid Res.,* **8:**429 (1967).

JONES, A. L., D. L. SCHMUCKER, R. D. ADLER, R. K. OCKNER, and J. S. MOONEY: A Quantitative Analysis of Hepatic Ultrastructure in Rats after Selective Biliary Obstruction, in R. PREISIG, J. BIRCHER, and G. PAUMGARTNER (eds), "The Liver: Quantitative Aspects of Structure and Function," Editio Cantor, Aulendorf, 1975.

KADENBACH, B.: Synthesis of Mitochondrial Proteins: Demonstration of a Transfer of Proteins from Microsomes into Mitochondria, *Biophys. Biochim. Acta.,* **134:**430 (1966).

KAYE, G. I., H. O. WHEELER, R. T. WHITLOCK, and N. LANE: Fluid Transport in the Rabbit Gallbladder. A Combined Physiological and Electron Microscopic Study, *J. Cell Biol.,* **30:**237 (1966).

KOGA, A.: Morphogenesis of Intrahepatic Bile Ducts of the Human Fetus, *Z. Anat. Entwickelungsgesch,* **135:**156 (1971).

LEBLOND, C. P. and B. W. WALKER: Renewal of Cell Populations, *Physiol. Rev.,* **36:**255 (1956).

LIN, C. and J. P. CHANG: Electron Microscopy of Albumin Synthesis, *Science,* **190:**465 (1975).

LOUD, A. V.: A Quantitative Stereological Description of the Ultrastructure of Normal Rat Liver Parenchymal Cells, *J. Cell Biol.,* **37:**27 (1968).

MAHLEY, R. W., R. L. HAMILTON, and V. S. LEQUIRE: Characterization of Lipoprotein Particles Isolated from the Golgi Apparatus of Rat Liver, *J. Lipid Res.,* **10:**433 (1969).

MALL, F. P.: A Study of the Structural Unit of the Liver, *Am. J. Anat.,* **5:**227 (1906).

MARVER, H. S., and R. SCHMID: The Porphyrias, in J. B. Stanbury, J. B. Wyngarden, and D. S. Frederickson (eds.), "Metabolic Basis of Inherited Disease," 3d ed., chap. 45, pp. 1087–1140, McGraw-Hill Book Company, New York, 1972.

MATTER, A. L. ORCI and C. ROUILLER: A Study on the Permeability Barriers between Disse's Space and the Bile Canaliculus, *J. Ultrastruct. Res.,* **11** (suppl) (1969).

MUELLER, J. C., A. L. JONES, and J. A. LONG: Topographical and Subcellular Anatomy of the Guinea Pig Gallbladder, *Gastroenterology,* **63:**856 (1972).

MYRON, D. R., and J. L. CONNELLY: The Morphology of the Swelling Process in Rat Liver Mitochondria, *J. Cell Biol.,* **48:**291 (1971).

NOVIKOFF, A. B.: Cell Heterogeneity within the Hepatic Lobule of the Rat, *J. Histochem. Cytochem.,* **7:**240 (1959).

NOVIKOFF, and E. ESSNER: The Liver Cell: Some New Approaches to its Study, *Am. J. Med.,* **29:**102 (1960).

NOVIKOFF, A. B., D. H. HAUSMAN, and E. PODBER: The Localization of Adenosine Triphosphate in Liver: In Situ Staining and Cell Fractionation Studies, *J. Histochem. Cytochem.,* **6:**61 (1958).

PACKER, L.: Relation of Structure to Energy Coupling in Rat Liver Mitochondria, *Fed. Proc.,* **29:**1533 (1970).

PETERS, T., B. FLEISCHER, and S. FLEISCHER: The Biosynthesis of Rat Serum Albumin. IV. Apparent Passage of Albumin through the Golgi Apparatus during Secretion, *J. Biol. Chem.,* **246:**240 (1971).

POPPER, H., and S. UDENFRIEND: Hepatic Fibrosis. Correlation of Biochemical and Morphologic Investigations, *Am. J. Med.,* **49:**707 (1970).

RAPPAPORT, A. M.: Anatomic Considerations, in Leon Schiff (ed.), "Diseases of the Liver," 3d ed, pp 1–49, J. B. Lippincott Company, Philadelphia, 1969.

RIGATUSO, J. L., P. G. LEGG, and R. L. WOOD: Microbody Formation in Regenerating Rat Liver, *J. Histochem. Cytochem.,* **18:**893 (1970).

SABOURIN, C.: Recherches sur l'anatomie normale et pathologique de la glande biliaire de l'homme, Alcan, Paris, 1888.

SASSE, D.: Chemorphology de Glykogensynthese und des Glykogengehalts wahrend der Histogenese der Leber, *Histochemie,* **20:**159 (1969).

SCHACTER, H., I. JABBAL, R. L. HUDGIN, and I. PINTERIC: Intracellular Localization of Liver Sugar Nucleotide Glycoprotein Glycosyltransferases in a Golgi-rich Fraction, *J. Biol. Chem.,* **254:**1090 (1970).

SCHIMKE, R. T., R. GANSCHOW, D. DOYLE, and I. M. ARIAS: Regulation of Protein Turnover in Mammalian Tissues, *Fed. Proc.,* **27:**1223 (1968).

SCHMUCKER, D. L.: Age-related Changes in Hepatic Fine Structure: A Quantitative Analysis, *J. Gerontol.* **31:**135–143 (1976).

SCHMUCKER, D. T., and A. L. JONES: Hepatic Fine Structure in Young and Aging Rats Treated with Oxandrolone: A Morphometric Study, *J. Lipid Res.,* **16:**143 (1975).

SCHREIBER, G., R. LESCH, V. WEINSSEN, and J. ZAHRINGER: The Distribution of Albumin Synthesis throughout the Liver Lobule, *J. Cell Biol.,* **47:**285 (1970).

STEINER, J. W., J. S. CARRUTHERS, and S. R. KALIFAT: The Ductular Cell Reaction of Rat Liver in Extrahepatic Cholestasis. 1. Proliferated Biliary Epithelial Cells. *Exp. Molec. Path.*, **1:**162 (1962).

STEINER, J. W., and J. S. CARRUTHERS: Studies on the Fine Structure of the Terminal Branches of the Biliary Tree. 1. The Morphology of Normal Bile Canaliculi, Bile Pre-ductules (Ducts of Hering) and Bile Ductules, *Am. J. Path.*, **38:**639 (1961).

TANDLER, B., R. A. ERLANDSON, A. L. SMITH, and E. L. WYNDER: Riboflavin and Mouse Hepatic Cell Structure and Function. II. Division of Mitochondria during Recovery from Simple Deficiency, *J. Cell Biol.*, **41:**477 (1969).

WANSON, J-C, P. DROCHMANS, C. MAY, PENASSE, and A. POPOWSKI: Isolation of Centrolobular and Perilobular Hepatocytes after Phenobarbital Treatment, *J. Cell Biol.*, **66:**23 (1975).

WEISSMAN, G.: Lysosomes, *New Eng. J. Med.*, **273:**1084 (1969).

WHEATLEY, D. N.: Binucleation in Mammalian Liver, *Exp. Cell Res.*, **74:**455 (1972).

WHEELER, H. O.: Secretion of Bile, in Leon Schiff (ed.), "Diseases of the Liver," 3d ed, pp. 84–102, J. B. Lippincott Company, Philadelphia, 1969.

WILSON, J. W., and E. H. LEDUC: Movements of Macrophages Studied with the Use of Thorotrast, *J. Natl. Cancer Inst.*, **10:**1348 (1950).

WISSE, E.: An Electron Microscopic Study of the Fenestrated Endothelial Lining of Rat Liver Sinusoids, *J. Ultrastruct. Res.*, **31:**125 (1970).

WOOD, R. L.: Evidence of Species Differences in the Ultrastructure of the Hepatic Sinusoid, *Z. Zellforsch.*, **58:**679 (1963).

The Pancreas

SUSUMU ITO

The human pancreas is a large retroperitoneal gland, often more than 20 cm long, lying on the posterior wall of the abdominal cavity behind the stomach. The *head* of the pancreas lies in the curve of the C-shaped duodenum and is joined by a slightly constricted region, or *neck,* to the *body,* or main part of the gland. The thin-tailed portion extends across the abdominal cavity to the spleen. The fresh pancreas is almost white, with a slight pink tinge owing to its vascularity. Unlike other abdominal organs, the pancreas lacks a well-defined capsule. Instead, the outer limit on its ventral aspect is a thin layer of connective tissue and peritoneal mesothelium. The gland is subdivided by delicate connective tissue septa into lobules of a size just visible with the naked eye. Blood and lymphatic vessels, nerves, and excretory ducts run in these septa.

The pancreas is both an exocrine and endocrine gland, and these functions are carried out by distinctly different groups of cells. Digestive enzymes are formed by acinar cells and are delivered by a duct system to the duodenum. Pancreatic hormones regulating carbohydrate metabolism are produced by the cells in the *islets of Langerhans,* which are clusters of endocrine cells embedded within the lobules of acinar tissue. The islets have no duct system; their products, like those of other endocrine glands, are released directly into the circulatory system.

THE EXOCRINE PANCREAS

HISTOLOGY OF THE EXOCRINE PANCREAS

The cells responsible for the enzyme-rich pancreatic secretions are the pancreatic *acinar cells,* serous-type cells which form the compound tubuloacinar or tubuloalveolar glands. Clusters of *acini* and their duct systems are separated by areolar connective tissue, which is continuous with that outlining the *pancreatic lobules* (Fig. 20-1). The acinus is composed of a single layer of pyramidal cells with their narrow apical ends bordering the lumen and their broad bases resting on a thin basement membrane and reticular connective tissue. The terminal portions of the pancreatic duct system extend into the acini so that the flattened duct cells are interposed between some of the acinar cells and the lumen. These duct cells within the acinus are known as the *centroacinar cells* (Fig. 20-2).

747

In the pancreas of the fasting individual, the apical portion of the acinar cells is laden with many refractile secretory granules, the *zymogen granules*. These possess acidophilic staining properties in routine histologic sections. The intensely basophilic basal portion of the cell appears lamellar or filamentous in favorable light-microscopic preparations (Fig. 20-2). Long before the biochemical nature of this basophilic material was known, it was named *ergastoplasm*. Its strong affinity for basic dyes is now known to be due to a high concentration of ribonucleoprotein. Inter-

spersed with the ergastoplasm are moderate numbers of filamentous mitochondria. A well-developed Golgi complex located in the supranuclear region may be stained by special silver- or osmium tetroxide–impregnation techniques. The precise location of the Golgi complex in the cell varies with the abundance of zymogen granules, being nearer the apex of the cell when few granules are present and supranuclear or lateral to the nucleus during phases in which the apical cytoplasm is filled with stored granules. The basally placed nuclei of the acinar cells are spherical and

FIGURE 20-1 Photomicrograph of human pancreas. Two islets of Langerhans and a number of small intralobular ducts are present in the acinar tissue. An interlobular duct is shown at the lower right. ×160.

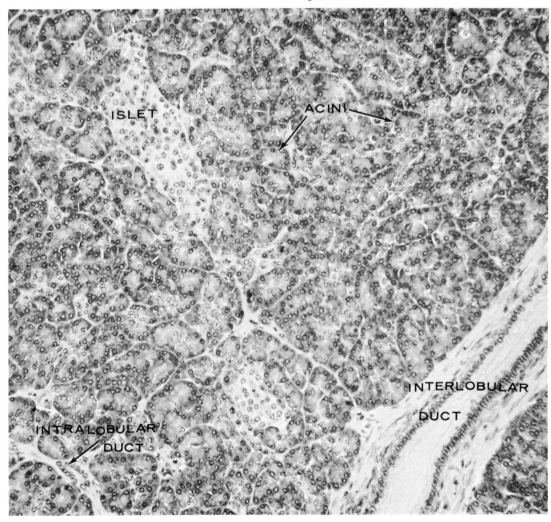

contain prominent nucleoli. Occasional cells are binucleate.

BLOOD VESSELS, NERVES, AND LYMPHATICS

The arterial blood supply to the pancreas is from the
celiac and superior mesenteric arteries, which send
branches into the gland along the ducts and in the
connective tissue septa. Veins generally accompany
the arteries and drain to the portal or the splenic vein.
The nerve supply arises from the celiac plexus; bundles of nerve fibers accompany the blood vessels,
finally terminating as fine branches on the acini (Figs.
20-7, 20-8). Myelinated nerves from the vagus are
also found in the interlobular connective tissue. Occasional Pacinian corpuscles may be found within the

pancreas. The distribution of the lymphatic system
with the organ remains to be elucidated.

FINE STRUCTURE OF THE PANCREATIC ACINAR CELL

The fine structure of the pancreatic acinar cells is
generally similar to that of other serozymogenic cells,
such as serous cells of the salivary glands and the
pepsinogenic cells of the gastric glands. Their common characteristics are the presence of an extraordinary abundance of rough endoplasmic reticulum (ER)
and the accumulation of zymogen granules.

The predominant organelle in the basal cytoplasm
of the pancreatic acinar cell is the rough ER, a membrane system of meandering tubules and flattened
cisternae which have numerous ribosomes attached to
the cytoplasmic surface (Figs. 20-3 and 20-4). Free
ribosomes are also found in abundance in the cytoplasmic matrix. Mitochondria with typical transversely
oriented cristae and varying numbers of dense intra-

FIGURE 20-2 Photomicrograph of human pancreas showing
several acini and an intralobular duct. Note the preservation of
fine cytologic detail in the acinar cells. The apical zymogen granules, the lightly stained supranuclear Golgi complex, and the striated appearance of the basal ergastoplasm are evident. Centroacinar and intralobular duct cells are lightly stained. Formalin
fixation, postosmicated, and Epon embedded. Toluidine blue stain.
×1120.

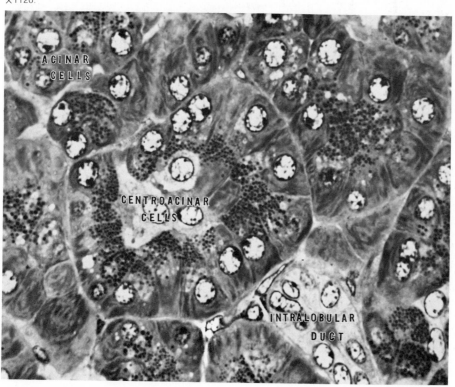

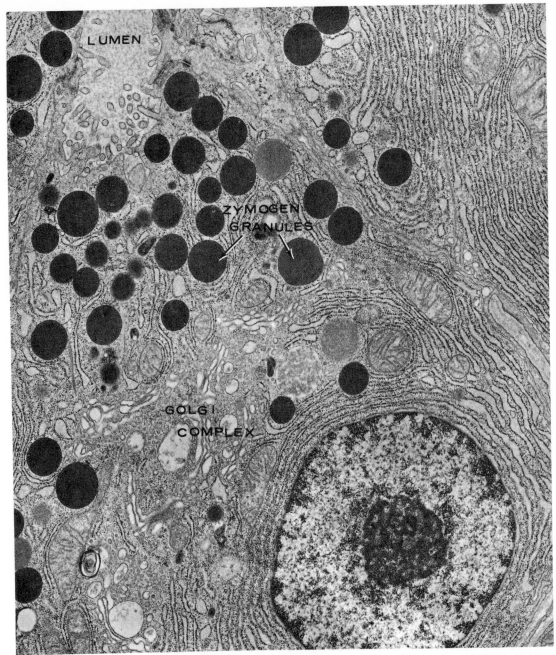

FIGURE 20-3 Electron micrograph of a human pancreatic acinar cell. The abundant granular endoplasmic reticulum and the store of dense zymogen granules are distinguishing features of this cell. In the supranuclear cytoplasm there is a prominent Golgi complex with zymogen granules in various formative stages. A profile of a zymogen granules whose contents have been discharged into the lumen is present at the apical border. A nucleus with a prominent nucleolus is present near the base of the cell. ×11,500. (All electron micrographs of the human exocrine pancreas were prepared from tissue blocks, courtesy of A. Like.)

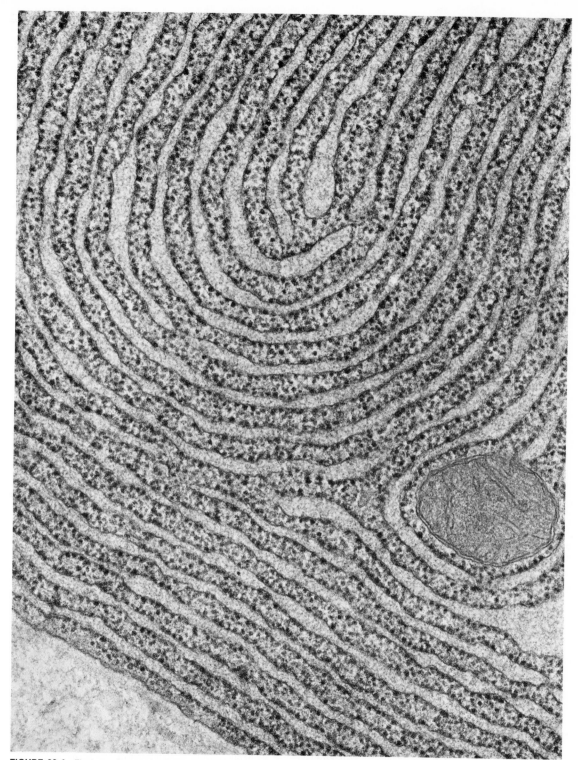

FIGURE 20-4 Electron micrograph of the basal cytoplasm of a human pancreatic acinar cell. Extensive lamellar arrays of ribosome-studded endoplasmic reticulum are characteristic features of these cells. The cisternae are filled with a flocculent precipitate of newly synthesized protein. A profile of a mitochondrion is included in the cytoplasm. ×65,000.

mitochondrial granules are sequestered between elements of the granular reticulum and along the lateral plasma membrane. Chromatin in the nucleus is generally dispersed, but there is a peripheral accumulation of chromatin adjacent to the nuclear envelope except at the nuclear pores. The outer, ribosome-studded membrane of the nuclear envelope is occasionally continuous with the endoplasmic reticulum. One or two prominent nucleoli are often located adjacent to the nuclear envelope. There are two distinctive zones in the nucleolus. One region, formed of granules resembling the cytoplasmic ribosomes, is arranged into coarse strands that form the nucleolonema; a second finely granular component, which is localized in the interstices, resembles chromatin in its structural appearance.

The extensive Golgi complex is formed of smooth-surfaced membranes arranged in lamellar arrays of flat cisternae with many associated small vesicles and larger vacuoles. Some of the Golgi vacuoles contain flocculent material of intermediate density; others have a dense substance similar to the zymogen granules. These are condensing vacuoles in transitional stages of zymogen granule formation. Direct continuity of the ER and the smooth-surfaced membranes of the Golgi complex are rarely, if ever, observed. However, continuities of the ER with smooth-surfaced vacuolar dilations associated with the Golgi complex have been reported. The relative infrequency of these connections suggests that they may be transitory. In addition to the components of the Golgi complex, one or two centrioles may be found in the cell center, but centrioles are more frequently observed in the apical cytoplasm just beneath the luminal plasma membrane.

Zymogen granules are generally concentrated in the apical cytoplasm just beneath the plasma membrane. The granules are variable in size, the largest measuring up to 1.5 μm in diameter. They are preserved as membrane-limited spherical granules whose density appears to vary with preservation technique. No ordered internal structure has been observed. The interstices between the granules are packed with ribosomes and ER membranes. When few or no granules are present, the rough ER and free ribosomes are distributed throughout the cell.

The luminal end of the cell has a few stubby microvilli coated with a thin layer of fine, radiating,

filamentous material. The plasma membranes of adjacent cells are fused into well-developed zonulae occludentes. The relatively straight lateral cell membranes are separated from one another by a narrow space of uniform width, joined by occasional desmosomes. A thin amorphous basement membrane, or lamina, with its associated collagen fibers, underlies the smooth-contoured base of the cell. The acinar cell cytoplasm also contains some dense, membrane-limited lysosomelike bodies, as well as a few multivesicular bodies.

THE DUCTS

Although the smallest ducts are not conspicuous in the usual histologic preparations, an extensive duct system permeates the organ. The apical borders of the acinar cells form the lumina of the acini. Unlike the salivary glands, in which the acini are found at the ends of the intercalated ducts, the pancreatic acinar cells tend to extend into the ducts, so some duct cells are apparently included in the lumen of the acinus and are therefore known as the *centroacinar cells*.

The fine structure of the centroacinar cells and the cells of the small ducts are similar (Figs. 20-5 and 20-6). Both have a sparse covering of microvilli on the free border, and the lateral cell membrane is fairly straight in the centroacinar cells. However, there is considerable interdigitation of intralobular duct cells. The cytoplasm appears empty, in contrast to the acinar cells. The duct cells have a few small mitochondria, a little Golgi complex, and only small amounts of endoplasmic reticulum.

Secretory ducts such as those in salivary glands are not found in the pancreas. The intralobular or intercalated ducts of the pancreas serve as tributaries to the larger *interlobular ducts* located in the connective tissue septa (Fig. 20-1). These interlobular ducts are formed by columnar cells, which appear similar to those of the smaller ducts but are intermingled with occasional goblet cells like those in the intestine. Argentaffin cells are also found in the simple columnar epithelium of the larger pancreatic ducts. The interlobular ducts join the main pancreatic duct, the duct of Wirsung, which traverses the entire length of the organ. Near the duodenum it runs along the ductus choledochus and either joins it or independently enters the ampula of Vater. An accessory duct, the duct of Santorini, located cranial to the main pancreatic duct, is also present. These large ducts are enveloped in a layer of dense connective tissue containing some

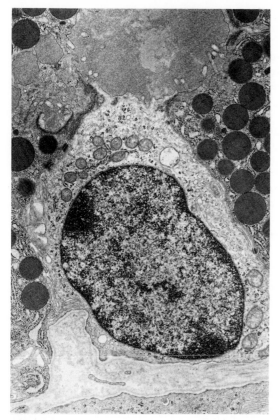

FIGURE 20-5 A low-power electron micrograph of a human centroacinar cell bordering the lumen of a pancreatic acinus. Note the low density of the centroacinar cell cytoplasm and the paucity of cytoplasmic organelles. A basal lamina underlies the duct and acinar cell. The interconnected zymogen granules of low density near the upper left corner are granules which may be discharging their contents into the lumen. ×10,000.

elastic fibers. Arteries, veins, and lymphatic vessels as well as sympathetic ganglion cells and nerves, which are mostly unmyelinated, are found in the connective tissue surrounding the ducts.

SECRETORY ACTIVITY

The pancreas normally releases its secretions into the intestine when chyme from the stomach enters the duodenum. Secretion may be stimulated experimentally by activation of the vagus nerve, by administration of drugs such as pilocarpine, or by injections of the intestinal hormones secretin or pancreozymin. The pancreatic secretions are highly alkaline, and their enzymes are activated when neutralized by the acidic gastric chyme.

The secretory mechanism of the pancreatic acinar cells studied by direct observations combined with the study of tissue sections prepared by special techniques led investigators to postulate that zymogen granules were formed in the basal ergastoplasm, condensed in the Golgi zone, and stored in the apical cytoplasm. More recently, studies using radioactive amino acids and light and electron-microscopic autoradiography, correlated with biochemical studies of cell fractions, have fully substantiated the early morphologic observations and interpretations.

On the basis of extensive morphologic and biochemical studies of various functional changes of the guinea pig pancreatic acinar cells, Siekevitz and Palade (1958) have postulated that the zymogen is synthesized by the ribosomes on the endoplasmic reticulum. The newly formed enzymes are then transferred to the lumen of the cisternae and, in the guinea pig pancreas, become visible as dense intracisternal granules. Although the mechanism for the transport of material is not clear, the zymogen is apparently transferred to the Golgi complex by an intermediary reticulum.

In the Golgi complex the zymogen is further concentrated in *condensing vacuoles* to the fully formed zymogen granules, which are enclosed in a smooth-surfaced membrane and stored in the apical cytoplasm. The morphologic process of zymogen secretion from the acinar cell is accomplished by the coalescence of the membrane limiting the zymogen granule with the apical plasma membrane. This results in the release of zymogen directly into the lumen.

Caro and Palade (1964) used a radioactively labeled amino acid [^{3}H]leucine and were able to localize specific sites of synthesis, concentration, and storage of zymogen by making autoradiographs of thin tissue sections and examining them in the electron microscope. It is interesting to note that all these studies using newly developed techniques substantiate the hypothesis made in 1875 by R. Heidenhain, who studied the cytology of the pancreatic acinar cells in various physiologic states.

The time period required for the synthesis of zymogen is quite short. Palade, Siekevitz, and Caro (1962) found that less than 45 min was necessary for a labeled amino acid to be secreted as a component of pancreatic juice. Using light-microscopic autoradiographs of incorporated [^{3}H]leucine, Warshawsky,

Leblond, and Droz (1963) showed that the mean life-span of a zymogen granule in the rat pancreas is about 47.7 min. The synthesis of zymogen begins in the ergastoplasm within 2 to 5 min and the product is found 15 min later in the Golgi complex. The enzymes are then stored or secreted from the apical cytolasm. Studies by Jamieson and Palade (1971) have shown that discharge of zymogen granules does not require continuous protein synthesis but depends on respiratory energy. The localization of the pancreatic enzymes chymotrypsin and carboxypeptidase in the zymogen granules was demonstrated histochemically by fluorescein-labeled antibody techniques.

The human pancreas secretes about 2 l of fluid per day. At least nine enzymes as well as water, bicarbonate, and salts are found in pancreatic juice. The presence of the proteolytic enzymes trypsinogen, chymotrypsinogen, and carboxypeptidase has been demonstrated in isolated zymogen granule fractions. Pancreatic amylase, an enzyme that breaks down

carbohydrate, has been found in both zymogen and soluble fractions. Also present in pancreatic juice are fat-splitting enzymes, lipase and lecithinase, and the nucleic acid–hydrolyzing enzymes ribonuclease and deoxyribonuclease. The distribution of some of the pancreatic enzymes within different acinar cells and zymogen granules as indicated by immunochemical and biochemical studies suggests that each zymogen granule contains all of the secretory proteins.

Experimental stimulation of pancreatic secretion by the intestinal hormone secretin elicits a bicarbonate-rich, watery secretion with little enzyme, which apparently comes from the intralobular and interlobular duct cells rather than the acinar cells. Further evidence for this secretory activity lies in the histochemical demonstration of carbonic anhydrase in the duct cells. Injections of a second hormone, pancreo-

FIGURE 20-6 Electron micrograph of a small intralobular duct. The cytoplasm of the duct cells is of low density and contains small mitochondrion and free ribosomes as well as granular and smooth-surfaced endoplasmic reticulum. Occasional cilia, as shown in the lumen, are present in the ducts. A small capillary with fenestrated endothelial cells is present in the adjacent connective tissues. ×13,000.

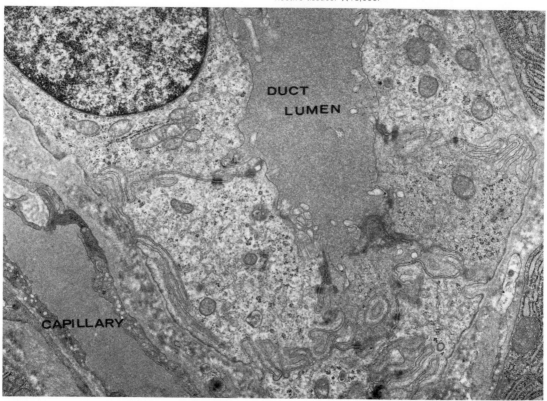

DUCT LUMEN

CAPILLARY

zymin, extracted from the duodenal mucosa, produce a flow of enzyme-rich pancreatic secretion originating from the acinar cells. The mechanism of the action of secretin and pancreozymin on the pancreas is not clear, but these hormones clearly play a major role in the control of enzyme secretion.

Even before the use of hormonal stimulation of

pancreatic secretion, physiologists had found that both stimulation of the vagus nerve and administration of pilocarpine produce an enzyme-rich secretion similar to that obtained with pancreozymin.

THE ENDOCRINE PANCREAS

The endocrine cells of the pancreas are found in scattered groups throughout the organ and are commonly designated as the *islets of Langerhans,* or simply as the pancreatic islets or islands. These occur as clusters of a few to hundreds of cells embedded in the acinar tissue (Figs. 20-1, 20-9 and Fig. 20-10, see color insert). Occasional single islet cells may be found among the exocrine secretory cells of the pancreatic acini. The distribution of islets is variable, but in humans they are more numerous in the tail of the organ. It has been estimated that approximately 1 million islets are present in a human pancreas.

The islet is highly vascular, with numerous capillaries that probably touch every endocrine cell. In contrast, the acinar tissue is rather poorly supplied with capillaries. This pronounced difference allows for the demonstration of the islets of Langerhans by perfusion with dyes.

In routine histologic preparations, the islet cells show no strikingly individual characteristics. They appear as islands of lightly stained cells (Fig. 20-9) surrounded by a thin layer of reticular fibers. The cells are smaller than those in the surrounding exocrine tissue, so the nuclei appear more closely packed. Appropriate fixation and staining techniques reveal the presence of several cell types. The two most common are the larger, flamed-shaped *alpha,* or A, cells which constitute about 20 percent and the smaller *beta,* or B, cells which constitute about 75 percent of the islet cells.

The A cells are sometimes absent in the smaller islets and when present tend to be located peripherally.

Both cell types contain characteristic secretory granules whose relative solubility originally distinguish A cells from B cells. The secretory granules of the A cells are preserved by alcohol or Formalin-containing fixatives, whereas the B cell granules are soluble in alcohol. If both types of granules are preserved by an appropriate fixative such as Zenker-Formol or Bouin's, differences in the staining affinities of the granules can be seen. With the Gomori aldehyde fuchsin method (Fig. 20-10, see color insert) the A cells contain red-staining granules and the B cell granules are deep-purple.

A third cell type encountered less frequently (about 5 percent) contains small granules with still different staining properties. These cells were first found in human pancreatic islets and designated *delta,* or D, cells. They are most numerous in primates but have been described in many other species. A staining characteristic of some of the D cell granules is their capacity to reduce silver nitrate to give the argentaffin reaction. In addition to these cells, a fourth type of agranular, clear cell, the *C* cell, has been observed in the guinea pig pancreas. The nature and significance of these infrequent cell types is unclear. Various possibilities, such as variations in the secretory cycle or degenerative stages of the A or B cells, have been suggested to explain the C and D cells.

FINE STRUCTURE OF THE ISLET CELLS

Osmium tetroxide fixation preserves the A and B cell secretory granules as dense, membrane-limited structures. The A cell granules are opaque and spherical. After aldehyde fixation an outer mantle of less-dense material fills the space between the dense core and the sac (Figs. 20-12 and 20-13). The structure of the A cell granules appears to be a relatively consistent characteristic among all mammals. The cytoplasm of the A cell contains a well-developed Golgi complex, a moderate amount of rough ER, and free ribosomes. A few small filamentous mitochondria are encountered in the cytoplasmic matrix, which has an overall low density when contrasted with the acinar cells (Fig. 20-9). The nucleus of the A cell tends to be deeply indented or lobulated.

The B cells contain variable numbers of granules (Fig. 20-11); which have distinct morphologic charac-

teristics in different species. In some mammals (rat, mouse, rabbit, guinea pig) the B cell contains granules that are generally similar in size but less opaque than those of the A cells. Furthermore, a large clear space is present between the B cell secretory granule and its limiting membrane. In other species (man, dog, cat, bat), the secretory granules are dense, crystalloid

FIGURE 20-7 The basal portion of a human pancreatic acinar cell with an adjacent nerve process containing several axons. The nerve contains numerous large dense cored vesicles as well as small clear vesicles. In the human pancreas, nerves have not been observed within the basement lamina. ×32,000.

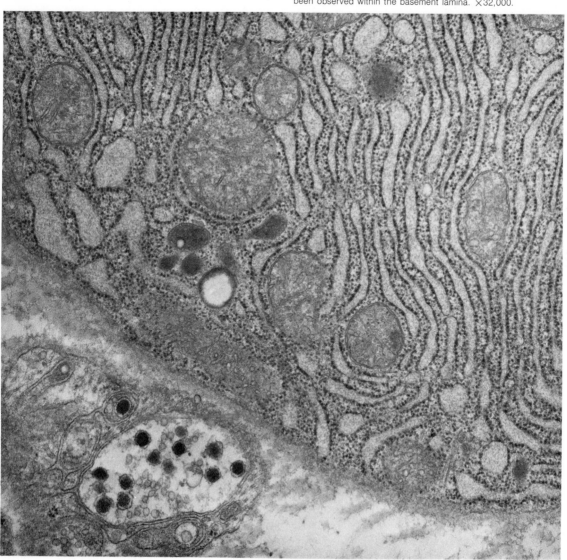

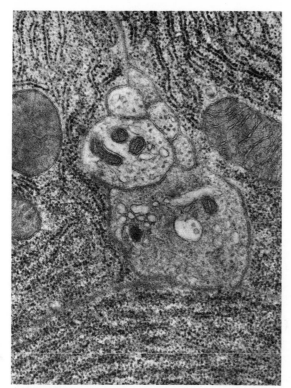

FIGURE 20-8 In the interstices between three adjacent bat pancreatic acinar cells, several axons are found in close contact with the epithelial cells. In the pancreas of certain species, nerve processes are found frequently within the basement lamina. ×30,000.

amounts of connective tissue may delineate the islet cells from the acinar cells and extend into the island. However, in many areas the plasma membranes of islet cells are closely apposed to the acinar cell membranes with no intervening basement lamina. Desmosomes are only rarely encountered joining islet cells. However, the cell membranes have folds that are interdigitated with adjacent cells or project into the intercellular space. Distinct basement laminae are always found bordering the base of the capillary endothelium and the adjacent islet cell. The endothelial cells of pancreatic capillaries in both acinar and islet tissues are the fenestrated type. Circular fenestrations are found in attenuated areas of the endothelial cell;

FIGURE 20-9 Photomicrograph of an islet of Langerhans and the surrounding acini in human pancreas. The different islet cell types cannot be distinguished in routine preparations. Hematoxylin and phloxine. ×380.

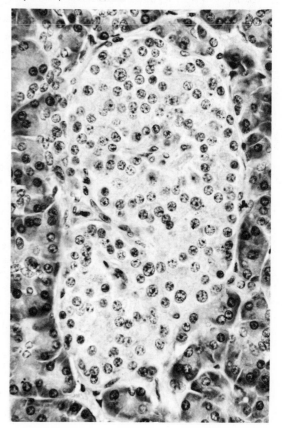

structures in a pale homogenous matrix, enclosed within a loosely fitting limiting membrane (Fig. 20-11). The B cell has a Golgi complex which is more prominent than that of the A cell and contains more rough ER and free ribosomes. The concentration of the reticulum, however, is lower than in the acinar cell. The granules in the B cell tend to be located between the round or ovoid nucleus and the plasma membrane bordering the capillary.

The D cell has not been extensively studied in many species, but it has been described in some as containing numerous membrane-enclosed granules of moderately low density (Fig. 20-14). Islet cells containing no characteristic granules, the C cells, have few organelles and the cytoplasmic matrix is of very low density. Some investigators regard the C and D cells as functional variants of either the A or B cells rather than as separate cell types.

A thin basement membrane or lamina and varying

758

they measure some 50 to 100 nm across and appear to have a thin diaphragm extending across the pore.

SECRETORY ACTIVITY

Histophysiologic studies on the islets of Langerhans have provided a growing understanding of this endocrine tissue. It is now clear that the islets produce the hormone *insulin,* which stimulates the deposition of glycogen in liver and skeletal muscle and also regulates glucose metabolism. Insulin is important for the

proper function of the enzyme hexokinase, which brings about phosphorylation of glucose during both the metabolic degradation of glucose and its incorporation into glycogen. When insulin is present in insufficient amounts or is inactive, glucose is not utilized properly. This causes a rise of the blood glucose level and the excretion of abundant and sweet urine, which is characteristic of diabetes mellitus.

FIGURE 20-11 Electron micrograph of portion of several islet cells in a human pancreatic islet. Parts of two beta cells containing numerous distinctive crystalline granules in a pale matrix and enclosed by a loose-fitting sac occupy much of this illustration. For comparison a fragment of an A cell is included at the upper right. Desmosomes are relatively infrequent between islet cells, but one is shown near the center of the figure. ×30,000. (Courtesy of A. Like.)

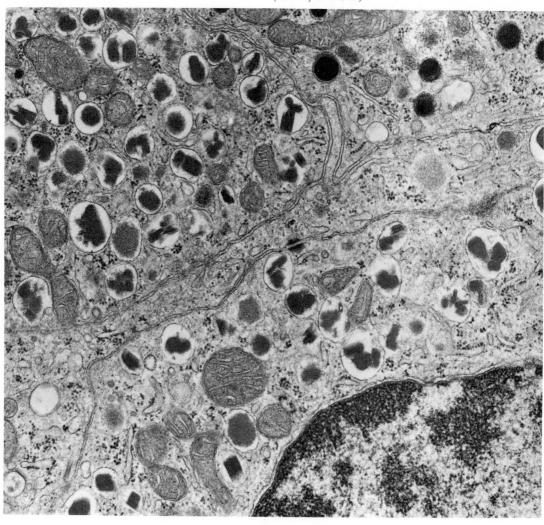

The discovery that the pancreas was involved in carbohydrate metabolism was the result of physiologic studies by Minkowski in the 1880s on pancreatectomized dogs. His assistant noted that flies were attracted to the urine, which was found to contain sugar. The hormonal nature of the islet cell secretions was clearly established by studies in which pancreatic ducts were ligated and in other experiments in which pancreatic tissue was implanted subcutaneously in animals that had been pancreatectomized. In neither of these experimental conditions did glycosuria occur, indicating that a necessary regulating factor was being secreted into the bloodstream by pancreatic cells.

The proof of the origin of pancreatic insulin was established when insulin was isolated from the whole pancreas. Early attempts to extract pancreatic hormones were unsuccessful because of the proteolytic action of the acinar cell enzymes. However, ligating

the pancreatic ducts caused degeneration of the acinar cells but no change in the islets. An extract of such organs was found by Banting et al. (1922) to contain a protein capable of alleviating diabetes mellitus. It was subsequently found that this hormone, insulin, was not inactivated by acid or alcohol, although the exocrine digestive enzymes were destroyed. By using these methods, the direct isolation of insulin from pancreatic tissue was possible.

Insulin is synthesized in the pancreatic islet by the B cell. Histologic examination of the remaining pancreas of animals made diabetic by removing a major part of the pancreas reveals a sequence of changes including degranulation of the cell, followed by hydropic degeneration which may accompany glycogen accumulation. Finally, there is complete degeneration of the B cells. Such cytologic alterations are interpreted as the result of pathologic hyperactivity of these cells. Similar changes in the B cells are obtained in

FIGURE 20-12 Electron micrograph of a portion of an A cell. The dense granules of the human alpha cells are embedded in a material of lower density, the mantal, and enclosed by a smooth membrane. Mitochondrion and granular endoplasmic reticulum are also present. ×31,000. (Courtesy of A. Like.)

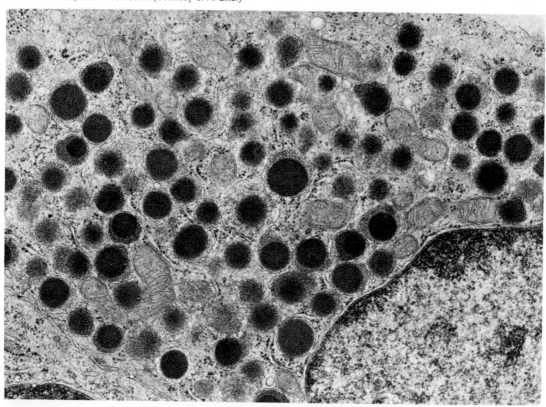

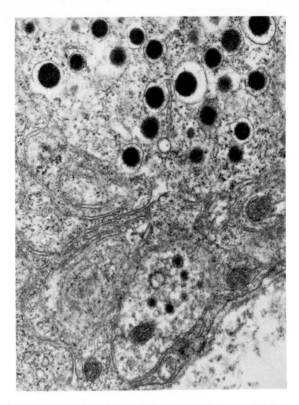

FIGURE 20-13 An electron micrograph of the basal portion of an A cell from a monkey pancreas. Unmyelinated axons are present between the basal lamina and the islet cell. ×30,000. (Courtesy of W. G. Forssmann.)

animals whose blood glucose concentrations have been experimentally elevated or who have been given excessive amounts of growth hormone.

Further study of islet function has been made possible by the drug *alloxan,* which produces a marked and permanent diabetes mellitus in experimental animals. After an initial increase in B granules, there is a degranulation of the B cells, followed by cell fragmentation. Although alloxan is specific for pancreatic B cells, it also damages other tissues; however, doses of alloxan sufficient to produce diabetes allow the other cells to recover.

FIGURE 20-14 Electron micrograph of a portion of a fetal human delta cell and part of an adjacent alpha cell. The granules of the cell type are of lower density, homogeneous composition, and enclosed by a tight-fitting membrane. ×25,000. (Courtesy of A. Like.)

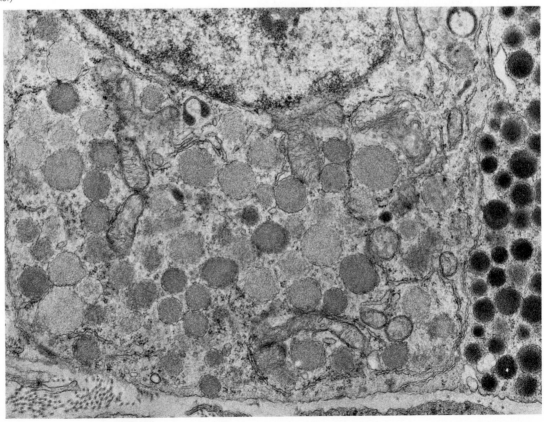

The prolonged administration of insulin results in a lowered blood glucose concentration, and the appearance of the B cells suggests that they are in a state of reduced secretory activity. There is an uncommon disease in humans, hyperinsulinism, which is due to a tumor of islet tissue in which B cells predominate and produce an excess of insulin with consequently reduced blood glucose levels.

The direct localization of insulin in the B cells has been accomplished with fluorescent antibody techniques and by the direct isolation and assay of these cells for insulin. Lacy and Williamson (1962) have calculated that each B cell of the rabbit contains 1.7 μU of insulin.

Evidence for the precise endocrine function of the A cell is less clear than for the B cell. However, there is good indication that the A cells are the source of *glucagon,* a hormone which affects sugar metabolism by accelerating liver glycogenesis and raising blood glucose. The localization of glucagon in the islet is suggested by the greater amount that can be isolated from the tail than from the head of the pancreas. Furthermore, the uncinate process of the dog pan-

creas is apparently devoid of A cells and no glucagon has been extracted from this region. Evidence for the origin of glucagon from the A cells is suggested by the undiminished amounts of glucagon extractable from the pancreases of alloxan diabetic rats and by immunofluorescent antibody studies which indicate that glucagon is localized in A cells.

In addition to insulin and glucogon secretion by pancreatic islet cells, there are some indications that gastrin may be present in either the A or the D cell, but the evidence is not conclusive. On the other hand, it is well established that there is a pancreatic tumor which produces excessive gastrin and results in high gastric acid secretion found in the Zollinger-Ellison syndrome. Another functional role of the islet cells is suggested by the recent immunocytochemical studies which have indicated that the D cell contains significant amounts of growth-hormone release-inhibiting hormone [also known as somatostatin (somatotropin-release inhibiting factor, SRIF)].

DEVELOPMENT OF THE PANCREAS

The pancreas arises in the human embryo during the fourth week of gestation as two separate outpocketings of the intestinal tube near the level of the common bile duct. These primordia, the dorsal and ventral pancreases, later meet and fuse (Fig. 20-15A and B). The dorsal portion enlarges much more rapidly and becomes the tail, body, and part of the head of the adult pancreas, and the ventral pancreas contributes to the remaining portion of the head. The duct of the ventral pancreas becomes the main outlet, which empties directly into the duodenum or into the common bile duct. The duct of the dorsal pancreas becomes the accessory pancreatic duct, which lies slightly cranial to the main duct and is smaller (Fig. 20-15C).

During development, the pancreas forms a ramifying system of tubules composed of a single layer of undifferentiated cells. These differentiate into *duct cells, acinar cells,* and *islet cells.* The duct cells retain some regenerative capacity in the adult organ. In addition to the differentiated duct cells in the adult pancreas, there are small tubular arrays of undifferentiated cells from which new acinar and islet cells will arise. Differentiated acinar tissues and islet cells are first found in the fetal pancreas during the third or fourth month of gestation.

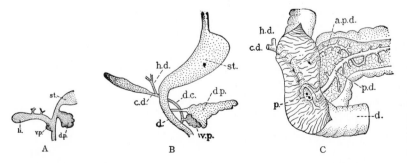

FIGURE 20-15 A and B. Diagram of the pancreas of human embryos, 10 and 15 mm. C. Dissection of duodenum and pancreas of adult human. a.p.d., accessory pancreatic duct; c.d. cyst duct; d., duodenum; d.c., ductus choledochus; d.p. dorsal pancreas; h.d., hepatic duct; li., liver; p., duodenal papilla; p.d., pancreatic duct; st., stomach; v.p., ventral pancreas.

REFERENCES

AMSTERDAM, A., and J. D. JAMIESON: Studies on Dispersed Pancreatic Exocrine Cells. II. Functional Characteristics of Separated Cells, *J. Cell Biol.*, **63:**10057 (1974).

BANTING, F. G. C. H. BEST, J. B. COLLIP, W. R. CAMPBELL, and A. A. FLETCHER: Pancreatic Extracts in the Treatment of Diabetes Mellitus, *Can. Med. Assoc. J.*, **12:**141 (1922).

BAUM, J. B., B. E. SIMMONS, R. H. UNGER, and L. L. MADISON: Localization of Glucagon in the Alpha Cells in the Pancreatic Islet by Immunofluorescent Techniques, *Diabetes*, **11:**371 (1962).

BECKER, V.: Histochemistry of the Exocrine Pancreas, in A. V. S. de Reuck and M. P. Cameron (eds.), "The Exocrine Pancreas," Ciba Foundation Symposium, Little Brown and Company, Boston, 1962.

BENCOSME, S. A., R. A. ALLEN, and H. LATTA: Functioning Pancreatic Islet Cell Tumors Studied Electron Microscopically, *Am. J. Path.*, **42:**1 (1963).

BENSLEY, R. R.: Studies on the Pancreas of the Guinea Pig, *Am. J. Anat.*, **12:**297 (1911).

CARAMIA, F.: Electron Microscopic Description of a Third Cell Type in the Islets of the Rat Pancreas, *Am. J. Anat.*, **112:**53 (1963).

CARO, L. G., and G. E. PALADE: Protein Synthesis, Storage, and Discharge in the Pancreatic Exocrine Cell. An Autoradiographic Study, *J. Cell Biol.*, **20:**473 (1964).

COVELL, W. P.: A Microscopic Study of Pancreatic Secretion in the Living Animal, *Anat. Rec.*, **40:**213 (1928).

DE DUVE, C.: Glucagon: The Hyperglycaemic Glycogenolytic Factor of the Pancreas, *Lancet*, **2:**99 (1953).

DIXIT, P. K., I. P. LOWE, C. B. HEGGESTAD, and A. LAZAROW: Insulin Content of Microdissected Fetal Islets Obtained from Diabetic and Normal Rats, *Diabetes*, **13:**71 (1964).

GOMORI, G.: Observations with Differential Stains on Human Islets of Langerhans, *Am. J. Path.*, **17:**395 (1941).

ICHIKAWA, A.: Fine Structural Changes in Response to Hormonal Stimulation of the Perfused Canine Pancreas, *J. Cell Biol.*, **24:**369 (1965).

JAMIESON, J. D., and G. E. PALADE: Condensing Vacuole Conversion and Zymogen Granule Discharge in Pancreatic Exocrine Cells: Metabolic Studies, *J. Cell Biol.*, **48:**503 (1971).

KRAEHENBUHL, J. P., and J. D. JAMIESON: Solid Phase Conjugation of Ferritin to Fab-Fragments For Use in Antigen Localization on Thin Sections. *Proc. Natl. Acad. Sci. USA*, **69:**1771 (1972).

LACY, P. E.: The Pancreatic Beta Cell: Structure and Function, *N. Engl. J. Med.*, **276:**187 (1967).

LACY, P. E., and J. R. WILLIAMSON: Quantitative Histochemistry of the Islets of Langerhans. II. Insulin Content of Dissected Beta Cells, *Diabetes*, **11:**101 (1962).

LAZAROW, A.: Cell Types of the Islets of Langerhans and the Hormones They Produce, *Diabetes*, **6:**222 (1957).

LIKE, A. A.: The Ultrastructure of the Secretory Cells of the Islets of Langerhans in Man, *Lab. Invest.*, **16:**937 (1967).

LIKE, A. A., and W. L. CHICK: Studies in the Diabetic Mutant Mouse. II. Electron Microscopy of Pancreatic Islets, *Diabetologia*, **6:**216 (1970).

MARSHALL, J. M.: Distributions of Chymotrypsinogen, Procarboxypeptidase, Desoxyribonuclease, and Ribonuclease in Bovine Pancreas, *Exp. Cell Res.*, **6:**240 (1954).

MUNGER, B. L., F. CARAMIA, and P. E. LACY: The Ultrastructural Basis for the Identification of Cell Types in the Pancreatic Islets. II. Rabbit, Dog and Opossum, *Z. Zellforsch.*, **67:**776 (1965).

OPIE, E. L.: Cytology of the Pancreas, in E. V. Cowdry (ed.), "Special Cytology," 2d ed., vol. 1, Paul P. Hoeber, Inc., New York, 1932.

PALADE, G. E.: Functional Changes in the Structure of Cell Components, in T. Hayashi (ed.), "Subcellular Particles," The Ronald Press Company, New York, 1959.

PALADE, G. E., P. SIEKEVITZ, and L. G. CARO: Structure, Chemistry and Function of the Pancreatic Exocrine Cell, in A. V. S. de Reuck and M. P. Cameron (eds.), "The Exocrine Pancreas," Ciba Foundation Symposium, Little, Brown and Company, Boston, 1962.

RENOLD, A. E.: Insulin Biosynthesis and Secretion—A Still Unsettled Topic. *N. Engl. J. Med.,* **283:**173 (1970).

SIEKEVITZ, P., and G. E. PALADE: A Cytochemical Study on the Pancreas of the Guinea Pig. I. Isolation and Enzymatic Activities of Cell Fractions, *J. Biophys. Biochem. Cytol.,* **4:**203 (1958).

SIEKEVITZ, P., and G. E. PALADE: A Cytochemical Study on the Pancreas of the Guinea Pig. II. Functional Variations in the Enzymatic Activity of Microsomes, *J. Biophys. Biochem. Cytol.,* **4:**309 (1958).

SJÖSTRAND, F. S.: The Fine Structure of the Exocrine Pancreas Cells, in A. V. S. de Reuck and M. P. Cameron (eds.), "The Exocrine Pancreas," Ciba Foundation Symposium, Little, Brown and Company, Boston, 1962.

THOMAS, T. B.: Cellular Components of the Mammalian Islets of Langerhans, *Am. J. Anat.,* **62:**31 (1937).

WARSHAWSKY, H., C. P. LEBLOND, and B. DROZ: Synthesis and Migration of Proteins in the Cells of the Exocrine Pancreas as Revealed by Specific Activity Determination from Radioautographs, *J. Cell Biol.,* **16:**1 (1963).

ZIMMERMANN, K. W.: Die Speicheldrüsen der Mundhöhle und die Bauchspeicheldrüse, in W. von Möllendorff (ed.), "Handbuch mikroskop. Anat. Menschen," vol. 5, pt. 1, Springer-Verlag OHG, Berlin, 1927.

The Respiratory System

SERGEI P. SOROKIN

The respiratory system consists of the lungs and a number of associated structures whose primary functions are to provide the living organism with oxygen from the air and to remove excess carbon dioxide from the bloodstream. The system is composed of three functional parts: a conducting portion, a respiratory region, and a ventilating mechanism. The *conducting portion* of the system includes the nasal cavity and associated sinuses, the nasopharynx, the larynx, the trachea, and the branching bronchial passages of the lungs. Collectively they warm, moisten, and filter the inspired air before it reaches the expansive *respiratory region* of the lungs, located distal to the bronchial tubes. There the cellular barrier between inspired air and bloodstream is sufficiently thin to promote rapid exchange of gases. An efficient musculoelastic mechanism moves air over the respiratory surface and forms a third functional part of the system. The components of this *ventilating mechanism* include the thoracic cage and its intercostal muscles, the muscular diaphragm, and the elastic connective tissue of the lungs. During inspiration, contraction of the muscles raises the ribs and lowers the floor of the thoracic cavity to increase its volume and to expand the lungs. During expiration, the muscles relax; elastic recoil of the expanded pulmonary tissue causes the thorax to contract. In forced expiration the natural recoil is abetted by contraction of the abdominal and external intercostal muscles, which decrease the volume of the thoracic cavity and lungs beyond their normal resting levels.

NASAL CAVITY AND SINUSES

The surfaces of the nasal cavity are covered by two types of lining: a *respiratory mucosa* that warms and moistens the air, and an *olfactory mucosa* that houses the receptors of smell. As the first segment of the conducting portion of the respiratory tract, the cavity is most fully developed in warm-blooded animals, where it is well separated from the oral cavity by the hard palate. The olfactory mucosa occupies a large proportion of the nasal lining of keen-scented animals such as carnivores and rooting ungulates; it is greatly restricted in primates and other forms that have a poor sense of smell. The respiratory mucosa is well developed in both the keen- and the feebly

765

scented. In the former, the mucosa is both more highly folded and more extensive in area; moistening the air enhances olfaction.

RESPIRATORY MUCOSA

The nasal cavity is divided into symmetric halves by the nasal septum (Fig. 21-1), which contains hyaline cartilage. Stratified squamous epithelium of the facial skin continues through the nostrils into the *vestibule*, beneath the projecting cartilaginous portion of the nose. Large hairs and associated sebaceous glands form the first defense there against the entry of particulate matter. Posteriorly the hair and glands become sparse, and the epithelium thins as it approaches the paired openings to the principal nasal chambers, located within the skull. These are smooth-sided along

FIGURE 21-1 Section through the nasal septum of a monkey, showing hyaline cartilage on the left and the richly glandular nasal mucosa on the right. Masson's trichrome stain. ×100.

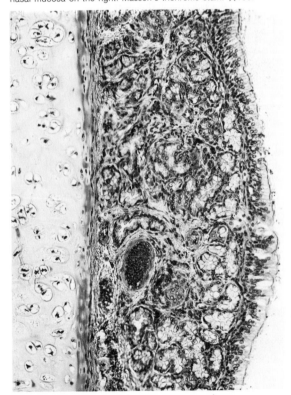

the septum but are convoluted laterally by turbinate projections from the underlying ethmoid and inferior turbinated bones, and each forms a narrow, ribbonlike passage for air. Their surfaces total some 160 cm^2 in humans and are coated with a mucous film. These anatomic arrangements help to promote turbulence in airflow; this assures the mucous film effective contact with the airstream. The epithelium beneath is pseudostratified, ciliated, and columnar. Goblet cells are abundantly but unevenly distributed within it, since they concentrate in sheltered regions. More exposed portions of the epithelium, such as that over the turbinates, may have small areas of transition to a stratified squamous lining. In fine structure, this epithelium resembles the epithelium of the trachea and bronchi described later.

Numerous branched, tubuloalveolar glands extend into the underlying connective tissue as invaginations of the epithelium. They resemble minor salivary glands, having short ducts and acini both lined by secretory cells. These vary widely in type within a mucous to serous range, and the cellular makeup of a typical gland varies with the species. In general, mucous cells occur nearer the openings of the glands along the ducts and acini, whereas serous cells occur more peripherally in the acini or in demilunes beyond them. The larger ducts occasionally contain a distinct columnar epithelium that separates the secretory cells from the surface lining of the nasal cavity, but the columnar cells lack basal striations and give no indication of participation in the secretory process.

Beneath the epithelium, the connective tissue is of fairly uniform composition until it blends into the periosteal and perichondrial layers of the nasal skeleton. Epithelium and glands are enveloped in a richly collagenous connective tissue. Mononuclear leukocytes may infiltrate the tissue freely or may occur as nodular aggregations.

Vascular Supply

The vascular supply to the nose is rich and has several unusual features. Although some differences in distributional pattern exist among mammals, the respiratory and olfactory mucosae usually have separate arterial supplies: the sphenopalatine and the ethmoidal arteries, respectively. Both vessels and their branches anastomose rather freely throughout their subdivisions. The main vessels to the respiratory mucosa lie next to the periosteum in a latticework pattern that becomes a close-meshed net as they run either obliquely or horizontally forward across the nasal sep-

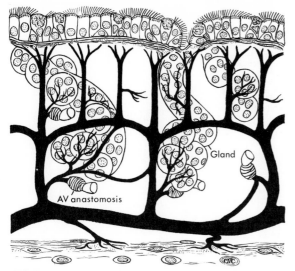

FIGURE 21-2 Arterial supply to the nasal mucosa. (After J. D. K. Dawes and M. M. L. Prichard. *J. Anat.,* **87:**311, 1953.)

tum and lateral walls. In contrast, arteries to the olfactory region spread out in a radial array. The main respiratory arteries send out superficial arcading branches; from them, other vessels run perpendicularly toward the surface, where they divide into arterioles that supply a network of capillaries just beneath the epithelium, and into others for the glands and the submucosal tissues. Arteriovenous anastomoses are common, particularly where the vasculature is richest, as in the path of the inspiratory stream and in the swell bodies described below (Fig. 21-2). These communicating vessels are tortuous; in their thick walls the medial smooth muscle has an epithelioid appearance, and the intima lacks an internal elastic membrane. As befits a secretory mucosa, the subepithelial and periglandular capillaries are fenestrated whereas the deeper ones are not. The veins are rather more conspicuous than the arteries, particularly where they lie over the arteries, as they do in humans, dogs, cats, and rabbits. There they exist as a superficial, fine-meshed plexus of small vessels and a deeper, coarser latticework of thick-walled tubes. These drain into larger veins at the anterior and posterior ends of the nasal cavity. In addition, a well-developed lymphatic system is present.

Over the middle and inferior turbinates the superficial venous plexus consists of cavernous, thin-walled vessels that lack muscular septa but otherwise resemble erectile tissue (Chap. 26). This is the region of the *swell bodies.* In humans and in other animals, blood flow is so regulated there that hourly periods of swelling occur alternately on the two sides of the nasal cavity, causing a reduction in airflow on the affected side and an upward deflection of the airstream on inspiration. Most of the respired air passes through the neighboring passage, giving the mucosa on the occluded side time to recover from desiccation and haply assisting the narial muscles in directing air to the olfactory region. This physiologic cycle is regulated autonomically. Engorgement results from constriction of the deeper veins and dilatation of the arterioles that feed the plexus through capillaries. Adrenergic fibers from the superior cervical ganglion form rich networks not only over the arteries and arterioles, as in other vascular beds, but over the veins as well, particularly in the swell bodies. They exert a tonic, vasoconstrictive action. Cholinergic nerves from the pterygopalatine ganglion promote vasodilatation and secretion by the glands. In the olfactory region, on the other hand, blood flow is not clearly affected by either sympatho- or parasympathomimetic agents.

Histophysiology

From the rear of the nasal cavity forward, the numerous circulatory loops each receive fresh arterial blood; but blood flow in the superficial vessels of each loop generally counters the flow of inspired air, and the whole forms a compound countercurrent system. Viewed from the surface, the small vessels are set in rows as in a heat exchanger. These are ranked most closely under surfaces most exposed to the inspiratory system, where glands are particularly abundant as well. In an engineer's terms, the nose is said to function like a scrubbing tower supplied with fresh fluid at successive levels. Despite a fractional-second contact time with the nasal mucosa, the inspired air is efficiently cleared of ozone, sulfur dioxide, and other water-soluble pollutant gases far better than it is cleared by the oropharynx. These gases are dissolved in the mucous carpet overlying the epithelium and are partially absorbed and partially carried off to the pharynx by ciliary action.

OLFACTORY MUCOSA

The olfactory mucosa of humans is limited to an area that covers some 500 mm^2 of the roof of the nasal

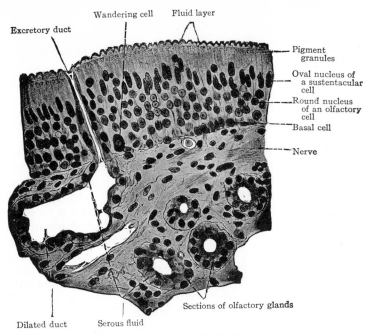

Excretory duct — Wandering cell — Fluid layer — Pigment granules — Oval nucleus of a sustentacular cell — Round nucleus of an olfactory cell — Basal cell — Nerve — Sections of olfactory glands — Dilated duct — Serous fluid

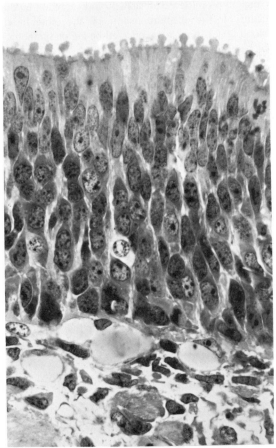

cavity and upper portions of the nasal septum. Compared with the respiratory mucosa, its pseudostratified columnar lining is taller, and the glands beneath are of a serous rather than mixed type (Fig. 21-3). The mucosa produces an ample fluid secretion in which odored substances are dissolved before being detected by cells of the epithelium. Three cell types predominate: *olfactory cells, sustentacular cells,* and *basal cells.* Olfactory cells are bipolar neurons. The others combine characteristics of epithelial and Schwann cells. The tall sustentacular cell is differentiated along secretory lines, whereas the short basal cell is undifferentiated and remains able to divide and to transform into either of the mature types. Special methods, such as silver impregnation or staining with methylene blue, are needed in order to distinguish the cells clearly by light microscopy. In routine sections identification is aided by a tendency for the round nuclei of olfactory cells to occur at a level between those of the basal cells and the ovoid nuclei of the supporting cells.

Individual olfactory cells within the epithelium respond differently to various odors; nonetheless these receptors all look alike. They are widest about the nucleus and from these taper into two processes, an apically directed *dendrite* and a centrally directed

FIGURE 21-3 (Top) Vertical section through the olfactory region of an adult human being. ×400. (Bottom) Olfactory epithelium in a neonatal rat. ×750.

axon. Unlike many neurons, the cell body contains little ergastoplasm, but a supranuclear Golgi apparatus and other organelles are present in moderation. The dendrite, approximately 1 μm in thickness, is crowded with microtubules that run along its length in parallel courses. Its apical end extends above the surface of the epithelium as a bulbous *olfactory knob,* which contains basal bodies, mitochondria, and profiles of agranular reticulum and bears a tuft of cilia. Among

different vertebrates the shape of this knob and the number of cilia present are highly variable characteristics of this cell. Frequently the knob measures about 4 μm high by 1.5 μm thick, and the cilia number 6 to 12 (Fig. 21-4). These have the dimensions and "9 + 2" axial structure of typical cilia for a few mi-

FIGURE 21-4 Olfactory epithelium, showing three-dimensional and ultrastructural aspects.

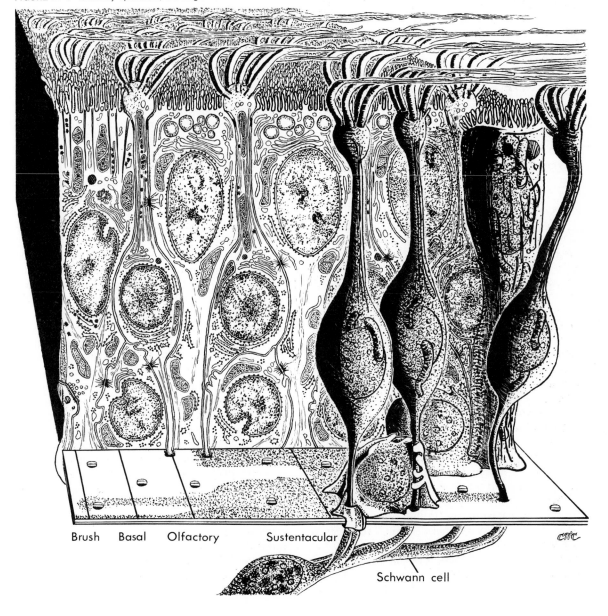

Brush Basal Olfactory   Sustentacular

Schwann cell

crometers, then abruptly narrow to half the usual diameter for the remainder of their length. Ciliary tubules within the distal segment change in configuration from doublets to singlets and gradually diminish in number. The shafts may be as long as 80 μm in cats, and the distal segment may be four or five times longer than the proximal segment in frogs. These measurements differ in other species. Olfactory cilia rarely exhibit motility. Their distal segments are too thoroughly enmeshed with other cilia and microvilli in the surface fluid to beat effectively. More certainly, they greatly increase receptor cell exposure to odorate substances.

Below the nucleus the olfactory cell becomes drawn into a threadlike axon. As its diameter approximates 0.2 μm, the process is just visible in the light microscope. It extends below the basal lamina to join axons from adjacent cells in forming small fascicles, which become invested by Schwann cells. The fascicles penetrate the cribriform plate of the ethmoid bone and become grouped into *fila olfactoria*. These lead into the ipsilateral member of the paired *olfactory bulbs*, where the axons synapse.

Among cells of the olfactory epithelium the sustentacular cells are the most numerous and most conspicuous. They differ in histochemical attributes from olfactory cells but share some of them, such as a capacity for reducing TPN (NADP), with basal cells and those of the glands beneath. These cells are rich in organelles, notably a supranuclear Golgi apparatus and a tightly compacted agranular reticulum. Together with numerous lipid-rich granules, the reticulum may fill the apical cytoplasm. Apart from lysosomes, other membrane-bounded granules are present. They give the cells a secretory complexion even if the granules differ in appearance from one species to another. Along the apical surface microvilli are prominent. Laterally the cells form the usual variety of junctional contacts with adjacent olfactory and sustentacular cells, but so-called gap junctions have not been observed. As a rule, these cells are spaced so as to separate adjacent olfactory cells. Moreover, they ensheath the dendritic and axonal processes of those neurons in mesaxons and in this respect resemble gliocytes. Metabolic exchanges evidently occur along the sustentacular-olfactory interfaces. Accordingly, the supportive function of these cells can be understood broadly. Toward the base of the epithelium, olfactory axons become ensheathed in processes from basal cells, only these are fingerlike rather than sheetlike and the wrapping is discontinuous (Fig. 21-4).

Beneath the olfactory epithelium the connective tissue contains the branched tubuloalveolar glands of Bowman and myelinated fibers of the trigeminal nerve, in addition to unmyelinated olfactory axons, Schwann cells, and the usual elements of connective tissue. Cuboidal cells of Bowman's glands contain secretory granules and discharge a serous fluid onto the olfactory surface by way of excretory ducts, which are lined by flattened cells (Fig. 21-3). The glands secrete continuously and provide fresh solvent for odored substances. The fibers of the trigeminal nerve terminate in slender processes that extend into the epithelium. Some of them synapse with nonciliated brush cells sparsely distributed there (Fig. 21-4) and elsewhere in the nasal and pulmonary linings. In the nose these cells possibly play a minor role in olfaction, for some trigeminal input reaches the olfactory bulbs. They may also provide sensory input for the sneeze reflex. Blood vessels to the olfactory region supply a rich subepithelial capillary plexus and a deeper one of veins. Lymphatics run among the veins, and the tissue blends into the subjacent perichondrium and periosteum.

Histophysiology

It has proved more difficult for humans to form concepts about olfaction than to conceptualize the processes of seeing and hearing. For one thing, they have no experience of olfaction to compare with their working knowledge of the other modalities gained from centuries spent in building optical devices, musical instruments, and the like. Accordingly, olfactory structure-function relations remain crudely understood. Notwithstanding, the olfactory cell is recognized as the primary receptor for smell, because only this cell type degenerates after sectioning of the olfactory nerves. Moreover, it resembles known sensory cells of the eye and ear in such details as the presence of some type of cilia at the apex, in the microtubular arrays between the apex and main body of the cell, and in the sheathing of its processes by other elements of the epithelium. If an odored substance is added to the surface fluid, this is reflected by a change in electrical potential recorded along the nerve. The change in potential is probably a summation of several activating and inhibitory discharges, including a negative potential representing the olfactory cell's initial response to stimulation and a positive potential associated with secretion by neighboring cells. Stimulation of the olfactory cell apparently results from depolarization of the plasma membrane covering distal portions of the cilia, for in extending through an often thick surface coating, these processes make first contact with the stimulating substance. In exceptional instances olfactory cells are not provided with cilia, but then the surface coating is thin and depolarization occurs on the microvilli.

It is not known precisely how the olfactory cells become stimulated, nor how collectively they are able to discriminate among a vast range of odors. Most vertebrate receptors seem to respond to a fairly wide range of substances. Insects possess an additional class of highly specific receptors for pheromones, which trigger stereotyped behavioral responses, but, although such responses are recognized as well in mammals, the receptors for them have not been identified in the olfactory epithelium. Clinical data provide evidence for less than 100 specific anosmias in humans; this is but one reason to believe that their olfactory cells respond to a limited number of "primary odors," with a range being perceived by differential action. Experimental evidence furthermore suggests that human olfactory discrimination often correlates with the shape of the stimulant molecules; this has led to a stereochemical theory of olfaction and a search for specific receptor proteins along the cell surface. Such a theory can account for the remarkable phenomenon of olfactory adaptation, whereby odors first noticed on entering a room are soon forgotten; but it must be conceded that the primary odors for humans may not be the same as those for another animal. Moreover, the theory must become reconciled to certain cases where sterochemically related compounds provoke dissimilar responses.

If the foregoing is uncertain, it is even less clear how olfactory neurons interact electrically with adjacent cells in the absence of gap junctions or other interfacial specializations considered prerequisite to electrical coupling. Nonetheless, signals are received from the epithelium and become partially integrated with other input in the cell bodies of the neurons before being transmitted along the axon. Axons from adjacent cells at first run in parallel but become intermixed as they enter the outermost layer of the olfactory bulb, so that the projection of the epithelium onto the bulb is not precisely topographic as it is in projections of the retina or cochlea on nuclei of the brain. The olfactory axons branch and synapse with dendrites of second-order neurons, termed *mitral* or

tufted cells, within spherical tangles of neuropil, termed *olfactory glomeruli*. Signals from about 1,000 olfactory cells converge on each second-order cell. In mammals each second-order cell sends its one main dendrite to a single glomerulus so that a given glomerular system represents a specific group of olfactory cells and can be so projected centrally. In the bulb, numerous subsidiary circuits connect neurons of the mitral series with smaller granule cells, as evidenced by the presence of dendrodendritic, dendroaxonal, and somatodendritic synapses between them. These circuits provide a basis for amplifying or inhibiting incoming signals and are abetted by feedback to the granule cells from higher centers. Recordings made from olfactory bulbs of human subjects seem to show that at this level odor quality is coded as patterns of frequency components, whereas odor detection is dependent on adequate signal strength and its characterization on still greater amplitude. From the bulbs, incoming signals are passed to third-order neurons in the olfactory cortex and nearby subcortical regions at the base of the forebrain. These higher centers and the olfactory bulbs interact directly or indirectly with more caudal parts of the brain, including the thalamus and hypothalamus. Olfactory sensations are represented bilaterally, owing to the presence of interbulbar fibers and cross connections at higher levels.

VOMERONASAL ORGANS

The vomeronasal (Jacobson's) organs are paired tubular structures located in the floor of the nasal cavity along each side of the septum. Their cavities are lined in part by an *accessory olfactory epithelium* and open by ducts either to the nasal or oral cavities. They are well developed in many mammals but in primates exist only during embryonic life. The accessory epithelium and the glands beneath resemble their counterparts in the olfactory mucosa, but accessory olfactory cells often lack cilia and their axons lead to small *accessory olfactory bulbs*, located one to a side. These are like olfactory bulbs of amphibians, which are simple in structure and do not possess segregated glomerular systems, as do the mammalian bulbs. The function of these organs is unknown; it is likely they are more involved than the olfactory mucosa with behavioral responses related to specific odors.

PARANASAL SINUSES

The paranasal sinuses are blind pockets that reach the nasal cavity through narrow openings. Their linings are continuous with the nasal mucosa and are similar in type, although less highly developed. Much of the epithelium is simple, ciliated, and columnar; the glands are smaller; and the connective tissue is reduced in amount. The sinuses contribute to the humidification of the nasal cavity. In keen-scented carnivores, portions of the sphenoidal and frontal sinuses may be occupied by ethmoturbinal bodies and serve as extensions of the olfactory area.

NASOPHARYNX

The pseudostratified ciliated columnar lining and glands of the nasal mucosa continue into the upper or nasal portion of the pharynx. With some interruption by stratified epithelium as the oropharynx and larynx are crossed, a similar covering is found in the remaining major conducting portions of the respiratory tract. In the pharynx, however, the mucosa becomes thinner and generally rests directly upon skeletal muscle, being separated from it by a broad elastic layer. Below the *fornix,* or roof of the pharynx, a zone of stratified columnar epithelium may extend for short distances as the lining undergoes transition to the noncornified, stratified squamous epithelium typical of the oral cavity and oropharynx. Ventrally, stratified squamous epithelium covers most of the nasal surface of the soft palate; laterally the ciliated epithelium extends downward around the openings of the eustachian tubes, which are similarly lined. The midline *pharyngeal tonsil* is located on the dorsal wall of the nasopharynx. Patches of stratified squamous epithelium are common on its surface, but pseudostratified columnar cells predominate. Ordinarily small, the tonsil may become quite large in childhood and together with lymphoid tissue near the auditory orifices constitute the *adenoids.* Stratified squamous epithelium is continued below the oropharynx into the laryngeal pharynx, where the respiratory tract becomes separated from the alimentary tract at the entrance to the larynx. During swallowing movements, food is excluded from the nasopharynx by the contraction of the pharyngopalatine muscles and the retraction of the uvula between them.

LARYNX

The larynx is a hollow, bilaterally symmetric structure framed by cartilages, bound together by ligaments and muscles, and located between the pharynx and the trachea. It acts primarily as a valve to prevent swallowed food from entering the lower respiratory tract, but it is a tone-producing instrument as well, and in humans it has important additional functions in the production of speech. The anatomic valve itself is termed the *glottis* and consists of a pair of lateral mucosal folds, the *vocal folds,* located partway inside the larynx. The size of the glottal aperture changes with circumstance. Partly open during quiet breathing, it widens to permit deep inspiration but closes prior to swallowing and before intrathoracic or intraabdominal pressures are raised. During phonation the aperture fluctuates rapidly between slightly open and fully closed positions.

GENERAL STRUCTURE

The larynx (Fig. 21-5) is based on a ring-shaped *cricoid* cartilage which rests upon the trachea. Above, the ventral and lateral walls of the larynx are framed largely by a shieldlike *thyroid* cartilage, which articulates with the side of the cricoid by means of two *inferior cornua* and with the hyoid bone by means of two *superior cornua.* A pair of pyramidal, *arytenoid* cartilages arise from the dorsocranial surface of the cricoid cartilage and delimit the dorsal wall. The summit of each is capped by a small *corniculate* cartilage. A midline

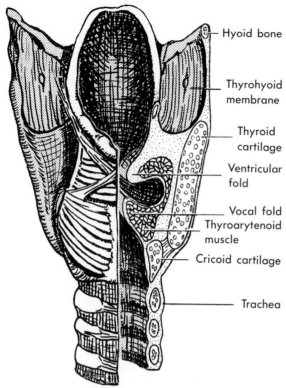

Labels on figure:
- Hyoid bone
- Thyrohyoid membrane
- Thyroid cartilage
- Ventricular fold
- Vocal fold
- Thyroarytenoid muscle
- Cricoid cartilage
- Trachea

FIGURE 21-5 Diagram of the human larynx showing the dorsal aspect on the left and a cutaway view of ventricular and vocal folds on the right. Approximately ×1.5.

epiglottis extends cranially from within the thyroid to define the ventral border of the laryngeal entrance, becomes attached to the hyoid bone, and thereafter ends as a clublike protuberance in the pharynx. These framing cartilages are linked to each other by means of striated *intrinsic muscles,* whose origins and insertions are confined to laryngeal structures. They are also interconnected by means of dense connective tissue, notably a sheetlike cricothyroid membrane and several thyrohyoid ligaments. The latter, together with the *extrinsic muscles,* help to attach the larynx to adjacent structures. In effect, the larynx is suspended from the hyoid bone and to some extent can slide up and down within a sleeve of connective tissue in accommodating itself to functional needs.

Within the larynx the mucosa is thrown into three pairs of lateral folds. The first pair stretches between the tips of the arytenoid cartilages and the epiglottis at the laryngeal entrance, frequently being stiffened by small *cuneiform* cartilages embedded within. These are the

aryepiglottic folds. The *ventricular folds,* or false vocal folds, are next, and the true *vocal folds* are last. Both of these may contain slight cartilaginous support, especially near their dorsal points of attachment, respectively to the ventricular and vocal processes of the arytenoids. Both insert on the thyroid cartilage ventrally. Above the vocal folds the laryngeal space (*vestibule*) is roughly triangular in cross section, and between vocal and ventricular folds the side walls recess to form the *laryngeal ventricles.* Below the vocal folds the lumen (*atrium*) gradually becomes cylindrical.

The Glottis

The glottal aperture is bordered by a pair of *vocal ligaments,* one to each side within the vocal folds, and from them it receives its configuration. The ligaments are bands of elastic connective tissue that extend from the arytenoid cartilage of each side to insert partly on a midline point on the thyroid cartilage (Fig. 21-7) and partly on portions of the cricothyroid membrane adjacent. The vocal folds also contain striated muscle fibers of the thyroarytenoid group, which lie lateral to the ligaments on each side and insert into the thyroid and arytenoid cartilages. Being suspended between these two cartilages, both of which articulate with the cricoid, each vocal fold is affected whenever the cartilages are moved. Since the intrinsic muscles interconnect the laryngeal cartilages, by their actions they serve to regulate the glottis. By the same token, they move the ventricular folds as well, though to a lesser extent. The principal actions to affect the glottal aperture are those that rock the arytenoids on the cricoid and those that rock and glide the thyroid on the cricoid. When the arytenoids are rotated outward (action of the posterior cricoarytenoid muscles), the glottis opens. Conversely, when they are rotated inward (lateral cricoarytenoids and interarytenoids), or when they are approximated in a gliding motion (arytenoid), it closes. When the thyroid is tilted forward (cricothyroids) or the cricoid is pulled backward (lateral cricothyroids and extrinsic cricopharyngeus) the vocal folds stretch, and when the thyroid is tilted backward (thyroarytenoids) they relax. Such muscular actions are related primarily to the valvular function of the glottis, for not all are essential to phonation. In phases of deglutition the larynx is moved principally by the extrinsic muscles. The intrinsic muscles nevertheless contribute to this process by drawing the arytenoid cartilages forward against the epiglottis to help close off the larynx (thyroarytenoids, aryepiglottics, and arytenoid).

HISTOLOGY

Epithelium and Glands

The mucosa of the larynx is continuous with that of the pharynx and the trachea and exhibits features of both. Stratified squamous epithelium from above extends partway into the larynx, over the aryepiglottic folds laterally and somewhat farther ventrally, where it covers the entire lingual side of the epiglottis and the upper half of its laryngeal aspect. It is also present at other points of wear, such as over the vocal folds and the arytenoid cartilages. Elsewhere this gives way to a pseudostratified, ciliated, columnar lining after passage through a transitional zone of stratified columnar epithelium. The pseudostratified epithelium and its associated glands resemble those of the trachea and bronchi and function similarly in conditioning the inspired air and in adding to the protective coating of mucus spread over the epithelial surface. Much of this is swept up to the larynx from the lower respiratory tract and in turn is driven into the pharynx by local ciliary action.

The laryngeal glands are small, branching, tubuloalveolar invaginations of the epithelium. They occur in groups and generally remain confined to the lamina propria. Exceptionally they may penetrate parts of the framing cartilages. Most frequently, as in humans, these deep excursions occur only in relation to the epiglottis and give that cartilage a uniquely pockmarked ap-

FIGURE 21-6 Cross section of the human larynx at the level of the ventricular folds. Muscles (arytenoideus and ventricularis portion of thyroarytenoideus) and glands are revealed by their reaction for succinic dehydrogenase. The ventricular appendixes extend between the folds and the thyroid cartilage (top of picture). ×10.

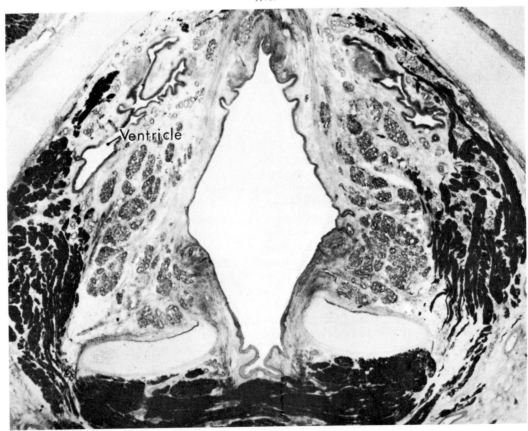

Ventricle

pearance. The glands are especially abundant along the rim of the aryepiglottic fold; these are *arytenoid glands*. Many occur as well in the ventricular folds (Fig. 21-6) and in the dorsal wall of the laryngeal ventricles. They are absent from the vocal ligaments and only gradually reappear toward the base of the vocal folds, whence they increase and eventually encircle the laryngeal

space at the level of the cricoid cartilage. Most of the glands produce a mucous secretion that stains less brilliantly with PAS and differs in other ways from the mucus of goblet cells. Accordingly, they can be considered *seromucous* glands, keeping in mind the limitations of the term. Like their counterparts in the nose and in conducting airways of the lungs, the laryngeal

FIGURE 21-7 Cross section of the human larynx at the level of the true vocal folds. The vocal ligaments are elevated above part of the laryngeal ventricles on each side. ×8.

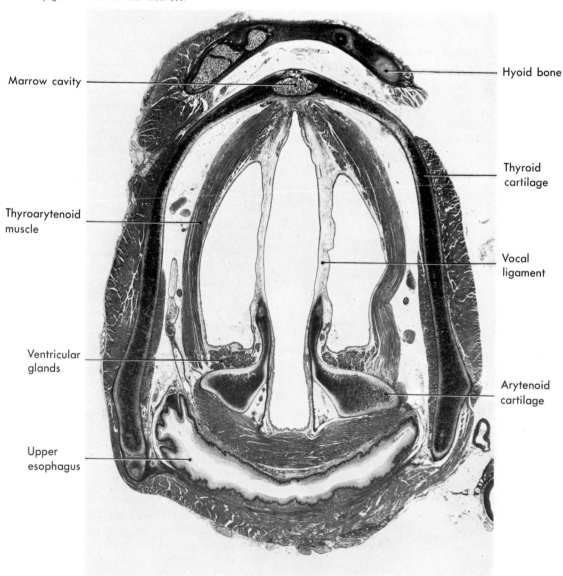

Marrow cavity

Thyroarytenoid muscle

Ventricular glands

Upper esophagus

Hyoid bone

Thyroid cartilage

Vocal ligament

Arytenoid cartilage

glands are regulated by unmyelinated nerves. These frequently penetrate the basal laminae of acini and ramify among the secretory cells as threadlike processes each bearing one or more swellings charged with predominantly clear (cholinergic) synaptic vesicles (Fig. 21-8). In addition to glands, a few taste buds occur at the base of the epiglottis.

Connective Tissue

Within the larynx the usual elements of connective tissue are combined in a great variety of textures. Beneath the epithelium this tissue is a rather loose lamina propria, but this becomes denser around solid structures and so is not everywhere distinct from the encircling submucosa. All cell types are represented, as are all the fibers, but elastic fibers are unusually abundant. These are heaviest in the glottis where they are bundled in parallel arrays to make up the vocal ligaments, which may be regarded as thickenings of the submucous cricothyroid membrane. The fibers of

FIGURE 21-8 Part of a seromucous acinus in the epiglottis of the little brown bat, showing an intraepithelial nerve ending with synaptic vesicles. ×12,000.

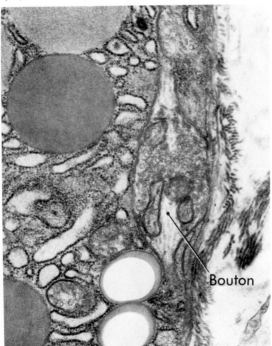

Bouton

this membrane diminish in size and number in caudal parts of the vocal folds; and in the lamina propria above the tissue becomes particularly loose so as to offer little resistance to edematous swelling. In humans the laryngeal connective tissue is unusually rich in *mast cells* which release histamine and other edema-producing agents during immediate-type hypersensitivity reactions (*anaphylaxis*). The laryngeal reaction often can be life-threatening, as are laryngeal infections, because both can lead to occlusion of the airway.

Small lymphoid nodules and migratory leukocytes frequently occur here as in all connective tissues close to the outside environment. Such nodules are rarely found near the glottis but become prominent below in the atrial part of the larynx. In capillaries supplying the epithelium and glands, fenestrated plaques appear in the endothelium at points where the vessels closely approach the basal laminae. The capillaries drain into venous plexuses situated more deeply. The lymphatic system is similarly arranged with a superficial network leading to a deeper plexus of larger vessels.

Cartilage

The laryngeal cartilages not only furnish examples of all the main histologic types of cartilage but illustrate some of the variations to be found within each type. Early in life all are hyaline cartilages. Later on, most of the cuneiforms and corniculates, part of the epiglottis, and the apices and vocal processes of the arytenoids become converted to elastic cartilage, and smaller portions of the epiglottis and the arytenoids become fibrocartilage. In sum, the larger structural cartilages remain hyaline, whereas the smaller ones become elastic. The fiber-containing cartilages of the larynx differ from each other most conspicuously in the patterns made by their fibrous networks. These follow lines of stress and may be curved and interlacing in the epiglottis but are straight and parallel where the vocal ligaments join the arytenoids. Certain differences are seen as well among the hyaline cartilages. For example, the capsular matrix is often more basophilic in the thyroid cartilage than in the others. However, any of the hyaline cartilages may ossify with age, and a marrow cavity may form inside the bone (Fig. 21-7). Among these variant cartilages the epiglottis stands out, for even though its cells unquestionably are chondrocytes, its matrix is sparse, variously admixed with other connective tissue cells and fibers, and closely intruded on by adjacent tissues. In some species it resembles *chondroid tissue* of lower vertebrates more than typical mammalian cartilage.

Muscle and Nerves

All the laryngeal muscle is cross-striated muscle, an unusual tissue to find in tubular viscera of vertebrates but present there as well as in adjacent portions of the esophagus. Functionally this muscle enables the larynx to carry out its specialized tasks. Phylogenetically it reflects the development of this region from the visceral skeletal system derived from splanchnic mesoblast and formed into cartilages and muscles of the mandibular, hyoid, and branchial arches. At first intended to expand and contract the pharynx for purposes of feeding and respiration, the muscles were later put to new uses as the branchial arches became transformed into the skeleton of the larynx. The intrinsic muscles seem to be composed of fiber types in the intermediate to red range, judging from criteria discussed in the chapter on muscle. The fibers are small and strongly reactive for the mitochondrial enzyme succinic dehydrogenase. Furthermore, electron micrographs of these muscles show that the mitochondria frequently occur in subsarcolemmal and interfibrillar chains. In bats, cricothyroid fibers additionally possess a highly developed sarcoplasmic reticulum. Such visible features might well help these muscles to achieve short refractory periods and rapid contractility, but alone they are an inadequate basis for predicting muscular performance. More certainly, physiologic characteristics of skeletal muscles are greatly influenced by their innervation.

The larynx is extensively represented in both sensory and motor cortex, and the muscles are under fine control. This is projected through the pyramidal system to motor neurons in the *nucleus ambiguus,* and signals reach the larynx through branches of the vagus nerve. One of these, the superior laryngeal nerve, innervates the cricothyroid muscle through its external branch. Other intrinsic muscles are controlled by the recurrent laryngeal nerve. Afferent impulses from the larynx initiate the cough reflex, mediate a general chemical sense, and influence reflex activity in swallowing. Sensory and secretomotor impulses are carried predominantly by the internal branch of the superior laryngeal nerve. It represents most of the region above the glottis and the subglottal region as well through communication with the recurrent nerve. Sensory input travels this path to cell bodies in the *nodose ganglion.* Sensation from part of the area of the epiglottis is carried to the *petrous ganglion* of the

glossopharyngeal nerve, whose domain is in the vicinity of the nasopharynx. Sympathetic innervation to the larynx is much as described in the section on the trachea. Owing to the small size of laryngeal motor units as well as to the widespread autonomic and sensory innervation of the region, laryngeal tissues are richly supplied with nerves. These are arranged in superficial and deep plexuses.

ROLE OF THE LARYNX IN PHONATION

Speaking and singing are characteristic human activities controlled by large segments of the human brain and effected principally by means of the larynx, other parts of the respiratory system, and structures in the mouth. In these activities, the mouth is relatively more important to speech and the larynx to singing. In both cases the glottis is the usual source of *voiced sound,* which is produced by the passage of air driven by elevated subglottic pressure through the closed vocal folds. These part intermittently to emit puffs of air, and this alternately compressed and rarefied air is delivered to the airways above, which act as resonating cavities. Voiced sound has a fundamental frequency determined by the mass of the vocal ligaments, their length, and their tension. This acoustic system has been likened to that of a reed organ pipe, where air is passed from a wind chest through the reed and into the organ pipe. In humans, however, the driving pressure, the pitch of the reed (glottis), and the size of the resonant cavity all are variable and not fixed. In singing, the larynx is called on to produce fundamental tones of greatly varied pitch, whereas for speech only a limited range is called for, centering around 125 cycles per second for men and around 225 for women. Moreover, certain sounds of speech, such as the *f* in fast, are not voiced but produced with an open glottis, whereas others, such as the *h* in hat, are produced by gradual closure, or aspiration. The resonant cavities are of importance because, depending upon their size and shape, they reinforce the fundamental tone and tones of higher pitch derived from the overtone series, beginning with a frequency of about 400 cycles per second. The laryngeal vestibule and the nasopharynx form a resonant cavity in the neck that automatically tunes itself to the frequency sung, because as the pitch is raised the larynx slides upward and shortens the cavity. The nasal cavity and sinuses are tuned to certain frequencies only, as their dimensions are fixed. The oral cavity is formed into a very finely tunable resonator regulated by movements of the tongue, the jaws, the soft palate, and the lips. It can be seen that speech sounds are generated principally in the mouth and not in the larynx; for spoken sounds can be whispered, and this is done with a partially open glottis. Roughly speaking, vowel sounds are steady-state sounds and consonants are transient ones, exceptions being the nasal sounds *m* and *n,* the rolled *r,* and the sustained *s.* Each vowel sound is characterized by a set of fixed pitches to which the oral resonator is tuned. This sound is excited by a laryngeal tone of equal or lower pitch. It is precisely when words are sung to high tones that the different requirements of singing and speech become clear; for if the laryngeal tone is higher than the ones needed to excite a certain vowel sound, the vowel cannot be pronounced correctly.

Glottic Structure Related to Phonation

It is believed that during phonation the edges of the closed glottis are driven apart by subglottic pressure but are drawn together again by a Bernoulli force and by *elastic recoil* of the vocal folds. This is the summation of the tension in stretched elastic fibers of the vocal ligaments and the tension exerted between antagonistic pairs of intrinsic muscles, principally the cricothyroids acting against the thyroarytenoids. Certain other muscles are involved as well, such as those acting to hold the folds together. The loudness of sound emitted from the larynx increases as the vocal folds are approximated, and when the glottis is closed,

further increases result largely from increases in subglottic pressure. It has been argued that the *vocalis* muscle, the part of the thyroarytenoid group that lies adjacent to the vocal ligament, influences both character and volume of laryngeal sound by helping to open the vocal folds during phonation. This argument is based upon claims that some of the vocalis fibers insert on the vocal ligaments instead of on the cartilages. Such claims have been disputed convincingly in the case of humans, although it is true some vocalis fibers insert into the cricothyroid membrane below the glottis. The argument remains a vital one in relation to the larynx of certain bats who use bursts of intense laryngeal ultrasound for purposes of echolocation.

On the whole, laryngeal muscles act more to alter the pitch and mode of vibration of the vocal folds than to initiate phonation or to amplify its intensity. Characteristically, these results can be achieved in more than one way. For example, the pitch of the laryngeal sound can be changed either by altering the tension, the length, or the mass of the vocal ligaments, or by causing only part of their length to vibrate. Similarly, by thinning out the edges of the glottal aperture the mode of vibration can be changed and the falsetto tone then results. All these changes require complex muscle action. In trained singers they seem to involve the intrinsic muscles more and extrinsic muscles less than they do in the case of vocal amateurs.

Human ventricular folds, pervaded by glands, are not well suited to phonation. They close over the closed glottis prior to coughing. Old-time singers made use of this action to initiate their vocal attack in a maneuver known as *coup de glotte.* In echo-locating bats, however, these folds may be as thin and flexible as the true vocal folds.

TRACHEA

The trachea, or windpipe, is a hollow tube originating at the base of the larynx and ending below at the *carina,* where it bifurcates to form the main airway, or *primary bronchus,* of each lung. Like the other conducting portions of the respiratory system, the trachea conditions the air as it passes to the lungs and provides protection from dust and airborne infection. It runs close to the ventral surface of the neck largely unstrengthened by neighboring tissues. Consequently, it would collapse during forceful inspiration, or on

inspiration against a closed glottis, were it not reinforced by a skeleton of cartilage embedded in its wall. This represents a part of the visceral skeleton of vertebrates, homologous to the fifth branchial arch of fish, and, like the laryngeal cartilages, adapted to new uses by terrestrial forms. To some extent, tracheal structures seem to reflect divergent *branchial* and *pulmonary* influences exerted on them during development. Although retaining a midline position and in large measure the bilateral symmetry associated with it, the trachea acquires a more radial plan of organization than that possessed by the larynx, and the tissues become arranged in concentric layers of mucosa, submucosa, an incomplete muscularis, and adventitia. This radial plan becomes fully developed in the bronchi and serves as the organizational basis for succeeding intrapulmonary airways.

HISTOLOGY

Epithelium and Glands

The tracheal mucosa closely resembles that of the nose and nasopharynx and is virtually identical with that in the lower part of the larynx and in the pulmonary bronchi. It is secretory, harboring many exocrine glands and being lined by a pseudostratified columnar epithelium in which *ciliated* and *mucous* cells predominate. This epithelium is taller in large mammals than in small ones. It may vary in appearance even among individuals of the same species, since it is sensitive to irritation and responds by increasing in height while its mucous cells and the glands beneath undergo hypertrophy. With more intense or prolonged irritation, portions of the epithelium may assume a stratified squamous form through a process of change termed *squamous metaplasia* by pathologists. This change is arguably within the epithelium's normal expressive range, since islands of stratified squamous cells normally occur in exposed parts of the pseudostratified lining of the upper airway and remain stable for a lifetime. In addition to ciliated and mucous cells, *basal* (short) cells stand out because their nuclei form a row close to the basement lamina to give the epithelium its apparently stratified appearance. These cells do not extend to the free surface and evidently serve as a reserve population for the epithelium. Other types of cells have minority representation but often escape notice completely because their distinguishing features are poorly resolved by light microscopy.

As seen by electron microscopy, at least six different cell types make up this laryngobronchial epithelium. Ultrastructural characteristics of these cells are illustrated in Fig. 21-9. The epithelium exhibits moderately high levels of activity for mitochondrial enzymes associated with oxidative phosphorylation and for lysosomal enzymes. Much of this activity is attributable to the ciliated and mucous cells. In ciliated cells the mitochondria tend to concentrate just below the apical cytoplasm which contains the ciliary basal bodies. The basal bodies are ranged in a single layer and number about 300 per cell. Each is a centriole that has

produced a cilium, and these extend from the basal bodies through the surface microvillous layer and into the lumen of the airway. At the base of these cells one sometimes sees one or two centrioles unassociated with cilia. The supranuclear region is occupied by the Golgi apparatus and various lysosomal elements, including a few large residual bodies. Ciliated cells have only moderate numbers of ribosomes, either free or attached to membranes of the endoplasmic reticulum, so that the appreciable cytoplasmic basophilia of this epithelium is ascribable in larger measure to the mucous cells. These resemble goblet cells of the small intestine and exhibit characteristics of protein-secreting cells: an extensive, cisternal ergastoplasm housed in the lower part of the cell, a supranuclear Golgi apparatus, and an apical cytoplasm charged with membrane-bounded but ofttimes coalescing mucous droplets. In these cells the centrioles usually are seen amidst the secretory material in the apical cytoplasm. When secretion occurs, the droplets are shed along with some of the cytoplasmic threads separating them. Thereafter the centrioles seem to become active in reconstituting the apical plasmalemma. A cell that has just released its secretion no longer is identifiable by light microscopy as a mucous cell and becomes another nonciliated cell in the epithelium. Collectively these are called *brush* cells, a term that recognizes their microvillous border as one of few distinctive features. Among this heterogeneous group a small number have been shown to possess epitheliodendritic (afferent) synapses with nerve processes that reach the cells from the underlying connective tissue (Fig. 21-9, brush$_1$). Consequently, these brush cells have been considered sensory receptors. They have numerous glycogen granules as well as a preponderance of agranular reticulum in their cytoplasm. In other brush cells, precursors of the basal bodies or intermediates in some other differentiative process may occur in the cytoplasm (Fig. 21-9, brush$_2$), indicating that these cells are immature and have recently replaced cells that have been cast off from the epithelium. Basal (short) cells often contain strands of a keratinoid material in the cytoplasm but otherwise appear even less differentiated than the immature brush cells.

Small-granule cells occupy a basal position in the epithelium along with the short cells. The designation small granule emphasizes the most conspicuous feature of these cells, a cytoplasm filled with small (1000 to 3000 Å) dense-cored granules, but the category includes a variety of cells belonging to two general classes, the first consisting of *neurosecretory cells* that produce catecholamines and the second encompassing the *polypeptide hormone secreting cells* of the body. Many cells in the first class are clearly neuronal in character, for example, the epinephrine- and norepinephrine-secreting cells of the adrenal medulla (Chap. 31). In the respiratory tract, members of this class possess epithelial characteristics but nonetheless remain rather conspicuously innervated. Several distinct varieties of the second class of cells occur in the epithelium lining both extrapulmonary and intrapulmonary air passages. They resemble some of the argyrophil or argentaffin endocrine cells of the ali-

mentary tract (Chap. 18), but the specific products and the distribution of specific cell types in the respiratory tract are imperfectly known. Both classes of cells are able to take up amine precursors and store the amines in cytoplasmic granules, a property they share with mast cells (Fig. 21-10).

Small-granule cells of the neurosecretory type are widely though sparsely distributed throughout the epithelium and glands of the respiratory system. They occur singly or else in small clusters; but in the extrapulmonary airways, they generally are solitary and appear columnar in shape, although they send slender granule-containing processes among the epithelial cells and along the basement lamina. Some of these contact and may synapse with small-granule cells of the endocrine type (Fig. 21-11), while others engage intraepithelial finger- or clublike structures interpretable as sensory nerve endings. The cells

FIGURE 21-9 Diagram showing ultrastructural characteristics of cells in the laryngobronchial epithelium.

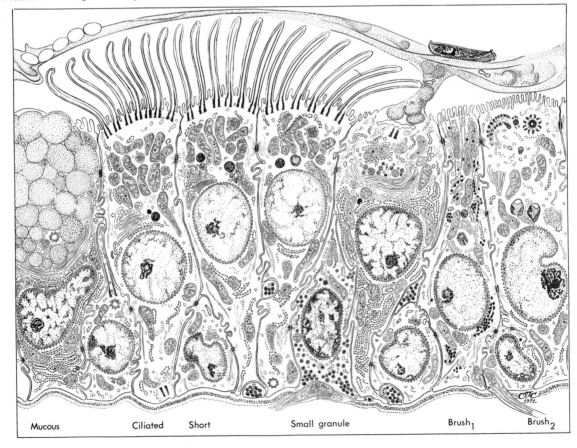

| Mucous | Ciliated | Short | Small granule | Brush₁ | Brush₂ |

themselves seem to be cholinergically innervated; for nerve processes, many bearing clear (*cholinergic*) synaptic vesicles frequently traverse the lamina propria beneath them en route to the epithelium. In the cell body, the Golgi apparatus is small and often lateral to the nucleus, while the approximately 1000-Å granules are concentrated in the basal cytoplasm. To judge from this kind of evidence, the cells participate as mediators in the integration of secretory processes. They are further described in the section on bronchioles as they occur in multicellular clusters.

Presumptively endocrine, small-granule cells occur singly among the cells of the epithelium. They tend to be more regularly columnar than the preceding cells, though they too have cytoplasmic processes, and they generally extend the full height of the epithelium. Among different members of the class, the gran-

FIGURE 21-10 Fluorescence resulting from uptake of L-dopa by small-granule cells of the upper tracheal epithelium of the rat. The section passes obliquely through the epithelium; an adrenergic nerve fiber fluoresces in the lamina propria beneath. ×364. (Work of R. Hoyt, Jr., A-W. El-Bermani, and S. Sorokin.)

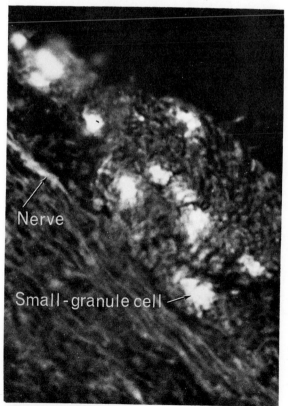

ules differ in mean diameter and in granular morphology as seen in electron micrographs. In some, as in the example illustrated, the Golgi apparatus is supranuclear, and the granules accumulate in the apical rather than the basal cytoplasm (Fig. 21-11).

The conducting airways also contain intraepithelial nerves. These are typical nervous processes containing parallel microtubular arrays along much of their length. They ramify throughout the lower part of the epithelium in potential spaces between the lateral surfaces of the cells. These spaces (Figs. 21-26, 21-27) open up somewhat when the cells become distended with fluid. More frequently they are obliterated, and adjacent cell membranes appear tightly interlocked. Epithelial elements including the small-granule cells are joined to each other on the sides by desmosomes and, where the cells reach the surface, by junctional complexes as well.

Tracheal glands share essential features and a certain variability as to cell type with the glands of the larynx and pulmonary bronchi (Fig. 21-12, *see color insert*). In humans they are mixed mucous glands with serous crescents, and they occur in far greater numbers than in the otherwise similar tracheas of the great apes. Around the tracheal lumen the glands generally extend into the submucosa. They are more highly developed dorsally where they may penetrate the muscularis to enter the adventitia. A more detailed discussion of the cell types in these glands will be found in the section on bronchi.

Connective Tissue

The connective tissue compartments of the trachea are not as well defined as they are in the walls of the alimentary tract (Chap. 18). This is especially true of small mammals where the total thickness of the tracheal wall is meager. In humans one distinguishes a lamina propria, a submucosa, and an adventitia. The lamina propria of the mucosa is a loose tissue containing interwoven collagenous and elastic fibers, many small vascular channels, and the usual fixed and wandering cells of connective tissue. The elastic fibers are joined into a continuous network in which the heavier fibers run in a predominantly longitudinal direction but are interconnected by slender fibrils (Fig. 21-13, *see color insert*). Peripherally these fibers become condensed into an *elastic membrane* that demarcates the lamina propria from the submucosa

(Fig. 21-21), which contains the distributing vessels and larger lymphatics of the tracheal wall. The submucosa has relatively fewer elastic fibers and more collagen than the propria; these fibers run in bundles among the glands and serve to bind the elastic network of the propria to the enveloping cartilaginous skeleton. The submucosa ends by blending into the perichondrium of the cartilages.

Cartilage

The tracheal cartilages are irregular, crescentic rings embedded in a fibrous connective tissue that forms a tube about the submucosa. There are 16 to 20 cartilages in humans. These are evenly spaced within the fibrous membrane, which normally is not fully stretched and so permits some tracheal movement. They sometimes branch, and adjacent cartilages

FIGURE 21-11 Endocrine type of small-granule cell in the laryngobronchial epithelium of *Myotis*. It is linked to other epithelial cells by conventional desmosomes (arrows) and passes over a process from a neurosecretory type of small-granule cell. ×11,700.

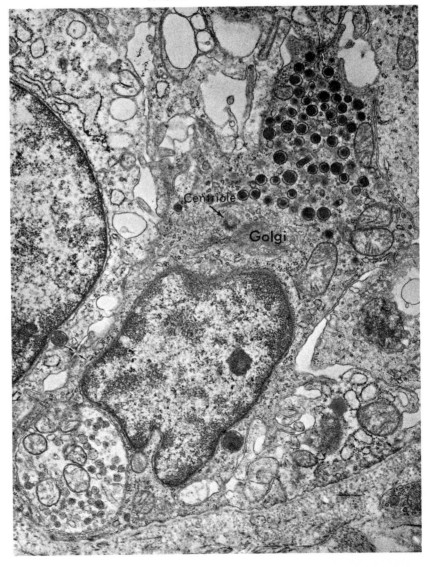

sometimes fuse with one another, but all are incomplete dorsally where the trachea contacts the esophagus. These gaps are bridged by fibrous tissue and bands of smooth muscle joining the ends of the cartilages. Near the tracheal bifurcation a few longitudinal muscle fibers run outside the transverse bands to link a number of the cartilages with the dorsal portion of the carinal ridge. This area receives additional support from the last cartilage, which extends under the bifurcation as well as around the sides of the trachea. In animals subject to unusually high transtracheal pressures, the tracheal skeleton may be modified in different ways. In seals the tracheal rings are supplemented by smaller cartilages embedded in the fibrous membrane, and the whole structure is stiffened; in bats the cartilages overlap each other like roofing tiles and provide additional buttressing at little cost in flexibility. Topographically, the tracheal skeleton occupies the innermost portion of the adventitia, but over the dorsum the muscularis takes up the corresponding part of the wall. Developmentally, the cartilage layer is distinct from the rest of the adventitia; the cartilages appear as independent chondrifications within a continuous, crescentic, cartilage-forming rudiment, which persists in adult life as the fibrous membrane. Histologically, the cartilages are hyaline but become fibrous with age. The perichondrium is virtually inseparable from the fibrous membrane and is thicker on the outer than on the inner surface of the rings. External to this region the adventitia becomes an areolar tissue rich in fat cells. It carries nerves and blood vessels to the trachea, receives its lymphatic drainage, and blends into tissues of the neck and of the mediastinum.

NERVES, BLOOD VESSELS, AND LYMPHATICS

The nervous, vascular, and lymphatic supplies to the trachea are independent of those to the lungs, although they resemble their counterparts in the walls of the larger pulmonary airways and function in concert with them. The trachea receives visceral afferent fibers and sympathetic and parasympathetic efferents. In its

innervation it differs from the pharynx or larynx principally in lacking a branchial motor component. The courses of individual fibers are all but impossible to trace because the sensory and autonomic nerves all contribute to plexuses formed about the viscera and while crossing them frequently exchange fibers. Rostral to the trachea such a plexus occurs in the lateral and dorsal walls of the pharynx, and caudally another (*pulmonary plexus*) occurs around the tracheal bifurcation. Some of the fibers in these networks end in the trachea. *Visceral afferent* fibers leave the trachea and adjacent structures through branches of the vagus nerve and travel to the nodose ganglion, or else they separate in the pharyngeal plexus and pass through the sympathetic trunk to reach cell bodies in the dorsal root ganglia of cervical and upper thoracic nerves. Cell bodies of preganglionic *sympathetic* efferents occur at upper thoracic levels of the spinal cord. Postganglionic fibers are said to originate from the three cervical ganglia and from the upper thoracic portion of the sympathetic trunk. Preganglionic *parasympathetic* fibers originate in the dorsal motor nucleus of the vagus and synapse with second-order neurons located in small tracheal ganglia embedded in the adventitia and submucosa. Fibers of all the foregoing types reach the tracheal wall chiefly from the left side through the left recurrent nerve, but some reach it from the right through the vagus and its right recurrent branch.

Tracheal tissues receive systemic blood through branches of the inferior thyroid arteries. These ramify in the submucosa and near the carina anastomose with bronchial arteries, which supply the walls of bronchi. Venous blood drains through the thyroid venous plexus and returns to the systemic circuit via the middle and inferior thyroid veins. Tracheal lymphatics lead out laterally to a few paratracheal nodes located beside the recurrent nerves, as well as to nodes of the superior deep cervical chain.

THE LUNGS

EXTERNAL FORM

The primary bronchi of the right and left lungs arise in the mediastinum from the bifurcation of the trachea.

They follow a short extrapulmonary course and together with the main pulmonary vessels and nerves enter the hilum of their respective lungs. These occupy the thoracic cavity which is smaller on the left than on the right owing to the position of the heart. Consequently, the right lung is always larger than the left and almost always is subdivided into a greater number of *lobes.* The lobes are separated from each other to varying degrees among different animal species but are confluent medially in the vicinity of the main bronchus. In humans there are three on the right lung and two on the left, but in many mammals the right lung has a fourth, infracardiac lobe extending between the heart and the diaphragm. Where the heart strongly inclines to the left, as in the insectivores, the left lung has but one lobe. Just as the lungs can be subdivided into lobes, the lobes can be subdivided into smaller units, termed *bronchopulmonary segments, subsegments,* and *lobules;* these are demarcated to varying degrees by fissures on the lobar surfaces. For all its varied appearance, the outward form of the lung imperfectly reflects its underlying structure, for a sheet of visceral pleura covers the surfaces. In providing an airtight capsule the pleura effectively conceals the system of airways together with associated respiratory tissue and vascular supplies that form the structural basis of the organ.

INTERNAL STRUCTURE

The lungs of birds and mammals are structurally the most complex of vertebrate lungs. Each is marvelously adapted to supply the large amounts of oxygen that these animals use; avian and mammalian lungs nevertheless differ basically from each other in the organization of conducting and respiratory regions. This chapter is concerned only with mammalian lungs, which share a single structural plan among all their prototherian, metatherian, and eutherian representatives. Wide variations on this plan nevertheless occur in some mammalian groups, especially among the marine mammals.

Each lung is organized fundamentally about its system of airways, metaphorically termed the *bronchial* tree. In this system the primary bronchus is a trunk that divides into a number of branches. These subdivide into smaller branches, and so on until tiny, thin-walled spaces are reached, where respiratory exchange takes place. In such an arrangement a given branch of the bronchial tree will ventilate a definite part of the respiratory surface. As a system of air conduits the bronchial tree is best visualized in casts

prepared by filling all but the last few generations of branches with latex or plastic casting materials, for then the branching pattern can be studied to advantage (Fig. 21-14). If the entire bronchial tree is cast, it takes on the form of the intact lung and appears solid.

The three-dimensional structure of the lungs is fully achieved by superimposing additional branching systems on the basic bronchial tree. The most important of these is the pulmonary vascular circuit consisting of the pulmonary arteries, capillaries, and veins (Figs. 21-15, 21-58, *color insert,* and 21-59, *color insert*). The arteries spread over the dorsolateral surfaces of the bronchial tree and follow its divisions precisely until in the respiratory region the vessels divide into capillaries. The bronchial arteries, pulmonary lymphatics, and nerves all follow the bronchial tree as closely as the pulmonary artery does; they also ramify along the pulmonary vessels and extend into the pleura. Pulmonary veins form at the boundaries between regions ventilated by adjacent bronchi and run within interfacial connective tissue to the main pulmonary veins, which are suspended from the ventral surfaces of the bronchi. A common adventitia of connective tissue invests the bronchial tree and associated blood vessels. It continues outward along the veins where it blends in with the surrounding septal tissue. At the surface this tissue becomes confluent with the connective tissue of the visceral pleura. The branching systems in the lungs thereby become bound together and linked through septa to capsular tissue at the surface. The larger of these septa run out to the lobar fissures and hence are *interlobar septa.* Others follow planes of separation between the segments of a lobe and are *intersegmental septa;* still others less regularly subdivide smaller parts of the lung.

Bronchopulmonary Segments

Clinical interest in the branching pattern of human lungs usually extends to the level of bronchopulmonary segments. These are supplied by branches of the lobar bronchi or by branches that immediately follow them; consequently segmental bronchi are third- or fourth-order branches. There are three segments in the right upper lobe, two in the middle, and five in the lower lobe. On the left there are five altogether in both divisions of the upper lobe and five in the lower lobe. From the preceding it can be seen that the segments carry their own arterial supply, which branches with the bronchi, and that they are bounded by connective tissue septa. At this level the bronchial tree rarely exhibits an unusual branching pattern. When anomalies occur, they do so at predictable sites, and the segmental artery is displaced along with the bronchus. This makes it feasible for surgeons to perform successful partial resections of the lungs in cases of serious pulmonary disease.

Branching of the Airways

The most typical mammalian lungs are adapted to fit comfortably within long, narrow, and deep thoracic

FIGURE 21-14 Cast of the left bronchial tree of a child, age 7 years, 10 months, in mediastinal view. 1–10, segmental bronchi; ×4a, displaced subsegmental branch, *, subsuperior bronchus of lower lobe. ×0.8. (Courtesy of E. A. Boyden and D. H. Tompsett.)

cavities such as many quadrupeds possess. In these the primary bronchi run caudally from the hilum toward the dorsomedial inferior angle of each lung. Secondary bronchi arise predominantly as outward-directed lateral branches of the primary bronchi. They also form a dorsal and a less complete ventral series and rarely an internal lateral one as well. The primary bronchus thereby serves as an axis for each lung. The secondary branches are largest cranially and smallest

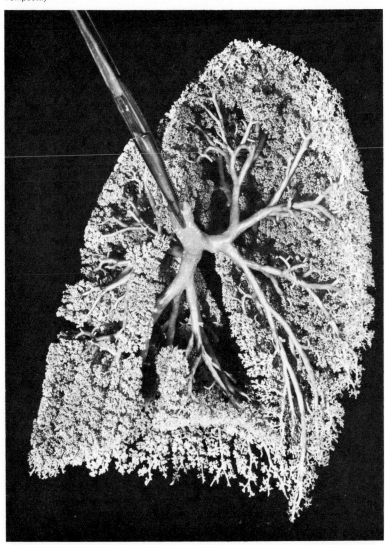

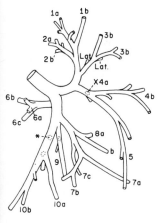

786

caudally. They are given off fairly regularly, the lateral branches in alternation with the dorsoventral sets. In humans the lungs are squeezed into a short, broad, and shallow thorax; accordingly, the pattern of bronchial branching is atypical. Informed opinion holds that the primary bronchi of humans are not true axial structures but give rise to three secondary bronchi in the right lung and two in the left. These become the lobar bronchi, and each develops its own pattern of branching.

Like the trachea, many of the subsidiary bronchi branch by unequal dichotomy, whereby the smaller of two diverging bronchi veers more from the path of its parent than the other. From this viewpoint, the bronchial tree consists of a sequence of unequal branchings that vary in number, depending on whether

counts are made in long or in short segments. In humans as many as 25 generations can be counted in the longest segmental bronchi, making the maximum number of divisions 27 or 28 starting from the primary bronchus. Nevertheless, because of the variation in size of bronchi belonging to the same branching order, and because of the variability in the number of generations between the trachea and the respiratory zone, the bronchial tree is not adequately described in this manner but yields more useful information when approached in other ways. These are discussed below.

The caliber of the airways and the angles of branching have been measured in bronchial trees of human and canine lungs. These data enable one to estimate patterns of airflow and the completeness of ventilation in various parts of the lung more accurately than is possible when calculations are based on abstract models. In these species the distance from the carina to the respiratory surface (the *bronchial path*

FIGURE 21-15 X-ray of autopsied left human lung showing pulmonary arterial tree as revealed after injection of contrast material. Compare pattern with that of the left bronchial tree (Fig. 21-14).

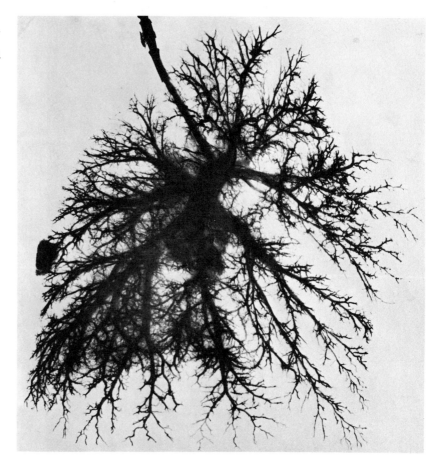

length) varies considerably in different parts of the lung. This inequality represents an accommodation of the bronchial tree to available space and is smaller in humans than in the long-chested dog, where the paths range from 2 mm to 12 cm, beginning with the base of the lobar bronchus. Other things being equal, bronchi of equal caliber have about the same number of terminal airways, and these lead to an approximately equal area of respiratory surface. Nevertheless, where the bronchial path is longer, its airways are of larger caliber than where the path is shorter; a lowered airway resistance is compensation for the long path. The main defect in this arrangement is that the respiratory surface at the end of these long pathways is exposed to a disproportionately large volume of residual air in the bronchial tree (the *anatomical dead space*), and under certain circumstances this may lead to unequal ventilation of ambient air in different regions of the lung.

As the bronchi bifurcate, the total cross-sectional area of the airway increases by a factor of about 1.3 in the first five generations and by somewhat more thereafter. If the total cross-sectional area is measured at successive distances from the carina, it is seen to reach a peak and then to decline. At first the increments due to branching predominate over the decrements due to termination of the smaller bronchial paths. Subsequently the terminations predominate. The effect of these anatomic arrangements is to make the conducting portions of the lungs as small as possible. In living specimens the airway is flexible and changes its configuration with each breathing cycle. It has been likened to a gradually expanding funnel on inspiration but to a cylinder during expiration, owing to changes in the diameters of distal bronchi (Fig. 21-16).

Along the distal half of a bronchial pathway the airways divide at regular intervals, often forking obtusely and always decreasing in caliber after branching. Farther along, a fairly abrupt transition leads to a region where branching is frequent and the branches are short and slender. In humans these patterns can be seen in bronchograms made after instilling radiopaque material in the bronchial tree. The coarser branching occurs at 0.5- to 1-cm intervals along an axial path of several centimeters; the finer branching occurs at intervals of 2 to 3 mm and extends about 1 cm farther (Fig. 21-17). The fine-meshed pattern is found in the distal part of all bronchial pathways whether they end deep in the lungs or near the pleural surface. By means of correlated histologic study it has been established that the final branches of this network are ter-

minal conducting airways. The respiratory portion of the lung begins immediately afterward, the region ventilated by one terminal radiating from the outlet for a distance of 2 to 5 mm.

The larger airways of the lungs are called *bronchi* and the smaller ones are called *bronchioles*. These are essentially anatomic terms but a fairly characteristic histologic appearance is associated with each. In humans the bronchi comprise some 9 to 12 generations, beginning with the primary bronchus and ending with airways having a caliber of approximately 1 mm. The bronchioles begin as branches of the smallest bronchi and in humans continue for up to 12 generations before ending as terminal bronchioles. A range is given because the number of bronchial and bronchiolar divisions vary, depending on the segment counted. Histologically, bronchi cannot be distinguished from bronchioles on the basis of a single characteristic. For example, it is often stated that bronchi contain cartilage in their walls whereas bronchioles do not. With such definitions one soon runs into terminologic difficulty: In the howling monkey and in many microchiropteran bats there is virtually no intrapulmonary cartilage (Fig. 21-18). On the other hand, in whales the cartilage extends to well beyond the conducting airways. In humans it is continued for varying distances along the part of the bronchial tree having the centimeter-branching pattern; the millimeter-branching airways are safely termed bronchioles.

Bronchi

For a short distance beyond their origin, extrapulmonary bronchi retain the structural organization of the trachea and a similar histologic appearance in the mucosa, submucosa, muscularis, and adventitia. Gradually two major changes become manifest. (1) the cartilaginous rings become less regular and (2) the muscularis develops into a complete ring of smooth muscle located between the submucosa and the cartilage. At first the bronchial cartilages only become shorter and narrower than those of the trachea, but not far beyond the hilum they become highly irregular in shape. Viewed in cross sections of the bronchi, the cartilages often seem isolated (Fig. 21-19), but viewed in three dimensions they remain part of a comprehensive skeletal framework. At bronchial bifurcations they are often saddle-shaped. Farther along the airway they become reduced to solitary

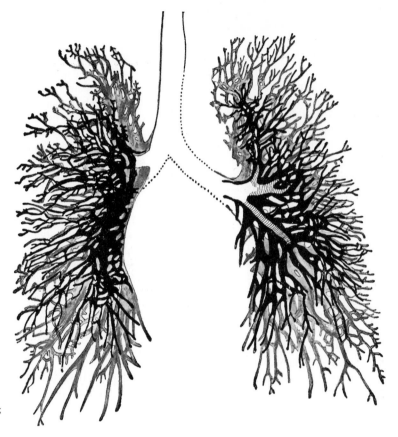

FIGURE 21-16 Bronchial tree. Tracings made from x-ray shadows. Gray, inspiration; black, expiration. (Work of C. C. Macklin.)

FIGURE 21-17 Centimeter and millimeter branching patterns in the peripheral airway. The end branches are terminal bronchioles. About natural size. (After L. Reid and G. Simon, *Thorax,* **13:**103, 1958.)

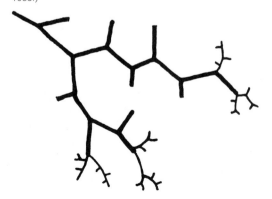

fragments. As in the trachea, the cartilages are hyaline, although parts of them are infiltrated with elastic fibers, especially in the smaller bronchi. The muscularis becomes a more prominent layer as the cartilages decline. It is made up of numerous fascicles of some 20 to 30 cells each (Figs. 21-18 and 21-20). These fascicles can be identified as separate entities, but in the bronchi they are closely packed into a continuous layer, and they all follow fairly similar circular or spiral courses about the airway. In the bronchi as in the trachea, the muscle fibers attach to each other as well as to the fibrous framework of the airway (Fig. 21-13). Some muscle fibers in the outer part of the muscularis are joined to the fibrous membrane that envelops the cartilages. This membrane also serves as an attachment for numerous fine elastic and collagenous fibers that cross the muscularis to join heavier fibrous networks in the connective tissue beneath the epithelium.

As the bronchial generations are traced, the airway gradually undergoes a change from a histologic appearance typical of bronchi (Fig. 21-19) toward one typical of bronchioles. With continued branching, the bronchial wall decreases in thickness, but all layers of the wall are not decreased proportionately. The disproportion alone accounts for most of the change in appearance. As the bronchi become smaller, the pseudostratified epithelium becomes lower. Connective tissue compartments internal to the muscularis become reduced in width. In small bronchi the lamina propria becomes so thin that the fibers of its elastic membrane lie immediately beneath the epithelium. The submucosa remains appreciably thick where it

FIGURE 21-18 Section of a bat's lung near the hilum showing the trachea and primary bronchi and part of the right lung. Glands are coextensive with the cartilage of the bronchial wall and in this species occur largely in the adventitia. Iron hematoxylin. ×30.

houses the acini of the bronchial glands. It contains branches of the bronchial arteries, which supply nutrient capillary beds for the airway. Near the hilum it contains the bronchial veins as well.

If the cells and collagenous fibers of an inflated lung are digested away, a skeleton of elastic tissue remains, perfect in its preservation of the outlines of the bronchial tree, the pulmonary alveoli, and the blood vessels (Fig. 21-22). In the airways the elastic skeleton comprises mainly the longitudinally oriented proprial fibers and elastic fibers in the fibrocartilaginous membrane of the inner adventitia (Figs. 21-12,

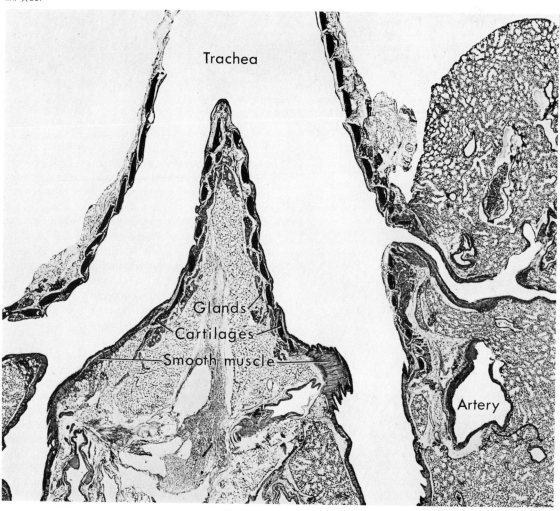

Trachea

Glands
Cartilages
Smooth muscle

Artery

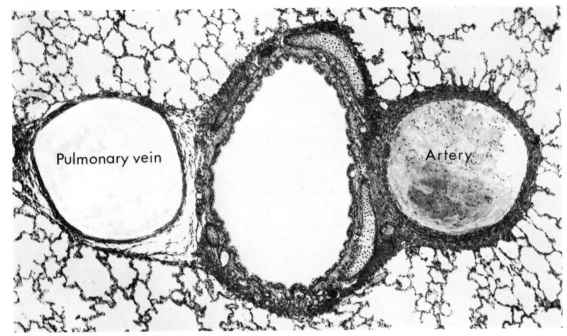

FIGURE 21-19 Cross section of a bronchus in a kitten. Mallory azan stain. ×85.

FIGURE 21-20 Adenosine triphosphatase activity in the lung of a beaver. The bronchial smooth muscle is strongly reactive at the cell margin (black) as is a small blood vessel in the space above. Gomori method, pH 9.4. ×350.

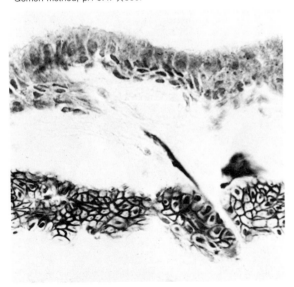

21-13, and 21-21). Submucosal fibers serve to suspend the mucosa from the outer layers of the airway and to support the blood vessels and glands within the submucosa. Consequently, these fibers take a more radial course overall than the proprial fibers. In the muscularis the fibers run in various, often circular, directions. Reticular fibers are distributed with the elastic fibers. They lie just beneath the epithelial basement lamina and form a delicate tracery around individual stromal cells. The coarser collagenous fibers are everywhere present in the connective tissues but are densest in the common investments of the major pulmonary septa, vessels, and bronchi.

Bronchial Glands

The bronchial glands closely resemble the numerous small glands located in the upper air passages. They are coextensive with the cartilaginous skeleton. Accordingly, along certain bronchial paths in humans they come as close as 2 to 3 cm from the pleura but approach less closely in other paths. In bats they scarcely extend beyond the hilum (Fig. 21-18). Surface mucous cells and these glands together produce the secretions that coat the surfaces of the airways. The relative contributions of the two sources differ

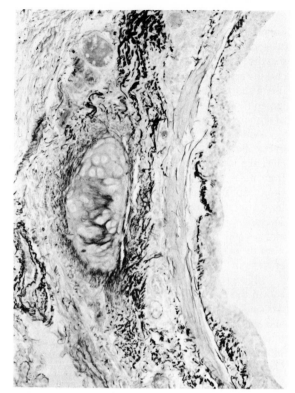

FIGURE 21-21 Cross section of a child's bronchus stained for elastic fibers. These are formed into an elastic membrane between the epithelium and muscularis, into a circular pattern in the muscularis, and into a longitudinal adventitial network. The cartilage is partly elastic. ×150.

small-granule cells similar to those in the surface epithelium and a number of unusual cell types that are inconspicuous in paraffin sections and, lacking mucoid droplets, are usually classified as serous cells. There is evidence that the human bronchial tree secretes several types of mucins; nevertheless, it is not certain whether the secretions are produced by one or by several different cell types. In the glands four acid glycoproteins are found—two sialomucins and two sulfomucins—and they are distributed differentially among the mucous cells. These cells resemble the surface mucous cells in fine-structural characteristics and in possessing secretory droplets that tend to coalesce. Since the surface cells of the larger airways produce sulfomucin and those more peripheral produce sialomucin, it would seem that all these products are made by cells similar in appearance. Nonetheless, in some species the bronchial glands possess still other mucoid cells. These have small secretory droplets like those in surface mucous cells of the gastric glands (Chap. 18). Even less is known about the serous cells

FIGURE 21-22 Thick section of a rat lung prepared to show the elastic fiber skeleton. Resorcin-fuchsin stain. ×80.

according to the species studied; this difference is compounded in the presence of chronic disease. As glands disappear from the airway, the surface mucous cells often increase in number. They are carried farther into the bronchial tree than the glands and end in the bronchioles. The glands are supplied by bronchial vascular beds furnished with fenestrated capillaries (Fig. 21-55). As described in the section on the larynx, glandular acini are penetrated by both sensory and secretomotor nerve endings. In contrast, the overlying pseudostratified epithelium has sensory but few motor endings. This difference may explain why the glands readily secrete after stimulation of parasympathetic nerves, whereas the surface cells respond more clearly to local irritation.

The major constituents of the glands are both mucous and serous epithelial cells, the myoepithelium, and at times some unspecialized, cuboidal lining cells in the larger ducts. Minor constituents include

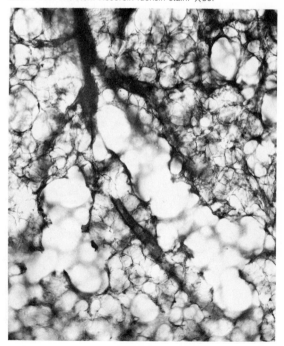

than the mucous cells, but among unusual cells grouped in this category, human glands have an acidophilic *oncocyte* and opossums have a *hydrotic* cell that seems capable of performing osmotic work. Stellate *myoepithelial* cells are found in the acini and partway up the ducts. They rest on the epithelial side of the basement lamina and encircle the secretory cells with their processes. They possess ultrastructural features of smooth muscle and by their contraction help to expel the contents from secreting glands (Fig. 21-23).

Bronchioles

At some point along any given bronchial path the airway, having lost its bronchial characteristics, gradually acquires new ones; the airway is then called a bronchiole (Fig. 21-24). It retains the radial organization of preceding passages but no longer is lined by a laryngobronchial type of epithelium, nor does it have cartilage, glands, or a continuous muscularis. New features are (1) a columnar epithelium in which a unique type of secretory cell displaces the mucous cell; (2) a proportional increase, compared with large bronchi, in the thickness of the muscularis; and (3) a separation of smooth muscle fascicles by connective tissue (Fig. 21-25). This effectively unites all connective tissue compartments of the bronchiolar wall into one investing mass.

Two major cell types, more of them ciliated than nonciliated, line the bronchioles (Fig. 21-26). The ciliated cells are similar to those in the bronchi except that they are shorter. The nonciliated *bronchiolar* cells give the epithelium its special character. These are tall, dome-shaped cells that protrude into the bronchiolar lumen to the tips of the cilia. Accordingly, in sections of bronchioles the epithelium has a scalloped contour.

As in many water-permeable epithelia, cytoplasmic leaflets extend from the lateral surfaces of both ciliated and nonciliated cells to intermingle with those from adjacent cells (Figs. 21-26 and 21-27). Moreover, capillary loops close to the basement lamina have discrete, fenestrated areas facing the epithelium. These features occur elsewhere along the conducting airways and in the body. They are a part of a mechanism to provide regulated water transport across the epithelium.

Reconstructions of the bronchiolar wall have shown the smooth muscle to be formed into a geodesic network. The separate fascicles of muscle branch and anastomose so that some fibers run circularly and others obliquely. Through this arrangement the force of contraction is exerted perpendicular to the wall. Owing to the comparative strength of the muscularis in the bronchioles, contractions are felt there more strongly than in the bronchi. Like muscles of the

FIGURE 21-23 Diagram showing a three-dimensional view of the acinus and duct of a bronchial gland. (Drawing by G. Pederson-Krag in S. Sorokin, *Am. J. Anat.,* **117:**311, 1965.)

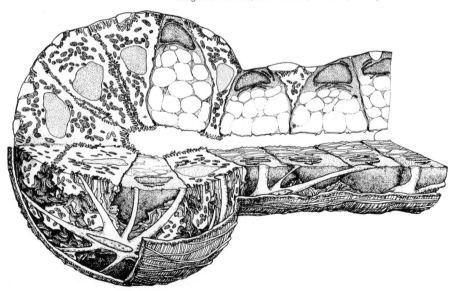

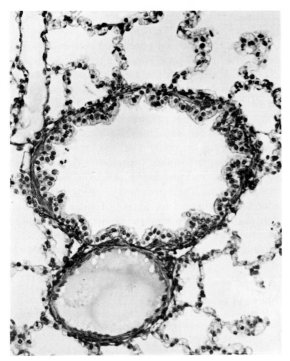

FIGURE 21-24 Bronchiole and small pulmonary artery in a kitten's lung. Mallory azan stain. ×125.

alimentary tract, those of the airway are activated by parasympathetic fibers and are known to undergo peristaltic movements. They participate in the cough reflex and increase bronchial tone in cold weather. They also relax during inspiration and contract at the end of expiration, thereby helping bronchial fiber systems to return distended airways to resting dimensions.

Bronchiolar Epithelial Cells

The basic organization of *bronchiolar cells* (Clara cells) gives them an unmistakable identity in the lungs of many mammals, even though striking interspecies differences may still be present in one or more of the cytoplasmic organelles. With a basal ergastoplasm and apical, membrane-bounded droplets, these cells can be classified as serous cells, but they contrast with others of this class in possessing an unusual abundance of agranular reticulum in the supranuclear and apical cytoplasm (Fig. 21-27). This predominates over the Golgi lamellae, the lysosomal particulates, the apical centrioles, and other normal features of the region. A granular reticulum, Golgi apparatus, and secretory granules are typical features of all cells man-

ufacturing proteins for export. In bronchiolar cells of mice, radioactively labeled leucine becomes incorporated into the granules after first passing through these organelles, and this suggests that proteins are included in the secretory product. Bronchiolar cells are among the more metabolically active cells in the lungs (Figs. 21-33 and 21-41). They have also been shown to incorporate into the granules both tritiated acetate and galactose, plausible precursors of lipid and polysaccharide, respectively. In several species the secretory droplets are like zymogen granules of other cells (Fig. 21-27); in rats they have a crystalline substructure; but in mice they appear electron-lucent (Fig. 21-28), as if rich in lipid. Mature granules in rats are said to be inactive for acid phosphatase and esterase, enzymes reactive in the bronchiolar cells' lysosomes, but very little positive information has been obtained about specific granule contents. Any full explanation of the functions of bronchiolar cells must account for the extensive agranular reticulum so regularly present. This organelle is well developed in cells substantially engaged in either cholesterol or carbohydrate synthesis, and experimental evidence rather confirms that the agranular reticulum of bronchiolar cells actively synthesizes both classes of compounds. In mice, both acetate and galactose appear in this cytoplasmic compartment; and in bats, glycogen accumulates against its cytoplasmic face (Fig. 21-28). An extensive agranular reticulum may also appear near the free surface of certain ion-segregating cells. It then possesses ion pumping sites and other characteristics of the plasmalemma, for in reality it is an extension of the surface. Such a reticulum usually exhibits many points of continuity with this surface, however; and these are not seen in bronchiolar cells. Material from both Golgi and agranular membranes is pinched off into the secretory granules, and they are slowly and individually released from the cells into the bronchiolar lumen (Fig. 21-27, inset). The surface fluid is rich in protein and also contains mucopolysaccharides and cholesterol, substances similarly present in secretions released in pulmonary alveoli (discussed under alveolar cells). To what extent alveolar and bronchiolar fluids are similar cannot be answered precisely, but it seems that surface tension-reducing lipid, abundant in alveoli, is relatively scarce in bronchioles.

In rodents, rabbits, and humans, bronchiolar cell mitochondria are unusually large, globose bodies with a voluminous matrix and few cristae (Fig. 21-28); tritiated acetate incorporation into such mitochondria is also high. In other species the mitochondria are more conventional in appearance.

Bronchiolar cells are present in a greater part of the bronchial tree of small as compared with large animals, probably because most of the branches are of small caliber. That is to say, bronchiolar cells will occur in airways if they are somewhat smaller than a millimeter in diameter. In chronic bronchitis the bronchioles are the main sites of obstruction by cellular debris and mucus; keeping this in mind, one might guess that secretions of bronchiolar cells serve to prevent this in normal subjects by providing proteo- or mucolytic enzymes and possibly nonenzymic substances to alter the stickiness of the secretions released higher up in the bronchial tree. These cells lie *distal* to the mucus-producing areas of the lungs just as serous cells generally are distal to mucous cells in glands, perhaps for a similar reason.

Compared with the nonciliated bronchiolar cells, the ciliated cells have longer microvilli, somewhat obscured by the cilia, the rudiments of a system of approximately (ca. 600-Å) tubular invaginations extending in from the apical surface, and rather large, sometimes extremely electron-dense lysosomal residual bodies (Fig. 21-27). These features arguably endow the ciliated better than the bronchiolar cells with whatever endocytotic capacity the epithelium has for both dissolved and finely particulate matter. This normally is small but experimentally demonstrable and a significant channel for uptake of airborne material deposited in the bronchioles under conditions where mucociliary clearance becomes impeded and material remains for some time on the surface. Some of this is

FIGURE 21-25 Longitudinal section of bronchiolar epithelium of a rat, showing ciliated and bronchiolar cells. Beneath the epithelium, bundles of smooth muscle are separated by connective tissue. Toluidine blue. ×1440.

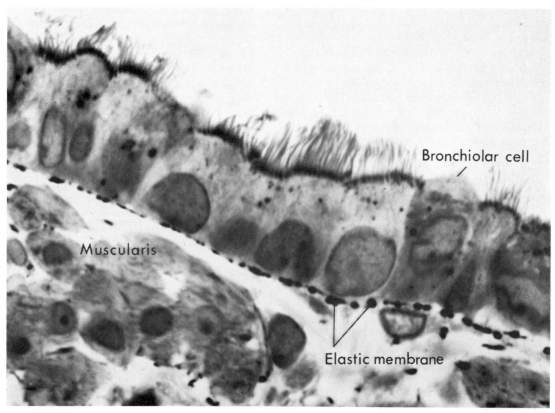

shunted into the lateral channels between cells and some reaches the connective tissue beneath.

Neurosecretory small-granule cells (previously described under tracheal epithelium) are usually organized into *neuroepithelial bodies* when they occur in small-caliber intrapulmonary airways, but in this grouped arrangement the cells have also been observed higher up the bronchial tree and distally as far as the pulmonary alveoli. In conventional histological sections, a keen observer might recognize them as a cluster of somewhat eosinophilic and columnar cells perhaps 8 to 10 cells wide, intercalated in the epithelium, and slightly bulging into the lamina propria. With staining techniques that delimit the intrapulmonary nerves, the cluster is argyrophilic, and the granules in the cells are faintly argentaffin. After exposure of freeze-dried sections to formaldehyde vapor and examination by fluorescence microscopy, the cells are

revealed by the yellow fluorescence of the biogenic amines stored in the granules. Like other types of small-granule cells, those of the neuroepithelial bodies convert exogenously administered amine precursors like deoxyphenylalanine by decarboxylation into dopamine, which is stored and gives off a telltale yellowish-green fluorescence. Individual outlines of the clustered small-granule cells are difficult to trace in electron micrographs; because, apart from extending fingerlike cytoplasmic processes beyond the cell body, the perinuclear cytoplasm itself interdigitates with adjacent cells in a complex manner. Cytoplasmic detail is more difficult to preserve in these cells than in other epithelial cells, and granule morphology varies somewhat according to the method of cell fixation, but the granules remain about 1000 Å in diameter and with their yellow fluorescence are nonetheless identifiable as stores principally of 5-hydroxytryptamine. The cells

FIGURE 21-26 Electron micrograph of bronchiolar epithelium of a bat, showing bronchiolar (upper left) and ciliated cells and the lateral interdigitations between cells. ×7000.

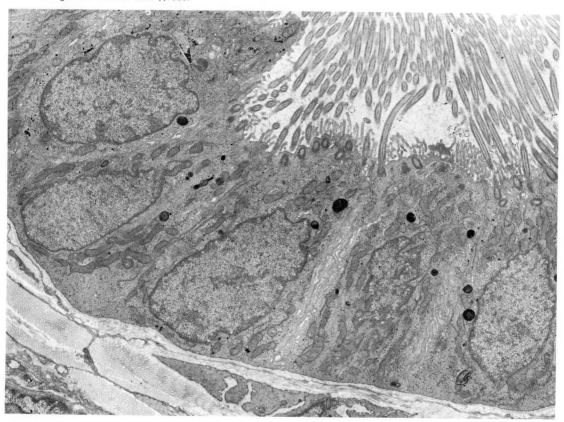

are reached by unmyelinated nerve fibers bearing clear synaptic vesicles. Synaptic contact between these cells and the nerves have been observed to occur at points where the vesicles are abundant in the nerve ending, but at the point illustrated (Fig. 21-29, open arrows) a conjectural "synapse" occurs where the nerve process is filled with mitochondria and has only a few vesicles. Deeper in the neuroepithelial body, sections frequently pass through unsheathed nerve processes,

which suggests that the cells in the cluster may be separately innervated. The general impression is that the small-granule cells are interposed between motor and sensory endings coming from the central nervous system and that their mode of operation is multifaceted. It has been proposed on the one hand that the cells respond to hypoxia in the airway by chemore-

FIGURE 21-27 Typical features of *bronchiolar cells* are a basal granular endoplasmic reticulum (GER), apical smooth reticulum (SER), and secretory granules, which are released at the free surface (inset). Intercellular channels and a large residual body (black) in a ciliated cell are also shown. Vampire bat. ×9450.

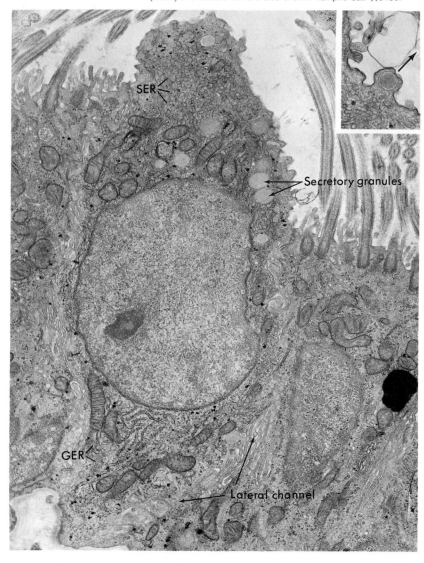

SER

Secretory granules

GER

Lateral channel

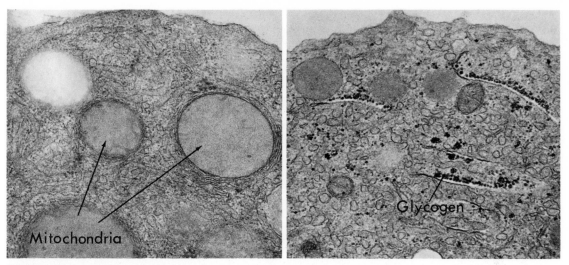

FIGURE 21-28 Detail of apical cytoplasm in bronchiolar cells of a mouse (left) and a bat (right). ×30,000.

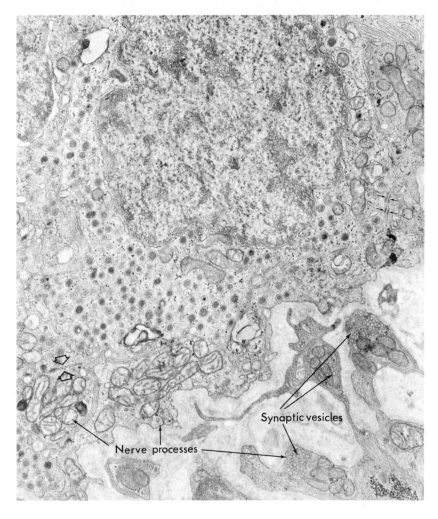

FIGURE 21-29 Small-granule cells of a bronchiolar neuro-epithelial body. Various unmyelinated nerves approach from below, and a mitochondria-rich process closely contacts one of the cells (open arrows), which all join adjacent epithelial cells by desmosomes (paired arrows). Vampire bat. ×12,000.

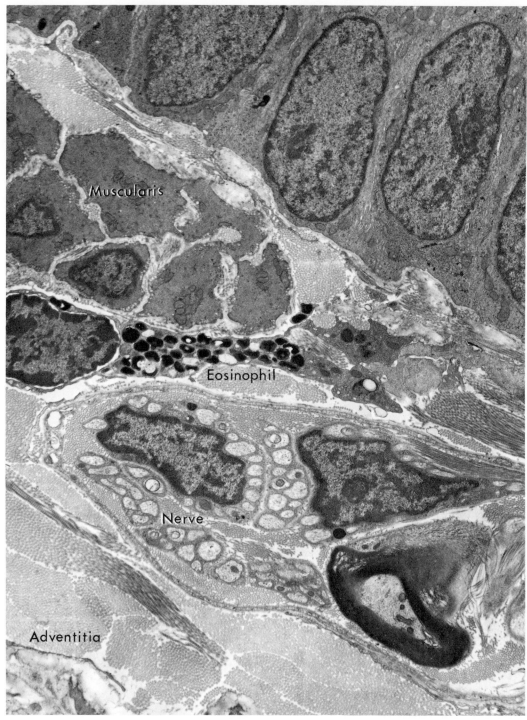

FIGURE 21-30 Electron micrograph showing bronchiolar connective tissue. A peribronchial nerve bundle carries a single myelinated axon and several small unmyelinated fibers wrapped in Schwann cell mesaxons. ×8000.

ception and a release of granules at the cell base. These may be circulated locally via the bronchial capillary plexus to affect airway smooth muscle, or else may be conveyed to the pulmonary veins via bronchopulmonary veins (discussed below under pulmonary circulation) to bring about venoconstriction and other more general effects. On the other hand, the cells may degranulate as well on stimulation by the central nervous system, and some of their effects may be on epithelial cells touched by their processes.

Apart from the preceding neuroepithelial cells, the bronchiolar epithelium has been reported to contain a presumably sensory brush cell like that figured in the trachea (Fig. 21–9, brush$_1$).

THE RESPIRATORY ZONE

Respiratory Bronchioles and Subdivisions

Each terminal bronchiole divides into two daughter branches called *respiratory bronchioles*. These resemble the terminal bronchiole in all but one respect: here and there the walls are interrupted by saccular outpocketings called *alveoli*, where respiratory gas exchange takes place (Figs. 21-31, 21-32, 21-33). At once possessing a respiratory surface and a bronchiolar structure, respiratory bronchioles are aptly

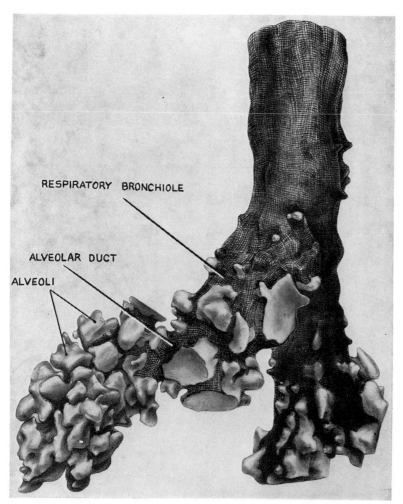

FIGURE 21-31 Cast model of a respiratory bronchiole with its subdivisions. Several alveolar ducts have been removed. The gradual onset of alveolarization along the bronchial path is clearly shown, although individual alveoli appear partly collapsed. The cross-hatching represents the approximate extent of the muscular coat in the airway. (From J. L. Bremer, *Carnegie Institute Contrib. Embryol.*, 1935.)

named. Subsequently the number of alveoli increase with each branching of the airway, and after about five divisions from the terminal bronchiole, the pathway ends in grapelike clusters of alveoli. As these branches are traversed, the fraction of the wall taken up by alveoli increases, until the wall becomes little more than a series of openings into the alveoli. At that point the branches still retain the appearance of a conduit and are called *alveolar ducts*. Farther on, the tubular sense is lost, and the remaining spaces are called, successively, *atria, alveolar sacs,* and *alveoli* (Figs. 21-34 and 21-36). The respiratory surface aerated by one terminal bronchiole is partitioned among the alveoli located all along the succeeding branches.

In adult humans there are normally three orders of respiratory bronchioles, and where they are not interrupted by alveoli, the walls are lined by a low columnar epithelium containing ciliated and bronchiolar cells. At the alveolar rim these cells become continuous with the thin alveolar lining. Beneath the

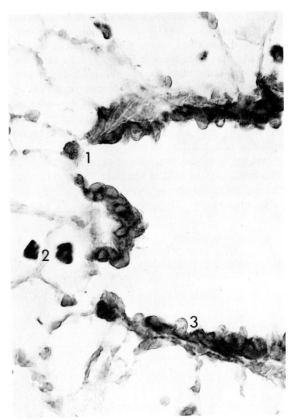

FIGURE 21-33 Respiratory bronchiole of a bat reacted for acid phosphatase. Ciliated cells and alveolar macrophages (2) are strongly reactive; great alveolar cells (1) and bronchiolar cells (3), less so. Burstone's method. ×200.

FIGURE 21-32 Respiratory bronchiole of a kitten. Note the low columnar epithelium on the left and the alveoli on the right. Mallory azan stain. ×125.

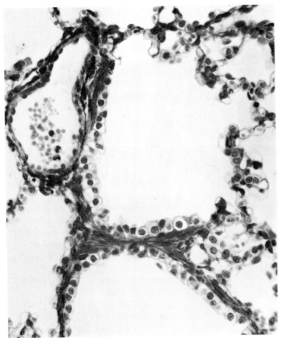

epithelium the muscularis remains prominent within an investment of connective tissue that contains vascular beds and pulmonary nerves (Fig. 21-30) and is carried into the alveolar walls. The respiratory bronchioles are followed by about two generations of *alveolar ducts*. Along their highly alveolated walls the ducts exhibit bronchiolar characteristics only in the few places where a group of columnar epithelial cells cover underlying bands of muscle and connective tissue. The muscle forms a terminal sphincter at the outlet of the last alveolar duct and almost always ends there (Figs. 21-35 and 21-36). Evidently because the bronchiolar and alveolar epithelia are closely related biologically, alveolar epithelial cells sometimes are admixed in the lining of the ducts. The alveolar ducts open into *atria*, which are vestibules communicating with the multilocular *alveolar sacs*. Occasionally one but usually two or more sacs arise from each atrium.

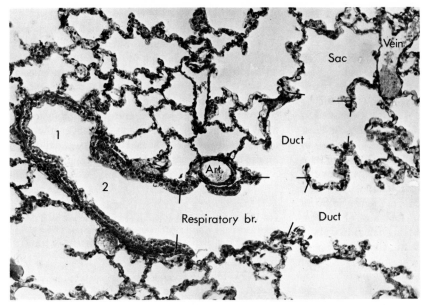

FIGURE 21-34 Terminal bronchial pathway in a kitten's lung. The two last bronchiolar orders (1,2), a short respiratory bronchiole, its pulmonary artery (Art.), and subsequent respiratory structures are shown. The alveolated passages may vary in overall proportions among different species. Mallory's azan. ×76.

FIGURE 21-35 Transition from the alveolar duct to the atrial space. Bronchiolar cells, a great alveolar cell, and a squamous alveolar cell are in continuity. The terminal muscle sphincter lies beneath. ×5000.

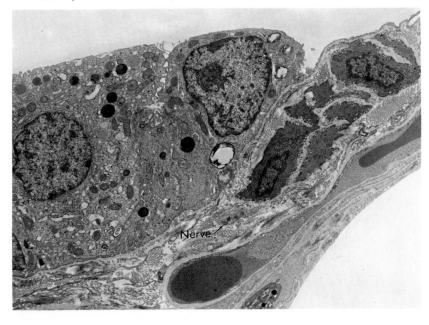

These are irregular cavities surrounded by pulmonary *alveoli*, which are the individual locules of the sacs. The alveoli are the smallest subdivisions of the respiratory tree. Within a given lung they are of fairly uniform size, but their dimensions are proportioned to the metabolic rate of the animal, being smallest (30 μm) in shrews and bats and largest (1,100 μm) in the large and sluggish Sirenia. In human beings, a total of some 300 million alveoli is divided between the lungs, and individual alveoli measure about 200 μm in diameter. Beyond the alveolar ducts the elastic fibers abandon their predominantly longitudinal course along the airway and form a complex network of fibers which come together to encircle the successive openings of atria, alveolar sacs, and alveoli.

Functional Respiratory Units

Those interested in pulmonary function have long sought to define functional subdivisions within the respiratory surface, aiming for an ideal unit that is at the same time modular and well defined anatomically. Such is the nonuniformity of the lungs that the ideal is unattainable, for it is one thing to find structurally similar units in this region, and it is another to find them uniform in size and shape. Moreover, the *average* size of these units is scaled up or down, depending on the animal possessing them. Among a wide range of mammals the size of such units is roughly com-

FIGURE 21-36 Diagram of the respiratory subdivisions in the lung, showing a respiratory bronchiole, alveolar ducts, and subdivisions. Smooth muscle (dark cells) ends in the alveolar ducts. The atria (circled) are spaces bounded by the termination of the alveolar duct, on one end, and the openings of the alveolar sacs, on the other. In addition, major features of the alveolar walls are presented.

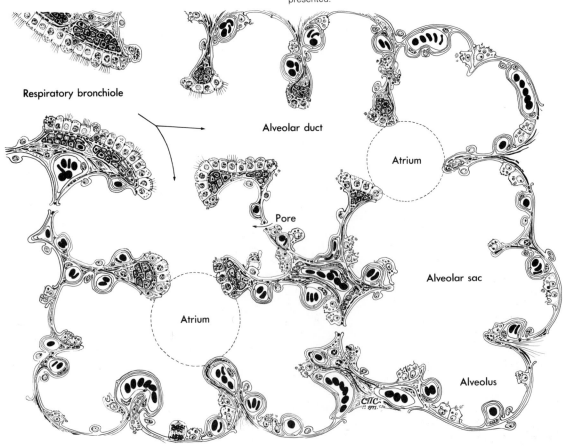

Respiratory bronchiole

Alveolar duct

Atrium

Pore

Atrium

Alveolar sac

Alveolus

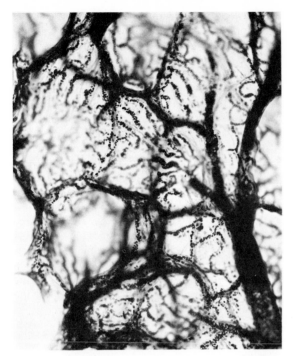

FIGURE 21-37 Thick section of adult human lung, showing the distribution of small blood vessels within the alveolar walls. ×125.

mensurate with lung volume, which is proportional to body weight, and with respiratory surface area, which varies linearly and directly with basal oxygen consumption. The best anatomic unit is the *acinus*, which is simply the terminal bronchiole and all its branches. In humans it has dimensions of millimeter size and is divided by its first-order respiratory bronchioles into two hemiacini. These differ in size and shape from each other and from those of other acini, the free variations on a simple pattern arising from a competition among branches for available space. A larger peripheral unit is the (secondary) *lobule,* supposedly formed by connective tissue septa passing into the lung from the pleura. Unfortunately, such septa are well defined only near the pleura and not deep within the lungs, and they do not demarcate equal volumes of lung. Consequently, this lobule has been redefined for the human lung in terms of the branching pattern in the peripheral airway (Fig. 21-17). It consists of a cluster of three to five acini whose terminal bronchioles arise close by one another at the end of a given centimeter-branching bronchial path. Such a unit

measures 1 to 2 cm^2 in volume and is of a convenient size for use in radiologic studies on patients.

Alveolar Organization

The alveolar wall is specialized toward promoting diffusion between external and internal environments. As at any exposed surface, an epithelium covers a vascularized connective tissue space, but in the alveolar wall the epithelial and connective tissue layers are both very thin, and the blood vessels form the richest capillary network in the body (Fig. 21-37). In details of organization these walls are similar in most mammalian lungs. Between adjacent alveoli a framework of elastic and collagenous fibers supports a meshwork of anastomosing pulmonary capillaries. The vessels are woven through the framework much as vines are woven through a trellis. In marine mammals, alveolar capillaries run in two beds, one on each of two adjacent alveolar surfaces, being separated from each other by a central connective tissue septum rich in cells and fibers, and from the alveolar air by a layer of epithelium. Through reduction in the connective tissue and through formation of extensive anastomoses, these capillary beds are rationalized by most other mammals into one system that serves adjacent alveoli. The connective tissue septum, having become thin and pliant, no longer occupies a distinctly central position but fills the interstices between the capillaries (Figs. 21-36 and 21-38). When alveoli abut against the pleura, the septa, or large blood vessels instead of against each other, the alveolar connective tissue blends in with the tissue of the adjacent structure. At such points only do alveoli contact lymphatic capillaries, for these vessels do not penetrate interalveolar septa except when the septa are rather thick, as in whales (Fig. 21-60).

The alveolar epithelium is inhomogeneous, consisting principally of attenuated *squamous alveolar* cells and pleomorphic *great alveolar* cells. The connective tissue beneath the epithelium makes up about a third of the thickness of the total air-blood barrier, which in rats averages about 1.5 μm with a range from 0.1 to several micrometers. Where the alveolar diffusion barrier is thinnest, the capillary loops press against the epithelium so that connective tissue is excluded and epithelium and endothelium are separated by only a submicroscopic basement lamina (Fig.

21-43). Compared with a single 1-μm micrococcus, this membrane does not present a formidable obstacle to invasion by microorganisms. Nonetheless, to judge by the absence of chronic inflammatory cells from the region, alveolar surfaces normally are not threatened by invasion. Credit for this falls on the *alveolar macrophages*, which move over surfaces coated by epithelial secretions and effectively police the alveoli. Capillaries within alveolar walls all belong to the pulmonary vascular circuit and do not have endothelial fenestrations (Fig. 21-54). Nevertheless, when the vascular compartment of the animal is overloaded and the filtration pressure rises, the pulmonary capillaries then leak fluid and small proteins through clefts between endothelial cells; these are held together by macular junctions that do not prevent passage of fluid around them. Excessive leakage into the alveoli is prevented by the alveolar epithelium, which possesses tight junctions and remains relatively impermeable until damaged.

Between the capillaries one or more small, slitlike *alveolar pores* can be seen in thick sections that have been fixed and dried in an expanded state (Fig. 21-39). These pores connect adjacent alveoli and are fully open in expanded lungs. They are then about 10 to 15 μm in diameter and are encircled by a few elastic and reticular fibers. These pores are the best known among several kinds of *accessory communications* between adjacent air spaces. Others exist at the levels of respiratory bronchioles and alveolar ducts, where short circuits can occur between the airway and alveoli of the same or of adjacent acini. Still others come into being as a result of aberrant branching within the acini, and they interconnect airways of adjacent bronchial paths either directly or indirectly. The latter provide relatively major intercommunications, perhaps through passages as large as 0.5 mm in diameter. These accessory channels normally may serve as a fine control in equalizing interacinar pressures, but the extent to which they are present varies greatly with the

FIGURE 21-38 Interalveolar wall in the lungs, showing the central connective tissue space in continuity with a pulmonary venule. ×7000.

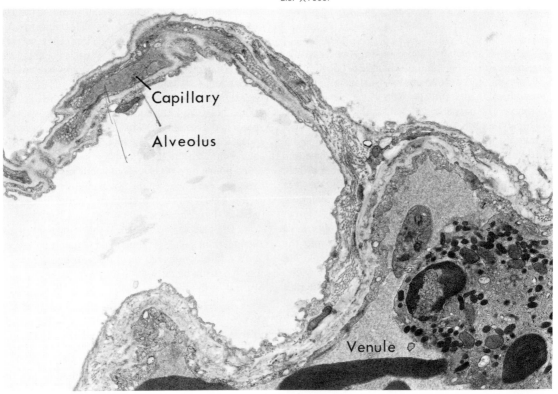

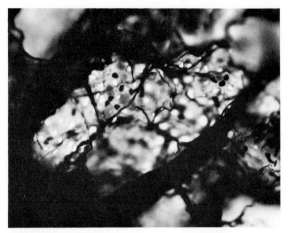

FIGURE 21-39 Thick section of human lung prepared to demonstrate pores between adjacent alveoli. The pores are seen as light spots, the alveolar nuclei as dark spots on the walls. ×250.

FIGURE 21-40 Light micrograph of a rat's lung showing bronchiolar epithelium (above) and respiratory tissue (below). Toluidine blue. ×400.

species. In canine lungs these paths are plainly evident; in humans they are apparent; but in pigs they are difficult to demonstrate. Where a terminal bronchiole is obstructed, the alveoli connected to it can be ventilated through these collateral channels. They may also serve as routes for the spread of pneumonia or neoplasm.

Alveolar Cells

There are three major types of cells in alveolar walls: endothelial cells of capillaries, squamous alveolar epithelial cells, and great alveolar cells. The capillaries resemble muscular capillaries and have been described above. By light microscopy the endothelial cells are difficult to distinguish from squamous alveolar cells because both are thin and elongate and their nuclei are small (Figs. 21-40 and 21-47). An alveolar

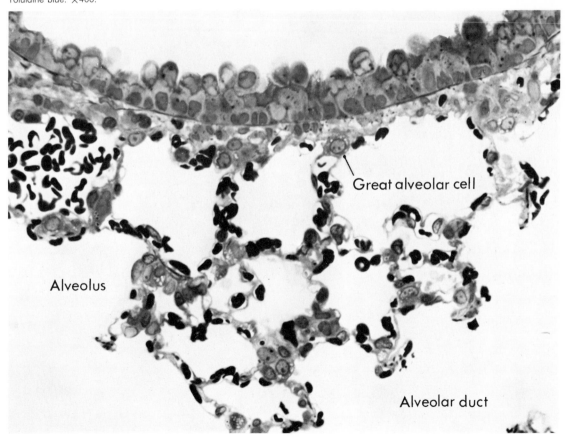

Great alveolar cell

Alveolus

Alveolar duct

brush cell of unknown function is a minor constituent of the epithelium.

Mast cells usually remain confined to the connective tissue surrounding the airways and blood vessels and follow the intrapulmonary course of these structures for varying distances according to the species. In rats these cells accompany the vessels through many generations of branching and appear in the visceral pleura as well. They closely approach the respiratory tissue but do not enter it. In guinea pigs they follow the vessels further and occasionally penetrate the interalveolar walls; this largely explains why anaphylaxis in these animals is centered in the lungs (Fig. 21-50, see color insert). Otherwise, the alveolar connective tissue normally contains only occasional fibrocytes, plasma cells, wandering leukocytes, and, rarely, a solitary smooth muscle fiber. Following severe challenge by

acute or chronic infection, however, the connective tissue space enlarges and receives a variety of inflammatory cells from the bloodstream.

Squamous alveolar epithelial cells (membranous pneumonocytes, type I cells, small alveolar cells, pulmonary epithelial cells) appear widely separated from each other because, beyond the perinuclear region the cytoplasm is abruptly attenuated (Fig. 21-42). Thereafter it extends over the basement lamina as a thin sheet and joins other epithelial cells making up the continuous alveolar lining. In many mammals the attenuated portions of the cytoplasm are so thin as to be below the resolving limit of the optical microscope (0.2 μm); in bats the layer may approach 250 Å, a thickness of little more than apical and basal plasmalemmae combined. For this reason a controversy

FIGURE 21-41 Frozen section of alveolar walls in a bat's lung reacted for diphosphopyridine nucleotide reductase. Great alveolar cells and the phagocytes are the most reactive cells present; they compare in reactivity with the epithelial cells of the airways. ×600.

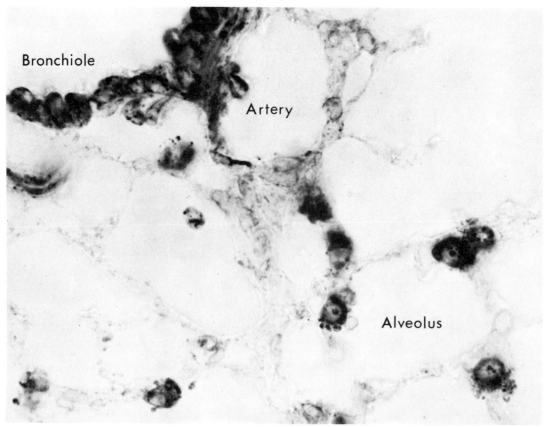

raged for years about whether or not a complete alveolar epithelium existed, but the question was resolved by electron microscopy. Squamous alveolar cells have inconspicuous metabolic activity as revealed histochemically (Fig. 21-41), and much of it must be directed toward maintaining surfaces so extensively exposed to alveolar air. These cells are rather deficient in ergastoplasm and other cytoplasmic organelles, but those present are distributed fairly evenly among perinuclear and peripheral regions. Micropinocytotic vesicles occur in small numbers at both basal and apical surfaces; and from the latter, short microvilli here and there extend into the alveolar space. Squamous cells are capable of using pinocytotic action to take up small amounts of protein from the alveoli; exceptionally they store protein aggregates within the cytoplasm. These cells are also able to ingest small amounts of inhaled particulate matter that reaches the alveolar surface, and they convey some of it across the epithelium by vesicular transport. Their main role is that of providing an intact surface of minimum thickness readily permeable to gases. The plasmalemmae of cells are the main barriers to diffusion in any multilayered biologic

membrane, but they are freely permeable to gases, which dissolve in lipids.

Great alveolar cells (granular pneumonocytes, type II cells, large alveolar cells, alveolar cells) carry out other epithelial functions. These pleomorphic cells often have a roughly cuboidal shape. They rest on the epithelial basement lamina, sometimes occupying niches between capillary loops and sometimes standing upright in twos and threes along the alveolar surface (Fig. 21-36). However they are mixed in the epithelium, they are joined to their neighbors by the same type of continuous tight junctions that bind all the epithelial cells together (Fig. 21-44). Great alveolar cells are identifiable in paraffin sections of lung because their nuclei are vesicular and relatively large and their cytoplasm appears vacuolated. At the light-microscopic level they stand out better in 1-μm plastic sections, and then the vacuoles are seen to be characteristic inclusions known as *multilamellar bodies* or *cytosomes* (Fig. 21-40).

Great alveolar cells have considerable metabolic capacity (Fig. 21-41) at a level equaled in alveolar regions only by alveolar macrophages. Within the

FIGURE 21-42 Squamous alveolar epithelial and neighboring cells in the alveolar wall. (Courtesy of E. Schneeberger.)

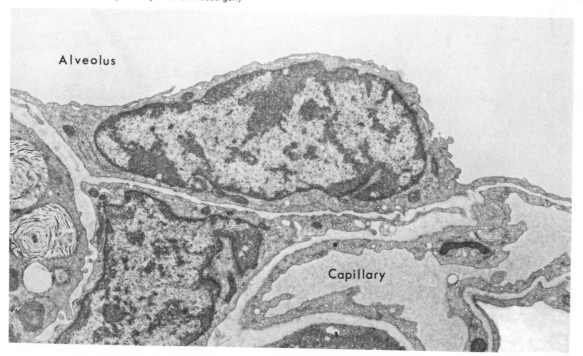

Alveolus

Capillary

cytoplasm this capacity is reflected by the presence of well-developed mitochondria, but a secretory function is indicated even more strongly by the presence of a loosely ordered granular endoplasmic reticulum, an extensive and widely dispersed Golgi apparatus, numerous multivesicular bodies, and the multilamellar bodies (Fig. 21-44). The latter range in size up to 1 μm and occur among forms transitional in appearance between multivesicular bodies and the cytosomes (Fig. 21-45). Multilamellar bodies give histochemical reactions for phospholipids, mucopolysaccharides, and proteins, including reaction for several lysosomal hydrolases which are also found in the Golgi lamellae and in the multivesicular bodies. The cytosomes are therefore synthetic products of great alveolar cells. By their appearance and retention of some lysosomal enzyme activity, they can be considered as homologues of residual bodies present in other cells, but unlike them they differ in content and in being secreted and not retained in the cytoplasm. Autoradiographic studies have shown that tritium-labeled leucine, galactose, and choline become incorporated in the cytosomes after first traversing synthetic centers in the cytoplasm. Great alveolar cells are the only pulmonary cells to incorporate considerable amounts of choline; this is a specific precursor of phosphatidyl-

choline, a surface-active component of alveolar secretions. Consequently, the multilamellar bodies of great alveolar cells are the source of this material in the lungs. Synthesis and release occur continuously, the bodies being extruded singly from the apical microvillous border of the cell. This secretion spreads over the alveolar surface and endows the extracellular coating with unusual surface activity. This is further described below.

The alveolar surface coating consists of lipid and aqueous phases and contains a detergent substance, termed *surfactant*, whose active principles are substances related to phosphatidylcholine. This material is interspersed with water molecules at the alveolar surface, thereby reducing their mutual cohesiveness and consequently reducing the surface tension at the air-fluid interface. In the presence of surfactant, the work of breathing is reduced because the alveolar surface tension that tends to collapse alveoli is reduced, and this requires a lessened inspiratory force to oppose it. Alveolar diameters are stabilized as well, since the surface tension is greater in small alveoli than in large ones, because of the greater curvature of the wall. Where two such alveoli are interconnected,

FIGURE 21-43 Electron micrograph of the alveolar membrane of a rat. The barrier between alveolar air and blood consists of a thin alevolar epithelium, a basement lamina, and the capillary endothelium. Within the endothelial cell a network of fine-caliber agranular reticulum occupies the space between two mitochondria (mi). Pinocytotic vesicles (pv) are seen in both epithelium and endothelium. ×15,000.

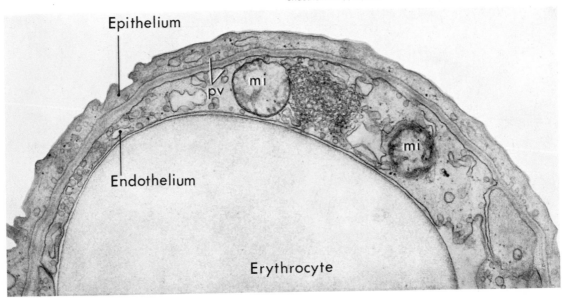

Epithelium

pv

mi

mi

Endothelium

Erythrocyte

the larger would expand at the expense of the smaller unless surface tensions were reduced. These are the problems faced by infants suffering from respiratory distress syndrome, frequently brought on by a deficiency in the great alveolar cells.

Although the presence of a surface-active alveolar coating is not doubted, it has been difficult to present good images of the material in electron micrographs, and the most successful ones to date have been made in lungs fixed by intravascular rather than intratracheal perfusion of tissue fixative. In the former technique the

extracellular lining is preserved as a superficial layer of phospholipids over a basal aqueous layer containing proteins and mucopolysaccharides. The upper layer consists of several lamellae each about 100 to 400 Å thick and resembles the crystalline phase of a polar lipid-water system. The lipid crystals (*tubular myelin*) fortuitously can be seen in continuity with released cytosomes (Fig. 21-46), to give visual confirmation that they are derived from these bodies. The basal

FIGURE 21-44 Great alveolar cell in the lungs of an opossum. (From S. Sorokin, *J. Histochem. Cytochem.*, **14**:884, 1966.)

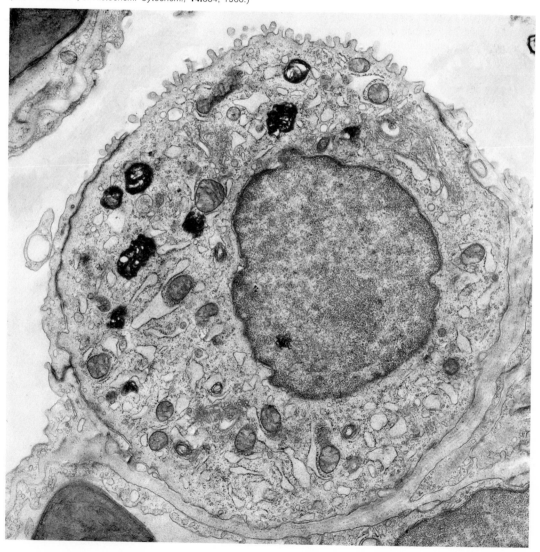

layer is of variable thickness, and the substances dissolved there may possess properties more broadly related to defense postures than to surface activity.

Alveolar Macrophages

Alveolar macrophages (alveolar phagocytes, dust cells) are preeminent among cells defending the respiratory region from contamination by microorganisms and inhaled particulate matter (Fig. 21-47). They have long been distinguished by their vigorous phagocytic activity, which is in strong contrast to the virtual absence of such activity by other alveolar cells. They are most unusual, however, because they regularly scavenge the *surface* of the epithelium. In general, macro-

phages rarely migrate over epithelial surfaces and almost never do so in the absence of significant inflammation in the connective tissue beneath. The metabolic capacity of these cells is considerable and diverse. This is well documented because alveolar macrophages can be washed out from the lungs through irrigation of the airway, and the resulting cell suspensions contain them in a high state of purity. In addition to possessing formidable aerobic oxidative capacity and a powerful intracellular digestive system (Fig. 21-33), these cells have a reserve synthetic capability that enables them to adapt their response to changing conditions.

In most respects, alveolar macrophages resemble

FIGURE 21-45 Sequence showing the development of cytosomes from small multivesicular bodies (mvb) through larger forms and on to secretion from the great alveolar cell. (From S. Sorokin, *J. Histochem. Cytochem.,* **14:**884, 1966.)

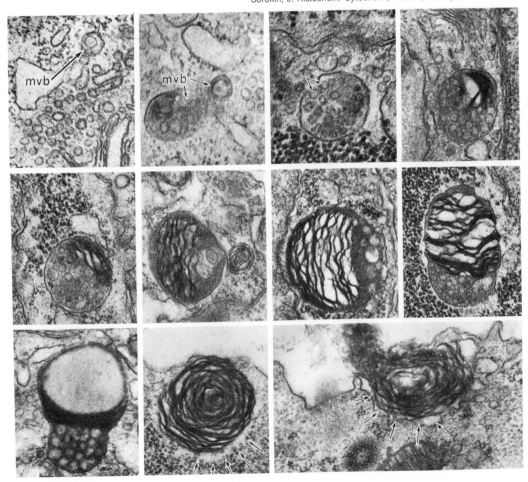

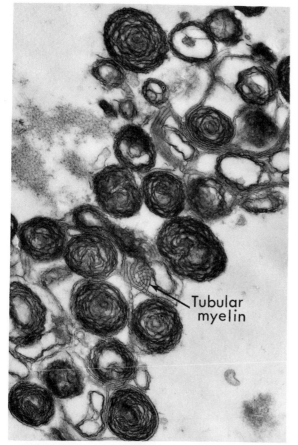

FIGURE 21-46 Accumulated secretions from great alveolar cells in a culture of rat lungs. Cytosomes are the source of tubular myelin present in alveolar surfactant.

macrophages from other parts of the body. A peripheral ectoplasm free of organelles and inclusions is filled with contractile myofilaments. A less fibrillar endoplasm within houses a euchromatic nucleus, the cytoplasmic organelles, and a great variety of dense bodies representing ingested matter enclosed within phagolysosomes (Fig. 21-48). If the cell had been migrating when fixed, the nucleus might be displaced toward the rear, the advancing end would be broad, and the trailing end would taper into a firm tail to provide purchase for the cell (Fig. 21-47). On the other hand, if the macrophage were examined in cell suspensions, it would be rounded and somewhat blebby at its outer margin. In migrating phagocytes, coated vesicles (acanthosomes) occur at points along the advancing edges. These indicate that alveolar macrophages take in solids or dissolved matter by

microendocytosis as well as by the more macroscopic processes of phagocytosis and pinocytosis; in this respect, the cells differ from neutrophilic granulocytes, which make use only of the latter. Phagocytosis involves formation and extension of pseudopodia, a process that draws on cellular mechanisms for motility; but although alveolar macrophages heartily ingest a great variety of particulate substances (Fig. 21-49, see color insert), they are less active than other phagocytes in moving about.

Within the cytoplasm the Golgi apparatus is well developed and surrounds a distinct, fibrillar centrosome, in which the centrioles reside. From them microtubules radiate into the cytoplasm and organize the surrounding organelles about the centrosome. The endoplasmic reticulum varies in extent with different phases of cellular activity, but the agranular reticulum usually predominates over the granular. Small rodlike mitochondria and free polysomes fill the available space. Pinocytotic and coated vesicles, phagosomes, a few multivesicular bodies, transitional lamellae between the agranular reticulum and the Golgi appara-

FIGURE 21-47 Macrophages in the alveolar space of a rat's lung. Toluidine blue. ×1000.

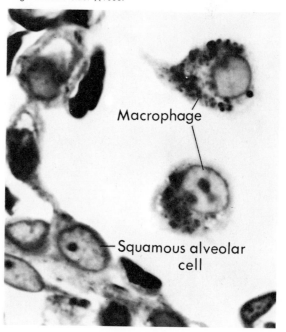

tus, primary lysosomes, and phagolysosomes of a great variety of sizes and shapes take up much of the space and give the cytoplasm a pronounced "digestive" character. The lysosomes sometimes have unusual configurations; these give alveolar macrophages of some animals a species-specific appearance. For example, in rabbits lysosomol bodies contain dense circular inclusions, whereas in cats they contain lamellated material often in a radial configuration. In humans and among several rodents, however, rounded or dumbbell-shaped primary lysosomes are admixed with larger phagolysosomes containing assorted alveolar debris (Fig. 21-48).

Notwithstanding the alveolar macrophage functions by ingesting particulate matter and digesting it, many fundamental facts about the cell and its life cycle remain unknown. The origin of the cell, the dynamics of its entrance and exit from the lungs, and the duration of its residence in alveolar walls and on the surface are imperfectly understood. Alveolar macrophages are able to divide, but many consider them a population in transit, capable of a few divisions at best. Various sources for these cells have been proposed, chiefly (1) hematopoietic tissues outside the lungs, (2) hematopoietic or connective tissues within the lungs, and (3) the alveolar epithelium, in particular the great alveolar cells. Recent experimental work has provided unequivocal evidence that at least some of the pulmonary macrophages are derived from hematopoietic cells. Under conditions where identifiable bone marrow cells are seeded into donor animals exposed to high doses of total body irradiation, it has been shown that all pulmonary macrophages originate from donor cells. Such seeding of the lungs is usually by cells with characteristics of monocytes, but in exceptional circumstances the seeded cells have proven to be morphologically indistinguishable from lymphocytes. In experiments that have employed total body irradiation, actively dividing populations of pulmonary cells would be compromised by the irradiation, and consequently any intrapulmonary source of the macrophages would decline. Among hypothetical intrapulmonary sources, the great alveolar cell remains a plausible but unfashionable one; for the cell is highly plastic and along with the pulmonary endothelial cell it behaves like a stem cell, dividing into one daughter cell that remains in place and into another that leaves the area. More likely intrapulmonary sources would be cells originally

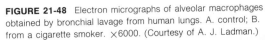

FIGURE 21-48 Electron micrographs of alveolar macrophages obtained by bronchial lavage from human lungs. A. control; B. from a cigarette smoker. ×6000. (Courtesy of A. J. Ladman.)

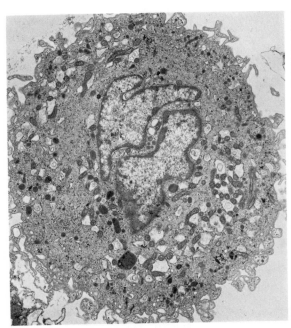
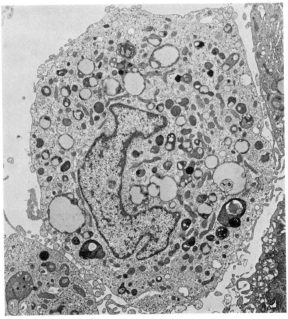

seeded from the bloodstream and left to develop a self-replenishing pool of mature macrophages for the lungs. Where the pool failed to maintain an adequate supply of cells, it could be renewed from time to time by further seeding from the bloodstream. In more acute emergencies, monocytes like neutrophils and other leukocytes could always be induced to cross the pulmonary capillaries to enter the interstitial tissues and the alveoli. Whether or not alveolar macrophages share a common origin with other macrophages of the body, they differ in enzyme content and levels of reactivity from blood-borne peritoneal macrophages of the same species. In particular, they differ from both peritoneal macrophages and heterophils in relying on oxidative phosphorylation to supply energy consumed during phagocytosis. These metabolic differences indicate that if alveolar macrophages are derived from the same itinerant precursors as other macrophages of the body, the precursors must undergo a period of adaptation in the lungs before they become full-fledged alveolar macrophages.

Dust-laden macrophages leave the alveolar surface by migrating or being slowly washed to the bronchial passages, where they are carried out to the pharynx and swallowed. While in transit, a number of them continue to pursue normal activities, such as scavenging the bronchial surface and dividing; others die and release their contents, some of which is cleared or reingested by other cells, and some of which may return to the lungs by passage through the bronchial epithelium.

Pulmonary connective tissue macrophages reside beneath the airway, around blood vessels, and in the pleura. Functionally they are distinct from alveolar macrophages, perhaps only because they are sheltered from direct exposure to airborne dusts and bacteria and not because of differences in metabolism; their position limits their mobility in any case, and they are the ultimate repository of uncleared particulate matter in the lungs. They have access to lymphatic pathways in the connective tissue and filter out material coming that way, as well as material entering the lungs from the bronchial arteries. A small part of the particulate matter deposited in the alveoli reaches these macrophages after it has crossed the intact or damaged alveolar epithelium to reach para-alveolar lymphatics (discussed under lymphatics), for it has not been demonstrated that sizable numbers of alveolar macrophages reenter the tissues once they have appeared on the alveolar surface.

PULMONARY CIRCULATION

The main blood supply to the lungs is furnished by *pulmonary arteries,* one for each lung. They carry high volumes of blood at low pressures ($^{25}/_5$ mm Hg) from the right side of the heart to pulmonary capillaries in the alveolar walls. These are drained by *pulmonary veins,* which carry oxygenated blood to the left side of the heart. *Bronchial arteries* are small derivatives of the thoracic descending aorta that carry blood at systemic pressure ($^{120}/_{80}$ mm Hg) to the walls of most of the airways (Fig. 21-51). *Bronchial veins* are present only near the hilum and form only accessory drainage from the bronchial wall. Consequently, most of the blood from the two arterial systems drains into the pulmonary veins, and the three vascular systems form one integrated circuit. As described in the section on the internal structure of the lungs, the arteries branch with the bronchial tree and hence alternate with the veins, which run in the septa between adjacent bronchi (Figs, 21-58 and 21-59, see color insert).

Pulmonary Vessels

From distributing vessels of the *pulmonary arterial system,* branches are sent to airway tissues beginning at the level of the respiratory bronchioles. Distal to the alveolar duct the artery branches; and from the level of the atrium, twigs are given off to the atria and a branch is sent to each alveolar sac. This divides into two, and the newly formed branches join the pulmonary capillary network (Fig. 21-37), whose mesh can be finer than the diameters of the capillaries forming it. Other features of this capillary bed have been described in the section on alveolar organization.

Venules drain the distal ends of the alveolar sacs. Pulmonary veins have four origins: from capillaries of the pleura, from alveolar ducts, from alveoli, and from the peribronchial venous plexus (Fig. 21-58). The veins draining the airway frequently occur at points where bronchi or bronchioles divide and are called *bronchopulmonary veins.* They provide the main channels for drainage of the bronchial arteries and consequently are the primary elements tying the pulmonary and bronchial circuits together. From these various origins, small vessels come together into veins that cross the respiratory tissue to enter larger caliber pulmonary veins situated in connective tissue septa

(Fig. 21-56); this is why in histological sections the smaller veins, in contrast to arteries, appear surrounded by alveoli and are separated by varying distances from the airway (Fig. 21-34). Occupying the boundary between regions supplied by adjacent bronchi—and hence adjacent arteries—the interfacial veins receive the drainage from both. Stated another way, the venous drainage of pulmonary segments or subsegments is always by more than one vein. Such medium to large vessels follow connective tissue planes of the lung, gathering into still larger veins, but continuing to receive small tributaries along the way. Eventually one trunk is formed for each lobe, and these come into relation with the artery and bronchus,

usually lying ventromedial to the bronchus while the artery lies dorsolateral. In human beings, the veins to the middle and upper lobes of the right lung usually combine into one vessel, so that two veins leave the lungs on either side of the heart. Exceptionally the three right lobar veins may enter the left atrium separately, while the pair from the left may enter by a single opening.

Bronchial Vessels

Usually two bronchial arteries are given off to the left lung and one is formed for the right. The left ones usually arise from the ventral aspect of the thoracic descending aorta, the cranial one just opposite the fifth thoracic vertebra in human beings, and the lower one just caudal to the left bronchus, which crosses ventral to the descending aorta. The right bronchial

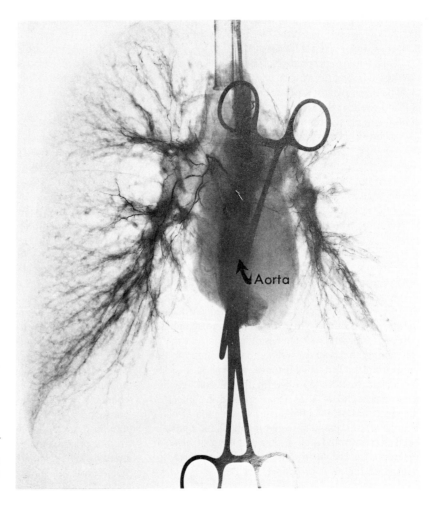

FIGURE 21-51 X-ray of autopsied human heart and lungs injected with contrast material to reveal the bronchial arterial system. The heart shadow overlies the descending thoracic aorta; from there the right bronchial artery (arrow) passes to the right bronchial tree; and on both right and left, the arteries branch with the bronchi.

Aorta

artery sometimes arises from the cranial left bronchial artery and sometimes from the first aortic intercostal, but the number and exact origins of all the bronchial arteries may vary, as may their intercommunication with nearby esophageal, pericardial, and even coronary circulations. On each side, the bronchial arteries run in the adventitia over the dorsal aspect of the bronchi, to end at the level of respiratory bronchioles. Along their course they send branches through the muscularis of the airway, giving off a capillary bed for the smooth muscle and another for the lamina propria. Deep to the latter venous plexuses are formed on

both sides of the muscularis. The outer one contains larger vessels that combine to form the bronchopulmonary veins. Beyond the respiratory bronchioles this system becomes supplied by branches of the pulmonary artery. Bronchial arteries also furnish blood to vasa vasorum of pulmonary arteries and veins (Fig. 21-56) and extend along interlobular septa to supply these areas as well as capillaries of the visceral pleura.

Bronchial veins are seen on the dorsal surface of

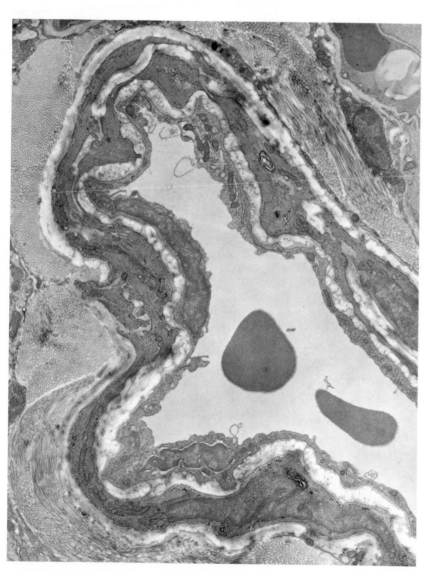

FIGURE 21-52 Pulmonary artery adjacent to a small intrapulmonary bronchus in a bat. The endothelium rests on an internal elastic membrane; the muscularis is only one cell layer thick but is infiltrated by (clear) elastic fibers, whereas the adventitia is collagenous. ×7200.

the extrapulmonary bronchi where they lie next to the bronchial arteries. They drain these structures as well as the visceral pleura and lymph nodes at the hilum. They become a single vessel on each side; on the right it empties into the azygous vein near its junction with the superior vena cava, and on the left it joins either the highest left intercostal or accessory hemiazygous vein.

Histology

Owing to reduced pressure in the circuit, pulmonary arteries and veins resemble each other more closely than do corresponding pairs of systemic vessels. The pulmonary vessels retain histological features of ar-

FIGURE 21-53 Section of rat lung stained for elastic fibers. A bronchus is cut in cross section above and a branch of the pulmonary artery lies below. A bronchial vessel (bron) is separated from the pulmonary artery by a lymphatic vessel (lym). Resorcin-fuchsin, lithium carmine, orange G. ×350.

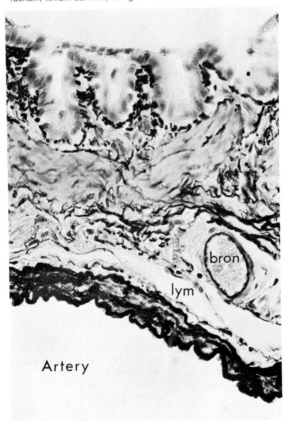

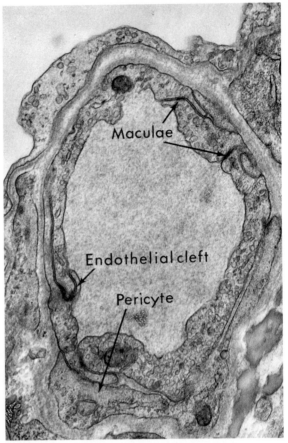

FIGURE 21-54 Alveolar capillary in an opossum's lung. ×12,180.

teries and veins, but among different species considerable variation occurs on both sides of the capillaries. The arteries have relatively more smooth muscle and elastic fibers than the veins and to their smallest divisions possess an internal elastic membrane. The veins contain a meshwork of predominantly longitudinally oriented elastic fibers at the intimal margin, moderate numbers of elastic fibers in the muscularis when this layer is occupied by smooth muscle, and variable amounts of them just external to it.

For some distance after they leave the heart, the pulmonary arteries remain elastic arteries, histologically comparable to the aorta and provided with elastic membranes encircling the intima and layered throughout the muscularis. Such vessels accompany major intrapulmonary bronchi of large mammals. In them the intima is multilayered and consists of an endothelium resting on a subendothelial connective

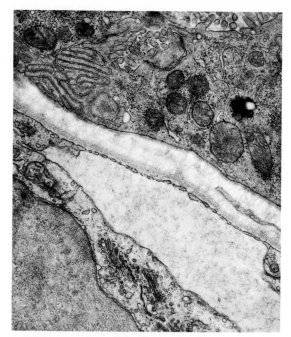

FIGURE 21-55 Endothelial fenestrations in a glandular capillary in the bronchial wall of an opossum. ×12,000.

tissue containing fibrocytes and relatively fine, longitudinally oriented fibers embedded in an abundant matrix. Just outside the circularly oriented muscularis, a number of smooth muscle bundles run longitudinally in the adventitia, which elsewhere contains fine, unmyelinated nerve processes and the vasa vasorum and is densely collagenous in texture. With branching of the arteries, intimal thickness and the number of elastic lamellae become reduced; a vessel with lamellae occupying the inner third of an otherwise well-elasticized muscularis might accompany a medium-sized bronchus. These are succeeded by vessels histologically closer to muscular arteries. In smaller mammals, the arteries of large bronchi have an intima composed only of endothelium and a single internal elastic membrane inside a muscularis richly layered with elastic fibers. These form a meshwork rather than fenestrated lamellae (Fig. 21-53); the fibers generally separate the smooth muscle fibers into layers, but they interconnect with each other and with an often denser meshwork of fibers at the boundary between muscularis and adventitia. The progressive thinning out of the arterial wall can be followed in the illustrations of kitten lung, beginning with a large bronchus and passing through bronchioles to respiratory bronchioles (Figs. 21-19,

21-24, 21-32, and 21-34). In small mammals the arteries throughout most of their length are relatively thin-walled musculoelastic arteries of the type described (Fig. 21-52). The endothelium of pulmonary arteries is composed of elongated cells that form overlapping junctions with one another and contain rather many smooth-surfaced micropinocytotic vesicles. The cytoplasm occasionally contains membrane-bounded secretory or absorptive granules, but these are more abundant in the endothelium of small pulmonary veins (Figs. 21-52 and 21-57). In contrast, the endothelial cytoplasm of certain bronchial arteries contains approximately 50-Å filaments in a dense matting sandwiched in between the apical and basal rows of pinocytotic vesicles. Histologically, bronchial vessels otherwise resemble other systemic blood vessels of comparable dimensions (Fig. 21-53).

Pulmonary capillaries are of the muscular, nonfenestrated type throughout, whereas bronchial capillaries are fenestrated, particularly in relation to the vascular beds supplying the glands, but also in relation to the airway epithelium, and especially to the bronchioles (Figs. 21-54 and 21-55). Here and there *pericytes* encircle both types of capillaries. For the most part they lie outside the endothelial basement membrane, but they extend processes inside, and these contact the endothelial cells for short distances (Fig. 21-54). The cytoplasm of these pericytes is filamentous in texture, and the cells are believed to function like smooth muscle; other pericapillary processes may belong to connective tissue macrophages.

Pulmonary veins of large animals sometimes prove difficult to identify in histological sections not only because the media contains considerable smooth muscle, but especially because sufficient elastic fibers are present to give the vein a crenelated appearance reminiscent of arteries seen in slides of material prepared with coagulating fixatives. Side by side, the vessels are easily distinguished (Fig. 21-19). It should be remembered that the venous adventitia is relatively thicker than the arterial, and it is always helpful to keep the anatomical course of these vessels in mind.

For short distances beyond their junction with the left atrium, the pulmonary veins of human beings have an adventitial coating of *cardiac muscle*. This spreads to the hilum in dogs, whereas in smaller mammals the muscle extends along intrapulmonary veins for varying distances to reach small veins less than 100 μm in

818

diameter in the smallest mammals. In these intra-pulmonary vessels the cardiac muscle occupies the media sometimes together with smooth muscle as in rats, and sometimes alone as in shrews and bats (Fig. 21-57); when this muscle occurs alone, the elastic fibers are heaviest beneath the intima, where they are formed into a coarsely porous lamella. The cardiac muscle is single-layered in small veins but multilayered in larger ones, and the cells resemble myocytes of the atrium (Chap. 7). During its development the muscle first appears in venous walls next to the heart and later spreads peripherally. It contracts slightly ahead of the heart and presumably functions as a dynamic valve in facilitating venous return.

Pulmonary venules have an endothelium like the endothelium of pulmonary capillaries, and the vessels have no muscularis (Fig. 21-38). It is thought that many exchanges taking place at the capillary level also occur in the venules; as in many capillaries, the endothelium of pulmonary capillaries and venules exhibit surface adenosine triphosphatase activity possibly associated with an active transmembrane transport mechanism, but in other respects these cells are not conspicuous metabolically (Fig. 21-41). Near the point where smooth or cardiac muscle joins the vessel wall and the venules become small veins, the endothelium rests upon a single mesh of elastic fibers supported by adventitial plies of dense collagenous connective tissue. The addition of muscle displaces the collagenous layer peripherally although a few threads of cytoplasm from fibrocytes remain interposed here and there between the elastic mesh and the muscle.

FIGURE 21-56 India-ink injection of bronchial arteries and pulmonary veins in the lungs of a vampire bat. A bronchopulmonary communication (large arrows) and injected vasa vasorum in the wall of the large vein (small arrows) are indicated. ×80.

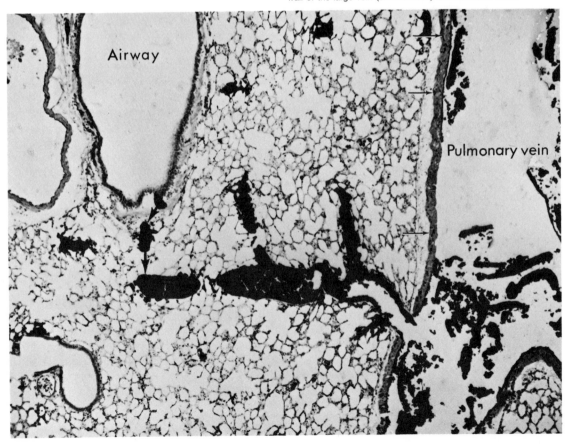

Functional Interrelationships

Several types of vascular anastomoses are found in the lungs. True anastomoses between bronchial and pulmonary arteries (Fig. 21-58, green) are found in the peribronchial tissue near small peripheral bronchi and in the pleura. These vessels are small and have well-developed muscular walls. From them bronchial arteriovenous shunts (Fig. 21-58, green stripes) branch off to the pulmonary veins, reaching them by way of the bronchopulmonary veins or by small peripheral pulmonary branches. These then are secondary anastomoses. Shortcuts are also to be found between parallel branches of bronchial arteries, and bronchial veins intercommunicate through the bronchial plexus. In healthy lungs the blood flow through

these shunts is of small magnitude, and it passes from the bronchial to the pulmonary circuit.

Sympathetic discharge produces little effect on the pulmonary circulation. Mechanical factors as well as the composition of the inspired gas influence it more clearly. Vasoconstriction and increased flow result from hypoxia. Once constricted, the vessels may be relaxed by parasympathomimetic action.

No proven chemoreceptors are known to exist in blood vessels of the lungs, but a glomus associated with the pulmonary trunk has been described. Histologically, it resembles the carotid body. It contains nests of epithelioid cells bound in connective tissue and richly supplied with blood from the pulmonary artery. Vagal and sympathetic fibers from the deep cardiac plexus provide innervation, but attempts to investigate glomar function have not given positive results.

FIGURE 21-57 Granule-rich endothelium and cardiac-muscle investment of a small pulmonary vein of the vampire bat. A simply folded intercalated disc (arrows) incorporating a close-gapped junction between cells (upper two arrows) is shown at the center of the field. ×21,200.

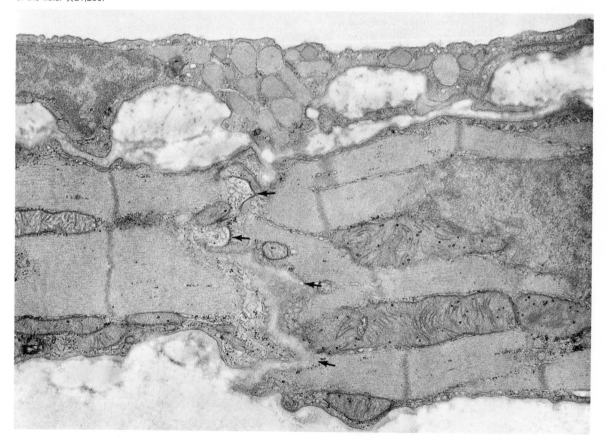

LYMPHATICS

The lymphatics of the lung are abundant and form a closed system. A superficial set lies in the visceral pleura; a deep one accompanies the bronchi and pulmonary vessels (Fig. 21-58, *color insert*). The sets interconnect at the hilum, where both enter the tracheobronchial lymph nodes. They also communicate near the origins of the pulmonary veins in the pleura and in the interlobar septa, which arise from the pleura (Fig. 21-61).

The lymphatic vessels may be compared to thin-walled veins. They exhibit abrupt changes in diameter and near the hilum frequently have valves. The walls of the larger vessels have three layers, the smaller have no media (Fig. 21-53), and the capillaries lack a continuous basement lamina but possess numerous anchoring filaments that tie into interstitial fibers. Lymphatic capillaries accompanying pulmonary arterioles and venules, as well as others present in pulmonary septa and bronchi, may closely approach adjacent alveoli; collectively they comprise the *paraalveolar lymphatics*, which drain their immediate surroundings as well as wick-away the more distant alveolar interstitium (Fig. 21-60). In humans and common domestic and laboratory mammals there are no lymphatic capillaries in interalveolar walls.

Within the lung, lymph flows centripetally along lymphatics of the bronchial tree and the pulmonary arteries and veins, being milked along by contraction of lymphatic smooth muscle, by inspiratory movements, and by pulsations of the blood vessels they entwine. At the bifurcations of bronchi, the fluid passes through lymphoid tissue, which is scarce in neonatal animals but gradually builds up in postnatal life. Pleural lymph reaches the hilar lymphatics either through the well-developed superficial channels (Fig. 21-62) or by way of the deep lymphatics.

NERVES

Fibers from both homolateral and contralateral vagus nerves and from the sympathetic chain contribute to

FIGURE 21-60 Interrelationships among blood vessels, lymphatics, and interstitium in pulmonary alveoli under resting conditions. Values for hydrostatic pressure (HP) and colloid osmotic pressure (OP) are given in mmHg. Capillaries of interalveolar walls may lose fluid to the interstitium, which has significant osmotic pressure and negative hydrostatic pressure but is virtually absent from sites of alveolar gas exchange. A tight epithelium impedes water loss to alveoli, but some water is available to secretory great alveolar cells. Venules may also lose water despite a low hydrostatic pressure within, for their endothelial cell junctions are apt to be more leaky than those of capillaries. The interstitium holds water like a gel, but it eventually drains into paraalveolar lymphatics.

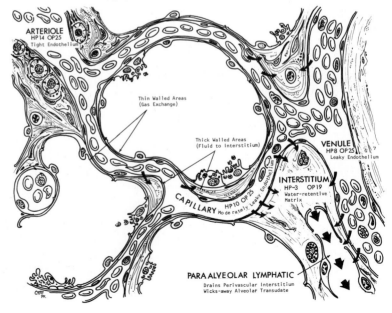

the posterior and smaller anterior pulmonary plexuses located at the hilum. From there fibers are sent to the bronchial tree, the blood vessels, and the visceral pleura. Nerves entering the lungs may at once become associated with the bronchi and blood vessels as in the rat, or else they may enter independently and shortly afterwards join pulmonary structures, as in primates; in entering the lung they occupy a space surrounded by the bronchus, the pulmonary artery, and the veins. Interspecies variation is also found in the exact intrapulmonary course of the nerves, although it generally conforms to the following pattern.

The main nerves to the bronchial tree travel together in bundles that run in the connective tissue outside the cartilage in rats, but in primates they run both superficial and deep to the cartilages. After these disappear, superficial and deep nerve bundles come together to form a single plexus deep in the adventitia,

and this extends to the respiratory bronchioles. Ganglion cells are associated with this system, being grouped into larger clusters in the hilar areas and into smaller ones or even solitary cells more peripherally (Fig. 21-64). These tend to occur near points of bundle branching. The nerves contain mixed fibers; perhaps a third of them are myelinated at the hilar level, but this proportion decreases as the bronchi are followed, because many of the myelinated nerves end in basketlike terminations on the ganglion cells. Each of these contributes a single unmyelinated axon to the nerve bundle. Peribronchial nerves in rats and primates are reactive for acetylcholinesterase and none exhibit fluorescence for catecholamines; accordingly, they are entirely cholinergic, and the bundles consist of both pre- and postsynaptic parasympathetic fibers.

Along its course the *peribronchial system* gives off fibers that ramify in a layer extending throughout the thickness of the bronchial smooth muscle (Fig. 21-63).

FIGURE 21-61 Injected specimen of adult human lung, showing the intercommunication between superficial and deep pulmonary lymphatics. [From J. Lauweryns, in S. C. Sommers (ed.), "Pathology Annual," vol. 6, p. 365, Appleton Century Crofts, New York, 1971.]

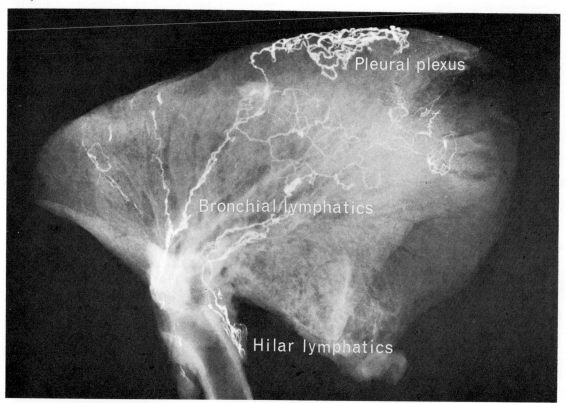

822

It also gives off others that do not communicate with the intramuscular layer but pass in between muscle bundles to reach the submucosa. The intramuscular layer is largely derived from the peribronchial nerves and consists of a tight-meshed plexus of unmyelinated, varicose fibers that are acetylcholinesterase-positive (Fig. 21-65). It is densest at bifurcations of bronchioles where contributions are received from nearby ganglion cells. The varicosities represent terminations to the bronchial smooth muscle (Chaps. 7 and 8); these contain clear synaptic vesicles, and the muscle can be considered to have an entirely cholinergic innervation.

A second system of nerves to the bronchial tree runs in close association with the bronchial arteries (Fig. 21-63). In rodents this *periarterial system* contains all the adrenergic fibers destined for the lung and only a few cholinergic fibers; in primates it also contains adrenergic fibers, but nearly half its fibers are cholinergic, and these largely branch off to join the intramuscular plexus. The adrenergic fibers form a

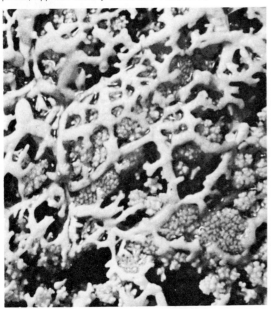

plexus that invests the bronchial artery and extends to other pulmonary vessels.

Superficial to the intramuscular plexus the submucosa is traversed by nerves having a number of different origins. Most exhibit varicosities along some part of their length and accordingly can be said to be terminal nerves of one kind or another. Those originating from the intramuscular plexus are thought to be postganglionic parasympathetic efferents. Other fibers originate from the peribronchial plexus, do not communicate with the intramuscular nerves, and extend in both longitudinal and circumferential directions in the submucosa. These unmyelinated fibers are cholinesterase-positive and are thought to be afferent terminals possibly associated with stretch receptors. The circumferential submucosal fibers eventually become single whence they lose their Schwann cell sheath and continue as naked processes beneath the epithelium. Among the unmyelinated nerves having this course in bats, some contain an abundance of both dense-cored (adrenergic) as well as clear (cholinergic) synaptic vesicles (Fig. 21-66), so that the classification of the nerve is not easily stated. In monkeys, a few *myelinated* fibers also run in the submucosa. The larger ones are acetylcholinesterase-negative and accordingly are deemed sensory, whereas the smaller ones are cholinergic and possibly preganglionic nerves to the neuroepithelial bodies. Sensory terminals have also been described in the smooth muscle layer and in intrapulmonary connective tissue septa; these are connected to large medullated fibers that run to the nodose ganglia of the vagus nerves.

The extent and character of intrapulmonary innervation beyond the respiratory bronchioles remains controversial; claims of an extensive innervation of alveolar ducts and alveolar walls are based primarily on studies using silver impregnation methods to reveal nerve bundles, but these methods are subject to the hazard of nonspecific staining of fine collagenous fibers which abound in these regions, and conclusions based on silver staining have not been confirmed by critical studies that identify nerves on the basis of acetylcholinesterase histochemistry or catecholamine fluorescence. An extensive innervation of respiratory tissue requires relatively large nerve bundles to supply it; as the main route of supply follows the bronchial axis, a rough assessment of the magnitude of innervation beyond can be made by examining the nerves surrounding the bronchiole and associated structures. It is, of course, also possible to reach respiratory tissue by nerves that follow the course of the blood vessels (below). Notwithstanding, at the bronchiolar level in bats, for example, peribronchial bundles typically contain but one myelinated axon and several smaller unmyelinated fibers enveloped in the cytoplasm of two or more Schwann cells; the whole is embedded in a collagenous matrix and surrounded by a perineurium (Fig. 21-30). These bundles and the unmyelinated nerve disappear before the airway loses its bronchiolelike wall structure and cuboidal epithelium, leaving only a few unmyelinated fibers of the intramuscular plexus to run in the connective tissue beneath, headed toward the terminal sphincter of smooth muscle (Fig. 21-35). At times a Schwann cell can be seen just deep to this sphincter, bearing a very few remaining processes after it has given off others to the overlying

muscle. In other species, electron micrographs reveal tiny unmyelinated nerve fascicles in walls of respiratory bronchioles and alveolar ducts. Immediately adjacent alveoli may be closely approached by these processes, but a general distribution of nerves in alveolar walls has not been convincingly demonstrated. In other words, few processes are left to innervate alveolar structures once all the smooth muscle in a given acinus has been provided for; whatever remains to be innervated through the peribronchial system is reached by the residual fibers, which continue to follow the course of the airway.

The innervation of bronchial and pulmonary arteries and pulmonary veins is predominantly by sympathetic fibers, but where cardiac muscle is present in the veins (Fig. 21-57), the myocardial portion is supplied by parasympathetic fibers. In the rat, the larger pulmonary arteries receive their adrenergic supply

FIGURE 21-63 Left. Hilar peribronchial nerve bundle in a rat's lung containing thick and thin fibers. Some extend toward the bronchial wall (right) where they join a plexus of varicose fibers. Methylene blue. ×259. Right. Periarterial nerve bundle spiraling about a bronchial artery and giving off fibers en route. The varicose plexus lies nearer the bronchiolar lumen (right). Methylene blue. ×122. (From A-W. El-Bermani, *Am. J. Anat.,* **137**:19, 1973.)

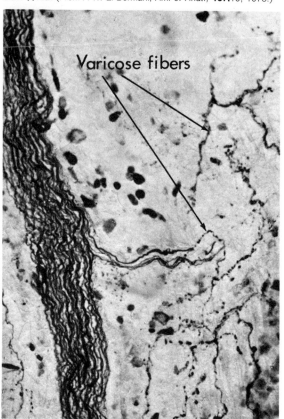

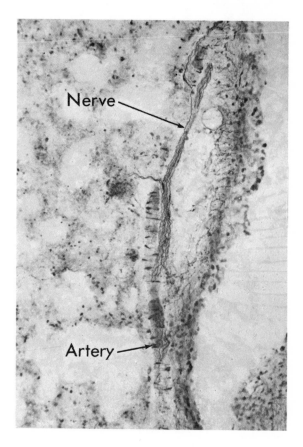

from branches of the plexus that surrounds the bronchial arteries; these are carried in with the vasa vasorum. The nerves are especially concentrated around bifurcations of the pulmonary arteries; and in the vessel walls, they ramify in a plexus located at the boundary between media and adventitia, from which a few branches penetrate the media. This plexus extends to the capillaries. Venules and the smallest veins of rats also receive adrenergic fibers derived from the distribution around the bronchial arteries; but in still smaller mammals, cardiac muscle displaces the smooth muscle in the corresponding veins, and a cholinergic

FIGURE 21-64 Frozen section of bat lung showing succinic dehydrogenase activity (dark gray) in tissues of the bronchial wall. Neurons of an adventitial ganglion are especially reactive. Left, bronchial epithelium; far right, alveoli including two reactive great alveolar cells. ×364.

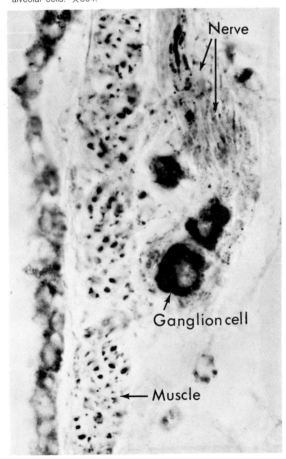

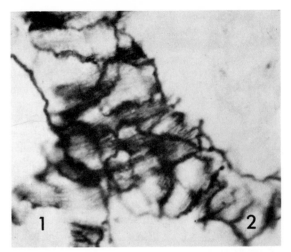

FIGURE 21-65 Acetylcholinesterase activity in varicose nerves of the intramuscular plexus of a rat's lung. The bronchiole branches into two (1,2), and bands of smooth muscle are faintly discernible in the background. ×250. (From A-W. El-Bermani, *Am. J. Anat.*, **137**:19, 1973.)

plexus replaces the adrenergic. Where only one layer of muscle occurs, this plexus lies just deep to it: but where the muscularis is multilayered in larger veins, the nerves run in among the cells.

The visceral pleura is innervated directly from the hilum as well as by nerves accompanying the bronchial arteries through pulmonary septa.

Stimulation of the vagus leads to contraction of the bronchial muscle and discharge of the glands. Sympathetic discharge, or administration of sympathomimetic agents, inhibits the vagus and dilates the bronchi. Three pulmonary vagal sensory receptors are currently well recognized by physiologists. They are viewed as mechanoreceptors because use is usually made of a distending stimulus to elicit their response: (1) *Slowly adapting stretch receptors* mediated by medullated fibers from intrapulmonary walls and increasingly active until cessation of inspiration; (2) *rapidly adapting mechano- and irritant receptors* carried by medullated fibers mainly from extrapulmonary airways and active in the cough reflex; and (3) juxtapulmonary capillary or *J receptors* carried by unmyelinated fibers from the respiratory zone. These respond to alveolar interstitial congestion and certain other kinds of irritation by promoting rapid, shallow breathing. The morphological form of all these receptors is still uncertain. Afferents from the visceral pleura and to some extent from the airway also carry pain. Intraepithelial nerves have been described in the sections on epithelium and glands.

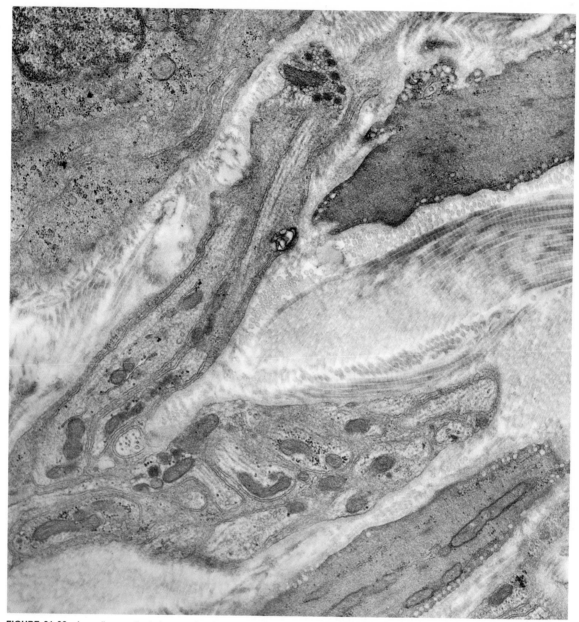

FIGURE 21-66 A small unmyelinated nerve sheathed by Schwann cell cytoplasm penetrates in between smooth muscle cells to enter the bronchiolar submucosa in a bat's lung. At this level a few processes branch off to run close to the base of the epithelium; one of them expands into a varicosity containing both clear and dense synaptic vesicles. ×11,600.

PLEURA

The *visceral pleura* is closely applied to each lung (Fig. 21-50). It is covered by a simple mesothelium whose cells are notable for the complexity of their junctions and the luxuriance of their brush border which is better developed in cells covering the ventral, caudal, and mediastinal surfaces than in those facing the ribs. They rest on a thin layer of dense fibrous tissue. Beneath lies the relatively thick connective tissue, rich in elastic fibers and sometimes rich in mast cells, that continues into the interlobar and interlobular septa of the lung. The dense pleural sheet effectively prevents leakage of air into the thoracic cavity. Pleural folds in the mediastinum may have several white patches (*Kampmeier foci*) where the pleural mesothelium is invaded by lymphocytes and macrophages. These may serve as windows on the thoracic cavity for immunologically competent lymphoid cells as well as points of embarkation for macrophages crossing onto the pleural surface. The *parietal pleura*, a thicker and less elastic membrane than the visceral pleura, contains fat cells. The vascular supply to the visceral pleura is derived from both pulmonary and bronchial circuits, the parietal supply is entirely systemic from vessels of the body wall.

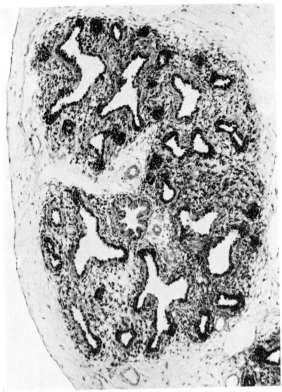

FIGURE 21-67 Section of a lobule from a 3.5-month fetal human lung, demonstrating glycogen (black). A central bronchiole is surrounded by tissue containing budding bronchial branches. These have cuboidal epithelium. Connective tissue surrounds the lobule; the parietal pleura is at the left. PAS method. ×125.

DEVELOPMENT OF THE LUNGS

The airways of the lung develop from a midline endodermal bud, the *laryngotracheal groove*, located on the floor of the pharynx between the sixth arches. This bud branches to form the two primary bronchi and their arboreous subdivisions. The larynx develops from adjacent pharyngeal structures. The future connective tissue adjacent to the pulmonary epithelium is derived from a relatively cellular mesenchyma, originally located next to the laryngotracheal groove. It accompanies the invading endodermal buds, which spread by rapid growth and division of component cells. These tissues advance amid a relatively acellular mesenchyma, which gives rise to the blood vessels, interlobar septa, pulmonary pleura, and cartilage. The growing tips, or *terminal buds*, of the expanding bronchial tree appear to be centers of much of the morphogenetic activity of the lungs, for they early reveal histochemical specialization and exhibit concentrated mitotic activity, apparently in response to inductive interaction between the endoderm and the mesenchyma. These phenomena account in some degree for the successive branching of the developing bronchial tree; however, differences between the configurations of right and left lungs become apparent early, and this argues for the simultaneous operation of higher-level genetic controls than may be necessary to regulate the preceding.

Fetal lungs have a glandlike structure. Their terminal portions are lined by a cuboidal epithelium (Fig. 21-67). Capillaries lengthen into loops that stretch overlying cells, and the epithelium begins to attenuate before the first breaths are drawn. Prenatal inspiratory movements and possibly contractions of smooth muscle in the bronchial tree help to shape the alveoli. At birth, lungs of various species differ greatly in histologic and histochemical maturity. It is not the presence of a thin alveolar epithelium so much as the development of an adequate pulmonary vasculature that is critical to the survival of premature infants. On this basis the extreme limit of viability has been placed at 4.5 months, but the chances of survival increase dramatically when alveoli appear.

Within a few hours after birth the lungs fill with air. At that time proprioceptive and other chemically mediated mechanisms produce a decrease in pulmonary vascular resistance and increase in blood flow. These effects are enhanced by the opening of new circulatory routes on expansion of the lungs. Some time later the *ductus arteriosus* closes, and the definitive pulmonary circuit comes into being.

In humans few nonrespiratory branches are added to the bronchial tree after birth; in dogs their

number may decrease. This is because alveolar formation is essentially a centripetal process superimposed on the centrifugal process that resulted in the laying down of the bronchial tree. The neonatal human lung contains shallow alveoli within a peripheral zone made up of clusters of thin-walled saccules. These alveoli enlarge in the immediate postnatal period as the terminal region is remodeled; septa grow in from the walls of the saccules, deepen the alveoli, and increase the respiratory surface. This is followed by the onset of retrograde alveolarization. As development proceeds, respiratory bronchioles become transformed into alveolar ducts, and bronchioles become respiratory bronchioles. The number of alveoli continue to increase until early adolescence, but the shorter bronchial pathways complete their development before then. The formation of accessory respiratory pathways at acinar and bronchiolar levels evidently is a by-product of this postnatal reorganization.

REFERENCES

ALLISON, A. C.: The Morphology of the Olfactory System in the Vertebrates. *Biol. Rev.,* **28:**195 (1953).

BARNETT, C. H.: A Note on the Dimensions of the Bronchial Tree, *Thorax,* **12:**175 (1957).

BOYDEN, E. A.: Development of the Human Lung, in V. C. Kelley (ed.), "Brennemann's Practice of Pediatrics," vol. 4, Chap. 64, Harper & Row, Publishers, Incorporated, New York, 1971.

BOYDEN, E. A.: The Structure of the Pulmonary Acinus in a Child of $6\frac{2}{3}$ Years, *Anat. Rec.,* **169:**282 (1971).

BOYDEN, E. A., and D. H. TOMPSETT: The Postnatal Growth of the Lung in the Dog, *Acta Anat.,* **47:**185 (1961).

BRAIN, J.: The Uptake of Inhaled Gases by the Nose, *Ann. Otol.,* **79:**529 (1970).

BRAIN, J. D., D. F. PROCTOR, and L. REID (eds.): "Respiratory Defense Mechanisms," Marcel Dekker, Inc., New York, 1977.

CAUNA, N., and K. H. HINDERER: Fine Structure of Blood Vessels of the Human Nasal Respiratory Mucosa, *Ann. Otol.,* **78:**865 (1969).

CHEVALIER, G., and A. J. COLLET: In vivo Incorporation of Choline-^{3}H, Leucine-^{3}H and Galactose-^{3}H in Alveolar Type II Pneumocytes in Relation to Surfactant Synthesis. A Quantitative Radioautographic Study in Mouse by Electron Microscopy, *Anat. Rec.,* **174:**289 (1972).

COURNAND, A.: Pulmonary Circulation, Its Control in Man, with Some Remarks on Methodology, *Science,* **125:**1231 (1957).

DANNENBERG, A. M., JR., M. S. BURSTONE, P. C. WALTER, and J. W. KINSLEY: A Histochemical Study of

Phagocytic and Enzymatic Functions of Rabbit Mononuclear and Polymorphonuclear Exudate Cells and Alveolar Macrophages, *J. Cell Biol.,* **17:**465 (1963).

DAWES, J. D. K., and M. M. L. PRICHARD: Studies of the Vascular Arrangements of the Nose, *J. Anat.,* **87:**311 (1953).

EL-BERMANI, A-W.: The Innervation of the Rat Lung. Acetylcholinesterase-containing Nerves of the Bronchial Tree, *Am. J. Anat.,* **137:**19 (1973).

EL-BERMANI, A-W., and M. GRANT: Acetylcholinesterase-positive Nerves of the Rhesus Monkey Bronchial Tree, *Thorax,* **30:**162 (1975).

FINK, B. R.: "The Human Larynx, A Functional Study," Raven Books, Abelard-Schuman Limited, New York, 1975.

FISCHER, H. H. BÖRSIG, and E. EDEN: Studien über den Bau des Bindegewebsgerüstes der Trachea bei verschiedenen Säugetieren, *Gegenbaurs Morphol Jahrb.,* **102:**227 (1962).

FLOREY, H., H. M. CARLETON, and A. Q. WELLS: Mucus Secretion in the Trachea, *Br. J. Exp. Path.,* **13:**269 (1932).

GODLESKI, J. J., and J. D. BRAIN: The Origin of Alveolar Macrophages in Mouse Radiation Chimeras, *J. Exptl. Med.,* **136:**630 (1972).

GOODRICH, E. S.: "Studies on the Structure and Development of Vertebrates," Dover Publications, Inc., New York, 1958.

HAM, A. W., and K. W. BALDWIN: A Histological Study of the Development of the Lung, with Particular Reference to the Nature of Alveoli, *Anat. Rec.,* **81:**363 (1941).

HAYEK, H. VON: Cellular Structure and Mucus Activity in the Bronchial Tree and Alveoli, in A. V. S. de Reuck and M. O'Connor (eds.): "Pulmonary Structure and Function," Ciba Foundation Symposium, Little, Brown and Company, Boston, 1962.

HEISS, R.: Der Atmungsapparat. in W. von Möllendorff (ed.), "Handbüch der Mikroskopischen Anatomie des Menschen," Springer-Verlag OHG, Berlin, 1936.

HONJIN, R.: Experimental Degeneration of the Vagus, and Its Relation to the Nerve Supply of Lung of the Mouse, with Special Reference to the Crossing Innervation of the Lung by the Vagi, *J. Comp. Neurol.,* **106:**1 (1956).

HONJIN, R.: On the Nerve Supply of the Lung of the Mouse, with Special Reference to the Structure of the Peripheral Vegetative Nervous System, *J. Comp. Neurol.,* **105:**587 (1956).

HUNG, K-S., M. S. HERTWECK, J. D. HARDY, and C. G. LOOSLI: Innervation of Pulmonary Alveoli of the Mouse Lung: An Electron Microscopic Study, *Amer. J. Anat.,* **135:**477 (1972).

KRAHL, V. E.: The Glomus Pulmonale: Its Location and Microscopic Anatomy, in A. V. S. de Reuck and M. O'Connor (eds.), "Pulmonary Structure and Function," Ciba Foundation Symposium, Little, Brown and Company, Boston, 1962.

KUHN, C., III, L. A. CALLAWAY, and F. B. ASKIN: The Formation of Granules in the Bronchiolar Clara Cells of the Rat. 1. Electron Microscopy, *J. Ultrastr. Res.,* **49:**387 (1974).

KUHN, C., III, and L. A. CALLAWAY: The Formation of Granules in the Bronchiolar Clara Cells of the Rat. II. Enzyme Cytochemistry, *J. Ultrastr. Res.,* **53:**66 (1975).

LAUWERYNS, J.: The Blood and Lymphatic Microcirculation of the Lung, in S. C. Sommers (ed.): "Pathology Annual," vol. 6, p. 365, Appleton Century Crafts, New York, 1971.

LAUWERYNS, J.: L'angioarchitecture du Poumon, *Arch. Biol.* (*Liege*), **75**(Suppl.):771 (1964).

LAUWERYNS, J. M., M. COKELAERE, P. THEUNYNCK, and M. DELEERSNYDER: Neuroepithelial Bodies in Mammalian Respiratory Mucosa: Light Optical, Histochemical and Ultrastructural Studies, *Chest,* **65:**(Suppl.): 22S (1974).

LELONG, M., and R. LAUMONIER: Histological and Histochemical Evolution of the Foetal Lung, in J. F. Delafresnaye and T. E. Oppé (eds.), "Anoxia of the New-born Infant, a Symposium," Charles C Thomas, Publisher, Springfield, Ill., 1954.

MACKLEM, P. T.: Airway Obstruction and Collateral Ventilation, *Physiol. Rev.,* **51:**368 (1971).

MACKLIN, C. C.: The Pulmonary Alveolar Mucoid Film and the Pneumonocytes, *Lancet,* **266:**1099 (1954).

MACKLIN, C. C.: Pulmonic Alveolar Vents, *J. Anat.,* **69:**188 (1935).

MACKLIN, C. C.: The Musculature of the Bronchi and Lungs, *Physiol Rev.,* **9:**1 (1929).

MILLER, W. S.: "The Lung," 2d ed., Charles C Thomas, Publisher, Springfield, Ill., 1947.

NEGUS, V.: "The Comparative Anatomy and Physiology of the Nose and Paranasal Sinuses," E. & S. Livingstone, Edinburgh, 1958.

OREN, R., A. E. FARNHAM, K. SAITO, E. MILOFSKY, and M. L. KARNOVSKY: Metabolic Patterns in Three Types of Phagocytizing Cells, *J. Cell Biol.,* **17:**487 (1963).

PATTLE, R. E.: Properties, Function and Origin of the Alveolar Lining Layer, *Proc. R. Soc. Lond.,* [*Biol*] **148:**217 (1958).

PETRIK, P., and A. J. COLLET: Quantitative Electron Microscopic Autoradiography of In Vivo Incorporation of ^{3}H-choline, ^{3}H-leucine, ^{3}H-acetate and ^{3}H-galactose in Non-ciliated Bronchiolar (Clara) Cells of Mice, *Am. J. Anat.,* **139:**519 (1974).

PFAFFMANN, C. (ed.): "Olfaction and Taste" Proceedings of the Third International Symposium, Rockefeller University Press, New York, 1969.

PROCTOR, D. F.: Physiology of the Upper Airway, in W. O. Fenn and H. Rahn, (eds.), "Handbook of Physiology," sec. 3, Respiration, vol. 1, p. 309, Waverly Press, Baltimore, 1965.

REID, L.: The Secondary Lobule in the Adult Human Lung with Special Reference to Its Appearance in Bronchograms, *Thorax,* **13:**110 (1958).

REID, L., and G. SIMON: The Peripheral Pattern in the Normal Bronchogram and Its Relation to Peripheral Pulmonary Anatomy, *Thorax,* **13:**103 (1958).

ROSS, R. B.: Influence of Bronchial Tree Structure on Ventilation in the Dog's Lung as Inferred from Measurements of a Plastic Cast, *J. Appl. Physiol.,* **10:**1 (1957).

SCHAEFFER, J. P.: The Mucous Membrane of the Nasal Cavity and the Paranasal Sinuses, in E. V. Cowdry (ed.): "Special Cytology," vol. 1, Paul B. Hoeber, Inc., New York, 1932.

SCHNEEBERGER, E., and M. J. KARNOVSKY: The Influence of Intravascular Fluid Volume on the Permeability of Newborn and Adult Mouse Lungs to Ultrastructural Protein Tracers, *J. Cell Biol.,* **49:**319 (1971).

SOROKIN, S.: The Cells of the Lungs, in P. Nettesheim, M. G. Hanna, Jr., and J. W. Deatherage, Jr. (eds.), "Morphology of Experimental Respiratory Carcinogenesis," CONF 700501, p. 3, U.S. Atomic Energy Commission, Oak Ridge, Tenn., 1970.

SOROKIN, S.: A Morphologic and Cytochemical Study on the Great Alveolar Cell, *J. Histochem, Cytochem.,* **14:**884 (1966).

SOROKIN, S., and J. D. BRAIN: Pathways of Clearance in Mouse Lungs Exposed to Iron Oxide Aerosols, *Anat. Rec.,* **181:**581 (1975).

SOROKIN, S., H. A. PADYKULA, and E. HERMAN: Comparative Histochemical Patterns in Developing Mammalian Lungs, *Dev. Biol.,* **1:**125 (1959).

TENNEY, S. M., and J. E. REMMERS: Comparative Quantitative Morphology of the Mammalian Lung: Diffusing Area, *Nature* **197:**54 (1963).

TOBIN, C. E.: Human Pulmonic Lymphatics, *Anat. Rec.,* **127:**611 (1957).

TOBIN, C. E.: Lymphatics of the Pulmonary Alveoli, *Anat. Rec.,* **120:**625 (1954).

WANG, N-S.: The Regional Difference of Pleural Mesothelial Cells in Rabbits, *Am. Rev. Resp. Dis.,* **110:**623 (1974).

WEIBEL, E.: Die Blutgelfässanastomosen in der menschlichen Lunge, *Z. Zellforsch,* **50:**653 (1959).

WEIBEL, E. R., and J. GIL: Electron Microscopic Demonstration of an Extracellular Duplex Lining Layer of Alveoli, *Resp. Physiol.,* **4:**42 (1968).

WOLSTENHOLME, G. E. W., and J. KNIGHT (eds.): "Taste and Smell in Vertebrates," J & A. Churchill, London, 1970.

The Urinary System

RUTH ELLEN BULGER

There are those who say that the human kidney was created to keep the blood pure, or more precisely, to keep our internal environment in an ideal balanced state. I would deny this. I grant that the human kidney is a marvelous organ, but I cannot grant that it was purposefully designed to excrete urine, or even to regulate the composition of the blood, or to subserve the physiological welfare of *Homo sapiens* in any sense. Rather I contend that the human kidney manufactures the kind of urine that it does, and it maintains the blood in the composition which that fluid has, because this kidney has a certain functional architecture: and it owes that architecture not to design or foresight or any plan, but to the fact that the earth is an unstable sphere with a fragile crust, to the geologic revolutions that for 600 million years have raised and lowered continents and seas, to the predacious enemies, and heat and cold, and storms and droughts, the unending succession of vicissitudes that have driven the mutant vertebrates from sea into fresh water, into desiccated swamps, out upon the dry land, from one habitation to another, perpetually in search of the free and independent life, perpetually failing for one reason or another to find it.[1]

INTRODUCTION

COMPONENTS OF THE URINARY SYSTEM

The normal human urinary system consists of two kidneys, two ureters, a bladder, and a urethra. The kidneys elaborate a fluid product called urine; the ureters, two fibromuscular tubes, conduct the urine to a single urinary bladder where the fluid accumulates for periodic evacuation via the single urethra which connects the bladder to the exterior.

KIDNEY FUNCTION

The kidneys make significant and sometimes vital contributions to several important functions:

1. The excretion of waste products of metabolism

2. The elimination of foreign substances and their breakdown products

[1] Homer W. Smith, "Studies in the Physiology of the Kidney," p. 66, University of Kansas, University Extension Division, Lawrence, Kans., 1939.

3. The maintenance of the extracellular fluid volume

4. The regulation of the amount and type of various salts to be retained or excreted by the body

5. The regulation of total body water

6. The control of acid-base balance

The kidneys carry out these various functions because of their architecture: gross, histologic, cytologic, and chemical. This particular architecture results from the modeling and remodeling that occurred during the long evolutionary process in which animals were subjected to varying environmental conditions. Three separate kidneys have developed during evolution: the pronephros, the mesonephros, and the metanephros. This evolutionary experience is repeated in each human embryo with the serial development of three separate kidneys and the subsequent degeneration of the first two during early embryonic life. In each of these kidneys there are filtering devices capable of developing a fluid which the adjacent tubules then modify. The filter has become more efficient and the tubule more complex during evolution.

Three separate physiologic processes are involved in the formation of urine by the adult metanephric kidney: (1) filtration, (2) secretion, and (3) reabsorption. The first step in the formation of urine is a *filtration* process in which an ultrafiltrate of plasma is created. The filtering membrane retains most large proteins within the blood, but a small amount of albumin (MW approximately 70,000) passes into the filtrate. As it passes down the tubule, the filtrate is altered by *secretion,* in which additional substances are moved by the lining cells of the tubule from the surrounding renal interstitium into the filtrate within the tubular lumen, and *reabsorption,* whereby substances are moved from the intratubular filtrate across the tubular cells back into the renal interstitium. The fluid that emerges at the end of the tubule is the net result of these three processes and is called *urine.*

Urine production in the mammalian kidney is a grossly inefficient process. In man, every 24 h 180 l of fluid are filtered by the renal corpuscles into the tubular lumens of the kidney, but normally only 1 or 2 l of urine are produced. The remainder of the filtered fluid is reabsorbed across the tubular epithelium to reenter the blood vascular system. This process requires a large expenditure of energy.

THE KIDNEY

The kidneys of man are paired, bean-shaped organs which lie in the retroperitoneal space on the posterior aspect of the abdominal cavity. The lateral border on each kidney is convex, and the medial border is concave. Normally one kidney is found on either side of the vertebral column, with their upper margins near the upper region of the twelfth thoracic vertebra. The upper poles lie closer to the vertebral column than the lower poles, and so the long axis of the kidney is parallel with the psoas muscles. The kidney is surrounded by a fibrous capsule and situated within a mass of fatty tissue.

The medial concave border is penetrated by a vertical slit called the *renal hilus.* Branches of the renal artery, vein, lymphatics, and nerves, as well as an expanded part of the ureter (called the *pelvis*), pass through the hilus to the renal parenchyma. The renal hilus communicates with a flattened cavity within the kidney called the *renal sinus.* Within the sinus, the expanded pelvis of the ureter branches into three or four major calyxes which in turn branch to form seven to fourteen minor calyxes. Loose connective tissue and fat tissue found within the sinus provide a region through which the vessels and nerves pass.

When the kidney is bisected into dorsal and ventral portions (Fig. 22-1), it can be seen to be divided into a cortex and a medulla. The cortex consists of a broad outer zone of dark red substance and projections which extend toward the renal sinus (called the *renal columns* because of their columnar profile in a section of kidney). The medulla is composed of a variable number of conical structures of lighter, striated appearance called *medullary pyramids.* They are situated with their bases adjacent to the outer zone of cortex, and their apexes project into the renal sinus. The apex of each medullary pyramid is capped by a funnel-shaped minor calyx. Urine produced by the kidney exits at the medullary apex and is funneled by a minor calyx into the remainder of the extrarenal collecting system.

The kidney is divided into units called *lobes*. One lobe consists of a conical medullary pyramid and the cortical substance which surrounds it like the cap of an acorn. The kidneys of some animals, such as rodents, consist of only one lobe (unilobar). However, multilobar human kidneys contain from six to eighteen lobes. During human fetal life, the lobes develop separately and are demarcated by deep clefts between them (Fig. 22-2). In postnatal life, however, these clefts are generally obliterated and the organ appears to have a smooth surface, although the lobes still exist within the kidney.

At intervals along the base of each medullary pyramid, striated elements called *medullary rays* penetrate into the cortex. Although they resemble the medullary substance because of their striated appearance, the medullary rays are considered part of the cortex. Each medullary ray forms the center of a small cone of renal parenchyma called a *lobule*.

An additional zonation can be seen in the gross

structure of the medulla, which is divided into an *outer zone* adjacent to the cortex and an *inner zone* including the medullary tip (which is called the *papilla*). The outer zone, in turn, consists of an outer and inner stripe. The zones seen grossly are a reflection of the differing morphologies of the regions of the renal secretory units and of their orientation within the kidney (Figs. 22-3 and 22-4).

FUNCTIONAL ANATOMY OF THE URINIFEROUS TUBULE

The functional unit of the kidney is the uriniferous tubule. Each kidney in man contains approximately one million of these units. The uriniferous tubule is composed of a long convoluted portion called the *nephron* and a system of *intrarenal collecting ducts*. Each of these segments was derived from a different embryologic primordium. The nephron developed from the metanephrogenic blastema (tissue from the caudal region of the urogenital ridge), whereas the

FIGURE 22-1 Gross anatomic appearance of a human kidney, at three-fifths its natural size. The tissue has been bisected to reveal elements of the internal structure. (From H. Braus, "Anatomie des Menschen." Springer-Verlag OHG, Berlin, 1924.)

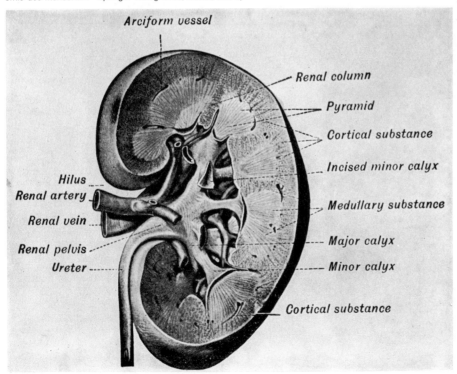

collecting ducts were derived from the ureteric bud (a diverticulum of the mesonephric duct). Despite this dual derivation, a gradual transition is seen in the structure and function at the junction of these two regions, so that the term *nephron* has recently been used synonymously with uriniferous tubule by some investigators. In this chapter, however, the term nephron will not include the intrarenal collecting ducts.

Nephron

The nephron is composed of several regions of diversified morphology, but all of them are characterized by cells that have an elaborate shape with numerous lateral interdigitating processes. The blind end of the

FIGURE 22-2 Photomicrograph showing one lobe of a metanephric kidney from a 6-month-old human fetus. The inset outlines the part of the kidney which appears in the photograph. The schematic diagram in the center of the lobe shows the position and arrangement of the renal tubules around a straight collecting tubule. ×18. (From B. M. Patten, "Human Embryology," 3d ed., McGraw-Hill Book Company, New York, 1968.)

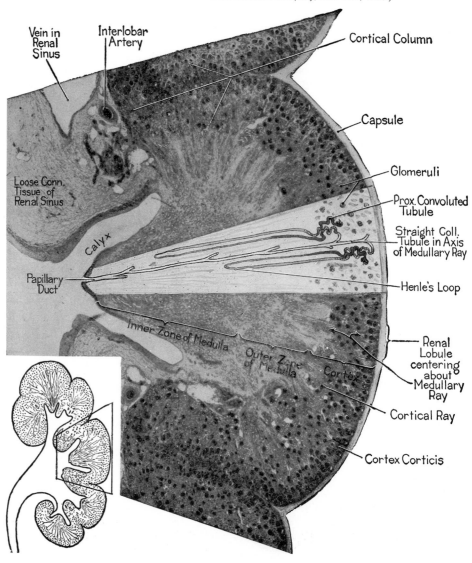

nephron is indented by a network of capillaries and supporting cells to form a filtering body called the *renal corpuscle.* In addition, the nephron consists of the following: (1) a neck, (2) a proximal convoluted tubule, (3) a straight region of the proximal tubule, (4) a thin limb, (5) a straight region of the distal tubule, (6) a macula densa region of the distal tubule, and (7) a distal convoluted tubule.

Nephrons are situated within the kidney in a characteristic position (Figs. 22-2 to 22-4) with the renal corpuscles and proximal convoluted tubules situated within the cortex. The straight portion of the proximal tubule, the thin limb segment, and the straight portion of the distal tubule form a looping

structure called the *loop of Henle,* which enters into the medullary pyramid by way of a medullary ray, forms a hairpin loop within the medulla, and returns to the cortex via the same medullary ray. As the straight portion of each distal tubule enters the cortex, it passes adjacent to its originating renal corpuscle, forming the macula densa of the distal tubule, and then continues as the distal convoluted segment.

Although all nephrons have these regions, two separate types of nephrons have been described. Presumably there is a continuum between the two types. The *cortical* nephrons are characterized by a renal corpuscle located in the peripheral region of the cortex and by a short loop of Henle which may lack a thin limb segment. The *juxtamedullary* nephrons are characterized by a larger renal corpuscle located in the cortex adjacent to the medulla, a longer convoluted

FIGURE 22-3 Scanning electron micrograph of a cross section from a rat kidney. The kidney can be divided into four radial zones: cortex (C); outer strip of the medullary outer zone (OS); inner strip of the medullary outer zone (IS): and inner zone of medulla with its papillary tip. The tip drains into the major calyx. ×30.

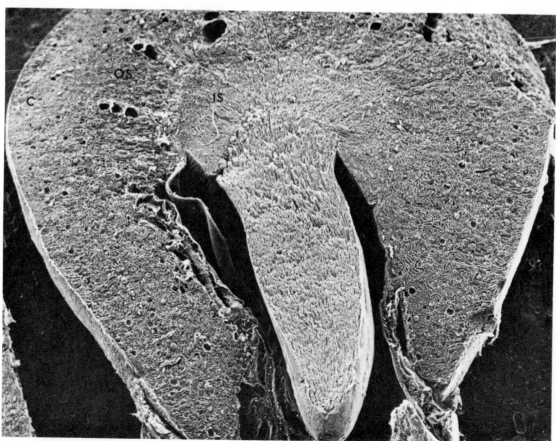

tubule, and a long loop of Henle with a lengthy thin limb segment. Even though the nephrons differ in length, each region of all nephrons tends to occupy a certain position in the kidney as a whole, causing the gross zonation described earlier (Fig. 22-3). For example, the thin limbs are seen in the inner stripe of the outer zone of the medulla and in the inner zone of the medulla, whereas the proximal and distal convoluted tubules are located only in the cortex (Fig. 22-4).

The nephrons empty into a complex system of collecting ducts. In human kidneys, the cortical nephrons tend to empty singly into a terminal collecting duct, whereas several juxtamedullary nephrons empty into an arched collecting duct which courses peripherally in the cortex and then enters the medullary ray. These cortical collecting ducts merge while traversing the medullary ray and medullary pyramid and empty

as several large collecting ducts at the apex of the medullary pyramid.

RENAL CORPUSCLE The nephron begins with a renal corpuscle located in the cortex and roughly oval in shape (Fig. 22-5). Estimates of their diameter in humans range from 150 to 250 μm. Each renal corpuscle consists of tufts of anastomosing capillaries and their supporting cells, which have developed within a double-walled capsule formed by half of the S-shaped bend in one end of the developing renal tubule. A renal corpuscle therefore has some resemblance to a balloon (the capsule) with a fist (the capillaries) punched into it. The outer wall of the capsule is called the *parietal* layer; the inner wall is the *visceral* (*glomerular*) layer. The space between the two walls of the

FIGURE 22-4 Schematic diagram of a cortical and a juxtamedullary nephron, showing the relationship of segments of the nephron to the zones of the kidney which can be seen grossly.

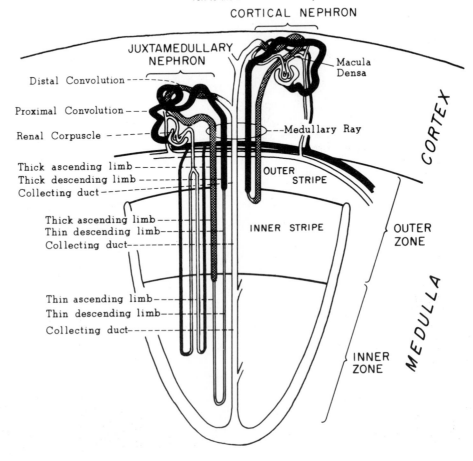

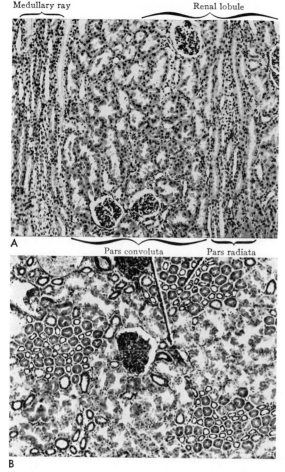

Medullary ray   Renal lobule

A

Pars convoluta   Pars radiata

B

FIGURE 22-5 Sections of kidney cortex cut perpendicular to the capsule in A and parallel to the capsule in B to show the medullary rays and the convoluted tubules which lie between them. ×80.

capsule is called *Bowman's space.* The epithelium of this visceral wall covers the anastomosing capillaries much like a glove covers each finger of a hand. Between the epithelium and the capillaries is an extracellular layer, the glomerular *basement membrane* (*basal lamina*).

At one region of the renal corpuscle, called the *urinary pole,* the parietal layer of capsular epithelium is continuous with the epithelium of the neck of the tubule (Fig. 22-6). Bowman's space is therefore continuous with the lumen of the remaining nephron, so that fluid formed by filtration within the renal corpuscle enters the lumen of the proximal convoluted tubule. Another region of the renal corpuscle located

roughly opposite the urinary pole is called the *vascular pole* (Fig. 22-7). It is marked by the point of entrance of the afferent arteriole and the exit of the *efferent* arteriole. The afferent arteriole enters the renal corpuscle and divides into four or more primary branches. Each of these branches becomes a network of anastomosing capillaries which forms a lobule. The lobule has a stalk or supporting region called the *mesangial region.* The capillaries within the lobules reunite to form the efferent arteriole which exits from the vascular pole. Since the efferent arteriole again breaks up to form a second capillary network, such an arrangement constitutes a portal system—an arterial portal system, in contrast to the venous portal system in the liver. The second capillary network surrounds the tubules and is therefore called the *peritubular capillary network.* Some authors describe a differing morphology at the vascular pole of juxtamedullary

FIGURE 22-6 Renal corpuscle of an epoxy resin section from a rat kidney, showing that Bowman's space is confluent with the proximal tubule lumen at the urinary pole (UP). Toluidine blue. ×520.

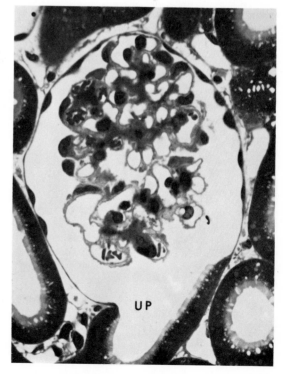

UP

nephrons (Ljungqvist, 1964). In their descriptions, the afferent arteriole is continuous with the efferent arteriole, and the capillaries to the renal corpuscle exit from the side of this arteriolar shunt. Because of the anatomy of the arterioles in the juxtamedullary region, if the renal corpuscle dies, an aglomerular vessel can form. These vessels have been called the *vasa rectae verae*.

The renal corpuscle therefore consists of the following parts: (1) the parietal epithelium of the capsule, (2) the visceral epithelium of the capsule, (3) the glomerular basement membrane (basal lamina), (4) the endothelium of the glomerulus, and (5) the intraglomerular mesangial region (Figs. 22-6 to 22-8). These will be considered in order.

The parietal epithelium of Bowman's capsule The parietal epithelium consists of a layer of simple squamous cells which bulge into Bowman's space in the region of their nuclei. They are polygonal in outline and rest on a thick basement membrane which in some cases appears to be multilayered. At the vascular

FIGURE 22-7 Renal corpuscle of an epoxy resin section from a rat kidney, showing the afferent and efferent vessels (arrows) at the vascular pole. ×320.

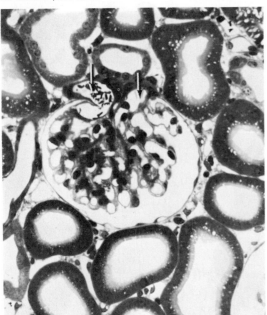

pole, the parietal epithelium is reflected to form the visceral layer.

The visceral epithelium of Bowman's capsule The visceral epithelium closely embraces the entire network of glomerular capillaries and consists of cells which have a complex shape. The cells, which are frequently called *podocytes*, do not rest on the basement membrane for long regions but tend to sit somewhat removed in Bowman's space. The cells have long primary processes called *trabeculae*. The trabeculae in turn branch to form secondary and tertiary processes. All three of these kinds of processes again branch to form thin, club-shaped terminal processes called *pedicels* (little feet) which interdigitate in a complicated manner with similar processes from adjacent cells. This is well demonstrated in a scanning electron micrograph taken by Arakawa (1970) (Fig. 22-9). The pedicels form a layer along the glomerular basement membrane. This elaborate interdigitation results in a extensive pattern of narrow slits between the pedicels. In electron micrographs, these slits seem to be bridged by a thin layer of material of unknown composition called the *filtration-slit membrane*, which is thinner than a cell membrane and appears to be similar to the diaphragms seen across the pores of fenestrated capillaries and across nuclear pores. The podocytes have nuclei which are large and irregular in shape and tend to be indented on one side in the region of the Golgi apparatus. They contain abundant protein secretory organelles, numerous fine filaments, and microtubules (Fig. 22-8).

Glomerular basement membrane (basal lamina) In adult human beings, the basement membrane is thick, with a mean diameter of approximately 320 to 340 nm (Jorgensen, 1966). It is thinner in very young children and in most experimental animals. The basement membrane stains with periodic acid–Schiff (PAS) reagent. It appears to contain a collagenlike protein and a mucopolysaccharide rich in sialic acid. It is composed of three layers: an electron-dense central layer, the lamina densa; and a less dense layer on either side, the lamina rara externa (adjacent to the glomerular podocytes); and a lamina rara interna (adjacent to the capillary endothelium). In the stalk region of each capillary loop, the basement membrane does not surround the entire endothelium but instead appears to be reflected with the glomerular epithelial cells from which it is presumably largely derived (Fig. 22-8).

Endothelium The endothelium consists of a simple squamous layer of fenestrated cells. The cells are extremely thin, except at the stalk region of the capillary where their nuclei bulge into the lumen. In this region the cells can have complex processes extending into the capillary lumen. The fenestrae of this particular endothelium differ from those found in the more typical fenestrated endothelium of the peritubular capillaries and of other regions of the body in that the pores appear to be more irregular in shape and larger

FIGURE 22-8 Electron micrograph from a renal corpuscle, showing capillaries (C), glomerular podocytes (P), with their small processes called pedicels (arrow), mesangial cells (M), and the glomerular basement membrane (BM). A portion of a parietal cell (PC) can be seen at the right. ×6100.

in size (approximately 50 to 100 nm in diameter) (Figs. 22-10 and 22-11). Although pores in fenestrated endothelium are generally bridged by a thin diaphragm, only a few of the fenestrae of the glomerulus are bridged by diaphragms. Both of these modifications (large-sized pores and few diaphragms) would increase the permeability of this endothelium. **Intraglomerular mesangial region** The mesangial or

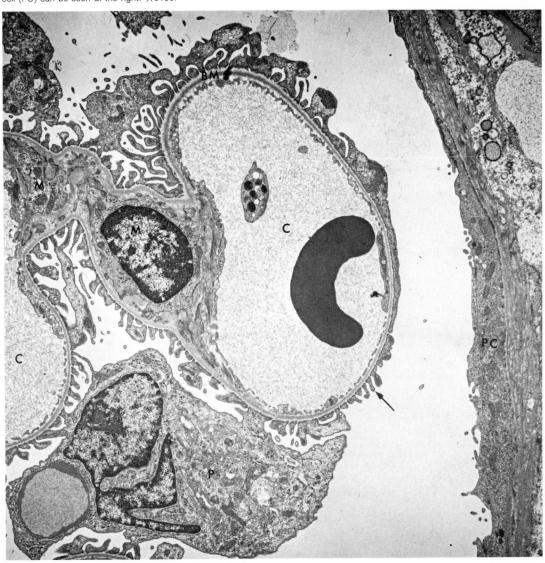

stalk region of the capillary tuft consists of a population of cells and the matrix material in which they are embedded. The cells appear similar to pericytes seen adjacent to vessels elsewhere in the body. Each cell contains a small, densely staining nucleus, fine filaments especially abundant along the cell membranes, and dense cytoplasmic plaques located along the cell membrane. The cells have long processes, some of which can penetrate the mesangial matrix underlying the capillary endothelium to come into contact with the endothelial cell. In some cases, these processes appear to project through the endothelium into the lumen of the capillary. The function of these mesangial cell projections is at present unknown. Mesangial cells are of particular importance because they have a propensity to divide in certain kidney diseases. The mesangial matrix appears to be an amorphous substance with less electron density than the lamina densa of the basement membrane. It appears to be continuous with the lamina rara interna. The mesangial cells appear to function by clearing the basement membrane of large proteins which have become lodged during filtration. The intraglomerular mesangial region

FIGURE 22-9 Scanning electron micrograph of a capillary loop from a normal rat kidney glomerulus, showing the processes of podocytes interdigitating along the surface of the capillary wall. ×4500. (Fig. 4, M. Arakawa, *Lab. Invest.,* **23:**489, 1970.)

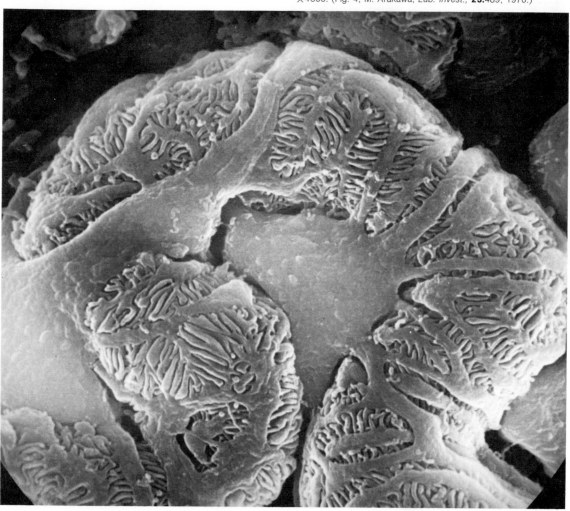

is continuous with the extraglomerular mesangial region (part of the juxtaglomerular apparatus) and in certain experimental circumstances can be seen to contain granulated cells like those of the extraglomerular mesangium.

Function of the renal corpuscle Because of its morphology, the renal corpuscle behaves as a filtering device which allows the passage of water and ions but retains large objects such as cells and even large protein molecules. Since a small amount of albumin penetrates the filter, it appears to be near the effective pore size of the filtration barrier. The barrier is com-

plex and, as can be seen in Fig. 22-11, consists of three morphologic structures: (1) the fenestrated endothelium, (2) the glomerular basement membrane, and (3) the slits between pedicels which are bridged by the filtration-slit membrane. Tracer molecules of various sizes have been used to determine the limits of the permeability of each of the barriers. The capillary endothelial pores limit the passage of red blood cells and other formed elements of the blood but allow the passage of a molecule such as ferritin (MW 450,000) (Farquhar et al., 1961). The basement membrane serves to restrict the passage of ferritin. Horseradish

FIGURE 22-10 Scanning electron micrograph showing a transected capillary loop. The podocytes (P) interdigitate along the capillary surface. Capillary fenestra are seen on the endothelial cell surface. ×17,200.

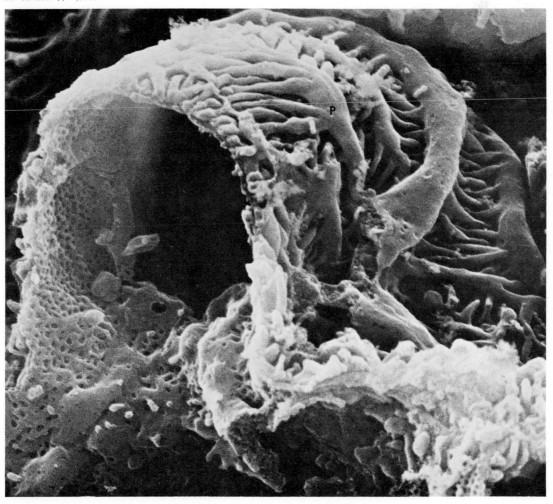

peroxidase (MW 40,000) penetrates the filtration-slit membrane (Graham and Karnovsky, 1966).

The maintenance of normal bloodflow conditions is also necessary for normal glomerular barrier function. In addition, loss of the negative charge from the capillary wall may be important in allowing proteinuria to develop.

Several morphologic features favor the production of a large volume of glomerular filtrate. The kidney has a large renal blood flow (approximately 20 to 25 percent of the cardiac output), and because of the vascular arrangement of the kidney, almost all the blood must pass through a renal corpuscle. In addition, a contractile efferent arteriole helps to maintain a high filtration pressure along the glomerular capillary bed. Also, as has been mentioned earlier, the endothelial pores are larger and the majority appear to lack a diaphragm. The complex shape of the podocytes increases the area of the intercellular channels through which the filtrate can pass to gain access to Bowman's space, and these are limited only by a thin diaphragm.

The pressure relationships of the renal corpuscle also favor filtration. Indirect techniques indicate that the hydrostatic pressure in the glomerular capillaries is nearly 90 mm Hg, whereas the opposing hydrostatic pressure of Bowman's space is only 15 mm Hg. The oncotic pressure within the capillaries is approximately 30 mm Hg, but almost no oncotic pressure is present within Bowman's space. The resulting glomerular filtration pressure is therefore equal to $(90 - 15) - (30 - 0)$, or 45 mm Hg.

Direct measurements of pressures can be taken using a mutant Wistar rat who has renal corpuscles visible on the surface. These measurements indicate that the glomerular pressures are lower than previously believed (Brenner et al., 1971); however, no evidence exists to show that the mutant glomeruli have normal pressures. In either case, the pressure results in an average of 180 l of glomerular filtrate being formed each 24 h in a normal human adult.

FIGURE 22-11 Electron micrograph of the filtration barrier from a rat renal corpuscle, showing a red blood cell (RBC) within a capillary lumen, an endothelial cell (E) with fenestrations, a basement membrane (BM), and a layer of interdigitating pedicels (Pe). ×71,700.

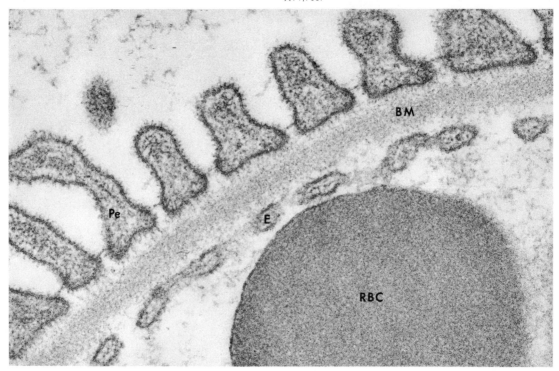

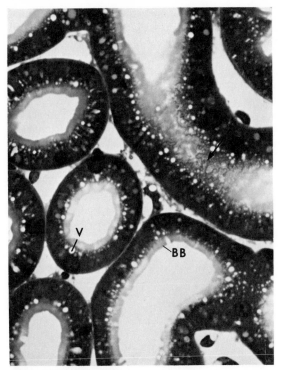

FIGURE 22-12 Profiles of proximal convoluted tubules in the cortex of a rat kidney embedded in epoxy resin. Note the brush border (BB) lining the lumen and the vacuoles (V) of the apical endocytotic apparatus. In the upper right-hand corner of the picture, the section cuts parallel to the surface of the cell in such a way that one can see the elaborate apical interdigitations of these cells (arrow). ×570.

NECK SEGMENT The transition region which connects the renal corpuscle with the proximal tubule is called the *neck segment*. It is not well developed in mammalian kidneys. The neck shows variation in structure and even in its presence in differing species. In rat kidneys, no neck segments are seen (Fig. 22-6), whereas in mouse kidneys, cells like those lining the proximal convoluted tubule have been observed to line the wall of Bowman's capsule. In human beings, however, certain nephrons have a short neck segment lined with simple squamous epithelium like the lining of the parietal wall of Bowman's capsule (Fig. 22-39). In cystinosis (a relatively rare inherited metabolic disease), these flattened epithelial cells extend for a greater length and constitute the Swan neck deformity (Darmady and Stranack, 1957).

PROXIMAL TUBULE The proximal tubule is composed of segments differing somewhat in their mor-

phology, histochemical reactions, and vulnerability to various toxins. Two of these are most frequently distinguished: a *proximal convoluted portion,* which constitutes the longest tubule in the cortex and hence the one most frequently seen in a random section; and a *straight portion (pars recta)* of the proximal tubule, which enters an adjacent medullary ray and turns toward the renal sinus to form the first part of the loop of Henle that penetrates into the medulla.

The lumen of the functioning proximal tubule is wide open in life because of the blood pressure. Anything that interrupts the blood supply to the organ will allow the proximal tubular lumens to collapse. To preserve the morphology of the living animal, an adequate filtration pressure must be maintained during fixation. This can be done by dripping the fixative on the kidney surface, by rapid freezing procedures, by microperfusion of single tubules, or by intravascular perfusion of fixative solutions.

Proximal convoluted tubule The proximal convoluted tubule is the longest and largest segment of the mammalian nephron, averaging approximately 14 mm in length and 30 to 60 μm in diameter. It is lined by a single layer of cells that have an elaborate shape, a well-developed microvillus (or brush) border along the lumen, an active endocytotic apparatus, and an abundant acidophilic cytoplasm (Figs. 22-12 to 22-21).

The cells exhibit an extensive system of lateral processes which interdigitate with corresponding lateral processes from adjacent cells. Large ridges extend the full height of the cell. More extensive but smaller interdigitating processes are also present in the apical region, and an especially prominent and elaborate system of primary and secondary interdigitations exist in the basal half of the cell (Fig. 22-16). These lateral interdigitating processes greatly increase the area of lateral cell membrane and form an extensive labyrinth of lateral intercellular spaces. The lateral processes are generally wide enough to contain one layer of large mitochondria which are oriented with their long axes from cell apex to cell base; this orientation causes the pattern of basal striations seen in the basal cytoplasm of well-fixed kidneys.

One of the major functions of the proximal tubule is to reduce the volume of glomerular filtrate by approximately 80 percent of its original volume, accomplished partly by active transport of sodium ions out of the proximal convoluted tubular cells into the lateral intercellular spaces by a Mg^+-dependent Na^+-K^+ activated ATPase pump presumably located within the lateral cell membrane. The abundant mitochondria located next to the lateral cell membranes provide the ATP for this transport. Because of the electric charge of the sodium ions pumped into the lateral space, chloride ions follow passively, and this accumulation of ions causes an osmotic movement of water into this labyrinthine system. The increased hydrostatic pressure thus created in the lateral spaces in turn forces fluid out through the porous basement membrane into the renal interstitium.

The brush border lining the luminal surface of the cells consists of long, closely packed, microvilli which are covered by the apical cell membrane (Fig. 22-14). An extracellular mucopolysaccharide coats these microvilli (Fig. 22-17). The microvilli of the proximal tubule appear to reabsorb amino acids and sugars in a manner similar to those of the intestinal striated border. Isolated segments obtained from rabbit renal cortex that are rich in brush border membrane contain a high concentration of two disaccharides and several ATPases (Berger and Sacktor, 1970). Similar prepa-

FIGURE 22-13 Electron micrograph of portions of three proximal convoluted tubules, showing the microvillus brush border (BB), the abundant endocytotic apparatus (EA), and the numerous elongated mitochondria (M) oriented perpendicular to the tubular basement membrane. ×3100.

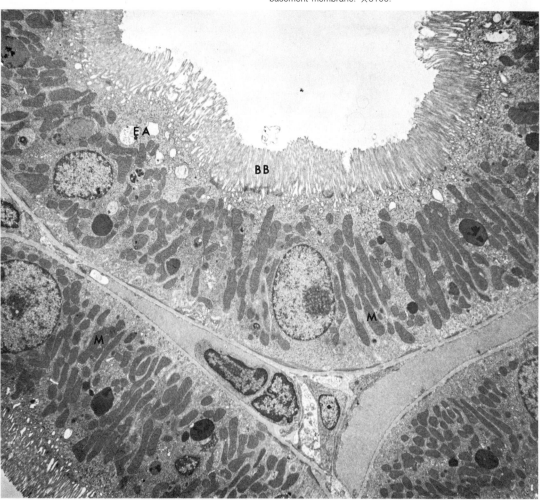

rations have also been shown to bind L-proline. This has been interpreted as evidence for the probable site of the initial step in the transtubular transport of the amino acid (Hillman and Rosenberg, 1970).

Although the glomerular filtrate contains only a low concentration of protein, the volume of filtrate is so large that several grams of protein are filtered each day (Fig. 22-18). The proximal tubule reabsorbs this filtered protein. The cell therefore contains a prominent endocytotic apparatus which includes the following components. (1) Tubular invaginations of the apical cell membrane are located between the bases of

the microvilli and extend down into the apical cytoplasm. The protein appears to be bound to the layer of fuzz (glycocalyx) radiating from the cell membrane (Fig. 22-19). (2) A series of small vesicles are thought to bud from the bases of the tubular invaginations and presumably to ferry the trapped protein molecules to the next component of the endocytotic apparatus. (3) Large apical vacuoles form by the fusion of the small vesicles (Fig. 22-20). (4) Condensing vacuoles condense the proteins. When tracer proteins such as horseradish peroxidase are injected into the vessels of a mammal, they are seen first within the lumen of the tubular invagination, second in the vesicles, third in

FIGURE 22-14 Electron micrograph of a proximal convoluted tubule, showing details of the microvillus brush border (BB), the endocytotic apparatus (EA), the numerous mitochondria (M) seen in the basal part of the cell, and the compartments formed by the lateral interdigitating processes from adjacent cells. ×9600.

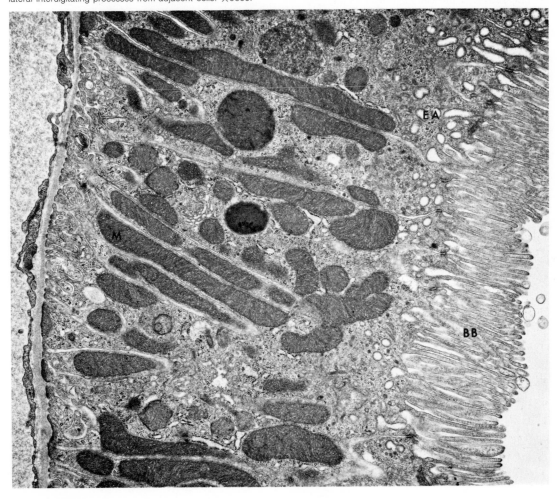

the apical vacuoles, fourth within the condensing vacuoles, and finally within lysosomes. Studies using horseradish peroxidase as a molecular tracer and the histochemical reaction for acid phosphatase as a lysosomal tracer when done simultaneously (Straus, 1964) have shown that within 60 min both the acid hydrolases and the absorbed protein can be seen within the same bodies. This presumably occurs by means of the fusion of primary or secondary lysosomes with elements of the endocytotic apparatus (Fig. 22-21). In general, proteins sequestered within lysosomes appear to be destined for breakdown into amino acids with their subsequent reuse by the animal. In the kidney, undigested residues within lysosomes can be released from the cell by fusion of the lyso-somal membrane with the cell membrane at the luminal surface.

The proximal tubular cells contain a large, round, centrally located nucleus with a prominent nucleolus. The Golgi apparatus lies in a supranuclear position and appears to consist of a large number of vesicles and membrane cisterns. Proximal tubular cells also contain microbodies (Fig. 22-22), with a dense matrix substance, often with a corelike nucleoid, and in some species platelike structures (marginal plates) along the surface. The bodies are frequently surrounded by the smooth endoplasmic reticulum (ER). Microbodies have been called peroxisomes (De Duve and Baudhuin, 1966) because they contain enzymes concerned with cellular metabolism of hydrogen peroxide. In addition, they may function in gluconeogenesis

FIGURE 22-15 Scanning electron micrograph of a proximal convoluted tubule. Note the apical brush border of microvilli and the elaborate lateral projections of cytoplasm. ×14,900.

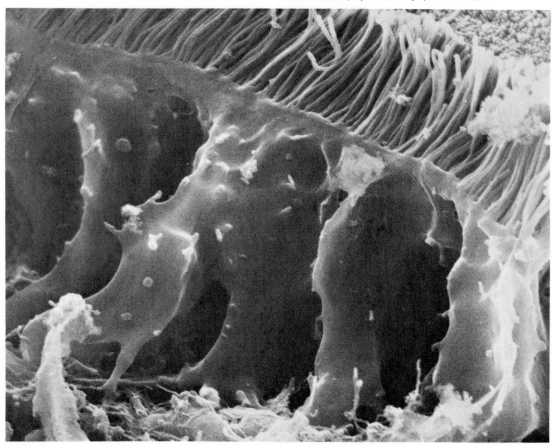

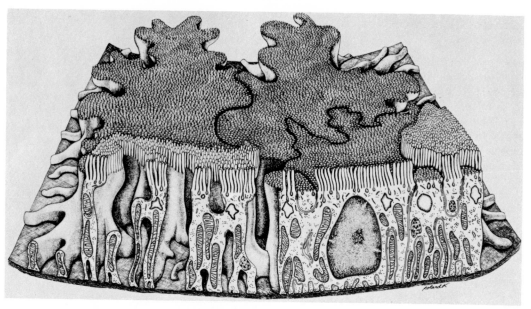

FIGURE 22-16 Diagram of a proximal convoluted tubular cell to show the elaborate interdigitations that occur between adjacent cells. Some interdigitating processes extend the full height of the cells, whereas smaller elaborate interdigitations occur in the basal and apical regions. (From Fig. 5, R. Bulger, *Am. J. Anat.,* **116:**237, 1965.)

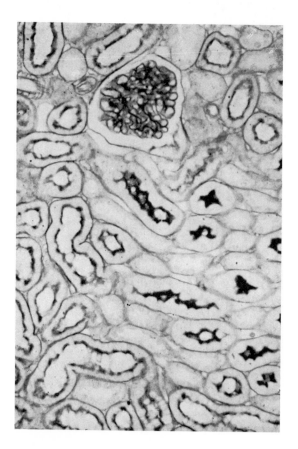

since it is well known that proximal tubular cells utilize fatty acids as an energy source. The proximal tubular cells are bound together by an extremely short tight junction and an intermediate junction. Desmosomes are only infrequently seen.

In addition to the functions already discussed, the proximal tubule reabsorbs bicarbonate by the secretion of hydrogen ions into the tubular lumen. This leads to the formation of carbonic acid, which breaks down into carbon dioxide and water. A number of exogenous organic acids (such as penicillin) and organic bases are actively secreted into the tubular fluid by the proximal tubule. The structure which accomplishes these functions has not been identified.

Straight part of the proximal tubule The straight part of the proximal tubule begins in the medullery ray and penetrates into the medulla for varying lengths, depending upon whether the nephron is of the cortical or juxtamedullary type. The straight part ends near the

FIGURE 22-17 PAS reaction in mouse kidney. A positive reaction is seen in the brush border of the proximal tubules and in the basement membranes of the tubules and of the renal corpuscle. ×300. (Courtesy of H. W. Deane.)

lower border of the outer stripe of the outer zone of the medulla where it abruptly changes into the cells of the thin limb of Henle's loop (Fig. 22-4).

The cells in the straight part of the proximal tubule are similar to those of the convoluted segment, but they appear to be lower in height and have a less elaborate shape (Fig. 22-23). The mitochondria, although still abundant, are smaller and more randomly distributed throughout the cell. The brush border is frequently well developed and PAS-positive. The cells contain fewer lysosomes and a less well-developed

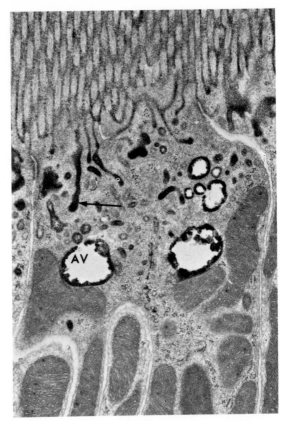

FIGURE 22-19 Electron micrograph of the apical region of a proximal convoluted tubular cell which was in the process of taking up horseradish peroxidase. The reaction product can be seen within the apical invaginations (arrow) formed by the apical plasma membrane and in apical vacuoles (AV). ×17,100.

FIGURE 22-18 Electron micrograph from a renal corpuscle of an animal that had received horseradish peroxidase prior to fixation. The dense reaction product can be seen in the capillary lumen (C) within the pores (P) of the endothelium and within the basement membrane (BM). The material is filtered into Bowman's space (BS). ×30,000.

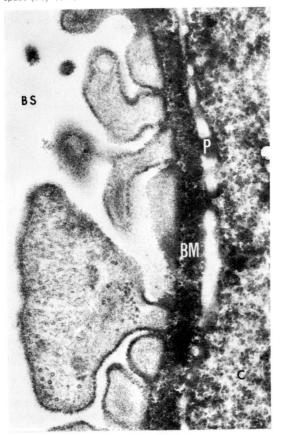

endocytotic apparatus. However, microbodies are more prominent in this region of the tubule.

THIN LIMB OF THE LOOP OF HENLE The thin limb segment can be short or absent in cortical nephrons and occurs largely on the descending limb, or it can be long, reaching far into the inner medulla in juxtamedullary nephrons, with both descending and ascending thin limb segments. In human nephrons, approximately 14 percent of the nephrons have long loops of Henle, whereas the remainder are cortical nephrons. The tubule is approximately 20 to 40 μm in diameter. The thin limb segment is lined by a thin squamous epithelium whose wall is approximately 1 to 2 μm in height (Fig. 22-24). Although the epithelium is therefore thicker than the endothelium, it is somewhat difficult to distinguish from endothelium in paraffin

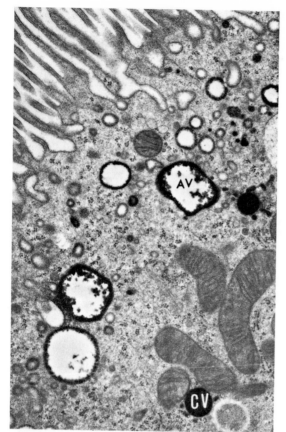

FIGURE 22-20 Electron micrograph of the apical region of a proximal tubular cell which was in the process of taking up horseradish peroxidase. The reactive product can be seen in apical vacuoles (AV) and in condensing vacuoles (CV) within the apical cytoplasm. ×13,700.

sections. In the region of the nucleus, the cell bulges into the lumen. Two types of thin limbs have been identified on the basis of the cell shape and the depth of their tight junctions in the rat (Schwartz and Venkatachalam, 1974). Type I thin limb demonstrates elaborate cellular interdigitations with shallow intercellular tight junctions. This structure would be compatible with a large passive ion permeability.

Type II thin limbs are characterized by noninterdigitating cells with a longer tight junction region. This type would be less likely to have a high passive ion permeability.

Type II thin limbs comprise those seen in the short loops of Henle and in the lower part of the descending thin limb of long loops of Henle.

The upper part of the descending thin limb of

long loops was of type I with elaborate interdigitations between cells. The ascending limb of the long loops was also characterized by type I cells but the interdigitations were less elaborate.

It was noted early that birds and mammals were the only two species whose nephrons had loops of Henle and were the only animals that could produce hypertonic urine. It was also noted that the fluid in the cortex was isosmotic with plasma, whereas there was an increasing osmotic concentration of the medulla as one approached the papillary tip. It was therefore postulated that the loop of Henle plays an important role in concentrating urine by serving as a countercurrent multiplier system.

FIGURE 22-21 Electron micrograph of the basal region of a proximal convoluted tubular cell that had taken up horseradish peroxidase 3 days prior to fixation. The reaction product can be seen within lysosomes (L) in the basal cytoplasm. ×11,500.

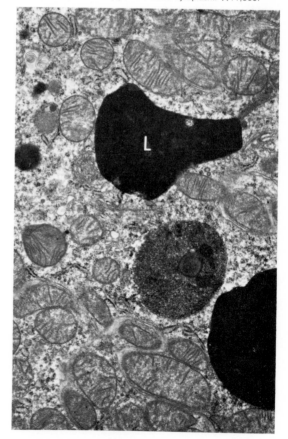

The loop of Henle is believed to function in the following manner. The ascending limb actively pumps ions from the tubular fluid into the extracellular space. In vitro work using rabbit kidney tubules indicates that the ion being actively pumped is chloride, with sodium ion following passively. In this region, the permeability to water appears to be low, so with the exit of the ions, the luminal fluid becomes hypotonic and the sodium chloride is trapped in the medullary interstitium. This hypothesis will be further discussed in the section Function of the Distal Nephron.

FIGURE 22-22 Electron micrograph showing microbodies (Mb) from a proximal convoluted tubular cell of a primate (Galago). The microbody is characterized by a single membrane surrounding it, a dense homogeneous matrix, dense bodies within the matrix, called nucleoids (N), and, in certain species, platelike structures along the edge of the body, called marginal plates (MP). ×50,400.

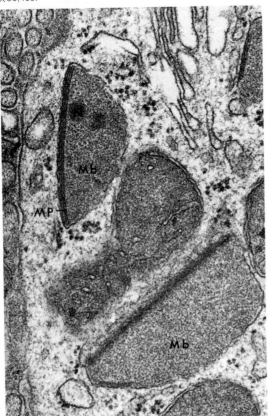

DISTAL TUBULE The distal tubule is composed of three regions: the straight part of the distal tubule (pars recta), the macula densa, and the distal convoluted tubule (Figs. 22-25 to 22-29).

Straight part of the distal tubule The straight part of the distal tubule begins near the border of the inner and outer medulla in a transition from the thin ascending limb. In some species such as rat, this transition appears to be fairly abrupt, and in others such as humans, it is gradual. The straight part of the distal tubule forms the third component of the loop of Henle and completes the looping structure by returning through the medulla and the medullary ray to the renal corpuscle from which the tubule arose. The cells of the ascending thick limb are extremely irregular in shape, with most of their interdigitations extending from the lumen to the basal region of the cell (Fig. 22-25). Although this straight part resembles the convoluted part of the distal tubule, the cells are shorter and therefore their nuclei bulge into the lumen. A few microvilli are seen along the cell surface. The lateral interdigitating processes contain numerous mitochondria which appear to be involved with the lateral cell membrane in the active transport of ions from the tubular luminal fluid that is present in this region. The permeability of the tubule to water is low in this region and therefore water does not become osmotically equilibrated and the luminal contents remain hypotonic to blood.

Macula densa As the distal tubule returns to the renal corpuscle of its origin, it runs adjacent to the efferent arteriole, the extraglomerular mesangium, and the afferent arteriole. In this region, the cells in the wall of the distal tubule are narrow and their nuclei are close together. In stained sections the nuclear accumulation causes a dense region, hence the name *macula densa* (Fig. 22-40). This association of the distal tubule with the two arterioles and the extraglomerular mesangium is called the *juxtaglomerular apparatus*, which will be discussed under that heading later in the chapter.

Distal convoluted tubule The distal convoluted tubule is shorter (approximately 5 mm) than the proximal tubule and hence fewer profiles are seen in a random section of the cortex. The diameter of this tubule is somewhat variable, being approximately 20 to 50 μm. The cells appear to be shorter, and more nuclei are seen in a cross-sectional profile than in the proximal tubule (Figs. 22-26 and 22-27), because, in part anyway, many cells are binucleate. Because the cells are short, distal tubules frequently have a larger

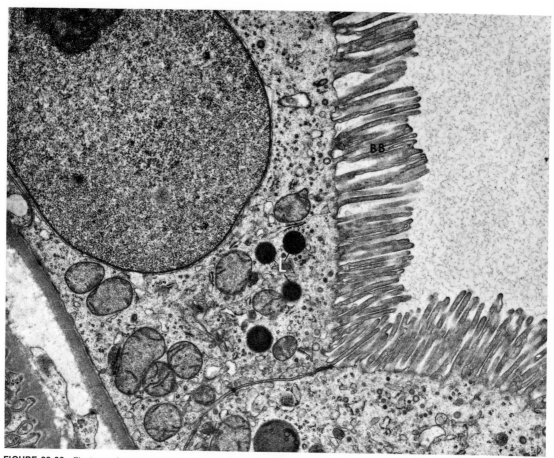

FIGURE 22-23 Electron micrograph of the straight part of the proximal tubule from a normal human kidney. The cells are of less elaborate shape, and the mitochondria are more circular in profile than in the convoluted portion. The brush border (BB) and lysomes (L) can be seen. ×16,000.

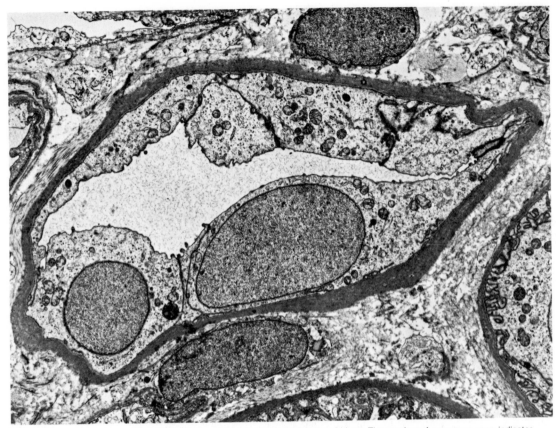

FIGURE 22-24 Electron micrograph of the thin limb segment from a normal human kidney. The number of processes seen indicates that the cells are elaborate in shape; however, human beings have a much simpler cell shape in this region than most experimental animals. ×9600.

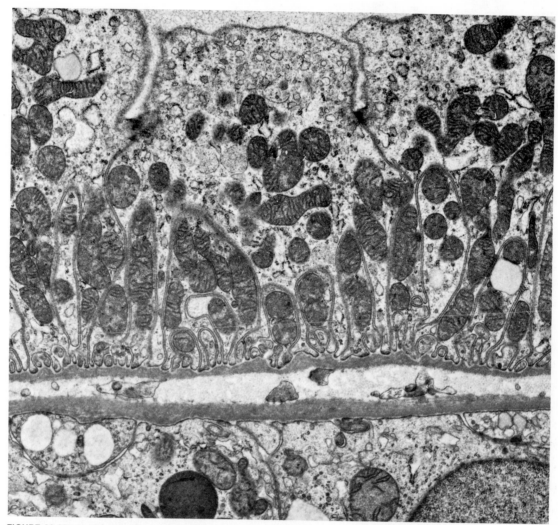

FIGURE 22-25 Electron micrograph of the ascending thick part of the distal tubule from a normal human kidney. The cells are highly interdigitated, and the lateral processes contain large mitochondria. ×12,800.

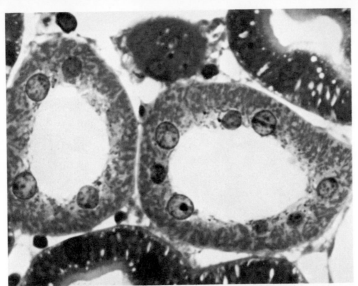

FIGURE 22-26 Light micrograph of two distal convoluted tubules from a rat kidney embedded in epoxy resin. The cells contain large mitochondria but lack a brush border. ×1000.

FIGURE 22-27 Electron micrograph of two distal convoluted tubular profiles, showing the large number of mitochondria contained in these cells and the few small microvilli which line the lumen but do not form a brush border. The nuclei lie in an apical position. ×2800.

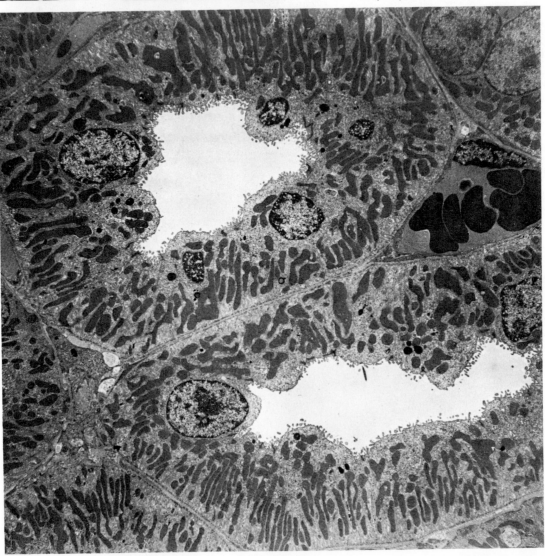

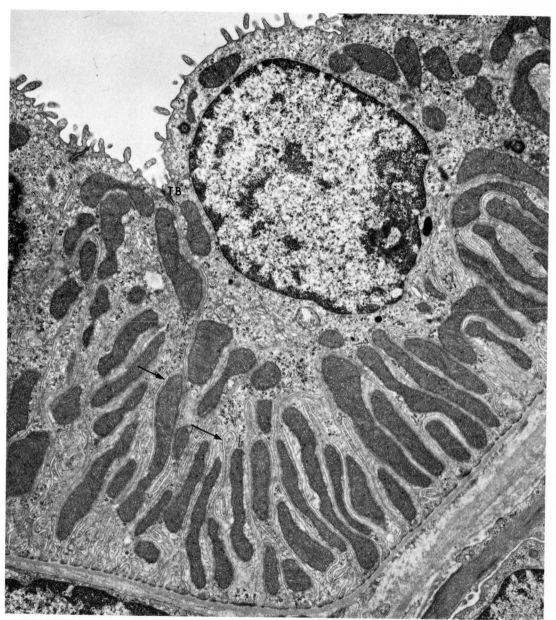

FIGURE 22-28 Electron micrograph of a distal convoluted tubule, showing the lateral intercellular labyrinth (arrows) formed by the inter-digitation of lateral processes in the basal region of the distal tubular cells. The large elongate mitochondria occupy these processes. The cell nucleus occupies an apical position. The cell surfaces are joined apical-laterally by prominent terminal bars (TB), and the apical cell membrane has only small microvilli. ×10,300.

luminal diameter than proximal tubules. The cells do not have a brush border, but a few luminal microvilli are seen. The endocytotic apparatus is not well developed; however, a few vacuoles and lysosomes can be seen within the cells. The cytoplasm appears somewhat less acidophilic than in the proximal tubule. In the basal region of the cytoplasm, lateral processes interdigitate with those from adjacent cells, forming an extensive lateral intercellular labyrinthine space like that seen in the proximal tubule (Fig. 22-28). The processes contain large mitochondria and form a pattern of basal striations similar to that seen in the proximal tubule. The active transport of sodium ions from the tubular filtrate can continue in this segment of the nephron. The nuclei appear to lie in the apical cytoplasm near the lumen. A continuous basement membrane surrounds the tubule.

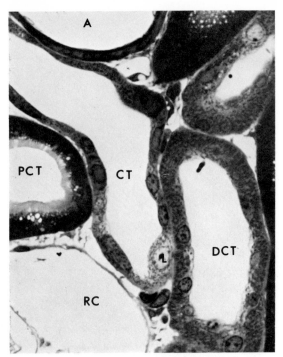

FIGURE 22-30 Light micrograph of a cortical collecting tubule (CT) from a rat kidney embedded in epoxy resin. Light (L) and dark (D) cells lining this tubule can be identified. Profiles of proximal (PCT) and distal (DCT) convoluted tubules, an arteriole (A), and a renal corpuscle (RC) can be seen. ×670.

FIGURE 22-29 Scanning electron micrograph of a distal tubule. This tubule is characterized by position in the kidney, lateral projections (P) which interdigitate with those from adjacent cells, and luminal microvilli and cilia (arrow). The microvilli appear to be most numerous along the cell borders (double arrow). ×2100.

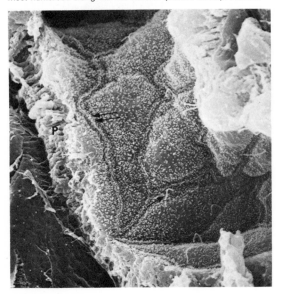

A gradual morphologic change is seen between the last region of the distal tubule and the collecting duct. The interdigitating processes of the distal tubular cells become less extensive. Intercalated (dark) cells similar to those described in the collecting duct appear in the latter region of the distal tubule.

Intrarenal Collecting Ducts

The collecting ducts can be divided into three regions: the initial segment found in the cortex (Figs. 22-30 to 22-34), the medullary segment found in the upper medulla, and the large papillary ducts in the apex of the papilla (Fig. 22-35). This division is somewhat arbitrary because there is a gradual transition in the form of the collecting ducts from their beginning to their end.

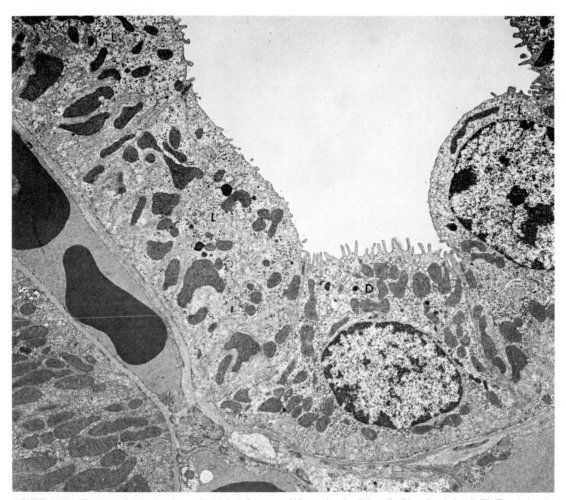

FIGURE 22-31 Electron micrograph of a cortical tubule from a rat kidney, showing light cells (L) and a dark cell (D). The dark cell is characterized by numerous mitochondria and an elaborate pattern of the apical cell membrane forming folds and microvilli. Abundant apical vesicles are also seen in the dark cell. ×5600.

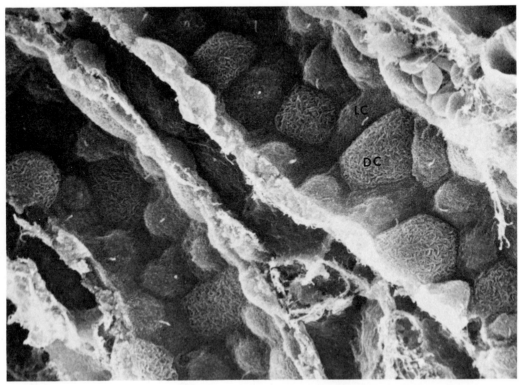

FIGURE 22-32 Scanning electron micrograph of two collecting ducts. The light cells (LC) have apical microvilli and a single cilium. The dark cells (DC) are characterized by branching irregular apical flaps and no cilia. ×1420.

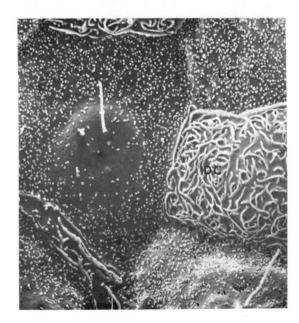

FIGURE 22-33 Scanning electron micrograph of the luminal surface of a cortical collecting duct. The dark cells (DC) and light cells (LC) can be identified by the type of surface specializations present. ×5000.

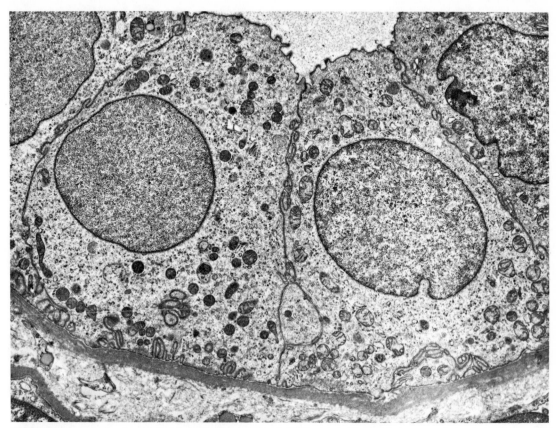

FIGURE 22-34 Electron micrograph of light cells from a human collecting tubule. These cells have a somewhat less elaborate contour to their cell membranes than do those of the rat. ×7700.

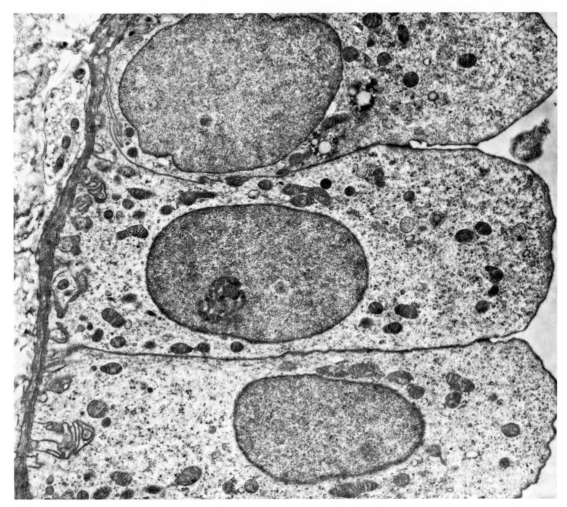

FIGURE 22-35 Electron micrograph of a medullary collecting tubule from a normal human kidney. Medullary collecting cells are taller than cortical ones but still contain some basal membranous infoldings and oval mitochondrial profiles. ×30,700.

INITIAL SEGMENT The initial segment includes the connecting portion from the distal convoluted tubule to the collecting tubules, which in cortical nephrons empties directly into a terminal collecting duct, and an arched portion formed by the confluence of several connecting pieces from juxtamedullary nephrons. The arched portion begins deep in the cortex and ascends and then turns to descend into a medullary ray. The number of nephrons which empty into arched collecting ducts prior to entrance into a terminal collecting duct versus those entering singly varies with the species. In humans both types occur.

Two types of epithelial cells line the collecting tubule (Figs. 22-31 and 22-33). The principal (light) cells are low cuboidal cells with well-defined cell margins; round, centrally placed nuclei; a fairly pale staining cytoplasm; and multiple, small, randomly oriented mitochondria. In electron micrographs, these cells are seen to have a few small microvilli and a basal cell region which contains some small, short, interdigitating processes as well as some tortuous infoldings of the basal cell membrane.

Interspersed between the principal cells are intercalated (dark) cells, which have a more intensely staining cytoplasm and contain more mitochondria located all around the nucleus. These cells have more microvilli on their luminal surfaces, and their apical cytoplasm contains a large number of vesicles. Dark cells are seen throughout the cortex and in some of the medulla but not in the papillary region. The dark cells are seen to vary in number with varying states of acid-base balance and may play a role in urine acidification (reviewed by Myers et al., 1966).

MEDULLARY COLLECTING DUCTS The medullary collecting ducts are similar in structure to the cortical ones, although the cells gradually increase in height (Fig. 22-34).

PAPILLARY DUCTS The convergence of the collecting tubules within the kidney leads to the formation of several large straight collecting tubules called *papillary ducts* (or *ducts of Bellini*) (Fig. 22-35). These large collecting ducts have a diameter of 200 to 300 μm. They empty their contents into the minor calyxes through small holes on the surface of the papillary apex. This surface is called the *area cribrosa* (Figs. 22-36 and 22-37).

FUNCTION OF THE DISTAL NEPHRON Since a gradual transition occurs in the function of the distal tubule and collecting duct, the two regions are often referred to as the distal nephron and are discussed together.

Concentration and dilution of urine (Fig. 22-38) The mammalian kidney can rid the body of water by producing a copious volume of dilute urine or conserve water by producing a small amount of concen-

trated urine. It manages this because it contains a countercurrent multiplier (the loop of Henle) and two countercurrent exchangers [the looping medullary vessels (vasa recta) and the large collecting ducts passing through the medullary interstitium].

The ascending limb of the loop of Henle pumps ions into the medullary interstitium from the tubular lumen. The water permeability of this region is low, so that osmotic equilibration does not occur. Because of the shape of Henle's loop, many of the ions are trapped within the medulla. This produces an increasingly hypertonic environment as the papilla of the medulla is approached. In human beings, the osmolarity of the interstitium may reach 1,200 milliosmoles per liter at the papillary tip. The collecting ducts again course through the medulla to empty at its apex. If they are permeable to water, the hypertonic environment of the medulla becomes a driving force to remove water from the tubular lumen by osmosis. The water permeability of the collecting ducts is controlled by an antidiuretic hormone (ADH). When blood levels of this hormone are high, the permeability of the collecting duct to water is increased and therefore water leaves the tubular fluid in the collecting duct by osmosis, producing a concentrated urine. The fluid entering the distal tubule is always hypotonic, and ions can continue to be pumped out of the distal tubular

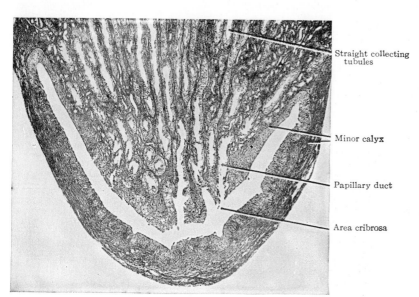

Straight collecting
tubules

Minor calyx

Papillary duct

Area cribrosa

FIGURE 22-36 Longitudinal section of the kidney papilla of a rhesus monkey, showing the area cribrosa and the wall of the minor calyx. ×40.

lumen. Therefore, when the titer of circulating ADH is low and the collecting duct permeability to water is decreased, a dilute urine will be produced.

Recently Kokko and Rector (1972) have proposed a new theory to explain the production of concentrated urine in which the papilla plays only a passive role. In this theory, the ascending thick segment provides the driving force by active reabsorption of chloride ions. Both the ascending and descending thin limbs act only as passive conduits with specific permeability properties. Their differing permeabilities to salts and urea allow the papilla to play a passive role in urine concentration.

Acidification of urine Although about half the bicarbonate ion is reabsorbed in the proximal tubule, the distal nephron still plays an important role in acid-base balance. It is the site of continued reabsorption of bicarbonate with resulting secretion of hydrogen ions, it is the site of secretion of hydrogen ion into the tubular lumen for buffering with anions of weak acids and of the acidification of the urine, and it is the site of conversion of ammonia to ammonium ions (although the ammonia might be produced elsewhere in the kidney).

Sodium-ion–potassium-ion exchange The distal nephron is also the site at which the hormone aldosterone stimulates sodium-ion reabsorption and potassium-ion secretion.

THE JUXTAGLOMERULAR APPARATUS

At the vascular pole of the renal corpuscle, a specialized portion of the distal tubule, the macula densa, comes into an intimate relationship with the afferent and efferent arterioles as well as with a pad of cells called the *extraglomerular mesangium* (Barajas, 1970; Barajas and Latta, 1967). Unmyelinated nerve endings are associated with these structures. These four entities (the afferent arteriole, the efferent arteriole, the macula densa, and the extraglomerular mesangium) constitute the juxtaglomerular apparatus (Figs. 22-39 and 22-40).

Modified smooth muscle cells in the wall of the afferent (and sometimes the efferent) arteriole in this region produce granules which can be identified by

FIGURE 22-37 Scanning electron micrograph of the papillary tip of a rat kidney. The large collecting ducts open onto this surface. ×300.

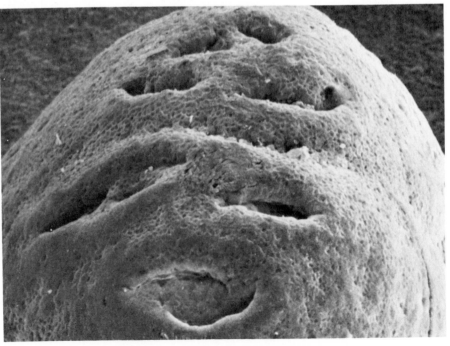

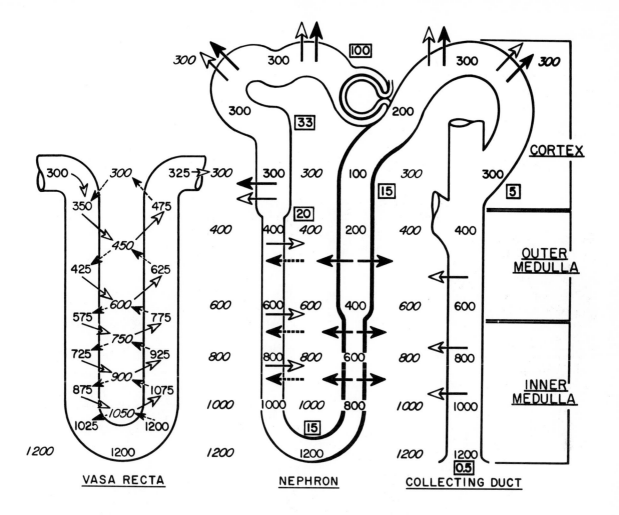

→ Na Active Transport
--→ Na Passive Diffusion
⇒ H₂O Passive Diffusion
☐ % Glomerular Filtrate Remaining at Each Level of Tubule

FIGURE 22-38 Summary of water and ion exchanges in the nephron during production of hypertonic urine, and of counter-current exchange across the vasa recta to preserve the osmolar gradient. Numbers represent concentration of urine, blood, and interstitium in milliosmoles per liter. Recent evidence indicates that active chloride transport and not active sodium transport is occurring in the ascending thick segment of the distal tubule of the rabbit. However, the active transport of this ion could establish the concentration gradient. In addition, the handling of the urea by the nephron also appears to be important in establishing the concentration gradient in the medullary interstitium. (Redrawn and modified from R. F. Pitts, "Physiology of the Kidney and Body Fluids." Year Book Medical Publishers, Inc., Chicago, 1963, courtesy of W. Roth.)

their staining properties and have been shown to contain the hormone renin (pronounced as in renal). These modified smooth muscle cells are called *juxtaglomerular cells*. Although the modified cells still contain intracellular filaments and dense bodies like other smooth muscle cells, they have more rough ER, a large Golgi apparatus, and a number of membrane-bounded secretory granules in various states of production, condensation, and storage (Fig. 22-41).

The *macula densa* comprises the cells lining the wall of the distal tubule between the ascending straight portion and the distal convoluted portion. The macula

FIGURE 22-39 Light micrograph of a juxtaglomerular apparatus from a human renal corpuscle showing the macula densa (MD), the afferent arteriole (AA), the efferent arteriole (EA), the extra-glomerula mesangium (EM), the intraglomerula mesangium (IM), the capillary loops (C), a neck region (N), and a proximal convoluted tubule (PCT). ×760.

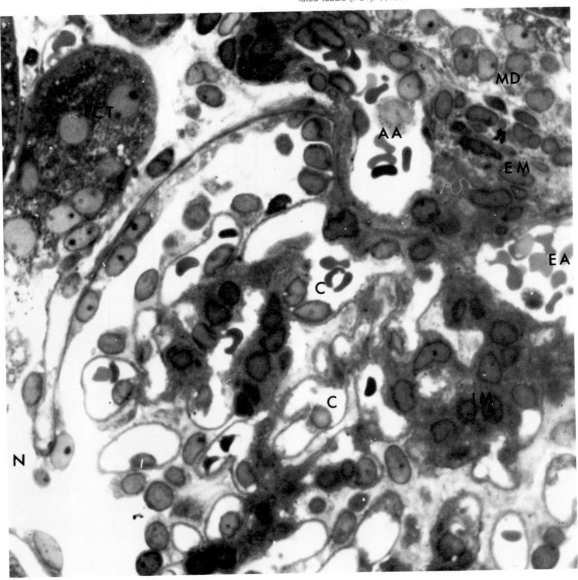

densa appears as a dense spot because the cells of this region are narrower than in adjacent portions of the tubule, and so the nuclei are closer together. In addition, the interdigitations generally seen in the basal cytoplasm of distal tubular cells are oriented parallel to the basement membrane instead of perpendicular to it. Some of these processes extend close to the juxtaglomerular cells and to the cells of the extraglomerular mesangium. The macula densa cells have mitochondria which appear shorter and more randomly oriented. The cells appear to be polarized toward the basal surface, and the Golgi apparatus is found lateral or basal to the nucleus. Because of its unique location, this region could be a sensing device of some parameter in the distal tubular fluid content and could affect the granulated cells in the arteriolar wall. The cells of the *extraglomerular mesangium* (sometimes called *Polkissen, Lacis cells,* or *polar cushion*) form a cushion of cells between the walls of the afferent and efferent arterioles. These cells resemble the intra-

glomerular mesangial cells with which they are contiguous. Although some of the cells contain granules, the majority are filled with fine intracytoplasmic filaments, dense attachment bodies at the cell membrane, and the usual organelles.

In response to a decrease in the extracellular fluid volume in an animal, the juxtaglomerular apparatus releases the enzyme renin, which acts on a plasma α-2-globulin, called *angiotensinogen,* and releases an inactive decapeptide known as angiotensin I. A converting enzyme, presumably located in the lung, converts angiotensin I to the octapeptide angiotensin II, which is the trophic hormone for the zona glomerulosa of the adrenal cortex and causes the release of aldosterone. Aldosterone then stimulates the distal nephron to reabsorb sodium ions in exchange for hydrogen or potassium ions. Since sodium is the major extracellular ion, its renal retention leads to an increase in the extracellular fluid volume of the animal. Angiotensin II is also a potent vasoconstrictor.

A local action for the renin-angiotension system also has been proposed in which the juxtaglomerular apparatus provides feedback control of the glomerular

FIGURE 22-40 Diagram of the juxtaglomerular apparatus redrawn and simplified from Fig. 22-39 to show the four elements of the juxtaglomerular apparatus as well as the position of the capillaries, mesangial cells, and epithelial cells of the renal corpuscle.

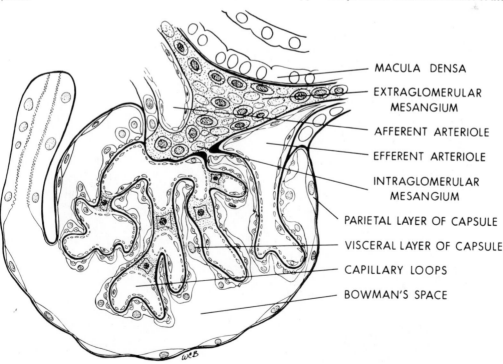

MACULA DENSA

EXTRAGLOMERULAR MESANGIUM

AFFERENT ARTERIOLE

EFFERENT ARTERIOLE

INTRAGLOMERULAR MESANGIUM

PARIETAL LAYER OF CAPSULE

VISCERAL LAYER OF CAPSULE

CAPILLARY LOOPS

BOWMAN'S SPACE

filtration rate on an individual nephron level. This feedback mechanism could be related to renal auto-regulation of blood flow (Thurau and Levine, 1971).

RENAL INTERSTITIUM

The cortical interstitium is small in normal animals. However, in a variety of disease processes the interstitium increases in volume and becomes fibrotic. Around the vessels, the interstitium is abundant (Swann and Norman, 1970). Two main cell types are seen within the cortical interstitium. The most frequently seen is the fibroblast. The second is a cell in the mononuclear series which, under certain circumstances, can be seen to contain a large number of phagocytic vacuoles and lysosomes. Fine collagen bundles traverse the cortical interstitium. Under normal circumstances, the interstitium also contains a fluid reabsorbate which is in transit from the lumen of the tubules to the capillaries.

In contrast, the interstitium of the medulla is

FIGURE 22-41 Electron micrograph showing juxtaglomerular cells from a rat kidney. The juxtaglomerular granules (Gr) can be seen within the cytoplasm of the modified smooth muscle cells. ×9300.

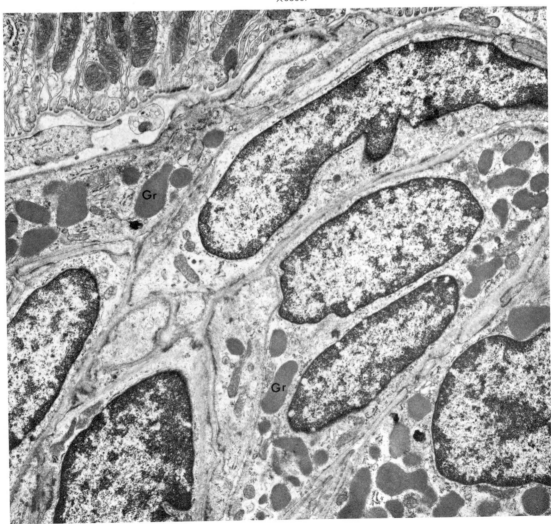

much more abundant; it contains a population of elongate interstitial cells whose long axes lie perpendicular to the long axes of the tubules in that region (Fig. 22-42). The cells are characterized by long, branching processes which come close to vessels and tubules and in some circumstances appear to encircle them. The most unique feature of these cells is that they contain a variable number of lipid droplets within their cytoplasm. In addition, the cytoplasm contains fine intracellular filaments, rough ER, numerous lysosomes, and other organelles. The cells appear to be partially surrounded by a layer of material which resembles basement membrane (external lamina) and also extends into the intercellular space around the cells, forming a network. Small bundles of collagen, flocculent material, and fine filaments (approximately 13 nm in diameter with an electron-lucent core) are seen within the intercellular matrix. Several functions have been proposed for these unique interstitial cells: (1) they elaborate the interstitial matrix; (2) they are contractile and presumably by contraction play a role in the concentration of urine; (3) they are phagocytic;

and (4) they produce the vasodepressor substances that have been isolated from the renal interstitium in certain animals, which are most likely prostaglandins E_2 and A_2 (Westura et al., 1970; McGiff et al., 1970; Muehrcke et al., 1970).

BLOOD VESSELS

Arteries

The *renal arteries* generally arise from the lateral region of the abdominal aorta at the level of the first and second lumbar vertebrae. Each artery runs downward and laterally and then usually divides into an *anterior* and *posterior division* before it reaches the renal hilus. The anterior division runs in front of the renal pelvis; the posterior division enters the renal sinus behind the renal pelvis. Although there appears to be variation in the next branching, five *segmental* branches are generally described. The anterior division branches into the upper, middle, and lower segmental arteries, and the posterior division becomes a posterior segmental artery. The fifth, or apical, segment can

FIGURE 22-42 Light micrograph of sections taken of the renal pyramid from a rat kidney, showing the horizontal, ladderlike array of interstitial cells located in this region. Epoxy resin section, toluidine blue. A, ×275; B, ×1100.

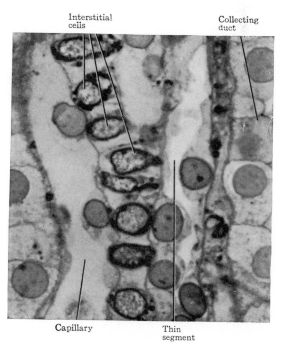

A

B

arise from either the anterior or posterior division or from branches of both divisions. While in the renal sinus, the segmental arteries branch to form interlobar arteries which enter the renal columns adjacent to the renal pyramids. At the base of the renal pyramid, the *interlobar* artery branches into many *arcuate arteries* that run across the base of the medullary pyramid near the cortico-medullary junction (Fig. 22-43). The arcuate arteries give off branches called *interlobular* arteries which course peripherally in the cortex midway between medullary rays (hence between renal lobules). As the interlobular arteries ascend, they give off *affer-*

ent arterioles which can serve one or more renal corpuscles. The afferent arteriole enters the renal corpuscle and forms several lobules of capillary networks. Anastomosis occurs between the capillaries in any lobule, but not between capillaries of adjacent lobules. The capillaries then converge to form the efferent arteriole which exits from the renal corpuscle at the vascular pole.

Postglomerular Capillary Circulation

The efferent arterioles leave the renal corpuscle and divide into a second capillary network (Fig. 22-43). The morphology of these capillaries differs, depending

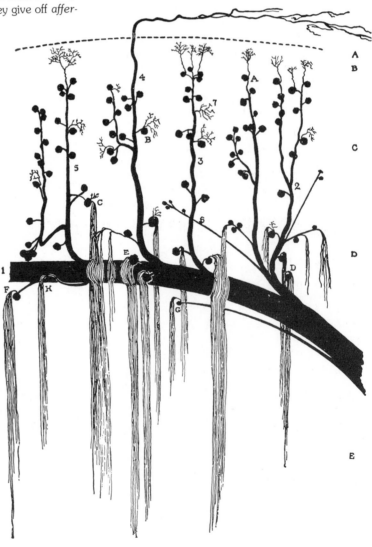

FIGURE 22-43 Diagram to represent the finer arterial distribution of the kidney. A. Capsule. B. Subcapsular zone. C. Cortex. D. Juxtamedullary zone. E. Medulla. The arcuate artery (1) gives off numerous interlobular arteries. The long, straight arteriolae rectae can be seen passing down into the medulla.

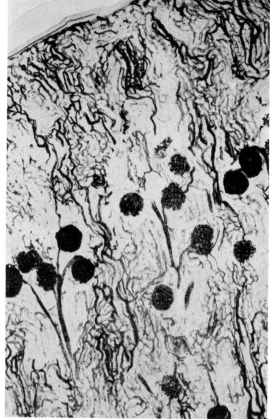

FIGURE 22-44 Arteries of the dog kidney were infused with a gelatin solution and therefore have visualized the interlobular arteries, the afferent arterioles, the glomerulus, the efferent arterioles, and the peritubular capillary anastomoses around the tubules. ×46.

FIGURE 22-45 Arteriolae rectae spuriae of a dog. Arteries were infused with colored gelatin. A. Radial section through the base of a renal pyramid, showing origin of tassels of arterioles at the junction of cortex and medullar. ×45. B. Transverse section of pyramid showing islands of arteriolae rectal spurial. ×42. (Courtesy of D. Fawcett.)

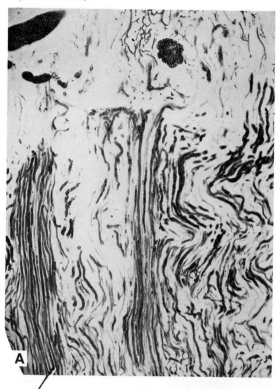

A

Arteriolae
rectae spuriae

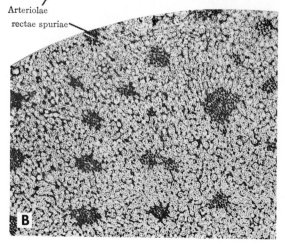

B

on whether the renal corpuscle is of the cortical or juxtamedullary type. The efferent arterioles from cortical nephrons are short and divide to form a tortuous *peritubular capillary network* supplying the associated convoluted tubules (Figs. 22-44 and 22-45). It appears that the blood in this capillary network flows rapidly in the direction opposite to that of the fluid in the tubular lumen (Steinhausen et al., 1970).

The majority of efferent arterioles from juxtamedullary nephrons divide to form several parallel unbranched vessels called the *arteriolae rectae spuriae* (Fig. 22-43). These vessels descend into the medullary pyramid, where they make a hairpin turn and ascend again in the region adjacent to the descending limb forming a vascular countercurrent exchanger (Fig. 22-46). The descending limbs are called *arteriolae rectae,* and the ascending limbs are called *venae rectae.* The walls of the arteriolar vessels in the outer medulla have a thicker endothelium (2 to 4 μm) than the walls of the ascending venous vessels. The venous vessels are lined by fenestrated capillaries. The vessels form capillary plexuses at various levels throughout the medullary pyramid. Blood flow through the medulla is much smaller in volume and slower in flow rate than that in the cortex, so that the inner medulla has a lower oxygen supply and derives most of its energy from glycolysis. The looping form of the vessels allows the osmotic gradient of the papilla to be maintained.

Veins

The venous supply in the kidney is quite irregular, and anastomoses occur between its vessels. Near the renal capsule, small venules drain in a starlike pattern, forming the stellate veins which, in turn, form the interlobular veins that course adjacent to the interlobular arteries and receive numerous tributaries from the cortical peritubular capillary network. The interlobular veins empty into the arcuate veins which extend across at the level of the cortico-medullary junction. The arcuate veins also receive blood from the venous branches of the vasae rectae. Interlobar veins are formed by the confluence of arcuate veins; these course adjacent to the medullary pyramid in company with the corresponding artery. The confluence of these vessels forms the renal vein. On the right side of the body, the renal vein is short, but on the left side of the body it is longer and receives blood from the gonadal, suprarenal, and inferior phrenic veins.

Lymphatics

Lymphatic vessels have been identified accompanying the larger renal vessels and appear to be more prominent around the arteries than around the veins. They have been identified along the interlobular, arcuate, interlobar, segmental, and renal arteries and veins (Kriz and Dieterich, 1970). In the region of the renal sinus, they converge into several large trunks which exit via the renal hilus. The lymph is then drained into nodes along the inferior vena cava and aorta. The lymphatics that accompany the interlobular vessels anastomose with a rich supply of lymphatics in the renal capsule and perirenal tissue. In addition, Rawson (1949), studying tumor penetration via renal lymphatics, identified lymph capillaries beginning at the tip of the medullary pyramid and extending peripherally to empty into lymphatic vessels at the base of the medullary pyramid. However, medullary lymphatics have not been clearly demonstrated in electron micrographs.

INNERVATION

Many autonomic nerve fibers which form the renal plexus accompany the renal artery and its branches to the kidney. The majority of these fibers are from the sympathetic division of the autonomic nervous system. The fibers are derived from cell bodies located mainly in the celiac and aortic ganglia. The sympathetic fibers innervate renal blood vessels to cause vasoconstriction. In addition, some authors believe that parasympathetic fibers of the autonomic nervous system derived from the vagus nerve also enter the kidney. Sensory fibers have been described as well. When these sensory fibers are cut, renal pain is blocked. Although numerous light microscopists describe nerve endings along the wall of the renal tubules and within the renal corpuscle, electron microscopists have not

FIGURE 22-46 Light micrograph of a cross section through a bundle of vasa recta (center) from the outer medulla of a human kidney. Note the patterned array with thick-walled descending limbs of the vasa recta (DL) being surrounded by thin-walled ascending limbs of the vasa recta (AL). The straight part of the distal tubule (D) and some thin limb sections (TL) can also be identified. ×420.

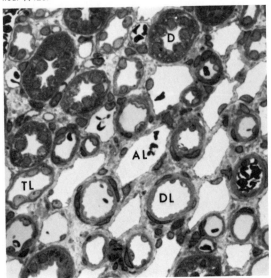

recognized them and have identified nerve endings only along the renal vessels, in the juxtaglomerular apparatus, and in the renal interstitium. Nerves have not been identified penetrating the basement membrane of any tubule or within the renal corpuscle. Since the nerve fibers to the kidney are cut during

renal transplantation, it is obvious that the kidney can function adequately without an extrinsic nerve supply.

EXTRARENAL COLLECTING SYSTEM

EXCRETORY PASSAGES

Urine is conveyed from the kidney to the bladder where it is stored. When the bladder becomes appropriately distended, the micturition reflex causes emptying of the bladder, and the urine leaves via the urethra. Urine is excreted through the minor calyxes (Fig. 22-47), the major calyxes, the renal pelvis, the ureter (Fig. 22-48), the bladder, and the urethra. The walls of all but the latter are similar in their basic

structure, being composed of an inner mucosal layer, a middle muscularis layer, and an external adventitial coat of connective tissue which binds the structure to the surrounding connective tissue. The upper portion of the bladder extends into the pelvic cavity and therefore is covered by parietal peritoneum and hence has a serosa. The thickness of the three layers of the wall increases from the minor calyxes to the bladder.

Mucosa

While the urine is being conveyed and stored within the extrarenal collecting system, only small changes

FIGURE 22-47 Light micrograph showing the wall of a minor calyx. The calyx is lined by transitional epithelium (TE), a lamina propria (LP), and muscularis (M).

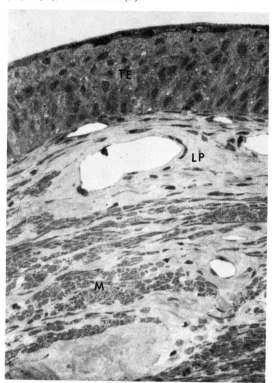

FIGURE 22-48 Light micrograph showing the wall of a dog ureter lined by transitional epithelium (TE), lamina propria (LP), muscularis (M), and a layer of adventitia (A) containing vessels. ×120.

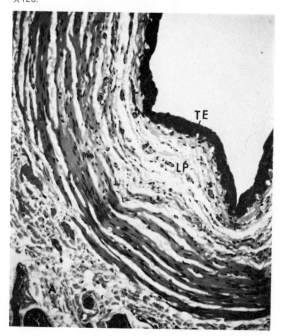

occur in its composition. A specialized lining layer called *transitional epithelium* along the lumen of the excretory passages and the bladder is responsible for this low permeability (Fig. 22-49). This intact epithelium seems to be a barrier to the rapid diffusion of salt and water. In addition, transitional epithelium gives a distensibility to the lining layer. The epithelium is generally said to be two to three cells thick in the minor calyxes, four to five cells thick in the ureter, and six or more cells thick in the empty bladder. The superficial cells of the transitional epithelium appear large and rounded and sometimes contain large polyploid nuclei in their superficial layer. When the epithelium is stretched, such as in the filling bladder, it becomes much thinner and the surface cells are stretched into a squamous layer. The distensibility of the transitional epithelium results not only from a change in shape of the cells from rounded to flat but also from certain other anatomic features. The surface

FIGURE 22-49 Light micrograph of part of the wall of a dog bladder, showing the transitional epithelium. (TE), the lamina propria (LP), and part of the muscularis (M). ×500.

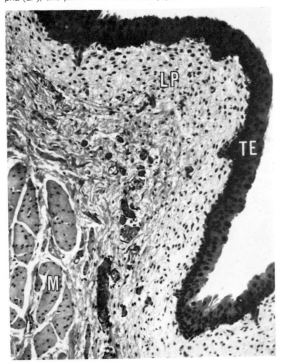

of the luminal cells is characterized by an irregular contour with small V-shaped indentations which penetrate into the cell (Figs. 22-50 and 22-51). The apical cytoplasm contains stacks of fusiform vesicles which are limited by a membrane of the same thickness as the apical plasma membrane (12 nm). It appears that the fusiform vesicles are formed from the surface membrane when the bladder is relaxing. This is demonstrated by placing a marker such as ferritin in the lumen of the bladder and observing its uptake into the fusiform vesicles (Porter and Bonneville, 1968). In addition, the epithelial cells beneath the surface appear to have numerous lateral interdigitations and projections which disappear during distension. Only a few small desmosomes are seen between the cells of the transitional epithelium.

Lamina Propria

The lamina propria is composed of a fairly dense layer of collagenous connective tissue which becomes somewhat looser in the lower region near the muscularis. There is no submucosa in the wall. When the excretory passages are empty, the mucosa is folded. When the organ is distended, the mucosa can be stretched flat; this folding allows for considerable increase in luminal diameter.

Muscularis

The muscular layer of the excretory passages usually consists of two layers of smooth muscle. Although the precise orientation of the muscle is complex, the inner layer appears to be oriented predominantly in a longitudinal fashion, whereas the outer layer is oriented predominantly in a circular fashion. In addition, the layers of smooth muscle differ from those of the gastrointestinal tract in that they are penetrated by connective tissue in such a manner that bundles of smooth muscle are seen.

The muscle layers are thinnest in the minor calyxes, but two layers of muscle are present (Fig. 22-47). The inner layer is attached to the base of the medulla and contains longitudinal fibers. The outer layer follows a more circumferential path with anterior and posterior loops which cross on the anterior and posterior sides of the calyx (Van den Bulcke et al., 1970). This layer extends higher up and forms a ring around the base of the medullary pyramid. The calyxes act as funnels whose walls contract in waves that move the fluid from the medullary pyramid into the renal pelvis.

The walls of the renal pelvis and the upper two-thirds of the ureter contain the same two layers of smooth muscle which continue to be found in bundles; however, they are thicker than in the walls of the calyxes. In the lower third of the ureter, an additional outer longitudinal layer of smooth muscle is found. Periodic peristaltic waves proceed down the ureter, forcing urine into the bladder. No definite pacemaker initiating these waves has been found.

The ureters pierce the bladder wall obliquely, and the inner longitudinal layer of smooth muscle inserts

into the lamina propria of the bladder. Because of the oblique course of the ureters through the wall of the bladder, their walls are pressed together as the bladder distends. The likelihood of urine refluxing into the ureters is therefore decreased.

BLADDER

The bladder is a reservoir for urine and varies in size and shape as it is filled (Fig. 22-49). Three layers of smooth muscle with complex orientation have been described in the thick wall of the bladder. The middle

FIGURE 22-50 Electron micrograph showing the transitional epithelium of a rat bladder. The large cells lining the apical surface are characterized by an irregular contour to their apical plasma membrane and by numerous fusiform vesicles within their cytoplasm. ×31,500. (Courtesy of F. Remington.)

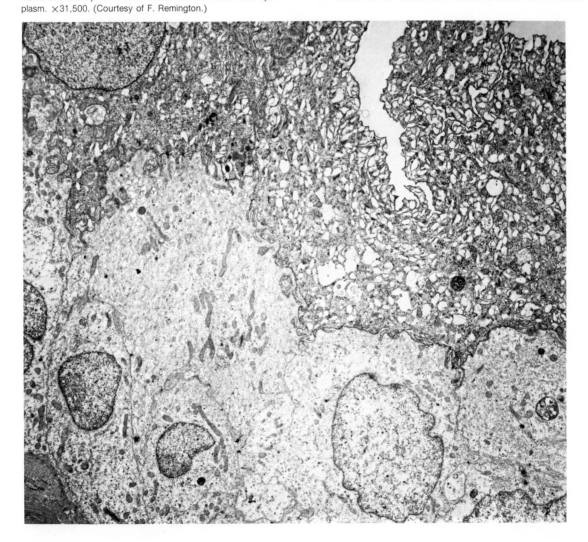

layer is the most prominent. Because of the tortuosity of the muscle, it is difficult to delineate clearly these various layers in a random histologic section. In the region of the trigone, an internal sphincter is formed by the orientation of smooth muscle around the opening of the urethra.

Blood Vessels

Blood vessels penetrate the walls of the excretory passages and enter the muscularis where they supply it with an abundant capillary network. A plexus is then formed within the lamina propria of the mucosa, and branches form a rich plexus of capillaries located just beneath the epithelium. In the deeper layers of the

FIGURE 22-51 Electron micrograph of the surface cell membrane of a transitional epithelial cell, showing the 120-Å thick apical plasma membrane (arrow) and similar membranes surrounding fusiform vesicles (V) in the cytoplasm. ×6600.

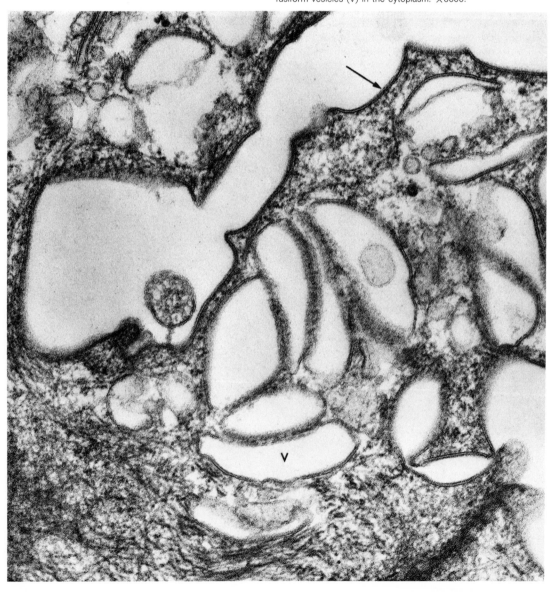

walls of the pelvis and ureters, abundant lymph vessels are seen accompanying these blood vessels.

Nerves

The bladder is supplied by both sympathetic and parasympathetic divisions of the autonomic nervous system. The sympathetic fibers traverse the inferior hypogastric plexus and form a plexus in the adventitia of the bladder wall, the *plexus vesicalis*. These sympathetic fibers appear to play little role in micturition. The preganglionic fibers of the parasympathetic division which supply the bladder arise from the spinal cord in the second, third, and fourth sacral levels. The fibers traverse to the bladder via the pelvic nerve and the inferior hypogastric plexus where they intermingle with the sympathetic fibers and synapse with ganglion cells located within the adventitia and muscularis of the bladder wall. These fibers are important for micturition. Afferent sensory fibers from the bladder traverse the pelvic and hypogastric nerves.

URETHRA

The urethra is a fibromuscular tube through which urine passes from the urinary bladder to the exterior. In the male, the urethra is long (approximately 20 cm) and also serves for the passage of seminal fluid during ejaculation. In the female, it is short (approximately 3 to 5 cm). Since the male and female urethra differ in structure, they will be considered separately.

Male Urethra

The male urethra can be divided into three segments. It begins at the neck of the bladder and extends through the prostate gland (prostatic portion), through the pelvic and urogenital diaphragm (membranous portion), and finally through the root and body of the penis to the tip of the glans penis (spongy, or anterior, part).

The *prostatic portion* of the urethra is approximately 3 to 4 cm in length. It extends through the prostate gland where multiple small prostatic ducts enter. On the posterior wall of the prostatic urethra, a conical elevation called the *veru montanum* (or *colliculus seminalis*) is located. A blind invagination called the *prostatic utricle* extends into the substance of the prostate at the summit of this region. The prostatic utricle is thought to represent a vestige of the fused caudal ends of the Mullerian or paramesonephric duct, which in the female form the uterus and most of the vagina. The ejaculatory ducts enter the urethra on

each side of the opening of the prostatic utricle. The urethra in this region is lined by transitional epithelium. The lamina propria is highly vascular. Two coats of smooth muscle bundles surround the mucosa in which the inner has bundles oriented longitudinally and the outer bundles are circular in orientation. The circular muscular bundles are a continuation of the thickened circular region at the bladder outlet, called the *internal sphincter* of the bladder.

The *membranous portion* of the male urethra runs from the apex of the prostate to the bulb of the corpus cavernosus penis, traversing the urogenital and pelvic diaphragms. It is therefore surrounded by striated muscle fibers which form the *external sphincter* of the bladder. The epithelium in this region is stratified or pseudostratified columnar.

The *spongy portion* (anterior) is approximately 15 cm long and extends through the bulb, body, and glans of the penis encased by the corpus cavernosum urethrae (spongiosum). The lumen of the urethra is dilated within the region of the bulb (intrabulbar fossa) and in the glans (novicular fossa). The epithelium lining most of the urethra in this region is pseudostratified columnar (Fig. 22-52), with patches of stratified squamous epithelium. In the novicular fossa the epithelium becomes stratified squamous. The ducts of the bulbourethral glands enter the spongy segment of the urethra. Mucus-secreting glands (glands of Littre) also empty into the urethra throughout its length. However, they are most frequently found within this spongy portion.

Female Urethra

The female urethra is relatively short, approximately 3 to 5 cm long. The lumen is crescentic in outline, and most of it is lined with stratified squamous epithelium (Fig. 22-53). Pseudostratified columnar epithelium may also be found. Within the epithelium some nests of mucus glands may be found. The lamina propria consists of a wide zone of vascular connective tissue which contains many thin-walled veins. The muscularis of the female urethra is similar to that in the bladder neck. An inner longitudinal layer of smooth muscle bundles is surrounded by a thicker layer of smooth muscle with circular orientation. The outer circular fibers are continuous with those in the internal sphincter of the urethra. The outer circular layer is reinforced with striated muscle fibers of the constrictor muscle of the urethra.

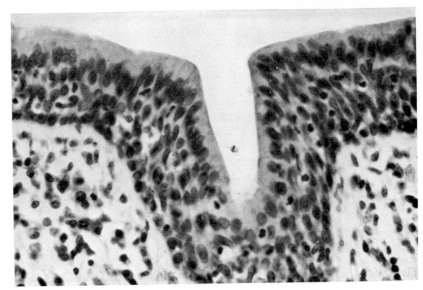

FIGURE 22-52 Pseudostratified epithelium lining the cavernous portion of the human male urethra. ×450.

FIGURE 22-53 Transverse section of the human female urethra. Picric acid–sublimate fixation ×10. (Von Ebner).

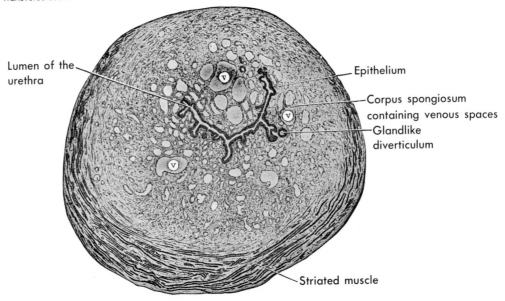

Lumen of the urethra

Epithelium

Corpus spongiosum containing venous spaces

Glandlike diverticulum

Striated muscle

REFERENCES

ARAKAWA, MASAAKI: A Scanning Electron Microscopy of the Glomerulus of Normal and Nephrotic Rats, *Lab. Invest.,* **23:**489–496 (1970).

BARAJAS, LUCIANO: The Ultrastructure of the Juxtaglomerular Apparatus as Disclosed by Three-dimensional Reconstructions from Serial Sections, *J. Ultrastruct. Res.,* **33:**116–147 (1970).

BARAJAS, LUCIANO, and HARRISON LATTA: Structure of the Juxtaglomerular Apparatus, *Circ. Res.,* **20, 21** (Suppl. II):15–28 (1967).

BERGER, SOSAMMA J., and BERTRAM SACKTOR: Isolation and Biochemical Characterization of Brush Borders from Rabbit Kidney, *J. Cell Biol.,* **47:**637–645 (1970).

BRENNER, BARRY M., JULIA L. TROY, and TERRANCE M. DAUGHARTY: The Dynamics of Glomerular Ultrafiltration in the Rat, *J. Clin. Invest.,* **50:**1776–1780 (1971).

BULGER, RUTH ELLEN: The Shape of Rat Kidney Tubular Cells, *Am. J. Anat.,* **116:**237–255 (1965).

BULGER, RUTH ELLEN, and BENJAMIN F. TRUMP: Fine Structure of the Rat Renal Papilla. *Am. J. Anat.,* **118:**685–722 (1966).

BULGER, RUTH ELLEN, FRANCES LEA SIEGEL, and ROBERT PENDERGRASS: Scanning and Transmission Electron Microscopy of the Rat Kidney, *Am. J. Anat.,* **139:**483–502 (1974).

CLARK, S. L., JR.: Cellular Differentiation in the Kidneys of Newborn Mice Studied with the Electron Microscope, *J. Biophys. Biochem. Cytol.,* **3:**349–362 (1957).

DARMADY, E. M., and F. STRANACK: Microdissections of the Nephron in Disease, *Br. Med. Bull.,* **13:**21 (1957).

DE DUVE, CHRISTIAN, and PIERRE BAUDHUIN: Peroxisome (Microbodies and Related Particles), *Physiol. Rev.,* **46:**323–357 (1966).

DU BOIS, A. M.: The Embryonic Kidney, in Charles Rouiller and Alex F. Muller (eds.), "The Kidney," vol. 1, pp. 1–59, Academic Press, Inc., New York, 1969.

FARQUHAR, M. G., S. L. WISSIG, and G. E. PALADE: Glomerular Permeability. I. Ferritin Transfer across the Normal Glomerular Capillary Wall, *J. Exp. Med.,* **113:**47 (1961).

GOTTSCHALK, C. W., and M. MYLLE: Micropuncture Study of the Mammalian Urinary Concentrating Mechanism: Evidence for the Countercurrent Hypotheses, *Am. J. Physiol.,* **196:**927 (1959).

GRAHAM, R. C., and MORRIS J. KARNOVSKY: Glomerular Permeability. Ultrastructural Cytochemical Studies Using Peroxidases as Protein Tracers, *J. Exp. Med.,* **124:**1123–1134 (1966).

HARPER, J. T., HOLDE PUCHTLER, SUSAN N. MELOAN, and MARY S. TERRY: Light-microscopic Demonstration of Myoid Fibrils in Renal Epithelial, Mesangial and Interstitial Cells, *J. Microscopy,* **91:**71–85 (1970).

HICKS, R. M., and B. KETTERER: Isolation of the Plasma Membrane of the Luminal Surface of Rat Bladder Epithelium, and the Occurrence of a Hexagonal Lattice of Subunits Both in Negatively Stained Whole Mounts and in Sectioned Membranes, *J. Cell Biol.,* **45:**542–553 (1970).

HILLMAN, RICHARD E., and LEON E. ROSENBERG: Amino Acid Transport by Isolated Mammalian Renal Tubules. III. Binding of L-proline by Proximal Tubule Membranes, *Biochim Biophys Acta,* **211:**318–326 (1970).

HOLLINSHEAD, W. HENRY: Renovascular Anatomy, *Postgrad. Med.,* **40:**241–246 (1966).

JORGENSEN, FINN: "The Ultrastructure of the Normal Human Glomerulus," Munksgaard, Copenhagen, 1966.

KOKKO, J. P., and F. C. RECTOR, JR.: Countercurrent Multiplication System without Active Transport in the Inner Medulla. *Kidney International,* **2:**214 (1972).

KRIZ, W., and H. J. DIETERICH: The Lymphatic System of the Kidney in Some Mammals. Light and Electron Microscopic Investigations, *Z. Anat. Entwicklungsgesch,* **131:**111–147 (1970).

877

LJUNGOVIST, S.: Structure of the Arteriole-Glomerular Units in Different Zones of the Kidney, *Nephron,* **1:**329–337 (1964).

MC GIFF, JOHN C., KEITH CROWSHAW, NORBERTO A. TERRAGNO, and ANDREW J. LONIGRO: IV. Renal Interstitial Cells: Prostaglandins and Hypertension Release of a Prostaglandin-like Substance into Renal Venous Blood in Response to Angiotensin II, *Circ. Res.,* **26:**1-121–1-130 (1970).

MOLLENDORFF, W. VON: Der Exkretionsapparat, "Handbüch der mikroskopischen Anatomie des Menschen," vol. 7 pt. 1. Springer-Verlag OHG, Berlin, 1930.

MUEHRCKE, ROBERT C., ANIL R. MANDAL, and FREDERICK I. VOLINI: IV. Renal Interstitial Cells: Prostaglandins and Hypertension. A Pathophysiological Review of the Renal Medullary Interstital Cells and Their Relationship to Hypertension, *Cir. Res.,* **26, 27:**1-109–1-119 (1970).

MYERS, CHARLES E., RUTH ELLEN BULGER, C. CRAIG TISHER, and BENJAMIN F. TRUMP: Human Renal Ultrastructure. IV. Collecting Duct of Healthy Individuals, *Lab. Invest.,* **15:**1921–1950 (1966).

OSVALDO, LYDIA, and HARRISON LATTA: The Thin Limbs of the Loop of Henle, *J. Ultrastruct. Res.,* **15:**144–168 (1966).

PITTS, R. F.: "Physiology of the Kidney and Body Fluids," Year Book Medical Publishers, Inc., Chicago, 1963.

PORTER, KEITH R., and MARY A. BONNEVILLE: "Fine Structure of Cells and Tissues," Lea & Febiger, Philadelphia, 1968.

RAWSON, A. J.: Distribution of the Lymphatics of the Human Kidney as Shown in a Case of Carcinomatous Permeation, *Arch. Path.,* **47:**283 (1949).

RHODIN, J.: Anatomy of Kidney Tubules, *Int. Rev. Cytol.,* **7:**485–534 (1958).

RICHET, G., J. HAGEGE, and M. GABE: Correlation between Bicarbonate Transfer and Morphology of Tubular Cells Distal to Henle's Loop in the Rat. *Nephion,* **7:**413–429 (1970).

ROUILLER, CHARLES: General Anatomy and Histology of the Kidney, in Charles Rouiller and Alex F. Muller (eds.), "The Kidney," vol. 1, pp. 61–156, Academic Press, Inc., New York, 1969.

SCHWARTZ, M. M., and M. A. VENKATACHALAM: Structural Differences in Thin Limbs of Henle: Physiological Implications. *Kidney International* **6:**193–208 (1974).

SMITH, H. W.: "The Kidney, Structure and Function in Health and Disease," Oxford University Press, New York, 1951.

SMITH, HOMER W.: "Studies in the Physiology of the Kidney," University of Kansas, University Extension Division, Lawrence, Kans., 1939.

SPERBER, I.: Studies on the Mammalian Kidney, *Zool. Bidrag. Uppsala,* **22:**249–431, 1944.

STEINHAUSEN, MICHAEL, GEORG-M. EISENBACH, and RAINER GALASKE: A Countercurrent System of the Surface of the Renal Cortex of Rats, *Pfluegers Arch. Europ. J. Physiol.,* **318:**244–258 (1970).

STRAUS, WERNER: Cytochemical Observations on the Relationship between Lysosomes and Phagosomes in Kidney and Liver by Combined Staining for Acid Phosphatase and Intravenously Injected Horseradish Peroxidase, *J. Cell Biol.,* **20:**497–507 (1964).

SWANN, H. G., and RICHARD J. NORMAN: The Periarterial Spaces of the Kidney, *Tex. Rep. Biol. Med.,* **28:**317–335 (1970).

THURAU, K., and D. Z. LEVINE: The Renal Circulation, in Charles Rouiller and Alex F. Muller (eds.), "The Kidney", vol. III, pp. 1–70, Academic Press, Inc., New York, 1971.

TISHER, C. C., R. E. BULGER, and B. F. TRUMP: Human Renal Ultrastructure. III. The Distal Tubule in Healthy Individuals, *Lab. Invest.,* **18:**655–668 (1968).

TISHER, C. C., R. E. BULGER, and B. F. TRUMP: Human Renal Ultrastructure. I. Proximal Tubule of Healthy Individuals, *Lab. Invest.,* **15:**1357–1394 (1966).

TRUETA, J., A. E. BARCLAY, P. DANIEL, K. J. FRANKLIN, and M. M. L. PRICHARD: "Studies of the Renal Circulation," Blackwell Scientific Publications, LTD., Oxford, 1947.

VAN DEN BULCKE, C., E. N. KEEN, and H. FINE: Observations on Smooth Muscle Disposition in the Urinary Tract, *J. Urol.,* **103:**783–789 (1970).

VENKATACHALAM, M. A., R. S. COTRAN, and M. J. KARNOVSKY: An Ultrastructural Study of Glomerular Permeability in Aminonucleoside Nephrosis Using Catalase as a Tracer Protein, *J. Exp. Med.,* **132:**1168–1182 (1970).

VENKATACHALAM, M. A., M. J. KARNOVSKY, H. D. FAHIMI, and R. S. COTRAN: An Ultrastructural Study of Glomerular Permeabilty Using Catalase and Peroxidase as Tracer Proteins, *J. Exp. Med.,* **132:**1153–1167 (1970).

WESTURA, EDWIN E., HARTMUT KANNEGIESSER, JAMES D. O'TOOLE, and JAMES B. LEE: IV. Renal Interstitial Cells: Prostaglandins and Hypertension. Antihypertensive Effects of Prostaglandin A$_1$ in Essential Hypertension, *Circ. Res.,* **26, 27:**1-131–1-140 (1970).

ZIMMERMANN, K. W.: Zur Morphologie der Epithelzellen der Saugetierniere. *Arch. Mikrobiol. Anat.,* **78:**199–231 (1911).

The Female Reproductive System

RICHARD J. BLANDAU

The female reproductive system (Fig. 23-1) is composed of an internal group of organs situated within the pelvis and consisting of the *ovaries,* the *oviducts* (also called *uterine* or *fallopian tubes*), the *uterus,* and the *vagina.* The external genitalia comprise the *mons pubis,* the *labia minora,* the *labia majora,* and the *clitoris.* The mammary glands, though not genital organs, are an important appendage to the reproductive system (see Chap. 24). The ovaries are paired organs situated on either side of the uterus, each 2 to 5 cm long, 1.5 to 3 cm wide, and 0.8 to 1.5 cm thick. The size of the ovaries varies greatly from week to week during each menstrual cycle or during pregnancy; this is related to the number and stage of development of the growing follicles and corpora lutea. To study the ovaries of any animal intelligently, it is important to know at which stage of the reproductive cycle they were removed.

The ovary is attached to the broad ligament by a double fold of peritoneum, the *meso-varium* (Figs. 23-1 and 23-2). The mesovarium is attached to the ovary only along one margin, the *hilum.* The *suspensory ligament* of the ovary (Fig. 23-1) is a fold of peritoneum which is directed upward over the iliac vessels and contains the ovarian vessels. The mesovarium and the suspensory ligaments often contain significant amounts of smooth muscle fibers whose rhythmic contractions, particularly at the time of ovulation, move the ovaries closer to the fimbriae of the oviducts.

SEXUAL MATURATION (PUBERTY)

The female sexual organs normally remain in an infantile state during approximately the first 10 years of life. In the succeeding 2 to 4 years there occurs a gradual enlargement of the reproductive organs, accompanied by growth of the breasts, changes in the contours of the body, and the appearance of axillary and pubic hair. This period of sexual development culminates in the appearance of the first menses (*menarche*) at an average age of 13.5 years. In a recent study of 30,000 menstrual cycles in women between 15 and 39 years of age, the average cycle length was 29 days with a standard deviation of 7.46 days. Mature reproductive

881

life, characterized by recurring menstrual cycles, lasts until about the forty-fifth to the fiftieth year of life. The human female then enters a period known as the *menopause* (also referred to as the *climacteric* or "change of life") during which reproductive cycles become irregular, lengthen, and eventually cease. Thereafter, in the *postmenopause* period, the reproductive organs are atrophic and functionless.

THE INTERNAL ORGANS

THE OVARIES

The ovaries are remarkable organs which store from the time of birth all the eggs the human female will ever have. They also secrete cyclically hormones that are essential for the postnatal growth and development of the secondary sex organs and the mammary glands.

Each ovary is covered by a continuous mesothelium composed of a single layer of cuboidal epithelium. Because of the tenuous attachment of this layer of cells to the underlying stroma, it is often brushed off in making the histologic preparation. Each ovary consists of an outer cortex and a central medulla (Fig. 23-2). The demarcation between these two areas is often indistinct (Fig. 23-3). Embedded within the loose connective tissue of the medulla are nerves, lymph vessels, and many large blood vessels. The arteries are often coiled and tortuous as they pass toward the cortical zone. This arrangement allows them to adapt readily during the phases of rapid ovarian enlargement, ovulation, and corpus luteum formation. The medulla may also contain remnants of a closed ductular system, the *rete ovarii*. These are small and irregularly arranged ducts, lined by a single layer of low cuboidal epithelium. Embryologically, they are ho-

FIGURE 23-1   Reproduction organs of the female human being.

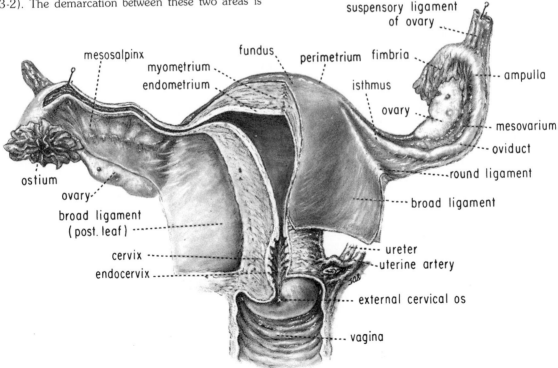

mologous to the *rete testes* in the male gonads. They have no function in the female, but on occasion they may become cystic.

The stroma of the cortex is composed of closely packed spindle-shaped cells (Fig. 23-3) arranged in irregular whorls except near the periphery where they form a dense, fibrous, collagenous connective tissue layer, the *tunica albuginea* (Figs. 23-2 and 23-3). Elastic fibers are few or absent. A few smooth muscle cells have been described as scattered in the cortical stroma and in the walls of preovulatory follicles in the ovaries of rats and monkeys. Contractions of the smooth muscles, particularly in the ovulatory follicles, may play a role in ovulation.

FIGURE 23-2 Unretouched photomicrograph of an ovary of the cat. Arrows point to the site of rupture of two ovarian follicles 1 h before the ovary was removed and fixed. ×12.

At the time of birth, in the human female 300,000 to 400,000 oocytes are embedded in the stroma of the cortex of both ovaries. Of these, only 420 to 480 may ovulate during the entire reproductive life of the individual and only about 5 percent of these will be fertilized. During each menstrual cycle, 15 to 20 follicles may grow to a considerable size (Fig. 23-3), but all of these except the one that will ovulate will degenerate. The majority of the remaining oocytes are destined to degenerate and disappear from the cortex by the process of *atresia,* which begins during the fetal period, is accentuated postnatally, and continues throughout the reproductive life span. More will be

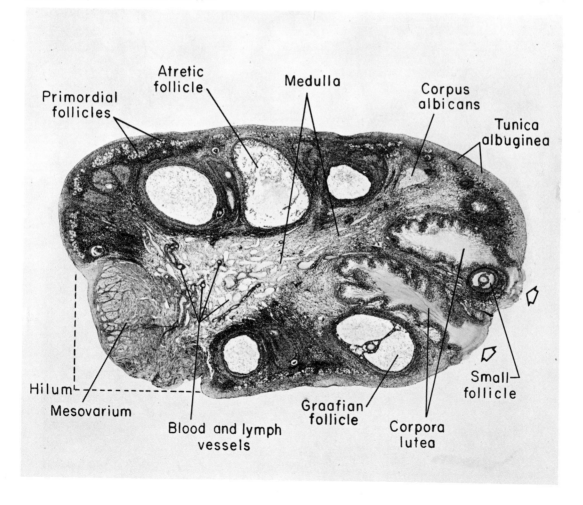

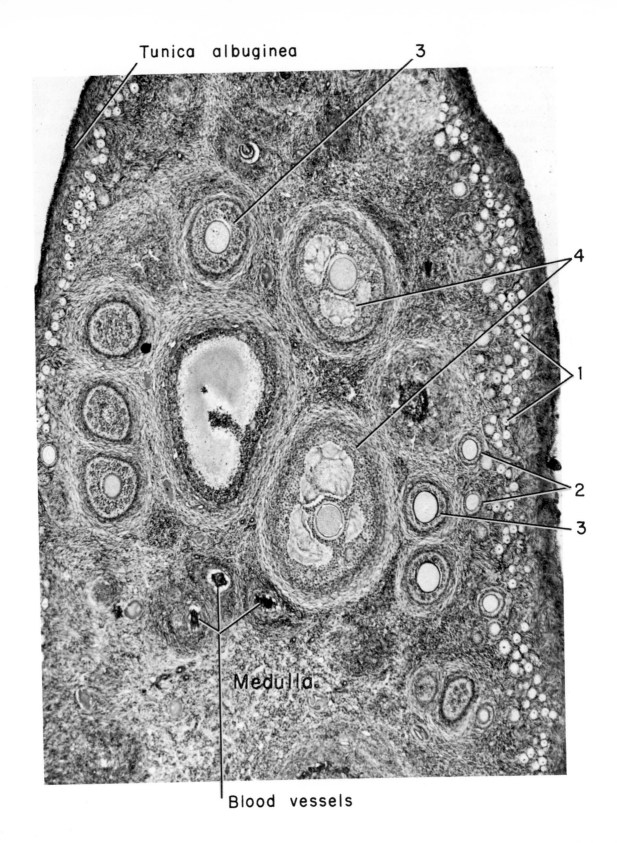

Tunica albuginea

3

4

1

2

3

Medulla

Blood vessels

FIGURE 23-3 Photomicrograph of a rabbit ovary showing (1) numerous primordial follicles with a single layer of flattened follicular cells, (2) unilaminar follicles with a single layer of cuboidal epithelium, (3) multilaminar follicles without antra, and (4) vesicular follicles with follicular antra. Note the increase in size of the egg as the follicle grows, and the presence of the zona pellucida in 2, 3, and 4. ×100.

FIGURE 23-4 Electron micrograph of a primordial follicle of a rabbit. Notice the oocyte surrounded by flattened follicular epithelium (FC) and the absence of zona pellucida. The cytoplasm of the oocyte contains some characteristic round mitochondria (M), a few strands of endoplasmic reticulum, and numerous free ribosomes. N, nucleus; NU, nucleolus; GA, Golgi apparatus. ×4500. (Courtesy of F. J. Silverblatt.)

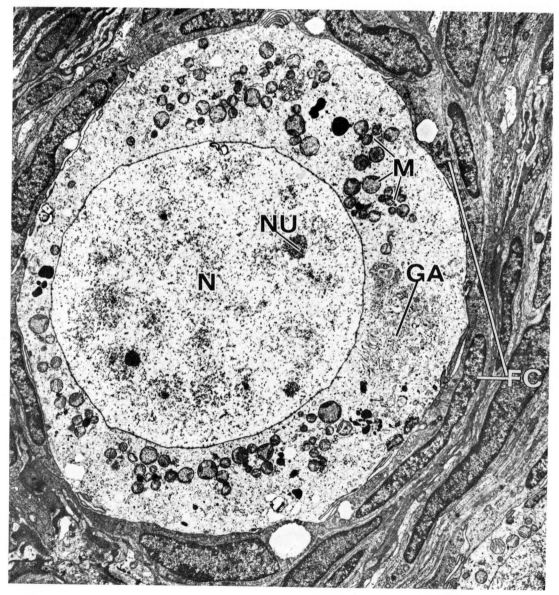

said concerning the various types of atresia later in this chapter.

Primordial or Unilaminar Follicles

The cortex of the ovary, particularly in the young female, contains large numbers of individual *primordial unilaminar* follicles (Fig. 23-3) consisting of a large oocyte enclosed in a single layer of cuboidal or columnar cells, resting on a basement membrane. A primordial follicle (Fig. 23-4) is composed of an oocyte and the follicular cells surrounding it, resting on a basement membrane. Because the oocyte is a cell of such large size (25 to 30 µm), its circumference may be surrounded by several flattened *follicular cells* in section. The plasma membranes of the oocyte and the follicular cells at this stage are relatively smooth, closely apposed to one another, and at certain places connected by desmosomes. The oocyte (Fig. 23-4) has a large vesicular nucleus with finely dispersed chromatin and one or more large nucleoli. The nuclear envelope bears well-developed pores. A well-developed Golgi apparatus with short tubular profiles may be located near the nucleus. The round mitochondria have typical cristae. The endoplasmic reticulum (ER) is represented by numerous small vesicles. The cytologic characteristics of the oocytes easily distinguish them from the follicular cells or any of the other cells in the cortical stroma (Fig. 23-3).

Growth of Follicles

As the oocyte begins to grow, the flattened follicular cells become cuboidal (Fig. 23-3) and proliferate rapidly to form a stratified epithelium. These are now

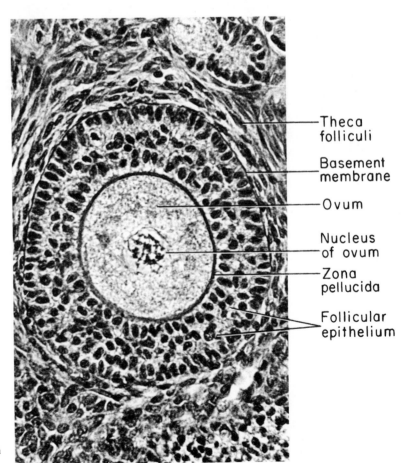

Theca
folliculi

Basement
membrane

Ovum

Nucleus
of ovum

Zona
pellucida

Follicular
epithelium

FIGURE 23-5 A multilaminar, growing follicle with a distinct basement membrane separating the follicular epithelium from the theca folliculi of a rabbit. ×350.

multilaminar primary follicles. They do not as yet have antra. The multilaminar epithelium rests on a distinct *basement membrane (membrana limitans externa)* (Fig. 23-5) which stains brilliantly with the PAS method. The basement membrane is exceptionally homogeneous and relatively highly polymerized, and it separates the *stratum granulosum* from the *theca interna* (Fig. 23-6). As the egg grows, a clear, refractile, highly polymerized membrane, the *zona pellucida (mucoid oolemma)* (Fig. 23-7), is interposed between the oocyte and the immediately adjacent follicular cells. The origin of the zona pellucida is uncertain; some believe it is formed from secretions of the follicular cells that immediately surround the egg, whereas other investigators suggest that peripheral Golgi bod-

ies in the oocyte itself have some function in its formation. The zona pellucida usually appears first in the unilaminar follicle with only a single layer of cuboidal or columnar cells.

As the zona pellucida appears, the plasma membrane of the oocyte forms numerous microvilli (Fig. 23-7) that extend into the zonal membrane. At the same time, irregularly arranged and sinuous cytoplasmic projections from the follicular cells (Fig. 23-7) penetrate the zona and make contact with the plasma membrane of the egg. Some follicle cell processes may penetrate deeply into the ooplasm of the oocyte. Thus, despite the presence of a rather thick zona pellucida (5 μm in the mature ovum), the egg and follicular cells maintain plasma membrane contact throughout the period of growth and until about the time of ovulation.

The Theca Cone

As the follicle begins to grow and becomes multilaminar, it tends to sink deeper into the cortical stroma, while the surrounding stromal cells become

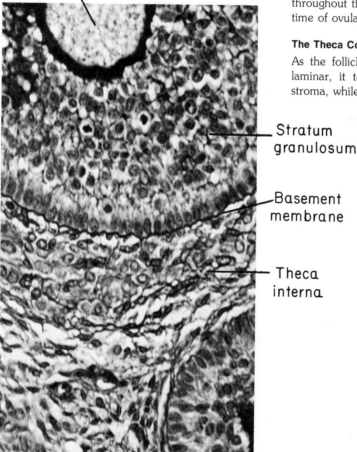

Egg

Stratum granulosum

Basement membrane

Theca interna

FIGURE 23-6 Section from a multilaminar follicle of a rabbit, showing the thickness of the basement membrane and the transformation of the theca interna into steroid-secreting cells. ×850.

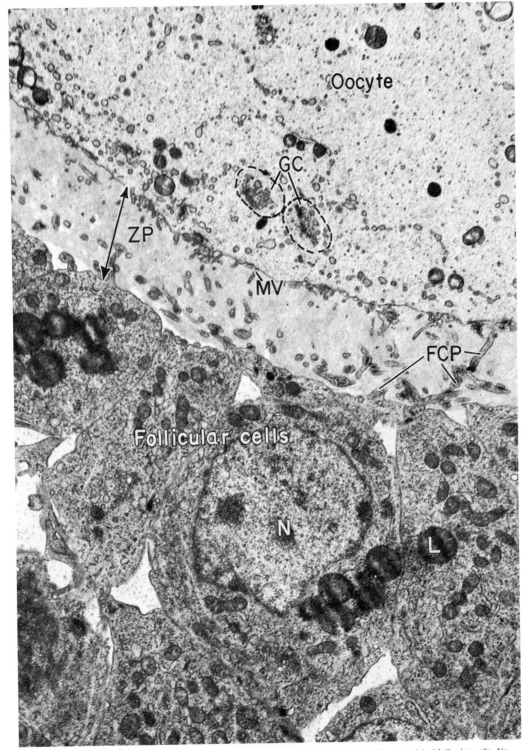

FIGURE 23-7 Electron micrograph of a peripheral sector of a mouse oocyte, its zona pellucida, and the associated follicular cells. Notice the numerous microvilli from the oocyte and the sinuous processes from the follicle cells penetrating the zona pellucida. ZP, zona pellucida, MV, microvillus; GC, Golgi complex; L, lipid; FCP, follicle cell processes; N, nucleus. ×7800. (Courtesy of D. L. Odor.)

arranged into a circumferential sheath to form the *theca folliculi* (Fig. 23-5). The growing follicle is then directed toward the ovarian surface by the formation of a wedge-shaped *thecal cone* (Fig. 23-8) whose details are not seen unless the follicle is sectioned in the proper plane. The directional movement of the thecal cone toward the surface moves the numerous oocytes stored in the cortex (Fig. 23-8) laterally so that they are not unduly compressed by the rapidly growing and expanding follicles. The stromal cells constituting the theca folliculi differentiate into an inner glandular and vascularized layer, the *theca interna* (Fig. 23-6), and an outer layer of connective tissue cells, the *theca externa*. The boundary between the

two thecal layers is indistinct, as is that between the theca externa and the surrounding stroma. The theca interna is composed of fibroblastlike cells which multiply to form a number of concentric layers of cells. In later stages of follicular growth these cells enlarge and differentiate into steroid-secreting cells. They appear either ovoid or spindle-shaped and have rounded nuclei. Lipid droplets are abundant and may be visualized, particularly if stained with fat stains. When the follicle ovulates, the thecal gland cells persist for only a short time before undergoing degeneration, and they soon disappear completely. Numerous small blood

FIGURE 23-8 The appearance of the theca cone in a growing follicle. Note how the primary oocytes are moved aside as the follicle expands toward the surface. ×300.

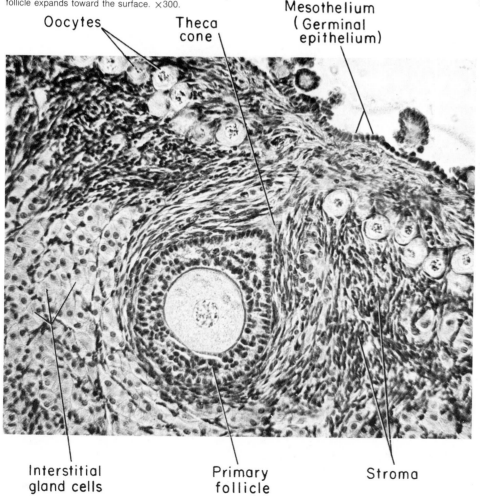

Oocytes

Theca cone

Mesothelium (Germinal epithelium)

Interstitial gland cells

Primary follicle

Stroma

vessels penetrate the theca externa to supply the complex vascular plexus of the theca interna (see Fig. 23-14B). Blood vessels do not enter the layers of follicular epithelium until after ovulation.

Development of the Vesicular Follicle

When the follicular cells have proliferated into 6 to 12 layers, there appear among them small lakes of follicular fluid which stain positively with the PAS reaction and are called the *Call-Exner bodies* (Fig. 23-9). They are thought to represent the precursors of follicular fluid. In some animals, such as the rabbit, the Call-

Exner bodies are numerous and much more obvious than in the ovarian follicles of women. The accumulations of follicular fluid enlarge and coalesce to form a fluid-filled cavity, the *follicular antrum* (Figs. 23-9 and 23-10). The *liquor folliculi* is a clear, viscid fluid rich in hyaluronic acid. In sectioned material it often has a granular appearance and stains a pale pink with the PAS method. An ovarian follicle with a completely formed antrum is described as a *secondary* or *vesicular* follicle. By the time antrum formation begins, the oocyte has attained its full size (125 to 150 μm in human beings) and is encompassed by a fully developed zona pellucida. The follicle continues to enlarge until it reaches a diameter of 8 to 10 mm or more (Fig. 23-11A and B).

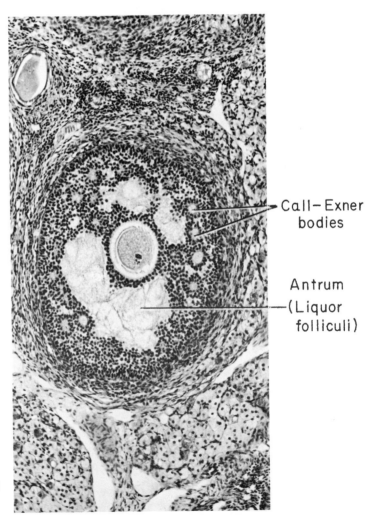

Call—Exner bodies

Antrum (Liquor folliculi)

FIGURE 23-9 A multilaminar, vesicular follicle of a rabbit in which the Call-Exner vacuoles are prominent. Fusion of these results in an enlarged antrum filled with follicular fluid. ×120.

The earliest phase of follicular growth which precedes antrum formation is not under hormonal control, whereas all the growth subsequent to and including liquor folliculi formation is dependent entirely upon the action of gonadotrophic hormones secreted by the adenohypophysis. The follicle has no endocrine function prior to the formation of an antrum, whereas after this event it becomes an endocrine body that secretes estrogens and, just before and after ovulation, both estrogens and progestins. In most vesicular follicles the egg, surrounded by several layers of follicular cells, assumes an eccentric position, giving an appearance of a small hillock protruding into the antrum (Fig. 23-11A). The follicular cells encompassing the egg constitute the *cumulus oophorus*. The zona pellucida is surrounded by a single continous layer of follicular cells, the *corona radiata* (Fig. 23-11B), which are anchored to the zona by cytoplasmic processes that penetrate the zona (Fig. 23-7).

The Preovulatory Follicle

The discharge of a mature ovum at ovulation results from a series of complex cytologic and growth changes within the egg itself and in the follicular and thecal cells surrounding it. Why only certain of the primordial follicles begin to grow and develop during any particular reproductive cycle is still a mystery.

In the human female, follicles require 12 to 14 days to reach maturity and attain the preovulatory stage. As the follicles reach their maximum size, they may occupy the full thickness of the ovarian cortex and bulge above the surface of the ovary (Fig. 23-11A).

Maturation Division of the Ovum

Before an egg can be fertilized, it is essential that its *diploid* number of chromosomes (46) be reduced to the *haploid* number (23). This process begins before the egg is discharged from the follicle and involves the

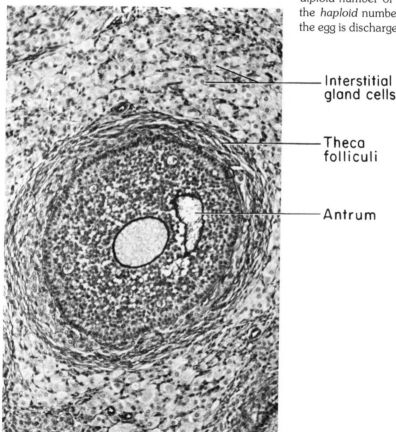

— Interstitial gland cells

— Theca folliculi

— Antrum

FIGURE 23-10 The early formation of an antrum, the concentric arrangement of the cells of the stroma to form the theca folliculi, and the arrangement and appearance of the interstitial gland cells of a rabbit ovary. ×100.

formation of the *first polar body* (Fig. 23-12), which results in the very unequal cytoplasmic division. In order to understand fully the various steps in this complex process, the reader is urged to review the process of meiosis.

In the human female, all the oocytes complete the earliest stages of meiosis during the fetal period, so that postnatally the chromosomes are in the *dictyo-*

tene, or "resting," stage of meiosis. They will remain in this stage throughout the reproductive life or until the oocyte begins the period of preovulatory growth, at which time the process of meiosis is resumed. In the formation of the first polar body, the *vesicular nucleus* or *germinal vesicle* moves to a position just beneath the *oolemma,* the plasma membrane of the egg (Fig. 23-12B); the chromatids, still attached at their chiasmata, condense and become visible at the microscopic level. The nuclear membrane disappears, and a spindle with fine spindle fibers is formed and assumes

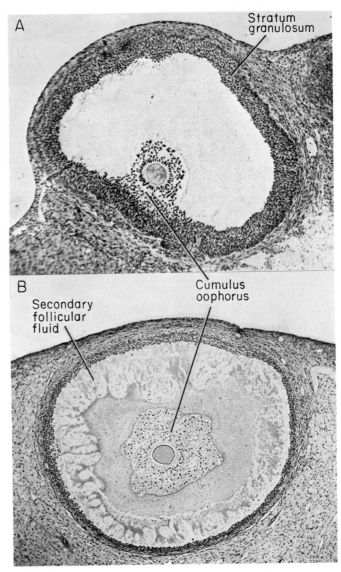

FIGURE 23-11 Photomicrograph of preovulatory follicles of (A) rat and (B) rabbit. Notice the separation of the cumulus oophorus from the stratum granulosum. Notice also the secretion of the secondary follicular fluid, especially in B.

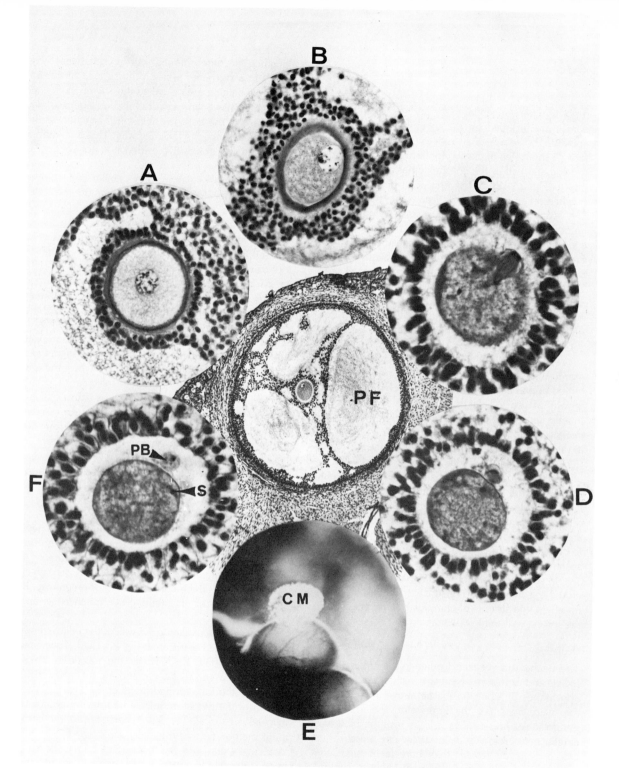

FIGURE 23-12 Stages in the formation of the first polar body in a preovulatory follicle (PF) of the rat. A. The centrally located vesicular nucleus at the beginning of the preovulatory growth phase. B. The movement of the nucleus to the periphery of the egg. C. Formation of the first polar body. D. Abstriction of the polar body vesicle and compacted chromosomes remaining within the egg. E. An ovulated follicle from a 16-mm motion picture. CM, cumulus mass. F. Section of this cumulus mass, showing the first polar body (PB) and the second maturation spindle (S), with the remaining chromosomes on the metaphase plate.

a position paratangential to the surface. The chromosomes are grouped on the metaphase plate of the spindle. The spindle then rotates 90° to the egg surface. A small bleb of clear cytoplasm is extruded from the egg and half of the chromosomes are discharged into it (Fig. 23-12C). The first polar body is quickly pinched off and comes to lie free within the perivitelline space (Fig. 23-12D). A second spindle forms immediately and the chromosomes remaining in the egg become arranged on the metaphase plate. This is the condition of the egg at the time of ovulation (Fig. 23-12E and F), and it has required approximately 8 to 10 h to attain this condition. The formation of the *second polar body* in the second meiotic division must await the transport of the ovulated egg into the ampulla of the oviduct and its penetration by a spermatozoon.

The size of the preovulatory follicle increases significantly during the 12 to 15 h prior to rupture, the period of *preovulatory swelling*. It involves (1) a rapid growth of the follicle itself, (2) the secretion of a thinner *secondary follicular fluid* (Fig. 23-11B) at an increased rate, and late in this phase (3) an increased inward folding of the stratum granulosum and theca (Fig. 23-11A; see also Fig. 23-15A). Changes occur also in the cumulus oophorus preparatory to freeing the ovum from the stratum granulosum. The intercellular cement anchoring the cumulus cells to one another depolymerizes so that they separate from one another (Fig. 23-11A and B). This separation appears to be related to the action of the luteinizing hormone secreted by the adenohypophysis.

In some animals the cumulus mass, with its enclosed egg, floats free within the antrum (Fig. 23-11B); in others, the strands of cumulus remain attached to the follicle wall until ovulation.

Ovulation

The mechanism of events leading to the rupture of the follicle and expulsion of the egg is still a mystery. The appearance of a bulging follicle above the surface of the ovary may give the impression that increasing intrafollicular pressure leads to its rupture. However, careful measurements of intrafollicular pressure just before ovulation reveals that there is no significant increase in pressure even at the moment of rupture. Approximately 30 min before a follicle ruptures, the stratum granulosum, the theca folliculi, and tunica albuginea become thinned out progressively (Fig. 23-13) in a restricted area on the surface of the follicle. This bulging area is called the *stigma* or *macula pellucida*. It has been suggested that collagenase may depolymerize the collagen fibers in the region of the stigma, weakening the follicular wall. This is an attractive theory, but conclusive evidence is not yet available.

Just before ovulation, a nipplelike cone bulges above the surface of the follicle. Its membranous covering appears similar to the basement membrane which separates the follicular cells from the theca. Within a few minutes, this membrane ruptures (Fig. 23-13D), expelling the ovum enclosed in the cumulus oophorus. This event is called *ovulation* (Figs. 23-13E and 23-14A), and the ovulated egg can now be termed the *gamete*. Ovulation has been observed many times in various living anesthetized laboratory animals and recorded cinematographically. In rats and rabbits a rather slow extrusion of the follicular contents was observed. The time between rupture of the stigma and discharge of the ovum averaged 72 s when the egg was preceded by some of the thin follicular fluid and 126 s when the cumulus oophorus was extruded first. In many mammals, including primates, the viscous follicular fluid is not completely expressed from the antrum during ovulation. It may remain adherent to the site of the stigma (Fig. 23-14A) until it is swept from the ovarian surface by the cilia lining the fimbriated end of the oviduct.

Formation of the Corpus Luteum

The ovulated follicle is transformed rapidly into a new, highly vascularized, glandular structure, the *corpus luteum* or *luteal gland*. It is called the *corpus luteum of ovulation* if pregnancy does not follow. If pregnancy ensues, it is called the *corpus luteum of pregnancy*. In pregnancy, the corpus luteum grows much larger and lasts longer.

Even before ovulation the wall of the follicle tends to become folded or plicated (Fig. 23-15A). The plicae are retained (Fig. 23-15B) as the follicle is transformed into a corpus luteum and are a characteristic feature of the fully formed luteal body. The transformation of the ovulatory follicle into a corpus luteum involves, first of all, the depolymerization of the basement membrane that originally separated the granulosa cell layers from the theca. This allows the connective tissue cells and blood vessels to invade the stratum granulosum (Fig. 23-16). The granulosa cells of the ovulatory follicle that will become the luteal cells

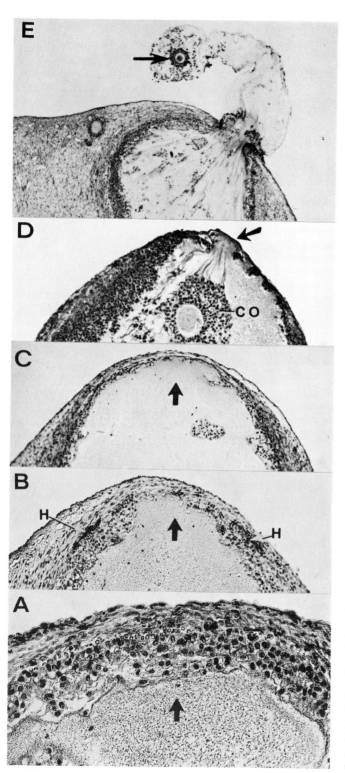

FIGURE 23-13 Stages in the formation of the stigma or macula pellucida in an ovulating follicle. A. Several hours before ovulation the stratum granulosum is still quite thick, as are the theca and tunica albuginea. B. One-half hour before ovulation hemostasis (H) appears in the region of the stigma. There is a significant thinning out of the follicular cells and stroma. C. A few minutes before rupture the follicular cells have almost disappeared, as has the stromal tissue in the region of the stigma. D. The stigmal cap lifts away and the free cumulus oophorus (CO) streams toward the opening. E. Ovulation is completed but the viscous antral fluid still adheres to the site of rupture.

of the corpus luteum begin to undergo cytomorphosis even before ovulation. The large preovulatory follicle secretes both estrogen and progesterone. Mitoses are seldom seen in the glandular parenchyma cells of the developing corpus luteum but are noted in the rapidly developing endothelium of the blood vessels which invade it.

The *luteal cells* enlarge and become polyhedral in shape and filled with lipid droplets (Fig. 23-17A). In ordinary histologic preparations the cytoplasm of the luteal cells contains numerous empty vacuoles whose lipid contents are dissolved out by the organic solvents used in processing the tissues. Several types of luteal cells have been described, but it is not known whether these are transition stages in the differentiation of a single cell type or represent distinct cell species. An interesting feature of the developing corpus luteum is the rapid invasion of the stratum granulosum with connective tissue elements and sprouts of capillary endothelium. The connective tissue forms a delicate reticulum supporting the luteal cells. A complex rete network of capillaries forms throughout the gland. With time, larger blood vessels are formed (see Fig. 23-14B). The formation of the vascular network in the developing corpus luteum is remarkably similar to that seen during the development of the vascular supply in any embryonic organ.

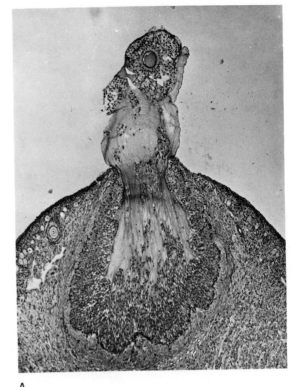

A

FIGURE 23-14A. Photomicrograph of an ovulation observed in situ in a living anesthetized rabbit. Immediately after ovulation, the ovary was fixed, removed, and cut in sections. PAS stain.

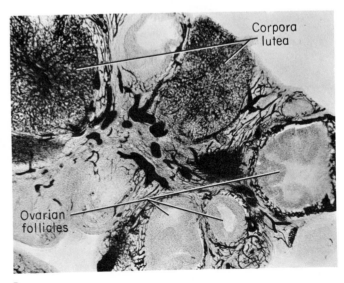

FIGURE 23-14B. Thick section of a rat ovary in which the blood vessels were perfused with carmine-gelatin. Notice also the rich vasculature of the corpora lutea.

Corpora lutea

Ovarian follicles

B

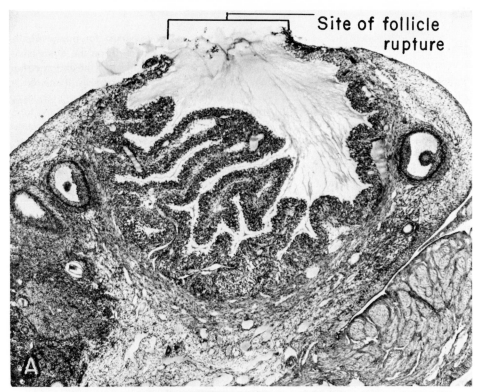

Site of follicle
rupture

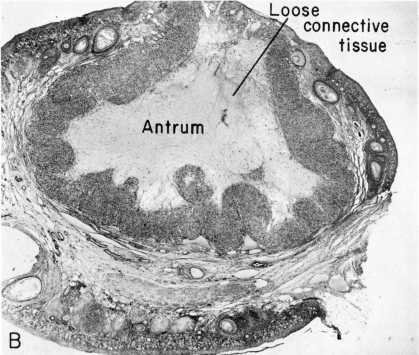

Loose
connective
tissue

Antrum

FIGURE 23-15 Photomicrograph of two stages in the development of the corpus luteum of the cat. A. The recent site of rupture as well as the remarkable foldings of the stratum granulosum. B. Several days later the luteal cells appear glandular and the antrum is being invaded by a loose connective tissue.

In electron micrographs of the corpus luteum, the luteal cells have mitochondria with tubular cristae and an abundant smooth ER so characteristic of steroid-secreting cells. The fully formed corpus luteum secretes both estrogens and progestins. If the egg is not fertilized, the corpus luteum lasts for about 14 days. With its demise (Fig. 23-17B), the rate of secretion of estrogens and progestins drops, and it begins to undergo involution. The luteal cells become filled with complex lipids and degenerate. With time, a hyaline intercellular material accumulates, and the former corpus luteum assumes the appearance of an irregular white, hyaline scar, the *corpus albicans* (Fig. 23-18).

The corpus albicans may persist for many months before it gradually disappears. If, on the other hand, the egg is fertilized and implants into the endometrium of the uterus, the corpus luteum persists. It enlarges to 2 to 3 cm to become the *corpus luteum of pregnancy*. During pregnancy, the corpus luteum remains functional for several months and then gradually declines up to full term. Involution is accelerated after delivery, leading to the formation of a corpus albicans. A corpus albicans formed from a corpus luteum of pregnancy may last for years.

Atresia of Follicles

As mentioned earlier, atresia, or degeneration of eggs and follicles, at all stages of follicular development is a prominent feature in the life of the ovaries. Large

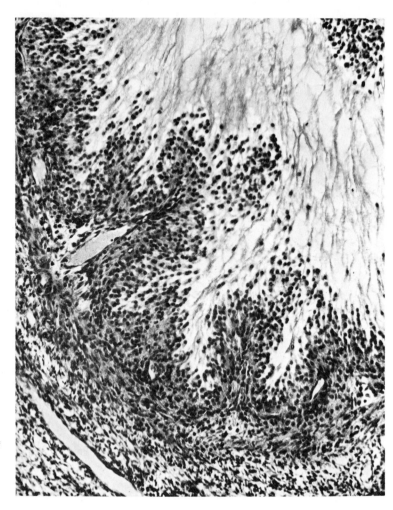

FIGURE 23-16 Section of the wall of a corpus luteum of a monkey one day after ovulation. Connective tissue and blood vessels are invading the stratum granulosum. ×100.

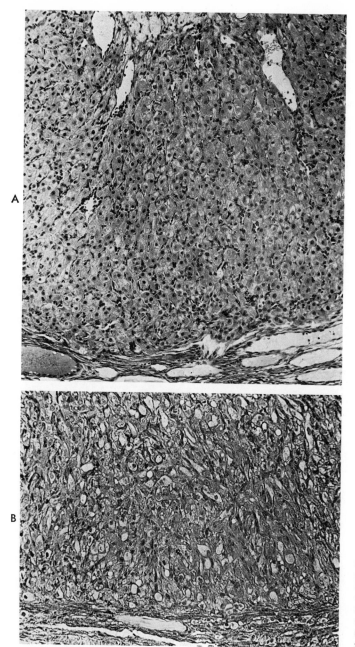

FIGURE 23-17 Corpus luteum at the peak of development and early degeneration in the monkey. A. Corpus luteum 8 or 9 days after ovulation. Cavity at top of picture. B. Corpus luteum first day of menstrual flow. Cells shrunken, extensive lipid vacuolation, nuclei pycnotic. ×95. (Courtesy of G. E. Corner.)

numbers of oocytes degenerate and disappear during the fetal and early postnatal periods. It has been proposed that a primary cause of atresia during these early periods is the disruption or loss of the follicular cells encompassing each oocyte. This suggests that if the life of the oocyte is to be maintained, the follicular cells must be in continuous and intimate contact with the plasma membrane of the egg. Among the groups of follicles that grow to a large size in each menstrual cycle, only one, as a rule, attains full maturity and ovulates. All the remaining large vesicular follicles and many of the smaller ones undergo atresia.

Atresia of a vesicular follicle may occur in many different ways (Fig. 23-19A, B, and C) but always with the usual signs of cell degeneration, such as pycnosis and chromatolysis of the nuclei and shrinkage and dissolution of the cytoplasm. The ooplasm cytolyzes, often leaving only the remnant of the zona pellucida (Fig. 23-19C) to mark the location of the ovum. Macrophage invasion of atretic follicles is a regular feature. The zona pellucida, composed of complex mucopolysaccharides, is more resistant, but eventually it, too, is broken down and engulfed by macrophages.

Occasionally, the basement membrane separating the follicular cells from the theca interna increases in thickness, assumes a corrugated hyalinelike appearance, and is then called the *glassy membrane*. In some atretic follicles the cells of the theca interna enlarge, become epithelioid (Fig. 23-19B), and may be arrayed in a radial or cordlike fashion. These cords of cells

may be separated from one another by delicate connective tissue fibers and a capillary network. The cells are often filled with lipid droplets, giving them an appearance of an old corpus luteum.

The Interstitial Gland

The origin, development, and endocrine function of the *interstitial gland* or *interstitial cells* of the ovary have been the subject of much confusion and controversy. In many mammals, such as the rabbit (Figs. 23-8 and 23-10) and women (Fig. 23-20), clusters or cords of large, epithelioid cells with cytology and vascularity typical of endocrine glands are dispersed in the cortical stroma. These are referred to collectively as the *interstitial gland* or *interstitial cells*. Cytologically, they resemble luteal cells to a remarkable degree.

The interstitial gland is present periodically in the ovary of the human female from before birth until well after the menopause. The interstitial cells are thought to originate from the cells of the theca interna of degenerating large secondary follicles or degenerating

FIGURE 23-18 Corpus albicans in human ovary.

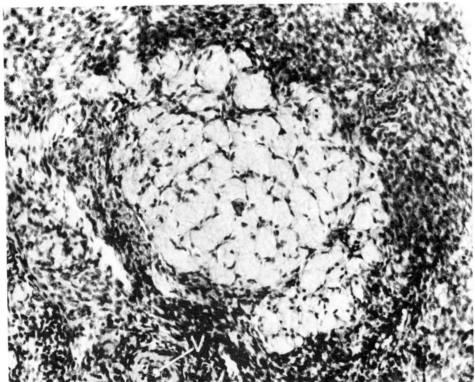
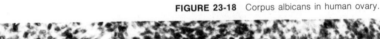

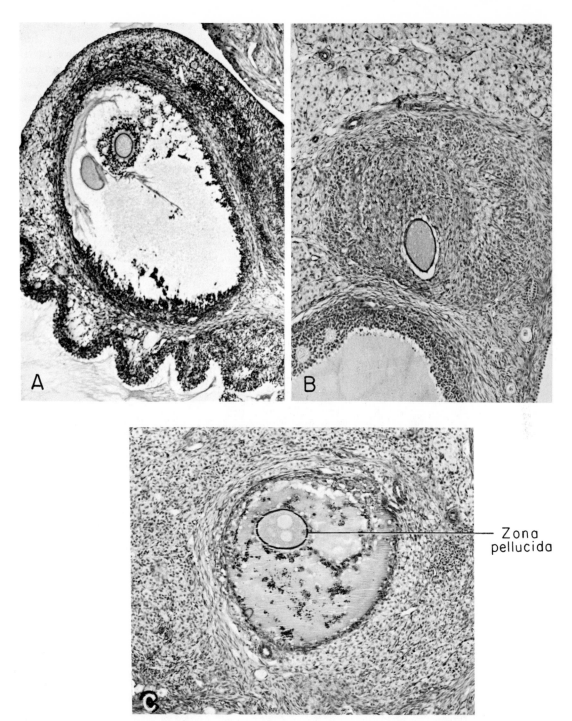

Zona
pellucida

FIGURE 23-19 Follicular atresia. A. Cat. B. Rabbit. C. Monkey. A. Large follicle cells of stratum granulosum and egg degenerating. B. Antrum filled with glandular-appearing cells, egg degenerated but zona pellucida still intact. C. Theca interna contributing to interstitial gland tissue; follicular cells cytolyzed and zona pellucida remains.

vesicular follicles of all sizes. The theca interna of the very large preovulatory follicles that are not destined to ovulate have already differentiated into functional thecal gland cells and therefore cannot be transformed into interstitial glandular tissue.

Differentiation of interstitial gland tissue is cyclic and is probably related to the rhythmic atresia of the various crops of vesicular follicles during the menstrual cycle or pregnancy. The role of the interstitial gland cells in normal ovarian physiology is yet to be completely defined. Studies on steroidogenesis in the ovarian stroma in women show that it principally synthesizes estrogens. In rabbits, on the other hand, interstitial cells are stimulated directly by gonadotrophins to synthesize and secrete 20α-OH-progesterone. Many believe that the interstitial gland plays a significant role in providing estrogens for the growth and development of the secondary sex organs during the prepubertal period.

Other groups of epithelioid cells may be found in the region of the hilum of the ovary and are called *hilus cells*. These cells are usually associated with vascular spaces and unmyelinated nerve fibers. They appear glandular, contain lipids, cholesterol esters, and lipochrome pigments and are identified best during pregnancy and at the onset of the menopause. Tumors or hyperplasia of the hilus cells usually leads to masculinization. Although the evidence is tenuous, it is suggested that these cells secrete steroids related to androgens.

Vessels, Nerves, Lymphatics

The ovaries have a rich blood supply from several sources (Fig. 23-14B). The principal arteries are the ovarian arteries which arise from the aorta below the level of the renal vessels. They travel a relatively long course through the infundibulopelvic ligaments to reach the ovaries. The ovarian arteries anastomose with the uterine arteries which are branches of the hypogastrics.

The veins accompany the arteries and often form

FIGURE 23-20 Mature interstitial gland tissue at $8\frac{1}{2}$ months of gestation in a woman. Notice the arrangement of the glandular cells and the nuclei of the capillary endothelium between the rows of cells. ×840. (Courtesy of H. W. Mossman.)

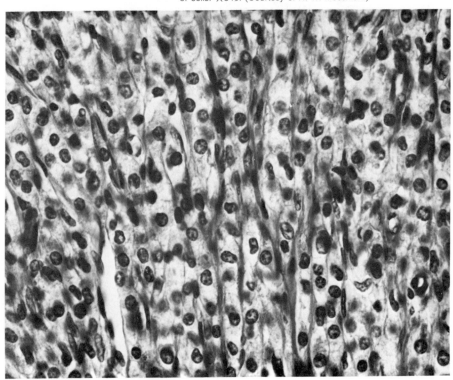

a complex plexus of vessels in the hilum. Of principal interest is the cyclic change and continuous reorganization of the vascular pattern of the ovaries as crops of follicles and corpora lutea grow, perform their function, and degenerate. Thus, with each cycle, an extensive blood and lymphatic system develops to support the growth and cytodifferentiation of various cells.

The ovary has a lymphatic system (Fig. 23-21) whose ubiquity and complexity are seldom appreciated. Large numbers of lymphatic vessels are organized around the developing follicles and corpora lutea. The extrinsic lymphatic drainage follows a course to the aortic, preaortic, and paraaortic lymph nodes in the pelvis.

In developing follicles, the lymphatics are arranged in a basketlike network within the theca folliculi but, like the blood vessels, do not penetrate into the

FIGURE 23-21 Diagram showing the arrangement of lymphatics within and around a corpus luteum, Graafian follicles, and stroma in the ovary of the ewe. (Courtesy of B. Morris.)

stratum granulosum. The corpora lutea, however, are heavily infiltrated by lymphatic vessels (Fig. 23-21). The lymphatic capillaries often have open intercellular junctions (Fig. 23-22) so that materials from the interstitial pores can readily enter the vessels. It has been shown in the ewe, for example, that coincident with the formation of the corpus luteum, lymph flow from the ovary increases significantly. It has been suggested that there may be an association between the synthesis and secretion of steroid hormones by the corpus luteum and an increase in capillary permeability.

Nerves

The nerves of the ovaries are derivatives of the ovarian plexus and uterine nerves. All vessels and nerves enter the ovary through the hilum. Most of the nerves are

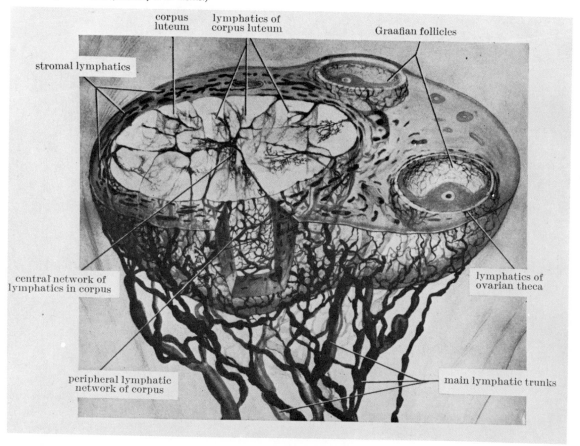

corpus luteum

lymphatics of corpus luteum

Graafian follicles

stromal lymphatics

central network of lymphatics in corpus

lymphatics of ovarian theca

peripheral lymphatic network of corpus

main lymphatic trunks

nonmyelinated and sympathetic and supply the muscular coats of arterioles. Some nonmyelinated fibers form plexuses around multilaminar follicles. Whether nerves are associated also with the generalized smooth muscle cells in the ovary is unknown. A few sensory nerve endings have been described in the ovarian stroma.

THE OVIDUCTS

The oviducts extend bilaterally from the uterus to the region of the ovary (Fig. 23-1). They provide the necessary environment for fertilization and segmentation of the egg until it attains the morula stage of development. The fertilized egg remains within the oviduct for a total of 3 days before it enters the uterus.

The oviducts in the sexually mature human female are 10 to 12 cm in length. They are suspended by a rather loose mesentery, the *mesosalpinx* (Fig. 23-23A and B), a derivative of the broad ligament. In the human, each oviduct may be divided into several linear segments distinguishable by gross examination and by study of transverse sections taken at different levels throughout the tube. These are the *interstitial* segment which pierces the uterine wall, the *isthmus* (Fig. 23-1) which constitutes approximately two-thirds of the oviduct, and the somewhat more dilated *am-*

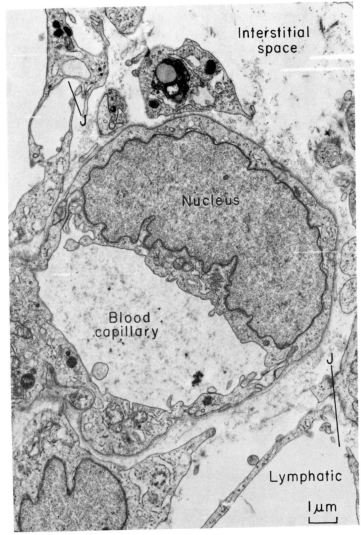

FIGURE 23-22 Low-power electron micrograph of a blood capillary and two adjacent lymphatics in the ovarian stroma of a rat. Notice the open junctions (J) (lines) in the endothelium of both lymphatics. ×8000. (Courtesy of B. Morris.)

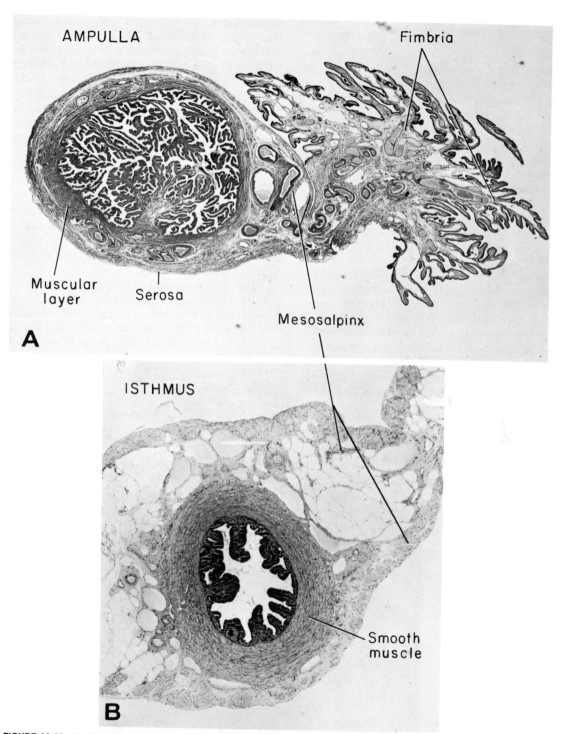

FIGURE 23-23 Photomicrograph through the ampulla (A) and isthmus (B) of the oviduct of a rabbit. In A, the section was cut to include some of the fimbria.

pulla (Fig. 23-1), which extends from the isthmus to the funnel-shaped orifice, the *infundibulum*. The free margin of the infundibulum is extensively folded and fluted, giving it a fimbriated or tentaclelike appearance (Figs. 23-1 and 23-23A). In many mammals the fimbriated end of the infundibulum embraces the ovary at the time of ovulation, almost completely enclosing it and forming the *ovarian bursa*. Such an intimate relationship of the fimbriae to the ovary has not been observed in the human female. The wall of the oviduct consists of a complex mucous membrane, a muscular layer, and, peripherally, a serosa.

The Mucosa

Throughout the length of the oviduct, the mucous membrane extends into the lumen in a linear system of complex folds which are elaborately branched, especially in the ampulla (Fig. 23-23A) where in a cross section they appear as a complex labyrinth of spaces. In the isthmus the folds are much less complex and are primarily simple, longitudinal ridges (Fig. 23-23B). The mucosal folds throughout the oviduct are quite thin and are composed of a surface epithelium of columnar cells resting on a lamina of connective tissue (Fig. 23-24). Many of the cells are ciliated and are interspersed among nonciliated cells that appear to be glandular (Fig. 23-24). The ciliated cells of the oviduct are most numerous on the fimbrial surface of the infundibulum, somewhat less so in the ampulla, and fewer still in the isthmus and interstitial segments. The cilia of the oviduct exhibit the basal body complexes and fibrillar arrangements typical of cilia elsewhere (Fig. 23-25).

The epithelium of the oviduct of the human female shows cyclic hypertrophy and atrophy during each menstrual cycle. The ciliated cells may vary in height from 30 μm at about the time of ovulation to 15 μm or less during the late luteal phase or shortly before the onset of menstruation. After the menopause, the epithelium is of the low cuboidal type and there are fewer ciliated cells.

The development of cilia in the oviduct is in some manner dependent on the presence of the ovary. In women born without ovaries, no ciliated cells develop and the mucosal folds are little more than broad ridges. In addition, it has been shown recently that removal of the ovaries from a sexually mature rhesus

FIGURE 23-24 Photomicrograph showing the ciliated and glandular cells of the surface epithelium of the ampulla of the oviduct of the monkey. (Courtesy of R. Brenner.)

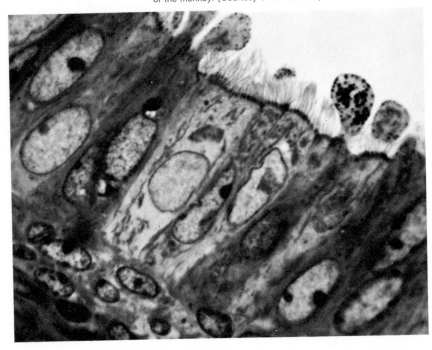

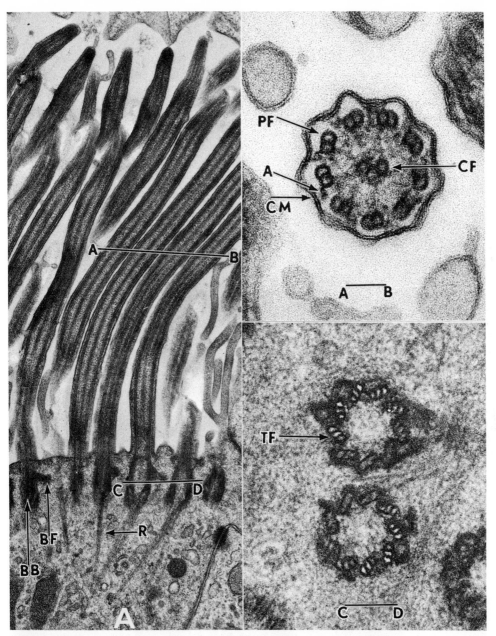

FIGURE 23-25A. Typical cilium and basal body complex. Each basal body (BB) has a basal foot (BF) and proximal rootlets (R). ×30,000. The line A–B through the cilia represents the transverse section seen on the upper right. The line C–D through the basal body represents the transverse section seen on the lower right. A–B. Cross section of a typical cilium. There are nine peripheral double fibrils (PF) and two single central fibrils (CF). A short projection or "arm" (A) is present on each peripheral doublet. The cilium is bounded by a ciliary membrane (CM). ×160,000. C–D. Cross sections of typical basal bodies. In each basal body there are nine peripheral triplet fibrils (TF) embedded in a dense material. The core of the basal body is much less dense and lacks central fibrils. ×130,000. (Courtesy of R. Brenner.)

monkey causes a dramatic atrophy of the oviduct epithelium with complete loss of cilia from the infundibulum and to a lesser extent from the ampulla. This phenomenon has not as yet been studied in the isthmus. If the castrate animal is injected with estrogens, the ciliated epithelium is completely restored. Experiments such as these demonstrate dramatically the processes involved in ciliogenesis and dependence of ciliated cells of the reproductive tract upon hormones for their full development and function.

The cilia of the fimbria all beat toward the ostium of the oviduct and play an important role in sweeping the ovulated eggs from the surface of the ovary and into the ampulla of the oviduct. Even though the mucosa of the ampulla is relatively well ciliated and all the cilia beat in the direction of the isthmus, it appears that egg transport through the ampulla is caused primarily by peristaltic muscular contractions. The role of ciliary beat in the ampulla is at present unknown.

After ovulation in the rabbit, the egg, embedded in the cumulus oophorus (Fig. 23-14A), is transported from the site of ovulation to the lower end of the ampulla in approximately 10 min. The ampulla is normally the site of sperm penetration and fertilization. From 15 to 18 h after fertilization, the egg has been freed of all its cumulus cells; it then moves into the isthmus where its transport is slowed, requiring approximately 2 days to reach the uterus.

It is usually assumed that all the cilia in the oviducts of mammals beat toward the uterus. It has been found recently, at least in the rabbit, that the ciliated cells on the surfaces of some of the longitudinal ridges in the isthmus of the oviduct beat in the direction of the ovary whereas others on adjacent ridges beat in the direction of the uterus. Whether currents set up by this alternate ciliary movement play any role in the passage of spermatozoa to the ampulla is unknown. It should be pointed out that the rate of passage of spermatozoa through the oviducts to the site of fertilization (the ampulla) is much too fast to be accounted for by their own motility. Although evidence is not complete, it appears that both muscular and ciliary activity are primarily responsible for the rapid movement of spermatozoa through the oviducts.

The mucous membrane of the oviduct rests directly upon the tunica muscularis with no intervening

FIGURE 23-25B. A surface view of a typical ciliated cell from the fimbria of the monkey oviduct as seen with the scanning electron microscope. (Courtesy Dr. Ruth Rumery.)

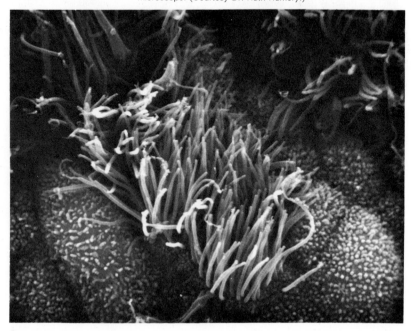

B

submucosa. The lamina propria of the mucous membrane is thin, consisting of a delicate, loose connective tissue extending into the folds and containing a few scattered muscle cells.

Muscularis

The muscularis of the oviduct consists, in general, of an inner circular or spiral layer and an external layer of rather poorly defined longitudinal fibers (Fig. 23-23A and B). There are no distinct boundaries between the two. A third, inner layer of longitudinal muscles has been described in the proximal isthmus in the oviducts of the human female. There is an obvious increase in the thickness of the circular muscle layers as the isthmus approaches the uterus. The peritoneal coat of the oviduct is covered by a thin serosa.

UTERUS

The human uterus is a hollow, pear-shaped organ with a thick muscular wall. It receives the oviducts and opens into the vagina through the cervical canal (Fig. 23-1). It lies in the pelvic cavity interposed between the bladder and rectum. Its size varies among non-pregnant women but average dimensions are length, 6.3 cm; breadth, 4.5 cm; and thickness, 2.5 cm. The expanded rostral portion is referred to as the *body* or *corpus uteri,* and the caudal portion, a part of which protrudes into the upper vagina, is the *cervix*. The cervical canal passes from the uterine cavity through the cervix and opens into the vagina. The opening visible from the vaginal vault is called the *external os* (Fig. 23-1). The term *fundus* refers to the dome-shaped upper portion of the body of the uterus from which the oviducts extend. The body of the uterus is flattened anteroposteriorly, and the lumen appears as a transverse slit. The cavity of the uterus is confluent with the lumina of the oviducts.

The wall of the uterus is composed of an internal layer, the *endometrium* (mucosa); a middle layer, the *myometrium* (muscularis); and an external layer, the *perimetrium* (serosa) (Fig. 23-1). It should be noted that the posterocaudal third of the uterus does not have a serosa, since this portion of the uterus lies below the peritoneal reflection. The connective tissue of the broad ligament at the lateral edges of the uterus is termed the *parametrium*.

Endometrium

Beginning at puberty, in the human, and continuing until the menopause, the uterine mucosa undergoes

cyclic changes in structure and secretory activity. The terminal event in each cycle is a partial destruction and sloughing of a portion of the endometrium, accompanied by some extravasation of blood, an event termed *menstruation*. The endometrium is a complex mucous membrane (Fig. 23-26). Its height varies from 1 to 7 mm, depending on the phase of the menstrual cycle. It consists of a simple columnar epithelium and a wide lamina propria, the *endometrial stroma*. It is firmly attached to the myometrium without any intervening submucosa. The stroma contains many simple tubular *uterine glands* (Fig. 23-26B) which open onto the surface of the mucosa, extend deep into the endometrial stroma, and end blindly near the muscularis. Occasionally, they are branched in the area adjacent to the myometrium. The epithelium lining the glands and that covering the surface appear identical. Occasionally, patches of ciliated cells may be seen either within the glands or on the surface epithelium facing the lumen. There is a basement membrane beneath the epithelium of both the glands and surface epithelium. The stroma in which the uterine glands are embedded resembles mesenchyme tissue (Fig. 23-26C); the cells are loosely arranged and stellate in appearance and often have oval nuclei.

The endometrium is usually divided into two layers or zones (Fig. 23-27), differing in their morphology and function: a *lamina basalis* or *basal layer* and a *lamina functionalis* or *functional layer*.

The basal layer is applied directly to the myometrium and occasionally may extend into small pockets in the muscularis (Fig. 23-26A and B at arrows). Dr. Carl Hartman once removed all the endometrial tissue from the uterus of a menstruating rhesus monkey by scrubbing it away with cotton swabs. At the end of the next menstrual cycle, he was surprised to find a completely regenerated endometrium. This was a dramatic demonstration of the regenerative capacity of the endometrium even from the bits of tissue tucked into the small pockets of the myometrium.

There is considerable variation in the thickness of the basal layer of endometrium. Its stroma is much more cellular and fibrous than that of the functional zone. The basal layer undergoes few obvious microscopic changes during a menstrual cycle and serves principally as a source of tissue for the cyclic regeneration of the functional layer. The functional layer rises from the basal layer toward the lumen of the uterus

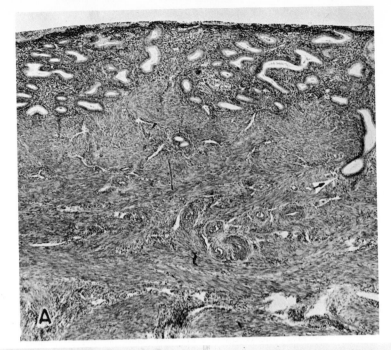

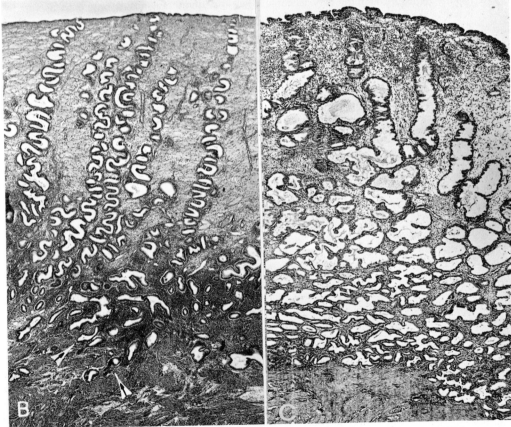

FIGURE 23-26 Photomicrograph of human endometrium during the menstrual cycle and pregnancy. A. Shedding of the stratum functionalis has been completed, and its regeneration has just begun. B. Early secretory endometrium. C. Gestational endometrium, fourteenth day of pregnancy. Notice the arrows pointing out stratum basalis tissue in crypts of myometrium.

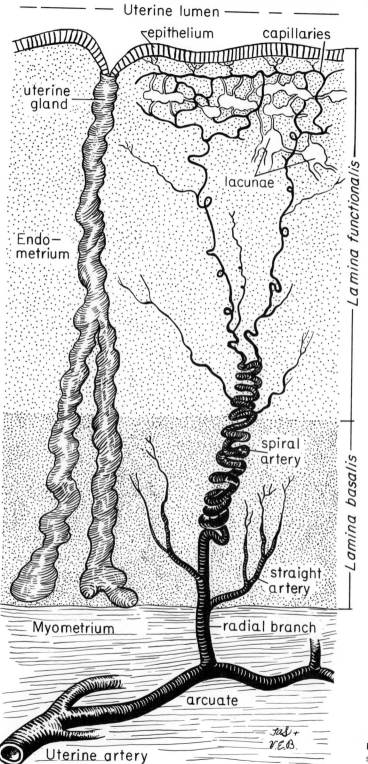

FIGURE 23-27 Diagrammatic representation of the glands and vasculature of the human endometrium.

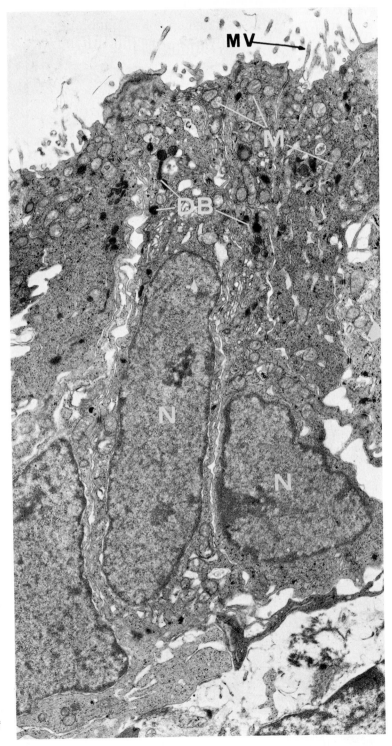

FIGURE 23-28 Electron micrograph of human epithelial cells during the early proliferative phase. N, nucleus; M, mitochondria; DB, dense bodies; MV, microvilli. ×10,500. (Courtesy of E. R. Friedrich.)

and is the site of the principal cyclic changes in the endometrium which prepare a bed for the fertilized ovum. The endometrial tissue, and particularly the functional zone, undergoes a constantly changing histologic picture which is related directly to the secretion of the various hormones by the ovary.

The epithelial cells during the early proliferative phase are tall columnar cells (Fig. 23-28) with numerous long, narrow microvilli extending from their surfaces. Their nuclei may be elongated or quite irregular in shape, their mitochondria are relatively small, and their Golgi complexes assume a supranuclear position. Many cells show cytoplasmic inclusions and granules of varying size and shape. At this stage in the cycle, glycogen is not discernible by electron microscopy. Dramatic changes in the cytology of cells (Fig. 23-29) are seen during the midsecretory phase, at the

time the corpus luteum is secreting actively. The mitochondria are larger and are surrounded by narrow tubules of rough ER. Large aggregates of glycogen, as well as numerous polyribosomes, are present. During the later secretory phase, the apical portions of the cells are filled with glycogen. The apical cell membrane becomes distended and ruptures, releasing glycogen and other cytoplasmic components into the lumen. During the premenstrual or degenerative phase (Fig. 23-30), the mitochondria are significantly smaller and lysosomes increase in number. Myelin figures or lipid droplets have formed within the remaining glycogen deposits.

A very elaborate and unique vascular system is

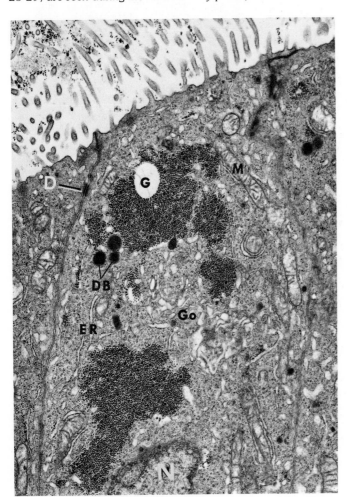

FIGURE 23-29 Electron micrograph of the apical cell portion of the midsecretory phase of human endometrium. Notice the large glycogen deposits (G), the slightly dilated Golgi structure (Go), and a few remaining dense bodies (DB). D, desmosome; ER, endoplasmic reticulum; M, mitochondria. ×11,400. (Courtesy of E. R. Friedrich.)

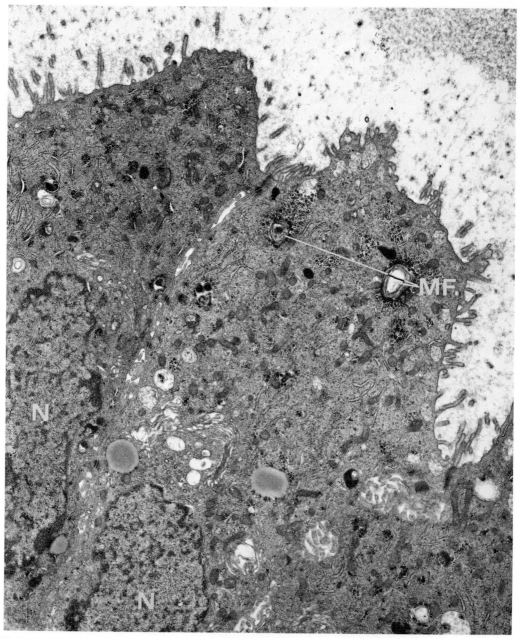

FIGURE 23-30 Premenstrual phase of human endometrium. Apical cell portions with small mitochondria and lysosomes; myelin figures (MF) forming within the glycogen deposits. ×11,400. (Courtesy of E. R. Friedrich.)

developed in anticipation of an implanting embryo, and this should be studied in some detail. The uterine artery gives off 6 to 10 *arcuate arteries* (Fig. 23-27) which extend between the outer and middle third of the myometrium and have *radial branches* inward to supply the endometrium. There may be 20 or more radial branches (sometimes called *submucous vessels*) from each arcuate artery. The *spiral arteries* (Fig. 23-27) are particularly characteristic of the endometrium. They pass through the basalis and extend into the functional zone. The proximal part of the vessel is an unchanging segment, whereas the distal end is subject to repeated degeneration and regeneration with each menstrual cycle. The typical development of the spiral arteries is dependent on a certain ratio of estrogens and progestins. Branches of the spiral vessels serve the tissues of the basalis as independent arteries or arterioles. These *straight arteries* (Fig. 23-27) are not subject to the actions of hormones.

As the spiral vessels traverse the functionalis, they divide into several terminal arterioles which frequently anastomose with one another. These, in turn, connect with a complex rete network of capillary units and *lacunas* (Fig. 23-27). The lacunas are very thin, dilated units which vary greatly in size. These structures are ordinarily not classified as part of the venous system but rather are terminal *ectatic capillaries* or *connecting lacunas* and are defined as part of the arterial vasculature. The venules and veins also form an irregular network with sinusoidal enlargements called *collecting lacunas* (Fig. 23-27). The lacunas are very thin, dilated phase of the cycle. The endometrial veins flow into a venous plexus concentrated at the basalis-myometrial border.

Cyclic Changes in the Endometrium

During a menstrual cycle, the endometrium passes through three successive phases which correspond to the functional activity of the ovary: The *proliferative* (or *follicular*) *phase* is concurrent with the growth of the follicles and estrogen secretion, the *secretory* (or *luteal*) *phase* coincides with the functional life of the corpus luteum, and the *menstrual phase* lasts through the period of menstrual bleeding.

PROLIFERATIVE PHASE During the proliferative phase, the endometrium increases in thickness from about 1 to 2 or 3 mm. The endometrial glands become longer and more numerous. Many mitoses may be seen throughout the epithelium and the stroma. The epithelial cells, particularly in the glands, become taller

and accumulate a considerable store of glycogen basal to the nucleus. No doubt other presecretory substances accumulate as well. The luminal surface of the epithelium is even and the cell membranes distinct and unbroken. The glands are either straight-walled or slightly wavy. They secrete a thin mucoid. The stroma during this time is rich in mucoid substance.

In the proliferative phase, the coiled arteries lengthen with the regrowth of the endometrium and extend through more than half its thickness. They are lightly coiled.

SECRETORY PHASE Remarkable modifications of the endometrium ensue within a day or two after ovulation has occurred. The glands become irregularly coiled and the glandular epithelium begins to secrete. The lumen of each gland becomes filled with a mucoid fluid rich in nutrients, particularly glycogen. The glycogen moves from a subnuclear position to the apical surface and, as described earlier, is discharged from the cells. The glands enlarge and often become sacculated, especially in the deeper third of the mucosa. The endometrium gradually becomes more edematous and may increase in thickness to 5 or 6 mm. This increase is primarily owing to swelling of the tissues rather than to proliferation of cells. The mesenchymatous cells of the stroma share in this edematous condition. During the luteal phase, the coiled arteries lengthen and become more spiral. Near the end of the cycle, rather characteristic decidual changes are often seen in the stromal cells.

MENSTRUAL PHASE Reduction in hormonal activity of the corpus luteum 4 to 5 days prior to the appearance of menstruation has a profound effect on the endometrium. Changes in the hemodynamics of blood flow in the functionalis are of primary significance in understanding the process of menstruation. The endometrium becomes ischemic and stops secreting. The functionalis shrinks, owing to loss of ground substance and water. The stromal cells become closely packed and densely stained. The lumina of the glands are reduced or obliterated in the general collapse of the endometrium. There is an intermittent constriction of the spiral vessels, resulting in reduced arterial and venous blood flow and stasis in the capillaries. Approximately 2 days after the endometrium begins its decline, the epithelium becomes disrupted, and blood, uterine fluid, and desquamated bits of the mucosa are sloughed from the functionalis and discharged via the vagina. This period of bloody vaginal discharge, lasting roughly 5 days, is termed the *menses*. The menstrual process begins with extravasation of blood from capillaries or from arterioles into the stroma. This blood forms small hematomas that coalesce and rupture onto the mucosal surface. Fragments of mucosa detach, leaving exposed stroma and naked vessels. The disintegrating functionalis becomes tattered and soaked with blood. Desquamation of tissue continues until the stratum functionalis is discarded.

Menstrual blood is both arterial and venous. Clotting is inhibited, and hemostasis is dependent upon vasoconstriction. Arterial bleeding is intermittent and brief, coincident with the period of relaxation of the coiled arteries, whereas bleeding from veins is a light but protracted seepage. The coiled arteries are shed piecemeal and more slowly than the neighboring stroma and glands, so they often protrude from the denuded surface of the menstruating endometrium. As the coiled portion is breaking up, contraction bands that occur beneath the coiled portion mark the extent of the arterial shedding. Small tufts of clotted blood fill the lumina at the tips of the coiled vessels. The straight arteries serving the stratum basalis do not become constricted during menstruation; hence, the stratum basalis remains well supplied with blood during the sloughing of the functionalis.

The functionalis is usually lost entirely, leaving only the basalis with the exposed blind ends of the glands. Elsewhere the mucosal surface is denuded and raw. With the cessation of hemorrhage and the concomitant initiation of the development of a new set of ovarian follicles, remnants of healthy uterine epithelium, particularly from the mouths of the glands, proliferate rapidly and provide the denuded areas with an epithelial covering.

THE GRAVID CYCLE After ovulation, it takes about 3 days for the fertilized ovum to reach the uterus. The zygote undergoes rapid embryonic growth and by the fifth day develops into a *blastocyst*. By the early part of the second week of the luteal phase, it becomes embedded in the uterine mucosa (*implantation, nidation*). At this time, the peripheral cellular elements of the blastocyst (the *chorion*) begin secreting a hormone known as *human chorionic gonadotrophin* (HCG) which helps sustain the life and function of the corpus luteum beyond the usual limits of a menstrual cycle. The growth of the endometrium is not interrupted; there is no menstrual flow, and this circumstance is commonly denoted as the first missed period. A secretory or progestational endometrium becomes a *gestational endometrium* (Fig. 23-26C) simply by the fact of pregnancy. It undergoes further progestational development during the early weeks of pregnancy.

The Cervix

The cervix uteri (Fig. 23-31) encloses the cervical canal, which is approximately 3 cm long and slightly distended in the middle portion. The mucosal lining of the cervix, the *endocervix,* is continuous with that of the body of the uterus (Fig. 23-1) but differs sharply in both its epithelium and underlying stroma. The mucous membrane, 3 to 5 mm thick, forms very complex, deep furrows or compound clefts called the *plicae palmatae* (Fig. 23-32). These folds run in longitudinal, transverse, and oblique directions and form a very irregular arrangement which may penetrate the entire thickness of the mucosa. This arrangement of folds is often misinterpreted as being a system of branching tubular glands of the compound racemose variety. The basic pattern, then, of the epithelium of the cervical canal is a complex system of clefts with accessory folds and tunnellike projections. The lining epithelium of the plicae palmatae consists of a single layer of tall, mucus-secreting cells. Some of the epithelial cells are ciliated, with the cilia beating toward the vagina. The height of the cells and the position of their nuclei vary with the time of the cycle and their secretory activity. During the proliferative and secretory phases, the epithelial cells synthesize mucus and other substances and package them in membrane-bounded vacuoles (Fig. 23-33). The cells laden with these materials stain poorly, and their nuclei are pushed to the base of the cells (Fig. 23-34). During active secretion, the nuclei rise to the center of the cells (Fig. 23-35) as the secreted mucus distends the lumina of the glands. Occasionally, some of the plicae become occluded and dilate with secretions. Such cysts are called *Nabothian follicles* (Fig. 23-31). The cervical canal is usually filled with mucus. The biochemical and biophysical characteristics of the mucus vary with the time in the cycle.

The mucosa of the cervix does not take part in the menstrual changes, so it is not sloughed. After the menopause, the mucosa shrinks, the glandular epithelium becomes gradually flattened, and the secretory activity is arrested. The subepithelial tissue of the human cervix is composed predominantly of a dense connective tissue. Smooth muscle makes up approximately 15 percent of the tissue with the distal portion of the cervix (partio vaginalis) containing no smooth muscle. The arrangement of the connective tissue and smooth muscle has a very complex pattern.

Myometrium

The musculature of the uterus forms a thick tunic that is composed of three muscle layers somewhat blended because of complex interconnecting bundles and interspersed by considerable connective tissue. Well-

defined muscle layers are not easily discernible over the body of the uterus. In general, the cells in the central portion of the muscularis are more circularly disposed, whereas those to either side tend to be directed obliquely or longitudinally. The middle region of the muscularis contains many large blood and lymphatic vessels (*stratum vasculare*). Over the cervix, the muscularis is layered in a relatively defined manner; there are an inner and outer longitudinal and a middle circular layer. Elastic fibers, though few and peripherally located in the uterus, are abundant in the outer wall of the cervix.

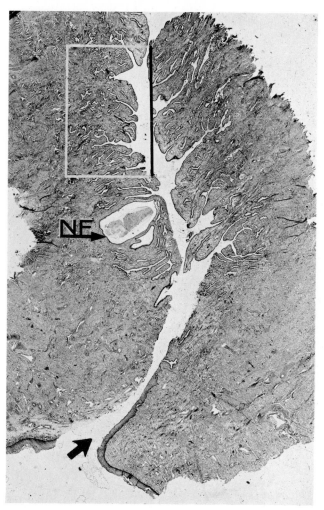

FIGURE 23-31 Longitudinal section of a human cervix uteri (proliferative phase of menstrual cycle). Arrow indicates lumen; NF, Nabothian follicle. Figure 23-32 is an enlargement of the rectangular box. H&E stain. ×9. (Courtesy of E. R. Friedrich.)

In the nonpregnant uterus the muscle cells are about 0.25 mm in length. During pregnancy, they increase in number and in size and may reach a length of 5 mm by the end of gestation, with a commensurate increase in cell thickness. New smooth muscle cells are added by differentiation from undifferentiated connective tissue cells and probably by division of preexisting smooth muscle cells. Since many of these remain after childbirth, the uterus does not revert to its virginal size. Other changes accompanying the distension of the pregnant uterus are increase in elastic tissue peripheral to the myometrium, striking growth of the blood vessels, and a thinning out of the muscle layers.

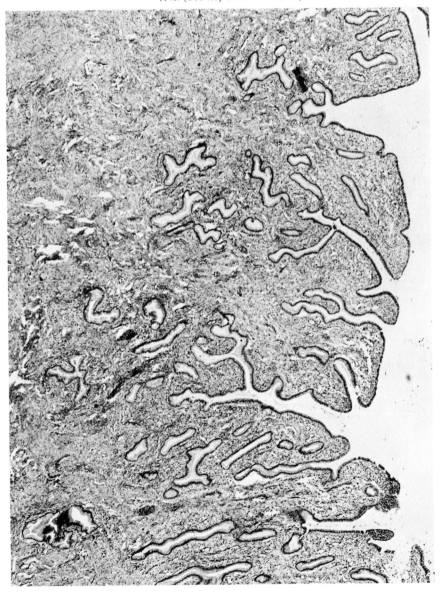

FIGURE 23-32 Enlargement of marked area in Fig. 23-31. Notice the arrangement and complex pattern of the plicae palmatae. ×40. (Courtesy of E. R. Friedrich.)

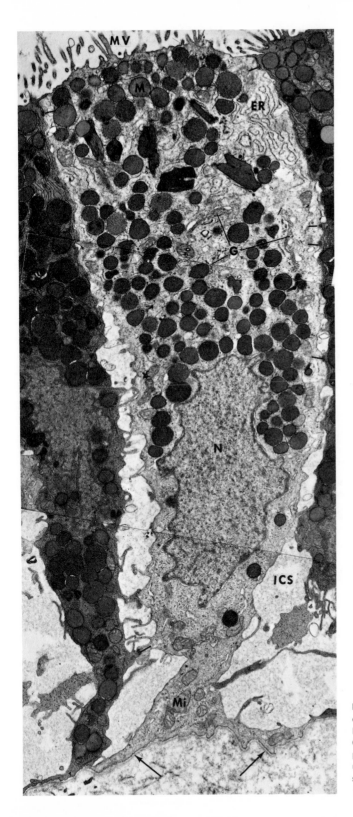

FIGURE 23-33 Electron micrograph of endocervical epithelial cells. ⟶, basement membrane; N, nucleus; G, Golgi complexes; ER, granular endoplasmic reticulum; M, mucous granules; MV, microvilli; ⟶, desmosomes; ICS, intercellular pores. ×9400. (Courtesy of E. R. Friedrich.)

Perimetrium

The pelvic peritoneum surrounding the uterine tubes and most of the uterus constitute their serosa. It extends from the sides of the uterus, forming the broad ligaments through which blood and lymph vessels and nerves reach the uterus on each side. The larger vessels are exceptionally tortuous.

Embedded in the perimetrium are the sympathetic ganglia and plexuses. The sympathetic supply to the uterus is derived from the hypogastric plexus, and the parasympathetic supply is by the way of rami from the second, third, and often the fourth sacral nerves. Large nerve trunks enter the uterus at the cervix and extend to all parts of the body and fundus. The musculature and blood vessels are abundantly supplied, and some fibers ramify in the endometrium, forming a network around the glands. Nothing is known about the significance of these fibers or what happens to them during the cyclic sloughing and regeneration of the superficial layer of the endometrium. No ganglia have been found within the wall of the uterus.

VAGINA

The vagina is a thick-walled fibromuscular tube that forms the lowermost segment of the reproductive tract and connects the uterus with the outside of the body. The wall consists of a *mucosa*, a *muscularis*, and a heavy covering of connective tissue. The lumen of the vagina is flattened anteroposteriorly. The mucosa is thrown into numerous transverse folds or *rugae* (Fig. 23-1).

FIGURE 23-34 Epithelium of human cervical glands. Cells laden with mucus. Notice the basal position of the nuclei. H&E stain. ×350. (Courtesy of E. R. Friedrich.)

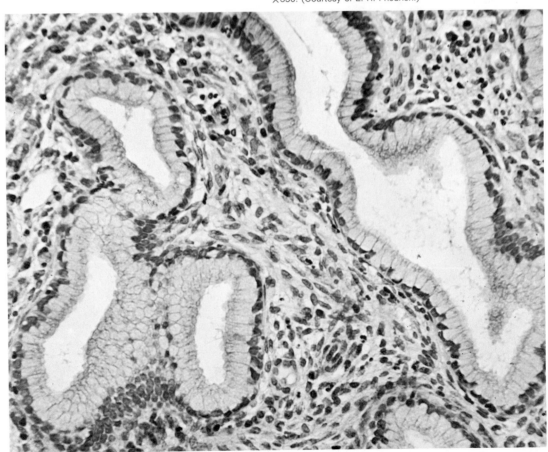

The mucous membrane consists of a stratified squamous epithelium many cell layers thick, resting on a papillated lamina propria (Fig. 23-36). Cells in the outer layers are greatly flattened and may contain keratohyaline granules, but they are not strictly cornified. At midcycle they all contain an abundance of glycogen. Some of the superficial layer of the vaginal epithelium may be shed at or near the time of menstruation (Fig. 23-37) and is referred to, in parallel with the uterine mucosa, as the *functionalis*.

The vagina is lubricated by mucus which originates from the cervix. There are no glands in the mucosa of the human vagina.

In the lamina propria subjacent to the vaginal epithelium, there is a wide band of rather dense fibrous connective tissue that is succeeded peripherally by a layer of loose connective tissue in which are

many blood vessels. Beyond this lies the muscle coat. Elastic fibers are plentiful beneath the epithelium and present sparingly elsewhere in the fibromuscular wall. Diffuse lymphoid tissue and solitary nodules (Fig. 23-36) are present occasionally in the mucous membrane. From these arise the lymphocytes which, along with granulocytes, invade the epithelium in large numbers in each menstrual cycle. The great accentuation in numbers, particularly of granulocytes before, during, and after menstruation, is apparent also in the vaginal smears.

The muscularis of the vagina is composed of an inner and an outer layer. In the outer portion there are bundles of longitudinal smooth muscle cells that are continuous with corresponding cells in the myometrium. Where the two muscle layers meet, the inner circular cells are interwoven with the outer longitudi-

FIGURE 23-35 Epithelium of human cervical glands in active secretion. Notice the change in the position of the nuclei and the secretory materials within the lumen. H&E stain. ×350. (Courtesy of E. R. Friedrich.)

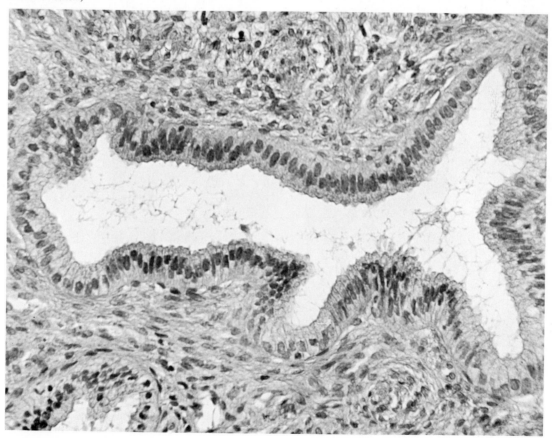

nal ones. Striated muscle cells form a sphincter around the introitus of the vagina.

The vagina has an external coat composed of a firm inner layer well supplied with elastic fibers and an

FIGURE 23-36 Photomicrograph of an oblique section through the vaginal wall of a monkey recovered a few hours after ovulation. Notice the lymph nodule (LN) in the submucosa. C is a cross section of a connective tissue core. Imagine the deep papilla at X cut in cross section.

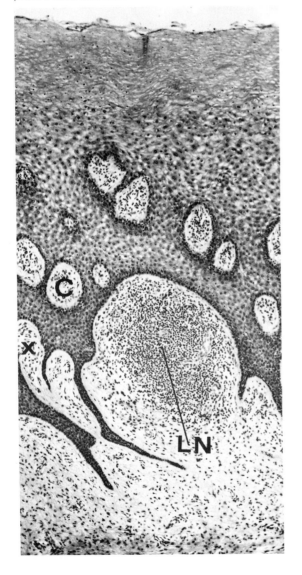

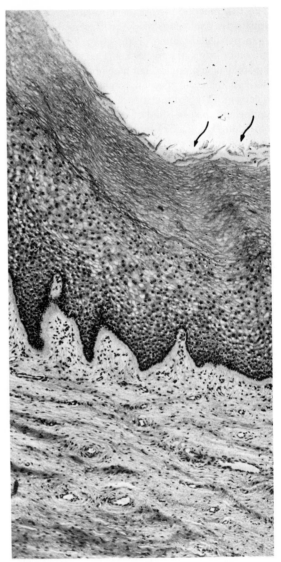

FIGURE 23-37 Photomicrograph of the vaginal mucosa in the fornix near the cervix in a monkey. Notice that the papillae are not as extensive. There is some peeling of the superficial layers (arrows) of stratified squamous epithelium. H&E stain. ×300.

outer layer of loosely arranged connective tissue which blends with that of surrounding organs.

Blood and lymphatic vessels are abundant in the wall of the vagina. The veins in the rugae are particularly numerous and large, and during sexual excitement they simulate erectile tissue. The vaginal wall receives myelinated and unmyelinated nerve fibers. The latter form a ganglionated plexus in the external fibrous coat and supply the muscularis and blood vessels. The myelinated fibers terminate in special sensory organs in the mucosa.

The surface cells of the vaginal epithelium undergo continuous desquamation and constitute the bulk of the cells seen in a vaginal smear. In subhuman primates and many lower forms, the free cells in the vagina vary in number, type, and form in a regular and predictable manner, correlating with events in the reproductive cycle. In women the vaginal epithelium varies little with the cycle, and smears are mainly useful in determining whether the vaginal mucosa is atrophic or under effective estrogen stimulation.

The glycogen stores in the superficial cells of the vaginal epithelium are fermented to lactic acid by certain acid-forming bacteria which thus influence the

pH of the vaginal fluid. The glycogen accumulation correlates with the amount of estrogen stimulation, being greatest at the time of ovulation. With diminished estrogen titer, as after ovulation, there is less glycogen formed and less broken down and so the pH of the vaginal fluid shifts toward alkalinity; this favors the development of infectious organisms such as staphylococci, *Escherichia coli,* trichomonas, and *Monilia albicans.* The ability of estrogen to reduce the vaginal pH and increase the thickness of the epithelial wall accounts for its effectiveness in the treatment of various vaginal infections that are especially common in children and postmenopaual women.

EXTERNAL SEX ORGANS (EXTERNAL GENITALIA)

These comprise the *labia majora* and *minora, clitoris,* and *vestibular glands.* The labia majora are homologous with the scrotum of the male. They are composed of skin and a thin layer of smooth muscle. In adulthood, the outer surface is covered with coarse pubic (genital) hair, with numerous sebaceous and sweat glands. The labia minora are devoid of hair, are covered by a stratified squamous epithelium, and enclose a highly papillated vascular core of loose connective tissue. Sebaceous glands, not connected with hair follicles, occur on both sides. Enhanced pigmentation is due to melanin granules in the deep strata of the epithelium.

The *clitoris* is an erectile body and is the homologue of the corpora cavernosa of the penis. It is mainly composed of two small cavernous bodies and a poorly developed *glans clitoridis.* The clitoris is covered with a thin layer of stratified squamous epithe-

lium overlying a vascular stroma with high papillae and containing many such specialized sensory nerve terminations as Meissner's corpuscles, Pacinian corpuscles, and Krause's end bulbs.

The *vestibule* is the space at the vaginal portal flanked by the labia. The epithelium differs from that of the vagina in possessing glands. The *lesser vestibular glands* secrete mucus and are situated mainly about the clitoris and urethral outlet. There is in addition a pair of *large vestibular glands* (*glands of Bartholin*), which are located in the lateral walls of the vestibule. They correspond to the bulbourethral glands of men and are similar in structure; they are the tubuloacinar type and are lined with columnar cells that produce a whitish, mucoid, lubricating fluid.

The *hymen* consists of fine-fibered vascular connective tissue covered on both sides with a mucous membrane similar to that of the vagina.

REFERENCES

BAKER, T. G., and L. L. FRANCHI: The Fine Structure of Oogonia and Oocytes in Human Ovaries, *J. Cell Sci.,* **2:**213 (1967).

BARTELMEZ, G. W.: Histological Studies on the Menstruating Mucous Membrane of the Human Uterus, *Carnegie Inst. Contrib. Embryol.,* **24:**141 (1933).

BASSETT, D. L.: The Changes in the Vascular Pattern of the Ovary of the Albino Rat during the Estrous Cycle, *Am. J. Anat.,* **73:**251 (1943).

BLACK, E.: Quantitative Morphological Investigations of Follicular System in Women, *Acta Endocrinol.,* **8:**33 (1951).

BLANDAU, R. J.: Biology of Eggs and Implantation, in W. C. Young (ed.), "Sex and Internal Secretions," 3d ed., vol. 2, chap. 14, p. 797, The Williams & Wilkins Company, Baltimore, 1961.

BLANDAU, R. J.: Ovulation in the Living Albino Rat, *Fertil. Steril.,* **6:**391 (1955).

BRENNER, R. M.: Renewal of Oviduct Cilia during the Menstrual Cycle of the Rhesus Monkey, *Fertil. Steril.,* **20:**599 (1969).

CORNER, G. W.: The Histological Dating of the Corpus Luteum of Menstruation, *Am. J. Anat.,* **98:**377 (1956).

CRISP, T. M., D. A. DESSOUKY, and F. R. DENYS: The Fine Structure of the Human Corpus Luteum of Early Pregnancy and during the Progestational Phase of the Menstrual Cycle, *Am. J. Anat.,* **127:**37 (1970).

DANFORTH, D. N.: The Fibrous Nature of the Human Cervix and Its Relation to the Isthmic Segment in Gravid and Nongravid Uteri, *Am. J. Obstet. Gynecol.,* **53:**541 (1947).

FLUHMANN, C. F.: The Glandular Structure of the Cervix Uteri, *Surg. Gynecol. Obstet.* **106:**715 (1958).

HAFEZ, E. S. E., and R. J. BLANDAU: The Mammalian Oviduct, "Comparative Biology and Methodology," The University of Chicago Press, Chicago, 1969.

HERTIG, A. T.: The Primary Human Oocyte: Some Observations on the Fine Structure of Balbiani's Vitelline Body and the Origin of the Annulate Lamellae, *Am. J. Anat.,* **122:**107 (1968).

HERTIG, A. T., and E. C. ADAMS: Studies on the Human Oocyte and Its Follicle. I. Ultrastructural and Histochemical Observations on the Primordial Follicle Stage, *J. Cell Biol.,* **34:**647 (1967).

JACOBSON, H. N., and O. NIEVES: Intrinsic Nerve Fibers of the Primate Endometrium, *Exp. Neurol.,* **4:**180 (1961).

MARKEE, J. E.: The Morphological and Endocrine Basis for Menstrual Bleeding, *Prog. Gynecol.,* **2:**63 (1950).

MARKEE, J. E.: Menstruation in Intraocular Endometrial Transplants in the Rhesus Monkey, *Carnegie Inst. Contrib. Embryol.,* **28:**220 (1940).

MORRIS, B., and M. B. SASS: The Formation of Lymph in the Ovary, *Proc. Roy. Soc. (London), Ser. B,* **164:**577 (1966).

MOSSMAN, H. W., M. J. KOERING, and D. FERRY, JR.: Cyclic Changes of Interstitial Gland Tissue of the Human Ovary, *Am. J. Anat.,* **115:**235 (1964).

ODOR, D. L.: The Temporal Relationship of the First Maturation Division of Rat Ova to the Onset of Heat, *Am. J. Anat.,* **97:**461 (1955).

PAPANICOLAOU, G. N.: The Sexual Cycle in the Human Female as Revealed by Vaginal Smears, *Am. J. Anat.,* **52:**519 (1933).

PRIBOR, H. C.: Innervation of the Uterus, *Anat. Rec.,* **109:**339 (1951).

RYAN, K. J., Z. PETERS, and J. KAISER: Steroid Formation by Isolated and Recombined Ovarian Granulosa and Thecal Cells, *J. Clin. Endocrinol. Metab.,* **28:**355 (1968).

RYAN, K. J., and R. V. SHORT: Formation of Estradiol by Granulosa and Theca Cells of the Equine Ovarian Follicle, *Endocrinology,* **76:**108 (1965).

SCHMIDT-MATTHIESEN, H.: "The Normal Human Endometrium," McGraw-Hill Book Company, New York, 1963.

STRASSMAN, E. O.: The Theca Cone and Its Tropism toward the Ovarian Surface, a Typical Feature of Growing Human and Mammalian Follicles, *Am. J. Obstet. Gynecol.,* **41:**363 (1941).

VICKERY, B. H., and J. P. BENNETT: The Cervix and Its Secretions in Mammals, *Physiol. Rev.,* **48:**135 (1968).

WITSCHI, E.: Migration of the Germ Cells of Human Embryos from the Yolk Sac to the Primitive Gonadal Folds, *Carnegie Inst., Contrib. Embryol.,* **32:**67 (1948).

The Mammary Gland

DOROTHY R. PITELKA

The mammary gland (*mamma*) is a compound tubuloalveolar gland of cutaneous origin. It is unique to the class Mammalia, and its function in infant nutrition is vital to most mammalian species. It is of extraordinary biological interest, inasmuch as its complex secretory product contains proteins, fats, and a sugar, all of which are organ-specific. Moreover, its major phases of development, function, and regression occur repeatedly in the adult female in response to a complex sequence of both internal (hormonal) and external (suckling) stimuli.

Mammae develop in pairs along embryonic *milk lines* running bilaterally from the axilla to the groin. A single pectoral pair is the rule for humans, but adventitious nipples or glands may appear elsewhere along the milk line. Each mamma consists of (1) the glandular epithelium, which is suspended in (2) subcutaneous connective tissue stroma within a more or less abundant bed of (3) adipose tissue, and (4) a *nipple,* or *teat,* where the gland's collecting ducts open to the skin surface. The epithelium is organized as a branching duct system terminating, when fully developed, in secretory *ductules* and *alveoli.* Contractile *myoepithelial cells* arranged in varying patterns surround the ductal and alveolar epithelium, within a continuous basement membrane that encloses the whole epithelial system.

GENERAL MORPHOLOGY AND HISTOLOGY OF THE ADULT GLAND

THE NIPPLE AND AREOLA

Fifteen to 20 independent excretory ducts (*lactiferous ducts, galactophores*), each leading from one of the lobes of the gland, open at the tip of the human nipple (Fig. 24-1). Packed among them are large sebaceous glands that often empty into the lactiferous ducts rather than at the surface. Keratinizing statified squamous epithelium, continuous with that of the skin, lines the outer parts of the lactiferous ducts, and horny cell debris usually plugs their openings. Among the epithelial cells of the outer parts of the lactiferous and sebaceous ducts, as well as the skin of the nipple and the surrounding *areola,* are variable numbers of dendritic melanocytes, giving these areas a darker pigmentation than the neighboring skin. Scattered over the areola are sebaceous glands, some sweat glands, and the clustered openings of *Montgomery glands,* once thought to be modified sebaceous glands but recently characterized as mammary glands equivalent in size and development to those opening on the nipple. The epidermis at the tip of the nipple is fissured and pitted externally; basally it interdigitates deeply with long dermal papillae (Fig. 24-1). The sides of the relaxed nipple are marked by circular wrinkles. Hair is absent from nipples and areola.

The dense collagenous connective tissue of the nipple and areola (Figs. 24-2 and 24-4) contains bundles of elastic fibers that fan out to attach to the

FIGURE 24-1 Galactophore opening at the tip of a human nipple. It is lined by keratinizing stratified squamous epithelium continuous with the nipple epidermis (Ep); the latter is deeply ridged externally and invaded basally by long dermal papillae (DP). The apparent bifurcation of the galactophore is probably the effect of oblique sectioning of a gently folded wall. At right are several sebaceous gland acini (SG). Hematoxylin and eosin. ×39. (Histological preparation courtesy of J. J. Elias.)

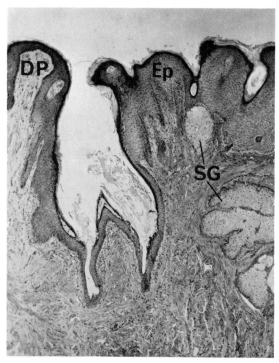

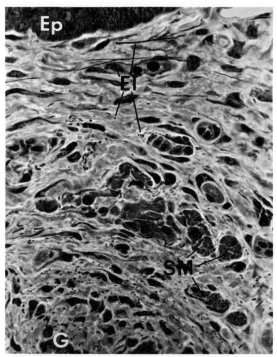

FIGURE 24-2 Connective tissue in the cross-sectioned nipple of a pregnant mouse. The basal cells of the nipple epidermis (Ep) appear at the top, and the tip of a fold in the galactophore (G) is just visible at the bottom. Elastic fibers (El) are numerous, oriented circularly near the epidermis and mainly longitudinally (seen in cross section as dense dots) elsewhere. Several smooth muscle bundles (SM) are cut in cross section. Epon embedment, Mallory's azure II-methylene blue. ×543.

overlying epidermis, particularly of the tip of the nipple. Abundant smooth muscle bundles, both radial and circular in arrangement, also attach to the overlying skin. Their contraction effects a wrinkling of the areola and erection of the nipple in response to cold, touch, or psychic stimuli.

Nipples and teats of other mammals are similar in basic structure (Fig. 24-3); erection of the nipple in many species aids the suckling young in grasping it. In ruminants, the complex of smooth muscles and elastic connective tissue may be responsible for sphincterlike closure of the teat canal, but such sphincters have not been demonstrated in the human nipple.

DUCT SYSTEM

From their openings at the tip of the human nipple (Fig. 24-1), the galactophores descend a short distance and then may branch into smaller lactiferous ducts, which

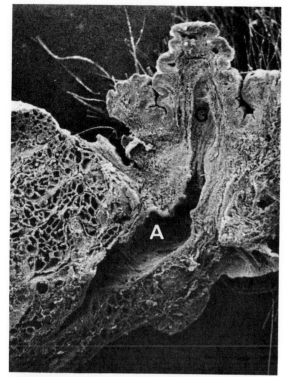

FIGURE 24-3 Nipple and adjacent tissues from a lactating mouse. The single galactophore (G), cut obliquely within the nipple, leads down into an expanded ampulla (A) below. Deep folds in the surface of the nipple allow for erection and elongation during suckling. The spongy material at the left is lobulo-alveolar tissue. Scanning electron micrograph; glutaraldehyde fixation, Freon critical-point drying. ×39. (Courtesy of M. K. Nemanic.)

radiate under the areola and expand as variably swollen ampullae, or *lactiferous sinuses* (Fig. 24-4), with folded walls. These in turn give rise to the branching smaller ducts leading ultimately in postpubertal females into the *lobules,* which are clusters of secretory alveoli.

The stratified squamous epithelium near the opening of the lactiferous duct shows a gradual transition to two approximately cuboidal layers in the lactiferous sinus. Through the remainder of the duct system, the superficial epithelial cells are columnar or cuboidal, with rather scant cytoplasm and a central, oval nucleus containing one or more nucleoli and scattered or marginal heterochromatin (Fig. 24-5). The basal layer consists of myoepithelial cells, smaller than the luminal cells and often more deeply stained, and with smaller and more contorted nuclei. They form a virtually continuous circumferential stratum in major duct

branches. The cells are spindle-shaped, oriented with the long axis of the duct, and frequently longitudinally ridged, giving the duct a characteristically serrated peripheral contour in cross or oblique section (Fig. 24-5).

As the duct system extends distally and its branches become smaller, the investment of myoepithelial cells becomes discontinuous and the cells begin to assume a stellate form, with long processes extending from a central perinuclear zone to form an open basket around the duct wall. The epithelial cells of distal ducts during pregnancy and lactation often enlarge and become slightly to fully secretory (Fig.

FIGURE 24-4 Lactiferous sinus under the areola of a woman in the eighth month of pregnancy. The wall of the sinus is wrinkled and folded. Around the deeply stained epithelium of the sinus is a layer of relatively cellular connective tissue. In the more peripheral, densely fibrous connective tissue are empty blood vessels and, at the left, some of the smooth muscle bundles (SM) that run under the skin of the areola. Hematoxylin and eosin. ×39. (Histological preparation courtesy of J. J. Elias.)

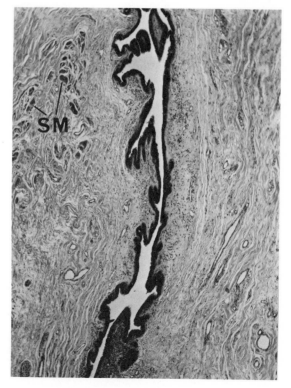

24-6); even in major ducts, occasional patches of secretory cells may appear.

ALVEOLI

The secretory unit of the mammary gland is the lobule. It consists of a cluster of alveoli around the single small duct that drains it and from which it originated (Fig. 24-7). Alveoli develop during pregnancy (or to a lesser and variable degree during postovulatory phases of the menstrual or estrous cycle) as blunt tubular or spherical outgrowths from the side or end of the duct. Their arrangement in lobular units is clearest when the gland is not fully developed (Figs. 24-7 and 24-8).

The alveolar wall is a single layer of epithelial cells, embraced by a loose network of myoepithelial cells with their long, slender processes. Until specific hormonal stimulation at some stage of pregnancy induces secretory differentiation, the epithelial cells resemble those of ducts. Upon stimulation, cytoplasmic volume increases and evidence of secretion becomes visible histologically in the form of vesicles in the cytoplasm and fat droplets in cells and lumen (Fig. 24-9). The extent of lobular differentiation at any given stage prior to or during pregnancy may vary widely within a single gland (Figs. 24-8 and 24-9) as well as among individuals and species.

FIGURE 24-5 Major duct from an adult virgin mouse; the lumen is at the top, connective tissue sheath (CT) below. Beneath the superficial epithelial layer (Ep) are myoepithelial cells (My), with smaller, more distorted, darkly stained nuclei; the basal surface of the myoepithelial layer is characteristically serrated. Epon embedment, Paragon stain. ×679.

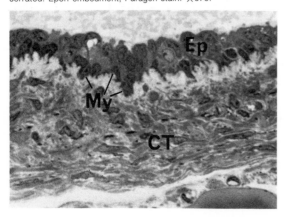

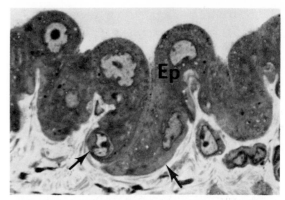

FIGURE 24-6 Distal duct from a lactating mouse. The lumen is at the top; connective tissue is at bottom. The folded wall consists of a discontinuous myoepithelial layer (arrows) and epithelial cells (Ep) that are much larger than those in major ducts. Epithelial nuclei are not noticeably different from those in Fig. 24-5, but the more abundant cytoplasm contains scattered, clear vesicles suggesting modest secretory activity. Epon embedment, Mallory's azure II-methylene blue. ×1261.

If nursing takes place, full secretory development is reached some days after parturition. In a lactating gland, alveoli are distorted by close packing and by the partial fusion of neighbors (Figs. 24-10 and 24-11); thus alveoli may drain into other alveoli within the lobule. Furthermore, cells of the terminal branches of the intralobular duct typically are fully secretory, so that these ductules are identifiable as drainage pathways only if one can follow their course for some distance (Fig. 24-10). The lactating lobule in histological section therefore has a spongy appearance, as of many irregular, intercomunicating chambers. Adjacent lobules in lactation are also close-packed, their limits indicated in section only by the connective tissue septa that bound them. When lactation ceases, lobules decrease greatly in size and many of them regress partially or completely, leaving a resting gland that again is predominantly ductal.

STROMA

Connective tissue of the mamma is basically of two types: variously dense, fibrous connective tissue enclosing the ducts and lobules and supporting the breast in its subcutaneous position; and loose, cellular connective tissue surrounding the ductules and alveoli within each lobule.

The dense, collagenous tissue of the nipple and the interlobar and interlobular septa in the adult gland

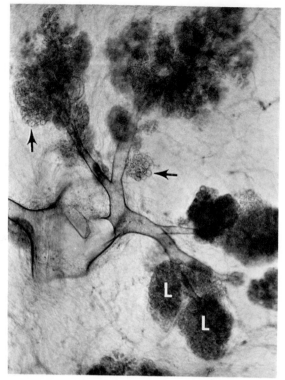

FIGURE 24-7 Persisting lobules in the resting gland of a 25-year-old woman who had had one child. A single terminal branch from a small duct enters each lobule (L). Bubblelike alveoli (arrows) can be distinguished at the edges of some lobules. 2-mm section in methylsalicylate, hematoxylin. ×20. (Courtesy of H. M. Jensen and S. R. Wellings.)

contains occasional elastic fiber bundles (becoming more abundant with age) and relatively few fibroblasts (Figs. 24-2, 24-4, and 24-8). In addition to the glandular parenchyma, it encloses blood and lymph vessels, nerves, and occasional histiocytes and mast cells. Peripherally, the septa merge with fibrous fascia that suspend the human breast from the sternum and pectoral muscle fascia and that connect via mammary ligaments with the overlying dermis. Within the supporting septa, each major lactiferous duct is surrounded by a sheath of concentrically layered fibroblasts, collagenous fiber bundles, and frequent elastic fibers (Figs. 24-2, 24-5, and 24-12). At the internal limit of the fibrous sheath, the basement membrane is a narrow, cell-free zone that contains the basal lamina of the epithelium and many collagenous fibers (Fig. 24-12). The sheath diminishes in thickness, density, and elastic fiber content as the duct divides into successively smaller branches.

Within lobules, frequent fibroblasts and abundant capillaries are enclosed in a loose collagenous network. At certain times associated with stages of menstrual or lactational cycles, lymphocytes, plasma cells, or macrophages may be present in large numbers.

Lobules of adipose tissue are also enclosed in the supporting stroma in most species, forming a special mammary fat pad. In rodents, the septa are relatively thin, and fat lobules interdigitate abundantly with lobules of glandular tissue; in bovine and human mammae, connective tissue is more abundant and separates most fat-cell tracts from epithelial lobules.

FIGURE 24-8 Relatively undifferentiated area of a human breast at 8 months of gestation. At the left is part of a lobe of adipose tissue (Ad); the edge of a cross-sectioned artery (Ar) is at the top right. Below it is a branching duct (D). Elsewhere are sections of smaller ducts and developing lobules (L). Thin-walled veins, lymph vessels, and arterioles are scattered throughout the abundant fibrous connective tissue. Immediately adjacent to ducts and within lobules, the connective tissue is more cellular, and the many nuclei at this low magnification create a densely stippled effect. Hematoxylin and eosin. ×34.

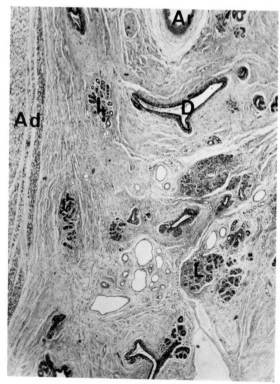

The mammary connective tissue increases in amount as ducts and blood vessels extend during pregnancy, but within lobules it appears to become attentuated as expanding alveoli, filling all available space, displace the stromal elements. Adipose cells may be progressively depleted of their fat stores in late pregnancy and lactation. They generally do not disappear even if fully depleted (Fig. 24-15) and can accumulate fat again after lactation ends.

CIRCULATION AND INNERVATION

The mamma is a skin gland, and its blood vessels and nerves are those of the skin where the gland is located. The human breast is supplied by the intercostal, lateral thoracic, and internal mammary (branch of the sub-

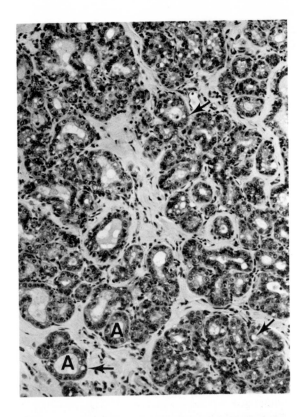

FIGURE 24-9 Another area of the same prelactating human gland as Fig. 24-8. Lobules here are well developed; and some of the alveoli (A) (or ductules—the two are not distinguishable) are enlarged; secreted material, including spherical residues of extracted fat droplets, fills the lumina, and some cells contain clear fat vacuoles (arrows). Hematoxylin and eosin. ×136. (Histological preparations for Figs. 24-8 and 24-9 courtesy of J. J. Elias.)

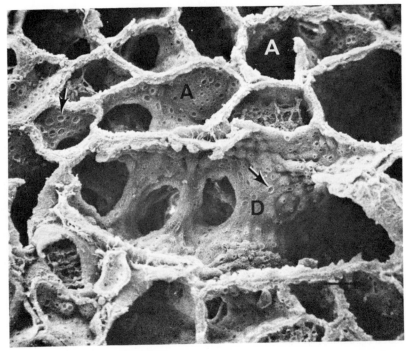

FIGURE 24-10 Mammary gland of a lactating mouse. In this scanning electron micrograph, close-packed alveoli (A) washed almost free of milk surround a small secreting ductule (D) with several openings. Secreting epithelium is distinguished by the flat craters (arrows) left by fat globules extracted during processing. Glutaraldehyde fixation, Freon critical-point drying. ×220. (From M. K. Nemanic and D. R. Pitelka, *J. Cell Biol.,* **48:**410, 1971.)

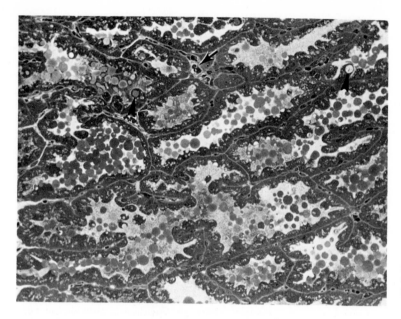

FIGURE 24-11 Mammary gland of a lactating mouse comparable to that in Fig. 24-10. Alveolar lumina contain spherical fat globules and finer particulate material. Within the cells are clusters of tiny, clear Golgi vesicles and some larger, round fat globules (arrowheads). The small blood vessels (for example, see arrow at top) and abundant capillaries between alveoli are identifiable by the presence of darkly stained erythrocytes. Epon embedment, Mallory's azure II-methylene blue. ×204.

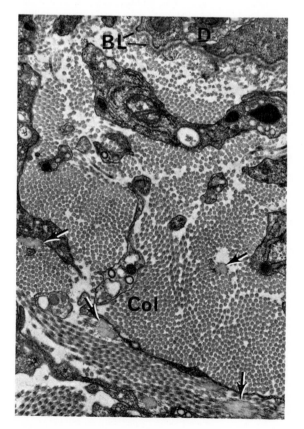

FIGURE 24-12 Connective tissue adjacent to a major lactiferous duct (D) of a midpregnant mouse. Most of the field is filled with large bundles of collagenous fibrils (Col); dispersed among them are several elastic fibers (arrows) and numerous fibroblast cell processes of various sizes. Close to the duct, the collagenous fibrils are more loosely and irregularly arrayed. Some of them appear to make contact with the basal lamina (BL). Electron micrograph. ×13,440.

clavian) blood vessels. The developing duct system, growing from the nipple within the connective tissue septa of the subcutaneous mammary fat pad, adopts the existing vascular system of the stroma, with the result that the mammary ducts and the blood vessels have different branching patterns. Thus, the same arterial supply serves the mammary gland and the overlying skin. Duct epithelium is separated from its blood supply by the thickness of its fibrous sheath, whereas growing end buds and secretory alveoli are more closely invested by capillary plexuses (Fig. 24-11).

Lymph flow from the lactating gland is high. Lymph capillaries are not present within the lobules, but fine lymph vessels surround them. Large lymphatics are frequent in the connective tissue septa; in the human, these lead mainly to the axillary lymph nodes.

Innervation of the mamma includes somatic sensory and sympathetic motor fibers. In the human breast, nonencapsulated, single or branching sensory end organs are numerous around the galactophores and in the dermis at the tip of the nipple; smaller numbers are associated with Montgomery galactophores on the areola. Such receptors in experimental animals are known during suckling to trigger the neuroendocrine reflex discharge of hormones responsible for milk ejection and for the maintenance of lactation. Histological evidence for sensory endings elsewhere in the gland is equivocal. However, receptors sensitive to intramammary pressure do exist; afferent discharges in mammary nerves of rabbits have been recorded after experimental increase in ductal fluid pressure.

The smooth muscles of the teat or nipple and areola are liberally innervated by sympathetic fibers, as are arteries and arterioles throughout the gland. In the species investigated, the rate of mammary blood flow is under nervous as well as hormonal control and is very labile. It increases sharply at parturition and remains remarkably stable from day to day during lactation under normal conditions but is readily diminished by stress. The consensus of recent investigators is that mammary myoepithelial and epithelial elements are not innervated.

THE CYTOLOGY OF SECRETION

To appreciate the special properties of the mammary gland's organization and ultrastructure, some familiarity with the nature of milk is necessary. The whole biological function of the gland is to provide, only at the proper time, a fluid that will meet all of the nutritional needs of the newborn young. The composition of milk is basically similar in all mammals; hence, it is not surprising that the internal structure of the gland differs very little among them.

MILK

Milk is a watery solution, or suspension, of proteins, lipids, carbohydrates, vitamins, salts, immunoglobulins, and a large number of other substances in small quantities. The predominant proteins, lipids, and carbohydrate are synthesized by the mammary epithelium and are unique to it; other components are synthesized there or are selectively transferred from the blood. The three major specific proteins are the abundant, nutritionally important caseins; α-lactalbumin, nutritional and also essential for lactose synthesis; and (at least in ruminants) β-lactoglobulin, the significance (other than nutritional) of which is unknown. Caseins are released from secreting cells mainly as micellar particles; the other two are released in solution. The major milk fats are neutral triglycerides. They are characterized by a higher proportion of short- and medium-chain and unsaturated fatty acids and a higher degree of molecular asymmetry than are found in other body fats; this composition causes the fats to remain liquid and mobile at body temperature. They are secreted as droplets surrounded by a coat that prevents coalescence. The disaccharide lactose, composed of glucose and galactose, is the major carbohydrate of most milks; it is released in solution. Certain classes of immunoglobulins are present in milk in varying amounts and in proportions differing from those in blood plasma. The intestinal epithelium in the newborn of many species—but not the human—can transfer some of these antibodies intact to the circulation. Unabsorbed immunoglobulins, especially IgA, serve an antimicrobial protective function in the infant's gut.

Milk is isosmolar with blood plasma. Since lactose is so abundant in milk as to be its major osmole, the transfer of osmotically active components from blood must be selectively controlled. Levels of Na, K, and Cl differ in the two fluids, and appear in milks of different species to be inversely related to lactose content. Calcium and phosphates, of great nutritional importance, are present in solution but are secreted in much larger quantities insolubly complexed with casein micelles. One or more iron-binding proteins are present in most milks, but the iron content is variable.

Caseins and several other milk proteins exhibit species-specific variations in composition; milk fats have characteristic species patterns of fatty acid composition and arrangement. Some species have little or no lactose, and a few have other oligosaccharides. Further species differences include variations in relative proportions. For example (Jenness), human milk is approximately 88 percent water, 4 percent fat, 1 percent protein, and 7 percent lactose; cow's milk has similar water and fat content but 3 percent protein and 5 percent lactose; and fur seal milk is 35 percent water, 53 percent fat, and 9 percent protein, with virtually no lactose. Some differences can be reasonably related to ecological considerations, state of development of the young at birth, or characteristic frequency of nursing, but others have no obvious explanation.

ALVEOLAR CELLS AND THE FORMATION OF MILK

Surface Characters

Like other active transporting epithelia, lactating mammary epithelium consists of a sheet of firmly joined, strongly asymmetric cells (Figs. 24-13, 24-14, and 24-18). Apical cell surfaces, facing the central lumen where milk is deposited, bear irregularly distributed microvilli, which tend to be longer and more numerous along cell borders than elsewhere. These borders are joined to one another laterally in a continuous mosaic. Below this zone of tight contact, contiguous lateral cell surfaces show varying contours: for part of their course, they are closely parallel and gently undulating; elsewhere they extend long, contorted cytoplasmic processes into intercellular spaces, or the

spaces may be closed and the processes compressed into interdigitating folds. The basal cell membrane is thrown intermittently into series of extensions and infoldings (Figs. 24-14, 24-15, and 24-18). This clearly increases the basal cell surface, although much less so than is the case in such water-transporting epithelia as the kidney proximal tubule. Evidence of pinocytosis at this surface is seen in the form of vesicles of various sizes in the subjacent cytoplasm and occasional membrane invaginations suggesting vesicle formation.

Inserted between the bases of epithelial cells are myoepithelial cell bodies or their slender processes (Figs. 24-14, 24-18, and 24-19); the latter can be seen indenting the basal surface of nearly every secretory cell. Myoepithelial membranes are studded with clusters of tiny, open plasmalemmal vesicles, similar to those characteristic of smooth muscle cells. Externally, a distinct, continuous basal lamina is present.

The structure that maintains continuous close contact of luminal cell borders is a tight-junction belt, or occluding zone (Figs. 24-14, 24-16, and 24-18), encircling every cell. Desmosomes are abundant in

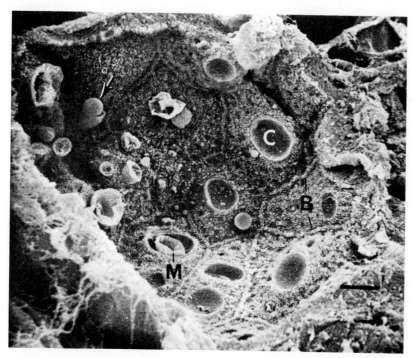

FIGURE 24-13 Luminal surface of an alveolus. The polygonal cell surfaces are thickly dotted with microvilli, and distinct rows of close-set microvilli mark the cell borders (B). Large, flat, empty craters (C) are left by extraction of large superficial fat droplets; in some instances the collapsed membrane envelope (M) remains; and in one case (arrow), a preserved fat globule still lies partly within the ruptured membrane. Scanning electron micrograph; glutaraldehyde fixation, Freon critical-point drying. ×1250. (From M. K. Nemanic and D. R. Pitelka, *J. Cell Biol.*, **48**:410, 1971.)

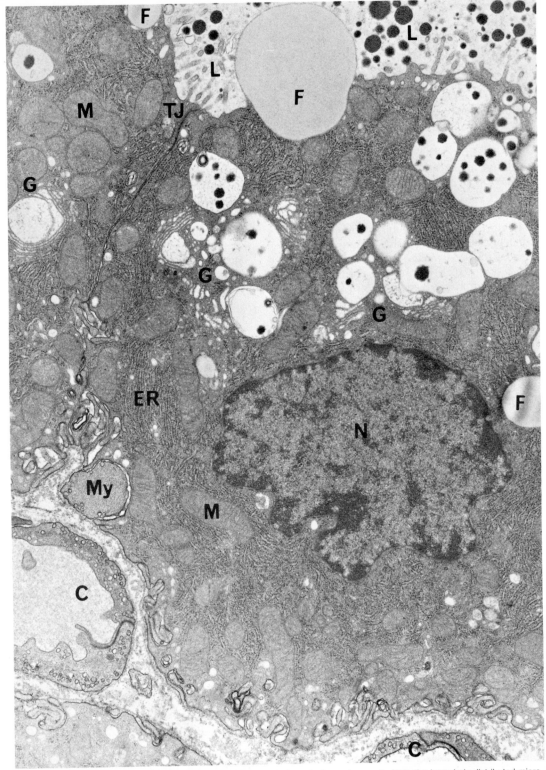

FIGURE 24-14 Typical mammary alveolar cells from a mouse at full lactation; electron micrograph. Note the irregularly distributed micro-villi on the luminal surface and the membrane convolutions at the basal surface. Very dense, round bodies in the lumen and secretory vacuoles are casein micelles. C, capillary; ER, rough endoplasmic reticulum; F, fat globule; G. Golgi complex; L, lumen; M, mitochon-drion; My, myoepithelial cell process; N, nucleus; TJ, tight junction. ×13,000.

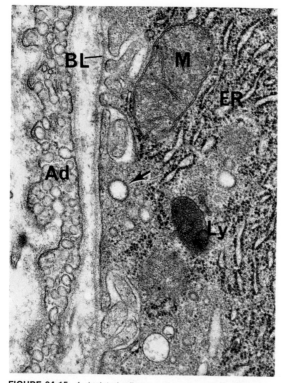

major ducts at all times and in alveoli during development, but there are few or none in lactating cells. Hence, the tight junctions here are essential to provide mechanical adhesion as well as to limit transepithelial permeability. As in other transporting epithelia, the occluding zone provides a permeability barrier by restricting diffusion of substances across the epithelium through intercellular spaces. Electron-opaque tracers such as lanthanum nitrate are unable to diffuse past it. More significantly, lactating mammary epithelium is impermeable to exogenous lactose and citrate, as well as to extracellular markers like sucrose and insulin. Although direct measurements are not available, its physiological and morphological properties are those of a relatively impermeable epithelium.

Gap junctions, thought to be the sites of direct transfer of ions and small molecules between cells in contact, are present rather frequently in or near the occluding zone and erratically elsewhere in mammary epithelium, linking epithelial and myoepithelial cells in all combinations.

FIGURE 24-15 A depleted adipose cell process (Ad), with contorted surface and abundant plasmalemmal vesicles crowding the visible cytoplasm, lies next to the base of an alveolar epithelial cell in a lactating mouse. A distinct basal lamina (BL) extends smoothly over the membrane convolutions of the alveolar cell; a less distinct lamina coats the fat-cell surface. Assorted vesicles are present in the alveolar cell; one (arrow) bears on its cytoplasmic surface a coat of short bristles often seen on pinocytic vesicles. M, mitochondrion; ER, cisternae of rough ER containing fine particulate material; Ly, probable lysosome. Electron micrograph. ×30,880.

FIGURE 24-16 Freeze-fracture replica of the occluding junction in lactating mouse mammary gland. Electron micrograph. Between the particle-studded lateral cell membrane, extending across the top of the picture, and the microvilli protruding into the lumen at the bottom is the network of gently undulating ridges and grooves. Meshes in the network are spindle-shaped next to the lumen and rounded abluminally. The number of ridges in any one transect of the band averages six to eight in lactating cells. At Cy, the fracture plane has left the membrane and passed through a projecting lip of cytoplasm. ×48,720. (From D. R., Pitelka et al., *J. Cell Biol.*, **56**:797, 1973.)

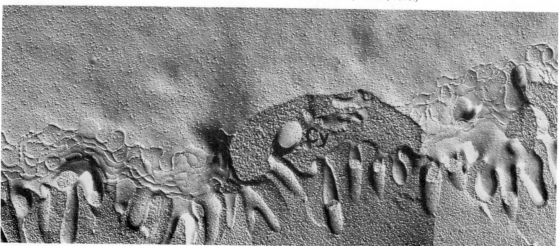

Cytoplasmic Structure and Function

The general architecture of the secreting mammary cell is that of any protein-synthesizing exocrine cell. It is dominated by flattened cisternae of rough endoplasmic reticulum (ER) filling most of the cytoplasm and by many Golgi complexes lateral and apical to the nucleus (Figs. 24-14 and 24-18). The Golgi region (Fig. 24-17) contains abundant microvesicles in addition to flattened proximal and inflated distal cisternae; the latter ultimately leave the Golgi complex and migrate to the surface as secretory vacuoles. Near the cell base are small, membrane-limited bodies with a dense matrix that presumably are lysosomes (Fig. 24-15). Activity of several lysosomal enzymes has been demonstrated biochemically and cytochemically in lactating cells. More complex lysosomal derivatives, apparently autophagic, are occasionally seen. Rod-shaped mitochondria are distributed through the cytoplasm and may be particularly abundant near the basal

cell surface (Fig. 24-14). Fat globules of various sizes are present in the cytoplasm of most cells, sometimes reaching 10 μm in diameter at the apical surface. In the dense cytoplasmic matrix are scattered microtubules, most frequent in the Golgi region, and filaments in small bundles or forming a mat of variable thickness beneath surface membranes. Smooth-membraned vesicles other than those of the Golgi complex are present chiefly near cell surfaces; there is no conspicuous smooth ER.

Caseins, α-lactalbumin, and other proteins synthesized on the ribosomes of the rough ER pass into the lumina of its cisternae, which become filled with fine particulate material of moderate electron density (Figs. 24-15 and 24-17). The transfer of this material to the Golgi complex is probably by migration of microvesicles, but this has not been demonstrated. Dispersed particles appear in the proximal, flat. Golgi cisternae and accumulate in inflated distal sacs. Con-

FIGURE 24-17 Golgi region of a lactating cell, showing abundant microvesicles (V) and a series of increasingly inflated Golgi cisternae (GC) containing dense particulate material or condensing granules. The cisternae of rough ER are filled with fine particulate material. Electron micrograph. $\times$40,600.

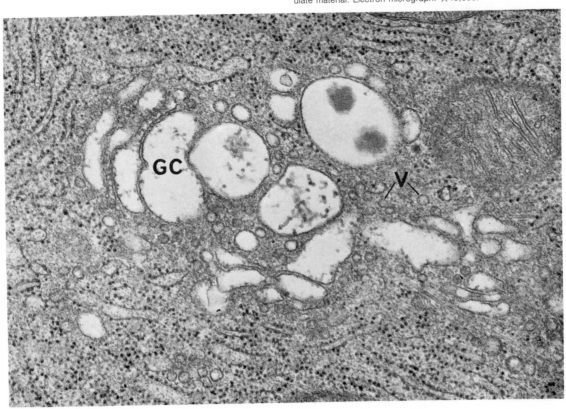

densation of most casein protein into dense micelles occurs here or during migration of the secretory vacuole to the cell surface. The micelles have a highly characteristic granular substructure and diameters up to 300 nm or more; a typical inflated vesicle encloses several of them (Fig. 24-14). The noncasein whey proteins, including α-lactalbumin, remain dissolved in the fluid filling the vesicle. Secretory vesicles reaching the apical plasmalemma fuse with it and release their contents to the lumen in a conventional exocytic process.

Milk fats contain, in various proportions, dietary fatty acids (mainly long-chain) from the blood and fatty acids (C4–C16) synthesized in mammary cells. Triglyceride synthesis occurs in the regions of the cell occupied by ER, where bound and free ribosomes are abundant, and at least some of the requisite enzymes are bound to ER membranes. Fat droplets appear in the cytoplasmic matrix, without any enclosing membrane. Increase in size occurs by accretion or fusion as the globule moves to the cell surface, where, by a mechanism not fully understood, it is extruded into the lumen (Fig. 24-14). The plasmalemma is carried out with it and pinches off behind it, enclosing it in a membrane envelope. In some instances, secretory vacuoles collect around the globule and may contribute their membranes to it directly during the pinching off. Fragments of cytoplasm are sometimes included within the envelope. Fat secretion thus contributes to the milk not only lipids and fat-soluble vitamins but membrane phospholipids, cholesterol, glycoproteins, and enzymes, plus cytoplasmic constituents in small amounts.

The discharge of bits of cytoplasm into the milk is a form of apocrine secretion. More extensive loss of apical cytoplasm or sloughing of whole cells may occur in late pregnancy or after weaning, and may be induced by mechanical milking, but has not been shown to occur on a large scale during normal lactation and suckling.

Lactose synthesis requires two proteins. One of these is a common galactosyl transferase in the Golgi membranes of many cell types; its usual function is to transfer galactose from UDP galactose to N-acetylglucosamine in the formation of glycoproteins. In the presence of the second protein, α-lactalbumin, the specificity of the galactosyl transferase activity changes so that glucose in low concentrations can serve as the galactose acceptor. Present evidence suggests that, since cytoplasmic membranes are impermeable to disaccharides, lactose draws water osmotically into the distal Golgi sacs—already containing casein—and they

swell. The result is that most of the volume of the secretory vacuole is occupied by fluid, in which the lactose, whey proteins, and other substances are dissolved.

Of the serum immunoglobulins, IgG is most abundant in the milk of species whose young can acquire passive immunity by absorbing it. Human infants obtain IgG by placental transfer before birth, and IgA is the major immunoglobulin in human milk. The mechanism by which mammary cells select immunoglobulin species from among those in the circulating blood or released by locally concentrated plasma cells is not known, nor is the means by which they are transported through the cells. Specific receptors on the basolateral membranes and transcellular transport via endocytic vesicles are likely possibilities. Secretory IgA is released into the milk (and other external secretions) as a dimer to which a component has been added during transit by the epithelial cells, the complex being more resistant than serum IgA to proteolysis and pH changes.

Membrane flux in the lactating cell is extensive and differs significantly from that in most secreting cells. Membrane is added as usual to the apical surface by exocytosis of secretory vesicles; in mammary cells, membrane is also extruded from the apical surface as fat globule envelopes. Whereas disassembly or recycling of excess surface membrane is necessary in other cells, totally new membrane constitutents must continually be synthesized by mammary cells to replace all of the membrane secreted with milk fat. Biochemical evidence for origin of apical surface membrane via the ER-Golgi system is particularly good in the case of mammary cells, where it has been drawn from comparisons of purified fat globule membrane with internal cytomembrane fractions (Keenan et al.).

Lactating tissue samples invariably include cells, or whole alveoli, that differ from the typical appearance; common variants include "light" cells with low matrix density, cells with inflated ER, and cells with little evidence of protein or fat synthesis. Some authors have attributed these to phased secretory cycles in individual or groups of cells, or to spontaneous cell degradation. Assessment of these possibilities is extremely difficult, however, because lactating tissue is particularly fragile and sensitive to mechanical, osmotic, or other damage. Always present are some preparative artifacts that may account for many morphological variants.

THE CYTOLOGY OF MILK EXCRETION

Milk secretion by lobuloalveolar tissue of the lactating mammary gland is slow but continuous. Suckling is intermittent, occurring only once a day in some species. In the intervals, milk accumulates, gradually inflating the alveolar lumina and seeping into the available ducts. The nursing infant, by its own action, can remove only that part of the milk lying in the ducts or sinuses near the nipple. The bulk of the milk in the ductal and alveolar lumina must be moved out into the larger ducts during nursing by contraction of myoepithelial cells. Milk excretion thus requires the myoepithelial network to eject milk from the blind terminal chambers of the gland and the ducts to contain it and channel it to the nipple.

MYOEPITHELIUM

Myoepithelial cells are distinguished by their basal position (they never abut on the lumen), their abun-

dant plasmalemmal vesicles, and their content of tracts of actinlike, parallel filaments 5 to 6 nm in diameter (Fig. 24-19). These tracts occupy the long cell processes of the alveolar myoepithelium (Figs. 24-14 and 24-18) and most of the basal cytoplasm, including the ridges, of ductal myoepithelium (Fig. 24-21). Irregularly distributed in islands within or around the filament tracts are cisternae of rough or smooth ER, small mitochondria, and ribosomes. Some filaments appear to insert in dense plaques under the cell membrane, and at these sites there often are hemidesmosomes (inset, Fig. 24-19) or simpler fibrillar connections to the basal lamina (Fig.

FIGURE 24-18 Schematic drawing of alveolar cells in a lactating mammary gland. Microvilli, concentrated along the cell borders, are shown in three-dimensional view on the apical surfaces. At the base of the cells, the basal lamina is indicated extending forward, with a branching myoepithelial cell process lying on it. Organelles are not drawn to scale.

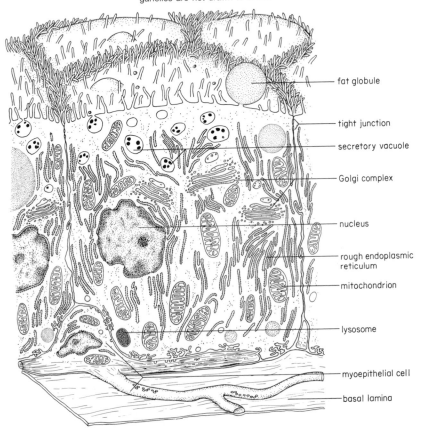

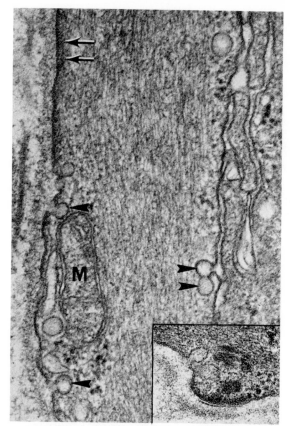

FIGURE 24-19 Myoepithelial cell process lying next to an alveolar cell on the right. Electron micrograph. At both edges of the myoepithelial process are plasmalemmal vesicles (arrowheads), most of them clearly open to the surface. Ribosomes and a mitochondrion (M) lie in islands in a cytoplasm otherwise occupied by parallel filaments. Under the cell membrane at upper left is a dense plaque (arrows); the space between the cell membrane and the basal lamina over this area is filled with filamentous material. ×60,000. Inset. A well-developed hemidesmosome at the surface of a differentiating myoepithelial cell from a 3-week-old mouse (same duct seen in Fig. 14-23). A typical hemidesmosome consists of a thin, dense plate outside the plasma membrane, filamentous material between it and the basal lamina, a dense plaque on the cytoplasmic side of the membrane, and two or three dense nodes associated with cytoplasmic filament tracts. Electron micrograph. ×62,080.

24-19). Nodes of a density similar to the plaques are scattered within the larger filament bundles. In ducts, the myoepithelial cells are attached to one another and to epithelial cells by desmosomes. In lactating alveoli, occasional gap junctions appear to be the only specialized junctions.

Myoepithelial contraction occurs in response to the hormone oxytocin in the milk-ejection reflex. Sensory stimuli from receptors in the nipple, or stimuli of sight and sound associated by conditioning with nursing, are conveyed to the hypothalamus, triggering release of oxytocin from the neurohypophysis into the blood. Myoepithelial contraction can be induced experimentally by oxytocin applied topically or injected, by mechanical or electrical stimuli, and by a variety of physiological and pharmacological agents known to induce contraction of smooth muscle. Contraction of myoepithelial cell processes embracing the alveoli and secretory ductules compresses their lumina, expressing the milk into the ducts. The contraction is accompanied or rapidly followed by a marked change in epithelial cell shape, from cuboidal or even squamus in engorged alevoli to pseudocolumnar, with the apical surface bulging far into the alveolar lumen (Fig. 24-20). The effects of contraction on duct shape are less clear. Milk inevitably drains from major ducts during tissue dissection; hence ducts in histological samples are usually empty and their walls folded. Ducts in milk-filled glands of living mice shorten and widen after oxytocin application. This increase in cross-sectional area could decrease resistance to milk flow, so that milk forced out of alveoli can continue down the ductal tree. Any significant increase in total ductal volume probably results from flattening of folds in the walls.

In the human and some other mammals without large gland cisterns, oxytocin release occurs in waves, evoking repeated myoepithelial response over a protracted suckling period.

DUCTS

The epithelial lining of major ducts consists of cells of unremarkable structure, showing little change during pregnancy and lactation. Both cells and nuclei often have convoluted surfaces; interdigitating processes between neighboring cells are abundant (Fig. 24-21). Apical surfaces bear microvilli that often are shorter than those of secretory cells. Prominent junctional complexes (Fig. 24-22), consisting of occluding junctions, intermediate junctions, and desmosomes, link epithelial cells at their apical borders; desmosomes and gap junctions are variably frequent elsewhere.

Cytoplasmic organelles—mitochondria, Golgi complexes, and rough ER—are sparse. Only filaments of various diameters appear more frequently than in secretory cells. The structure of the major ducts is thus

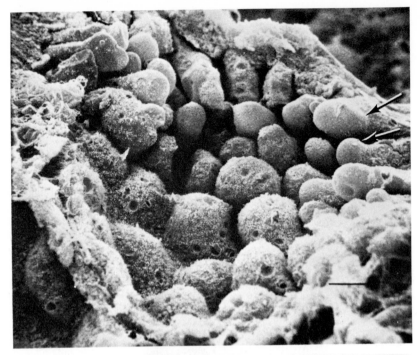

FIGURE 24-20 Luminal surface of a contracted alveolus in a lactating mouse mammary gland. Scanning electron micrograph. Most of the cells bulge deeply into the lumen. Apical membranes are covered with microvilli and fat craters except where large subsurface fat droplets occupy the apical bulge; here the membranes become smooth (arrows). Compare the cell shapes here and in the more inflated alveoli in Figs. 24-10 and 24-13. Glutaraldehyde fixation, Freon critical-point drying. ×1250. (From D. R. Pitelka et al., *J. Cell Biol.,* **56:**797, 1973.)

FIGURE 24-21 Major lactiferous duct from a lactating mouse. As compared with secretory alveolar cells, ductal epithelial cells have a small cytoplasmic volume. They bear typical microvilli on their apical surfaces and many irregular processes extending from their lateral and basal surfaces (arrows) and interdigitating with those of adjacent epithelial and myoepithelial cells. In the myoepithelial cell (My) layer, cell bodies occupy angular basal protrusions and in addition have peripheral ridges and valleys, with the result that the duct profile in cross section appears serrated at both low and high magnification. Nuclei of both epithelial and myoepithelial cells have irregular contours. Electron micrograph. ×7275.

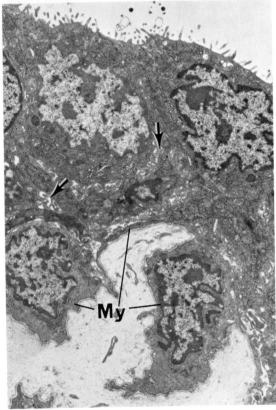

consistent with their function as conduits and storage spaces, mechanical integrity and flexibility being the most important requirements. There is no evidence that the mammary ducts are capable of selective reabsorption of any constituent of the secreted fluid, as are those of some other exocrine glands.

In the lactating gland, gradations in a number of characteristics associated with secretion appear between the typical major duct cells at one extreme and the fully developed ductular and alveolar cells at the other. Increasing prominence of the synthetic and secretory organelles, decrease and disappearance of desmosomes, progressive development of the basal membrane convolutions in epithelial cells, increasing discontinuity of the myoepithelial layer, and thinning of the connective tissue sheath are evident, but not all in parallel, as the ducts approach their intralobular endings.

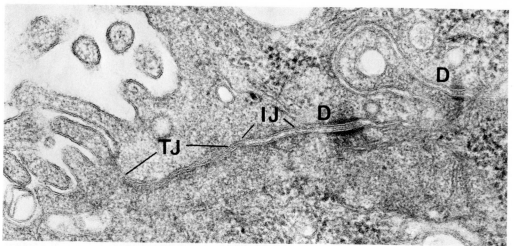

FIGURE 24-22 Junctional complex linking cells in a major mammary duct from a lactating mouse. Electron micrograph. The outer leaflets of the cell membranes are fused at several points in the tight junction (TJ). Next to this are a poorly developed adhering, or intermediate, junction (IJ), a distinct desmosome (D), and farther along the interdigitating membranes, a smaller desmosome. A meshwork of filaments occupies the cytoplasm adjacent to the junctional zone in the cell at the bottom. ×64,000.

MAMMARY DEVELOPMENT AND ITS HORMONAL CONTROL

MORPHOGENESIS AND CYCLIC DIFFERENTIATION

The human embryonic milk line, a low ectodermal ridge extending from forelimb to hind limb in the 9-mm embryo, regresses caudally but thickens in the thorax to form a solid epithelial bud by the end of the second month. Relatively little development occurs in the next 3 months. A 13-week anlage examined with the electron microscope by Salazar and Tobon consisted of a solid mass of undifferentiated epithelial cells, beginning to form small branches in the upper dermal mesenchyme. The cells ultrastructurally resembled those of the neighboring epidermis. During the second trimester of gestation, continued proliferation and branching produce the 15 to 20 major duct rudiments, which bifurcate and develop lumina. Luminal epithelial cells are cuboidal to columnar and well polarized, with apical microvilli and junctional complexes; basal cells include some undifferentiated ones and some distinct myoepithelial cells. The dermal mesenchyme surrounds the growing buds with more or less concentrically oriented cellular and fibrous layers. During the next 3 months, ducts elongate and branch, reaching the subcutaneous connective tissue. The nipple is first apparent as an external prominence at about 20 weeks. In the last trimester, its superficial cells are sloughed and the deeper cells form the keratinized, stratified, squamous lining of the galactophores.

The sequence of prenatal development is similar in other mammals. Mammary anlagen differentiate in embryos of both sexes; and in the human and some other species, similarity in kind and rate of development continues after birth until the approach of puberty. In the male mouse and rat, the stalk between the growing rudiment and the epidermis ruptures at about the time fetal androgens begin to appear; the gland rudiment persists and develops further, but the nipple is lacking. Castration in either sex, or growth of rudiments in organ culture without hormones, results in female-type development (Kratochwil).

A brief burst of ductal proliferation occurs in glands of both sexes in the human and some other species at birth, accompanied by secretion of a fluid called witch's milk. Hormonal stimulation is presumably the cause, but whether of fetal or maternal origin is unknown.

Mammary growth from birth to the approach of puberty usually parallels body growth. The histology and ultrastructure of the established ducts are essentially as in the adult gland, with a luminal epithelial lining surrounded by a myoepithelial layer. At growing tips or new branching points, cell proliferation may create multilayered thickenings. In the wake of active growth, cells gradually become aligned in two layers and the basal ones differentiate as myoepithelial cells (Fig. 24-23).

At some time prior to the appearance of other external signs of puberty in females, growth in all tissues of the mammary gland accelerates, and the duct system proliferates more or less extensively through the connective tissue septa of the mammary fat pad. With the onset of ovarian cycles, further ductal growth may occur during the first several preovulatory phases. Postovulatory phases are characterized by varying degrees of ductular or alveolar development; in the human and some other mammals with relatively long luteal phases, the general pattern of lobule development may be laid down in the postpubertal nulliparous female. Further proliferation may occur in succeeding cycles, but this is followed by corresponding regression, and the ducts remain well spaced within the stroma. Cyclic ultrastructural changes have been described in ductule cells in the adult human gland, modest secretory differentiation appearing during the luteal phase. Individual variation is great, however.

During pregnancy, ductal elongation and branching resume, and lobuloalveolar development fills the stroma between ducts. Epithelial cell proliferation continues through pregnancy and into lactation. When first formed, alveolar cells resemble those of small ducts. The various signs of preparation for lactation—growth in cytoplasmic volume; quantitative increase in cytoplasmic RNA, rough ER, Golgi membranes, and mitochondria; rise in synthetic enzyme levels; and accumulation of secretory products in cells and lumina—occur in different sequences and at different relative times in the gestation span in different species. By the end of pregnancy, there is usually a considerable but not maximal development of the morphological secretory apparatus (Fig. 24-24), the

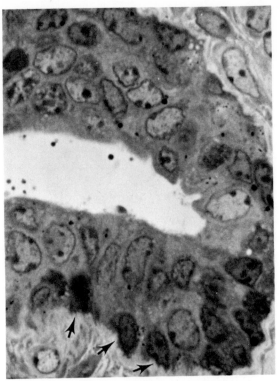

FIGURE 24-23 Major duct in the gland of a 3-week-old mouse. The epithelium in the upper half of this cross section adjoins a branching site and appears multilayered. The epithelium in the lower half is predominantly double-layered, the basal layer of cells showing the smaller nuclei, increased density, and serrated external surface characteristic of ductal myoepithelium (arrows). Epon embedment, Mallory's azure II-methylene blue. ×1455.

enzyme complement characteristic of lactation is present, and lumina are engorged with fat and protein. Milk available to the nursling during the first day or so is mainly that accumulated before birth. It is called colostrum; its antibody content is exceptionally high, and its composition is more similar to blood plasma than is that of typical milk, probably owing to leakiness of occluding junctions in the prelactating epithelium. Soon after parturition, the rates of all secretory activities rise rapidly, the permeability of the junctions drops, and typical milk appropriate for the needs of the young is secreted.

REGRESSION AND INVOLUTION

Lactation can be terminated and regression induced at any time by the cessation of nursing, but under natural conditions the size and secretory activity of the gland

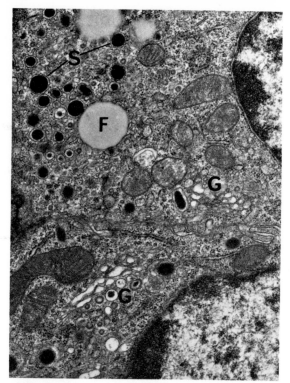

FIGURE 24-24 Supranuclear cytoplasm in two alveolar cells from a midpregnant mouse. Ribosomes are abundant, rough ER is sparse. Fat droplets (F) are present, and secretory vesicles (S) are numerous but small, each containing a single dense protein granule and little fluid. Golgi complexes (G) are evident, but their cisternae are not conspicuously inflated. Electron micrograph. ×19,400.

Many of these vacuoles enclose aggregates of protein particles, some perhaps taken up from the lumen, and the contents lose the characteristic structure of casein micelles (Fig. 24-25). Cytoplasmic organelles soon are seen in stages of degradation within vacuoles. Finally, degenerating cells and debris apparently are removed by macrophages or other phagocytic cells. As a result of these processes, whether abrupt and drastic in premature regression or more gradual during normal weaning, some secretory cells revert to a resting stage while others—the majority in many species—are destroyed. Myoepithelial cells and the basal lamina generally persist, condensing around the remaining epithelium.

Senile involution of the human breast typically begins well before menopause with gradual reduction of lobular tissue, especially peripherally. Ultimately,

FIGURE 24-25 Alveolar cells in a mouse gland 24 h after removal of the young. The mother had nursed the pups for 3 weeks, approximately a normal span. There has been little regression of ER or Golgi complex, but grossly swollen and fused secretory vesicles are present (S), and some possible autophagic vacuoles have appeared (AV). In the lumen is a cellular structure that may represent sloughed cytoplasm, containing a vacuole packed with caseinlike granules. Electron micrograph. ×5820.

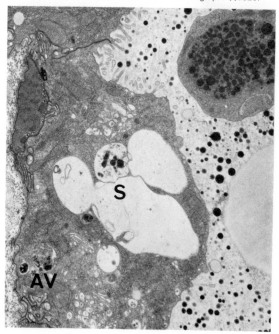

decline slowly as the growing young resort increasingly to other foods. The histology and ultrastructure of regression have been most extensively examined in laboratory animals—usually mice—after abrupt premature removal of the young. In these cases, secretion continues for a day or more and the glands become greatly distended with milk. There follows a period in which several processes appear to play a role. Rupture of some cells and alveolar walls releases cytoplasm into the lumen and luminal contents into the interstitial spaces. How much of this is the mechanical result of handling glands already under the tension of abnormal engorgement is unknown. Autophagic and perhaps heterophagic activity becomes intense in the mammary epithelium. The concentrations of several lysosomal enzymes increase following removal of young, and these levels persist while other enzymatic activities decline. Large cytoplasmic vacuoles appear.

with advancing age, almost all the finer ducts and alveoli disappear (Fig. 24-26) and the connective tissue becomes thickened and hyaline. Local abnormal configurations of ductal or alveolar tissue may be frequent in breasts of postmenopausal women or of old females of other species.

HORMONES

Hormonal control of mammary growth and activity is known to be of paramount importance. The kinds and sequences of hormones involved have been extensively studied in experimental animals by administration of hormones to intact animals, by extirpation of endocrine organs and replacement of specific hormones, or by hormone induction of differentiation in

FIGURE 24-26 Breast of a 52-year-old woman showing persistence of ducts but involution of almost all alveoli; only tiny, shrunken lobular structures remain (arrows). A 2-mm section in methylsalicylate; hematoxylin. ×5.6 (Courtesy of H. M. Jensen and S. R. Wellings.)

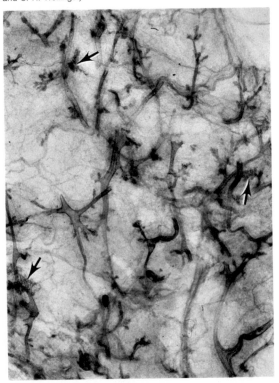

organ culture. Because of species differences, variations in experimental technique, and the prohibitive difficulty of identifying all the synergistic and antagonistic hormonal and metabolic actions that may come into play in a normal animal, the picture that emerges is neither clear nor complete, but certain effects are generally recognized.

Ovarian steroid hormones stimulate mammary growth at puberty and during pregnancy. Estrogens are considered to promote ductal growth and estrogen plus progesterone to promote lobuloalveolar development. Essential to these effects are the hypophyseal protein hormones prolactin and growth hormone. The placenta secretes estrogen, progesterone, and mammogenic hormones; these can replace or augment the effects of ovarian steroids and hypophyseal prolactin during pregnancy. Also involved in mammary maintenance and growth, directly or in synergism with the other essential hormones, are adrenal corticoids, insulin, and thyroid and parathyroid hormones.

Appropriately scheduled increase in quantity of glandular tissue is thus assured by the actions of hormones also effective in regulating ovarian and uterine cycles. Apart from growth itself, the events of intracellular differentiation during pregnancy and the activation of lactogenesis at parturition require specific and coordinated control that appears largely dependent on hormone combinations and sequences. The onset of active lactation is accounted for, in part at least, by an abrupt fall in progesterone level at the end of pregnancy. Progesterone has been shown to block the production of α-lactalbumin and to inhibit a stimulatory effect of estrogen on circulating prolactin levels. Estrogen, prolactin, and corticosteroids in the circulation increase in late pregnancy after a period of low activity; injection of glucocorticoid or prolactin or both can initiate lactation in pregnant animals.

Hormonal requirements for the maintenance of milk secretion also vary considerably among species. Prolactin is probably universally necessary, and adrenal corticoids usually are, whereas the ovarian steroids are not required and may even be inhibiting. The continuing availability of the requisite hormones is governed by neuroendocrine mechanisms. Sensory stimuli of suckling lead to release of several hormones from the anterior pituitary (as well as of oxytocin from the posterior pituitary), the most important being prolactin and ACTH. A complex of releasing and inhibiting factors in the hypothalamus mediates these responses.

BREAST CANCER

Pathological states affecting the human mammary gland include microbial infections, endocrine malfunctions causing abnormal lactation, congenital anomalies in size, shape, or number of glands, and a large number of forms of abnormal growth. The latter range from chronic mild proliferation and sloughing of ductal epithelium, occurring in many premenopausal breasts, through a variety of benign, localized tumors, to cancer. In both incidence and mortality, breast cancer is the major cancer in women; the lifetime probability of developing it is about 7 percent for a woman born in the United States.

Tumor development can affect both the epithelial and the connective tissues of the breast, and the transformation to malignancy (progressive growth with invasion of surrounding tissues or metastasis to other sites) may involve either tissue. Pure connective tissue cancers (*sarcomas*) are rare, however; most breast cancers—and more than 85 percent of all human cancers—are of predominantly epithelial origin (*carcinomas*). They vary widely in growth rate and in the extent of loss of cell and tissue differentiation (*anaplasia*). Many malignant breast tumors are believed to originate with proliferation of duct lining cells. These are contained for variable periods within the duct, gradually filling its lumen. Subsequent growth may take the form of extension of ductlike tubules or solid cords of epithelium through the surrounding connective tissues, or cells may migrate singly or in groups out of the duct wall to infiltrate among stromal elements. Ultrastructural studies have shown frequent discontinuities in the basal lamina associated with such infiltration, but it is not known whether these permit or are created by the cell movement.

Metastases in the lungs, brain, bone, or other sites are the most common direct causes of death. Clumps of cells dislodged from the tumor are carried by the lymph and blood circulation until they lodge in a small vessel and grow in the new site.

Research on breast tumorigenesis relies heavily on the mouse and rat as experimental models. Mammary tumor incidence approaches 100 percent in females of inbred mouse strains regularly selected for this character and infected with murine mammary tumor virus (MuMTV). These mouse tumors are mainly epithelial and typically show some alveolar organization (Fig. 24-27). They grow progressively in the subcutaneous connective tissue, retaining a normal or hypertrophied basal lamina between epithelial and stromal elements, and eventually lead to host death through circulatory failure or infection. They metastasize frequently to the lungs (Fig. 24-28), and rarely to other sites; the metastatic tumors resemble the primary ones.

MuMTV is an RNA virus of distinctive structure, the mature form of which is produced almost exclusively in mammary epithelial cells. It consists of a dense, RNA- and protein-containing nucleoid within a loose envelope; the latter is derived from the cell membrane but bears an MuMTV-specific coat of glycoprotein spikes (Fig. 24-29). Like the other RNA tumor viruses (*oncornaviruses*) that cause leukemia and related diseases in a number of animals, MuMTV contains a characteristic high-molecular-weight RNA and, among several proteins and enzymes, a reverse transcriptase, or RNA-directed DNA polymerase, which produces a DNA copy of the RNA genome. There is evidence that oncornavirus DNA may be integrated in the nuclear genome of the host cell and replicated at subsequent cell divisions. Certain MuMTV strains are transmitted congenitally; most are also transmitted in milk. Infection of the young and subsequent tumorigenesis require, in addition to the virus, inherited susceptibility and adequate hormonal stimulation. Oncornavirus production does not destroy the host cell, and the mechanism by which the virus may ultimately cause some of the infected cell population to escape from normal growth controls is not known. Mammary tumor development may be hastened in MuMTV-carrying mice or induced in presumably MuMTV-free mice by administration of exogenous hormones, particularly estrogen or prolactin. Established tumors usually do not require hormones for further growth, however.

No mammary tumor virus has been demonstrated in rats, and spontaneous mammary cancer is rare; some strains, however, are highly susceptible to mammary tumor induction by hormones or chemical carcinogens. Their tumors are often responsive to endocrine treatment, as are some kinds of human tumors.

Because of the proven link between oncornaviruses and mammary or some other cancers in experimental animals, recent years have seen an inten-

946

sive search for a viral agent in human breast cancer. In numerous studies, particles with morphological or biochemical resemblance to MuMTV have been reported from human milk, tumor tissues, or culture fluid from breast cell cultures; but these, although apparently widespread, have not been abundant or consistent enough in distribution to demonstrate correlation with the occurrence of breast cancer, nor has production of the particle by the human tissue been proved in most cases. Recently, McGrath and his colleagues isolated a virus with several properties of MuMTV from a human breast carcinoma cell line and showed it to replicate in these cells. In this and some other work, antigenic relations between a suspect particle and MuMTV has been suggested by immunologic tests. Thus it appears that one or more viruses of the oncornavirus type may be present, and perhaps common, in human populations. If such a virus should prove to be an essential factor in breast cancer devel-

opment, the disease might ultimately be preventable by vaccination or drug treatment. That virus infection alone could not be sufficient for cancer development appears certain; even in highly biased laboratory conditions, viral carcinogenesis requires a coincidence of other factors. Endogenous viruses with oncornavirus properties but without known pathogenicity have been found in many animal species.

Other possible factors in human breast carcinogenesis are suggested by epidemiological studies. Genetics or environment or both appear to be significant: breast cancer incidence is much higher in North America and Northern Europe than in most of Asia and Africa. It is higher among whites than among blacks in the United States, but Japanese populations

FIGURE 24-27 Mammary tumor in a mouse. Electron micrograph. A small lumen (L) is almost filled with microvilli and dense, spherical particles of mammary tumor virus. Tumor cell nuclei are roughly ovoid, with frequent indentations; they contain one or more nucleoli and conspicuous marginal heterochromatin. The cytoplasmic volume is relatively small, similar to that in normal duct cells. The usual cytoplasmic organelles are present but not abundant. One of the cells contains clusters of intracytoplasmic incomplete virus particles (arrow). ×9135.

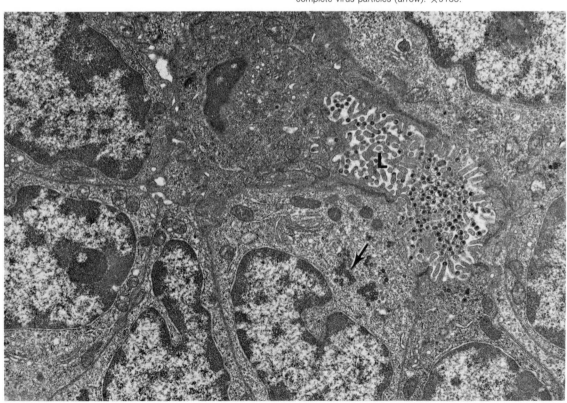

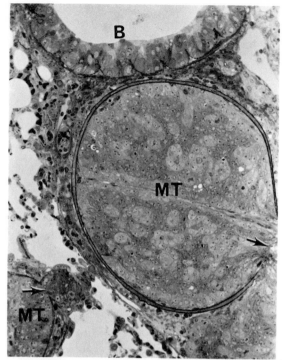

FIGURE 24-28 Metastatic mammary tumor tissue (MT) within two arterioles in a mouse lung; part of a bronchiole (B) is seen at the top and partially collapsed pulmonary alveoli at the left and bottom. The arteriolar tunica media, with its darkly stained elastic lamellae, is stretched by the tumor mass, and both arterioles have ruptured (arrows), permitting the tumor to expand into the pulmonary tissues. Epon, Mallory's azure II-methylene blue. ×193.

spond to addition of hormones or to their deletion by endocrinectomy. Demonstration of specific hormone receptors in cells of the tumor may be useful in predicting hormone response. Other treatments for breast cancer include drugs and irradiation; immunological methods are also being explored. Reduction of mortality rests primarily on diagnosis and treatment of a tumor before it has spread beyond the breast. Improvement in histological or biochemical techniques for identifying premalignant lesions is therefore a continuing research goal.

FIGURE 24-29 Mammary tumor virus particles in a mouse tumor. The particles are released by budding through the cell surface; in this electron micrograph, two immature particles (arrows) are still attached to microvilli. The free mature virus particle consists of a nucleoid, with a dense center and a thin, dense wall, positioned eccentrically within a rather loose membrane envelope. The envelope is derived from the cell's plasmalemma but bears surface spikes of viral glycoprotein. ×79,540. Inset. A negatively stained virus particle, showing the coating of spikes in face view and in profile. Electron micrograph. ×145,500.

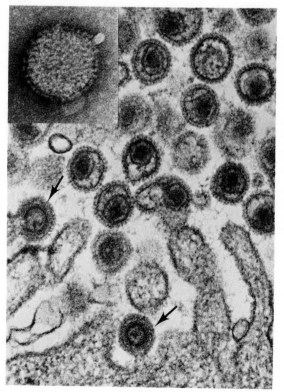

in this country have higher incidences than in Japan. Close blood relatives of breast cancer patients have a higher probability of developing the disease than unrelated controls; this is not attributable to milk transmission of an infective agent, as the great decline in breast feeding over the past 50 years has not been accompanied by a significant decline in breast cancer incidence. Reproductive physiology probably plays a role. The most complete current statistics indicate that the age of a woman at her first childbirth is related to her breast cancer risk. For a woman bearing her first child at the age 30, the risk is about the same as that for a nulliparous woman and about twice as high as that for a woman bearing her first child before the age of 20.

Hormone therapy for breast cancer has been developed empirically and on the basis of data from experimental animals. Some human tumors are unresponsive to any hormone manipulation; others re-

REFERENCES

BAUMAN, D. E., and C. L. DAVIS: Biosynthesis of Milk Fat, in B. L. Larson and V. R. Smith (eds.), "Lactation," vol. II, p. 31, Academic Press, Inc., New York, 1974.

BEER, A. E., R. F. BILLINGHAM, and J. HEAD: The Immunologic Significance of the Mammary Gland, *J. Invest. Dermatol.,* **63:**65 (1974).

COLE, P.: Epidemiology of Human Breast Cancer, *J. Invest. Dermatol.,* **63:**133 (1974).

COWIE, A. T.: Overview of the Mammary Gland, *J. Invest. Dermatol.,* **63:**2 (1974).

COWIE, A. T., and J. S. TINDAL: "The Physiology of Lactation," Edward Arnold (Publishers) Ltd., London, 1971.

CROSS, B. A., and A. L. R. FINDLAY: Comparative and Sensory Aspects of Milk Ejection, in M. Reynolds and S. J. Folley (eds.), "Lactogenesis: the Initiation of Milk Secretion at Parturition," p. 245, University of Pennsylvania Press, Philadelphia, 1969.

CUTLER, M.: "Tumors of the Breast," J. B. Lippincott Company, Philadelphia, 1962.

DABELOW, A.: Die Milchdrüse, in "Handbuch der mikroskopischen Anatomie des Menschen," vol. III/3, p. 277, Springer-Verlag OHG, Berlin, 1957.

EBNER, K. E., and F. L. SCHANBACHER: Biochemistry of Lactose and Related Carbohydrates, in B. L. Larson and V. R. Smith (eds.), "Lactation," vol. II, p. 77, Academic Press, Inc., New York, 1974.

ELIAS, J. J., D. R. PITELKA, and R. C. ARMSTRONG: Changes in Fat Cell Morphology during Lactation in the Mouse, *Anat. Rec.,* **177:**533 (1973).

FALCONER, I. R., and J. M. ROWE: Possible Mechanism for Action of Prolactin on Mammary Cell Sodium Transport, *Nature* (*Lond.*), **256:**327 (1975).

FANGER, H., and H. J. REE: Cyclic Changes of Human Mammary Gland Epithelium in Relation to the Menstrual Cycle. An Ultrastructural Study, *Cancer,* **34:**574 (1974).

GIRARDIE, J.: Histocytomorphologie de la Glande Mammaire de la Souris C3H et de Trois Autres Rongeurs, *Z. Zellforsch.,* **87:**478 (1968).

GOULD, V. E., J. MILLER, and W. JAO: Ultrastructure of Medullary, Intraductal, Tubular and Adenocystic Breast Carcinomas: Comparative Patterns of Myoepithelial Differentiation and Basal Lamina Deposition, *Am. J. Pathol.,* **78:**401 (1975).

GROSVENOR, C. E., and F. MENA: Neural and Hormonal Control of Milk Secretion and Milk Ejection, in B. L. Larson and V. R. Smith (eds.), "Lactation," vol. I, p. 227, Academic Press, Inc., New York, 1974.

HAAGENSEN, C. D.: "Diseases of the Breast," 2d Ed., W. B. Saunders Company, Philadelphia, 1971.

HELIMINEN, H. J., and J. L. E. ERICSSON: Studies on Mammary Gland Involution I-III, *J. Ultrastruct. Res.,* **25:**193 (1968).

HELMINEN, H. J. and J. L. E. ERICSSON: Effects of Enforced Milk Stasis on Mammary Gland Epithelium, with Special Reference to Changes in Lysosomes and Lysosomal Enzymes, *Exp. Cell Res.,* **68:**411 (1971).

HOLLMANN, K. H.: Cytology and Fine Structure of the Mammary Gland, in B. L. Larson and V. R. Smith (eds.), "Lactation," vol. I, p. 3, Academic Press, Inc., New York, 1974.

JENNESS, R.: Biosynthesis and Composition of Milk, *J. Invest. Dermatol.,* **63:**109 (1974).

KEENAN, T. W., D. J. MORRÉ, and C. M. HUANG: Membranes of the Mammary Gland, in B. L. Larson and V. R. Smith (eds.), "Lactation," vol. II, p. 191, Academic Press, Inc., 1974.

KRATOCHWIL, K.: In Vitro Analysis of the Hormonal Basis for the Sexual Dimorphism in the Embryonic Development of the Mouse Mammary Gland, *J. Embryol. Exp. Morphol.,* **25:**141 (1971).

LEIGHTON, J.: "The Spread of Cancer," Academic Press, Inc., New York, 1967.

LINZELL, J. L.: Some Observations on the Contractile Tissue of the Mammary Glands, *J. Physiol.,* **130:**257 (1955).

LINZELL, J. L.: Mammary Blood Flow and Methods of Identifying and Measuring Precursors of Milk, in B. L. Larson and V. R. Smith (eds.), "Lactation," vol. I, p. 143, Academic Press, Inc., New York, 1974.

LINZELL, J. L., and M. PEAKER: Mechanism of Milk Secretion, *Physiol. Rev.,* **51:**564 (1971).

LINZELL, J. L., and M. PEAKER: Changes in Colostrum Composition and in the Permeability of the Mammary Epithelium at about the Time of Parturition in the Goat, *J. Physiol.,* **243:**129 (1974).

MAYER, G., and M. KLEIN: Histology and Cytology of the Mammary Gland, in S. K. Kon and A. T. Cowie (eds.), "Milk: the Mammary Gland and its Secretion," vol. I, p. 47, Academic Press, Inc., New York, 1961.

MCGRATH, C. M., P. M. GRANT, H. D. SOULE, T. GLANCY, and M. A. RICH: Replication of Oncornavirus-like Particles in Human Breast Carcinoma Cell Line MCF-7, *Nature (Lond.),* **252:**247 (1974).

MONTAGNA, W., and E. E. MACPHERSON: Some Neglected Aspects of the Anatomy of Human Breasts, *J. Invest. Dermatol.,* **63:**10 (1974).

NANDI, S., and C. M. MCGRATH: Mammary Neoplasia in Mice, *Adv. Cancer Res.,* **17:**353 (1973).

NEMANIC, M. K., and D. R. PITELKA: A Scanning Electron Microscope Study of the Lactating Mammary Gland, *J. Cell Biol.,* **48:**419 (1971).

OZZELLO, L.: Electron Microscopic Study of Functional and Dysfunctional Human Mammary Glands, *J. Invest. Dermatol.,* **63:**19 (1974).

PITELKA, D. R., S. T. HAMAMOTO, J. G. DUAFALA, and M. K. NEMANIC: Cell Contacts in the Mouse Mammary Gland. I. Normal Gland in Postnatal Development and the Secretory Cycle, *J. Cell Biol.,* **56:**797 (1973).

PORTER, J. C.: Hormonal Regulation of Breast Development and Activity, *J. Invest. Dermatol.,* **63:**85 (1974).

RICHARDSON, K. C.: Contractile Tissues in the Mammary Gland with Special Reference to Myoepithelium in the Goat, *Proc. R. Soc. Med. Lond. (Biol)* **136:**30 (1949).

SAACKE, R. G., and C. W. HEALD: Cytological Aspects of Milk Formation and Secretion, in B. L. Larson and V. R. Smith (eds.), "Lactation," vol. II, p. 147, Academic Press, Inc., New York, 1974.

RAYNAUD, A.: Morphogenesis of the Mammary Gland, in S. K. Kon and A. T. Cowie (eds.), "Milk: the Mammary Gland and its Secretions," vol. I, p. 3, Academic Press, Inc., New York, 1961.

SALAZAR, H., and H. TOBON: Morphologic Changes of the Mammary Gland During Development, Pregnancy and Lactation, in J. B. Josimovich, M. Reynolds, and E. Cobo (eds.), "Lactogenic Hormones, Fetal Nutrition, and Lactation," p. 221, John Wiley & Sons, Inc., New York, 1974.

SCHLOM, J., R. MICHALIDES, D. KUFL, R. HEHLMANN, S. SPIEGELMAN, P. BENTVELZEN, and P. HAGEMAN: A Comparative Study of the Biologic and Molecular Basis of Murine Mammary Carcinoma: A Model for Human Breast Cancer, *J. Natl. Cancer Inst.,* **51:**541 (1973).

SIMMONS, R. L., and A. RIOS: Differential Effect of Neuraminidase on the Immunogenicity of Viral Associated and Private Antigens of Mammary Carcinomas, *J. Immunol.,* **111:**1820 (1973).

STOLFI, R. L., R. A. FUGMANN, L. M. STOLFI, and D. S. MARTIN: Synergism Between Host Anti-tumor Immunity and Combined Modality Therapy Against Murine Breast Cancer, *Int. J. Cancer,* **13:**389 (1974).

TANNENBAUM, M., M. WEISS, and A. J. MARX: Ultrastructure of the Human Mammary Ductule, *Cancer,* **23:**958 (1969).

TOBON, H., and H. SALAZAR: Ultrastructure of the Human Mammary Gland. II. Postpartum Lactogenesis, *J. Clin. Endocrinol. Metab.,* **40:**834 (1975).

TUCKER, H. A.: General Endocrinological Control of Lactation, in B. L. Larson and V. R. Smith (eds.), "Lactation," vol. I, p. 277, Academic Press, Inc., 1974.

WAUGH, D. and E. VAN DER HOEVEN: Fine Structure of the Human Adult Female Breast, *Lab. Invest.,* **11:**220 (1962).

WELLINGS, S. R., H. M. JENSEN, and R. G. MARCUM: An Atlas of Subgross Pathology of the Human Breast with Special Reference to Possible Precancerous Lesions, *J. Natl. Cancer Inst.,* **55:**231 (1975).

WOESSNER, J. F., JR.: The Physiology of the Uterus and Mammary Gland, in J. T. Dingle and H. B. Fell (eds.), "Lysosomes in Biology and Pathology," vol. I, p. 299, North-Holland Publishing Company, Amsterdam, 1969.

The Human Placenta

HELEN A. PADYKULA

The placenta is a transient organ characteristic of mammals that mediates physiologic exchange between the mother and the developing embryo-fetus. It is important at the outset to understand that the placenta has both fetal and maternal parts and is, therefore, composed of cells of two different genotypes. This is a biologic situation with important immunologic implications, since the placental-fetal complex may be viewed as "a natural allograft resistant to rejection." The following general definition, derived from Mossman's (1937) monograph, is a useful one to remember. The placenta consists of "an intimate apposition or fusion of the fetal membranes with the uterine mucosa for the purpose of carrying out physiological exchange." To understand what a placenta is in morphologic terms, it is thus essential to know the structure of the extraembryonic membranes and also of the progestational uterine endometrium.

The functions of this maternal-fetal complex are manifold. The placenta must serve temporarily as a fetal lung, kidney, intestine, and probably as a fetal liver as well; furthermore, it is a complex endocrine organ. In their gonadotropic, lactogenic, and metabolic effects, placental protein hormones resemble closely those of the gonadotropins and growth hormone of the anterior pituitary. Oxygen and nutrients are transferred across the placenta from the maternal blood to the fetal blood; carbon dioxide and various metabolic waste products are transported in the reverse direction. The placental association places the fetal bloodstream in close proximity to the maternal bloodstream, but normally these two bloodstreams do not mix. They are separated by tissue layers called the *placental barrier.*

The placenta varies considerably in its morphology among the orders of mammals. This diversity makes it quite unique when compared with organs such as the lung, kidney, or liver, which are relatively similar among different mammals. Placental diversity has phylogenetic significance which is most likely related to the evolutionary modifications that occurred in the vertebrate extraembryonic membranes as they were modified for intrauterine development. In this chapter the discussion is limited to the human placenta. However, it should be emphasized that thorough understanding of the placenta of primates is derived only through a knowledge of comparative placentation (Mossman, 1937; Amoroso, 1952; Steven, 1975) and going even farther back phylogenetically, through a knowledge of the development of birds and reptiles. The reader is advised to review the structure and function of the extraembryonic membranes of the chick and pig as well as the histophysiology of the primate uterus (see standard texts of embryology and Chap. 23). The most complete collection of human placental specimens ever gathered together may be studied in an excellent monograph by Boyd and Hamilton (1970), which is a rich source of information on placental morphology.

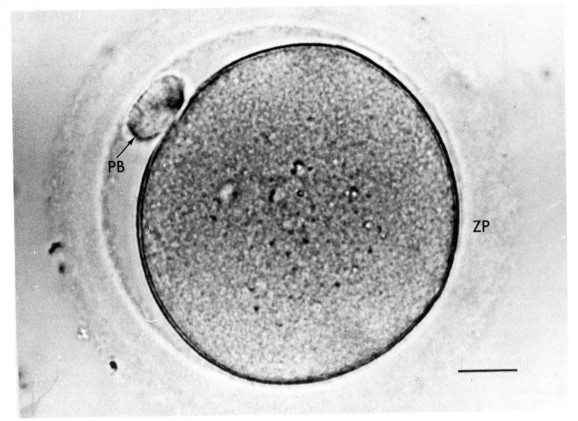

PB

ZP

FIGURE 25-1 A living human secondary oocyte cultured in pyruvate Krebs-Ringer medium. Under in vitro conditions, human oocytes obtained from ovarian follicles proceed with meiosis, form the first polar body (PB), and mature to the metaphase II stage. The cumulus cells have been removed; the zona pellucida (ZP) is present. Scale marker, 20 μm (From J. F. Kennedy and R. P. Donahue, *Science*, **164**:1292, 1969).

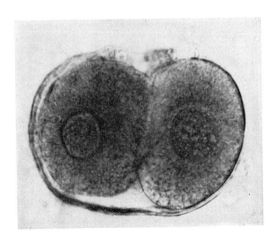

Viviparous animals, when compared with oviparous forms, have relatively small ova that contain little stored nutrient. The human ovum, as it is shed from the graafian follicle, is 100 to 150 μm in diameter and is surrounded by a thick glycoprotein coat, the *zona pellucida* (Fig. 25-1) and a variable number of corona radiata cells. Fertilization occurs in the ampulla of the fallopian tube. As the newly formed zygote passes through the fallopian tube, it undergoes holoblastic cleavage (Fig. 25-2) and forms a solid mass of cells called the *morula*. Between 84 and 96 h after ovulation, the morula enters the uterus, fluid begins to accumulate among the cells, a central cavity appears, and the *free blastocyst* is formed (Fig. 25-3). The blastocyst exists free in the uterine secretions for approximately 3 days, since the youngest attached

FIGURE 25-2 Two-cell stage of the human zygote, probably 1-$\frac{1}{2}$ to 2-$\frac{1}{2}$ days old, obtained from the fallopian tube. The zona pellucida still surrounds the blastomeres. ×400. (Courtesy of A. T. Hertig and J. Rock.)

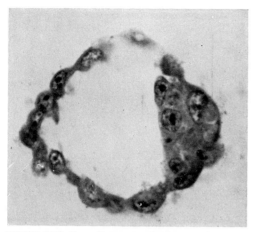

FIGURE 25-3 Normal human free blastocyst approximately 4-½ days old obtained from the uterine cavity. Observe the layer of primitive trophoblastic cells surrounding the blastocyst cavity, and the inner cell mass located at one pole (to the right). The zona pellucida has almost completely disappeared. ×600. (Courtesy of A. T. Hertig and J. Rock.)

human blastocyst is estimated to be 7½ days of age (Fig. 25-5).

The human blastocyst, like that of most mammals, is nearly spherical (Fig. 25-3). The precursor of the parenchyma of the placenta, the *trophoblast* ("nutritive layer"), makes a precocious appearance as a thin layer of extraembryonic cells that surrounds a fluid-filled cavity and a mass of embryo-forming cells (the inner cell mass) located at one pole of the inner surface of the trophoblast. The trophoblast is the outer component of the *chorion*, the outermost extraembryonic membrane. At implantation the zona pellucida is shed, and the blastocyst begins to implant in the highly glandular progestational uterus at approximately day 21-22 of the menstrual cycle. Currently the biology of the mammalian blastocyst is an area of intensive investigation considered to be related to the development of effective fertility control (see Blandau, 1971). Human differentiation has been achieved in vitro from the fertilization of preovulatory oocytes to the blastocyst stage.

IMPLANTATION

The human blastocyst usually implants on the upper posterior wall of the body of the uterus near the midsagittal plane. As the trophoblastic cells come into contact with the uterine epithelium they proliferate and soon form an attachment to the uterine wall (Fig. 25-4). As we trace placental differentiation, it will become evident that the trophoblast forms the parenchyma of the fetal placenta and that it is the regulatory component of the placental barrier.

The blastocyst of the rhesus monkey begins to implant on the ninth day after fertilization (Fig. 25-4). The trophoblastic cells proliferate rapidly in a coronal area at the embryonic pole of the blastocyst, and several points of attachment to the uterine epithelium are established. In the rhesus monkey the trophoblast forms desmosomal association with the uterine epithelium. This intimate ultrastructural association suggests that the uterine epithelium does not recognize the genetic "foreignness" of the trophoblast.

The youngest known attached human blastocyst

(approximately 7½ days) is shown in Fig. 25-5.[1] The local surface epithelium has disappeared, and the trophoblast is in contact with the connective tissue. The trophoblast, which is in the form of a thick plate, has differentiated into the *syncytiotrophoblast*, a multinucleated cytoplasmic mass or syncytium which arises by the fusion of separate cells of the *cytotrophoblast*. Intact superficial maternal capillaries are in close association with the primitive syncytial trophoblast of this early implant.

The human embryonic complex undergoes *interstitial implantation*; it sinks into the endometrial connective tissue and becomes enclosed by it. By the eleventh day the interstitial position is achieved and

---

[1] Our knowledge of early human development is derived primarily from the important studies of A. T. Hertig and J. Rock. For a comprehensive bibliography of their work, see the paper by Hertig, Rock, and Adams published in 1956. See also O'Rahilly's (1973) survey of the Carnegie collection of human embryos of the first 3 weeks of development.

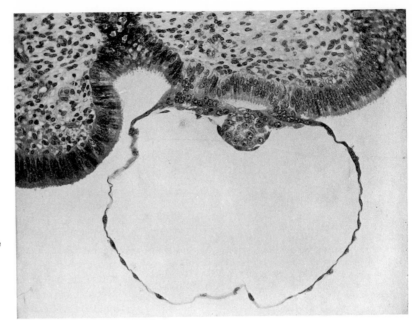

the uterine epithelium covers over the site (Figs. 25-6 to 25-8). A view of the endometrial surface at the implantation site of a normal 11-day human embryo is shown in Fig. 25-6. The embryonic complex resides in a slightly raised, glistening, translucent area, a little less than 1 mm in diameter, surrounded by a bright red area which reflects a modification of blood vessels in the adjacent stroma. Microscopic examination of

sections of this 11-day implant reveals that rapid growth and differentiation of the trophoblast has occurred around the entire circumference (Fig. 25-8). At this time two types of trophoblast are clearly evident: an inner layer of primitive cytotrophoblast composed of individual cells and a broad outer layer of primitive syncytial trophoblast. The syncytium now possesses spaces called *lacunae* that contain maternal blood.

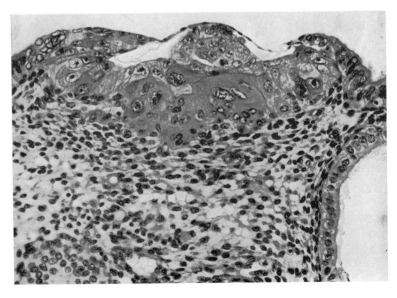

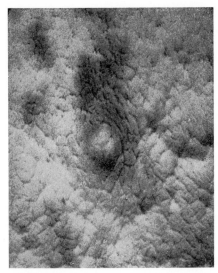

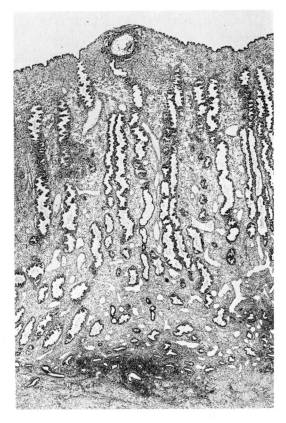

FIGURE 25-6 Surface view of the human endometrium and implantation site on the eleventh day of development. Sections through this specimen are shown in Figs. 25-7 and 25-8. ×8. (Courtesy of A. T. Hertig and J. Rock.)

FIGURE 25-7 (Right) Section through an 11-day human implantation site in the 25-day secretory endometrium. The invading blastocyst has achieved an interstitial position, being located immediately below the endometrial surface. The whole expanse of the endometrium is evident with its dilated, coiled glands heavy with secretion. See Fig. 25-8 for enlargement of the implantation site. ×20. (Courtesy of A. T. Hertig and J. Rock.)

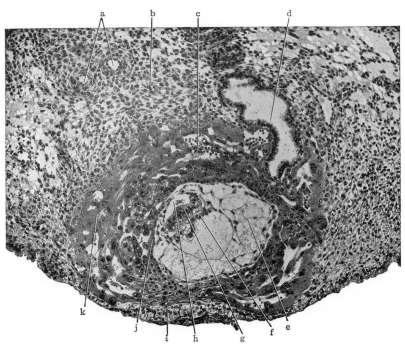

FIGURE 25-8 Section through an 11-day human implantation site in the 25-day secretory endometrium. Within the syncytial trophoblast (k) is an intercommunicating network of lacunar spaces that contain some maternal blood (c). The bilaminar embryonic germ disc is apparent in the center of the implant, with the amniotic cavity above and the yolk sac cavity below. Above the embryo and to the right is an enlarged secretory endometrial gland (d), whereas above and to the left the edematous stroma contains a coiled artery (a,b). e, exocoelom; f, endoderm forming part of the yolk sac; g, ectodermal embryonic shield; h, amniotic cavity enclosed by amnion which is delaminating in situ; i, repairing endometrial epithelium; j, cytotrophoblast. ×100. (Courtesy of A. T. Hertig and J. Rock.)

The lacunae communicate with each other and with maternal sinusoids and veins: these vascular connections allow the initiation of the maternal circulation. The presence of the placental hormone, *human chorionic gonadotrophin* (HCG), in the maternal circulation at this time provides evidence that a functional maternal vascular connection has been established. Data obtained recently on the rhesus monkey indicate that this first rise in circulating chorionic gonadotropin "rescues the corpus luteum" by stimulating ovarian progesterone secretion which maintains gestation until progesterone production by the placenta commences near the twenty-third day of pregnancy (Atkinson et al., 1975). This early endocrine activity by the trophoblast also provides a convenient basis for early recognition of pregnancy in human beings.

At this early stage of development, two extra-embryonic membranes, not involved in the formation of the human placenta, are also being differentiated (Fig. 25-8). The *amnion* is a domelike membrane that encloses a fluid-filled cavity over the embryonic plate. At this time the embryonic disc is bilaminar and consists of a thick plate of ectoderm and a thin ventral layer of endoderm. The *yolk sac* is attached to the ventral surface of the embryonic disc; its cavity is lined dorsally by the primitive endoderm and elsewhere by a layer of flattened cells. The confluent spaces in the loose extraembryonic mesenchyme surrounding the yolk sac represent the exocoelom. Although the yolk sac is involved in placentation in subprimate mammals, it never establishes contact with the chorion in man (Fig. 25-12). The human yolk sac plays an important role as the initial site of fetal blood cell formation (see Chap. 11).

ESTABLISHMENT OF THE PLACENTAL VILLI AND CIRCULATION

The third week of pregnancy (days 14 to 21) is a period of intense trophoblastic growth and differentiation, a time when the significant placental relationships are established. By the fifteenth day the maternal circulation through the syncytial trophoblast becomes fully functional, as lacunae become large and confluent and connect with endometrial spiral arteries as well as with the veins. Cords of trophoblast, called *primary chorionic villi,* begin to extend outward from the surface of the chorion, owing to rapid proliferation of the cytotrophoblast, which provides a fundamental cellular mechanism for expansion of the fetal placenta. After the fifteenth day, mesenchyme appears in the proximal attached portions of the cords and extends progressively toward their growing distal ends (Fig. 25-9). As mesenchyme forms in the cores of the villi, they are gradually converted from primary chorionic villi into *secondary villi.* Each secondary villus contains a core of mesenchyme surrounded by a continuous sheath of cytotrophoblast which is covered, in turn, by a mantle of syncytial trophoblast. The maternal blood flows through large intercommunicating spaces that have arisen from the confluence of the lacunae of the primitive syncytium, which are now referred to collectively as the *intervillous space* (Fig. 25-10). The surface of the syncytiotrophoblast is bathed directly by

circulating maternal blood at this early time in gestation.

The distal tips of the secondary villi are now solid columns (*cytotrophoblastic cell columns*) that unite peripherally to form the *trophoblastic shell* (Figs. 25-10 and 25-11), which encloses the entire implant and is the outermost frontier of embryonic tissue. It is composed principally of cellular trophoblast but also contains irregular strands of peripheral syncytial trophoblast, some of which penetrate quite deeply into the endometrium and make contact with the uterine blood vessels. The arrangement of the cytotrophoblast in the columns and shell provides a mechanism for lengthening the villi and for circumferential expansion of the fetal placenta. Recent electron microscopic examination of this early penetration of the endometrial stroma indicates that fetal trophoblastic cells come into direct contact with maternal decidual cells (altered stromal cells). This intimate intermingling of cells with different genotypes is of considerable interest immunologically and has been designated for now as the "deciduotrophoblastic complex" (Tekelioglu-Uysal et al., 1975). Later in pregnancy, the cytotrophoblast proliferates in localized areas on some villi, creating the *cytotrophoblastic cell islands* (Fig. 25-27).

Embryonic blood vessels appear in the cores of

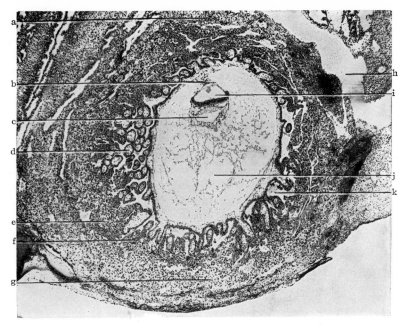

FIGURE 25-9 Section through a 16-day human implantation site. Observe the embryonic shield with the amniotic cavity (i) above it and the yolk sac cavity (c) below it. The dark chorion encloses the large exocoelom (j) and is connected to the embryo by the mesodermal body stalk (b). Secondary villi containing cores of mesoderm and angioblasts are differentiating (d). Peripheral to these is a lamina composed largely of cytotrophoblast, constituting cell columns (f) and the developing trophoblastic shell (e). Surrounding the latter is the decidua. Below, separating the implant from the uterine cavity, is a broad zone of decidua capsularis (g). a, decidua basalis; k, intervillous space; h, dilated maternal venous sinus. ×30. (Courtesy of A. T. Hertig and J. Rock.)

FIGURE 25-11 Section through the 18- to 19-day human placental site. The curved germ disc has differentiated to the stage of Hensen's node and the primitive groove. The yolk sac (ys) contains blood islands. The body stalk (bs), which is partly penetrated by an endodermal diverticulum, connects with the chorionic mesoderm. Secondary placental villi (v) are evident; their distal ends are solid masses of cytotrophoblast that fuse peripherally to form the trophoblastic shell (ts). ×15. (Courtesy of A. T. Hertig and J. Rock.)

FIGURE 25-10 Section through the placenta of a rhesus monkey of the twenty-ninth day of gestation. Secondary chorionic villi are visible; each villus consists of a core of mesoderm surrounded by a darkly stained mantle of cytotrophoblast and syncytium which borders the intervillous space (is) through which maternal blood circulates. The tips of the villi extend downward as columns of cellular trophoblast (primary villi). The distal ends of these trophoblastic cell columns (tc) unite on the periphery of the growing placenta to form the trophoblastic shell (ts). The latter merges indistinctly with the underlying decidually transformed endometrium (d). g, uterine gland. Iron-hematoxylin stain. ×5.

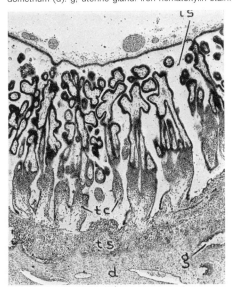

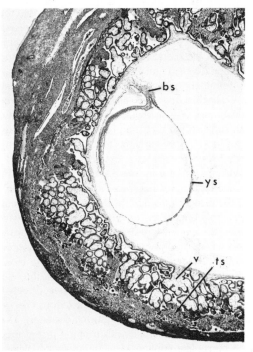

the villi and form the *tertiary* placental villi. The primordium of the umbilical cord also makes its appearance through the formation of the *body stalk* (Fig. 25-11), which is the homolog of the allantoic stalk in other groups of mammals. The mesodermal primordium connects the caudal part of the embryonic shield with the chorion to form a *chorioallantoic placenta.* By subsequent differentiation and elongation, the body stalk forms the *umbilical cord* that contains *umbilical vessels.* The newly formed blood vessels of the placental villi thus become connected through the umbilical vessels with the embryonic heart; toward the end of the third week, fetal blood begins to circulate in the capillaries of the villi. The placental villi are now supplied by both maternal and fetal blood, and physiologic exchange is thereby greatly facilitated.

The allantoic stalk of most mammals contains an endodermal diverticulum of the hindgut which in association with the allantoic mesoderm forms the allantoic sac. In humans and monkeys the endodermal diverticulum of the hindgut remains rudimentary and microscopic (Fig. 25-11).

PLACENTAL (CHORIONIC) VILLI

The structural and functional unit of the human fetal placenta is the *stem* villus with its branches which become increasingly abundant as pregnancy proceeds. It brings the fetal bloodstream close to the maternal blood for physiologic exchanges. At the same time, the villous structure creates a tremendous absorptive surface that facilitates transport. Each stem villus with its branches has a separate fetal blood supply; this unit has been designated as a *fetal cotyledon.*

The stem villus or fetal cotyledon originates at the *chorionic plate* (Fig. 25-30A, B, see color insert). During pregnancy each stem villus subdivides longitudinally at its distal end to create villi of a second and third order. These, in turn, form still smaller branches, some terminating in the trophoblastic shell (basal plate) and called *anchoring villi.* Investigators disagree on the number of fetal cotyledons; Boyd and Hamilton (1970) suggest that their number decreases from approximately 320 in early gestation to 60 at term, whereas Freese (1974) states that there are 120 to 240 (see Wilkin, 1965, for further discussion). Besides the elaboration of the fetal absorptive surface, the significance of the fetal cotyledon resides in its separate fetal blood supply and in its topographic association with the maternal spiral artery (Fig. 25-30B). In the rhesus monkey it is generally agreed that each fetal cotyledon is aligned with the opening of one spiral artery. However, in the human placenta only about half the fetal cotyledons are aligned with spiral arteries (Freese).

The size and shape of the fetal cotyledons change steadily as branching continues during gestation. The cotyledons directly aligned with a spiral artery may have a barrel-like configuration (tambour of Wilkin) that encloses a central cavity devoid of villi (Fig. 25-13A and B). The possible significance of this hollow cotyledonary form will be pursued later in the discussion on placental circulation.

As the villi differentiate, they become longer and highly branched. They are described by some investigators as resembling trees rooted in the chorionic plate, with branches extending into the intervillous space (Figs. 25-12 and 25-30A). At term, approximately 11 m^2 of surface area have been differentiated on the placental villi; this calculation does not include the further amplification created by microvilli on the free trophoblastic surface.

The morphology of the villi has been difficult to interpret at the microscopic level, since only pieces of the branches are seen in sections (Fig. 25-14). The total surface area for transport is expanded by an increase in the number of terminal villi coupled with a decrease in their diameter. Scanning electron microscopy is providing a promising new approach to analysis of the progressive differentiation of the villous tree (Fig. 25-15). The *terminal* (or free) villi extend freely into the intervillous space and contain sinusoidal capillaries.

In the early placenta the villi occur all over the surface of the chorion (Fig. 25-12). Basally, in association with the thick well-vascularized endometrium, the villi branch elaborately and grow in length. They constitute the *chorion frondosum* and eventually give rise collectively to the gross discoidal form of the definitive placenta. The endometrial connective tissue in this region is called the *decidua basalis.* Over the outer chorionic wall, which bulges toward the uterine cavity, the villi are much shorter and there, by the third month of gestation, the villi and the associated *decidua capsularis* dwindle, leaving the *chorion laeve*. As the fetus enlarges and its membranes expand, the chorion laeve eventually fuses with the *decidua vera* of the opposite uterine wall, thereby obliterating the uterine cavity. Consult a textbook of mammalian embryology for illustration of these relations.

The villus of the early placenta has a loose mesenchymal core covered by two layers of trophoblast (Figs. 25-16 to 25-19). (Figs. 25-17 and 25-19, see color insert.) The inner or cytotrophoblastic layer is composed of large *Langhans' cells* that have large nuclei and a slightly basophilic cytoplasm. Overlying the Langhan's cells is a more basophilic layer of relatively thick syncytiotrophoblast. Mitoses occur in the Langhans' layer but not in the syncytium; in vivo isotopic labeling of dividing nuclei with [³H]thymidine has established that in the rhesus monkey the Langhans' cytotrophoblast produces the syncytium through cell fusion (Fig. 25-18). The Langhans' cells decrease

FIGURE 25-12 Normal human gestation sac at 40 days, carefully separated and removed from the uterus. The chorion laeve has been removed to reveal the relationships of the embryo with the extraembryonic membranes. The embryo is most immediately enclosed by the amnion. The chorionic membrane encloses the exocoelom into which the small yolk sac extends. The placental villi project outward from the chorionic plate: at this early stage, the villi are diffusely distributed over the entire chorionic surface. ×3.5. (Carnegie Institution of Washington.)

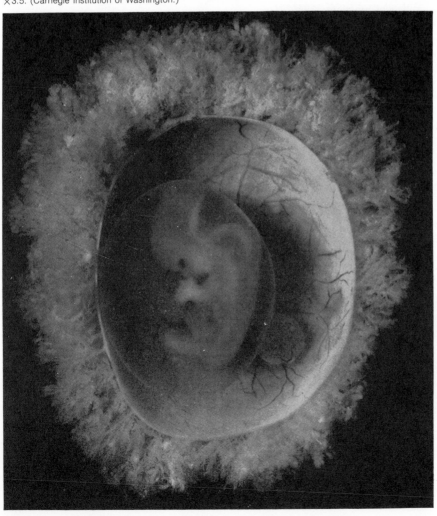

in number after the fifth month of pregnancy; at term, relatively few remain. Thus, the Langhans' layer is a germinal bed of cells that multiply, transform, and then fuse with the syncytium to cause its expansion. These germinal cells store a considerable amount of glycogen during the first 4 to 6 weeks of gestation; thereafter the glycogen store diminishes.

The undifferentiated state of the Langhans' cells is evident also in their ultrastructure (Fig. 25-26). Free ribosomes are common in the cytoplasm, whereas rough endoplasmic reticulum is relatively sparse; the Golgi complex is well developed. The mitochondria are larger than those of the syncytium. The Langhans' cells are associated with each other and with the syncytium by desmosomes and tight junctions; their basal surfaces rest on the basal lamina. Transitional cells with ultrastructural characteristics occur intermediate between those of Langhans' cells and syncytium, and evidence of cell fusion between these transitional cells and the syncytium has been obtained. Remnants of fusion are represented in the syncytial cytoplasm by fragments of cell membranes, desmosomes, and even intercellular spaces. Thus, the multinucleate condition of the syncytiotrophoblast originates in the same manner as that of skeletal muscle fibers, that is, by the fusion of initially separate cells.

The placental syncytium is a remarkable structural differentiation (Figs. 25-16 through 25-21). By its position and prevalence, it must be the chief regulator of transport and is also most likely the site of synthesis of both the steroid and protein placental hormones (see below). The syncytiotrophoblast is a continuous layer of multinucleated cytoplasm that forms a complete covering over the multitudinous villi. A significant structural-functional point is the apparent absence of intercellular space in this absorptive surface. All substances entering or leaving the fetal blood must therefore pass through the syncytial cytoplasm. This

FIGURE 25-13 Isolated human fetal cotyledons. A. The fetal vasculature was injected with a plastic material. The elaborate branching of the stem villus is evident. The dark central area (S) represents the intracotyledonary space (or central cavity). B. A highly coiled maternal uteroplacental (spiral) artery is aligned with the entrance to the intracotyledonary space. The fetal villi appear as a white mass here. (From Freese, 1974.)

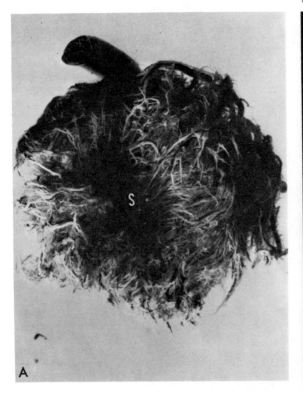

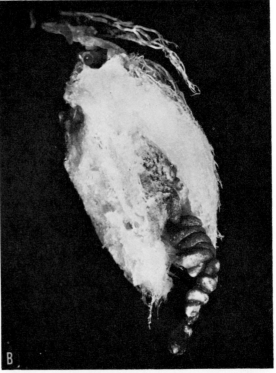

layer, which is thick early in gestation, becomes progressively thinner as gestation advances (Fig. 25-22), although regional differences in the thickness of the syncytium exist in the maturing placenta. As the Langhans' layer becomes discontinuous, the syncytium comes increasingly in contact with the basal lamina.

The free surface of the syncytium interacts directly with the maternal blood and is modified into a profusion of highly pleomorphic microvilli (Fig. 25-21). In addition, the syncytial surface is extended by larger projections in the form of ridges that are studded with microvilli. The elaborate and irregular form of the surface projections suggests tremendous mobility of the superficial cytoplasm. Some are pseudopods and contain cytoplasmic organelles; others consist of clublike microvilli. Like the conspicuous microvillous

borders of the small intestine and proximal tubule of the kidney, this placental border is rich in alkaline phosphatase activity. Between the microvilli are small, bristle-coated pits or caveolae which may be involved in macromolecular uptake. Relatively large tabs of syncytium, such as that illustrated in Fig. 25-19, often project into the intervillous space. In normal pregnancy, such nucleated syncytial sprouts are liberated into the intervillous space and enter the maternal venous system. They get as far as the maternal pulmonary capillaries but apparently do not enter the systemic arterial system. Later in pregnancy, even whole villi are released into the maternal circulation (Ramsey, 1973). The significance of this remarkable phenomenon is unknown.

A conspicuous feature of the nuclei of the syncytiotrophoblast is their tendency to clump close together (Figs. 25-19 and 25-32). They are usually located in the basal cytoplasm and are larger in younger stages than in later stages of gestation. Vacuolation

FIGURE 25-14 Human placental villi at 10 weeks (A) and at term (B). Both photomicrographs were taken at the same magnification. Note that as gestation proceeds, the branches of the villous tree become progressively finer and more numerous. Also, the placental barrier becomes thinner and fetal capillaries come in close apposition to the trophoblastic cover. Compare with Fig. 25-15. H&E. ×100.

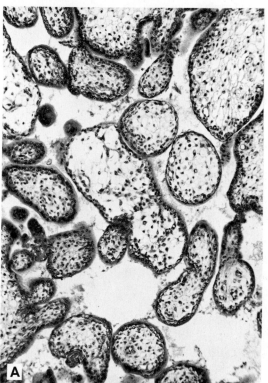
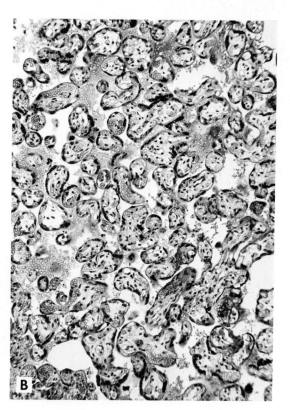

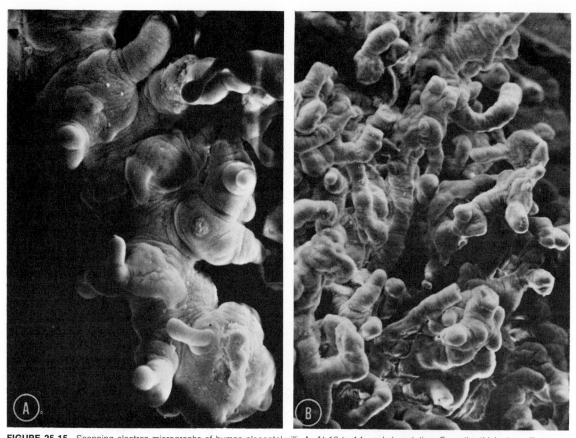

FIGURE 25-15 Scanning electron micrographs of human placental villi. A. At 10 to 14 weeks' gestation. From the thick stem villus, smaller branches are originating. B. Term placenta. Note the profusion of slender villi. (From B. F. King and D. N. Menton, *Am. J. Obstet. Gynecol.,* **122:**8248, 1975.)

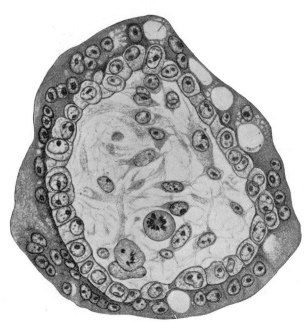

FIGURE 25-16 Cross section of a young human placental villus, showing an axial mesenchymal core surrounded by the two-layered trophoblastic epithelium composed of an inner cellular layer of Langhan's cells (cytotrophoblast) and an outer layer of syncytium (syncytial trophoblast). Vacuoles of various sizes occur in the syncytium. ×550. (Courtesy of W. J. Hamilton and R. J. Gladstone.)

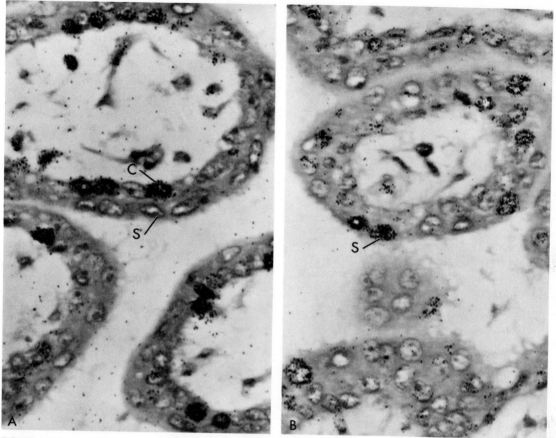

FIGURE 25-18 Radioautographs showing the incorporation of tritiated thymidine into the placental villi of the rhesus monkey. A. One hour after intravenous injection of [³H]thymidine, only the nuclei of the cytotrophoblastic (C) or Langhans' cells are labeled. B. However, 48 hours after such an injection, a high percentage of syncytiotrophoblastic (S) nuclei carry the label. ×600 (Courtesy of A. R. Midgley and G. B. Pierce.)

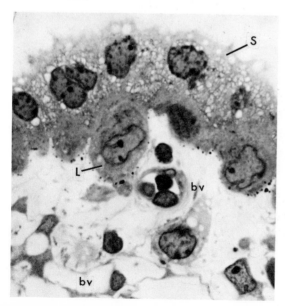

FIGURE 25-20 Human placental villus at 10 weeks. The cytoplasm of the syncytiotrophoblast (S) appears vacuolated. The nuclei of the syncytium have a heavier chromatin pattern than those of Langhans' cells (L). Fetal blood vessels (bv) are generally not closely apposed to the trophoblast. Plastic section, 2 μm, toluidine blue. ×600.

of the cytoplasm is common during the first 3 months (Fig. 25-20), but the ultrastructural basis of this has not been adequately defined. The superficial cytoplasm, especially in the early syncytium, is distinctly acidophilic; the ultrastructure of this region shows a concentration of smooth-surfaced vesicles of various sizes and tubules that are presumably components of the smooth endoplasmic reticulum. In contrast, the basal and perinuclear cytoplasm is intensely basophilic (Fig. 25-19), reflecting a high concentration of both free ribosomes and rough ER, whose cisternae are often dilated (Fig. 25-21) and contain a moderately dense material. This elaborate system of rough-surfaced membranes suggests that this trophoblastic region is involved in the synthesis of proteins for export,

such as the placental protein hormones, HCG, human chorionic somatomammotropin (HCS), and perhaps human chorionic thyrotropin (HCT) (see below). Golgi complexes are distributed at intervals in the syncytium. Slender filamentous mitochondria that have both lamellar and tubular cristae occur throughout the cytoplasm. Glycogen is stored in the syncytio-

FIGURE 25-21 Electron micrograph of the human placenta at 4 months' gestation. The two trophoblastic layers are evident; the syncytiotrophoblast (S) is attached to the subjacent germinal cytotrophoblast or Langhans' cells (L) by desmosomes (D). The Langhans' cells lie on the basal lamina (arrow). A thin layer of connective tissue intervenes between the trophoblastic complex and the underlying blood vessel (BV). The free surface of the syncytium is modified into an irregular microvillous border. The superficial cytoplasm of the syncytium contains vesicles and irregularly shaped vacuoles. Rough endoplasmic reticulum is abundant in the syncytium but relatively sparse in the Langhans' cells. The undifferentiated cytoplasm of the Langhans' cells contains many free ribosomes. G, Golgi complex. ×15,000. (Courtesy of A. C. Enders.)

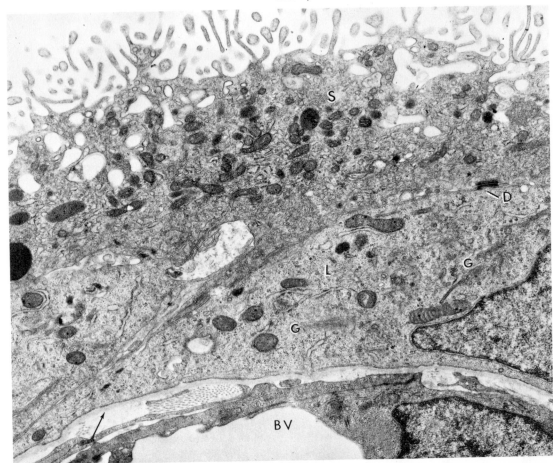

trophoblast only during the first month and disappears by the end of the second month.

Both endocytosis and exocytosis are most likely well developed in the syncytiotrophoblast and may be, for example, related to the transport of maternal antibodies to the fetal blood and to the secretion of HCG and HCS into the maternal blood. This two-way intrasyncytial traffic offers challenge to analysts. Ultrastructural evidence suggests that the syncytium possess endocytic mechanisms for protein uptake comparable to those of other mammalian systems involved in antibody transport, such as the neonatal small intestine and visceral yolk sac placenta. Such cellular systems are involved in bulk uptake of proteins, and they possess conspicuous lysosomal systems. Current evidence indicates that the lysosomal

system (as judged through ultrastructural localization of acid phosphatase) is represented primarily in the form of multivesicular bodies (Fig. 25-23A and B). An endocytic vesicle containing absorbed protein probably fuses with a multivesicular body, the material is processed, and various secondary derivatives, including dense bodies, are formed. These observations represent the first concrete steps to sort out the various populations of cytoplasmic granules limited by smooth membranes that form a conspicuous feature of the syncytium.

A significant cytochemical feature of the syncytium is the presence of numerous birefringent, sudanophilic droplets throughout gestation. These lipid droplets have cytochemical properties similar to those of steroid-producing cells of the gonads and adrenal cortex. These cytochemical comparisons have long suggested that the syncytium may be responsible

FIGURE 25-22 Diagram of the human placental barrier near term. The maternal blood (MB) is separated from the fetal blood (FB) by the syncytiotrophoblast (S), occasional Langhans' cells (L), basal lamina of the trophoblast (bl), fetal connective tissue (CT), basal lamina (bl) of the fetal capillary, and the fetal endothelium (E). (Courtesy of A. C. Enders, 1965.)

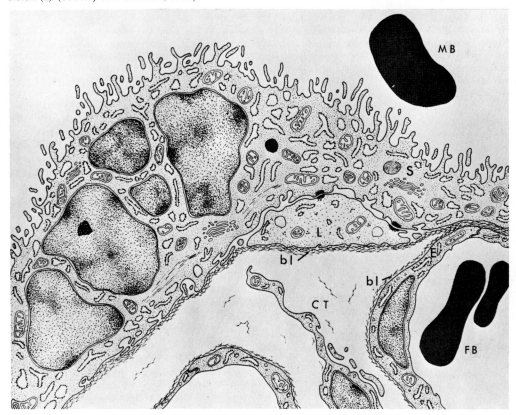

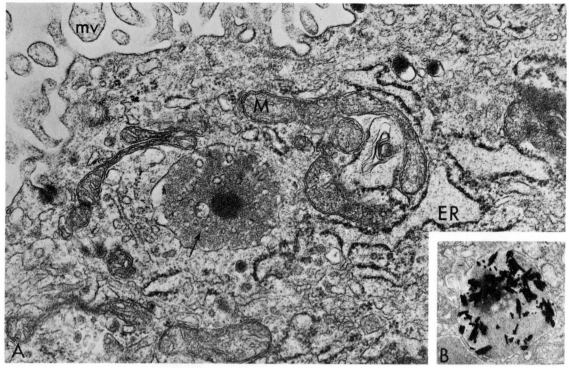

FIGURE 25-23 Multivesicular bodies in the human syncytiotrophoblast. A. A multivesicular body (arrow) contains a dark nucleoid. Note also the abundant rough endoplasmic reticulum (ER), mitochondria (M) with lamellar and tubular cristae, and microvilli (mv). ×30,000 (From Martin and Spicer, 1973.) B. Acid phosphatase activity in the multivesicular bodies. (From L. H. Hoffman and D. L. Di Pietro, *Am. J. Obstet. Gynecol.,* **114:**1087, 1972.)

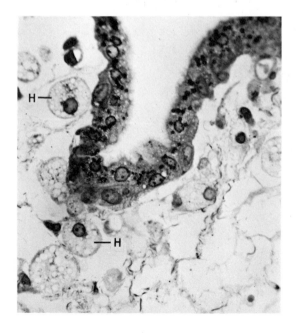

for the secretion of the placental steroids, estrogen and progesterone. This suggestion has been given more substance by the localization within the villous trophoblast of Δ^5-3β-hydroxysteroid dehydrogenase, an enzymic complex involved in the biosynthesis of steroid hormones. Furthermore, during the first trimester, the mitochondria of the syncytium have both tubular and lamellar cristae, another feature associated with steroid-producing cells.

The stroma of the villi is initially a loose mesenchyme which becomes more densely collagenous with advancing gestation. Two types of cells occur in this fetal connective tissue, fibroblasts and a unique cell type called the *Hofbauer cell.* The fibroblasts possess

FIGURE 25-24 Human placental villus at 10 weeks. The two-layered trophoblast rests on a rather loose mesenchymal stroma. The highly vacuolated Hofbauer cells (H) are located within a loose meshwork of reticular fibers, and mesenchymal or fibroblastic cells. See Fig. 25-25. Plastic section, 2 μm, toluidine blue. ×450.

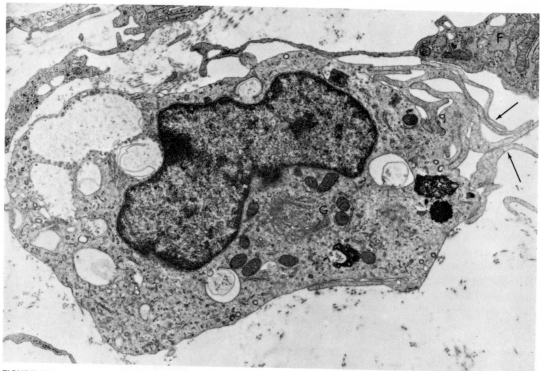

FIGURE 25-25 Electron micrograph of a Hofbauer cell in the human placenta at 3 months' gestation. The Hofbauer cells have ultrastructural features resembling those of tissue macrophages. The cell surface appears highly mobile, with broad cytoplasmic extensions (arrows) suitable for engulfing materials. Vacuoles of varying size and content are conspicuous, along with some dense bodies. G, Golgi complex; F, fibroblast. ×9000. (Courtesy of A. C. Enders.)

the usual ultrastructural features of this cell type in other organs where they are known to be the elaborators of the precursors of collagen fibrils and ground substance. The Hofbauer cells are large, elliptical, and vacuolated and have an eccentrically placed nucleus. They are most numerous in the early placenta (Fig. 25-24). Ultrastructural and cytochemical evidence suggests that they are similar to macrophages (Fig. 25-25). Although the specific function of the Hofbauer cells is unknown, they may participate in the removal and remodelling of the extracellular stromal material that would necessarily occur in relation to the lengthening and branching of the villi.

Branches of the umbilical arteries and vein course through the stroma of the stem villi and their branches (Figs. 25-30A and B, and 25-31). The terminal (free) villi possess an anastomosing network of capillaries that are sinusoidal in dimension; they may exceed 50 μm in diameter (Fig. 25-32). These wide vessels allow an unusually small decrease in the blood pressure from the umbilical artery to the umbilical vein.

JUNCTION OF MATERNAL AND FETAL TISSUES

The region of confrontation between fetal and maternal tissues is interesting from an immunologic point of view, since cells of two different genotypes are in intimate association. It is the region of placental attachment. Nothing is known abut the cohesive forces that bind the trophoblast to the decidua here. At birth this region of attachment will become the region of separation as the *deciduate placenta* is shed.

In the early placenta the outermost fetal tissue, the trophoblastic shell, is formed by the fusion of solid columns of cytotrophoblast at the distal tips of the secondary villi (Fig. 25-10). The trophoblastic shell comes into close association with the *decidua,* which is the designation for the endometrium of the pregnant uterus and, in actuality, means the modified endometrial stroma. The cells of the two genotypes intermingle here, and it is difficult to distinguish between them in a routine light microscopic preparation. Recent ultrastructural observations at 20 to 40 days of pregnancy demonstrate that maternal decidual cells are in part in direct contact with the fetal trophoblastic cells. Furthermore, lymphocytes are present near this deciduotrophoblastic complex. From the time of implantation a peculiar extracellular material called *fibrinoid* accumulates around the fetal cytotrophoblasts (Figs. 25-26 to 25-28); the term fibrinoid describes a group of substances related to fibrin. In later development, this junctional intermingling of maternal and fetal cells is referred to as the *basal plate.* During the second half of pregnancy, the basal plate thins out.

The cellular relationships in the basal plate are incompletely described and remain a challenge to specialists in the subject. Efforts to identify the Y chromosome, in the case of a male fetus, hold promise of distinguishing between the trophoblastic and decidual components. During interpretation it is useful to remember that the decidual cells are derivatives of the uterine connective tissue, whereas the trophoblastic cells are epithelial derivatives held together by

FIGURE 25-26 Human placenta at term, showing the composition of the basal plate at two different magnifications. The upper part of each photomicrograph shows the basal plate, whereas the lower part contains placental villi (v) and the intervillous space (IV). In the basal plate, the peripheral or basal cytotrophoblastic cells (PC) possess conspicuous cytoplasmic basophilia, a major cytochemical feature of this cell type. Note also that these epithelial cells are embedded in fibrinoid (F). Maternal blood is evident in the intervillous space, and the fetal sinusoids are packed with erythrocytes. Note in B that syncytium (S) clothes the fetal aspect of the basal plate. Eosin-methylene blue. A, ×100; B, ×450.

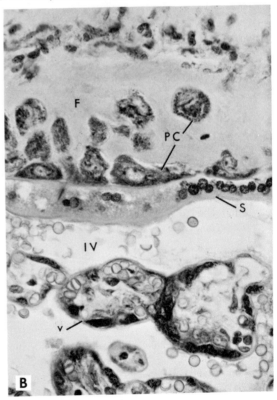

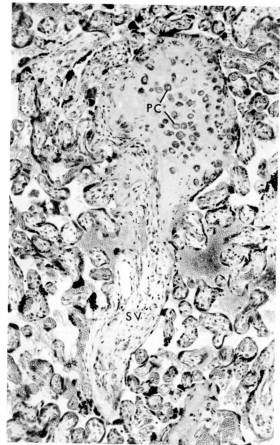

FIGURE 25-27 Human placenta at term, showing a portion of a stem villus (SV) with an associated island of cytotrophoblast (PC). The large stem villus occupies the center of the photomicrograph and is surrounded by numerous sections through the finely branched villous tree. The trophoblastic cells of the island stain darkly because of their high cytoplasmic content of ribonucleo-protein. Eosin-methylene blue. ×100.

cells and lutein cells, occur in the basal trophoblasts at term (Fig. 25-29); this enlargement of cellular surface area suggests intensive involvement in transport activities. The basal cytotrophoblastic cells later in gestation contain fine glycoprotein granules. To some investigators, these cells bear some resemblance to the gonadotrophin-secreting basophils of the anterior pituitary and thus might be the producers of chorionic gonadotrophin. The basal plate has also been identified as a probable site for the production of relaxin. Investigators attempting to localize the site of secretion of HCG by immunohistochemical procedures have usually used only samples of the villous portion of the placenta. Most of these studies identify the syncytium as the probable synthesizer of both HCG and HCS. Further work must still be done to establish with certainty the sites of origin of the protein hormones. Since the cytotrophoblastic cells of the basal plate, cell columns, and cell islands have the cytologic features that synthesize protein for export, they should be studied further.

The separated uterine surface of the delivered placenta shows elevated convex subdivisions of *maternal cotyledons* (lobes) that are demarcated by grooves. *Placenta septa* which project into the intervillous space occur at these intercotyledonary grooves of the basal plate. Investigators disagree about whether these septa are maternal or fetal in origin or whether they have a dual origin. Attempts to distinguish maternal from fetal cells by identifying female sex chromatin, or the Y chromosome of a male fetus, have not yet resolved this controversy.

The nature of the immunologic relationship of the trophoblast with the uterine epithelium and then with decidual cells is of considerable theoretical and practical importance. Also, once maternal circulation is established, the maternal blood cells in the intervillous space are washed against the fetal syncytium. Early embryonic tissue is antigenic and the uterus is immunologically competent, yet gestation proceeds to term without rejection by the mother. Considerable effort is being directed toward the possibility that extracellular coats, such as the cell coat (glycocalyx) of the epithelia, or extracellular deposits, such as fibrinoid, may constitute an immunologic barrier. In addition, the antigenicity of the trophoblast is generally described as weak or masked.

desmosomes (Fig. 25-28). It is significant that these peripheral and basal cytotrophoblastic cells differ considerably in their ultrastructure and cytochemistry from the Langhans' cytotrophoblast on the villi. Their cytoplasm is strongly basophilic (Fig. 25-26) and contains a well-developed rough ER (Fig. 25-28), whereas the Langhans' cell cytoplasm is faintly basophilic and has little rough ER (Fig. 25-21). "Intracellular canaliculi," comparable to those of gastric parietal

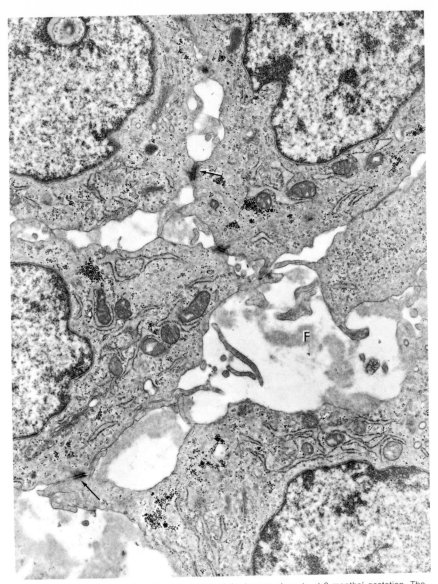

FIGURE 25-28 Electron micrograph of the cytotrophoblastic cells of the basal plate of the human placenta at 3 months' gestation. The basal cytotrophoblastic cells are joined together at intervals by desmosomes (arrows); also large intercellular spaces contain a relatively amorphous dense material called fibrinoid (F). Conspicuous components of the cytoplasm are rough endoplasmic reticulum, mitochondria, Golgi complex, and glycogen particles. ×15,000. (Courtesy of A. C. Enders.)

PLACENTAL CIRCULATION

The gross anatomy of the placenta reflects strongly the vascular arrangement. A pattern of blood flow through the *definitive discoidal placenta* was illustrated by Ramsey and Harris (1966) (Fig. 25-30A, color insert).

More recently, a somewhat modified interpretation has been presented by Freese (Fig. 25-30B, color insert). The two *umbilical arteries* are continuous with the fetal internal iliac arteries and carry blood rich in

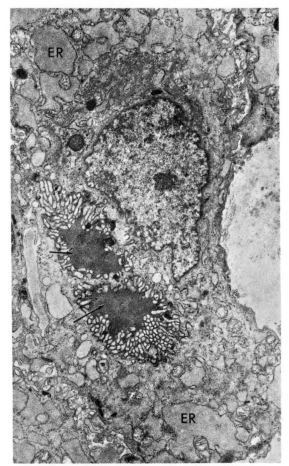

growing tips of the villi and thus the volume of the capillary bed increases steadily during pregnancy. Each fetal cotyledon with its ramifications is autonomous. To keep pace with the growing fetus, fetal cotyledons increase in weight and length instead of spreading the area of placental attachment.

The circulation of maternal blood commences during the second week; the fetal circulation is established by the end of the third week. The vascularity becomes increasingly rich on both maternal and fetal sides. Early in pregnancy, the fetal capillaries lie in a central position in the vilus, but as pregnancy advances, these thin-walled, anastomosing, endothelial tubes with their large lumina come to lie just beneath the surface of the trophoblast (Fig. 25-32). The venous blood is returned from the multitude of terminal villi through a system of veins that accompany the arteries. These lead eventually to the single *umbilical vein* that carries oxygenated blood back to the fetus where it connects with the ductus venosus. The fetal circulation through the placenta is maintained by a pressure head;

FIGURE 25-29 Cytotrophoblastic cell from the basal plate in the human term placenta. Two intracellular canaliculi (arrows) are surface specializations of the basal cytotrophoblastic cells. Note also the abundant expanded rough endoplasmic reticulum (ER). ×8000. (M. Uehara, T. Hando, and S. Takeuchi, *Acta Obstet. Gynaecol. Jap.,* **19:**102, 1972.)

FIGURE 25-31 Branches of the stem villi in the human placenta at term. In the branches of the stem villus (SV) at the right, a fetal artery and vein course through its core. In addition, a branch point is evident in this stem villus. Eosin-methylene blue. ×100.

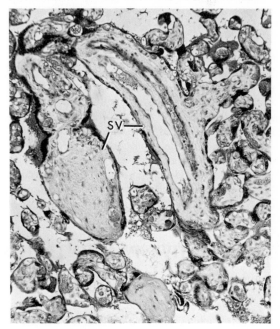

carbon dioxide from the fetus to the placenta. In the chorionic plate they divide into numerous placental arteries that spread fanwise; from these radial trunks, vertical branches are given off which ramify into the stem villi (fetal cotyledons) and their numerous branches. The configuration of the fetal cotyledon has been depicted as treelike (Fig. 25-30A) or barrel-shaped (Figs. 25-30B and 25-13). The branching form of the villus is followed by the blood vessels (Fig. 25-32). The fetal arteries branch and rebranch to break up finally into the *sinusoidal capillary bed* of the smallest villi (Fig. 25-32). Throughout gestation, newly formed capillaries invade the syncytial buds on the

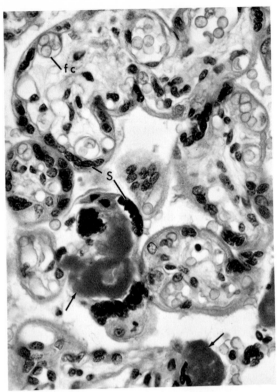

FIGURE 25-32 Human placental villi at term. Fetal sinusoidal capillaries (fc) are now closely apposed to the syncytiotrophoblast (S). The stroma is denser than in early gestation. Hyalinization of the villi is evident (arrows). In certain areas the nuclei of the syncytium are crowded together and form dense clusters. Eosin-methylene blue. ×450.

it has been demonstrated in the fetal lamb that at term the pressure gradient between the umbilical arteries and umbilical vein is approximately 65 mm Hg. The placental capillary pressure is much above that of other capillary beds and also exceeds the pressure in the maternal intervillous space. The umbilical arteries, as well as the sinusoidal capillaries, have large lumina, and this keeps the pressure high.

Maternal blood enters the intervillous space through open-ended *uteroplacental arteries* (endometrial spiral arteries) that penetrate the basal plate.

At the point of entry the arteries have terminal dilations. These are the remarkably modified coiled arteries of the nonpregnant endometrium which have been rebuilt from invading cytotrophoblasts. The tunica media is largely replaced by trophoblast. It is interesting that the trophoblast does not, however, invade the uteroplacental veins.

There is often one arterial entry opening at the center of a fetal cotyledon (Fig. 25-30B). Where such alignment occurs, there is an intracotyledonary villous-free space that would offer low resistance to the pulsatile flow of maternal arterial blood. Where such alignment is absent, the fetal cotyledon lacks a central cavity (Freese, 1974).

The maternal blood from the uteroplacental artery spurts into the intervillous space in fountainlike jets. It has been assumed that the force of this pulsatile jet stream sweeps aside the free terminal villi, especially near the point of arterial entry (Fig. 25-30A). According to another interpretation, the jet stream may be directed into a central, villous-free cavity of the fetal cotyledon (Fig. 25-30B). Since the maternal arterial blood pressure is considerbly greater than that in the intervillous space, the arterial stream is driven toward the chorionic plate; then as the pressure of the stream decreases, lateral dispersion occurs. Lateral dispersion has been visualized in living pregnant rhesus monkeys by x-ray cinematographic means. The blood then falls back in a fountainlike spray to bathe the extensive surface of the syncytiotrophoblast, and exchanges between the two bloodstreams occur. Finally it drops back into venous openings that are distributed along the basal plate. The venous pressure is lower than that of the intervillous space; thus differences in the blood pressure of the arteries, intervillous space, and veins control the maternal circulation in the placenta. The maternal and fetal bloodstreams move in more or less opposite directions, but investigators tend to agree that countercurrent flow does not occur, at least in the primate placenta. Further functional interpretation must, however, await agreement on the three-dimensional form of the human stem villus and its branches.

COMPARATIVE PLACENTATION

The human placenta may be described as *hemochorial, villous, discoidal,* and *deciduate.* To understand the meaning of this classification, it is necessary to appreciate comparative placentation, a topic beyond the scope of this chapter. Detailed information on comparative placentation can be found in the works of Grosser (1927), Mossman (1937), Amoroso (1952), Wislocki and Padykula (1961), and Steven

(1975). Briefly, however, the yolk sac and allantois fuse with the chorion in different mammals to form various placental relations. In human beings, only a chorioallantoic placenta is formed. The chorioallantoic placentas of mammals can be classified according to gross form or on the basis of the histologic structure of the placental barrier. The gross form is related to the distribution of villi (or lamellae) over the surface of the chorion. The early human placenta starts out with the villi quite uniformly distributed over the outer surface of the chorion; this gross arrangement is described as a *diffuse placenta* (Fig. 25-12). It differentiates into a definitive form that is discoidal in shape, that is, the villi are arranged in the form of a disc (Fig. 25-30). Other gross forms are cotyledonary (ruminants) or zonary (carnivores).

The histologic classification introduced by Grosser is based on the microscopic structure of the placental barrier. Grosser's classification is derived from the number of maternal tissue layers that inter-

vene between the maternal and fetal circulations (Fig. 25-33) and thus has functional implications. When the chorion is apposed to an intact (epithelial) endometrium, this relation is described as *epitheliochorial* (for example, pig, horse). In the *syndesmochorial* placenta (ruminants), the uterine epithelium is destroyed, leaving the connective tissue stroma exposed to the trophoblast. In the *endotheliochorial* placenta (for example, carnivores) most of the connective tissue surrounding the maternal capillaries is destroyed, thus placing the trophoblast in close association with the maternal endothelium. In the *hemochorial* placenta (for example, bats, higher primates, some insectivores, and rodents), the maternal blood comes into direct contact with the chorionc villi or lamellae through the loss of the maternal capillary endothelium. In this type of placenta the endometrium becomes transformed into decidua and is partially destroyed. At birth there may be considerable bleeding (in humans and monkey) as the *deciduate* placenta is shed. Although Grosser's scheme is generally useful and valid, ultrastructural observations have indicated that it is an oversimplification from the morphologic point of view (see Fig. 25-33) and thus most likely from a functional point of view as well.

FIGURE 25-33 Chorioallantoic barriers of sow, sheep, cat, and humans near full term. This reinterpretation of Grosser's classification indicates that the differences in the widths of the various types of placental barriers may not be as great as is generally believed. The fetal capillaries (fc) and maternal capillaries (mc) are heavily outlined. In the human placenta, the maternal capillaries have been eroded, and the maternal blood circulates through the intervillous space. In the epitheliochorial placenta of the sow and in the syndesmochorial placenta of the sheep, the fetal capillaries penetrate deeply into the trophoblast, and the maternal capillaries push into the overlying tissue. These morphologic modifications decrease significantly the distance between the two bloodstreams. Furthermore, the placental barriers of the sheep and cat are practically identical with respect to the number of layers separating the two bloodstreams. (prepared by G. B. Wislocki in consultation with E. C. Amoroso.)

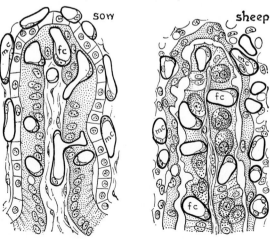
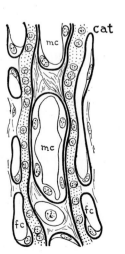
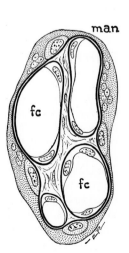

THE HUMAN PLACENTAL BARRIER

Early in implantation the hemochorial nature of the human placental barrier is established, as maternal blood circulates through the lacunae lined by syncytium (Fig. 25-8). As the villi form and expand, the thickness of the barrier decreases progressively as the Langhans' cells disappear, the syncytium flattens into a thin layer, and the sinusoidal capillaries assume a position closer to the basement membrane. The barrier is thus composed entirely of fetal tissue. The branches of the villous tree become progressively smaller and more numerous (Fig. 25-14). Concomitant with this progressive structural change, there may be alterations in permeability to many substances.

The placental barrier at term varies in its thickness; it can be as thin as 2 μm but with some areas as thick as 60 μm. Evidence is gathering that regional differences may exist along the barrier. A substance passing from the maternal blood to the fetal blood first encounters the free surface of the syncytium, which is highly modified to form a multitude of pleomorphic microvilli and other surface projections. Recent cytochemical analysis indicates the presence of a special surface coat along the free surface. Small molecules presumably are transferred through the plasma membrane of these elaborate evaginations to enter the syncytium. Uptake of macromolecular substances may occur through pinocytosis, since invaginations of the plasma membrane are frequent and in close association with small vesicles. The pathway of absorption through the syncytium is unknown. Although membrane-limited droplets have been reported in the syncytium, it is not known whether they represent absorption or secretion, since the abundant endoplas-

mic reticulum of the syncytium may be involved in both activities. The ultrastructure of the syncytium is quite similar to that of thyroid follicular cells, which are also involved in the two-way traffic of secretory and absorptive functions.

The basal surface of the syncytial trophoblast borders on either Langhans' cells or on the epithelial basal lamina directly; the latter relation becomes more common as gestation proceeds (Fig. 25-22). At term the basal cytoplasm is modified to form narrow infoldings as well as footlike processes. Associated with these invaginations there are often relatively large irregular gaps between the syncytium and the epithelial basement lamina. This structural amplification of the basal surface may be related to transport from the fetal toward the maternal blood. The epithelial basal lamina rests on a thin layer of connective tissue, and occasionally the processes of fibroblasts may intervene between the epithelium and the capillary. The endothelial cells rest on their own basal lamina, with their junctions closely apposed. Pinocytotic vesicles occur on both surfaces of the endothelial cells. In some regions the connective tissue layer may be obliterated and the two basal laminae become closely apposed or fused.

Thus, at the ultrastructural level, the three-layered hemochorial placental barrier becomes further subdivided into at least five ultrastructural layers: syncytium, trophoblastic basal lamina, connective tissue layer, endothelial basal lamina, and endothelium. Since it is known that there is considerable regulation of the substances transferred between the two bloodstreams, the mechanism of regulation must be distributed among these ultrastructural layers.

FUNCTIONS OF THE PLACENTA

The transport activities of the placenta are complex because the numerous materials required for the synthesis of fetal tissues must be transferred and the waste products of fetal metabolism removed. In general, small molecules cross more readily than larger ones. The building blocks for proteins, phospholipids, and polysaccharides are transferred from the maternal blood to support the synthesis of the macromolecules in the fetus. A well-known exception to this is the transfer of antibodies across the human placenta; the

transmission of passive immunity is a prenatal event in humans and depends on the placental capacity to transport intact protein molecules. Some current thinking is being directed toward the possibility of transplacental passage of antigens and consequent effects on fetal immunologic abilities.

Although it is generally believed that gases pass by means of simple diffusion, evidence indicates that the arrangement of the microcirculation is a major factor in placental gas exchange. In the human placenta the free-flowing maternal blood cascading over the villous branches of the fetal cotyledon presents a strong challenge to physiological interpretations of transport activities. Glucose transport into placental cells is believed to occur by facilitated diffusion. The regulation in the amount of glucose that crosses the placental barrier is illustrated in the example of the diabetic mother. Her high blood glucose results in some increase in fetal blood sugar, but the fetal level is always considerably less than the maternal level. Amino acids are normally more concentrated in fetal blood than in maternal blood. This reflects the action of specific active transport mechanisms in the placenta. Of the various components of the placental barrier, the one that is most likely involved with the mechanism of regulation is the syncytium.

The trophoblast resembles the hepatic parenchyma in its wide range of both anabolic and catabolic activities. For example, it has been shown that placental tissue can synthesize fatty acids and steroids from acetate or pyruvic acid. It performs conversions of substrate; for example, andogens are converted to estrogens and glucose to fructose. It is not surprising that the placenta exhibits great biochemical complexity, since it performs the multiple functions usually associated with the lungs, kidneys, anterior pituitary, ovaries, liver, and intestinal mucosa of the adult organism.

The placenta is a multipotential endocrine gland that can perform some of the functions of the anterior pituitary and ovary. In some species, including humans, the ovaries can be removed quite early in pregnancy without affecting its course; the placental steroids maintain an appropriate gestational environment. Three protein placental hormones mimic certain functions of the adult pituitary, human chorionic gonadotrophin (HCG), human chorionic somatomammotropin (HCS), and human chorionic thyrotropin (HCT). HCG is a glycoprotein hormone with inherent FSH and LH activities; although its full role remains to be defined, HCG stimulates initial production of estrogen and progesterone by the corpus luteum of early pregnancy. HCS [also known as human placental lactogen, (HPL)] is a single polypeptide chain that is remarkably similar to human growth hormone (HGH) in molecular weight and in the number and sequence of amino acids. Both HGH and HCS have growth-promoting and lactogenic, as well as metabolic, effects, which has led to the suggestion that HCS is the growth hormone of pregnancy. The placenta has all the enzymatic machinery needed to

synthesize progesterone from acetate or cholesterol but lacks two enzymes needed for estrogen synthesis; however, these are present in the fetal adrenal and possibly the fetal liver. Estrogen is therefore synthesized by the integrated endocrine activity of the *feto-placental unit*. The concept of the feto-placental unit was introduced in 1962 by Diczfalusy who defined it as follows: "the fetus and placenta form a functional unit to carry out biosynthetic reactions together, which the placenta *per se* or the fetus *per se* are incapable of completing."

Immunocytochemical procedures have shown that HCG and HCS are localized almost exclusively in the syncytiotrophoblast of the placenta. Thus, there is a strong possibility that the syncytium is the site of synthesis of both of these protein hormones, although available evidence indicates that the basal cytotrophoblast should still be considered as a possible site of origin. Demonstration of the presence of HCG in the rough endoplasmic reticulum of the syncytium provides evidence that it is synthesized there (Dreskin et al., 1970). Most investigators believe that the syncytiotrophoblast is also the site of synthesis of progesterone and estrogen. The occurrence in the syncytium of the special lipid droplets and mitochondria with tubular cristae, which are characteristic of steroid-synthesizing cells of the gonads and adrenals, as well as the presence of Δ^5-3β-hydroxysteroid dehydrogenase, supports this possibility. A troublesome ultrastructural point, however, is the relatively inconspicuous smooth ER in the syncytium; this organelle is characteristically abundant in other steroid-synthesizing cells, such as those of the gonads and adrenal. Cytochemical evidence thus suggests that the syncytiotrophoblast may be capable of synthesizing not only protein but steroid hormones as well, and this unique possibility deserves further exploration. Moreover, these endocrine synthetic mechanisms in the trophoblast endow the fetus with a certain capacity for autonomous control of the gestational milieu. The extraordinary autonomy of the placenta is well expressed in the following quotation. "The placenta is a unique organ—an allograft resistant to immunological destruction and functioning to a large extent autonomously, independent of homeostatic regulatory mechanisms in the mother."[2]

---

[2] J. Ginsburg, *Ann. Rev. Pharmacol.*, **11**:387, 1971.

Biologists have considered the placenta as a major factor in the forces which initiate birth. It has been suggested that the placenta undergoes age changes as gestation proceeds. The principal morphologic age changes in the human placenta are the accumulation of fibrin and fibrinoid and the hyalinization of the syncytium (Figs. 25-28 and 25-31) (see review by Wislocki, 1956). However, it is not at all certain that these changes limit placental function. There is some evidence of waning physiologic activity near term, but on the whole it has been difficult to pinpoint the functional changes as being related to senescence. As fetal organs differentiate and acquire their characteristic functions, it is possible that the placenta may relinquish some of its activities. However, interrelations between placental differentiation and fetal differentiation are incompletely defined. The concept of the feto-placental unit, which rests primarily, so far, on evidence related to steroid metabolism, is an important step in this direction. The life-span of the human placenta is normally less than 266 days. Thus the placenta provides an interesting model for studying differentiation, since kaleidoscopic changes in morphology, function, and chemical composition occur in a relatively short time.

UMBILICAL CORD

The human umbilical cord is a translucent, glistening, white "rope" of tissue that is fetal in origin. It extends from the umbilicus to the placenta and reaches a length of 35 to 50 cm at term. It consists of two *umbilical arteries* and one *umbilical vein* embedded in an abundant mucous connective tissue (Fig. 25-34, see color insert). It is covered by an epithelium which is initially single-layered and becomes stratified late in gestation. In transverse sections, the arteries usually appear constricted, whereas the vein is generally open. The umbilical cord and its peculiar blood vessels usually exhibit torsion; there is an average of 11 spiral turns, with the number being proportional to the length of the cord. From the umbilicus to the placenta, the caliber of the blood vessels increases, but the vein normally remains larger than the arteries.

Mucous connective tissue is highly characteristic of the umbilical cord. In this specialized stroma, the ground substance is unusually abundant. This slippery, gelatinous material, rich in mucopolysaccharide, is also called *Wharton's jelly*. It fills the relatively large intercellular spaces that are located among the interlacing bundles of collagenous fibers. The intense metachromasia of Wharton's jelly suggests the presence of sulfated polysaccharide (Fig. 25-34; see color insert). Collagen fibers are plentiful, but elastic and reticular fibers are scarce except in the umbilical vessels. The cells of this connective tissue are a primitive form of fibroblast, which are stellate in shape in collapsed cord and elongate in distended cord. They resemble fibroblasts ultrastructurally but have usually thick bundles of microfilaments (Parry, 1970). In routine preparations, the outlines of these cells are difficult to recognize, and only their nuclei are evident. Like many other embryonic cells, they have a rich store of glycogen. Fetal autonomic nerve fibers occur in the cord, but their terminations have not been determined.

The *umbilical arteries* are peculiar in their structure. Their relatively thick muscular walls are heavily impregnated with metachromatic ground substance. Unlike muscular arteries elsewhere, they do not have an elastica interna. Instead, their walls contain a diffuse network of elastic fibers which is especially dense beneath the intima. The arteries have a thick muscular coat, but there is lack of agreement about the arrangement and number of layers of smooth muscle fibers. There is no elastica externa, and the tunica adventitia is replaced by mucous connective tissue.

The wall of the *umbilical vein* is quite muscular, being composed of intermingled longitudinal, oblique, and circular smooth muscle fibers. Its elastic component is less conspicuous than that of the umbilical arteries; elastic fibers are limited to an elastica interna which is a primary feature used to distinguish the vein from the arteries. The smooth muscle cells of both umbilical arteries and vein are rich in glycogen.

The human umbilical cord is a derivative of the body stalk (Fig. 25-11), which is considered to be the homolog of the allantoic mesoderm. The endodermal component of the allantois extends the entire length of the cord as a slender epithelial tube. At birth, however, it is represented by only a strand of epithelial cells in the vicinity of the umbilicus. In addition, the stalk of the yolk sac, surrounded by an extension of the body cavity, occurs in the umbilical cord in early development. This stalk contains the endodermal vitelline duct and the vitelline vessels enclosed in a slender strand of mesoderm. The loop of intestine from which the yolk stalk originates may also extend into the cord; ordinarily it is retracted into the abdomen by the time of birth; if it is not, umbilical hernia results. Usually the stalk of the yolk sac and its vitelline vessels, together with the coelom of the cord, have been obliterated some time before birth, so that no traces of them remain in the cord.

REFERENCES

AHERNE, W., and M. S. DUNNILL: Morphometry of the Human Placenta, *Br. Med. Bull.,* **22:**5 (1966).

AMOROSO, E. C.: Placentation, in A. S. Parkes (ed.), ''Marshall's Physiology of Reproduction,'' vol. 2, chap. 15, Longmans, Green & Co., Ltd., London, 1952.

ATKINSON, L. E., J. HOTCHKISS, G. R. FRITZ, A. H. SURVE, J. D. Neill, and E. KNOBIL: Circulating Levels of Steroids and Chorionic Gonadotropin During Pregnancy in the Rhesus Monkey, with Special Attention to the Rescue of the Corpus Luteum in Early Pregnancy, *Biol. Reprod.,* **12:**335 (1975).

BLANDAU, R. J. (ed.): ''The Biology of the Blastocyst,'' The University of Chicago Press, Chicago, 1971.

BOYD, J. D., and W. J. HAMILTON: ''The Human Placenta,'' W. Heffer & Sons, Ltd., Cambridge, England, 1970.

CRAWFORD, J. M.: Vascular Anatomy of the Human Placenta, *Am. J. Obstet. Gynecol.,* **84:**1543 (1962).

DAWES, G. S.: ''Foetal and Neonatal Physiology,'' Year Book Medical Publishers, Inc., Chicago, 1968.

DICZFALUSY, E.: Endocrine Functions of the Human Fetus and Placenta, *Am. J. Obstet. Gynecol.,* **119:**419 (1974).

DRESKIN, R. B., S. S. SPICER, and W. B. GREENE: Ultrastructural Localization of Chorionic Gonadotropin in Human Term Placenta, *J. Histochem. Cytochem.,* **18:**862 (1970).

EDWARDS, R. G., C. W. S. HOWE, and M. H. JOHNSON (eds.). ''Immunobiology of Trophoblast,'' Cambridge University Press, England, 1975.

ENDERS, A. C.: Formation of the Syncytium from Cytotrophoblast in the Human Placenta, *Obstet. Gynecol.,* **25:**378 (1965).

ENDERS, A. C.: Fine Structure of Anchoring Villi of the Human Placenta, *Am. J. Anat.,* **122:**419 (1968).

ENDERS, A. C., and S. J. SCHLAFKE: Cytolgical Aspects of Trophoblast-Uterine Interaction in Early Implantation, *Am. J. Anat.,* **125:**1 (1969).

ENDERS, A. C., and B. F. KING: The Cytology of Hofbauer Cells, *Anat. Rec.,* **167:**231 (1970).

FINN, C. A.: The Biology of Decidual Cells, *Adv. Reprod. Physiol.,* **5:**1 (1971).

FREESE, U. E.: Vascular Relations of Placental Exchange Areas In Primates and Man, in L. Longo and H. Bartels (eds.), ''Respiratory Gas Exchange and Blood Flow in Placenta,'' Department of Health, Education and Welfare Publication (NIH) 73-361 (1974).

GROSSER, O.: ''Früenentwicklung, Eihautbildung und Plazentation des Menschen und der Saügetiere,'' Bergmann, Munich, 1927.

HARRIS, J. W. S., and E. M. RAMSEY: The Morphology of Human Uteroplacental Vasculature, *Contrib. Embryol.,* **38:**45 (1966).

HERTIG, A. T., J. ROCK, and E. C. ADAMS: A Description of 34 Human Ova Within the First 17 Days of Development, *Am. J. Anat.,* **98:**435 (1956).

LOBEL, B. L., H. W. DEANE, and S. L. ROMNEY: Enzymic Histochemistry of the Villous Portion of the Human Placenta from Six Weeks of Gestation to Term, *Am. J. Obstet. Gynecol.,* **83:**295 (1962).

MARTIN, B. J., and S. S. SPICER: Multivesicular Bodies and Related Structures of the Syncytiotrophoblast of Human Term Placenta, *Anat. Rec.,* **175:**15 (1973).

MARTIN, C. B., JR., and E. M. RAMSEY: Gross Anatomy of the Placenta of Rhesus Monkeys, *Obstet. Gynecol.,* **36:**167 (1970).

MIDGLEY, A. R., JR., G. B. PIERCE, JR., G. A. DENEAU, and J. R. G. GOSLING: Morphogenesis of Syncytio-trophoblast in Vivo: an Autoradiographic Demonstration, *Science,* **141:**349 (1963).

MOSSMAN, H. W.: Comparative Morphogenesis of the Foetal Membranes and Accessory Uterine Structures, *Carnegie Inst. Contrib. Embryol.,* **26:**129 (1937).

O'RAHILLY, R.: Developmental Stages in Human Embryos. Part A. Embryos of the First Three Weeks (Stages 1–9), *Carnegie Institute,* Publication 631, 1973.

PARRY, E. W.: Some Electron Microscope Observations in the Mesenchymal Structures of Full Term Umbilical Cord, *J. Anat.,* **107:**505 (1970).

RAMSEY, E. M.: Placental Vasculature and Circulation, in R. O. Greep (ed.), "Handbook of Physiology," vol. 3, pt. 2, sec. 7, chap. 47, American Physiological Society, Washington, D.C., 1973.

STEPTOE, P. C., R. G. EDWARDS, and J. M. PURDY: Human Blastocysts Grown in Culture, *Nature (Lond.),* **229:**132 (1971).

STEVEN, D. H. (ed): "Comparative Placentation, Essays in Structure and Function," Academic Press, New York, 1975.

TEKELIOGLU-UYSAL, M., R. G. EDWARDS, and H. KISMISCI: Ultrastructural Relationships Between Decidua, Trophoblast, and Lymphocytes at the Beginning of Human Pregnancy, *J. Reprod. Fertil.,* **42:**431 (1975).

WILKIN, P.: Organogenesis of the Human Placenta, in R. L. DeHaan and H. Ursprung (eds.), "Organo-genesis," chap. 30, Holt, Rinehart and Winston, Inc., New York, 1965.

WISLOCKI, G. B.: Morphological Aspects of Ageing in the Placenta, *Ciba Found. Colloq. Ageing,* **2:**105 (1956).

WISLOCKI, G. B., and H. S. BENNETT: Histology and Cytology of the Human and Monkey Placenta, with Special Reference to the Trophoblast, *Am. J. Anat.,* **73:**335 (1943).

WISLOCKI, G. B., and H. A. PADYKULA: Histochemistry and Electron Microscopy of the Placenta, in W. C. Young (ed.), "Sex and Internal Secretions," 3d ed., vol. 2, chap. 15, The Williams & Wilkins Company, Baltimore, 1961.

WYNN, R. M.: Fine Structure of the Placenta, in R. O. Greep (ed.), "Handbook of Physiology," vol. II, pt. 2, sec. 7, chap. 42, American Physiological Society, Washington, D.C., 1973.

The Male Reproductive System

MARTIN DYM

GENERAL FEATURES

The male reproductive system (Fig. 26-1) consists of the primary sex organs, the two testes, and a set of accessory sexual structures. The testes function both as an exocrine gland that produces the male germ cells and an endocrine gland that produces the male sex hormone, testosterone. This hormone is responsible for germ-cell production, growth and function of the accessory male sex organs, and the development of other attributes of masculinity, such as beard, deep voice, and strong musculature. The accessory sexual organs include: (1) the copulatory organ, the penis; (2) a complicated set of tubules which lead from the testes to the penis; and (3) an associated group of glands, referred to as the male accessory glands, that contribute fluid secretions to the semen upon ejaculation. In the adult human male, each testis is an ovoid organ weighing approximately 12 g. Its average dimensions are 4.5 cm in length, 2.5 cm in breadth, and 3 cm in the anteroposterior diameter. The testes are suspended in the scrotum and are invested anteriorly and laterally by a serous cavity, the tunica vaginalis, derived from the peritoneum (Fig. 26-2).

Immediately deep to the tunica vaginalis, the testis is covered with a thick fibrous capsule, the tunica albuginea. The inner aspect of the tunica albuginea, the tunica vasculosa, consists of loose connective tissue and contains the large blood vessels of the testis. At the posterior margin of the testis, the tunica albuginea thickens and is projected into the interior of the gland as the mediastinum testis. Ducts, blood vessels, lymphatics, and nerves enter or leave the testis through the mediastinum.

From the mediastinum, delicate connective-tissue septa pass into the interior of the organ subdividing it into about 250 lobules. Each testicular lobule contains one to four sperm-producing, convoluted seminiferous tubules. The connective tissue spaces occupying the intervals between the seminiferous tubules are filled with the blood vessels, lymphatics, nerves, macrophages, fibrocytes, lymphocytes, and Leydig cells—the endocrine cells responsible for testosterone production.

The seminiferous tubules form coiled loops that empty at both ends into the rete testis, a series of epithelial-lined channels within the mediastinum. Spermatozoa and testicular fluid produced within the tubules pass into the ductuli efferentes and epididymis via the rete testis (Fig. 26-3). Anastomoses and branching of the seminiferous tubules are common in man.

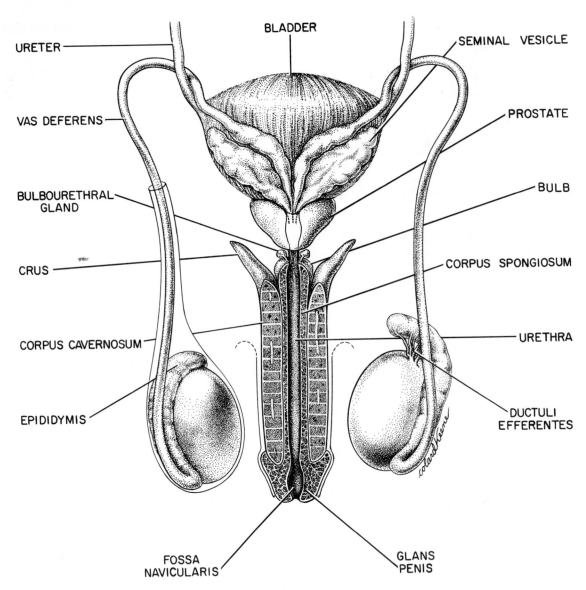

URETER

BLADDER

SEMINAL VESICLE

VAS DEFERENS

PROSTATE

BULBOURETHRAL GLAND

BULB

CRUS

CORPUS SPONGIOSUM

CORPUS CAVERNOSUM

URETHRA

EPIDIDYMIS

DUCTULI EFFERENTES

FOSSA NAVICULARIS

GLANS PENIS

FIGURE 26-1 Posterior view of the human male reproductive system.

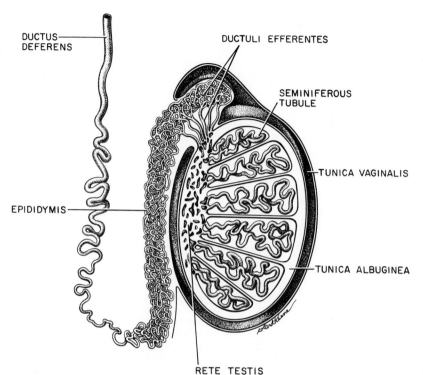

DUCTUS DEFERENS

DUCTULI EFFERENTES

SEMINIFEROUS TUBULE

TUNICA VAGINALIS

EPIDIDYMIS

TUNICA ALBUGINEA

RETE TESTIS

FIGURE 26-2 Diagram demonstrating the seminiferous tubules and the excurrent duct system of the human testis.

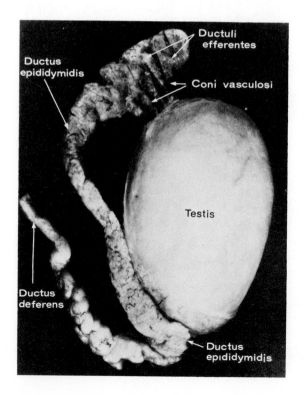

Ductuli efferentes

Ductus epididymidis

Coni vasculosi

Testis

Ductus deferens

Ductus epididymidis

FIGURE 26-3 Photomicrograph of a human testis and its excurrent duct system. ×1.35. (Courtesy of A. F. Holstein.)

Occasionally the tubules may terminate blindly at one end. Uncoiled, each seminiferous tubule can measure up to 80 cm in length and 150 to 250 μm in width. In man, the combined length of the tubules in one testis is approximately 255 m.

VASCULAR AND NERVOUS CONNECTIONS TO THE TESTIS

It is a distinctive feature of mammals that the testicular artery becomes highly convoluted as it approaches the testis and is surrounded by the venous pampiniform plexus, a thermoregulatory device for precooling arterial blood. Some branches of the testicular artery enter the testis through the mediastinum, whereas others pass over the periphery of the testis in the tunica vasculosa. Arterioles enter the septula from both the mediastinum and the periphery. Branches leave the septula and form capillary plexuses around the con-

voluted seminiferous tubules. Veins accompany the arteries. Lymphatic vessels are numerous in the tunica albuginea and extend along the tubules. The testes have both a vasomotor and a sensory innervation. Nerves from the spermatic plexus form a net in the deeper part of the tunica albuginea and from there reach the walls of the tubules and the Leydig cells. The blood vessels and nerves do not penetrate into the seminiferous epithelium.

BOUNDARY LAYERS OF THE SEMINIFEROUS TUBULES

The seminiferous tubules of common laboratory rodents are bounded by a constant number of clearly defined cellular and acellular layers (Fig. 26-4). Adjacent to the seminiferous epithelium is its basal lam-

FIGURE 26-4 Electron micrograph of the rat's tunica propria. Deep to the basal lamina, collagen fibrils are seen in transverse section. The myoid cells (peritubular contractile cells) are characterized by densely packed filaments and pinocytotic vesicles. Note the endothelium of a lymphatic sinusoid adjacent to the external glycoprotein coat of the myoid cell. ×27,270. (From M. Dym and D. W. Fawcett, Biol. Reprod., **3**:308–326, 1970.)

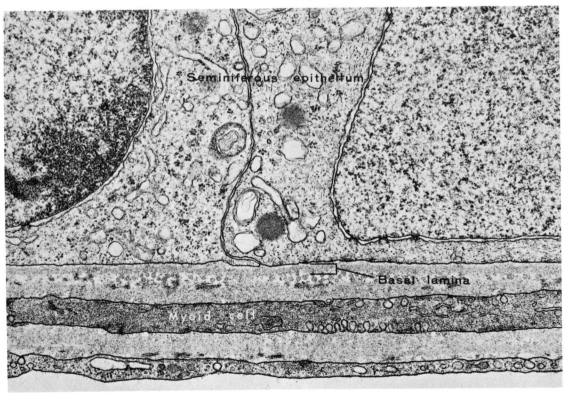

ina. Outside this is a clear zone containing fibrils of varying orientation. Peripheral to the thin collagenous reticulum is a layer of flattened cells, the myoid cells, followed by a layer containing lymphatic endothelial cells. Collectively, the structures surrounding the epithelium may be referred to as the tunica propria or the limiting membrane. In monkeys and humans, the seminiferous tubules are ensheathed by a basal lamina adjacent to which are found collagen fibrils and multiple layers (three to five) of flattened myoid cells (Fig. 26-5). The myoid cells (peritubular contractile cells) contain many extremely fine cytoplasmic filaments believed to be actin and therefore contractile. Recent work has demonstrated that these filaments will combine with heavy meromyosin.

Individual seminiferous tubules are known to contract in vitro and it is likely that the myoid cells are responsible for these rhythmic movements. In addition to maintaining the integrity of the seminiferous epithelium, the myoid cells may assist in the propulsive movements of sperm and testicular fluid from the seminiferous tubules to the rete testis. In many instances of male infertility the boundary layers of the tubules become greatly thickened.

SEMINIFEROUS EPITHELIUM

The seminiferous tubules are lined by a highly complex and specialized stratified epithelium, termed the

FIGURE 26-5 Electron micrograph of the myoid cells surrounding a human seminiferous tubule. ×20,000. (Courtesy of M. H. Ross).

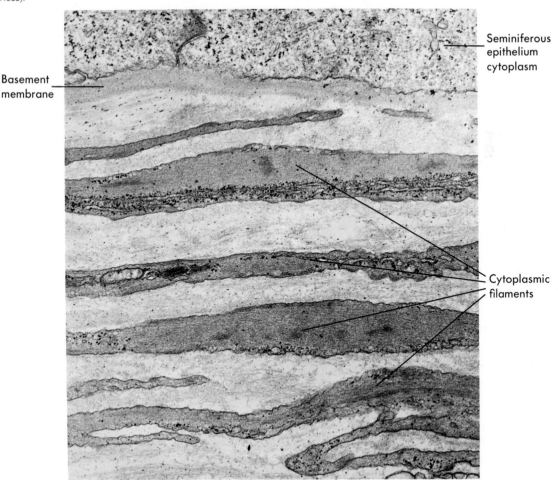

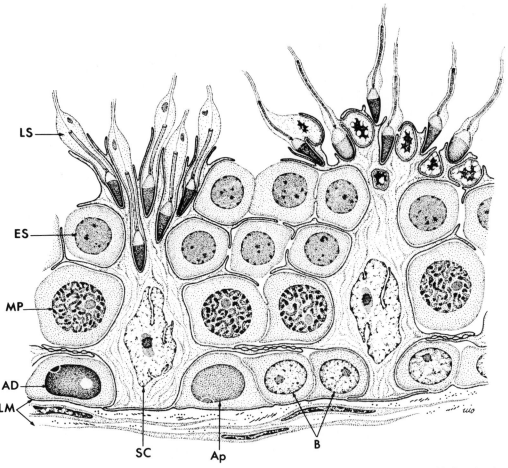

FIGURE 26-6 A drawing of the seminiferous epithelium showing the relation of the Sertoli cells and germ cells. Middle pachytene spermatocytes (MP); early spermatids (ES); late spermatids (LS); A dark spermatogonium (AD); A pale spermatogonium (AP); limiting membrane (LM); Sertoli cell (SC); B spermatogonia (B). (Courtesy of Y. Clermont).

seminiferous or germinal epithelium. In the adult, this epithelium is composed of two populations of cells: (1) a nonproliferating population of supporting cells, the Sertoli cells; and (2) a proliferative population of germ cells that migrates continuously from the periphery of the tubule to the luminal free surface. The germinal elements consist of successive generations of cells arranged in well-defined concentric layers within the epithelium. These include, from the periphery

to the lumen of the tubule, spermatogonia, spermatocytes, and immature and mature spermatids (Figs. 26-6 and 26-7).

FIGURE 26-7 A schematic drawing of the six stages (cell associations) of the cycle of the seminiferous epithelium in man. Sertoli cell, Ser; dark and pale type A spermatogonia, Ad and Ap; type B spermatogonia, B; preleptotene spermatocyte, Pl; leptotene spermatocyte, L; zygotene spermatocyte, Z; pachytene spermatocyte, P; primary spermatocyte in division, Im; secondary spermatocyte, II; spermatids in various steps of differentiation, Sa, Sb, Sc, Sd; residual bodies, RB. (From Y. Clermont, *Am. J. Anat.,* **112**:35, 1963.)

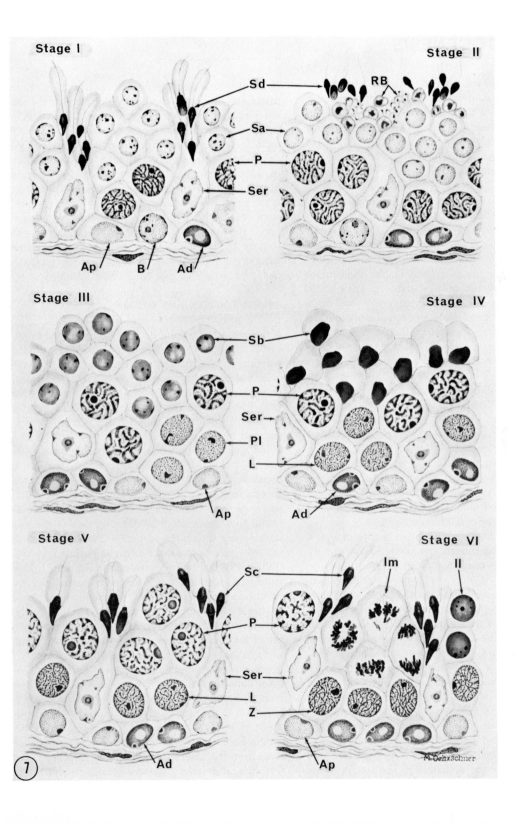

SPERMATOGENESIS

Spermatogenesis refers to the process whereby the spermatogonial stem cells at the base of the seminiferous tubules divide and differentiate to give rise ultimately to spermatozoa at the luminal free surface.

SPERMATOGONIA AND STEM-CELL RENEWAL

On the basis of nuclear staining three classes of spermatogonia have been described in men: (1) dark type A (Ad) spermatogonia; (2) pale type A (Ap) spermatogonia; (3) type B spermatogonia (Figs. 26-6 and 26-7). Generally, the spermatogonia are approximately 12 μm in diameter and border the limiting membrane of the seminiferous tubules. Their nuclei are round or slightly ovoid, approximately 6 to 7 μm in diameter, with nucleoli usually attached to the nuclear envelope. The Ad spermatogonium has a nucleus containing a deeply stained, finely granulated chromatin, while the Ap cell possesses a nucleus showing a finely granulated but pale-stained chromatin. Frequently, a large pale-staining nuclear vacuole is found within the type A dark cell. Type B spermatogonia are characterized by spherical nuclei containing large clumps of chromatin adjacent to the nuclear envelope and a centrally located nucleolus. The cytoplasm of the spermatogonia stains lightly, has a faint granular texture, and may possess a crystal of Lubarsch, approximately 1.0×7.0 μm. This inclusion is composed of closely packed parallel arrays of dense filaments interspersed with dense granules.

In rodents, four successive generations of type A spermatogonia have been described: A_1, A_2, A_3, A_4. The type A_1 cells divide by mitosis to give rise to type A_2; the type A_2 in turn yield type A_3, which finally produce type A_4 spermatogonia. Type A_4 spermatogonia divide and give rise to intermediate (In) spermatogonia which in turn yield type B cells. The latter spermatogonia (In, B) are the differentiated elements, committed to the production of spermatocytes. In addition, a group of spermatogonia is present in the seminiferous epithelium which rarely divides or have a very long cell-cycle time. These have been referred to as "reserve" stem cells (Ao).

For spermatogenesis to continue indefinitely, without exhausting the supply of spermatogonia, some type A spermatogonia must serve as stem cells and give rise to other type A stem cells. The identity of the stem cells in the seminiferous tubules has still not been fully clarified. Some investigators believe that the undifferentiated type A_4 spermatogonia serve as stem cells; others believe that the long cycling population of cells, the type Ao, are in fact the stem cells (As).

In man and monkeys, 3 h after a single injection of ^{3}H-thymidine, the type Ad spermatogonia remain unlabeled, thus indicating that they are not actively undergoing mitosis. The Ad may be the "reserve" stem cells or the long-cycling spermatogonia population in the primates and perhaps sporadically give rise to type Ap spermatogonia in order to maintain their numbers at normal levels. The type Ap spermatogonia divide by mitosis to give rise to type B cells.

SPERMATOCYTES AND MEIOSIS

Meiosis is a type of nuclear division restricted to gametes, that is, spermatocytes and oocytes, wherein the number of chromosomes characteristic of somatic cells, the diploid number (2n), is halved to the haploid number (1n). For this reason meiosis is termed a reduction division. The haploid nuclei of the gametes unite and the diploid number of chromosomes is restored in the process of fertilization. The fertilized ovum and all its descendents except the gametes divide by mitotic division, and the diploid number is therefore maintained in somatic cells. Meiosis has the second major function of providing genetic variation by the exchange of segments of homologous chromosomes and the random selection of one of the two homologues during the reduction division.

Meiosis involves two successive nuclear divisions with one division of chromosomes (Fig. 26-9). Preleptotene spermatocytes produced as a result of the mitotic divisions of the type B spermatogonia closely resemble the parent type B cells, although their nuclei are somewhat smaller. They are located at the periphery of the tubule and are frequently in direct contact with the basal lamina of the epithelium (Fig. 26-7). Soon after their formation the preleptotene spermatocytes duplicate their DNA in preparation for the first meiotic division, which reduces the number of chromosomes to the haploid condition. After the incorporation of nucleotides and other substances for DNA synthesis, the preleptotene spermatocytes migrate away from the basal lamina. The lengthy prophase of this division involves extensive rearrangement of the chromatin as the cells progress through leptotene, zygotene, pachytene, and diplotene stages.

In the leptotene stage the chromosomes are evident as thin and delicate filaments. This is followed by

zygotene, where pairing of homologous chromosomes occurs (synapsis). As the cells enter pachytene, the chromosomes become shorter and thicker and each one splits into two chromatids, attached by a centromere. There is a marked increase in nuclear and cellular volume as the cells progress through the pachytene stage. It is also at this stage that an exchange of genetic material occurs between pairs of homologous chromosomes.

During synapsis, as the homologous chromosomes pair, unusual tripartite structures become visible in the nucleus (Fig. 26-8). They are composed of

FIGURE 26-8 An electron micrograph of a rat pachytene spermatocyte. Portions of five synaptonemal complexes (A, B, C, D, and E) can be seen. Inside the sex vesicle (Sv), portions of the X and Y chromosomes are seen. (Courtesy of A. Hugenholtz.) *Inset.* Five synaptonemal complexes (A, B, C, D, and E) shown in the electron micrograph are depicted in this drawing, based on serial sectioning of the entire nucleus. Each complex represents a set of paired chromosomes, has a centromere (Ce), and is attached with both ends to the nuclear envelope. A is the longest pair of chromosomes and C and E are nucleolar- bearing (No) chromosomes. The sex vesicle (Sv) contains the cores of the X and Y chromosomes. (Courtesy of P. B. Moens.)

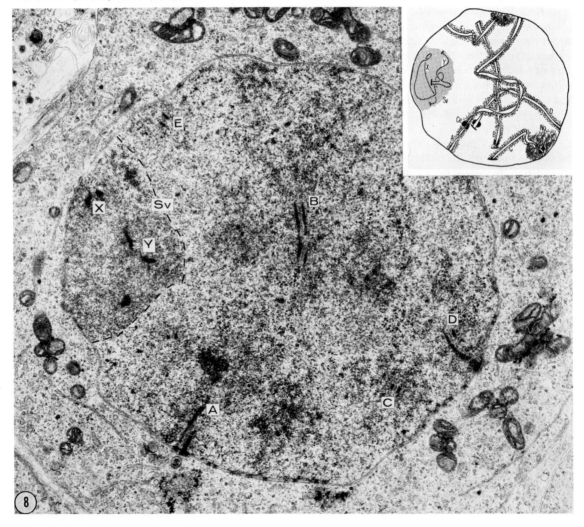

two dark parallel bands separated by a clearer interval in which a thin dense line is found. These structures are called synaptonemal complexes and are typically found in zygotene and pachytene spermatocytes. Each of the complexes actually represents a pair of homologous chromosomes and is attached at both ends to the nuclear envelope. The homologous paired chromosomes, termed a bivalent, therefore consist of four chromatids. The pachytene stage is very long, occupying about 16 days in humans; these cells are therefore visible in most cross sections of seminiferous tubules.

After the pachytene stage, the two chromosomes of each bivalent separate sufficiently to become visible (diplotene stage), but at certain points along their length they remain attached. These attachment sites are termed chiasmata. The final stage of prophase of the first meiotic division is called diakinesis. Here the chromosomes of each bivalent pair move further apart, thicken even more, and stain very deeply; the synaptonemal complexes disappear, signifying that crossover is complete.

At the end of prophase, after the dissolution of the nuclear envelope, the two bivalents (four chromatids) align themselves at the equatorial plate in metaphase I. During anaphase I the daughter chromatids of each homologue, united by their centromeres, move to opposite poles. In contrast to mitosis, the centromeres of the first meiotic division do not divide. Anaphase I and telophase I quickly follow and two new cells, namely, the secondary spermatocytes, are formed, each containing the haploid number of chromosomes.

Secondary spermatocytes (8 to 9 μm) are much smaller than primary spermatocytes and in addition to size differences may be identified in sections by their spherical nuclei containing pale-stained granular chromatin. Since they have a relatively short duration (8 h), they are infrequently found in sections of seminiferous tubules. The secondary spermatocytes quickly enter the prophase of the second maturation division without duplicating their DNA. During metaphase II, the chromosomes line up on the equatorial plane; whereas in anaphase II, the centromeres divide and each chromatid moves to the opposite pole in a manner identical to that seen in mitosis. After telophase II, the young spermatids are formed, each containing the haploid number of chromosomes (Fig. 26-9).

SPERMATIDS AND SPERMIOGENESIS

Spermiogenesis refers specifically to the differentiation of the newly formed spermatids to mature spermatids just prior to their release into the tubule lumen. The major features of this extraordinarily complex process involve elaboration of the acrosome from the Golgi

---

FIGURE 26-9 The stages of meiosis I and II shown schematically. A pair of homologous chromosomes, one dark and the other light, is followed through meiosis I. Then chromatids of a daughter cell are traced through meiosis II. The events are as follows:

Prophase I. Leptotene: The chromosomes become apparent as thin linear structures. Zygotene: Homologous chromosomes line up and pair with one another point to point (synapsis). Pachytene: With pairing completed, the chromosomes become shorter and thicker, and each longitudinally splits into chromatids, the centromere remaining single. The four chromatids of the two chromosomes constitute a bivalent. Chromatids from each of the homologous chromosomes may cross over one another, forming a chiasma. Diplotene: The chromosomes further shorten and broaden; they also coil. Homologous chromosomes begin to move apart but are held together at the chiasma. Diakinesis: The chromosomes become broader, thicker, more tightly coiled; they move further apart.

Metaphase I. The chromosomes are on the equatorial plate.

Anaphase I. The chromosomes diverge, exchanging chromosomal segments at the site of the chiasma.

Telophase I. Each chromatid pair, joined by a single centromere, lies in a daughter cell. The chromatids uncoil and lengthen to some extent.

Chromatids in the left-hand daughter cell pass through the following stages in meiosis II:

Prophase II. This stage is transient and possibly absent, since the chromatids may move directly to metaphase II.

Metaphase II. Chromatids become shorter, broader, and coiled. The centromere divides.

Anaphase II. Chromatids separate and move to opposite poles.

Telophase II. Each of the chromatids is now a daughter cell.

Thus in the course of these two divisions the four chromatids forming the bivalent of prophase I are separated, first into two daughter cells of telophase I, each containing two chromatids (4n → 2n), and then into two daughter cells again in telophase II, each containing one chromatid (2n → 1n). A total of four daughter cells is produced, each having the haploid (1n) number of chromosomes. In a male individual four sperms are produced; in a female, one ovum and three polar bodies. On fertilization the diploid (2n) number is restored.

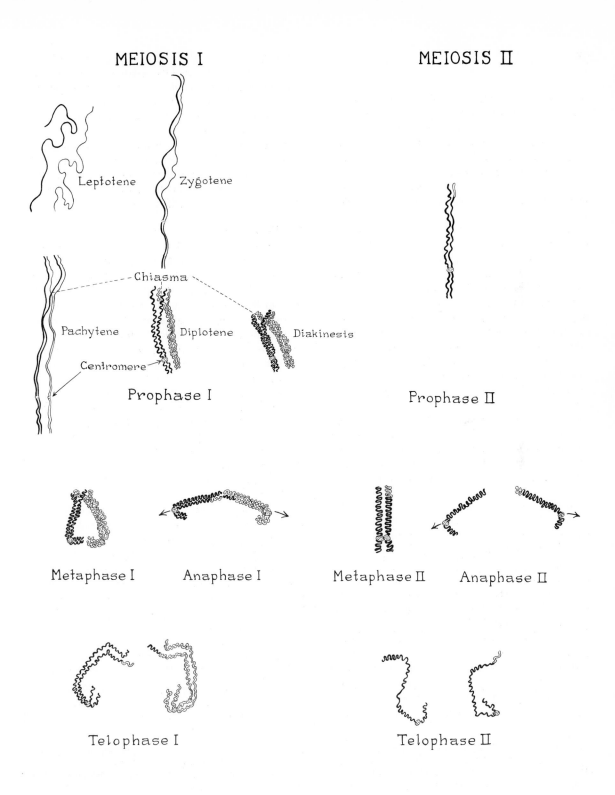

MEIOSIS I

MEIOSIS II

Leptotene Zygotene

Chiasma

Pachytene Diplotene Diakinesis

Centromere

Prophase I

Prophase II

Metaphase I Anaphase I

Metaphase II Anaphase II

Telophase I

Telophase II

apparatus, condensation and elongation of the nucleus, formation of a motile flagellum, and extensive shedding of cytoplasm. The factors responsible for these dramatic nuclear and cytoplasmic changes are still poorly understood.

It is convenient for descriptive purposes to subdivide spermiogenesis into four successive phases: Golgi, cap, acrosome, and maturation (Figs. 26-10 to 26-12).

Golgi Phase

The newly formed spermatids closely resemble the secondary spermatocytes from which they are derived although their nuclei are somewhat smaller (5 to 6 μm). The cytoplasm is pale-stained and contains a juxtanuclear Golgi complex. Perinuclear mitochondria, a pair of centrioles, free ribosomes, smooth endoplasmic reticulum, and a few lipid droplets characterize the cytoplasm. An irregularly shaped basophilic mass, the chromatid body, is also visible. An early sign of spermatid differentiation is the appearance of periodic acid Schiff positive granules in the region of the Golgi apparatus (Fig. 26-10). These proacrosomic granules, rich in glycoprotein, soon coalesce within a membrane-bounded acrosomic vesicle, containing a single large granule, the acrosomic granule, that becomes closely applied to the nuclear envelope. The acrosomic granule appears to be surrounded by the less-dense acrosomic vesicle. The vesicle and granule continue to enlarge through further contributions from the surrounding Golgi substance. There are numerous communications between the extensive smooth endoplasmic reticulum and the Golgi complex. The position of the acrosomic region on the nucleus identifies the anterior pole of the spermatid. During this phase of spermatid development, in many species, the mitochondria suddenly migrate toward the periphery of the cytoplasm to lie very close to the plasma membrane. In 1 μm sections of epon-embedded seminiferous tubules, examined with the light microscope, the spermatid plasma membrane appears thickened and somewhat irregular as a result of the close association of the mitochondria.

While the acrosomic granule and vesicle are being elaborated, the two cylindrical centrioles, situated at right angles to each other, move from a position near the nucleus to the periphery of the cell opposite the forming acrosome (Fig. 26-12). Formation of the characteristic axoneme of the sperm tail (nine peripheral doublets plus a central pair of microtubules) is initiated by the distal centriole which is now oriented perpendicular to the cell surface. The centrioles migrate back to the nucleus along the long axis of the cell without interrupting the formation of the microtubular core of the tail. The proximal centriole attaches itself to the caudal pole of the nucleus (implantation fossa) while the distal centriole continues to induce the production of the flagellum (Fig. 26-13).

Cap Phase

During this phase a head, or acrosomic, cap develops from the acrosomic vesicle and granule and spreads eventually to overlie the entire anterior one-half of the nucleus (Figs. 26-10 and 26-12). The acrosomal cap, derived through reshaping of the membrane of the acrosomal vesicle, consists of an outer and inner acrosomal membrane enclosing the acrosomal contents. Between the nuclear envelope and the inner acrosomal membrane there is the formation of a granular-filamentous material. Furthermore, in the region of the acrosome, the nuclear envelope loses its nuclear pores and appears denser, possibly because of chromatin condensation on its inner aspect. The chromatoid body migrates to the region of the centrioles and appears to surround the origin of the flagellum near the distal centriole.

Acrosome Phase

The main characteristics of this phase are the orientation of the anterior pole of the spermatid nucleus (acrosomic region) toward the base of seminiferous tubules and the elongation and condensation of the nucleus itself (Fig. 26-11). The spermatid cytoplasm is displaced toward the luminal region of the seminiferous tubules. In this manner the acrosomal region of

FIGURE 26-10 Electron micrographs of successive steps in the development of the acrosome in monkey spermatids. During early spermiogenesis (*a*) a small forming acrosomic vesicle (arrowheads) is visible in the juxtanuclear Golgi (G) region. The acrosomic granule (white asterisk) soon forms within the vesicle and both migrate to the nuclear envelope (*b*). Gradually the acrosomic vesicle (arrowheads) spreads to cap more than one-half of the nuclear surface (*c, d, e,* and *f*). The acrosomic granule appears to redistribute and form the acrosomal contents (F). Note the well-developed smooth endoplasmic reticulum (ER) and its intimate association with the Golgi complex. *a, b,* and *c,* ×11,000; *d, e,* and *f,* ×8700; *d* and *e* were slightly retouched. (From M. Pladellorens and M. Dym.)

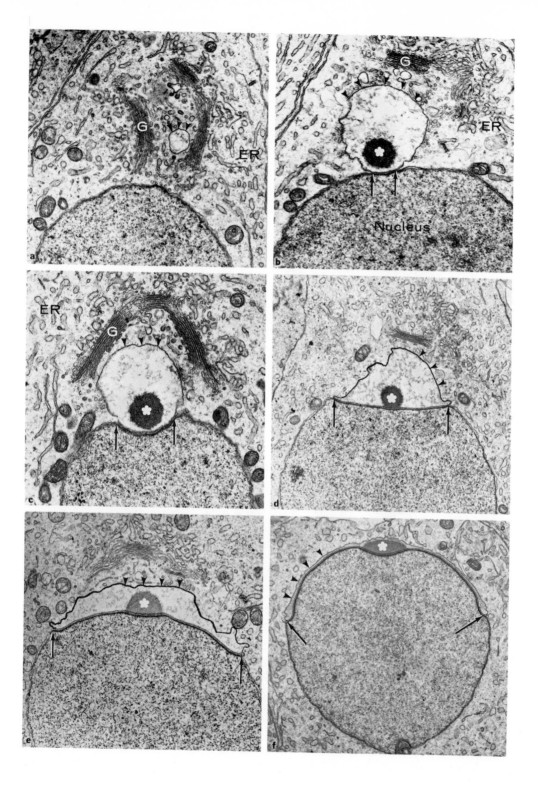

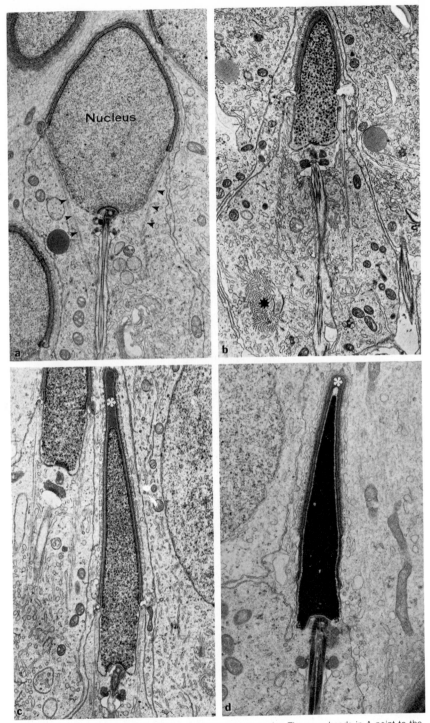

FIGURE 26-11 Nuclear condensation and elongation are demonstrated in these electron micrographs. The arrowheads in A point to the manchette. Note the unusual pattern of endoplasmic reticulum (black asterisk) in *b*. The white asterisks demonstrate the apical segment of the acrosome. *a, b, c,* and *d* approximately ×8000. (From M. Pladellorens and M. Dym.)

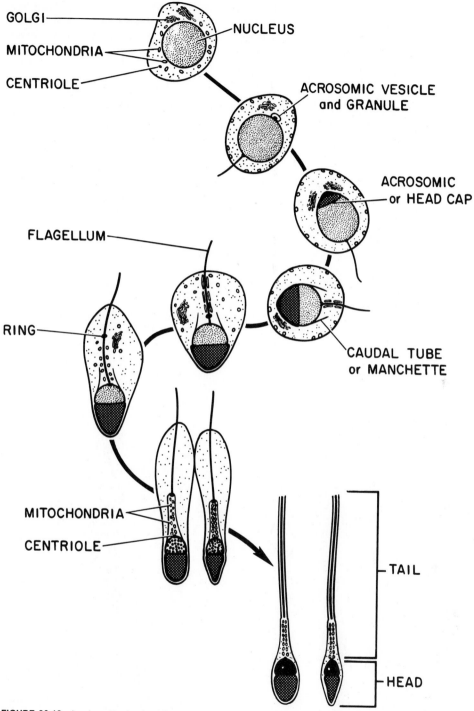

GOLGI

MITOCHONDRIA

CENTRIOLE

NUCLEUS

ACROSOMIC VESICLE and GRANULE

ACROSOMIC or HEAD CAP

FLAGELLUM

RING

CAUDAL TUBE or MANCHETTE

MITOCHONDRIA

CENTRIOLE

TAIL

HEAD

FIGURE 26-12 A schematic drawing of spermiogenesis in the human. (Modified from Clermont and Leblond, *Amer. J. Anat.,* **96:**229, 1955.)

the nucleus closely approximates the plasma membrane and the cell becomes somewhat elongated. The nuclei begin to progressively flatten and elongate while the DNA granules enlarge and become uniform in size and evenly dispersed, except for some clear spaces. These vacuoles mostly disappear, and in the final stages the nuclei assume a homogeneous appearance, stain very deeply, and are devoid of visible substructure (Fig. 26-11).

The Golgi complex detaches itself from the anterior pole of the nucleus and migrates freely in the cytoplasm when the acrosome ceases growing. At about the same time, cytoplasmic microtubules are assembled and form a cylindrical sheath that attaches itself to the caudal pole of the nucleus close to the posterior margin of the acrosome cap. This is called the manchette, or caudal, tube, the function of which remains unknown (Figs. 26-11 and 26-12).

In the region of the implantation fossa there are modifications in the centriolar apparatus which result in the formation of the neck region or connecting piece of the spermatozoa (Fig. 26-14). As the tail differentiates further, there is also the formation of nine longitudinally oriented coarse fibers along the

flagellum adjacent to the microtubules. These nine columns of dense fibers are firmly united to nine segmented columns in the connecting piece of the neck (Fig. 26-14).

The annulus, a ringlike structure near the centrioles, migrates down the flagellum. The mitochondria which up to now were dispersed in the spermatid cytoplasm line up along the coarse fibers of the flagellum from the neck region to the annulus (Fig. 26-16). This portion of the tail is called the midpiece. As the mitochondrial migration ends, the caudal tube disappears. Distal to the midpiece a fibrous sheath develops to surround the nine longitudinally oriented coarse fibers (Fig. 26-15). The plasma membrane of the spermatid follows closely the contours of the developing flagellum.

Maturation Phase

The main features of this phase are the pinching off and phagocytosis of the residual spermatid cytoplasm

FIGURE 26-13 Electron micrographs showing the early development of the spermatid tail. In *a* the centrioles have migrated to the cell surface. The distal centriole appears to induce the formation of the 9 + 2 axoneme (*b* and *c*). Finally, the proximal member of the pair of centrioles migrates to the implantation fossa (arrowheads) at the caudal pole of the nucleus (*d*). ×10,000. (From Bloom and Fawcett, "*A Textbook of Histology*," 10th ed., Saunders, Philadelphia, 1975.)

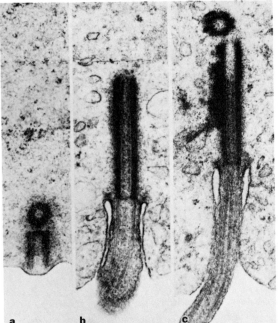

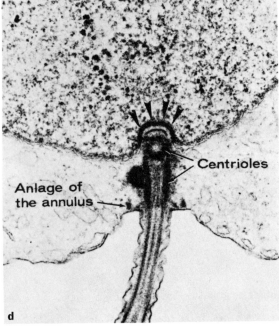

Centrioles

Anlage of
the annulus

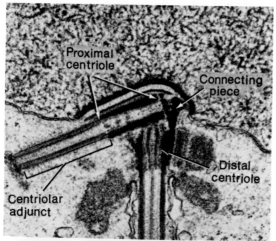

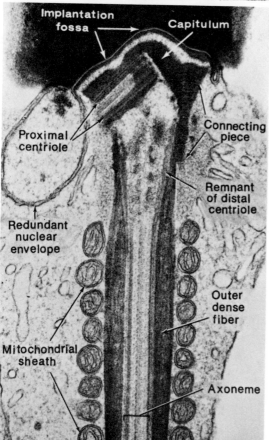

by the Sertoli cells. Finally, the Sertoli cells engineer the release of the late spermatids into the tubule lumen. In some species there may be further condensation of the nucleus and shape alterations in the acrosome during this final phase of spermiogenesis.

THE SPERMATOZOON

The mature human spermatozoon is approximately 60 μm long and may be subdivided into two major parts, the head and the tail. The principal components of the head are the acrosome and the nucleus. Segments of the tail, in order of their proximity to the head, are designated the neck, the middle piece, the principal piece, and the end piece (Figs. 26-17, 26-18, see color insert, and 26-19).

The head, which consists mostly of nucleus, has a flattened pyriform shape and is 4.5 μm long, 3.0 μm wide, and 1 μm deep. The condensed nucleus is a compact mass of chromatin that appears very dense and homogeneous in electron micrographs. The acrosome overlies the anterior two-thirds of the nucleus like a cap and contains glycoprotein and numerous lysosomal enzymes that are probably important in fertilization. In some species the acrosome projects well beyond the anterior tip of the nucleus and has a volume many times that of the nucleus. In the human, however, the acrosome is relatively small and closely follows the nuclear contours.

The neck region consists of a pair of centrioles and nine segmented columns (connecting piece) that appear to merge with the nine outer dense fibers of the rest of the tail. The middle piece, a segment about 5 to 7 μm long and a little over 1 μm thick, extends from the neck to the annulus. It contains the proximal portion of the characteristic 9 + 2 flagellum, the nine coarse fibers, and the circumferentially oriented mitochondria. The mitochondria adhere tightly to the coarse fibers and are packed very close to each other in a helical arrangement.

FIGURE 26-14 These electron micrographs demonstrate the neck region of the developing spermatids. The segmented connecting piece appears to be continuous with the outer dense fibers. During further development, the centriolar adjunct and the distal centriole disappear. A, ×14,560; B, ×20,800. (From W. Bloom and D. W. Fawcett, A Textbook of Histology, 10th ed, W. B. Saunders Co., Philadelphia, 1975.)

The principal piece, extending from the annulus nearly to the end of the tail, forms the main portion of the flagellum and is about 45 μm in length. The axoneme and the nine longitudinally oriented dense fibers are enclosed in a sheath of circumferential fibers that extend the length of the principal piece. These fibers are semicircular in shape and end on opposite sides in two longitudinal columns, which are really thickenings of the sheath. The circumferential fibers branch and anastomose. The end piece is simply the terminal segment (5 μm) of the flagellum, in which the central microtubular complex is bare.

It is well established that large clusters of similar types of germ cells differentiate simultaneously within the seminiferous tubules. This very precise synchronous development may be partially attributed to the fact that germ cells in the same step of differentiation are con-

FIGURE 26-15 Transverse and longitudinal sections through the middle piece, principal piece, and end piece of guinea pig spermatozoa. The internal core of the middle piece consists of a central pair of microtubules, the axoneme (AF), surrounded by nine peripheral pairs of microtubules and nine outer course fibers (OCF). MS, mitochondrial sheath. In the principal piece the circumferential fibers (CF) of the sheath are continuous with the apposed longitudinal columns (LC). P, plasmalemma. All similar magnifications. (Courtesy of D. W. Fawcett.)

Middle piece   Principal piece   End piece

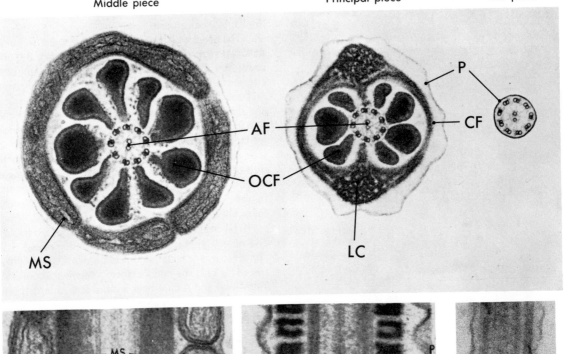
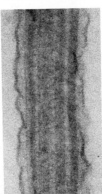

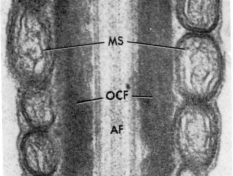
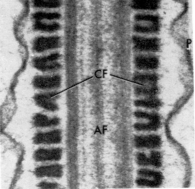

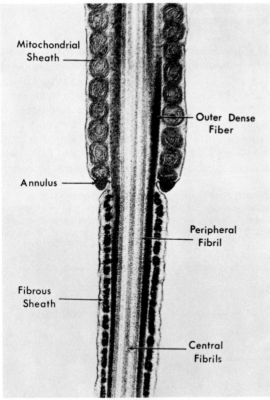

Mitochondrial
Sheath

Outer Dense
Fiber

Annulus

Peripheral
Fibril

Fibrous
Sheath

Central
Fibrils

FIGURE 26-16 An electron micrograph demonstrating the annulus at the junction of the middle and principal pieces of the spermatozoon. ×33,000. (Courtesy of D. W. Fawcett.)

nected to one another by intercellular bridges, that is, cytokinesis is incomplete. These bridges are enduring structures that persist until the late spermatids are released into the tubule lumen as free spermatozoa (Fig. 26-20).

In rodents, clusters of 16 or more type A_1 spermatogonia may be interconnected by cytoplasmic bridges. These cells divide a total of eight times during spermatogenesis, and if the progeny of all divisions remains joined, upward of 4000 spermatids might be found interconnected. These theoretical maximum numbers are in fact never achieved, since numerous germ cells degenerate during normal spermatogenesis. In the human, the clusters of synchronously developing germ cells are much smaller; therefore, far fewer germ cells are joined by cytoplasmic bridges.

The cytoplasmic bridges appear to form during mitosis as a result of incomplete cytokinesis. They are usually 2 to 3 μm in width and are locally reinforced or

stiffened by a layer of dense material on the inner or cytoplasmic surface (Fig. 26-22). Bridges are usually not evident in routine histological sections of paraffin-embedded material, but they may be seen with the light microscope in 1-μm plastic sections of material fixed and embedded for electron microscopy (Fig. 26-21). In the thinner plastic sections there is less superimposition of structure and one can utilize more effectively the resolving power of the light microscope and obtain images of surprising clarity.

The occurrence of bridges among spermatogonia has implications for stem-cell renewal in the testis. It is likely that once incomplete cytokinesis of the type A stem spermatogonia has been initiated, then all linked daughter cells must be equally commited to progressive differentiation; means that when two completely separate type A spermatogonia result from a type A mitotic division, the cells probably remain as stem cells.

CYCLE OF THE SEMINIFEROUS EPITHELIUM

Examination of the seminiferous epithelium in all mammals, including humans, reveals that the germ cells are not arranged at random but are organized into well-defined cellular associations. For instance, in a particular region of the seminiferous tubules, late spermatids at a given step in spermiogenesis occur only in specific combination with early spermatids, spermatocytes, and spermatogonia at respective steps of their development (Figs. 26-23 and 26-24). These groupings of cells succeed one another in any given area of the seminiferous tubules and the sequence repeats itself indefinitely. Each recognized cell grouping represents a stage in the cyclic process and the series of successive stages occurring between two appearances of the same cellular association, in a given area of the seminiferous tubule, is defined as the cycle of the seminiferous epithelium. The number of such stages in a cycle is constant for any given species; the rat has 14 (Fig. 26-25), the guinea pig and monkey 12, and man 6 (Fig. 26-26); the stages are designated by Roman numbers.

If it were possible to continuously examine in the living animal a portion of a seminiferous tubule, all 14 stages (in the rat) would occur in succession in that particular region, and the series (cycle) would repeat itself time after time. During the duration of one cycle, a type A_1 spermatogonium in stage VIII would evolve to a preleptotene spermatocyte in the same stage; the preleptotene cell would differentiate to a pachytene cell; the pachytene would become a step 8 spermatid and the step 8 spermatid, a step 15 spermatid. Thus, it is obvious that there are four to five successive generations of germ cells within the seminiferous epithelium and that the development of any single generation occurs concomitantly with the development of the earlier and later generations. The cells in each generation are all at precisely the same step of development.

In all mammals examined, except humans, a given cellular association occupies a relatively long length or segment of the seminiferous tubules. Each such segment corresponds to a stage of the cycle of the seminiferous epithelium and is numbered accordingly. The segments are disposed along the tubule in consecutive order to form what is termed, somewhat inaccurately, the wave of the seminiferous epithelium. Each wave consists of the complete series of segments represent-

FIGURE 26-17 Drawings of the head and neck regions of human spermatozoa. The left drawing depicts the oval outline seen in a frontal view; the right drawing is of a section perpendicular to the left one and depicts the pyriform shape of the spermatozoon. (From H. Pedersen and D. W. Fawcett, Functional Anatomy of the Human Spermatozoa, in E. S. E. Hafez (ed) "Human Semen and Fertility Regulation in the Male," Mosby, St. Louis, 1976.)

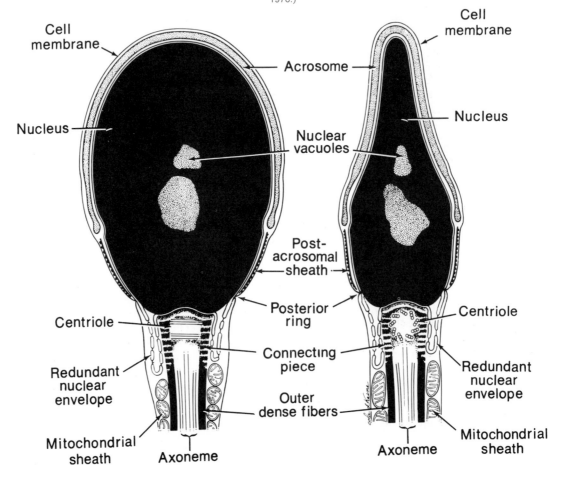

ing the recognized cellular associations for that species (Fig. 26-27). The segments are disposed distally along the seminiferous tubule in descending order and form a continuous succession of waves. Rats, for example, have an average of 12 waves per tubule. The descending order in the sequence of segments applies to both limbs of the tubular arches, reading distally from the rete testis. The continuous successions of waves in each limb meet distally near the midpoint of the arch. At this point, designated the site of reversal, the order of sequence of segments reverses. The reversal is owing to the shift in the direction of progression from distal to proximal along the tubule. At points where the seminiferous tubules branch, the continuity of the descending order is not broken.

In distinguishing between waves and cycles of the seminiferous epithelium, it is important to bear in mind that the cycle refers to changes taking place over

a period of time in a given area of the seminiferous tubule, whereas the wave refers to the distribution of different cellular associations along the length of the tubule.

The average length of each tubular segment correlates roughly with the relative duration of the corresponding cellular association or stage of the cycle. In rats, the several segments in a wave vary in average length from 0.4 to 3.2 mm, and the stages they represent vary from 6 to 63 h. However, there is no strict proportionality between segmental length and duration of the stages of the cycle. For example, in rats, segment VI has a length equal to about 2 percent of the wave, whereas the duration of stage VI is 9.2 percent of the cycle. The length of segments and waves varies considerably, but the duration of the stages and of the cycle is constant.

FIGURE 26-19 A schematic drawing of the mammalian spermatozoon, as revealed by electron microscopy, showing transverse sections at different locations along its length. (Slightly modified from W. Bloom and D. W. Fawcett, "A Textbook of Histology," 10th ed.)

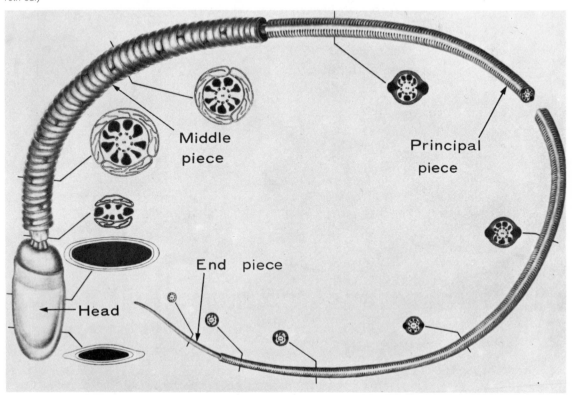

Middle piece

Principal piece

End piece

Head

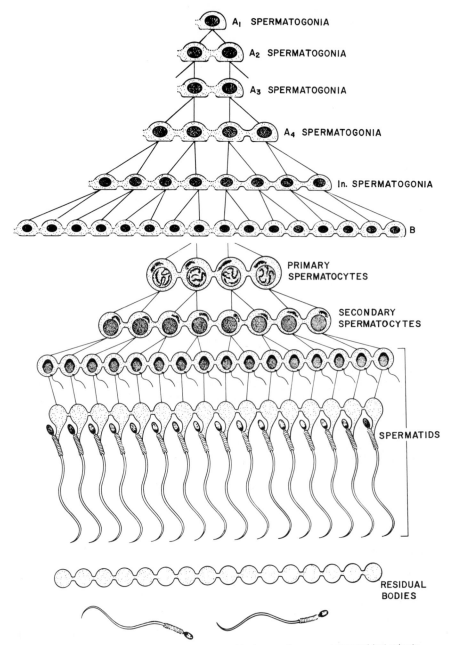

FIGURE 26-20 A model depicting intercellular bridges connecting the germ cells. Individual spermatozoa are separated just prior to their release into the tubule lumen. For the sake of simplicity, the cells are shown in linear array. (From M. Dym and D. W. Fawcett, *Biol. Reprod.,* **4:**195–215, 1971.)

In subhuman primates and in lower species a particular cell association occupies an extensive area along the length of a seminiferous tubule (up to 10 mm); therefore, any tubule cross section examined with the light microscope will usually reveal the same cellular association throughout (Fig. 26-28). In human seminiferous tubules, each cellular association occupies a very small area along the length of a seminiferous tubule. Indeed, each patchlike cellular grouping does not even extend around the circumference of the tubule; cross sections of human seminiferous tubules frequently thus reveal two to four cellular associations (Figs. 26-28 and 26-29). Humans, therefore, do not

exhibit a wave of the seminiferous epithelium. However, the fundamental pattern of the cycle of the seminiferous epithelium is as characteristic of humans as of other mammalian species.

DURATION OF SPERMATOGENESIS

Preleptotene spermatocytes are the most advanced germ cells in the human testis to incorporate tritiated thymidine in preparation for the DNA synthesis of the first meiotic division. One hour after a single injection of ^{3}H-thymidine the preleptotene spermatocytes in stage III of the cycle were labeled (Fig. 26-26). As the cells progressed through leptotene, zygotene, and pachytene stages, the pachytene spermatocytes in the same stage of the cycle demonstrated the label 16 days later. As expected, after a further 16 days, round

FIGURE 26-21 Light micrograph depicting at least eight type B spermatogonia in the rat connected by intercellular bridges. ×1200. (From M. Dym and D. W. Fawcett, *Biol. Reprod.*, **4**:195–215, 1971.)

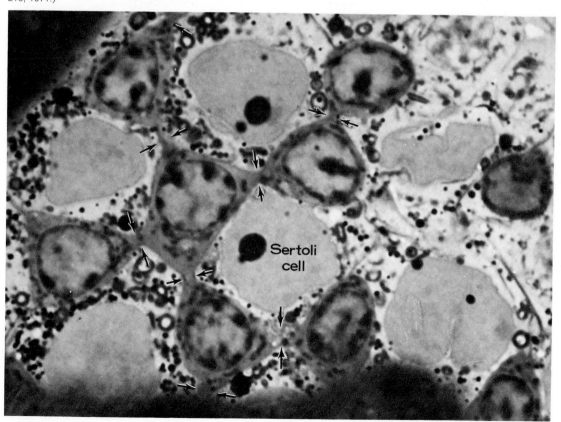

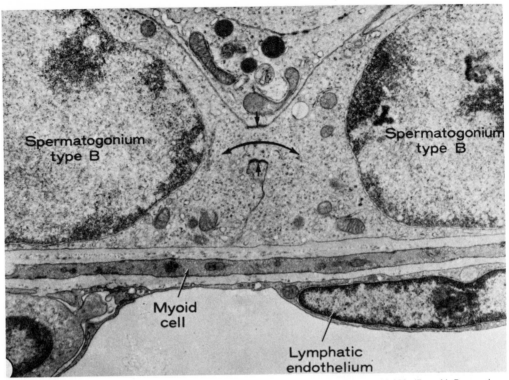

FIGURE 26-22 Electron micrograph of two type B spermatogonia connected by an intercellular bridge. ×11,000. (From M. Dym and D. W. Fawcett, *Biol. Reprod.,* **4:**195–215, 1971.)

FIGURE 26-23 and 26-24 Light micrographs of rat seminiferous tubules showing germ cells in various steps of development. The schematic drawings on the left depict the stage of the cycle of the seminiferous epithelium. ×600. (Schematic drawing taken from M. Dym and Y. Clermont, *Am. J. Anat.,* **128:**265–282, 1970.)

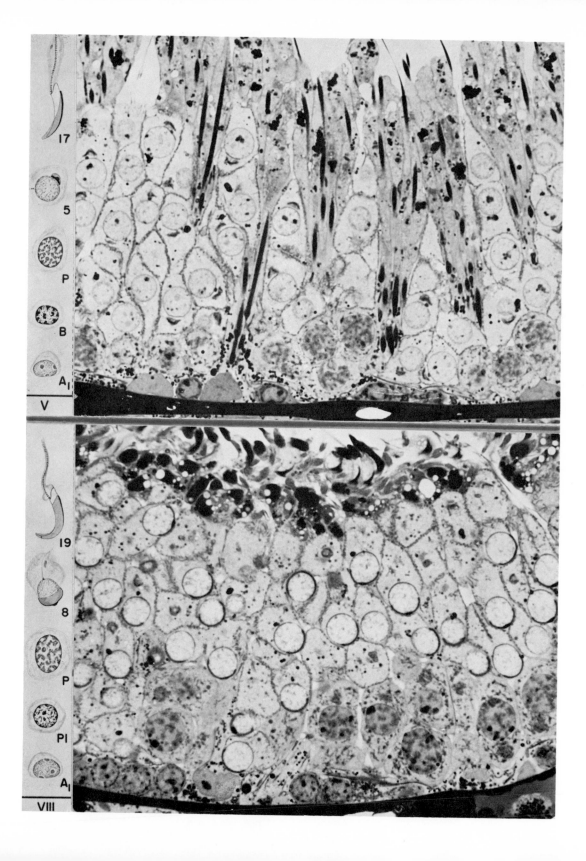

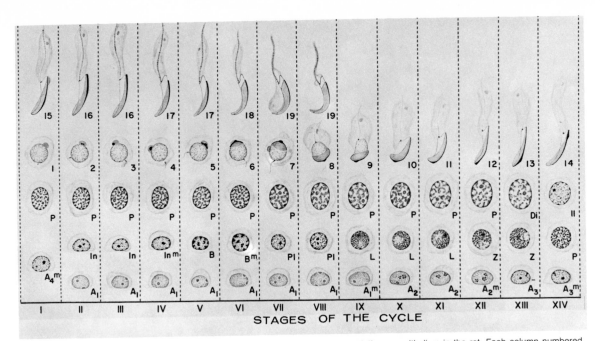

STAGES OF THE CYCLE

FIGURE 26-25 The cellular composition of the 14 stages of the cycle of the seminiferous epithelium in the rat. Each column numbered with a roman numeral shows the cell types present in one of the cellular associations found in cross sections of seminiferous tubules. The cellular associations or stages of the cycle succeed one another in time in any given area of the seminiferous epithelium in the rat. Following cellular association XIV, cellular association I reappears, so that the sequence starts over again. The stages of the cycle were identified by means of 14 of the 19 steps of spermiogenesis (numbers 1 to 19). These steps were defined by the changes observed in the nucleus and in the acrosomic structure (acrosome and head cap seen applied to the surface of the nucleus) in sections stained with the PA-Schiff-hematoxylin technique. Letters: A_1, A_2, A_3, and A_4 represent four generations of type A spermatogonia; In, intermediate spermatogonia: B, type spermatogonia; the subscript m next to a spermatogonium indicates occurrence of mitosis; P1, preleptotene spermatocyte; L, leptotene spermatocyte; Z, zygotene spermatocyte; P, pachytene spermatocyte; II, secondary spermatocyte. (From M. Dym and Y. Clermont, *Am. J. Anat.,* **128:**265–282, 1970.)

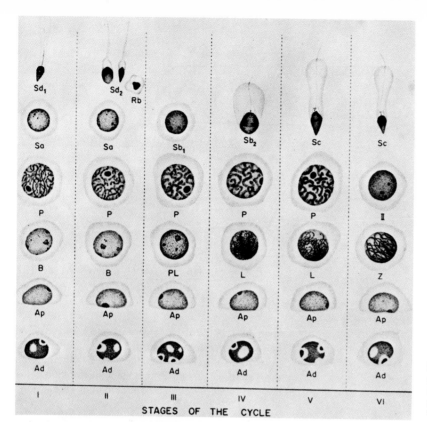

FIGURE 26-26 The six stages or cellular associations in humans. See Fig. 26-7 for a description of lettering. (Courtesy of Y. Clermont.)

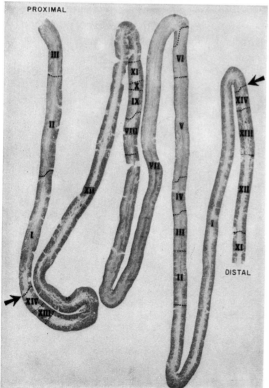

FIGURE 26-27 An isolated seminiferous tubule of rat testis, showing a wave of the seminiferous epithelium. Fourteen segments representing the 14 stages of the cycle of the seminiferous epithelium are arranged in continuous numerical and distally descending order to form a so-called wave. The limits of the wave are indicated by arrows. Note the difference in lengths of the several segments and the variability in length of segments of a given type (compare segments I, II, and XII) (From Fig 7 B. Perey, Y. Clermont, and C. P. Leblond, *Am. J. Anat.,* **108:**55, 1961.)

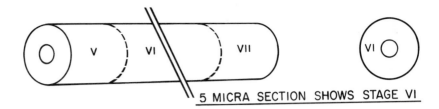

5 MICRA SECTION SHOWS STAGE VI

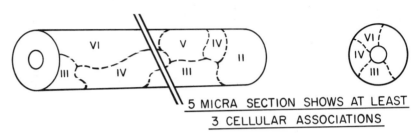

5 MICRA SECTION SHOWS AT LEAST
3 CELLULAR ASSOCIATIONS

FIGURE 26-28 Diagrammatic representation of the major difference in the organization of the seminiferous epithelium between humans (lower) and most subhuman species (upper). In humans the cell associations occupy small patchlike areas along the length of the tubule. In the subhuman species each cell association occupies a more extensive area along the length of the tubule.

FIGURE 26-29 Photomicrograph showing in a single cross section of a seminiferous tubule four different and well demarcated stages of the cycle of the seminiferous epithelium ×40. (From Y. Clermont, *Am. J. Anat.* **112**:50, 1963.)

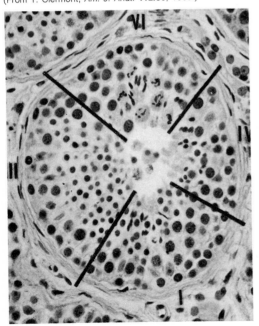

spermatids in the stage III were labeled; and finally, 16 days later, mature spermatids retained the label, just prior to their release into the tubule lumen. From these studies it was determined that the duration of the cycle in humans occupied an interval of 16 days and that the time taken for spermatogonia to evolve into spermatozoa is about 64 days. The duration of the cycle and the duration of spermatogenesis are constant and species-specific. Furthermore, it cannot be altered by hormone withdrawal or by other deleterious actions on the testis. Either the germ cells differentiate at their normal speed or they degenerate and die.

STRUCTURE AND FUNCTION OF SERTOLI CELLS

The Sertoli cells are nondividing tall columnar elements which extend from the base of the seminiferous epithelium to the tubule lumen (Fig. 26-30). This elaborate cell type consists of a narrow portion resting on the basal lamina, an intermediate portion which provides lateral processes around which the spermatocytes and spermatids are arranged, and apical projections which enclose the late spermatids, just prior to

FIGURE 26-30 Diagram illustrating the fine structure of the Sertoli cell and the cellular tight junctions separating adjacent Sertoli cells. The occluding junctions between Sertoli cells subdivide the seminiferous epithelium into two compartments: a *basal compartment* containing the spermatogonia, preleptotene and leptotene spermatocytes, and an *adluminal compartment* containing the more advanced spermatocytes and spermatids. (After M. Dym and D. W. Fawcett, *Biol. Reprod.*, **3**:308–326, 1970.)

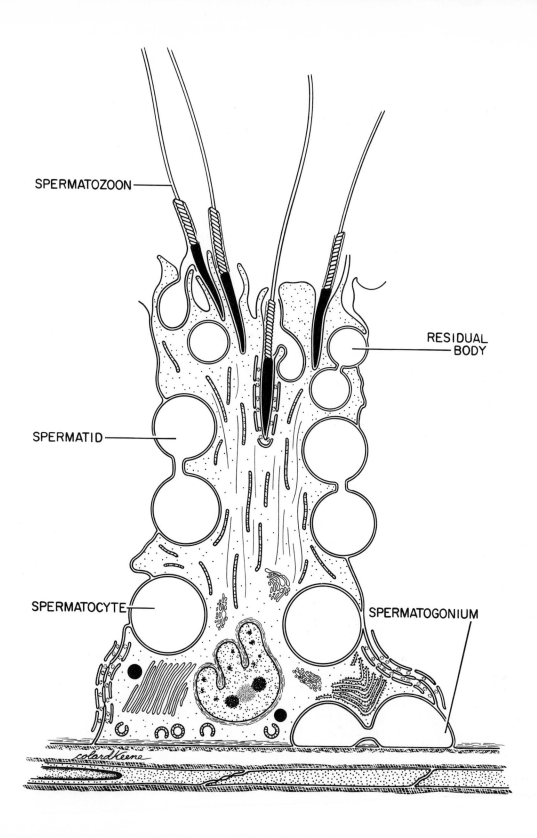

SPERMATOZOON

RESIDUAL BODY

SPERMATID

SPERMATOCYTE

SPERMATOGONIUM

colordKeene

their release into the tubule lumen. The basal portion of the cell is voluminous and is characterized by an irregularly shaped nucleus and abundant profiles of smooth endoplasmic reticulum (Fig. 26-31). Lipid droplets, thin filaments, glycogen granules, numerous spherical and elongated mitochondria exhibiting transverse cristae of orthodox lamellar configuration and a very large well-developed Golgi complex are also evident. Isolated patches of rough endoplasmic reticulum are present and occasionally several such cisternae can be found arranged circularly around a single lipid droplet. Membrane-limited bodies of various sizes, shapes, and densities, and in humans only, inclusion bodies of Charcot-Böttcher are other characteristic features of the basal cytoplasm (Fig. 26-32). The latter are irregularly shaped filamentous structures about 20 μm long and 1 μm wide. The intermediate and apical portions of the columnar Sertoli cells contain rod-shaped mitochondria and longitudinally oriented microtubules and filaments. The Sertoli cell nucleus is large and is characterized by a homogeneous nucleoplasm and a distinctive tripartite nucleolus (Fig. 26-33). A sheath of fine cytoplasmic filaments completely surrounds the Sertoli cell nucleus and separates it from other organelles. Near the base of the seminiferous epithelium, adjacent Sertoli cells are joined by tight junctions. These are frequently found overlying the spermatogonial population and early spermatocytes and are characterized by subsurface filaments, hexagonally packed, and cisternae of endoplasmic reticulum subjacent to the filaments (Fig. 26-34).

Because the germ cells develop in the microenvironment provided by the Sertoli cells, it is possible that the full control of germ-cell differentiation is mediated by the Sertoli cell. The various functions which may be ascribed to the Sertoli cell are listed below:

Support and Nutrition of Germ Cells

On the basis of shape and strategic position within the seminiferous epithelium, it has been suggested that the Sertoli cell provides nutrients for the avascular germinal epithelium. Although it is likely that the Sertoli cell transports nutrient material from the capillaries to the germ cells, no direct evidence exists for this function.

Release of Late Spermatids into the Tubule Lumen

It has been suggested that the Sertoli cells engineer the release of late spermatids into the tubule lumen. They may also be involved in the movement of germ cells from the basal lamina to the tubule lumen. Recent work has shown that the Sertoli cell filaments contain actin and are therefore probably contractile.

Steroidogenic Function

An early step in the synthesis of testosterone is the side-chain cleavage of cholesterol to form the C_{21} steroid pregnenolone (Fig. 26-35). In vitro studies on cultured Sertoli cells have demonstrated that the enzymes required for this cleavage are not present in Sertoli cells. Therefore, it may be concluded that de novo synthesis of testosterone does not occur in the Sertoli cells. On the other hand, under certain experimental conditions, the Sertoli cell is able to convert C_{21} steroids such as pregnenolone and progesterone to testosterone, but this role may not be significant in normal spermatogenesis.

Phagocytosis

It is well known that during the normal process of spermatogenesis, numerous germ cells degenerate at specific stages of the cycle of the seminiferous epithelium. In addition, as late spermatids are released into the tubule lumen, the residual cytoplasm is shed and retained within the seminiferous epithelium. The Sertoli cells effectively phagocytize these vast numbers of degenerating entities, but the mechanism by which this is accomplished remains obscure.

Secretory Function

If the ductuli efferentes are ligated in experimental animals, the testis soon swells and becomes turgid. This increase in weight and size of the organ is attributed to a continuous production of fluid by the Sertoli cells plus a lack of a normal egress route. In addition to fluid secretion, the Sertoli cells elaborate a specific protein referred to as androgen-binding protein (ABP). This protein is found within the lumen of the seminiferous tubules and proximal portion of the excurrent duct system of the testis. It appears to be under dual control of follicle-stimulating hormone (FSH) and testosterone. The role and importance of ABP is still under investigation, but it may serve as a means of concentrating testosterone within the seminiferous epithelium, thereby providing the high local concentrations necessary for spermatogenesis.

FIGURE 26-31 Electron micrograph of the basal portion of a monkey Sertoli cell. Note the filamentous zone surrounding the nucleus (arrowheads) and the abundant agranular reticulum. ×8190. (From M. Dym, *Anat. Rec.*, **175**:639–656, 1973.)

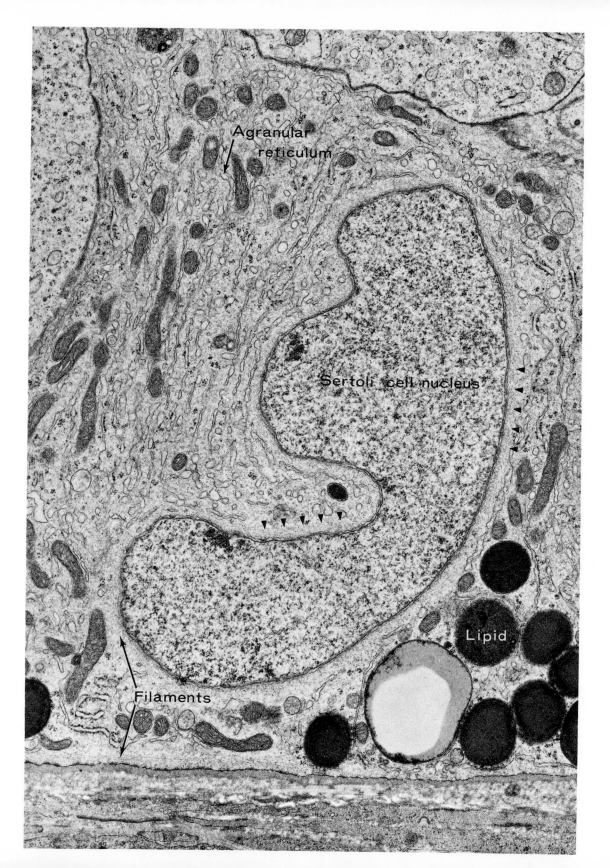

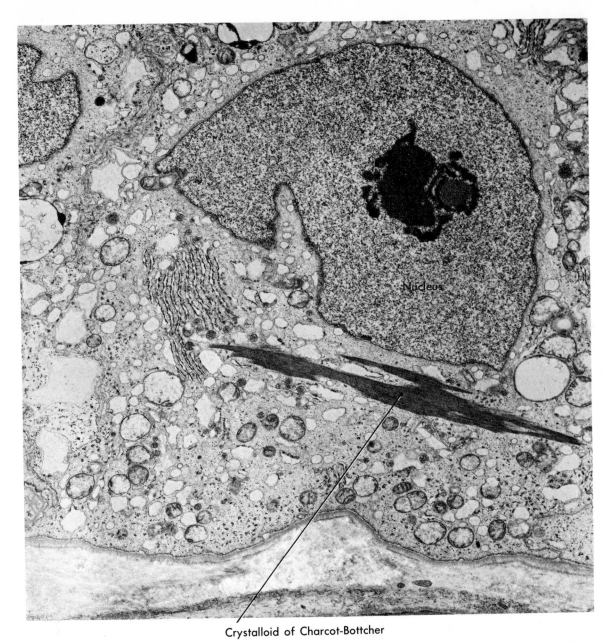

Nucleus

Crystalloid of Charcot-Bottcher

FIGURE 26-32 Electron micrograph of a human Sertoli cell. The fine structure is similar to that found in other species except for the presence of annulate lamellae and crystalloids of Charcot-Böttcher. ×10,000. (Courtesy of M. J. Rowley.)

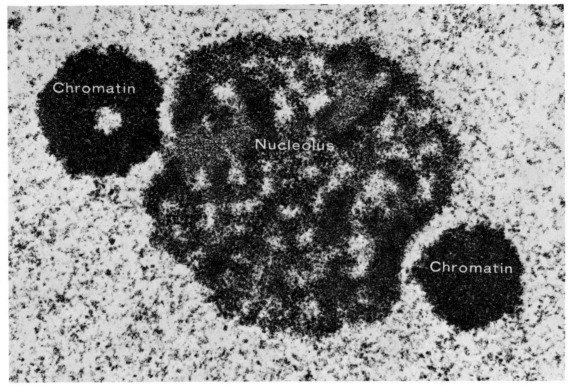

FIGURE 26-33 The tripartite nucleolar complex of Sertoli cells is depicted in this electron micrograph. The nucleolus proper is surrounded by two satellite bodies of perinucleolar chromatin. ×48,000.

FIGURE 26-34 Electron micrograph of a Sertoli-Sertoli intercellular junction. Tight junctions (arrowheads) and 90-Å "narrow" junctions (arrows) are apparent. Subsurface cisternae of endoplasmic reticulum (asterisks) are separated from the cell surface by bundles of filaments that are hexagonally arranged. ×63,000. (From M. Dym and D. W. Fawcett, *Biol. Reprod.*, **3:**308–326, 1970.)

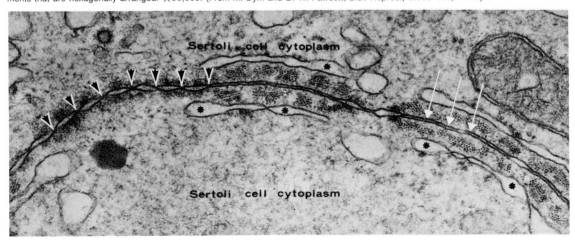

Cell-to-cell Communication

Gap junctions, exhibiting 20-Å interspaces, are located between adjacent Sertoli cells. A central pore in the junctional complex extends between the connected cells and permits ions and small molecules to pass from cell to cell. In this manner one Sertoli cell may communicate with its neighbor. This may partially explain the synchrony in the wave that is observed among adjacent segments of the seminiferous tubules.

Role of the Sertoli Cell in the Blood-Testis Barrier

Tight junctions between adjacent Sertoli cells delimit two compartments within the seminiferous epithelium (Fig. 26-30): (1) a *basal compartment* between the junctional complexes and the basal lamina containing the spermatogonia, preleptotene and leptotene spermatocytes, and (2) an *adluminal compartment* between the junctions and the tubule lumen containing the more mature spermatocytes and spermatids. Circulating plasma proteins are excluded from the lumen of the seminiferous tubules and it is likely that the Sertoli-Sertoli junctional complexes are the morphological site of the barrier (Figs. 26-36 and 37).

The subdivision of the seminiferous epithelium into two compartments may be important for a number of reasons. The germ cells in the basal compartment synthesize DNA and, as such, they have direct access to blood-borne substances associated with this process. On the other hand, soon after the spermatocytes are formed, they migrate from the basal compartment to the specialized environment of the adluminal compartment. Meiosis and spermiogenesis are processes unique to the testis, which may require the special milieu provided by the Sertoli cells. In addition, the tight junctions may permit the accumulation of high concentrations of androgen-binding protein within the epithelium. Finally, haploid germ cells contain antigens which are "foreign" to the body. The barrier may serve to isolate these proteins from the general circulation, thereby preventing an antibody response. The full biological significance of the blood-testis barrier remains to be elucidated. Certain

FIGURE 26-35 A schematic representation of the steps in the conversion of acetate to testosterone. All the enzymes are present in the microsomal fraction except for the cholesterol side-chain cleaving enzymes which are found in the mitochondria.

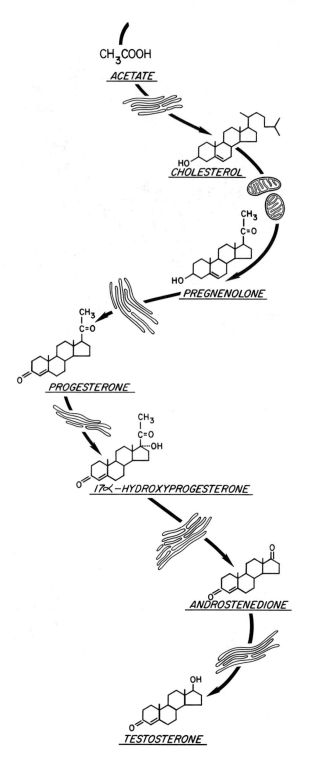

amino acids and ions are found in very high concentrations in the lumina of the seminiferous tubules, whereas cholesterol is excluded. These latter observations cannot be explained simply by the presence of junctions between Sertoli cells.

INTERSTITIAL TISSUE, LYMPHATICS, AND LEYDIG CELLS

The seminiferous tubules are bound together by the interstitial tissue which consists of loose connective

FIGURE 26-36 Light micrograph of several seminiferous tubules showing the distribution of vascularly injected horseradish peroxidase. The black reaction product is present in the interstitial tissue and surrounds the seminiferous tubules. No peroxidase is found inside the lumen of the seminiferous tubules. ×180. (From M. Dym, *Anat. Rec.,* **175:**639–656, 1973.)

tissue septa in which there are lymphatic vessels, capillaries, arterioles, venules, fibrocytes, macrophages, mast cells, lymphocytes, and Leydig cells (Fig. 26-38). In rodents the lymphatic capillaries have an unusually large lumen and lie among the tubules (Fig. 26-39). Leydig cells appear to be directly exposed to the lymph. In primates lymphatics are more typical, discrete vessels (Fig. 26-40). The interstitial lymphatics drain into those of the rete testis which, in turn, form the two or three large vessels of the spermatic cord.

The clusters of Leydig cells are located in the angular spaces among the seminiferous tubules and are frequently associated with blood vessels. These

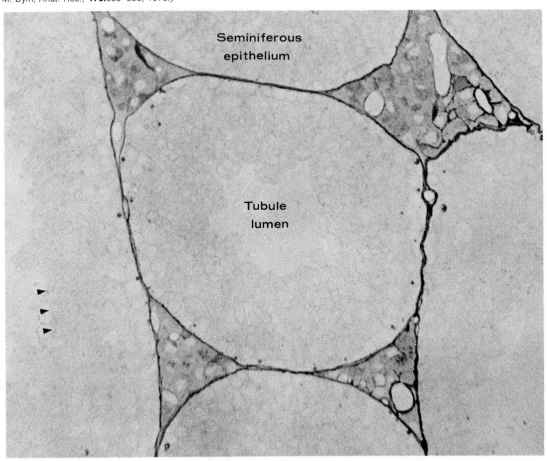

Seminiferous epithelium

Tubule lumen

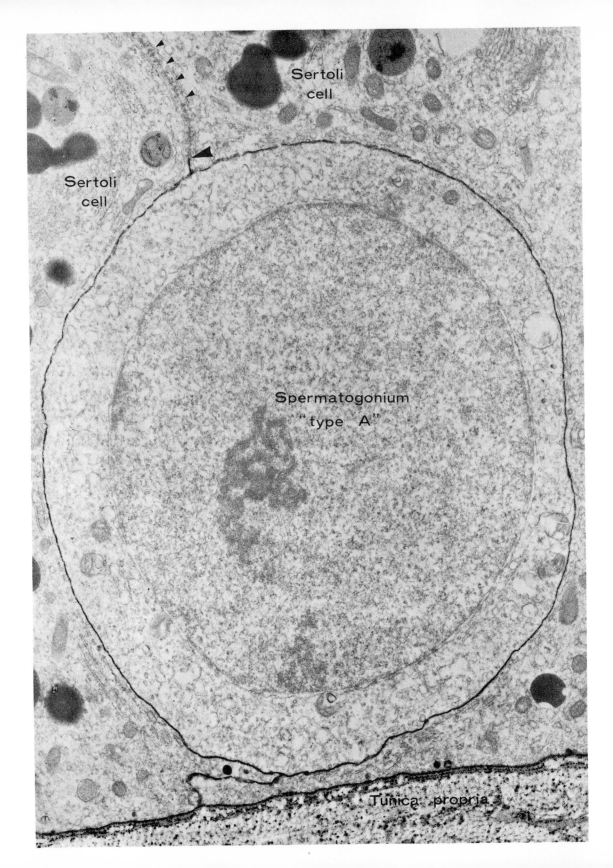

Sertoli cell

Sertoli cell

Spermatogonium "type A"

Tunica propria

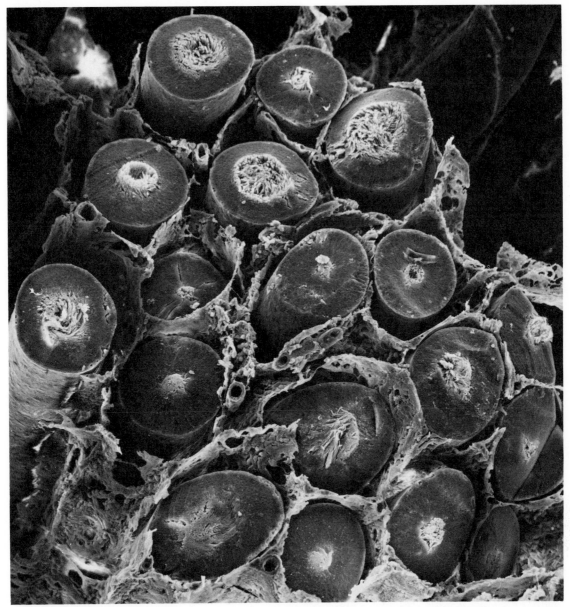

FIGURE 26-38 A scanning electron micrograph of a portion of a rat's testis showing a number of seminiferous tubules in transverse section. The interstitial tissue is seen among the tubules. ×33. (Courtesy of A. K. Christensen.)

FIGURE 26-37 An electron micrograph of a monkey spermatogonium surrounded by lanthanum nitrate. The lanthanum was perfused into the monkey's testis with the fixative. The junctional complexes between Sertoli cells (arrowheads) above the spermatogonium prevent the electron-opaque tracer from deeper penetration into the seminiferous epithelium. ×11,000. (From M. Dym, *Anat. Rec.*, **175:**639–656, 1973.)

cells have a spherical or irregularly polyhedral shape and are about 20 μm in diameter. Occasionally fusiform or elongated cells are found. The nuclei are usually rounded and the cell surface is characterized by numerous small microvilli. The most prominent cytoplasmic organelle is the abundant smooth endoplasmic reticulum (Fig. 26-41). This feature is characteristic of steroid-secreting cells. Mitochondria, patches of rough endoplasmic reticulum, a well-developed large Golgi complex, a pair of centrioles, and lipid droplets are also located within the acidophilic cytoplasm. Lipochrome pigment granules are abundant, especially in older men, and are seen as heterogeneous conglomerations of dense granules.

In humans, conspicuous cytoplasmic crystals of Reinke are characteristic features (Fig. 26-42). These are of inconstant occurrence among individuals and among the cells of a given individual. The crystals vary widely in size and form but are often rectilinear and may be 20 μm long and 3 μm thick. The angles may be sharp or rounded. The crystals are composed of macromolecules about 50Å in diameter, which being evenly spaced at about 190 Å present a highly ordered pattern of internal structure.

FIGURE 26-39 An electron micrograph of an interstitial region in the rat's testis. The close association of the Leydig cells to the blood vessels is seen. The Leydig cells appear to be directly exposed to lymph in the lymphatic sinusoids. Note the microvilli at the surface of the Leydig cells. ×3000. (Courtesy of R. Vitale.)

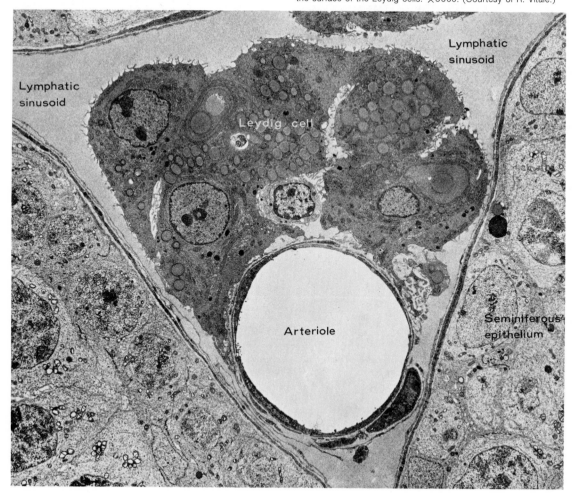

By the use of histochemical techniques, the Leydig cells have been shown to contain cholesterol, ascorbic acid, lipases, esterases, leucylamino peptidase, succinic dehydrogenase, cytochrome oxidase, and 3-B-ol dehydrogenase. Recent work has shown that the Leydig cells secrete glycoprotein for export. The Leydig cells produce testosterone from the precursor cholesterol. Most of the enzymes necessary for this conversion are located within the smooth endoplasmic reticulum, although the cholesterol side-chain cleavage enzymes are located in the mitochondria.

HORMONAL CONTROL OF SPERMATOGENESIS

In addition to producing spermatozoa, the testis secretes into the blood stream an androgenic steroid

FIGURE 26-40 A light micrograph of the interstitial region of a monkey's testis. A small capillary is located below a larger lymphatic vessel. A few Leydig cells are noted adjacent to the seminiferous tubule below. ×450.

hormone, testosterone, which is essential for puberal development, spermatogenesis, and structural and functional maintenance of the male accessory organs. In fact, testosterone probably acts on most tissues and organs in the body. The Leydig cells are responsible for secretion of the testicular androgenic hormone (Fig. 26-43).

The characteristic structure and endocrine function of the interstitial cells are sustained and controlled by the hypophyseal gonadotropic hormone LH (luteineizing hormone) also known as ISCH or interstitial cell-stimulating hormone. In the absence of LH, the interstitial cells undergo severe atrophy and cease producing testosterone. The completely atrophic Leydig cell is spindle-shaped, the amount of cytoplasm is greatly reduced, and the nucleus is smaller

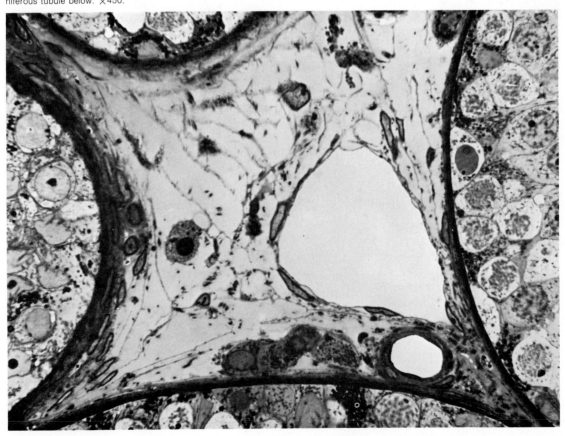

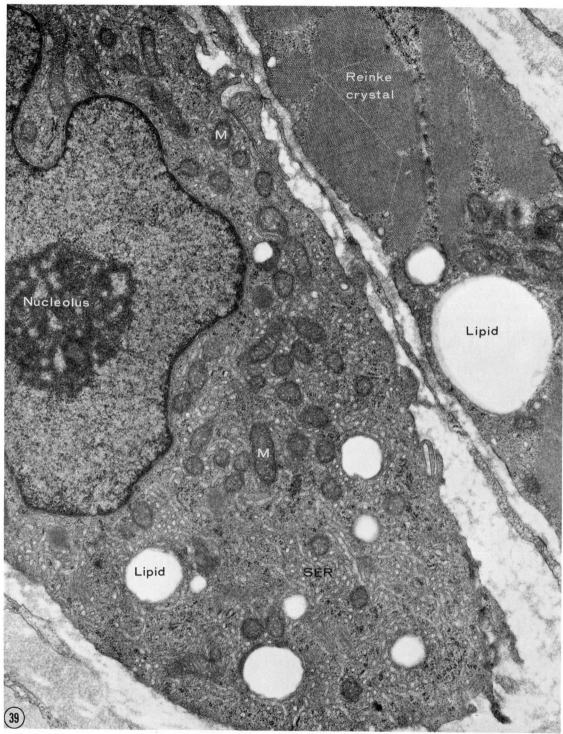

FIGURE 26-41 An electron micrograph of human Leydig cells. The cytoplasm is characterized by smooth endoplasmic reticulum (SER), lipid droplets, partially extracted, and numerous mitochondria (M). A Reinke crystal is also noted. ×17,640. (Courtesy of A. K. Christensen.)

and pycnotic looking. The lipid droplets also disappear.

Very high concentrations of testosterone adjacent to the seminiferous tubules are required to maintain spermatogenesis in the adult; however, lower peripheral levels will maintain secondary sex characteristics and male libido. Lowered circulating levels of testosterone will result in an increased release of LH from the pituitary and an increased production of testosterone by the Leydig cell.

The role of LH in the male, therefore, is clear. It stimulates the Leydig cells to produce testosterone, which is required for spermatogenesis. Testosterone alone can maintain spermatogenesis, male libido, and the accessory glands following hypophysectomy in experimental animals. This appears to indicate that FSH is not required for male reproductive function. However, much biochemical data has accumulated indicating that the Sertoli cell is the primary target for FSH in the testis. When FSH is administered to im-

FIGURE 26-42 Electron micrograph of a crystal of Reinke found in a Leydig cell of a human testis. ×16,400. (Courtesy of M. J. Rowley.)

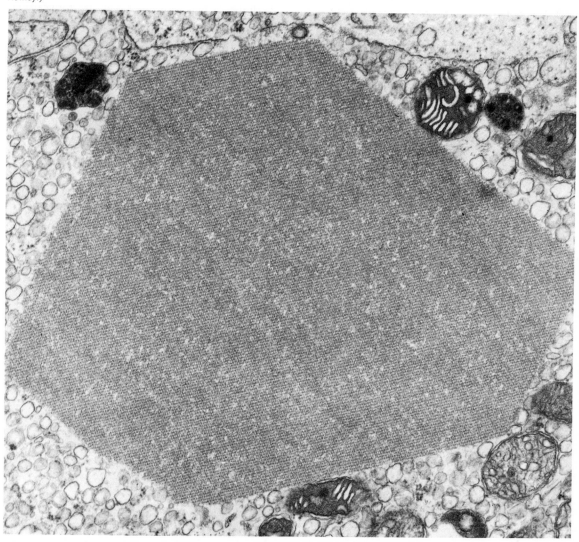

mature rat testes, there is (1) a binding of FSH to receptors present on the plasma membrane of the Sertoli cell; (2) a stimulation of the membrane-bound adenylate cyclase and a concomitant increase in the intracellular accumulation of cyclic AMP; and (3) an activation of cyclic AMP-dependent protein kinases and an eventual increase of protein synthesis. Other work has demonstrated that the Sertoli cells respond to FSH by increasing the secretion of androgen-binding protein. Autoradiographic studies with labeled FSH demonstrated that this hormone is localized to the Sertoli cells. Thus, it is obvious that there are many important actions of FSH on the seminiferous tubules at the biochemical level; however, it has proved difficult to assign a definitive requirement for this hormone in the biological process of spermatogenesis. No doubt more work will be carried out in this area.

FACTORS INFLUENCING TESTICULAR FUNCTION

Heat

The germinal cells in the seminiferous tubules are particularly susceptible to injury by temperatures above that of the scrotum, which in men is 1.5 to 2.5°C lower than that of the abdominal cavity. When the testes of mature male animals are surgically re-

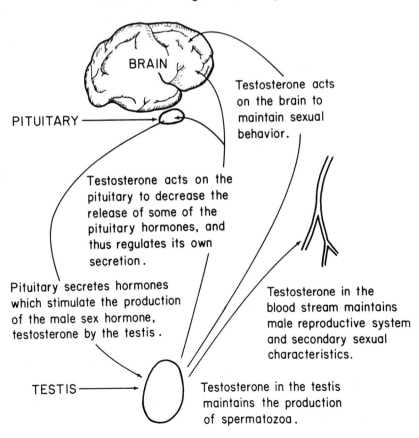

HORMONAL CONTROL OF MALE REPRODUCTIVE FUNCTION

Feedback Regulation System

BRAIN

PITUITARY

Testosterone acts on the brain to maintain sexual behavior.

Testosterone acts on the pituitary to decrease the release of some of the pituitary hormones, and thus regulates its own secretion.

Pituitary secretes hormones which stimulate the production of the male sex hormone, testosterone by the testis.

Testosterone in the blood stream maintains male reproductive system and secondary sexual characteristics.

TESTIS

Testosterone in the testis maintains the production of spermatozoa.

FIGURE 26-43 Diagrammatic representation of the hormonal control of male reproductive function. (Courtesy of A. Bartke.)

tracted into the abdomen, the seminiferous epithelium degenerates. The Sertoli cells are not reduced in number nor does this procedure cause an early impairment of the androgenic function of the Leydig cells, as shown by the fact that the accessory sexual organs are maintained at normal adult size for at least 6 to 8 months, after which they may gradually become smaller. In addition to tubular injury at body temperatures, fevers are well known to induce temporary infertility. Frequent immersions in hot baths or close-fitting, tight trousers may also result in a reduction of sperm numbers in the ejaculate.

Cryptorchidism

Ten percent of newborn males have testes which are not fully descended into the scrotum. This condition is referred to as cryptorchidism. Most of these descend spontaneously; however, if this does not occur, surgical intervention is usually carried out at around 5 years of age. Beyond the age of 5 there is evidence that irreversible changes occur. A prolonged residence of the testis within the abdomen results in progressive degeneration of germ cells. If the testis is not in the scrotum at puberty, spermatogenesis is likely never to occur. Beyond the age of 30, fibrosis takes place which frequently impairs Leydig cell function. At this age the abdominal testis may also develop neoplastic changes and must therefore be removed.

Irradiation

Dividing populations of cells are very sensitive to radiation. Graded doses of ionizing radiation, administered directly to human testes, evoke correspondingly graded biologic responses resulting in an eventual denuding of the germinal epithelium and a reduction in sperm count. In general, the lower the dosage, the less dramatic is the cell loss and the more rapid the recovery. However, even a few rads will destroy a significant number of the spermatogonial population.

Age

After the age of 55, spermatogenesis decreases very gradually, although the Sertoli cells and Leydig cells appear unaltered. There is also an increase in the number of abnormal, nonviable sperm in the ejaculate. However, men in their 80s and 90s still have adequate spermatogenesis with sperm counts within the normal range. Provided that they are physically fit, they can father children.

Vasectomy

After ligation of the vas deferens (vasectomy) the seminiferous tubules continue to produce spermatozoa at normal levels. The fate of these sperm in vasectomized men remains an enigma. In some species after vasectomy, spermatozoa are resorbed in the male reproductive tract or stored in cysts and distended portions of the epididymis. In the human and monkey, epididymal macrophages appear to be involved in the sperm resorption. Since spermatozoa possess antigens which are foreign to the body, this resorption may result in the production by the immune system of circulating antisperm antibodies. These immunoglobulins can immobilize and destroy the sperm upon contact. The antibodies do not penetrate the seminiferous tubules because of the effective blood-testis permeability barrier. However, evidence is accumulating that these high-molecular-weight proteins can enter the lumen of the rete testis and epididymis and possibly affect the fertilizing capacity of spermatozoa in these regions. This may partially explain why men who have reanastomoses of the vas deferens, after vasectomy, may possess normal numbers of sperm in their ejaculate but sperm that appear incapable of fertilizing the egg.

EXCURRENT DUCT SYSTEM OF THE TESTIS

TUBULI RECTI AND RETE TESTIS

The convoluted seminiferous tubules within a given testis lobule are arranged mainly in the form of loops (Fig. 26-44), each end of which joins the rete testis (Fig. 26-45, see color insert). As the seminiferous tubules approach the rete there is a gradual depletion of the germinal elements until the tubules are lined only by Sertoli cells. This portion of the tubule without germ cells is very short and ends in an abrupt transition to the simple cuboidal epithelium characteristic of the tubuli recti. The tubuli recti, or straight tubules, are confluent with the rete testis. The rete testis consists of a series of channels or interconnected chambers lined by simple cuboidal or low columnar epithelium within a bed of highly vascular loose connective tissue. The luminal surface of the epithelial cells is covered with short microvilli and a single long flagellum (Fig. 26-46). In most mammalian species the rete occupies an axial position in the testis extending from the ductuli efferentes at the upper pole of the testis to the lower pole (Fig. 26-44). The seminiferous tubules release their contents into the axial rete at many points along its entire length. In men, the rete testis is present in the posterior portion of the testis within the mediastinum; in rats, mice, and hamsters, the rete is located in a superficial position immediately deep to the tunica albuginea (Fig. 26-45, see color insert)

DUCTULI EFFERENTES

In men 10 to 15 ductules, the ductuli efferentes (Fig. 26-47, see color insert), emerge from the mediastinum and connect the rete testis with the ductus epididymidis. Each ductulus efferens is coiled into a cone-shaped mass in the head of the epididymis. The epithelium consists of alternating patches of tall and low columnar cells. Two cell types are present, the ciliated and the nonciliated cell (Fig. 26-48). Both contain abundant supranuclear granules and most of the common cellular organelles. The cilia beat in the direction of the epididymis and may assist in the movement of sperm. The nonciliated cells are absorptive in function and bear numerous microvilli on their free surface. In addition to acting as a conduit for sperm, the ductuli efferentes absorb most of the fluid produced within the seminiferous tubules.

The epithelium of the ductuli is surrounded by a layer of circular, smooth muscle several cells thick. It is significant that from the ductuli efferentes to the urethra the sperm duct has a muscular coat. Once spermatozoa have been carried to the ductuli efferentes by the flow of luminal fluid, their further transport is assured by muscular action. The muscle layer thickens toward the ductus epididymidis. Among the muscle cells there are elastic fibers which, like those of the ductus epididymidis and ductus deferens, first appear at puberty.

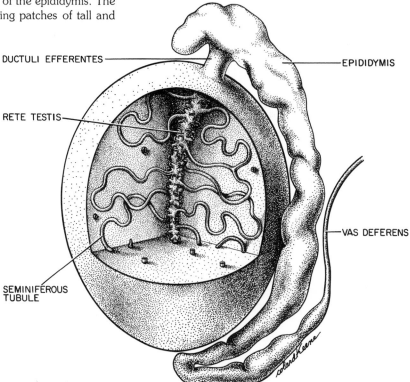

DUCTULI EFFERENTES

EPIDIDYMIS

RETE TESTIS

VAS DEFERENS

SEMINIFEROUS TUBULE

FIGURE 26-44 Drawing of a monkey's testis and epididymis demonstrating the axial rete in the central core of the testis. Seminiferous tubules empty into the rete at many points along its length.

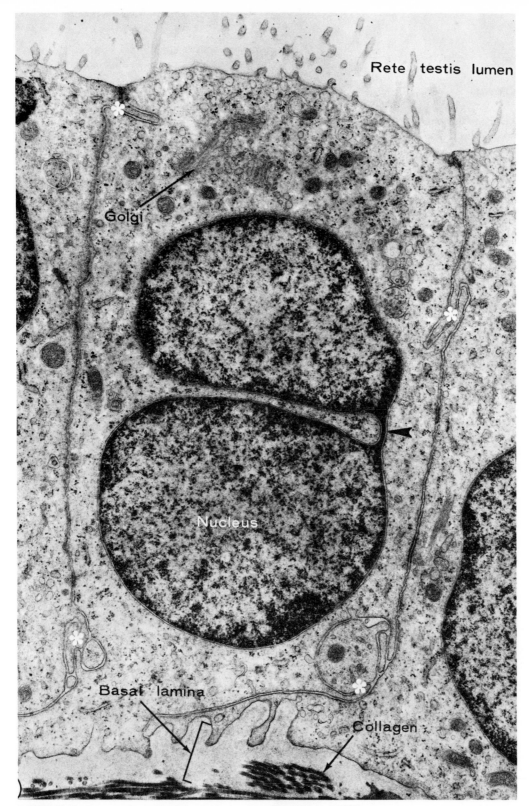

Rete testis lumen

Golgi

Nucleus

Basal lamina

Collagen

FIGURE 26-46 Electron micrograph of the monkey's rete testis epithelium. ×7500.

DUCTUS EPIDIDYMIS

The ductus epididymis in mammals is a highly tortuous tube 4 to 5 m in length. The coils of this duct together with the entwining vascular connective tissue, smooth muscle, and surrounding tunic form the epididymis. The epithelium is pseudostratified columnar and rests on a basal lamina and a thin lamina propria encircled by the smooth muscle, with the fibers oriented circularly. The muscle layer is very thin over most of the length of the tube, but it thickens markedly and longitudinal fibers appear near the ductus deferens. Outside the muscle layer, loose connective tissue is molded about the duct and constitutes the interstitium of the epididymis. Blood vessels, lymphatic vessels,

and nerves occur in the fibrous stroma. The nerves form a thick myenteric plexus with autonomic ganglia in addition to perivascular nets. The plexus is more highly developed in the vas deferens and seminal vesicles.

For descriptive purposes the epididymis may be subdivided into three portions: head, body, and tail (Fig. 26-49). The segment of the head into which the ductuli efferentes empty is called the initial segment. Spermatozoa leaving the testis exhibit weak, random, circular motion and are incapable of fertilizing ova. On the other hand, sperm taken from the tail of the epididymis have a strong unidirectional motility and are able to fertilize ova. Thus, it is clear that the sperm require the epididymal environment to become ma-

FIGURE 26-48 Light micrograph of a transverse section through a ductus efferens in a monkey. Both the ciliated and nonciliated cells are densely packed with granules. ×650 (Courtesy of A. S. Ramos, Jr.)

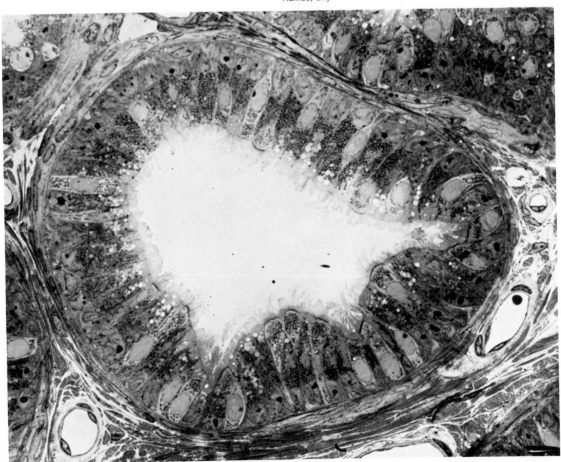

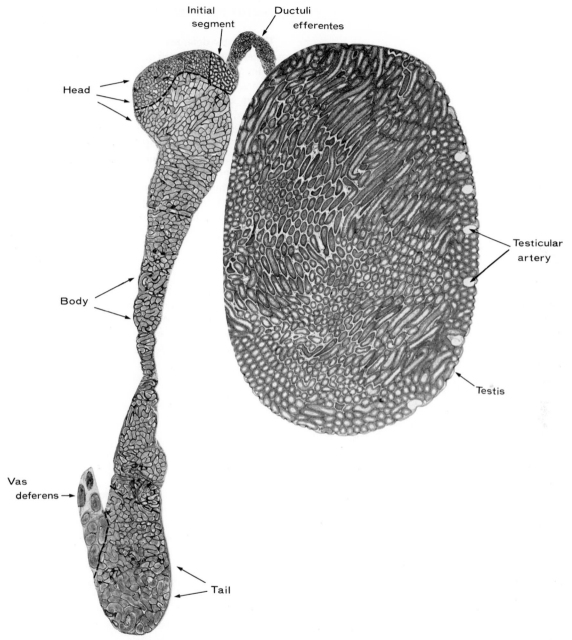

FIGURE 26-49 Photographic montage of the rat's testis and epididymis. The ductuli efferentes empty into the "initial segment" of the epididymis. Note the morphological differences in the epididymal duct along its length. ×6.75.

ture; furthermore, this maturation is androgen-dependent. The mechanism by which the epididymis induces the functional maturation of spermatozoa is now under intensive investigation. It is known that the epithelium secretes glycerylphosphorylcholine, carnitine, sialic acid, glycoproteins, and possible steroids into the tubule lumen.

It is not surprising that various segments of the epididymis exhibit different morphological characteristics, since the respective regions perform various functions. For example, the head region absorbs fluid and particulate matter readily; the tail acts as a sperm reservoir and can contract forcefully upon appropriate nervous stimulation.

The epididymal duct is lined by tall columnar cells resting on a well-defined basal lamina (Fig. 26-50). The luminal free surface of the epithelium bears long nonmotile microvilli (stereocilia), the height of which decreases from 80 μm in the head region to 40 μm in the tail. The principal cell is the most abundant and is characterized by an impressively large supranuclear Golgi complex and abundant profiles of rough endoplasmic reticulum in the basal cytoplasm. The apical cytoplasm contains numerous micropinocytotic vesicles, multivesicular bodies and lysosomes, lipid droplets, coated vesicles, and mitochondria. The nucleus in the head region is cigar-shaped with the long axis parallel to the long axis of the cell. Nuclear membrane infoldings are present in the distal part of the head and in the body and reach a maximum in the tail region where most nuclei have very bizarre shapes.

Small, round cells containing spherical nuclei are found at the base of the epididymal epithelium insinuated among the principal cells. These basal cells contain few organelles and appear lightly stained in electron micrographs. The function of the basal cells remains obscure. Intraepithelial lymphocytes are located at all levels in the epithelium. In rodents and monkeys they represent about 2 percent of the total cell population. The ultrastructure of these cells closely resembles that of thoracic duct lymphocytes.

DUCTUS DEFERENS

The ductus deferens is a thick-walled tube that is continuous with the tail of the epididymis and extends to the prostatic urethra. Near the prostate the lumen widens and appears as a spindle-shaped enlargement, the ampulla. At the distal end of the ampulla the duct is joined by the duct of the seminal vesicles. From this point it continues to the urethra as the ejaculatory duct (Fig. 26-1). The wall of the ductus deferens is composed of three well-defined layers, the mucosa, muscularis, and adventitia.

The mucosa protrudes into the lumen in several low longitudinal folds (Fig. 26-51). The epithelium is similar in structure to, but not as tall as, that in the epididymis. Some of the columnar cells are exceedingly rich in mitochondria. Nonmotile stereocilia are present on the free surface of the cells and frequently they are matted together and form cones. The stereocilia tend to disappear toward the ampulla. A thin basal lamina is present. The lamina propria is very dense, largely because of a heavy infiltration of elastic fibers. The vas deferens is surrounded by a three-layered, smooth muscle coat 1 to 1.5 mm thick. The fibers of the inner and outer layers are arranged longitudinally and those of the middle layer circularly. The adventitia is composed of a fibrous covering of the muscle layer and loose connective tissue, which blends with that of contiguous structures.

AMPULLA OF THE VAS DEFERENS

The longitudinal folds in the mucosa of the ductus deferens extend into the ampulla, where they increase in height and become branched. The ampulla has a wide lumen and its muscular coat is thinner, with less distinct layers, than elsewhere in the ductus deferens. The longitudinal muscle layers separate into long strands which terminate toward the ejaculatory duct. The epithelium of the ampulla is pseudostratified columnar similar to the rest of the vas. Glandular diverticula showing evidence of secretion extend deep into the surrounding muscle layer.

FIGURE 26-50 Schematic drawing of the principal and basal cells (A) in the human epididymis. Note the following changes from the head (A) to the tail regions (E): decreased epithelial height; decreased height of stereocilia; increased nuclear membrane infoldings. (Courtesy of A. S. Holstein.)

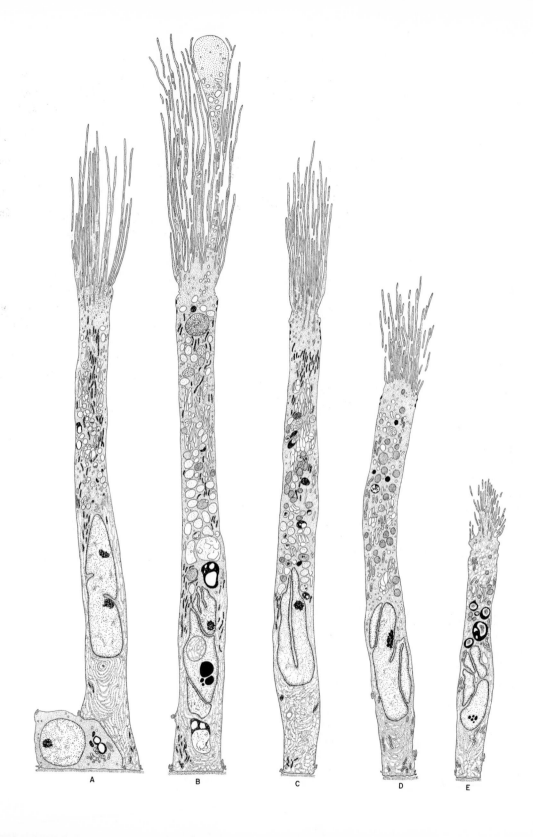

A   B   C   D   E

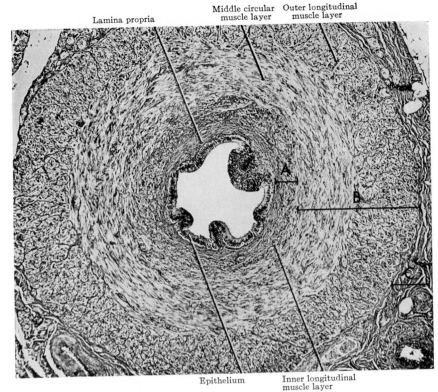

Lamina propria   Middle circular   Outer longitudinal
                  muscle layer   muscle layer

Epithelium   Inner longitudinal
              muscle layer

FIGURE 26-51 Photomicrograph of a transverse section of the human ductus deferens. A, mucosa; B, muscularis; C, adventitia. ×50.

EJACULATORY DUCT

The portion of each ductus deferens which extends from the ampulla to the urethra is reduced in width and receives the duct of the seminal vesicle. The conjoined duct is known as the ejaculatory duct. These ducts, 1 cm in length, penetrate the prostate gland and open into the prostatic urethra on a thickened portion of the urethral mucosa known as the colliculus semi-nalis, or verumontanum. The mucous membrane, cast into numerous thin folds, forms glandular diverticula, similar to, but less elaborate than, those in the ampulla. The epithelium is pseudostratified or simple columnar.

MALE ACCESSORY SEX ORGANS

SEMINAL VESICLES

The seminal vesicles arise as outgrowths from the vas deferens distal to the ampulla. They develop into elongated, hollow organs 5 to 10 cm long, whose walls are packed with small, saclike evaginations. The proximal extremity of each vesicle joins the vas deferens to form the ejaculatory duct (Fig. 26-1). Each vesicle is honeycombed by thin primary folds of mucosae which extend deep into the lumen. These branch and anas-tomose into secondary and tertiary folds which join to form numerous irregular chambers, all of which communicate with the large central lumen. This arrangement increases the surface area of the secretory epithelium. The folds are covered with a pseudostratified epithelium consisting of tall columnar, nonciliated cells that reach the luminal surface, and basal cells identical with those seen elsewhere in the excurrent duct (Fig. 26-52). The secretory cells have a single ovoid nucleus and contain numerous granules,

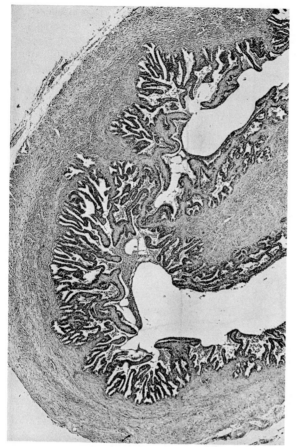

FIGURE 26-52 Longitudinal section of a diverticulum of a human seminal vesicle. ×27.

clumps of lipochrome pigment, and some lipid droplets.

The lamina propria contains many elastic fibers. A layer of smooth muscle consisting of inner circular and outer longitudinal fibers and an external sheet of loose connective tissue complete the wall of the seminal vesicle.

Fine structural observations on the epithelium of the seminal vesicles reveal characteristics usually identified with active secretion of protein. The cytoplasm is packed with rough endoplasmic reticulum, some channels of which appear to communicate with the very prominent supranuclear Golgi apparatus. The apical cytoplasm exhibits large vacuoles containing dense secretory granules.

The abundant secretion formed in the seminal vesicles is a viscid material with a whitish yellow color. This gland produces a substantial portion of the whole

ejaculate and contains many reducing substances. Prostaglandins were first discovered in sheep seminal vesicles and these glands are frequently used to study the mechanism of prostaglandin secretion. The most important free sugar produced is fructose, and an analysis of this compound in semen may be used to evaluate the secretory activity of the gland. The height of the cells and their functional activity are dependent upon the action of testosterone. After castration, the seminal vesicles shrink and cease forming fluid and the epithelium is reduced to low cuboidal.

PROSTATE

The prostate, like the seminal vesicles, is a major secretory contributor to the seminal plasma. It is a compact musculoglandular organ, 20 g in weight, in contact with the inferior surface of the bladder (Fig. 26-1). The prostate surrounds the first portion of the urethra as it leaves the bladder and consists of three groups of glands arranged somewhat concentrically around the urethra (Fig. 26-53). The smallest are the periurethral mucosal glands. This area of the prostate is involved in the production of nodular hyperplasia but is not related to the main function of the prostate or to the origin of cancer. The periurethral glands are separated from the true prostate by a mass of smooth muscle tissue. Previous descriptions subdivided the true prostate into (1) submucosal glands and (2) main prostatic glands (Fig. 26-53). Cancer of the prostate originates in the true prostate, mainly from the "peripheral zone." The prostate consists of 30 to 50 tubuloalveolar glands opening directly into the prostatic urethra through 15 to 30 ducts. The ducts of the mucosal glands open at various points into the urethra, whereas those of the true prostate open onto the posterolateral urethral sinus near the verumontanum. In each lobe the glands are embedded in a markedly fibromuscular stroma which aids in the ejaculatory discharge of the prostatic fluid.

The glandular epithelium in the prostate is normally simple columnar or pseudostratified (Fig. 26-54). Basal cells resting on the basal lamina are insinuated among the columnar cells. Near the urethra the lining of the epithelium changes to the transitional type characteristic of the bladder and prostatic urethra. Histochemically, the prostatic epithelium is remarkable for the abundance of acid phosphatase.

The prostatic secretion is a colorless fluid, pH 6.5, rich in proteolytic enzymes. The most potent one is fibrinolysin which plays a role in the liquefaction of semen. Zinc, citric acid, and acid phosphatase also occur in high concentrations in prostatic fluid. The latter two products provide a reliable and sensitive test for the assessment of prostatic function.

As seen by electron microscopy, the prostatic epithelial cells possess luminal microvilli and an abundance of rough endoplasmic reticulum, except in the region of the Golgi complex (Fig. 26-55). Apically the cisternae of the endoplasmic reticulum membranes are moderately distended. Numerous vacuoles containing secretory granules are a common feature of the apical cytoplasm. Castration changes are marked by a reduction in height of the epithelial cells and a loss of the secretory products. These and other cellular changes are reversed by the administration of testosterone.

In the prostatic alveoli, especially of older persons, there are concretions of various forms, 0.2 to 2 mm in diameter; in sections they may exhibit concentric layers and show double refraction with polarized light

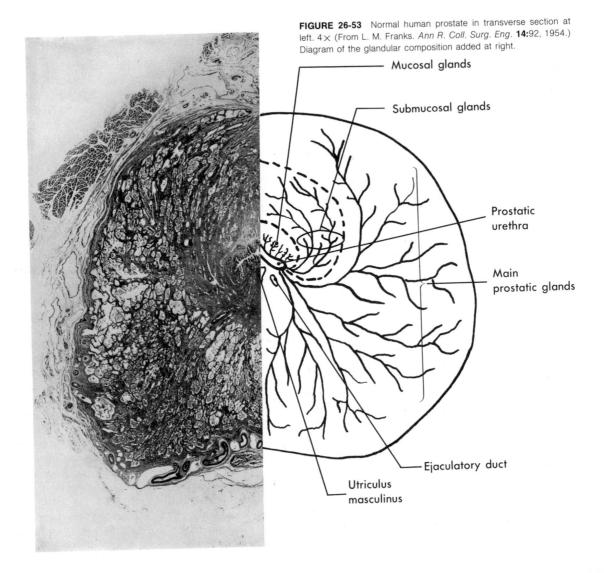

FIGURE 26-53 Normal human prostate in transverse section at left. 4× (From L. M. Franks. *Ann R. Coll. Surg. Eng.* **14**:92, 1954.) Diagram of the glandular composition added at right.

Mucosal glands

Submucosal glands

Prostatic urethra

Main prostatic glands

Ejaculatory duct

Utriculus masculinus

(Fig. 26-56). These structures are believed to be condensations of secretory material and are probably deposited around fragments of cells. The larger concretions sometimes obstruct the prostatic ducts and cause distension of the gland. Octahedral crystals also occur in the prostatic secretion.

The prostate is surrounded by a fibroelastic cap-

sule with some smooth muscle fibers on its inner aspect. These muscle fibers connect with others that penetrate between the prostatic lobules. In many rodents one pair of the lobes of the prostate, the coagu-

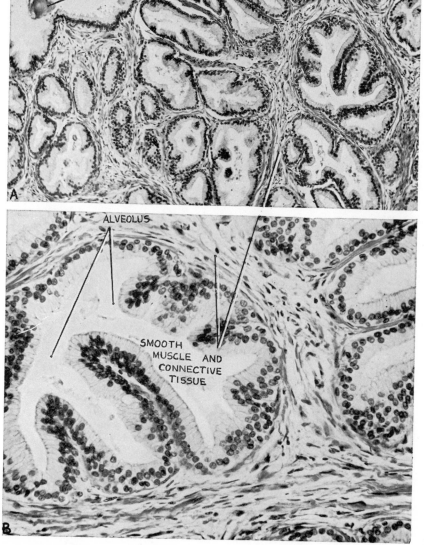

FIGURE 26-54 Human prostate. A. Note fibromuscular stroma. ×90. B. Note simple columnar epithelium, few basal cells, secretion in lumen. ×275.

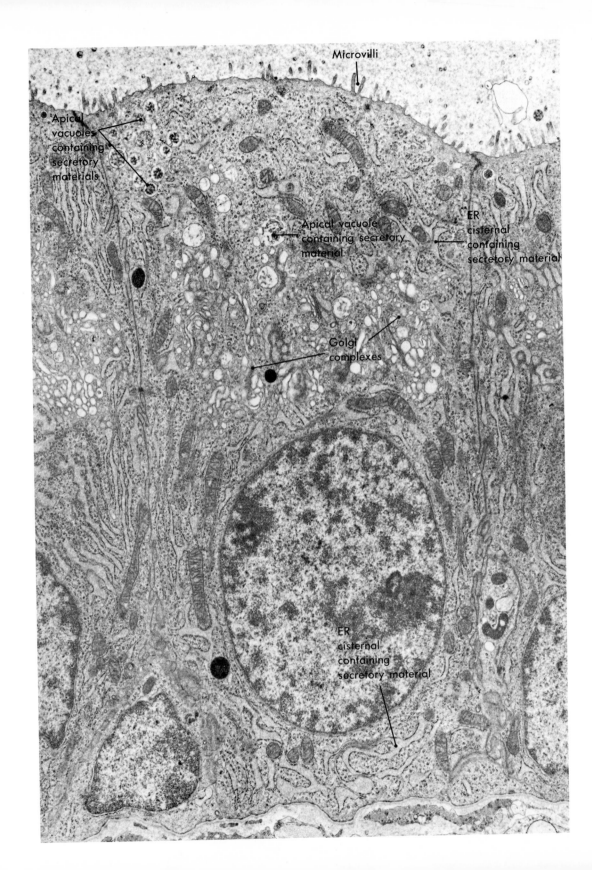

Microvilli

Apical
vacuoles
containing
secretory
materials

Apical vacuole
containing secretory
material

ER
cisternal
containing
secretory material

Golgi
complexes

ER
cisternal
containing
secretory material

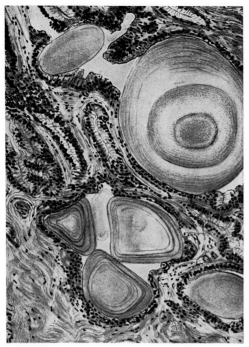

FIGURE 26-56 Section of the human prostate, showing concretions. ×90.

cleus. At the peak of secretion, the cells appear to be filled with mucus and have their nuclei flattened against the basal lamina. Basket cells may also be found. The glands are divided into small lobules by septa composed of connective tissue and skeletal muscle. The excretory ducts are lined with simple columnar epithelium, except near the urethral orifice where it becomes pseudostratified columnar. The coating of the ducts is made of fibrous tissue and a thin layer of smooth muscle. The secretory product is a clear, viscous, mucouslike substance composed of galactose, galactosamine, galacturonic acid, sialic acid, and a methylpentose. It is poured into the urethra under erotic stimulation and probably acts as a lubricant.

PENIS

The penis is an elongate organ consisting principally of the urethra and three parallel cavernous bodies (Figs. 26-1 and 26-58). The paired corpora cavernosa penis are placed dorsally, and beneath them in the midline is

FIGURE 26-57 Section through part of a lobule of the bulbourethral gland. (Stieve.) ×90.

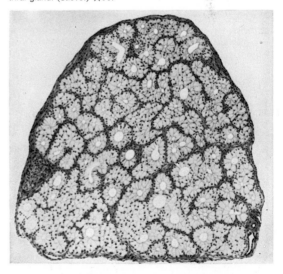

lating gland, is differentiated to supply a secretion which coagulates the seminal fluid in the vagina, forming a plug.

The utriculus masculinus is a small pouch on the dorsal wall of the urethra that opens on the verumontanum between the orifices of the two ejaculatory ducts.

BULBOURETHRAL GLANDS

The two bulbourethral glands, or Cowper's glands, are pea-sized structures situated one on each side of the urethral bulb and connected with the penile urethra by fairly long ducts (Fig. 26-1). These are compound tubuloalveolar glands; the end pieces may be rounded sacs or simple tubes (Fig. 26-57). The cells of the simple epithelium vary greatly in height and appearance. In the resting state, they are columnar with granular cytoplasm and have a clear spherical nu-

FIGURE 26-55 Columnar cells of the epithelium of ventral prostate of a 28-day-old rat. These cells possess enlarged Golgi complexes, dilated cisternae of rough endoplasmic reticulum, and vacuoles containing dense secretory material. ×12,000. (Courtesy of C. J. Flickinger.)

the single corpus cavernosum urethrae (spongiosum) that originates as an expanded portion, the bulbous urethrae, and terminates as the glans penis, a structure at the end of the penis having the appearance of a blunted cone. The urethra lies in the center of the spongiosum. A dense, fibroelastic connective tissue layer, the tunica albuginea, binds the three cavernous bodies together and also provides an attachment to the skin over the shaft of the penis. The deepest fibers of this tunic are organized as a capsule around each cavernous body. Those surrounding the corpora cavernosa penis fuse in the midline to form a septum in the penis which becomes incomplete distally. The albuginea enclosing the spongiosum is thinner and contains circularly arranged smooth muscle fibers and more elastic fibers than that of the paired cavernous bodies.

The cavernous bodies are composed of true erectile tissue that increases in size by filling with blood and changing from a flaccid to a rigid state, thereby producing an erection of the penis. These bodies are honeycombed by a complex network of venous spaces separated by trabeculae. The trabeculae are lined with typical vascular endothelium and have connective

FIGURE 26-58 Cross section of the penis of a 23-year-old man. The septum between corpora cavernosa penis is incomplete. Section is from distal one-third of the organ (Stieve) ×2.5.

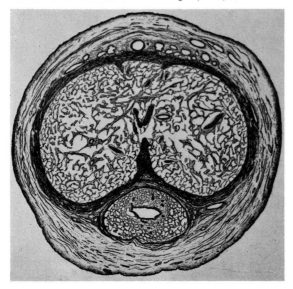

tissue and smooth muscle in the wall. Blood enters these spaces from two sources: from capillaries in the walls of the trabeculae that drain into the spaces; but more importantly for the purpose of erection, from the terminal branches of arteries which course through the walls of the trabeculae and empty directly into the spaces. These are the helicine arteries, so called because they are coiled and twisted in the flaccid penis. They have heavy muscular walls, with subendothelial thickenings of the longitudinal muscle fibers that partly occlude the lumen. The veins draining the cavernous bodies have such thick walls that they resemble arteries; they contain abundant columns of inner longitudinal muscle fibers that make the lumen crescentic or star-shaped. The erectile tissue of the glans penis consists only of convolutions of large veins, and it does not reach the same state of rigidity as the shaft of the erect penis.

Recent studies of the vascular events associated with the process of erection and detumescence of the penis have clarified our understanding of these important processes (Fig. 26-59). The presence of arteriovenous (AV) anastomoses between the deep artery of the penis and the peripheral venous return has been reaffirmed. Hemodynamic experimental work in humans has shown that blood flow into the cavernous spaces of 20 to 50 ml per min will produce erection without the necessity of postulating a venous-closing mechanism. Since parasympathetic activity on the AV complex is required to increase blood flow to the cavernous spaces, it is suggested that concomitant sympathetic activity produces contraction of arterioles supplying the rest of the penis. This combined autonomic interplay assures a rigid intromittent organ through which sperm can be discharged into the vaginal vault. Relaxation of such autonomic activity after sexual excitement reduces blood flow to the cavernous spaces and shunts most of the blood to the peripheral venous vessels, thereby returning the penis to its flaccid condition.

The skin of the penis is thin, elastic, fat-free, and somewhat more deeply pigmented than that covering the body. Coarse pubic hairs are present at the root of the organ; elsewhere over its shaft there are only lanugo hairs. At the forward end of the penis, the skin is attached to the corona of the glans and forms a circular fold, the prepuce (foreskin) that overlies the glans. The inner surface of the prepuce differs from the skin elsewhere on the penis by having a thinner epidermis and being free of sebaceous and sweat glands (the skin of the glans is glabrous). Over the body of the penis there is a subcutaneous layer of smooth muscle fibers which is continuous with the tunica dartos of the scrotum. On the corona glandis, sebaceous glands occur in the absence of hair follicles.

The penis is abundantly supplied with spinal, sympathetic, and parasympathetic nerve fibers. The sensory fibers of the medullated spinal nerves (dorsal

nerves of the penis) terminate in many types of sensory endings; as tactile corpuscles in the papillae of the dermis, as end bulbs of Krause and Pacinian corpuscles in the superficial connective tissue, and as genital corpuscles found in or near the cavernous

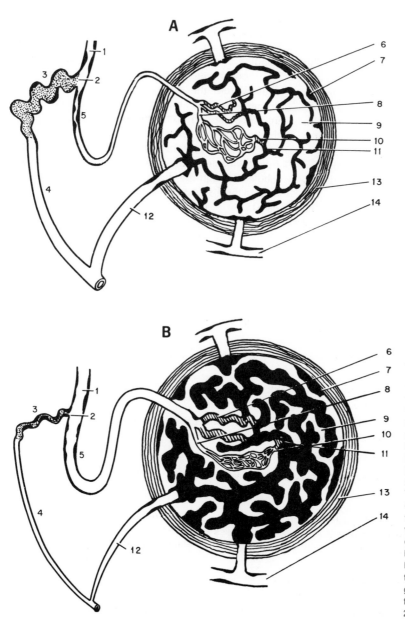

FIGURE 26-59 Vascular relationships of the human penis. A. In the flaccid state, blood flows toward the corpora cavernosa in the deep artery of the penis (1). This vessel possesses intimal cushions which tend to regulate blood flow. Almost all the blood passes directly into (2) an arteriovenous anastomosis (3) which is usually dilated in this state and connects with efferent veins (4). Minimal amounts of blood pass to the corpora cavernosa. At a point inside the corpora this artery (5) divides into two branches, the helicine artery (6) that empties almost immediately into the blood spaces of the erectile tissue (7, 11) and the nutritive artery (8) of the trabeculae (9) which, after breaking up into a capillary network re-forms into a small vein (10) and empties into the cavernous space (11). Cavernous spaces are drained by veins which have internal cushions (12, 14). These pierce the tunica albuginea (13) and constitute the efferent venous return. B. During erection, blood flow in the deep artery of the penis (1) increases. The opening (2) of the arteriovenous anastomosis (3) is reduced by active vasoconstriction resulting in a slight dilated artery (5) passing through the tunica albuginea (13) into the cavernous body. The helicine arteries (6) dilate the cavernous spaces (7) fill with blood while the nutritive vessel (8) and its venous junction (10) with the cavernous space (11) become compressed. Blood flow leaving the cavernous body (12, 14) is not reduced despite the internal structure of these emergent veins. (Adapted and modified from G. Conti, *Acta Anat.*, **5**:217–262, 1952.)

bodies. Free sensory endings also occur. The sympathetic and parasympathetic nerves are a continuation of the prostatic plexus and supply the numerous smooth muscles of the trabeculae and the cavernous blood vessels. The glans is peculiar in that it has no receptors for light touch, warmth, or cold; however, cylindrical end bulbs of Krause are present.

SEMEN

This secretion consists of spermatozoa suspended in a complex fluid derived from the accessory sex glands which empty into the excurrent duct system. The ejaculate is about 3 ml in volume and contains approximately 200 to 300 million spermatozoa. In humans, three main glandular systems contribute successively to the ejaculate. The first portion comes from the prostate gland and is a thin, milky emulsion that is slightly acid. In addition, the acid phosphatases are mainly derived from the prostate. The second portion comprises the secretions from the testes, ductus epididymidis, and ductus deferens and therefore contains the highest concentration of spermatozoa. The third portion possesses the highest concentration of fructose, a substance specific for the seminal vesicles and a prime energy source for motile sperm. Prostaglandins, a family of biologically active lipids found in high concentrations in human seminal plasma, are derived from the seminal vesicles. Their biological properties as regulators of smooth muscle activity may influence sperm transit in the male and the female and the implantation process.

The average transit time of human spermatozoa from their release into the lumen of the seminiferous tubules through the ductular system to their appearance in the ejaculate is 12 days (with a range of 1 to 21 days).

REFERENCES

General References

BRANDES, D.: "Male Accessory Sex Organs. Structure and Function in Mammals," Academic Press, New York, 1974.

GORLAND, M.: "Normal and Abnormal Growth of the Prostate," Charles C Thomas, Springfield, Illinois, 1975.

HAMILTON, D. W., and R. O. GREEP (eds.): Male Reproductive System, Sec. 7, Endocrinology, vol. 5, in "Handbook of Physiology," American Physiological Society, Washington, 1975.

JOHNSON, A. D., W. R. GOMES, and N. L. VANDEMARK (eds.): "The Testis." vol. 1, Development, Anatomy and Physiology; vol. 2, Biochemistry; vol. 3, Influencing Factors. Academic Press, New York, 1970.

MANN, T.: "Biochemistry of Semen and of the Male Reproductive Tract," Methuen and Co., London, 1964.

STEINBERGER, E.: Hormonal Control of Mammalian Spermatogenesis, Physiol. Rev., **51**:1 (1971).

Specific References

BARTKE, A., M. E. HARRIS, and J. K. VOGLMAYR: Regulation of Testosterone and Dihydrotestosterone Levels in Rete Testis Fluid. Evidence for Androgen Biosynthesis in Seminiferous Tubules In Vivo, in F. S. French, V. Hansson, E. M. Ritzen, and S. N. Nayfeh (eds), "Hormonal Regulation of Spermatogenesis," Plenum Press, New York, 1975.

CHRISTENSEN, A. K.: Leydig cells. Sec. 7, Endocrinology, vol. 5, Male Reproductive System, in D. W. Hamilton and R. O. Greep (eds), "Handbook of Physiology," Amer. Phys. Soc., Washington, 1975.

CHRISTENSEN, A. K., and D. W. FAWCETT: The Fine Structure of Testicular Interstitial Cells in Mice. Amer. J. Anat., **118**:551 (1966).

CLERMONT, Y.: The Cycle of the Seminiferous Epithelium in Man. Amer. J. Anat., **112:**35 (1963).

CLERMONT, Y.: Renewal of Spermatogonia in Man. Am. J. Anat., **118:**509 (1966).

CLERMONT, Y.: Two Classes of Spermatogonial Stem Cells in the Monkey (Cercopithecus Aethiops). Am. J. Anat., **126:**57, (1969).

CLERMONT, Y.: Kinetics of Spermatogenesis in Mammals: Seminiferous Epithelium Cycle and Spermatogonial Renewal. Physiol. Rev., **52:**198 (1972).

CLERMONT, Y., and E. BUSTOS-OBREGON: Re-examination of Spermatogonial Renewal in the Rat by Means of Seminiferous Tubules Mounted "in toto." Am. J. Anat., **122:**237 (1968).

CLERMONT, Y., and S. C. HARVEY: Effects of Hormones on Spermatogenesis in the Rat, in "Endocrinology of the Testis," Ciba Foundation Colloquia on Endocrinology, **16:**173 (1967).

CLERMONT, Y., and C. P. LEBLOND: Spermiogenesis of Man, Monkey, Ram and Other Mammals as Shown by the "Periodic Acid-Schiff" Technique. Amer. J. Anat., **96:**229 (1955).

CONTI, G.: L'érection du Pénis Humain et Ses Bases Morphologico-Vascularies. Acta Anat., **14:**217 (1952).

DE KRETSER, D. M., K. J. CATT, and C. A. PAULSEN: Studies on the In Vitro Testicular Binding of Iodinated Luteinizing Hormone in Rats. Endocrinology, **88:**332 (1971).

DORR, L. D., and M. J. BRODY: Hemodynamic Mechanisms of Erection in the Canine Penis. Amer. J. Physiol., **213:**1526 (1967).

DYM, M.: The Fine Structure of the Monkey (*Macaca*) Sertoli Cell and Its Role in Maintaining the Blood-Testis Barrier. Anat. Rec., **175:**639 (1973).

DYM, M.: The Fine Structure of Monkey Sertoli Cells in the Transitional Zone at the Junction of the Seminiferous Tubules with the Tubuli Recti. Am. J. Anat., **140:**1 (1974).

DYM, M.: The Mammalian Rete Testis—A Morphological Examination. Anat. Rec., **186:**493 (1976).

DYM, M., and Y. CLERMONT: Role of Spermatogonia in the Repair of the Seminiferous Epithelium Following x-Irradiation of the Rat Testis. Am. J. Anat., **128:**265 (1970).

DYM, M., and D. W. FAWCETT: The Blood-Testis Barrier in the Rat and the Physiological Compartmentation of the Seminiferous Epithelium. Biol. Reprod., **3:**308 (1970).

DYM, M., and D. W. FAWCETT: Further Observations on the Numbers of Spermatogonia, Spermatocytes, and Spermatids Connected by Intracellular Bridges in the Mammalian Testis. Biol. Reprod., **4:**195 (1971).

FAWCETT, D. W.: The Mammalian Spermatozoon. Develop. Biol., **44:**395 (1975).

FAWCETT, D. W.: Ultrastructure and Function of the Sertoli Cell, in sec. 7; Endocrinology, vol. 5, Male Reproductive System. D. W. Hamilton and R. O. Greep (eds.), "Handbook of Physiology," Amer. Phys. Soc., Washington, 1975.

FAWCETT, D. W., and M. H. BURGOS: Studies on the Fine Structure of the Mammalian Testis. II. The Human Interstitial Tissue, Amer. J. Anat., **107:**245 (1960).

FAWCETT, D. W., P. M. HEIDGER, and L. V. LEAK: Lymph Vascular System of the Interstitial Tissue of the Testis as Revealed by Electron Microscopy. J. Reprod. Fertility, **19:**109 (1969).

FAWCETT, D. W., and R. D. HOLLENBERG: Changes in the Acrosome of Guinea Pig Spermatozoa during Passage through the Epididymis. Z. Zellforsch., **60:**276 (1963).

FAWCETT, D. W., and D. M. PHILLIPS: Observations on the Release of Spermatozoa and on Changes in the Head during Passage through the Epididymis. J. Reprod. Fertility Suppl., **6:**405 (1969).

FLICKINGER, C. J.: Ultrastructural Observations on the Postnatal Development of the Rat Prostate. Z. Zellforsch., **113:**157 (1971).

FRENCH, F. S., and E. M. RITZÉN: Androgen Binding Protein in Efferent Duct Fluid of Rat Testis. J. Reprod. Fertility, **32:**479 1973).

HAMILTON, D. W.: Steroid Function in the Mammalian Epididymis. J. Reprod. Fertil. (Suppl.), **13:**89 (1971).

HAMILTON, D. W.: Structure and Function of the Epithelium Lining the Ductuli Efferentes, Ductus Epididymis, and Ductus Deferens in the Rat, in sec. 7, Endocrinology, vol. 5, Male Reproductive System, D. W. Hamilton and R. O. Greep (eds.), "Handbook of Physiology," Amer. Phys. Soc., Washington, 1975.

HELLER, C. G., and Y. CLERMONT: Kinetics of the Germinal Epithelium in Man. Recent Prog. Hormone Res., **20:**545 (1964).

HELLER, C. G., M. F. LALLI, and M. J. ROWLEY: Factors Affecting the Testicular Function in Man. "Pharmacology of Reproduction," vol. 2, Pergamon Press, New York (1968).

HOLSTEIN, A. F.: Morphologische Studien am Nebenhoden des Menschen, in "Zwanglose Abhandlungen aus dem Gebiet der normalen und pathologischen Anatomie," hrsg. von W. Bargmann u. W. Doerr. Stuttgart, G. Thieme (1969).

HUCKINS, C.: The Spermatogonial Stem Cell Population in Adult Rats. I. Their Morphology, Proliferation and Maturation, Anat. Rec., **169:**533 (1971).

KORMANO, M., and H. SUORANTA: Microvascular Organization of the Adult Human Testis, Anat. Rec., **170:**31 (1971).

LAM, D. M. K., R. FURRER, and W. R. BRUCE: The Separation, Physical Characterization and Differentiation Kinetics of Spermatogonial Cells of the Mouse. Proc. Nat. Acad. Sci., **65:**192 (1970).

LEBLOND, C. P., and Y. CLERMONT: Spermiogenesis of Rat, Mouse, Hamster and Guinea Pig as Revealed by the Periodic Acid-Fuchsin Sulfurous Acid Technique. Amer. J. Anat., **90:**167 (1952).

MASON, K. E., and S. L. SHAVER: Some Functions of the Caput Epididymis. Ann. N.Y. Acad. Sci., **55:**585 (1952).

MCNEAL, J. E.: The Prostate and Prostatic Urethra: A Morphological Synthesis. J. Urol., **107:**1008 (1972).

MEANS, A. R., J. L. FAKUNDING, C. HUCKINS, D. J. TINDALL, and R. VITALE: Follicle Stimulating Hormone, the Sertoli Cells and Spermatogenesis, in "Recent Progress Hormone Research," Academic Press, New York, 1976.

MOENS, P. B.: Mechanisms of Chromosome Synapsis at Meiotic Prophase. Internat. Rev. Cytol., **35:**117 (1973).

NEWMAN, H. F., J. D. NORTHRUP, and J. DEVLIN: Mechanism of Human Penile Erection. Invest. Urol., **1:**350 (1964).

NICANDER, L.: Studies on the Regional Histology and Cytochemistry of the Ductus Epididymidis in Stallions, Rams and Bulls. Acta Morph. Neerl. Scand., **1:**337 (1958).

ORGEBIN-CRIST, M. C.: Studies on the Function of the Epididymis. Biol. Reprod. (suppl.), **1:**155 (1969).

PEREY, B., Y. CLERMONT, and C. P. LEBLOND: The Wave of the Seminiferous Epithelium in the Rat. Amer. J. Anat., **108:**47 (1961).

ROOSEN-RUNGE, E. C.: The Process of Spermatogenesis in Mammals. Biol. Rev., **37:**343 (1962).

ROWLEY, M. J., J. D. BERLIN, and C. G. HELLER: The Ultrastructure of Four Types of Human Spermatogonia. Z. Zellforsch., **112:**139 (1971).

ROWLEY, M. J., F. TESHIMA, and C. G. HELLER: Duration of Transit of Spermatozoa through the Human Male Ductular System. Fertil. Steril., **21:**390 (1970).

SETCHELL, B. P., and G. M. H. WAITES: The Blood-Testis Barrier, in sec. 7, Endocrinology, vol. 5, Male Reproductive System, D. W. Hamilton and R. O. Greep (eds.), "Handbook of Physiology," Amer. Phys. Soc., Washington, 1975.

SOHVAL, A. R., Y. SUZUKI, J. L. GABRILOVE, and J. CHURG: Ultrastructure of Crystalloids in Spermatogonia and Sertoli Cells of Normal Human Testis. J. Ultrastruct. Res., **34:**83 (1971).

STIEVE, H.: Mannliche Genitalorgane, in vol. 7, pt. 2, W. von Möllendorff (ed.), "Handbuch mikroskopischen Anatomie des Menschen," Springer-Verlag OHG, Berlin, 1930.

ZAMBONI, L., R. ZEMJANIS, and M. STEFANINI: The Fine Structure of Monkey and Human Spermatozoa. Anat. Rec., **169:**129 (1971).

The Hypophysis

NICHOLAS S. HALMI AND GWEN C. MORIARTY

INTRODUCTORY REMARKS ON ENDOCRINE TISSUES

The *endocrine glands* are also known as *ductless glands* or *glands of internal secretion*. Their parenchymal cells manufacture specific products, termed *hormones,* which they usually secrete into the bloodstream. Hormones act as chemical regulators of the functions of specific tissues elsewhere in the body or of the somatic cells in general. The specific structure affected is spoken of as the *target organ* of the hormone concerned. The endocrine glands constitute one of the great coordinating mechanisms of the body, the other being the nervous system. The two systems are intimately linked in their functions. The focus of neuroendocrine integration is the adenohypophysis, which regulates a number of target glands (thyroid, adrenal cortex, gonads) and is in turn controlled by "release" and "inhibitory" factors (hypophyseotropic hormones) produced in hypothalamic neurons and conveyed to the adenohypophysis through blood vessels. Both the nervous and the endocrine system participate in the maintenance of a steady physiologic state and are therefore described as having a *homeostatic* or *homeokinetic* role.

The glands which are universally recognized as endocrine glands are the hypophysis, thyroid, parathyroids, adrenals (each consisting of medulla and cortex), gonads, and islets of the pancreas. The placenta, when present, also elaborates hormones. Some other organs (intestine, kidney) have endocrine functions in addition to their dominant activity. The number of hormones produced by the endocrine glands ranges from one (testis) to nine (hypophysis).

Endocrine glands have no ducts, so their cells secrete into vascular channels. Most endocrine glands are primarily composed of parenchyma and blood vessels, with relatively little stroma. The parenchymal cells are usually polyhedral epithelial cells, arranged with at least one surface abutting upon the wall of a blood or lymph vessel. Their cytoplasm generally contains either clear vacuoles filled with lipid material or granules that are denser than the cytoplasm and have specific affinities for certain dyes. The presence of these cytoplasmic inclusions is not, however, a necessary condition for the elaboration of hormones. Cells which produce steroid hormones (for example, those of the adrenal cortex) contain lipid droplets; those whose products are peptide or protein hormones (such as the cells of the anterior pituitary lobe) have secretion granules in their cytoplasm. The abundance of these droplets or granules correlates better with the amounts of hormones stored than with their secretion rate.

1039

The endocrine glands have an exceptionally rich blood supply; the thyroid and adrenals are among the most vascular tissues in the body. This is a reflection of their intense metabolic activity and of the fact that the bloodstream both supplies the materials from which hormones are synthesized and carries away the released hormones.

HYPOPHYSIS (PITUITARY GLAND)

GROSS STRUCTURE AND SUBDIVISIONS

The hypophysis lies at the base of the brain, to which it is linked by a stalk, the *infundibular stalk.* In human beings, the stalk is long and slants forward from the brain to the hypophysis. The hypophysis is flattened on the superior surface and is distinctly elongated in the transverse plane. Average measurements of the gland are 1.3 cm (transverse) × 1 cm (sagittal) × 0.5 cm (vertical). It weighs less than 1 g in adults, being somewhat heavier in females than in males. The hypophysis undergoes some enlargement during pregnancy and may weigh up to 1.5 g in multiparae. The hypophysis in human beings, as in most mammals, rests in a depression in the sphenoid bone, the *sella turcica.* The dura mater of the brain extends across this bony depression as a diaphragm, the *diaphragma sellae,* and is reflected over the surface of the hypophysis to form a fibrous connective tissue capsule which is fused with the periosteum lining the sella.

By gross inspection, the hypophysis is seen to consist of two lobes. The anterior lobe is pinkish and composed of soft, friable glandular tissue; the posterior lobe is white, more fibrous, and firmer. On microscopic examination, other structural components of the hypophysis are revealed (Fig. 27-1). A small portion, connected with and extending upward from the anterior lobe, surrounds the pituitary stalk in a collar-like fashion, forming the *pars tuberalis.* Between the two major parts of the hypophysis lies a thin cellular partition termed the *intermediate lobe,* or *pars intermedia.* The hypophysis is attached to the brain by means of the infundibulum, consisting of an elongated *infundibular stem* and the so-called median eminence, which contains the *infundibular recess* of the third ventricle. The infundibular stem thickens beneath the diaphragma sellae and continues as the button-shaped *pars nervosa,* or *infundibular process.* The stem attaches to the brain at the median eminence. The pars nervosa, stem, and median eminence constitute the neurohypophysis (see Fig. 27-1). In human beings, the median eminence is poorly developed, and the pars nervosa is intimately fused with the pars intermedia. This gland is structurally so complex that the terms *anterior lobe* and *posterior lobe,* though well established in the literature of endocrinology and eminently useful because they indicate the two most important functional parts of the hypophysis, do not encompass the entire gland. A much-used classification of the structural components of the whole hypophysis is given in Table 27-1. The infundibular stem and the pars tuberalis which surrounds it constitute the *hypophyseal stalk.*

HISTOGENESIS OF THE HYPOPHYSIS

The adenohypophysis and the neurohypophysis have different embryologic origins. The former arises as an invagination (Rathke's pouch) of the lining of the future oral cavity, whereas the nervous component develops as a downgrowth (infundibulum) from the floor of the diencephalon (Fig. 27-2A).

The two anlagen are closely situated and soon establish contact. The stem of tissue connecting the nervous lobe to the brain is retained in the adult as the core of the pituitary stalk. The attachment of Rathke's pouch to the roof of the oral cavity is lost early in embryonic life, but rudiments are sometimes found as a cellular strand in the sphenoid bone and as a nest of glandular tissue, known as the *pharyngeal pituitary,* at the site of origin in the nasopharynx. The pharyngeal

TABLE 27-1 DIVISIONS OF THE HYPOPHYSIS

MAJOR DIVISION	SUBDIVISIONS
Adenohypophysis	Pars tuberalis Pars intermedia—intermediate lobe Pars distalis—anterior lobe

Neurohypophysis	Pars nervosa or infundibular
	    process—posterior lobe
	Infundibulum
	    Infundibular stem
	    Median eminence (of tuber cinereum)

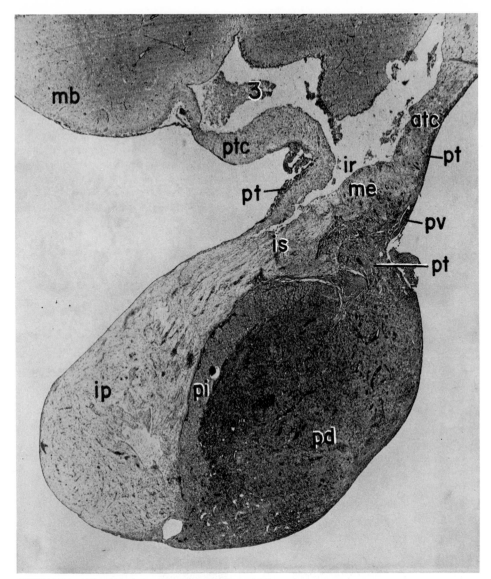

FIGURE 27-1 Midsagittal section through a rabbit hypophysis that is in connection with the hypothalamus. This shows the pars distalis (pd), the pars intermedia (pi), the infundibular process or pars nervosa (ip), the infundibular stem (is), the pars tuberalis (pt), a portal vessel (pv), the median eminence (me), anterior and posterior portions of the tuber cinereum (atc and ptc), the third ventricle (3) with its infundibular recess (ir), and the mammillary body (mb). Azan.

pituitary may produce functional pituitary tumors. At least one hormone (growth hormone) has been identified in its cells.

Figure 27-2 illustrates well what happens as the development of Rathke's pouch proceeds. It aligns itself early against the rostral surface of the infundibulum and develops into three separate glandular portions: (1) the rostral wall of the pouch, which thickens very markedly to form the pars distalis; (2) the caudal wall, which becomes a very thin layer of cells that fuses with the neural outgrowth and is known as the pars intermedia; and (3) the bilateral thickenings of the wall on the dorsolateral aspects of Rathke's pouch, which form two hornlike extensions that pass around the infundibular stem, one on each side, forming a collar of tissue, the pars tuberalis.

BLOOD SUPPLY OF THE HYPOPHYSIS

The hypophysis derives its blood supply from two sets of arteries: inferior hypophyseal arteries that arise from the internal carotids and supply mainly the pars nervosa, and several superior hypophyseal arteries emanating from the internal carotids and from the posterior communicating artery of the circle of Willis. The superior arteries feed a capillary plexus in the pars tuberalis which gives off capillary loops that penetrate the median eminence and infundibular stem. This plexus is drained by portal vessels that pass down the pars tuberalis and supply the capillaries in the pars distalis. The portal vessels are so called because, like the portal vein of the liver, they are interposed between two sets of capillaries, one in the pars tuberalis and infundibular stem, and another in the pars distalis. In addition, a set of short inferior hypophyseal arteries feeds the outer layer of the pars distalis. Another artery which bypasses the portal sysem arises from the superior hypophyseal arteries and supplies posterior portions of the pars distalis. It is called the loral artery. Anastomoses between the capillaries of the pars nervosa and those of the anterior lobe exist but are not abundant. The blood supply of the pars distalis ex-

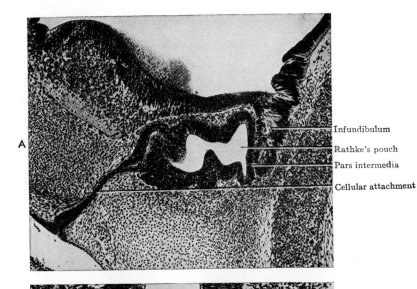

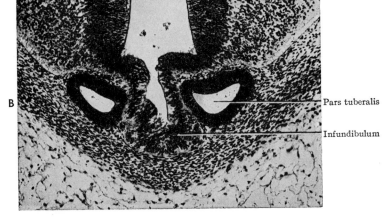

FIGURE 27-2 Development of the human hypophysis. A. A 17-mm embryo. Midsagittal section through the bulbous end of Rathke's pouch and the adjacent infundibulum. The cellular strand marks the point of origin of the epithelial component of the hypophysis. B. Median section through the hypophysis of a midterm fetus. Pars tuberalis points to lateral extensions of Rathke's pouch, which later become obliterated. The pars tuberalis is formed by the walls of these recesses. (Courtesy of B. Romeis.)

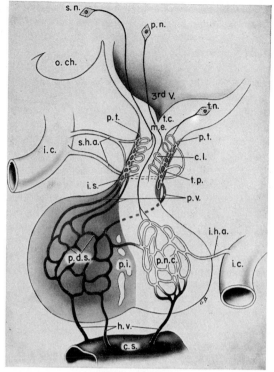

FIGURE 27-3 Diagram of the hypophyseal blood supply. The following structures are labeled: optic chiasm (och), supraoptic nucleus (sn), periventricular nucleus (pn), third ventricle (3d v), tuberal nuclei (tn), tuber cinereum (tc), median eminence (me), pars tuberalis (pt), tuberal plexus (tp), capillary loops from tuberal plexus (cl), internal carotid (ic), superior hypophyseal arteries (sha), infundibular stem (is), portal vessels (pv), pars distalis capillaries (pdc), pars intermedia (pi), pars nervosa capillaries (pnc), inferior hypophyseal artery (iha), hypophyseal veins (hv), and cavernous sinus (cs). (Drawing by G. Buckley.)

plains why an outer shell and the portions lying close to the pars nervosa are the only ones surviving complete interruption of the portal vessels. The venous drainage of both the pars distalis and the pars nervosa is by way of hypophyseal veins that empty into the cavernous sinus (Fig. 27-3).

The hypophyseal "portal circulation" is a remarkably constant feature throughout the vertebrate groups. Although the hypothalamic and hypophyseal blood supplies are separate except for a few capillary anastomoses, the portal vessels provide the morphologic basis for the regulation of the anterior lobe by the hypothalamus. Hypothalamic nerve fibers end around the capillary loops in the infundibular stem, and substances that have traveled along them (neurohormones, hypophyseotropic factors) are released there into the bloodstream; the blood, thus enriched, is carried to the pars distalis by the portal vessels, and the neurohormones can then influence the cells of this part of the adenohypophysis. The hypophyseal portal circulation provides the vascular part of what is called the *neurovascular link* between the hypothalamus and the pituitary (see section on Hypothalamic Regulation).

NERVE SUPPLY OF THE HYPOPHYSIS

Nerve fibers originating from hypothalamic cells are an integral part of the neurohypophysis and are discussed in that context. Nerve fibers of the infundibular stalk do not appear to extend into the pars distalis, but in some mammals nerve fibers leave the pars nervosa to terminate about cells of the pars intermedia. Although some postganglionic sympathetic and possibly also parasympathetic nerve fibers can be found in the adenohypophysis, there is no evidence that their function is anything other than vasomotor.

ADENOHYPOPHYSIS

In spite of its small size, the adenohypophysis elaborates seven hormones: growth hormone (GH, or somatotropin, STH), prolactin, thyrotropin (TSH), the gonadotropins (LH and FSH), adrenocorticotropin (ACTH), and the precursor of melanocyte-stimulating hormone (MSH), lipotropin (LPH).

MICROSCOPIC STRUCTURE

Pars Tuberalis

The pars tuberalis forms a collar of cells 25 to 60 μm thick around the neural stalk. It is thickest anterior to the stalk and frequently incomplete on the posterior aspect. The cells are arranged in short cords or globular clusters and occasionally as small follicles. Nests of squamous cells are often found in or around the pars tuberalis. They were believed to give rise to tumors (craniopharyngiomas), but such groups of squamous cells are seldom seen in children, whereas craniopharyngiomas are most commonly discovered during the second decade of life.

Pars Intermedia

In most species this portion of the adenohypophysis is quite distinct. It is lacking in some mammals (for example, whales) and in birds. In such animals, a dural septum separates the pars distalis from the pars nervosa. In human beings, the pars intermedia is rudimentary and is composed of chromophobic and basophilic cells. These often surround colloid-filled cysts and merge imperceptibly with those of the pars distalis. Sometimes a remnant of Rathke's cleft persists; in such cases the pars intermedia cells are those posterior to the lumen. The cells lining follicles may be ciliated. A unique feature of the human gland is the

invasion of the pars nervosa by basophilic (specifically β_1) cells similar to those in the pars distalis (Fig. 27-4A). Such displaced cells may be quite numerous or altogether absent. Tubular (salivary type) glands surrounded by loose lymphoid tissue (Fig. 27-4B) can often be seen in the pars nervosa next to the pars intermedia.

Pars Distalis

The pars distalis forms about 75 percent of the hypophysis. The cells in the pars distalis are arranged mainly in cords between which are large-bore capillaries. Some cells appear to be in clusters and others in twisted cords; and still others form small, well-defined follicles whose lumina may contain colloid. There is very little connective tissue in any part of the hypophysis, and in the pars distalis only a light meshwork of reticular fibers is present. These are entwined around the basement membranes of the cells and the capillaries (Fig. 27-5).

FIGURE 27-4 Portions of the human pars nervosa. A. Basophilic cells of the anterior lobe (top) invading the pars nervosa. Masson's trichrome. B. Salivary-type glands (t) surrounded by lymphocytes in the pars nervosa. Note a blood vessel (v) and a large intermediate lobe cyst (ic). Gomori's trichrome.

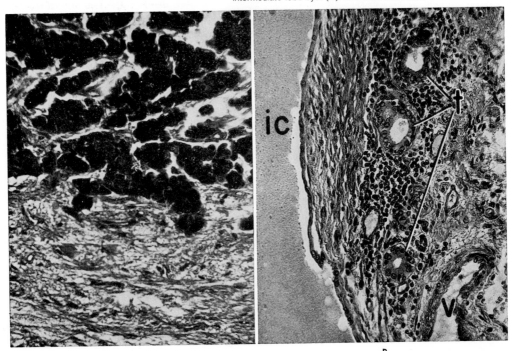

A   B

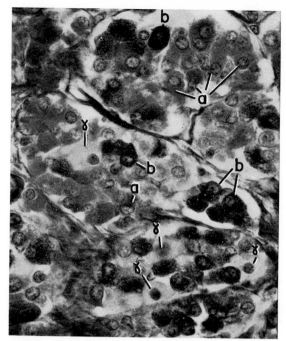

FIGURE 27-5 Portion of a human pars distalis. Note reticular fibers dividing cell nests; see also acidophils (a), basophils (b), and γ cells (γ). PAS-hematoxylin–orange G.

introduced a number of new nomenclatures since Romeis's treatise was published. This and the extension of his terminology to species other than human beings have created much confusion. The most significant developments achieved with refined staining techniques since Romeis's book was published are the following: (1) with aldehyde thionin-PAS-orange G, his β cells can be broken down into two categories: the PAS-red β_1 cells and the aldehyde thionin-blue β_2 cells; (2) in the hypophyses of lactating women, two types of acidophils can be distinguished with erythrosin-orange G or carmoisine-orange G: the orangeophilic cells that correspond to the α cells and the erythrosinophilic (carmoisinophilic) cells that are the same as the pregnancy cells of earlier authors (η cells of Romeis). An even more important recent advance, achieved with the use of immunocytochemistry, has been the identification of the cell types of the human hypophysis as the source of specific hormones, so that a functional nomenclature is now applicable to them. Table 27-2 shows the correspondence of functionally and tinctorially differentiated cell types in the human pars distalis.

Among the *acidophils* of the human hypophysis, Romeis's α type usually predominates. These cells are located preferentially in posterolateral parts of the lobe; they are smaller than most basophils and rounded. The granulation may vary from sparse to extremely dense. The granules are small and highly refractile. The α cells stain immunohistochemically for GH (STH) (Fig. 27-6A). Acidophils of another type, less numerous, quite variable in shape, and apparently wedged between adjacent cells, cannot be distinguished tinctorially, but they are revealed by immunocytochemistry as the source of prolactin (Fig. 27-6B). When they enlarge in response to elevated levels of estrogen (as in pregnancy, and continuing into lactation), the hyperplastic prolactin cells (pregnancy cells, η cells) become erythrosinophilic and carmoisinophilic while maintaining their immunoreactivity for prolactin (Fig. 27-6C). The functional significance of the generally inconspicuous ϵ cells described by Romeis is not clear.

The commonest *basophils* are of the β_1 type. Such cells are most numerous in the central, anterior part of the lobe. They are generally larger than the average α cell and usually ovoid. The intensely PAS-reactive granules in the cytoplasm of β_1 cells are

The classic nomenclature distinguishes three main types of cells in the pars distalis: *acidophils, basophils,* and *chromophobes.* These were said to constitute about 40, 10, and 50 percent of the anterior lobe cells, respectively, but more recent observations by both light and electron microscopy have shown that chromophobes are much less numerous and largely supportive elements (follicular cells) forming a network within the parenchyma. "Basophil cells" is a misnomer, since these cells are actually characterizd by blue staining of their granules with the aniline blue component of triacid stains such as Mallory's. However, an alternative term, "mucoid," which is based on the fact that basophils are periodic acid-Schiff (PAS) positive, has not gained wide acceptance. The nomenclature of Romeis (1940) takes into account that with appropriate stains the classic cell types can be further broken down into distinct entities. Romeis thus distinguished between α and ϵ acidophils, β and δ basophils, γ cells (which were previously regarded as chromophobes but which appear to be a distinct kind of basophil), and undifferentiated or degranulated chromophobes. Unfortunately, different authors, using a variety of fixatives and staining procedures, have

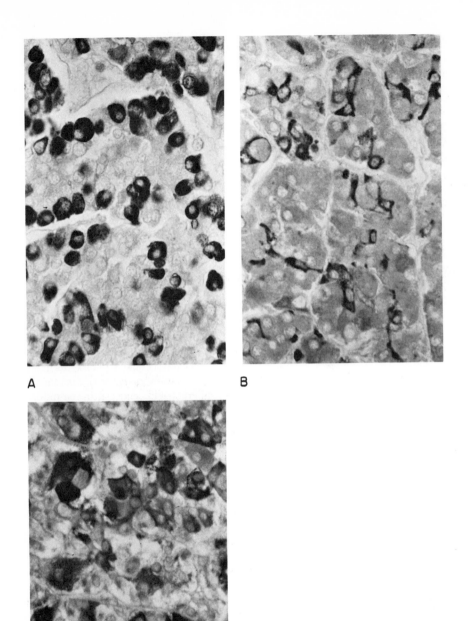

FIGURE 27-6 Human anterior hypophyseal lobes immunocyto-chemically stained by the unlabeled antibody peroxidase-antiperoxi-dase (PAP) complex method. A. GH cells in a normal hypophysis. B. Prolactin cells in the same hypophysis. C. Hypertrophic, hyperplastic prolactin cells from the hypophysis of a lactating woman. A and B: 400; C: 250. (Rearranged from N. S. Halmi, J. A. Parsons, S. L. Erlandsen, and T. Duello, *Cell Tiss. Res.*, **158:**497, 1975.)

TABLE 27-2 CORRESPONDENCE OF IMMUNOCYTOCHEMICALLY IDENTIFIED FUNCTIONAL CELL TYPES IN THE HUMAN PARS DISTALIS WITH THOSE DIFFERENTIATED BY TINCTORIAL MEANS

FUNCTIONAL NOMENCLATURE	ROMEIS-EZRIN GREEK-LETTER NOMENCLATURE	CLASSICAL NOMENCLATURE
Somatotrops or GH cells	α	⎤
Lactotrops or prolactin cells (resting)	?	Acidophils
Lactotrops or prolactin cells (pregnancy, lactation)	η	⎦
Cortico-lipotrops or ACTH/LPH cells	β_1	⎤
Thyrotrops, or TSH, cells	β_2, γ	Basophils
Gonadotrops, or FSH/LH cells	$\delta, \gamma?$	⎦
Poorly granulated cells of all varieties	Chromophobes	⎤ Chromophobes
Follicular cells	Chromophobes	⎦

usually numerous. Immunocytochemically the β_1 cells stain for both ACTH and βMSH, but it seems that the reaction for the latter is due to the presence of the larger precursor molecule of βMSH, βlipotropin (βLPH). Therefore, the proper designation of β_1 cells, called ACTH/MSH cells by Phifer et al. (1974), is ACTH/LPH cells. The strongly aldehyde thionin-positive β_2 cells are usually angular. Their granulation appears quite coarse. These cells are often confined to the anterocentral portions of the pars distalis (Fig. 27-7). Immunocytochemistry has shown that they contain TSH. At least some of the γ cells (Fig. 27-5) are also immunoreactive for TSH. Another type of "basophil" cell in the anterior lobe is represented by

Romeis's δ basophils. These are generally smaller than the β_1 cells, round, and often sparsely granulated. They are more frequent than β cells in lateral parts of the lobe, and quite variable in size; some of the larger cells of this type are hard to distinguish from γ cells. Their granules, which stain with aldehyde thionin, are said to be lysosomes rather than true secretion granules (those are finer, not visible under the light microscope, and very prone to postmortem autolysis). Immunocytochemical studies have located both FSH and LH in δ cells. Since there is no evidence for separate FSH and LH cells, δ cells can be collectively called FSH/LH cells or gonadotrops (Fig. 27-8). The γ cells are large, have few PAS-positive granules but

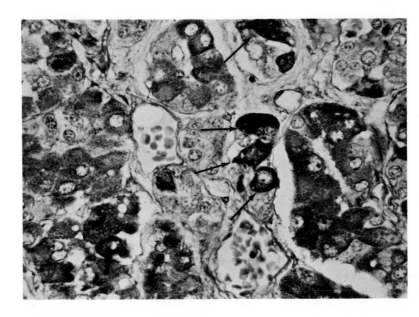

FIGURE 27-7 Anteromedian portion of a human pars distalis stained with aldehyde thionin–PAS–orange G. The ACTH/LPH (β_1 cells), stained with PAS, are those with variable gray granulation. The angular or irregularly shaped TSH (β_2) cells, stained with aldehyde thionin, appear dark (arrows).

sometimes many colloid droplets, and show a prominent Golgi image (Fig. 27-5). It is questionable whether they are a separate cell type: they may be morphologically distinct but functionally heterogeneous.

True *chromophobes* (other than follicular cells) are much less common than counts based on conventionally stained material indicate, if they indeed exist. Most of the apparently chromophobic cells certainly have a few specific granules. It is commonly believed that the cells of the pars distalis show cyclic secretory activity, that is, that they first accumulate and then release their specific granules. "Chromophobes" may therefore be transitionally degranulated cells. Since large shifts in the distribution of granulated cells may occur and mitoses are infrequent in the anterior lobe, the apparent chromophobes are the probable reservoir from which more fully granulated cells of different types originate.

ULTRASTRUCTURE OF
THE ADENOHYPOPHYSEAL CELLS

Because of the limited availability of well-preserved human material, our knowledge of the ultrastructure of the pars distalis of human beings is still somewhat sketchy.

Among the *acidophils,* the α or GH cells resemble those of more extensively studied species such as the rat quite closely. Their granules are densely packed and average 350 nm in diameter. The rough endoplasmic reticulum is well developed. The *prolactin cells* in the resting state have not been well studied with the electron microscope. The enlarged prolactin cells in pregnancy and lactation (η cells) are characterized by relatively sparse granules which, like those in the prolactin cells of the rat, may be quite large (over 600 nm in maximal diameter) and often irregularly shaped. The rough endoplasmic reticulum is exceptionally well developed in these cells. In tumors arising from prolactin cells, the granules are sometimes small, but their mode of extrusion from the cell is unique: they leave parts of the cell not adjacent to capillaries ("misplaced exocytosis").

Among the *basophils,* the ACTH/LPH cells (β₁ cells) are round or ovoid, with granules at random throughout the cytoplasm. Granule size overlaps so much with that of GH cells that distinction on this

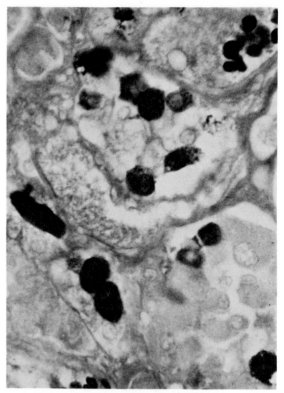

FIGURE 27-8 Gonadotropic cells of human adenohypophysis immunocytochemically stained with antibody against LH. Unlabeled antibody-PAP complex method. Staining of red blood cells is a result of their peroxidase activity and not an immunocytochemical reaction.

basis is tenuous. The two cell types can be readily distinguished, however, by electron-microscopic immunocytochemistry. ACTH/LPH cells often contain large lipids droplets. A feature unique to them is the presence, in the cytoplasm, of a small number of fibers about 60 to 80 Å in diameter. These can become much more numerous in pathologic states (see Crooke cells below). Immunostaining reveals a single set of granules reactive for ACTH and βMSH (because of the βLPH content) in the ACTH/LPH cells (Figs. 27-9 and 27-10). In contrast to the human ACTH/LPH cells, the ACTH cells in the pars distalis of the rat are stellate, with ovoid granules mostly in the periphery. The *TSH* (β₂) cells have, like those of the rat, the smallest secretory granules of all hypophyseal cells (150 nm or less across) (Fig. 27-9). The *gonadotropic* (δ) cells have granules intermediate in size between those of GH and TSH cells. Their electron

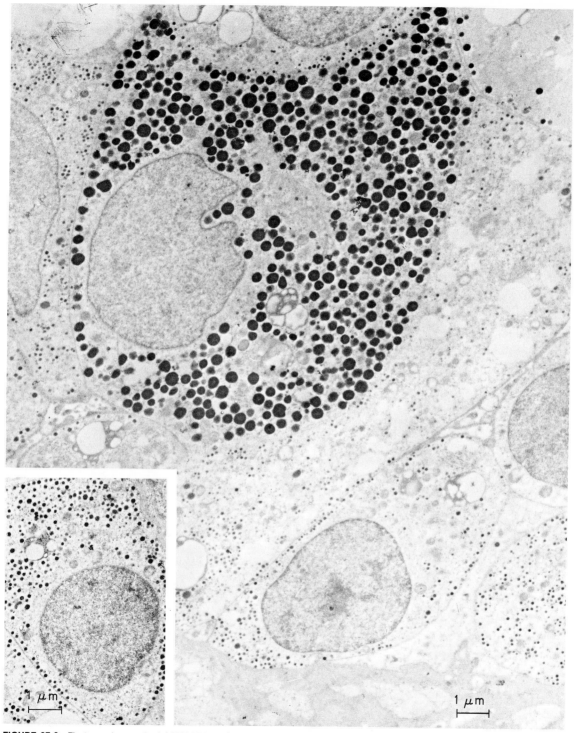

FIGURE 27-9 Electron micrograph of ACTH/LPH cell (upper part of field) whose granules were immunocytochemically stained with antibody against $^{17-39}$ACTH. Unlabeled antibody-PAP complex method. The adjacent cells with considerably smaller, unstained granules are TSH cells. The inset (lower left) shows the granules of TSH cells immunocytochemically stained with antibody against the hormone-specific β chain of TSH. (The glycoprotein hormones of the pituitary, TSH, FSH and LH, share a virtually identical α chain.)

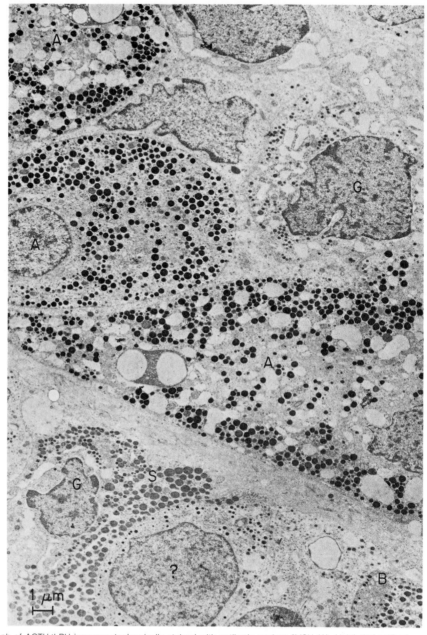

FIGURE 27-10 Electron micrograph of ACTH/LPH immunocytochemically stained with antibody against βMSH (A). Unlabeled antibody-PAP complex method. Also shown are an unstained growth hormone cell (S) and gonadotrops (G).

density is quite variable. These cells often contain lipid droplets and lysosomes (Fig. 27-11). The γ *cells* are characterized by few secretory granules and an abundance of smooth endoplasmic reticular sacs. They resemble the hypertrophic-hyperplastic TSH cells in the pituitary of hypothyroid rats ("thyroidectomy cells").

The *follicular cells* are stellate or elongated, and their apexes may join together to line small spaces filled with homogeneous colloid, into which they extend microvilli.

HISTOCHEMISTRY OF THE ADENOHYPOPHYSIS

The basophilic cells of the adenohypophysis, including the γ cells, can be best defined as the cells whose secretory granules give a positive PAS reaction after digestion with amylase; that is, they contain glycoproteins. These granules, which usually appear coarse, must correspond to aggregates of those seen under the electron microscope. Recent studies of thin sections from glutaraldehyde-fixed human pituitaries have shown scattered PAS-positive granules in most nonbasophilic cells too. Basophilic cells are (at least in the rat) the source of glycoprotein hormones (TSH, gonadotropins). It is therefore likely that these hormones contribute to the PAS-positive nature of their granules. In human beings, however, the cells with the most markedly PAS-reactive granules, the β_1 cells, produce the simple peptides ACTH and βLPH. The colloid droplets seen in hypophyseal cells are intensely PAS-positive and sudanophilic, and they may contain a lipid pigment. Intercellular colloid also stains with PAS. Basophilia due to rough ER is found in the cytoplasm of anterior lobe cells. It is most pronounced in active acidophils.

HISTOPHYSIOLOGY OF THE ADENOHYPOPHYSIS

Hormones Produced by Different Cell Types

Since the adenohypophysis is known to produce a number of hormones and contains several cell types, many efforts have been made to identify the cellular source of individual hormones. Even before the immunocytochemical studies, whose success has permitted the functional classification of human adenohypophyseal cell types (Table 27-2), much light was shed on the function of pituitary cell classes by (1) bioassays of different parts of large hypophyses in

which cell types are unevenly distributed, and (2) attempts to correlate typical histologic changes in various physiologic or pathologic states, and, under experimental conditions, with altered hormone storage or secretion. Since target organ hormones act back on the cells that produce the tropic hormones, experimental changes in the levels of target gland hormones have been especially useful in eliciting characteristic responses in the hypophysis. Experimentally induced or spontaneously arising tumors of individual cell types often produce an excess of the hormone normally elaborated by these cells, and have thus furnished important information on the cellular sources of different hormones.

Growth Hormone (GH, Somatotropin, STH)

GH is a simple protein that enhances body growth after birth. Its absence results in *pituitary dwarfism;* its oversecretion in childhood leads to *gigantism* and during adult life to *acromegaly* (enlargement of hands, feet, mandible, and viscera). In addition to the immunocytochemical staining of α cells for GH (Fig. 27-6A), the origin of GH from these cells is attested to by the occurrence of α cell tumors (adenomas) in gigantism or acromegaly. The production of GH by acidophils in the hypophyses of animals is supported by several observations: (1) the GH acidophils in rats lose their granules after thyroidectomy, and the animals' growth stops concomitantly; small doses of thyroid hormones restore both the pituitary GH cells and growth; (2) in a strain of dwarf mice, the hypophysis is severely deficient in acidophils; and (3) GH is found predominantly in "acidophilic" regions of the bovine hypophysis.

Prolactin

Prolactin is a simple protein that promotes mammary development and lactation. It also participates in the maintenance of corpora lutea in rodents, whose prolactin has therefore been called *luteotropin (LTH)*. In the pituitary of a number of species (for example, rabbit, cat), staining with azocarmine and orange G reveals two types of acidophils, carmine cells and orange cells. The former are consistently prominent when prolactin secretion is enhanced (Fig. 27-12, see color insert). As indicated, the human "resting" prolactin cell does not stain differentially, except by immunocytochemistry (Fig. 27-6B), but the hyper-

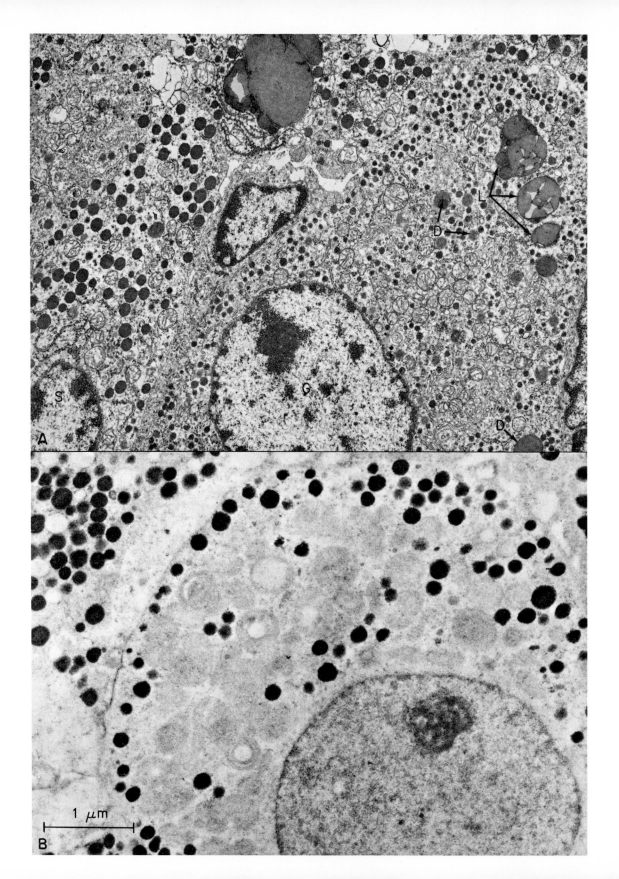

trophic, hyperplastic, and hyperactive prolactin cell in pregnancy and lactation (Fig. 27-6C) does. Human pituitary tumors composed of prolactin cells may cause milk flow (galactorrhea) not associated with postpartum lactation. Preliminary evidence suggests that apparently nonfunctional adenomas of the human hypophysis classified as "chromophobic" often contain immunoreactive and ultrastructurally identifiable prolactin cells, and may be accompanied by high levels of prolactin in blood, without other clinical signs.

Thyrotropin (Thyroid-stimulating Hormone, TSH)

This glycoprotein hormone stimulates many functions of the thyroid. In human beings with primary thyroid failure, hypersecretion of TSH is accompanied by the appearance of large, lightly granulated basophils containing colloid droplets. These are said to be derived from TSH (β_2) cells. Conversely, in Graves' disease, a condition characterized by hypersecretion of thyroid hormones in response to a nonpituitary thyroid stimulator, their negative feedback effect on the TSH cells of the pituitary causes these to regress. In thyroidectomized rats, the TSH cells become enlarged, hyperplastic, and degranulated. TSH stores in the hypophyses of such rats fall, while circulating TSH levels rise. Excess thyroid hormone given to rats cause involution of pituitary TSH cells accompanied by decreased storage and diminished secretion of TSH. TSH-producing adenomas of the thyrotrops occur in mice after destruction of their thyroid with radioactive iodine. A few TSH-producing β_2 cell adenomas in man have also been described, mostly in people who had primary failure of the thyroid.

Gonadotropins: Follicle-stimulating Hormone (FSH) and Luteinizing Hormone (LH)

FSH, a glycoprotein, stimulates the growth of ovarian follicles past the primordial stage and activates the spermatogenic epithelium of the testis. LH, also a glycoprotein, is necessary for ovulation and the secretion of estrogen by the follicle; it also stimulates the Leydig cells of the testis to secrete androgen. In human beings, the most convincing proof for the identity of gonadotrops (FSH/LH cells) is immunocytochemical (Fig. 27-8). These cells regress during pregnancy, when placental estrogen exerts a negative

feedback effect on them, and are usually small and few in childhood, when gonadotropin secretion is at a low level. However, they do not show the expected hypertrophy and hyperplasia after the menopause, when secretion of gonadotropins is elevated. This is in contrast to the marked enlargement and multiplication of gonadotrops in castrated rats. Whereas there is as yet no evidence for separate FSH and LH cells in man, such cells can be readily distinguished in seasonal breeders such as bats, in which the two hormones are secreted at different times.

Adrenocorticotropin
(Adrenocorticotropic Hormone, ACTH)

ACTH is a polypeptide containing 39 amino acids. ACTH stimulates the adrenal cortex to secrete glucocorticoids such as cortisol. In human beings ACTH has been immunocytochemically localized in anterior and posterior lobe β_1 cells with anti-[1-39]ACTH or antiserum against the biologically inactive C-terminal sequence of the molecule ([17-39]ACTH) (Fig. 27-9). The latter has the advantage of circumventing immunoreactivity due to MSH or LPH, which share a number of amino acids with the N-terminal portion of ACTH, and the disadvantage of not necessarily demonstrating biologically active ACTH. Spontaneous hypersecretion of ACTH, which leads to adrenal cortical hyperplasia and hypercortisolism (Cushing's disease), is often associated with relatively small "basophilic" (β_1 cell) tumors of the hypophysis. If a patient with Cushing's disease is bilaterally adrenalectomized, his pituitary sometimes develops relatively large tumors. These were believed to be chromophobic, but electron microscopy has shown that they are composed of sparsely granulated β_1 (ACTH/LPH) cells. Such tumors secrete large amounts of both ACTH and βLPH. Further, Cushing's disease or administration of glucocorticoids leads to a pathognomonic alteration of the β_1 cells (those outside the tumor if one is present): their granules are in part or totally replaced by PAS-negative material that is homogeneous under the light microscope (Crooke's hyalin change, Fig. 27-13) and revealed by the electron microscope as being due to a

---

FIGURE 27-11 A. Conventional electron micrograph of a gonadotrop (G) from a normal human hypophysis. Note relatively small granules of variable size and electron density, several lipid droplets (L), and dense bodies (D). Portions of a GH cell (S) show the larger size of its secretion granules. (Courtesy of Dr. S. S. Schochet, Jr.) B. Secretion granules of a gonadotrop immunocytochemically stained with antibody against the β chain of FSH. Unlabeled antibody-PAP complex method. The unevenness of the outline of the granules is due to the ring-shaped PAP complex molecules deposited on them.

great increase in the normally present but sparse fibrils characteristic of ACTH/LPH cells. Crooke's change is seldom seen in posterior lobe basophils. Its functional significance is obscure, but it undoubtedly reflects the effects of the negative feedback of excess glucocorticoids on the cells that secrete ACTH.

Melanocyte-stimulating Hormone (MSH)

MSH is a polypeptide whose structure partially overlaps with that of ACTH. It occurs in two forms, α and βMSH. The human hypophysis contains no αMSH and the precursor molecule, βLPH, instead of βMSH. MSH causes dispersal of melanin in the melanophores of amphibians. Its physiologic role in mammals is not clear, although injection of large doses of MSH into human beings does cause hyperpigmentation. In species with a distinct pars intermedia, MSH is produced in that part of the hypophysis. In human beings, β_1 cells of pars distalis and pars nervosa alike stain immunocytochemically with antibody against βMSH, owing to their βLPH content (such antibodies do not distinguish between βMSH and βLPH) (Fig. 27-10). Bioassays of human hypophyses have shown MSH-like activity (which βLPH possesses) paralleling basophil cell content in the pars nervosa, but very little bioactive ACTH. It is conceivable, therefore, that the β_1 cells in the posterior lobe contain biologically inactive C-terminal ACTH fragments demonstrated with antibodies against [17-39]ACTH, rather than bioactive ACTH.

HYPOTHALAMIC REGULATION OF THE ADENOHYPOPHYSIS

Many of the functions of the adenohypophysis depend on its connections with the hypothalamus. Furthermore, some of the negative feedback effects of target gland hormones on the respective tropic hormones are mediated by way of the hypothalamus. In rats, hypophyses transplanted under the kidney capsule show total or substantial loss of gonadotropic, thyrotropic, and adrenocorticotropic function. The basophils in such grafts are decreased in number and size or are absent. When such transplants are placed back under the median eminence and reestablish normal vascular connections, their structural and functional integrity returns. More or less selective interference with the secretion of various hypophyseal hormones can be achieved by appropriately placed hypothalamic lesions. These functional changes are accompanied by corresponding morphologic alterations of the adenohypophysis. It is likely that circumscribed hypothalamic regions produce specific substances that govern the release (and also the production) of different hypophyseal principles. These factors must reach the adenohypophysis via the portal vessels. The thyrotropin-releasing hormone (TRH) has been chemically identified as pyroglutaminyl-histidyl-prolineamide and synthesized, as have the decapep-

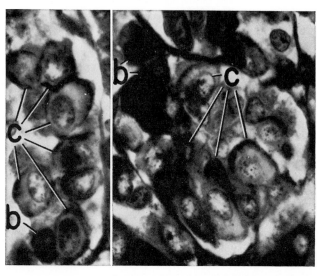

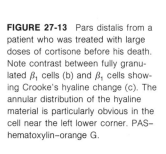

FIGURE 27-13 Pars distalis from a patient who was treated with large doses of cortisone before his death. Note contrast between fully granulated β_1 cells (b) and β_1 cells showing Crooke's hyaline change (c). The annular distribution of the hyaline material is particularly obvious in the cell near the left lower corner. PAS–hematoxylin–orange G.

tide that releases gonadotropins (Gn-RH, LH-RH) and a 14-amino acid inhibitor of GH secretion (somatostatin). Prolactin secretion seems to be tonically inhibited rather than stimulated by the hypothalamus, although TRH releases prolactin as well as TSH. Transplanted pituitaries of rats are eventually transformed so as to consist largely of acidophils of the prolactin-producing type. In such animals, corpora lutea are maintained much beyond the normal physiologic limit. Even tissue cultures of pituitary cells secrete prolactin and respond to estrogen, which is also a stimulus to prolactin production in vivo. The

intermediate lobe also seems to be restrained by the hypothalamus. Section of the hypophyseal stalk or transplantation of the adenohypophysis in amphibians leads to hyperplasia of the isolated pars intermedia and to blackening of the skin due to enhanced production of MSH. The regulation of βLPH secretion in human beings is different: βLPH and ACTH are generally released in parallel, both being under predominantly stimulating hypothalamic influences.

NEUROHYPOPHYSIS

The neurohypophysis secretes two hormones into the systemic circulation: *vasopressin* (antidiuretic hormone, ADH) and *oxytocin*. In addition, it is in this part of the pituitary that the "release" and inhibitory hypophyseotropic factors which regulate functions of the adenohypophysis are discharged into the portal vascular system that feeds the pars distalis.

STRUCTURE

The neurohypophysis is a complex of structures that include the axon terminations of secretory nerve cells of the hypothalamus. The neurosecretory cells are distinct from other neurons in that their axons do not terminate upon other nerve cells or upon other effector cells but store the secretory product and release it into the bloodstream. Neurosecretory cells which conform to this definition, and which produce secretory material with similar staining characteristics, have been described in many arthropods, as well as in the hypothalamus of vertebrates. Although their staining characteristics are similar, and although similar elementary granules of the order of 100 to 300 nm have been identified in these cells with the electron microscope, a variety of physiologic activities has been linked to the neurosecretory systems of the different species studied.

Developing from the floor of the diencephalon behind the optic chiasma, the *infundibulum* (median eminence and infundibular stem) and the *pars nervosa* at first contain the continuation of the cavity of the third ventricle (infundibular recess). This cavity is usually obliterated during development, except for remnants lined by ependymal cells. Following this

obliteration, the hilar or central portion of the pars nervosa is formed by a densely packed bundle of nonmyelinated fibers known as the *hypothalamohypophyseal tract* (Fig. 27-14). The number of these fibers, estimated by Rasmussen to be at least 50,000, was thought by him "to be out of all proportion to the cellular content of the neural lobe, and to the amount of epithelium in pars tuberalis, pars infundibularis and pars intermedia."

The origins of the nerve fibers of the hypothalamohypophyseal tract have been precisely determined by experients in animals in which the hypophyseal stalk was sectioned. The resultant interruption of the nerve fibers in the infundibular stem is followed by chromatolysis and retrograde degeneration of their nerve cell bodies in the supraoptic and paraventricular nuclei of the hypothalamus, in more scattered nerve cells caudally in the tuber cinereum, and in the suprachiasmatic nuclei of rodents. There is evidence from animal experiments that nerve fibers arising from cell bodies in the infundibular and tuberal regions (*tuberohypophyseal tract*) terminate mainly in the median eminence, whereas nerve fibers originating in the supraoptic and paraventricular nuclei (*supraopticohypophyseal tract*) end mostly in the pars nervosa. In human beings, however, the median eminence is not prominently developed and does not have the characteristic neurohypophyseal structure seen in other vertebrates, including lower primates. The nerve endings of the human tuberohypophyseal tract and of some of the fibers of the supraopticohypophyseal tract can be found around the capillary loops in the infundibular stem.

The hypothalamohypophyseal tract branches as it

enters the hilum of the pars nervosa, and the branches are dispersed to form the core of the irregular lobules of which the pars nervosa is composed. An analysis of the structure of the pars nervosa of a primitive mammal, the opossum, has revealed the fundamental plan of the neurohypophyseal lobule (Fig. 27-15). In the "typical" lobule, the central core of nerve fibers extends to the margin of the lobule as parallel arrays of blindly ending nerve-fiber terminals, the *palisade zone*. The lobule is surrounded by a *septal zone* of loose collagenous tissue containing a rich network of capillary vessels, which in some fashion receive the secretory products contained in the nerve terminals.

FIGURE 27-14 The primate neurohypophysis. Sagittal section of the neurohypophysis of a cynomolgus monkey, in situ in meninges and sella turcica. Protargol silver stain shows rostral and caudal contributions to the hypothalamohypophyseal tract, which sweeps from the infundibulum into the pars nervosa; ot, optic tract; III, third ventricle; me, median eminence; tub, pars tuberalis; i, pars intermedia; pd, pars distalis; pn, pars nervosa; s tr, supraopticohypophyseal tract; t tr, tuberohypophyseal tract; d, diaphragma sellae; ds, dorsum sellae. ×12. (Bodian.)

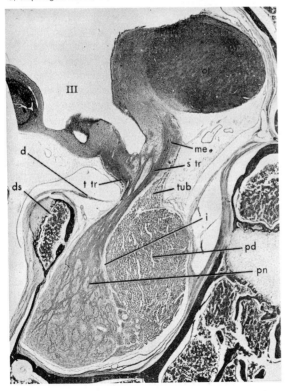

Among the nerve fibers are dispersed the dominant intrinsic cells of the neurohypophysis, the neuroglialike *pituicytes*, whose short processes often extend out to the septal zone between the nerve terminals. They have been described in detail by Romeis (1940), who emphasized the occurrence of a variety of pituicytes and a variety of inclusions within them. In most mammals, including human beings, the lobular pattern is greatly distorted, but careful inspection may reveal "typical" lobules as well as lobules so modified as to appear "inverted," with a central rather than peripheral septal or vascular zone.

In about 5 percent of human hypophyses, aggregates of large, round cells with coarse PAS-positive granules can be seen in the neurohypophysis. The origin and significance of these so-called choristomas are not known.

A histologic key to the role of the neurohypophysis was supplied by the finding of Bargmann (1966) that the abundant gelatinous material in the pars nervosa could be selectively stained and shown to be present not only in the pars nervosa but also in the nerve fibers of the hypothalamohypophyseal system. In some mammals the stainable material is also readily demonstrable in nerve cell bodies in the hypothalamus. By means of certain stains (chrome alum hematoxylin, aldehyde fuchsin, or aldehyde thionin after permanganate oxidation), this *neurosecretory substance* (Figs. 27-13 and 27-14) is stained a brilliant blue or purple. Thickenings, outpocketings, and terminals of the axons in the hypothalamohypophyseal tract, the so-called *Herring bodies* (Fig. 27-16), have similar staining characteristics. Evidence for the relation of the neurosecretory substance to the active principles of the neurohypophysis was obtained by the demonstration that the substance can be depleted by certain osmotic stimuli, such as salt ingestion or water deprivation, which have an antidiuretic effect (Fig. 27-17). Moreover, depletion of the stainable substance is concomitant with depletion of the antidiuretic activity of extracts of the pars nervosa. Immunocytochemical findings supporting Bargmann's concepts regarding the relationship of neurosecretory substance and neurohypophyseal hormones will be discussed below.

FINE STRUCTURE

Electron-microscopic observations have revealed that electron-dense, membrane-bounded granules of the order of 100 to 300 nm, contained within axons and axon terminals in the neurohypophysis, disappear in

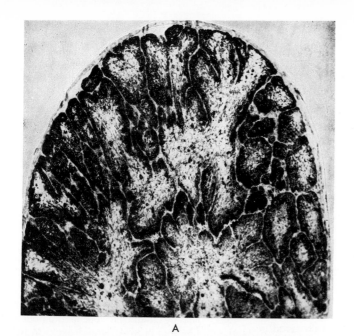

A

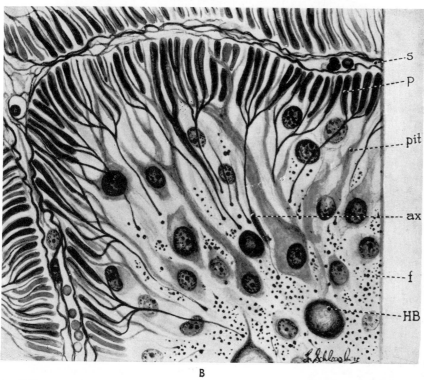

B

FIGURE 27-15 Opossum neural lobe. A. Low-power view. The lobules are outlined by the dense staining of the palisade zone surrounding the pale hilum of each lobule. Note deeply stained Herring bodies in the hilum of each lobule. Chrome alum-hematoxylin. ×70. B. Schematic representation of the histologic organization of a neural lobe lobule. Nerve fibers of the hypophyseal tract (f), pituicyte cell bodies (pit), and three Herring bodies (HB) are shown in the hilum of the lobule (lower right). Surrounding this, the palisade zone (p) is seen to be formed by rodlike nerve fiber terminals containing the stained neurosecretory substance. Although light micrographs have suggested that the nerve-fiber terminals are coated with neurosecretory substance, electron micrographs indicate that the granules which probably represent neurosecretory substance are confined within the plasma membrane of the axon terminals. The central core of the cylindrical axon terminals often contains a cluster of neurofilaments which may represent the axon terminal as seen in silver impregnations at the light-microscopic level. Interspersed among axon terminals are pituicyte fibers which extend to the vascular-collagenous septal layer (s). Axon (ax). (Bodian.)

response to and are restored by the same stimuli which cause depletion and restoration of the neurosecretory substance and of posterior lobe hormones, respectively. Electron-microscopic studies of the secretory process in the neurohypophysis have revealed that neurosecretory granules are found only within the cytoplasm of nerve cells, and especially in the nerve-fiber terminals (Fig. 27-18), where they can be stained immunocytochemically for hormones (for example, ADH, Fig. 27-19) and their associated carrier peptides, the neurophysins. Other fibers contain smaller granules (50 to 80 nm) reminiscent of membrane-bounded granules found in adrenal medulla (catecholamine granules) (Fig. 31-16) and in adrenergic nerve endings. In addition to neurosecretory granules, smaller vesicles (30 nm) have also been observed in the nerve-fiber terminals in the pars nervosa. These resemble synaptic vesicles. The specific granules of the posterior pituitary have been isolated in relatively pure form by centrifugal sedimentation in a fraction containing most of the hormone of the gland. Some evidence was obtained that ADH and oxytocin are stored in different granules.

In light-microscopic preparations stained with

FIGURE 27-16 Neurosecretion-laden fibers of the human infundibular stem are shown in contact with or near Herring bodies (dark, irregular blobs). Aldehyde thionin after permanganate oxidation. ×160.

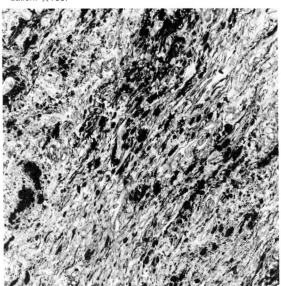

silver, the Herring bodies are revealed as greatly expanded axon portions, containing a more densely stained core. In electron-microscopic preparations (Fig. 27-18), the core appears as a densely osmiophilic mass of tightly packed concentric membranes, or it may contain a number of smaller laminated bodies. The peripheral axoplasm contains numerous neurosecretory granules that are usually more electron-opaque than those seen in the palisade-zone terminals. Depletion of granules of Herring bodies by means of osmotic stimulation is more difficult to achieve than is the depletion of those in the palisade zone.

HISTOCHEMISTRY

The localization of the active principles of the neurohypophysis by chemically specific methods rests upon the finding that both ADH and oxytocin (which were synthesized by du Vigneaud) are octapeptides which contain cystine, as do the carrier peptides (neurophysins) to which they are linked. Histochemical techniques for the disulfide groups of cystine (for example, performic acid Alcian blue) have been successfully applied to the demonstration of neurosecretory substance. The selectivity of chrome alum hematoxylin and of other staining methods for the neurosecretory substance also appears to be based on these disulfide groups.

HISTOPHYSIOLOGY

Of the two hormones of the neurohypophysis, *vasopressin* was named after its pharmacologic blood-pressure-raising effect; the term *antidiuretic hormone (ADH)* is preferable since it refers to a physiologic function of the hormone: it makes the distal convoluted tubules and collecting ducts of the kidney permeable to water and thereby enables the solute pool in the renal medulla to cause water absorption from these ducts. In the absence of ADH, a large volume (sometimes 20 l per day or more) of dilute urine is voided (diabetes insipidus). *Oxytocin* (the spelling should be ocytocin) is named after the effect relatively large doses of this hormone have on the parturient uterus: by enhancing contractions the hormone "speeds up birth." Whether or not this is a normal physiologic function of the hormone is questionable. However, oxytocin is known to play a role in the evacuation of the lactating breast. It squeezes milk

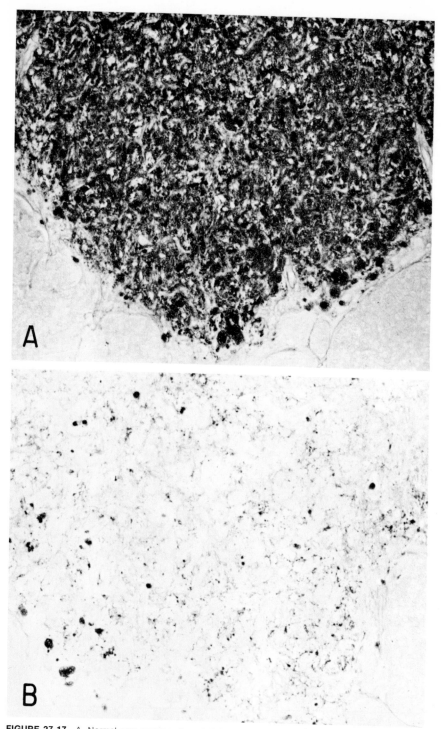

FIGURE 27-17 A. Normal pars nervosa of a rat. It is loaded with neurosecretory substance. B. Pars nervosa of a rat which had received a 2.5 percent sodium chloride solution instead of drinking water for 4 days. Note almost complete disappearance of the neurosecretory substance. Aldehyde fuchsin after permanganate oxidation. ×160.

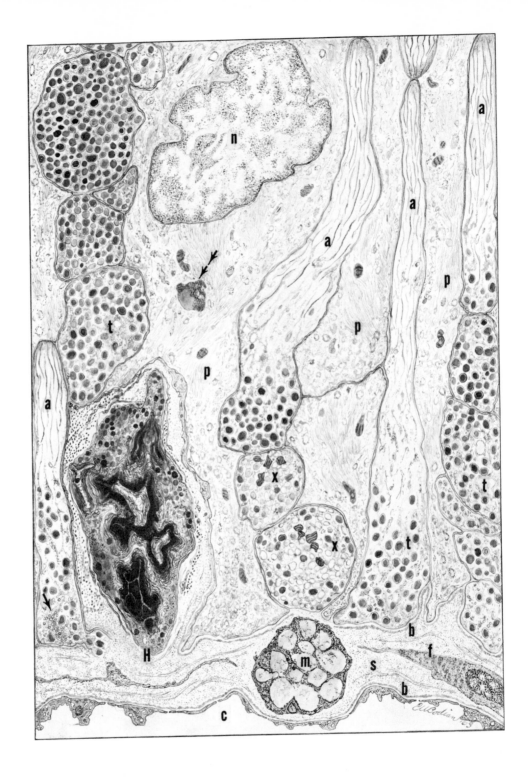

from mammary alveoli by causing contraction of the myoepithelial cells surrounding them.

Although it was originally believed that the hormones of the neurohypophysis are produced by pituicytes, which were thought to be stimulated by the fibers of the hypothalamohypophyseal tract that terminate around them, the prevalent view is that of Bargmann, who first suggested that the hormones are manufactured in the perikarya of the supraoptic and paraventricular nuclei and travel with the axoplasmic flow along the axons arising from these, to be discharged at or near the nerve endings in the posterior lobe. Section of the pituitary stalk or removal of the posterior lobe alone does not cause permanent diabetes insipidus: the median eminence in experimental animals subjected to these procedures is readily transformed into a miniature infundibular process. ADH and oxytocin are extractable from the hypothalamus, not only the neurohypophysis, although in small amounts. The classic observations of Fisher, Ingram, and Ranson (1938), who produced diabetes insipidus by placing lesions in the hypothalamus of cats, are easily explained: by severing the hypothalamohypophyseal tract before it reaches the neurohypophysis, such lesions prevent the normal flow of hormones to their site of delivery into the blood and even cause retrograde degeneration of the nerve cells in the supraoptic and paraventricular nuclei. There is evidence that the former contains about equal amounts of ADH and oxytocin, and the latter more oxytocin than ADH, but less than there is in the supraoptic nucleus. ADH and oxytocin are apparently produced in separate cells, since, as shown in Fig. 27-20, different cells stain immunocytochemically with antibodies against ADH or oxytocin. The same cells can be demonstrated with antibodies against ADH-associated and oxytocin-associated neurophysin, respectively. According to Sachs et al. (1969) the hormones are synthesized as larger molecules encompassing both the

hormones and their associated neurophysins. These precursor molecules are cleaved into neurophysin and hormone as they travel toward the nerve terminals with the axoplasmic flow. ADH and oxytocin in the neurosecretory cell processes are linked to their respective neurophysins by noncovalent bonds and in a 1:1 molar ratio. In several species, two neurophysins (I and II) have been found, and in some a third (neurophysin III). In the rat, neurophysin I is associated with ADH and neurophysin II (and III) with oxytocin. The convection of the neurophysin-hormone complexes to the neurohypophysial axon terminals seems to occur with the aid of neurotubules. Hormone content and the density per area of neurosecretory granules (which also contain neurophysins) correlate well if measured along the hypothalamohypophyseal tract, or during dehydration experiments (Fig. 27-17).

An instructive experiment of nature is a strain of rats (Brattleboro strain) which have hereditary diabetes insipidus. In these, the cell that would ordinarily produce ADH and neurophysin I are immunocytochemically negative for both, whereas those that manufacture oxytocin and neurophysin II are immunocytochemically and functionally normal.

Release of ADH and oxytocin (which can occur independently) takes place when the neurosecretory granules are extruded by exocytosis at the nerve terminals: the contents enter the perivascular spaces and there quickly lose their electron density. Only in exceptional circumstances does stainable neurosecretory material appear in the blood vessels. When oxytocin or ADH are discharged, the appropriate neurophysins are also released into the circulation. The most descriptive nomenclature applied to human neurophysins is based on the stimuli which cause their secretion: the neurophysin linked to oxytocin is, like

FIGURE 27-18 Diagram illustrating, at the electron-microscopic level, the principal features of organization of the zone of hormone transfer in the opossum. Capillary lumen (c) lined by endothelium with abundant vesicles indicating active pinocytosis, and numerous "pores"; septal zones (s), composed of collagen space, bounded by basement membranes (b), and separating palisade axon terminals (t) from endothelium. Septal zone contains fibroblasts (f) and mast cells (tip of mast cell shown at m). Isolated depleted palisade terminals (x) occur in the normal animal, unassociated with an increase of synaptic microvesicles. Such vesicles (arrow) typically occupy the tips of palisade terminals near the septal zone. Axons (a) are generally free of neurosecretory granules, which occur almost wholly within the expanded palisade axon terminals. Axons and palisade axon terminals are interspersed with pituicytes and their processes (p), which may extend down to the septal zone. Pituicytes occasionally contain dense inclusions (double arrow). Nucleus of pituicyte (N). Herring bodies (H) are axon terminals apparently formed by development of a central cavity, which becomes surrounded by densely packed membranous lamellae. The cytoplasmic matrix is only in the hilum of pars nervosa but as far distally as the border of the septal zone, where they may be surrounded by membranous processes of the pituicytes. Approximately ×8,000. (Bodian.)

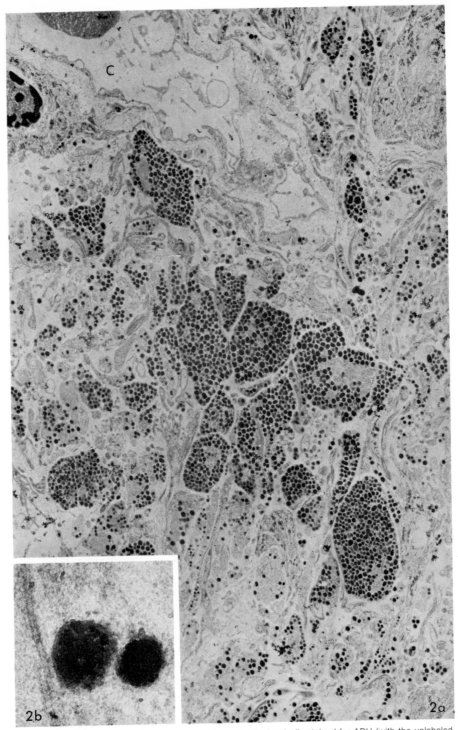

FIGURE 27-19 Electron micrograph of the posterior pituitary of a guinea pig, immunocytochemically stained for ADH (with the unlabeled antibody-PAP complex method). ADH is confined to the neurosecretory granules in axons and nerve terminal. The inset shows that the round PAP complex molecules corresponding to the sites of ADH storage are strictly limited to the neurosecretion granules. ×8400; Inset ×110,000. (From A. J. Silverman, and E. A. Zimmerman, *Cell Tiss. Res.*, **159**:291, 1975.)

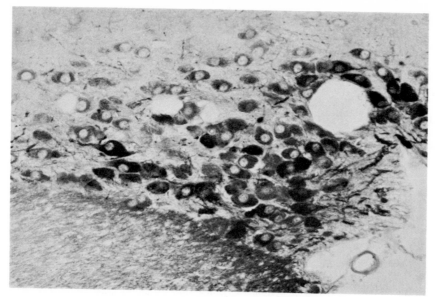

A

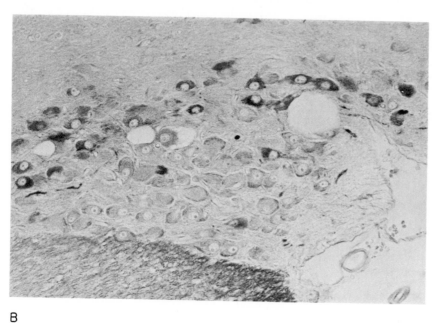

B

FIGURE 27-20 Supraoptic nucleus of a rat, stained immunocytochemically for ADH (A) and oxytocin (B). Note the dissimilar distribution of the perikarya containing these hormones. (Courtesy of Dr. E. A. Zimmerman.)

hormone itself, released in response to estrogen and hence is called estrogen-stimulated neurophysin; that attached to ADH is secreted, along with ADH itself, after the administration of nicotine, and therefore is called nicotine-stimulated neurophysin. The role of the small synapticlike vesicles in the nerve endings of the hypothalamohypophyseal tract is not clear: some believe they are remnants of the membranes of neurosecretion granules; others believe that they produce acetylcholine which is involved in hormone discharge. The release of hormones occurs in response to impulses which travel along the axons of neurosecretory cells. What role, if any, the pituicytes play in the discharge of neurohypophyseal hormones is obscure.

The physiologic stimuli for ADH secretion are an increase in plasma osmolality and a decrease of blood volume in certain pressure-sensitive portions of the vascular system. The perikarya of the supraoptic and paraventricular nuclei themselves may be osmoceptors, since they are in unusually intimate contact with capillaries. The question arises why secretion of neurohypophyseal hormones cannot occur into such hypothalamic capillaries themselves. It may be pertinent that the hypothalamus has and the neurohypophysis lacks a blood-brain barrier: the hypothalamus does not whereas the neurohypophysis does stain with vital dyes injected into animals. It is conceivable that the blood-brain barrier permits the passage of the constituent amino acids of the peptide hormones but prevents the entry of these hormones into blood after their synthesis, whereas this is not impeded in the neurohypophysis. ADH discharge also occurs in response to stressful stimuli or upon electrical excitation of the hypothalamus. Oxytocin is released after stimulation of the nipple, as by suckling, or after vaginal distension. These stimuli are conveyed to the hypothalamus along neural pathways.

It is believed that the hypophyseotropic release and inhibitory factors, through which the hypothalamus exerts control over the adenohypophysis, are elaborated in the perikarya of scattered hypothalamic neurons and then travel to the capillaries of the median eminence and the infundibular stem along the axons of the tuberohypophyseal tract, much as described for the hormones released into the systemic circulation in the infundibular process. Some of the fibers of the supraopticohypophyseal tract also end along capillary loops in the median eminence and stalk. Fibers from both tracts occasionally end along the processes of specialized ependymal cells in the median eminence which are called tanycytes. The tanycytes have their cell bodies near the third ventricle, and they span the entire width of the median eminence, with their processes terminating near the capillaries of the superior portal plexus. Some investigators believe that the tanycytes transport neurosecretions from nerve fibers (and possibly the cerebrospinal fluid) to the portal vascular system. Several workers have found them immunoreactive for neurophysin. The nerve fibers containing gonadotropin releasing hormone (Gn-RH, LH-RH) have been identified immunocytochemically, as have those carrying the inhibitor of GH release, somatostatin. The location of the perikarya from which these fibers originate has been more difficult to assess by immunocytochemical means, but cell bodies containing somatostatin have been convincingly demonstrated in the anterior part of the hypothalamus. It has been suggested that ADH or neurophysin released into the portal circulation from nerve terminals of the supraopticohypophyseal tract may be involved in the regulation of the secretion of ACTH and possibly that of other pars distalis hormones.

REFERENCES

General

DANIEL, P. M.: The Anatomy of the Hypothalamus and Pituitary Gland, in L. Martini and W. F. Ganong, (eds.), ''Neuroendocrinology,'' vol. 1, pp. 15–80, Academic Press, Inc., New York, 1966.

FAWCETT, D. W., J. A. LONG, and A. L. JONES: The Ultrastructure of Endocrine Glands, *Recent Progr. Horm. Res.*, **25**:315–380 (1969).

GANONG, W. F., and L. MARTINI (eds.): ''Frontiers in Neuroendocrinology,'' Oxford University Press, New York, 1976.

MEITES, J. (ed.): "Hypophysiotropic Hormones of the Hypothalamus: Assay and Chemistry," The Williams & Wilkins Company, Baltimore, 1970.

ROMEIS, B.: Hypophyse, in W. von Möllendorff (ed.), "Handbuch der mikroskopischen Anatomie des Menschen," vol. 6, pt. 3, Springer-Verlag OHG, Berlin, 1940.

Adenohypophysis

BAKER, B. L.: Functional Cytology of the Hypophysial Pars Distalis and Pars Intermedia, in R. O. Greep and E. B. Astwood (eds.), "Handbook of Physiology," sec. 7, vol. 4, pt. 1, pp. 45–80, American Physiological Society, Washington, D.C., 1974.

EZRIN, C., and S. MURRAY: The Cell of the Adenohypophysis in Pregnancy, Thyroid Disease and Adrenal Cortical Disorders, in J. Benoit and C. da Lage (eds.), "Cytologie de l'Adénohypophyse," pp. 183–200, Editions du C. N. R. S. (no. 128), 1963.

HALMI, N. S.: The Current Status of Pituitary Cytophysiology, N. Z. Med. J., **80:**551–556 (1974).

HALMI, N. S., J. A. PARSONS, S. L. ERLANDSEN, and T. DUELLO: Prolactin and Growth Hormone Cells in the Human Hypophysis: A Study with Immunoenzyme Histochemistry, Cell Tiss. Res., **158:**497–507 (1975).

HERLANT, M., and J. L. PASTEELS: Histophysiology of Human Anterior Pituitary, Meth. Achievm. Exp. Path., **3:**250–305 (1967).

MORIARTY, G. C.: Adenohypophysis: Ultrastructural Cytochemistry. A Review, J. Histochem. Cytochem., **21:**855–894 (1973).

NAKANE, P.: Classifications of Anterior Pituitary Cell Types with Immunoenzyme Histochemistry, J. Histochem. Cytochem., **18:**9–20 (1970).

PHIFER, R. F., A. R. MIDGLEY, JR., and S. S. SPICER: Immunohistologic and Histologic Evidence that Follicle-Stimulating Hormone and Luteinizing Hormone are Present in the Same Cell Type of the Human Pars Distalis, J. Clin. Endocrinol., **36:**125–141 (1973).

PHIFER, R. F., D. N. ORTH, and S. S. SPICER: Specific Demonstration of the Human Hypophyseal Adreno-cortico-Melanotropic (ACTH/MSH) Cell, J. Clin. Endocrinol., **39:**684–692 (1974).

PHIFER, R. F., and S. S. SPICER: Immunohistochemical and Histologic Demonstration of Thyrotropic Cells of the Human Adenohypophysis, J. Clin. Endocrinol., **36:**1210–1221 (1973).

PHIFER, R. F., S. S. SPICER, and D. N. ORTH: Specific Demonstration of Human Hypophysial Cells Which Produce Adrenocorticotropic Hormone, J. Clin. Endocrinol., **31:**347–361 (1970).

PURVES, H. D.: Cytology of the Adenohypophysis, in G. W. Harris and B. T. Donovan (eds.), "The Pituitary Gland," vol. 1, pp. 147–232, University of California Press, Berkeley, 1966.

TIXIER-VIDAL, A., and M. G. FARQUHAR (eds.): "The Anterior Pituitary," Academic Press, Inc., New York, 1975.

Neurohypophysis

BAKER, B. L., W. C. DERMODY, and J. R. REED: Distribution of Gonadotropin-Releasing Hormone in the Rat Brain as Observed with Immunocytochemistry, Endocrinology, **97:**125–135 (1975).

BARGMANN, W.: Neurosecretion, Int. Rev. Cytol., **19:**183–201 (1966).

BINDLER, E., F. S. LA BELLA, and M. SANWAL: Isolated Nerve Endings (Neurosecretosomes) from the Posterior Pituitary. Partial Separation of Vasopressin and Oxytocin and the Isolation of Microvesicles, J. Cell Biol., **34:**185–205 (1967).

CHRIST, J. F.: Nerve Supply, and Cytology of the Neurohypophysis, in G. W. Harris and B. T. Donovan (eds.), "The Pituitary Gland," vol. 3, pp. 62–130, University of California Press, Berkeley, 1966.

FISHER, C. V., W., R. INGRAM, and S. W. RANSON: Diabetes Insipidus and the Neurohumoral Control of Water Balance: A Contribution to the Structure and Function of the Hypothalamicohypophysial System, J. W. Edwards, Publisher, Incorporated, Ann Arbor, Mich., 1938.

SACHS, H., P. FAWCETT. TAKABATAKE, and R. PORTANOVA: Biosynthesis and Release of Vasopressin and Neurophysin, *Recent Progr. Horm. Res.,* **25:**447–491 (1969).

SCHARRER, B.: Neurohumors and Neurohormones: Definitions and Terminology, *J. Neurovisc. Rel.* (suppl.), **9:**1–20 (1969).

SILVERMAN, A. J., and E. A. ZIMMERMAN: Ultrastructural Immunocytochemical Localization of Neurophysin and Vasopressin in the Median Eminence and Posterior Pituitary of the Guinea Pig, *Cell Tiss. Res.,* **159:**291–301 (1975).

SLOPER, J. C.: The Experimental and Cytopathological Investigation of Neurosecretion in the Hypothalamus and Pituitary, in G. W. Harris and B. T. Donovan (eds.), "The Pituitary Gland," vol. 3, pp. 130–288, University of California Press, Berkeley, 1966.

ZIMMERMAN, E. A., R. DEFENDINI, H. W. SOKOL, and A. G. ROBINSON: The Distribution of Neurophysin-Secreting Pathways in the Mammalian Brain, *Ann. N.Y. Acad. Sci.,* **248:**92–111 (1975).

The Pineal Gland

W. B. QUAY

An endocrine status for the pineal gland (pineal body or epiphysis cerebri) has gained additional supporting evidence in recent years. However, the functional importance of the pineal gland in human beings is far from clear. No tissue or cellular activity has been shown to depend in all circumstances on either the presence of the pineal gland or its suggested secretory products. Instead, experimental studies utilizing laboratory mammals indicate that the pineal's endocrine role is as an intermittent mediator of time changes in some physiological rhythms, particularly some of those that are approximately daily (circadian) or seasonal or that relate to reproductive periodicity. It is probably mostly owing to the complex temporal nature of pineal activity that physiological investigations of its functions have often provided inconsistent or contradictory results.

The mammalian pineal gland is a single median structure that develops from the posterior part of the diencephalic roof. Superficially its dorsal median origin from diencephalic neural ectoderm resembles the ventral median diencephalic origin of the neurohypophysis. However, beyond this embryological parallel, the presence of neuroglia in both and the similarly endocrine functions, the pineal gland and neurohypophysis have little in common. Mammalian pineal glands lack neurosecretory axon terminals and neurohemal hormone storage and release systems, such as dominate the microstructure of the neurohypophysis.

Evolutionarily, the pineal gland is unique among the endocrine glands of vertebrate animals for the magnitude and diversity of its morphological remodeling. The pineal complex of organs in many lower vertebrates (cyclostomes, fishes, and some amphibians and reptiles) is dominated by photosensory and eyelike structures with afferent ganglionic connections to the brain. Within several different groups of higher vertebrates (turtles, snakes, birds, and mammals), separate but similar evolutionary changes have occurred, leading to a more or less solidly parenchymatous and primarily endocrine rather than sensory pineal organ. All direct photosensory capacity and all the primitive afferent pineal neural connections with the brain have been lost in adult mammals insofar as is known at this time. On the other hand, the amount and biochemical differentiation of the mammalian pineal's endocrine secretory tissue, made up of unique pinealocytes, have increased.

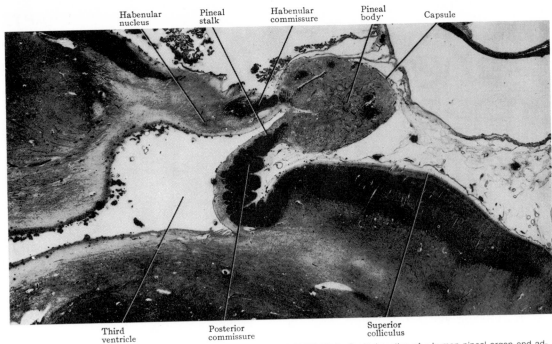

Habenular nucleus   Pineal stalk   Habenular commissure   Pineal body·   Capsule

Third ventricle   Posterior commissure   Superior colliculus

FIGURE 28-1 Sagittal section of a human pineal organ and adjacent structures of the dorsal junction of diencephalon (left) and mesencephalon (right). Loyes iron-hematoxylin technique for myelin. ×8. (Courtesy of P. I. Yakovlev.)

DEVELOPMENT AND HISTOGENESIS

The human pineal gland arises early during the second month of embryonic life. Although it is a single median structure in the adult (Fig. 28-1), in the embryo it often has two parts, an anterior and solid one from the region of the habenular commissure, and a posterior and hollow one originating from a sacklike evagination of the diencephalic roof between the habenular and posterior commissures. Cellular proliferation is earlier and greater in the anterior part. Clear differentiation of human pineal cells into pinealocytes and glial cells is not possible until about the150th day of development. Neuroepithelial proliferations forming the pineal parenchyma consist at first of cords and follicles of cells, which become invested by embryonic mesoderm. Pineal neuroepithelial cells give rise to parenchymal cells or pinealocytes and to neuroglial cells (Fig. 28-2). During later development most signs of parenchymal cords and follicles are lost, to be replaced

by lobules composed mostly of pinealocytes. Intervening septa and trabeculae of stromal tissue are derived mostly from embryonic mesoderm or meningeal mesenchyme with more limited cellular contributions from neural crest and vascular systems (Fig. 28-2).

From postnatal to adult ages, mammalian pineal growth is mainly by hypertrophy of the pinealocytes and secondarily and variably by increase in glial and stromal cells and their products. In human beings, this is seen most clearly in the variable, but usually increasing, width with age of the interlobular connective tissue septa (Fig. 28-3). Neither notable increase in pinealocyte numbers nor pineal regeneration has been demonstrated in situ in any adult mammal, excluding the abnormal cellular capacities in pineal tumors and some heterotopic transplants. Thus pineal growth and regenerative abilities resemble those of the central nervous system.

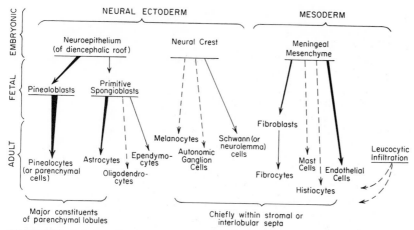

FIGURE 28-2 Developmental origins of cells found in mammalian pineal glands. Relative thickness of arrows for cellular descents are intended to suggest relative numbers of cells in the different lines. Dashed arrows signify cell types and origins that are variable in relation to pineal region, species, age, or pathological processes.

STRUCTURE AND COMPOSITION

Adult human pineal glands, measuring 5 to 8 mm in length and 3 to 5 mm in width, are covered by a thin but compact connective tissue capsule, which is externally continuous with meningeal (pial and arachnoid) tissues. Basally the gland is attached to the brain by a stalk, containing in humans an extension of the third ventricle, the pineal recess (Figs. 28-1 and 28-4). The pineal stalk also contains nerve fibers from the adjacent habenular and posterior commissural regions. These are generally considered to be merely nerve-fiber loops, pulled out developmentally with the basal pineal tissue in which they are embedded. Although they are usually viewed as without either synaptic relations or functional significance within the pineal gland, recent neurophysiological findings have reopened the question of their possible importance. Pineal innervation is thought to be exclusively autonomic, with the endocrine functioning of the pinealocytes depending on their sympathetic innervation. Pineal sympathetic fibers consist both of small fascicles entering the capsular surface in many places along with small blood vessels and of a *nervus conarii* penetrating the posterior pole of the organ, following the fusion of its bilateral component trunks ascending intracranially along the tentorium cerebelli on each

side. These trunks originate from the superior cervical sympathetic ganglia, but it is possible that some of the contributing postganglionic nerve-cell bodies lie more peripherally and intracranially.

Pineal blood supply is by small arteriolar branches from offshoots of the two posterior choroid arteries. Each of these in turn originates from the posterior cerebral artery on the same side. Shortly after penetration of the capsule, pineal arterioles lead into a capillary network, which permeates to the interior of the organ. Ultrastructural fenestration of the capillary endothelium is reported in some species. Perivascular spaces or poorly defined channels occur along and outside the capillary walls. Sympathetic nerve processes and cytoplasmic terminations of pinealocyte processes often lie in or close to these perivascular spaces and their intercellular extensions (Fig. 28-5). The degree to which these components are invested by a basal lamina, connective tissue, and glial cell cytoplasm varies among species of mammals. Vascular drainage of the pineal is by venules that course beneath the capsule before passing through the adjacent meningeal tissue, to drain eventually into larger veins or dural venous sinuses of the vicinity. In human beings, this means primarily the great cerebral vein (of Galen).

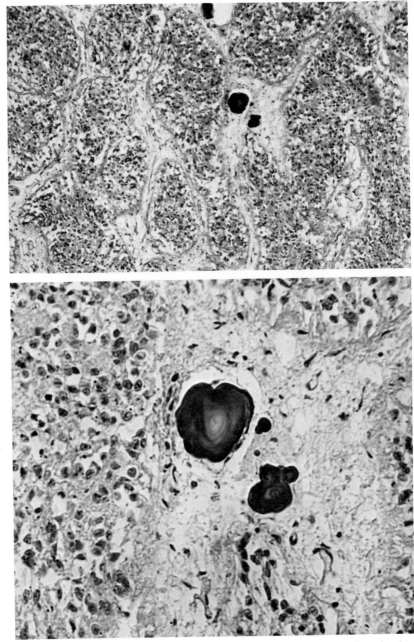

FIGURE 28-3 Low (above) and intermediate (below) power views of human pineal tissue stained with acid alum hematoxylin and eosin. A distinct lobulation of the parenchyma and concretions in the stroma are seen. (From a 78-year-old woman; death due to cardiovascular disease and myocarditis.)

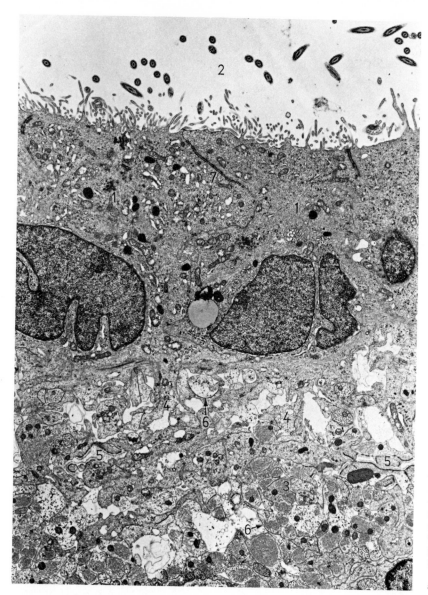

FIGURE 28-4 Ependymal cells (1) covering the proximal or ventricular surface of the pineal organ (squirrel monkey) where it faces on the pineal recess (2), an extension of the third ventricle. Ependymal cilia and microvilli are seen in the recess. Below the ependymal cells filamentous glial processes (3) intermingle with processes of the ependymal cells (4). Nearby are extracellular spaces (5) lined by a basal lamina, and in continuity with the perivascular space. Tight junctions (6) occur between glial cell processes, and a junctional complex (7) joins the ependymal cells. ×6324. (Courtesy of H. Wartenberg and Springer-Verlag.)

The pineal's anatomical position is critical in relation to intracranial venous drainage, lying close to the union of outflow from the deep cerebral veins with the median and deep dural venous sinuses. Pineal tumors often impede or divert this outflow by compressing it against the splenium of the corpus callosum.

PINEALOCYTES

Pinealocytes, or pineal parenchymal cells, constitute the majority of the cells seen within the lobules, and are specific to pineal tissue (Fig. 28-6). A large, often polymorphic and deeply creased, nucleus containing one to several large nucleoli and associated chromatin masses is characteristic (Figs. 28-5 and 28-7). Like neurons, pinealocytes often have two or more cytoplasmic extensions or processes, numerous cytoplas-

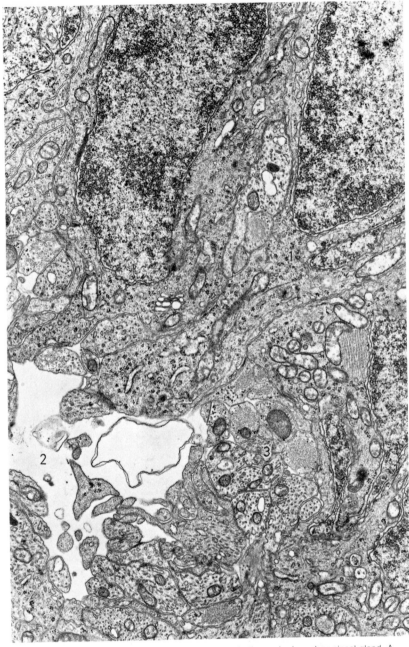

FIGURE 28-5 Structural interrelations of cell processes in the vicinity of an intercellular space in the squirrel monkey pineal gland. A short cytoplasmic process from a pinealocyte (1) courses toward the space (2); nerve (3), glial, and pinealocyte processes are intermingled. ×13,950. (Courtesy of H. Wartenberg and Springer-Verlag.)

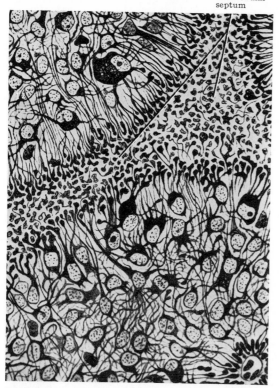

Interlobular
septum

FIGURE 28-6 A classical and semidiagrammatic interpretation of the organization of pinealocytes within a small region of the adult pineal organ, based upon metallic impregnations and light microscopy. Parts of two parenchymatous lobules are shown. In each, polymorphic pinealocytes have club-shaped processes often terminating in the vicinity of small vessels in the interlobular tissue. (After Del Rio-Hortega.)

mic cisterns, microtubules, vesicles of several kinds, organelles for active oxidative metabolism and protein synthesis, and at least portions of structures usually associated with synaptic contacts in central nervous or retinal tissues. The cytoplasmic extensions of the pinealocytes sometimes include shorter and thinner types that terminate within the group of adjacent cells, and longer, thicker types that terminate within or close to the perivascular space. Within the swollen, clublike endings of the latter processes are found vesicles and grumose or dense bodies that are sometimes suggestive of containing presecretory cell products (Fig. 28-8). Pinealocyte mitochondria are notable for their relatively great number or concentration in the perikaryon, their polymorphism and frequently great size (to 4 μm in length in the rat). Various mitochondrial inclusions have been described, especially in pinealocytes of adult or old animals; these include concentrically lamellated bodies, clusters of osmiophilic granules within the mitochondrial matrix, dense intracristal layers, and dense-cored microcylinders 270 to 330 Å wide.

It remains unclear whether in human beings and other mammals the pinealocytes constitute one or more cell types or subtypes, or whether variations in their cytoplasmic density ("light" and "dark" pinealocytes of electron microscopists) and other characteristics pertain only to differences in phase or level of activity in a single cell type.

HISTOCHEMISTRY AND HISTOPHYSIOLOGY

Pineal specific products are biochemically of two kinds, indoleamines and peptides or proteins. Melatonin (5-methoxy-N-acetyltryptamine), best-known and most-studied of pineal indoleamine products, has been proposed as a pineal hormone, with effects most often described in reproductive and nervous tissues. Although melatonin can cause rapid blanching of some amphibian skin, a property useful in bioassays, it has little if any effect on mammalian pigment cells. In domestic fowl, and presumably in mammals as well, melatonin's detection in the blood depends both on the presence of the pineal gland (melatonin is not detectable in pinealectomized animals) and on the

time of day. In human blood plasma, a material with biological and chemical characteristics of melatonin follows a 24-h rhythm, showing detectable and peak levels during the night only. In laboratory mammals, other links and controls in the series of events leading to melatonin's synthesis and release in pineal tissue have been defined experimentally. The profound daily rhythmicity in pineal biosynthetic and metabolic activity appears to be under sympathetic control through the agency of norepinephrine and cyclic-AMP (adenosine 3',5'-monophosphate). Cellular localizations and daily changes in norepinephrine and serotonin, a precursor of melatonin, have been described from the use of the fluorescence histochemical technique of Falck and Hillarp for catecholamines such as norepinephrine (green fluorescent product) and tryptamines such as serotonin (yellow fluorescent product). By this and other methods, pineal synthesis of serotonin and related compounds is seen to be localized to the pinealocytes, whereas norepinephrine is restricted to the sympathetic nerve fibers and endings.

Much less is known about pineal peptides and proteins and their cellular origins. However, increasing attention is being directed to these as possibly including hormonal products. Arginine vasotocin, usually considered an evolutionarily primitive octapeptide hormone of the neurohypophysis, is found and apparently synthesized in adult mammalian pineal glands as well. There are also pineal-specific peptides whose composition and significance are as yet poorly known.

Pineal glands from humans and some ungulate mammals often contain calcareous concretions, known also as corpora arenacea, acervuli, psammoma bodies and brain sand (Fig. 28-3). These seem to be glial or stromal in origin as well as localization, and they do not differ structurally or chemically from such deposits in a wide variety of other tissues. Their primary microcrystalline structure resembles that of

FIGURE 28-7 Pinealocytes of the squirrel monkey pineal gland. Pinealocyte nuclei (1) here are frequently deeply creased and have peripherally placed nucleoli. Cytoplasmic processes of the pinealocytes include some that are dendritelike (2) and some that are neuritelike (3). ×8184. (Courtesy of H. Wartenberg and Springer-Verlag.)

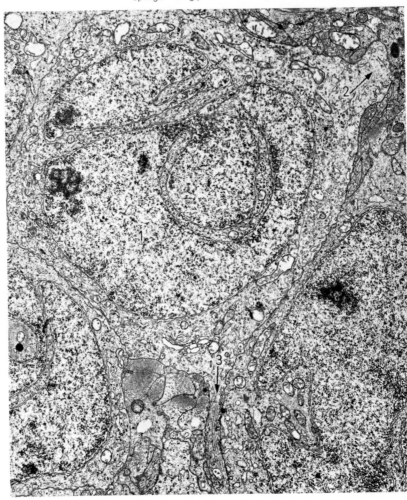

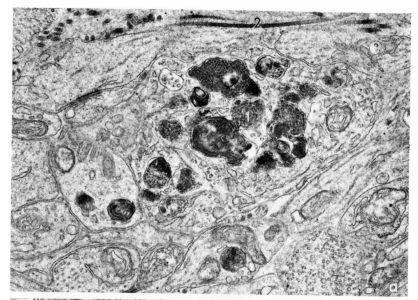

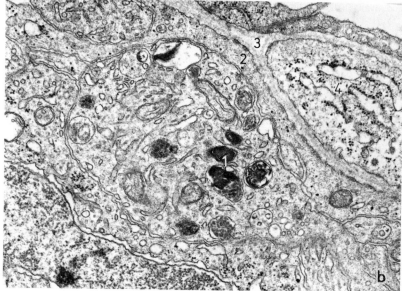

FIGURE 28-8 Structural relations of the terminations of pinealocyte processes in primate (monkey) pineal glands. (Courtesy of H. Wartenberg and Springer-Verlag.) A. Group of pinealocyte terminations within the perivascular space of the rhesus monkey. Dense bodies (1) inside the pinealocyte endings are considered by some investigators to represent a secretory product. Outside the endings are occasional collagen fibers (2). Terminations are intermingled here with glial cell processes and nerve fibers. ×18,600. B. Pinealocyte termination in a squirrel monkey, containing dense bodies (1), and separated by a glial cell sheet (2) from the perivascular space (3). A pericyte (4) lies within the latter and close to capillary endothelium at the top right. ×24,100.

hydroxyapatite. It has been shown that their occurrence in some human pineal glands is not associated with decrease in melatonin-forming (hydroxyindole O-methyltransferase) or several other kinds of important enzymes. Thus the presence of such concretions in a particular pineal gland cannot be necessarily construed as diagnostic of reduced or impaired pineal function. The prevalence of corpora arenacea in human pineal glands increases with age, and is most useful to the radiologist in providing an intracranial landmark in radiograms. Various other histological and cytological features of the human pineal gland change or increase during either youth or older age. But there is wide individual variation in these occurrences, even in pineal glands from the eighth or ninth decades of life. In summary, recent ultrastructural and biochemical studies are in accord with the belief that pineal functional activity follows postnatal differentiation and continues into adult and older ages in humans and most other mammals.

REFERENCES

ALTSCHULE, M. D. (ed.): "Frontiers of Pineal Physiology." The M.I.T. Press, Cambridge, Mass., 1975.

ARIETI, S.: The Pineal Gland in Old Age, *J. Neuropathol. Exp. Neurol.*, **13:**482 (1954).

AXELROD, J.: The Pineal Gland: A Neurochemical Transducer, *Science,* **184:**1341 (1974).

BLOOM, F. E., and N. J. GIARMAN: The Effects of p-Cl-phenylalanine on the Content and Cellular Distribution of 5-HT in the Rat Pineal Gland: Combined Biochemical and Electron Microscopic Analyses, *Biochem. Pharmacol.,* **19:**1213 (1970).

HÜLSEMANN, M.: Development of the Innervation in the Human Pineal Organ: Light and Electron Microscopic Investigations, *Z. Zellforsch.,* **115:**396 (1971).

ITO, T., and S. MATSUSHIMA: Electron Microscopic Observations on the Mouse Pineal, with Particular Emphasis on Its Secretory Nature, *Arch. Histol., Jap.,* **30:**1 (1968).

KAPPERS, J. A.: The Mammalian Pineal Organ, *J. Neurovisc. Relat.,* **9**(Suppl.):140 (1969).

KAPPERS, J. A. and J. P. SCHADE (eds.): Structure and Function of the Epiphysis Cerebri, *Prog. Brain Res.,* **10** (1965).

KITAY, J. I., and M. D. ALTSCHULE: "The Pineal Gland," Harvard University Press, Cambridge, Mass., 1954.

KLEIN, D. C., and G. R. BERG: Pineal Gland: Stimulation of Melatonin Production by Norepinephrine Involves Cyclic AMP-mediated Stimulation of *N*-Acetyltransferase, in P. Greengard and E. Costa (eds.), "Role of Cyclic AMP in Cell Function," Raven Books, Abeland-Schuman, Limited, New York, 1970.

MACPHEE, A. A., F. E. COLE, and B. F. RICE: The Effect of Melatonin on Steroidogenesis by the Human Ovary in Vitro, *J. Clinc. Endocrinol. Metab.,* **40:**688 (1975).

PAVEL, S., I. DUMITRU, I. KLEPSH, and M. DORCESCU: A Gonadotropin Inhibiting Principle in the Pineal of Human Fetuses: Evidence for its Identity with Arginine Vasotocin, *Neuroendocrinology,* **13:**41 (1973/4).

PELHAM, R. W., G. M. VAUGHAN, K. L. SANDOCK, and M. K. VAUGHAN: Twenty-four-hour Cycle of a Melatonin-like Substance in the Plasma of Human Males, *J. Clin. Endocrinol. Metab.,* **37:**341 (1973).

QUAY, W. B.: Cytochemistry of Pineal Lipids in Rat and Man, *J. Histochem. Cytochem.,* **5:**145 (1957).

QUAY, W. B.: "Pineal Chemistry in Cellular and Physiological Mechanisms." Charles C Thomas Publishers, Springfield, Ill., 1974.

QUAY, W. B.: Pineal Canaliculi: Demonstration, Twenty-four-hour Rhythmicity and Experimental Modification, *Am. J. Anat.,* **139:**81 (1974).

REITER, R. J.: Pineal Regulation of Hypothalamicopituitary Axis: Gonadotrophins, "Handbook of Physiology," vol. IV, pt. 2, chap. 41, p. 519, American Physiological Society, Washington, D.C., 1974.

RODIN, A. E., and R. A. TURNER: The Perivascular Space of the Pineal Gland, *Tex. Rep. Biol. Med.,* **24:**153 (1966).

TAPP, E., and M. HUXLEY: The Histological Appearance of the Human Pineal Gland from Puberty to Old Age, *J. Pathol.,* **108:**137 (1972).

WARTENBERG, H.: The Mammalian Pineal Organ: Electron Microscopic Studies on the Fine Structure of Pinealocytes, Glial Cells and on the Perivascular Compartment, *Z. Zellforsch.,* **86:**74 (1968).

WOLSTENHOLME, G. E. W., and J. KNIGHT (eds.): "The Pineal Gland," Ciba Found. Symp., 1971.

WURTMAN, R. J., J. AXELROD, and D. E. KELLY: "The Pineal," Academic Press, Inc., New York, 1968.

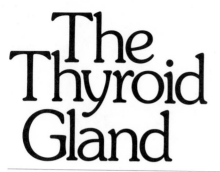

The Thyroid Gland

LOIS W. TICE

Although the thyroid is classified as an endocrine gland, its cells perform both exocrine and endocrine secretory functions in the process of manufacture and release of thyroid hormone. Recognition of their dual function provides a key to understanding thyroid histology. In the exocrine phase of secretion, thyroid follicular cells synthesize and secrete thyroglobulin, a large glycoprotein (MW 660,000). This is stored extracellularly in the interior of the thyroid follicles where it is partially iodinated. In the endocrine phase of secretion, stored thyroglobulin is taken up by the follicular cells and broken down to active thyroid hormones. These are then released into the blood and lymph. The active hormones are iodinated amino acids, L-thyroxine (tetraiodo-L-thyronine) and 3,5,3'-triodo-L-thyronine. They function to stimulate metabolism, particularly oxidative metabolism, and have important effects on maturation (brain development and amphibian metamorphosis, for example). In addition, the thyroid in mammals contain C cells (parafollicular cells or light cells). These cells produce another hormone, calcitonin or thyrocalcitonin, which acts to lower blood calcium.

ORIGIN AND DEVELOPMENT

The parenchyma of the thyroid gland is of entodermal origin, and arises by a median down-growth of the base of the tongue. The developing gland is connected to its point of origin by the thyroglossal duct which usually becomes obliterated during later development, but which may give rise to persisting structures such as the pyramidal lobe, thyroglossal cysts or thyroid tissue within the tongue (lingual thryoid). The thyroid may include branchial pouch derivatives such as parathyroid glands and C cells. However, transplantation experiments have shown that C cells originate in the neural crest and migrate into the ultimobranchial body during development. Remnants of the ultimobranchial body also produce ultimobranchial tubules (Fig. 29-1) or follicles lined by stratified squamous epithelium. Other unusual types of follicles containing, for example, ciliated cells have been observed in some species. In nonmammals the ultimo-branchial body may remain a separate organ.

    The proliferating mass of embryonic thyroid cells breaks up into small cords and sheets of

1077

cells. Only late in development do recognizable thyroid follicles with follicular lumina appear. The appearance of follicles with stored colloid seems to coincide with the onset of mature function and iodination of thyroglobulin. With the appearance of follicular lumina containing extracellular stored colloid, the cells around it become arranged into a single continuous layer surrounded by basement membrane. The cell layers together with the colloid which they enclose are called *follicles;* they constitute the basic functioning unit of the adult thyroid gland. They are variable in shape and range in humans from 50 to 900 μm in diameter.

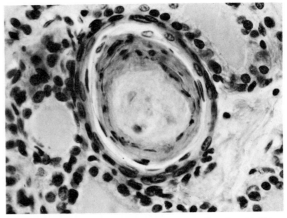

FIGURE 29-1 Ultimobranchial tubule in a normal rat thyroid. This is the oval cross section of a closed tube lined by stratified squamous epithelium. The lumen contains desquamated cells with pycnotic nuclei, and debris. (Courtesy of C. P. Leblond.)

GROSS STRUCTURE

In human beings the thyroid gland normally weighs from 15 to 30 g. It consists of two lateral lobes connected by an isthmus which lies close to the second and third tracheal rings. It is located near the shield-shaped thyroid cartilage of the larynx, from which it takes its name. It is surrounded by a fibrous capsule from which connective tissue septa may extend into the interior of the gland, separating it into lobules. The follicles are separated by a loose connective tissue, the stroma, containing blood vessels, nerve fibers, and lymphatics. Its rich blood supply is via the superior and inferior thyroid arteries. Smaller arteries within the gland may have intimal thickenings or endothelial cushions. These break up into an extensive capillary network which comes into close contact with the basement membranes of the capillaries. A network of lymphatic vessels is also found between the follicles. These drain into larger vessels beneath the capsule and ultimately into cervical or retrosternal lymph nodes.

Small nerve bundles enter the thyroid together with the larger blood vessels. These are primarily postganglionic sympathetic fibers which originate in the middle and superior cervical ganglia, although cholinergic fibers are also contributed by the recurrent laryngeal branch of the vagus. Many of these fibers synapse on blood vessels and are therefore probably vasomotor in function. In some species (mouse and human) nerve fibers are also found which terminate in close contact with the follicles themselves. The physiologic function of these fibers is not known in normal animals. In animals in which pituitary function has been suppressed, sympathetic stimulation can lead to effects which mimic the effects of TSH, thyroid-stimulating hormone.

LIGHT MICROSCOPIC HISTOLOGY

In the light microscope, the thyroid follicle is the dominant feature of the gland. This consists of a cuboidal (in humans) epithelium which forms a continuous cell layer around the central mass of colloid (Fig. 29-2A). The colloid is amphoteric, staining with both acidic and basic dyes. Because it contains thyroglobulin, a glycoprotein, it is PAS-positive. The relative height of the epithelial cell layer and the relative size of the mass of colloid depend on the activity of the follicle as well as in the species studied. When the gland is inactive, the mass of colloid is large and the cells around it flattened (Fig. 29-2C). In hyperactive

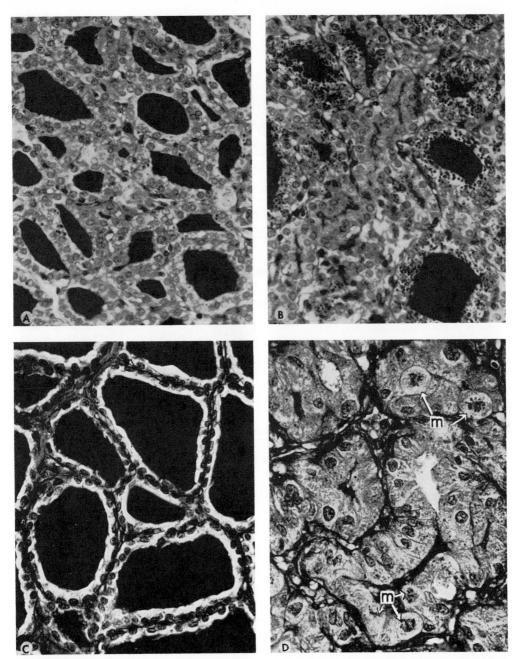

FIGURE 29-2 Rat thyroid in normal and experimental states. A. Normal thyroid. Note ''cuboidal'' follicular cells and a few intracellular colloid droplets. B. Thyroid 3½ h after intravenous injection of 250 mU of thyrotropin. Many follicles contain only traces of colloid. Intracellular colloid droplets are abundant in the follicular cells of follicles which have larger amounts of colloid in their lumina. C. Thyroid several weeks after hypophysectomy. Note distension of lumina by colloid, which shows some shrinkage in the periphery. The follicular cells are flat. D. Thyroid of a rat that was fed an iodine-deficient diet for several weeks and then injected for 10 days with the thiocarbamide propylthiouracil. The collapsed lumina contain little colloid. The follicular cells are tall columnar; several mitoses (m) can be seen. The capillaries are engorged. All sections stained with PAS-hematoxylin. (A and B from S. H. Wollman, *J. Cell Biol.,* **21:**191, 1964.)

states the cells are tall and may be in mitosis, and the mass of colloid is relatively small (Fig. 29-2D). In normal animals an intermediate situation is seen, and there is considerable variation in activity existing from follicle to follicle, with a corresponding variation in histologic appearance.

Two kinds of epithelial cells are present in the follicles—typical follicular epithelial cells and parafollicular or C cells (Fig. 29-3). The follicular cells, unlike the parafollicular cells, show a definite polarity in the arrangement of their organelles. The nucleus at the base of the cell varies in shape depending on the height of the follicular epithelium. It is relatively flat in squamous epithelial cells and round or ovoid in columnar cells. In flattened epithelia the Golgi apparatus may be displaced to one side of the nucleus, whereas in cuboidal or columnar epithelial cells it lies above it. Mitochondria are found throughout the cytoplasm, which varies in its basophilia depending on the state of activity of the cells. Colloid droplets may be present, particularly after TSH stimulation. Rarely, degenerating cells with pyknotic nuclei (colloid cells of Langendorff) are observed.

Parafollicular cells (often called C cells because of their calcitonin secretion) are relatively uncommon and may occur singly or in groups. They have no obvious polarity and never contain colloid droplets. They are larger than follicular cells and their cytoplasm appears pale with many staining methods;

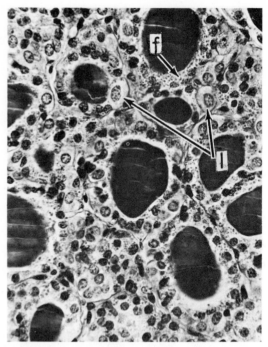

FIGURE 29-3 Normal rat thyroid. Note differences between follicular cells proper (f), which contain numerous colloid droplets, and the larger C cells (light cells) (l), which do not. PAS-hematoxylin stain. (Courtesy of C. P. Leblond.)

hence their other name of light or clear cells. They may stain intensely with silver impregnation techniques, probably because of their catecholamine content.

ULTRASTRUCTURE

In the electron microscope the follicular colloid is homogeneous or faintly reticular with a moderate electron density. It is bounded by the follicular cells which have microvilli at their apical border (Figs. 29-4, 29-5 and 29-8A). The microvilli tend to vary in height depending on the functional activity of the cell (Fig. 29-5). Between the microvilli, bristle-coated pits are sometimes observed. The tight junction at the apical end of the lateral plasma membrane forms a continuous seal between adjacent follicular cells. This probably functions to prevent leakage of the antigenically active thyroglobulin from the lumen of the follicle. Desmosomes, gap junctions, and interdigitations of the lateral plasma membranes of adjacent cells are

also present. The basal plasma membrane has many infoldings.

The nucleus of the follicular cells varies in height depending on the height of the cell. In active cells the nucleolus may be prominent. Long filamentous mitochondria are randomly distributed. Ribosomes and polysomes are scattered through the cytoplasm.

Many ultrastructural features of thyroid follicular cells are typical of cells producing protein for export. Cisternae of rough-surfaced endoplasmic reticulum, usually distended, are found throughout the cytoplasm and are largely responsible for its basophilia. The well-organized Golgi apparatus lies between the nucleus and the apical end of the cell or may be dis-

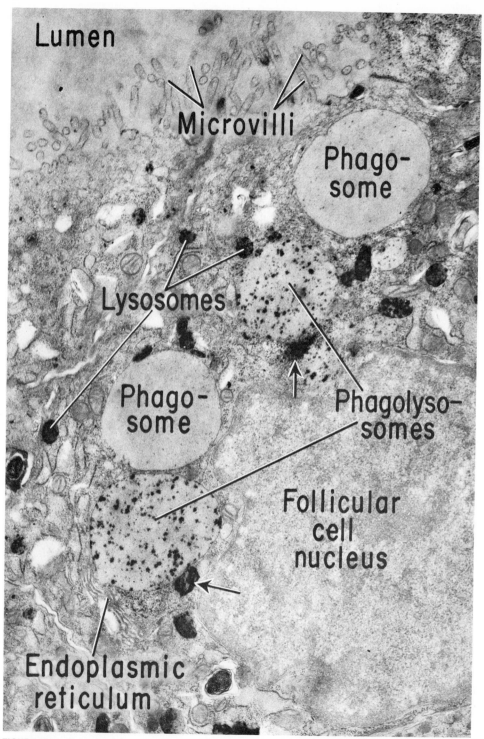

FIGURE 29-4 Electron micrograph of the apical portion of a follicular cell stained for acid phosphatase. Note the presence of the enzyme in the darkly stained lysosomes, some of which are closely attached to the much larger colloid droplets (phagosomes) (arrows). The two large droplets with irregular black speckling are phagolysosomes, whose colloid has become intermingled with lysosomal contents, as demonstrated by the irregular staining for acid phosphatase. ×20,000. (From S. H. Wollman, *J. Cell Biol.*, **25:**593, 1965.)

placed laterally. The apical cytoplasm contains many small vesicles. Some of these are bristle-coated. Others have a moderately electron dense homogeneous content and have been shown to empty their contents into the follicular lumen. The *apical vesicles* are probably the means by which thyroglobulin is transported from the Golgi apparatus to the follicular lumen.

Other organelles appear to function in thyroglobulin retrieval from the follicular lumen, its subsequent digestion, and the ensuing endocrine secretion of thyroid hormone. In occasional cells, *pseudopods* are seen—projections of the apical plasma membrane into the follicular lumen (Fig. 29-8B). These pseudopods sequester bits of colloid, and their membranes then fuse to form intracellular *colloid droplets* or

phagosomes which then sink into the apical cytoplasm of the follicular cells. The colloid droplets (Figs. 29-4 and 29-5B) are relatively large cytoplasmic bodies, with a homogeneous, moderately electron dense content bounded by a membrane. *Lysosomes*—small, often homogeneous, dense bodies bounded by a single limiting membrane—appear to fuse with the colloid droplets to form larger phagolysosomes during colloid digestion (Fig. 29-4). Coated vesicles formed from coated pits also participate in protein uptake by thyroid cells, but their quantitative importance in colloid resorption has not been evaluated and is probably quite small.

The follicular cells lie on a homogeneous basement membrane with a delicate network of collagen fibrils beneath it. The abundant capillary network, often with fenestrated endothelial cells, comes in close contact with the basement membrane and its associated fibrils.

FIGURE 29-5 Rat thyroids incubated in a medium for demonstration of peroxidase activity. A. Three weeks after hypophysectomy. The flattened follicular cells (FC) are at the top of the figure. Beneath them are the basement membrane (B) and narrow processes of connective tissue cells. A blood vessel (BV) with an endothelial cell nucleus is at the bottom of the figure. The follicular cells have peroxidase activity in the nuclear envelope (ne) and in a few flattened cisternae of rough-surfaced endoplasmic reticulum (R). The small Golgi apparatus (g) is relatively inactive. No peroxidase activity is present at the cell apexes. ×15,950. B. This rat was hypophysectomized for 3 weeks and then given TSH for 2 days before autopsy. The follicular lumen (L) is at upper right, the basement membrane (B) at lower left. The nuclear envelope of the follicular cell has intense peroxidase activity. RER cisternae (RER), now somewhat expanded, have greatly increased in number. These, and some vesicles and lamellae of the expanded Golgi apparatus (g), are peroxidase-positive. A few peroxidase-positive apical vesicles are present near the cell apex. Some peroxidase activity is also present in the follicular lumen (*). Note the colloid droplets (C) and lysosomes (L). ×16,250.

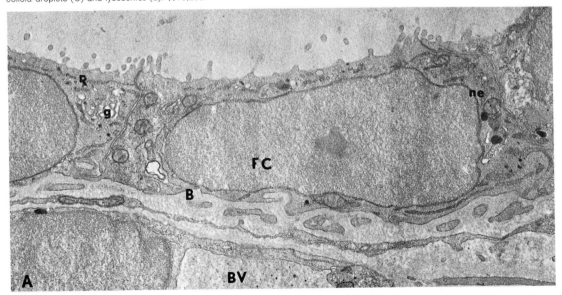

C CELLS

Although parafollicular cells (Fig. 29-6) may occur in groups outside the thyroid follicles, others are enclosed within the basement membrane of the follicles. In this location they are never in contact with the follicular colloid, although the cytoplasm of the intervening follicular cells may be very attenuated. They vary widely in shape and may have cell processes which sometimes seem to extend toward nearby capillaries. They have large, pale nuclei and abundant narrow cisternae of rough-surfaced endoplasmic reticulum which sometimes form whorls or spirals. Nearby is their extensive Golgi apparatus.

The predominant ultrastructural feature of parafollicular cells is their small secretory granules 1000 to 1800 Å in diameter (Fig. 29-6A). In well-fixed cells these have a finely granular content separated from

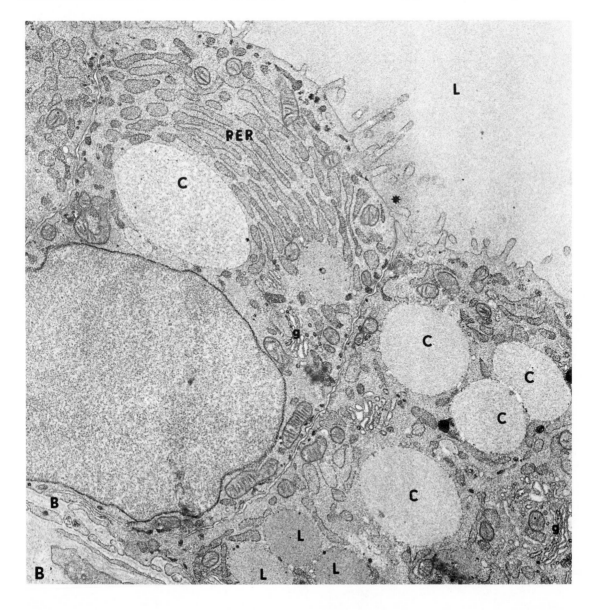

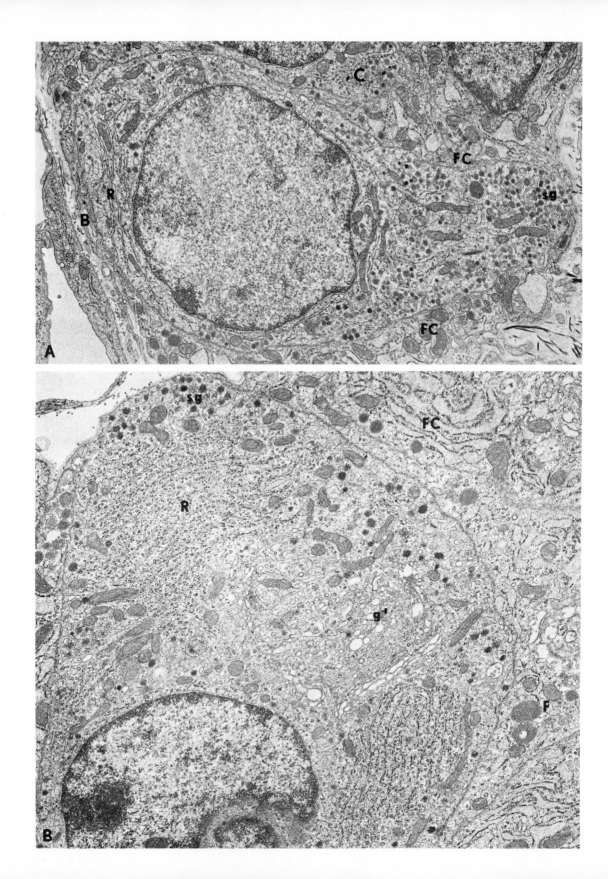

the membrane by a clear space. The granules appear to be formed by budding off of lamellae of the Golgi apparatus, and transitional forms between the Golgi apparatus and secretory granules may be seen in many cells. Their long mitochondria are randomly distributed.

HISTOCHEMISTRY AND HISTOPHYSIOLOGY

Many cytochemical and autoradiographic studies have been directed to the question of where in thyroid cells various events occur in the synthesis of thyroglobulin and its breakdown into an active thyroid hormone. As we have noted earlier, it is convenient to separate the two phases of secretion, the exocrine phase in which thyroglobulin is secreted apically into the colloid, and the endocrine phase, in which resorbed colloid is broken down into active thyroid hormone and secreted into the blood. However, it must be emphasized that in the living thyroid cell, both phases of secretion take place simultaneously.

THYROGLOBULIN SYNTHESIS AND SECRETION

To begin with, iodide and amino acids are actively transported into the follicular cells via the basal plasma membrane. Autoradiographic studies have shown that thyroglobulin protein precursors are synthesized in the rough-surfaced endoplasmic reticulum (RER) (Fig. 29-7), and some of the carbohydrate residues (mannose) are added. Further carbohydrate residues (galactose and fucose—the terminal carbohydrate residue of one carbohydrate side chain) are added in the Golgi apparatus, and the uniodinated molecule is assembled. The thyroglobulin, as yet uniodinated, is then transported via apical vesicles to the follicular lumen where it is added to the colloid mass.

Concurrently, a peroxidase, thyroperoxidase, is synthesized by the follicular cells and is transported to the follicular lumen via the same route (RER, Golgi, apical vesicles) and is also released into the follicular lumen (Fig. 29-5). This enzyme, like other peroxidases, can iodinate proteins, and thyroperoxidase is responsible for iodination of thyroglobulin. Iodination apparently occurs only in the follicular lumen (Fig. 29-9) despite the probable coexistence of the two proteins within the same organelles in the follicular cells. The reason for the absence of intracellular iodination is not known. (This situation reminds us of fetal thyroid, where iodination of thyroglobulin appears to begin concomitantly with the appearance of follicular lumina.) The process of iodination has been intensively studied. It appears to involve the oxidation of iodide to a higher valence state, but the details of its mechanism are still in doubt. Iodotyrosyl groups couple within the thyroglobulin molecule to produce peptide-linked hormone (iodothyronyl) groups. This is the storage form of thyroid hormone.

FIGURE 29-6 A. Parafollicular cell from normal mouse thyroid. This cell lies within the basement membrane (B) of the follicle and is flanked by another C cell (C) and by follicular cells (FC). The somewhat elongated cell contains long mitochondria, narrow RER cisternae (R), and many small moderately electron dense secretory granules (sg). The Golgi apparatus is not included in the section. ×10,000. B. Mouse C cell 4 h after the start of hourly calcium injections. Note the surrounding follicular cells (FC). Only a few secretory granules (sg) are observed, and these tend to be peripherally placed. RER cisternae (R) are abundant, and the prominent Golgi apparatus (g) has an unusually large number of associated vesicles. ×12,800.

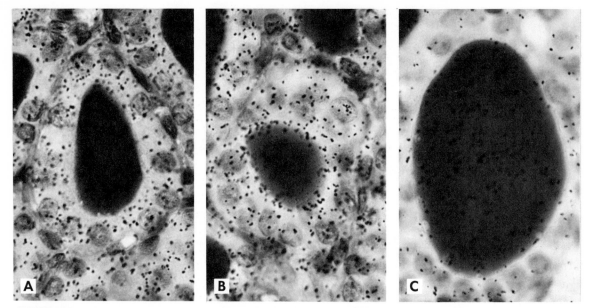

FIGURE 29-7 Radioautographs of thyroids from rats killed at various time intervals after the injection of [³H]-labeled leucine. The dark grains indicate the locations of proteins (largely thyroglobulin) synthesized from the labeled leucine. A. At 30 min, the grains overlie the cytoplasm of the follicular cells. They are located throughout the cell but are scarce at the apical edge in contact with the colloid. No grains are over the colloid. B. At 4 h, the grains predominate in the apical end of the cells. C. At 36 h, the grains are distributed uniformly over the colloid. All three sections are counterstained with PAS-hematoxylin. (Courtesy of N. J. Nadler, K. Harrison, and C. P. Leblond.)

SECRETION OF THYROID HORMONE

The second phase of thyroid secretion involves the re-uptake of thyroglobulin by the follicular cells and its breakdown to active hormone. The production of pseudopods and colloid droplets has been described above. This process may require the participation of microtubules and microfilaments since it is inhibited by colchicine and cytochalasin B. Subsequently, lysosomes fuse with colloid droplets to form phagolysosomes, large bodies which contain cytochemically demonstrable acid-phosphatase and esterase, classical marker enzymes for lysosomes (Fig. 29-4). It is presumed that the lysosomes, which also contain a protease active at acid pH, contribute their enzymes to the colloid droplet and that the acid proteases are responsible for the breakdown of thyroglobulin. Iodotyrosine precursors which make up most of the iodine in thyroglobulin are enzymatically deiodinated, releasing their iodine to be reused by the cells. The details of the process by which the active hormones are subsequently released from the cell are not well understood, but it is assumed that they diffuse from the base of the follicular cell into the blood and lymph.

C CELLS

As befits their neural crest origin, C cells have much of the biochemical machinery of the sympathetic neuron or the adrenal medulla. Fluorescence microscopy and autoradiographic studies have shown that they take up catecholamines or their amino acid precursors, decarboxylate the precursors to catecholamines, and store them together with their protein hormone, calcitonin, in a reserpine-sensitive granule. Cytochemi-

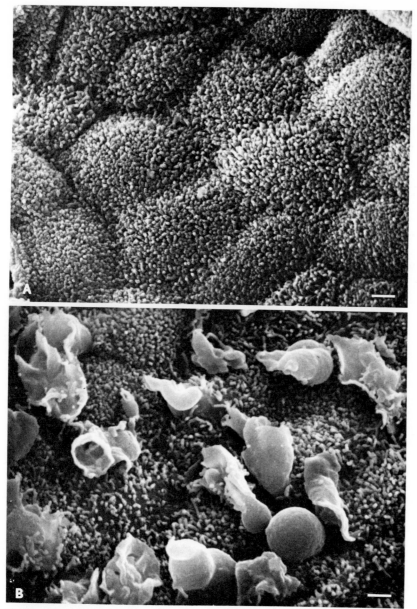

FIGURE 29-8 Scanning electron micrographs of the apical surfaces of thyroid follicular cells. The glands were fixed and subjected to critical point drying. A. Microvilli cover the apical surface of unstimulated thyroid follicles from a hypophysectomized rat for 24 h. Each cell appears to be slightly elevated in its center. The depressed regions mark the boundary between adjacent cells. ×499. B. Thyrotropin (TSH) elicits these large apical pseudopods in many follicles within 5 to 20 min in hypophysectomized animals. Pseudopods evidently form as broad flat lamellae which curl up and overlap, engulfing droplets of colloid; the pseudopods then assume a globular form, retract into the cell, and disappear from the apical surface. Under these conditions, new pseudopods are continually initiated for approximately 1 h and cells of a given follicle tend to respond synchronously. Responding cells generally display a single pseudopod and individual pseudopods usually engulf multiple droplets of varied sizes. ×4914. (Micrographs courtesy of Dr. B. K. Wetzel.)

cally, they also contain monamine oxidase, an enzyme capable of oxidizing cytoplasmic catecholamines. When experimental animals are injected with calcium, the cells rapidly degranulate (Fig. 29-6B), and con-comitantly blood calcitonin levels increase. Degranulation, together with loss of catecholamine-induced fluoresence, can also be produced more slowly in animals fed diets high in vitamin D_2. The primary effect of calcitonin is to inhibit the resorption of bone calcium salts. This results in a fall in blood calcium levels.

REGULATION OF THE THYROID ACTIVITY

The pituitary hormone TSH is the most important regulator of thyroid activity, although as noted earlier, sympathetic activity may also mimic TSH effects under circumstances in which TSH secretion is minimal or absent. The pituitary-thyroid axis appears to form a feedback loop, for elevated blood levels of thyroid hormone act to suppress TSH secretion. In part, this appears to be a direct pituitary effect; and in part, pituitary function is affected by suppression of hypothalamic production of a thyroid-releasing hormone (TRH).

Because of this feedback loop, the thyroid gland may appear hyperactive when blood levels of circulating thyroid hormone are normal or low. Iodine deficiency, or administration of drugs which interfere with production of thyroid hormone, lead to increased TSH production and this in turn results in a hyperactive gland. Conversely, administration of thyroxine can suppress TSH secretion with the consequence that the thyroid gland comes to resemble the gland seen after hypophysectomy.

The mode of action of TSH appears, at least in part, to be via a specific TSH receptor. When TSH combines with the receptor, adenyl cyclase is activated and intracellular levels of cyclic AMP increase. TSH stimulation can be mimicked by cyclic AMP or by dibutyryl cyclic AMP.

The morphological effects of TSH are best studied in hypophysectomized or thyroxine-suppressed animals. All follicles and cells do not respond at the same rate to the hormone, possibly because of local variations in blood flow. Within a short but variable time (usually a few minutes but depending on the species studied) after TSH administration, pseudopods are observed, followed by the appearance of intracellular colloid droplets (Fig. 29-2B). Lysosomes migrate apically from their former position at the base of the cell. Lysosome migration and pseudopod formation do not appear to be interdependent, since migration of lysosomes can still be observed when pseudopod formation has been inhibited. Exocytotic release of apical vesicles is also observed after TSH

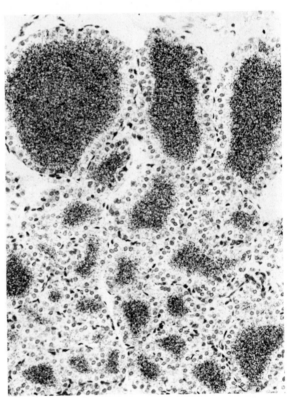

FIGURE 29-9 Radioautograph of the thyroid of a rat which had received ^{125}I-labeled iodide in its drinking water long enough to have its body iodine stores labeled to the same specific radioactivity (that is, the same number of counts per minute per unit mass of iodine). In this condition of so-called radioisotopic equilibrium, the distribution of radioactivity reflects that of nonradioactive iodine faithfully. Note that essentially all the blackening of the emulsion due to the radioactive iodine is over the colloid in the lumina rather than in the follicular epithelium. ×240. (From S. H. Wollman, *Endocrinology,* **81:**1074, 1967.)

administration. Thyroid blood flow increases. Later there are signs of increased synthetic activity by the follicular cells. Synthesis of both thyroglobulin and thyroperoxidase (Fig. 29-5) appears to be TSH-stimulated. Eventually, if stimulation is prolonged, increased cell division and hyperplasia of the gland occur (Fig. 29-2D).

REFERENCES

ANDROS, G., and S. H. WOLLMAN: Autoradiographic Localization of Radioiodide in the Thyroid Gland of the Mouse, *Am. J. Physiol.*, **213:**198–208 (1967).

BROWN-GRANT, K.: Regulation of TSH Secretion, in G. W. Harris and B. T. Donovan (eds.), "The Pituitary Gland," vol. 2, pp. 235–269. University of California Press, Berkley, 1966.

DUMONT, E.: The Action of Thyrotropin on Thyroid Metabolism, *Vitam. Horm.*, **29:**289–412 (1971).

EKHOLM, R. and L. E. ERICSON: The Ultrastructure of the Parafollicular Cells of the Rat, *J. Ultrastruct. Res.*, **23:**378–402 (1968).

HEIMANN, P.: Ultrastructure of Human Thyroid: A Study of Normal Thyroid, Untreated and Treated Diffuse Toxic Goiter, *Acta Endocrinol. [Suppl.] (Kbh.)*, **53:**110 (1966).

LOEWENSTEIN, J. E., and S. H. WOLLMAN: Distribution of ^{125}I and ^{127}L in the Rat Thyroid Gland during Equilibrium Labeling as Determined by Autoradiography, *Endocrinology*, **81:**1074–1085 (1967).

NADLER, N. J., S. K. SARKAR, and C. P. LEBLOND: Origin of Intracellular Colloid Droplets in the Rat Thyroid, *Endocrinology*, **71:**120–129 (1962).

NADLER, N. J., B. A. YOUNG, and C. P. LEBLOND: Elaboration of Thyroglobulin in the Thyroid Follicle, *Endocrinology*, **74:**333–354 (1964).

PITT-RIVERS, R., and W. R. TROTTER (eds.): "The Thyroid," Butterworth & Co. (Publishers), Ltd., London, 1964.

SELJELID, R., A. REITH, and K. F. NAKKEN: The Early Phase of Endocytosis in the Rat Thyroid Follicle Cell, *Lab. Invest.*, **23:**595–605 (1970).

STRUM, J. M., and M. J. KARNOVSKY: Cytochemical Localization of Endogenous Peroxidase in Thyroid Follicular Cells, *J. Cell Biol.* **44:**655–66 (1970).

TAYLOR, S. (ed.): "Calcitonin: Procedings of the Symposium on Thyro Calcitonin and the C Cells," Heinemann Educational Books, Ltd., London, 1968.

WETZEL, B. K., S. S. SPICER, and S. H. WOLLMAN: Changes in Fine Structure and Acid Phosphatase Localization in Rat Thyroid Cells Following Thyrotropin Administration, *J. Cell Biol.*, **25:**593–618 (1965).

WHUR, P., A. HERSCOVICS, and C. P. LEBLOND: Radioautographic Visualization of the Incorporation of Galactose-^{3}H and Mannose-^{3}H by Rat Thyroids in vitro in Relation to the Stages of Thyroglobulin Synthesis, *J. Cell Biol.*, **43:**289–311 (1969).

WOLLMAN, S. H., S. S. SPICER, and M. S. BURSTONE: Localization of Esterase and Acid Phosphatase in Granules and Colloid Droplets in Rat Thyroid Epithelium, *J. Cell Biol.*, **21:**191–201 (1964).

WOLLMAN, S. H., and I. WODINSKY: Localization of Protein-bound I^{131} in the Thyroid Gland of the Mouse, *Endocrinology*, **56:**9–20 (1955).

The Parathyroid Gland

ROY O. GREEP

NUMBER, LOCATION, AND ORIGIN

The parathyroid glands in humans are paired and are usually four in number, but there may be only two glands or as many as six in an individual. One pair of glands is generally located on the dorsal surface of the lateral lobes of the thyroid gland; the other pair may lie anywhere from just caudal to the lower pole of the thyroid to the anterior or posterior mediastinum. The parathyroids are brownish ovoid bodies, 6 to 7 mm long by 2 to 3 mm thick and weighing, in the adult, about 35 mg each. The variability in number and location of the parathyroid glands and the prevalence of aberrant glands may become matters of critical importance when, as in states of hyperparathyroidism, the location and removal of pathologic parathyroid tissue are necessary. Whereas most mammals, such as humans have a superior and inferior pair of glands, the rat and mouse have only the superior pair. In the rabbit the superior (or internal) pair is embedded in the thyroid gland but the inferior (or external) pair lies free in the surrounding tissue.

MICROSCOPIC STRUCTURE

The human parathyroid has a thin external connective tissue capsule from which very fine trabeculae extend into the body of the gland, forming poorly defined irregular lobules, which are further partitioned into sheets or cords by finer septa. In this fibrous stroma are found large blood vessels, nerves, lymphatics, and fat cells. Beginning at puberty, an increasing number of fat cells come to occupy the stroma, until 50 to 80 percent of the gland volume is occupied by fat (Fig. 30-1). The gland cells themselves are enmeshed in reticular fibers which also support a rich network of capillaries. The nerves end mainly on the vascular elements and are not believed to influence the endocrine functions of the parathyroid glands. At one point on their surface the cells abut on a capillary into which the parathyroid hormone is presumably emptied. Cell polarity in the normal human parathyroid is not evident.

Two varieties of parenchymal cells—*chief* cells and *oxyphil* cells—are readily identifiable in the adult human parathyroid gland (Fig. 30-1). It will be well to keep in mind, however, that the finding of numerous transitional cells by electron microscopy has raised the possibility that these are not different cells but cytologic modifications of a single type of parenchymal cells.

CHIEF CELLS

The chief cells are considerably more numerous than the oxyphil cells. By light microscopy they have a round, centrally located nucleus with one or two nucleoli. The main distinguishing feature is their water-clear and apparently empty cytoplasm, although electron microscopy shows that they contain the usual cytoplasmic organelles such as mitochondria, Golgi apparatus, and endoplasmic reticulum (ER), as well as varying numbers of glycogen granules and lipid droplets (Fig. 30-2). Cells relatively depleted of glycogen are thought to be in active secretion, whereas more abundant glycogen is suggestive of an inactive storage phase. Several workers have described coated granules or vesicles of varying electron density tentatively thought to contain the secretory product parathyroid hormone (PTH) (Fig. 30-3), probably identical to argyrophilic granules seen earlier by light microscopy. These coated granules have been observed inside mitochondria and free in the cytoplasm of chief cells, oxyphil cells, and adjacent endothelial cells lining the parathyroid capillaries. Their distribution suggests that they are being secreted into the bloodstream, but their relationship to the secretion of parathyroid hormone has not been established. Localized lamellar arrays of rough ER probably account for the basophilic bodies seen by histologic means. Lipid vacuoles occur singly or in large, round, membrane-bounded bodies containing lipid vacuoles of various dimensions (Fig. 30-2). Other lipid bodies probably representing lipofuscin, the autofluorescent wear-and-tear pigment, are present.

OXYPHIL CELLS

The oxyphil cells are mostly larger than chief cells, their cytoplasm is strongly eosinophilic, and they have relatively small nuclei which may appear pycnotic. They are usually much fewer in number than chief cells and may occur singly, in nests, or in sizable nodules. The oxyphil cells do not appear until immediately prior to or at the time of puberty and become

FIGURE 30-1 Photomicrograph of a normal adult human parathyroid gland showing groups of cords, sheets, and acini of chief cells separated by a stroma containing numerous fat cells. Oxyphil cell nodules (O) are also seen among the chief cells. H&E. × 130 (Courtesy of S. I. Roth.)

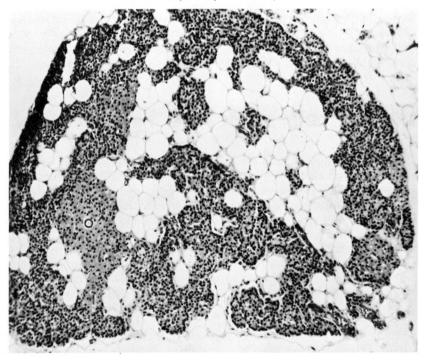

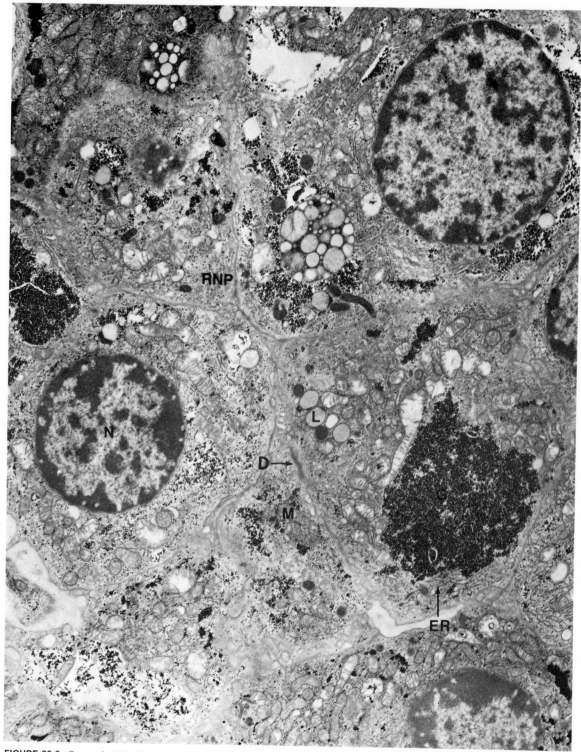

FIGURE 30-2 Group of chief cells from a normal human parathyroid gland. Note the variation in abundance of glycogen and number of mitochondria. G, glycogen; L, lipid; D, desmosome; M, mitochrondria; N, nucleus; RNP, ribonucleoprotein; ER, endoplasmic reticulum. (Courtesy of R. J. Weymouth and H. R. Seibel.)

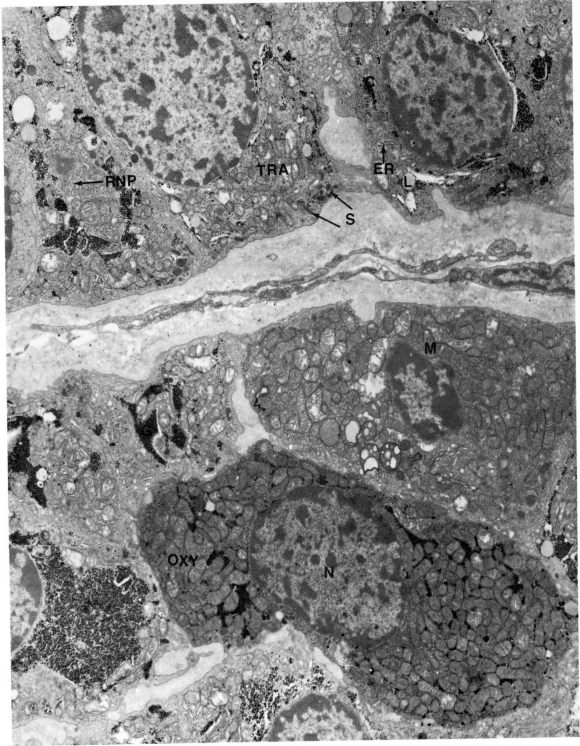

FIGURE 30-3 Oxyphil cell in a normal human parathyroid gland shown in comparison with chief cells and a transitional cell. Note the range in density of mitochondria and the presence of glycogen in granules. OXY, oxyphil cell; C, chief cell; TRA, transitional cell; S, secretory material. (Courtesy of R. J. Weymouth and M. N. Sheridan.)

somewhat more abundant in old age. Thus far, oxyphils have been found in only two other species, macaque monkeys and cattle and in the latter, not in the young.

The most striking feature of the oxyphils is that by histochemical or ultrastructural observations the cytoplasm is seen to be tightly packed with large mitochondria (Fig. 30-3). Some glycogen granules, bits of ER, and pigment are interspersed between the mitochondria.

TRANSITIONAL CELLS

Cells with intermediate characteristics which appear to be transitional between chief cells and oxyphils are abundant. Such cells show wide variation in number of mitochondria and content of glycogen granules (Fig.

30-3). The classification of the parenchymal cells of the human parathyroid gland into chief and oxyphil cells was based on histologic criteria. Recent electron-microscopic observations tend to favor the concept that there is only one parenchymal cell type, the chief cell. All others, including the oxyphil, represent modifications of the chief cell. This concept is supported also by the fact that during the first years of life, only chief cells are present.

Desmosomes connect the plasma membranes of both chief and oxyphil cells. The plasma membranes of adjacent cells are generally smooth, although areas of extensive interdigitations do occur. Intercellular spaces vary in extent and may contain glycogen.

ENDOCRINE FUNCTION

Parathyroid hormone (PTH) has been purified and the complete covalent structure determined. It is a straight-chain peptide containing 84 amino acids and has a molecular weight of 9,563 daltons.

The amino acid sequence of PTH obtained from bovine, porcine, and human glands differs in a few of the 84 residues. Evidence is available indicating that the hormone is synthesized as a larger precursor peptide with a molecular weight of 11,500 to 13,000 daltons (Hamilton, et al., 1971; Kemper et al., 1972 and 1975; and Wong and Lindall, 1975). This has been termed pro-PTH and is believed to be cleaved in the gland to yield the native (1-84) secretory form of PTH. (For a review, see Gray et al., 1974.) A fragment of the amino-terminal portion of the native molecule (2-27) and synthetic 1-34 PTH possess significant biological activity suggesting that the amino-terminal portion of the native molecule is important for the expression of its hormonal activity.

The parathyroid hormone serves the vital function of maintaining the calcium content of the blood plasma at an optimal and nearly constant level (10 mg per 100 ml). This is necessary for normal neuromuscular activity. Following removal of the parathyroids in humans and many other mammals, blood calcium falls and neuromuscular irritability increases, eventuating in tetany and often death. The acute signs, but not all the long-term effects, of hypoparathyroidism are ameliorated by any treatment which will elevate

the blood calcium to normal levels. Injections of calcium salts are immediately effective, and extracts of the parathyroid glands of domestic animals afford relief within a few hours through increased mobilization of calcium from the skeletal depots—an effect brought about by an action of parathyroid hormone on osteocytes and osteoclasts, leading to increased bone resorption, and also by stimulation of the renal tubular reabsorption of calcium ions.

Parathyroid hormone also has an important regulatory influence on the concentration of blood inorganic phosphate. Excessive secretion of parathyroid hormone leads to a reduction in blood phosphate, and hypoactivity leads to an increase. These changes are mediated by an effect of the hormone on the kidney. This induced drain of phosphate through the urine is referred to as the *phosphaturic action* of the parathyroid hormone. Work with pure parathyroid hormone has conclusively demonstrated that the calcemic and the phosphaturic responses are owing to a single hormone. It is well established that the parathyroid hormone acts directly on the kidney tubules to promote the reabsorption of calcium and inhibit the reabsorption of phosphate from the urine.

The parathyroid hormone, acting systemically, can effect the bones and erupting teeth. Thus, overactivity of the parathyroid glands may lead to osteitis fibrosa cystica, a condition characterized by excessive loss of bone tissue with replacement by fibrous connective tissue. In hypoparathyroidism, the calcification of developing bones and teeth may be seriously impaired. Some of the systemic effects are a result of the direct action of parathyroid hormone on bone and kidney cells, whereas others stem indirectly from resulting changes in the plasma concentration of calcium and phosphate. A direct effect of the parathyroids on bone was suggested by the production of local erosion under grafts of parathyroid glands onto the surface of bones and conclusively demonstrated by showing that parathyroid hormone stimulates bone resorption in tissue culture.

The functional activity of the parathyroid glands is regulated by the concentration of calcium ions in the blood plasma. Approximately half the blood calcium is in ionic form and half is bound. Lowering of the ionic calcium acts as a feedback mechanism, stimulating the parathyroids to secrete more hormone; and if sustained, this will result in an enlargement of the glands. Conversely, when the blood ionic calcium is elevated, as by the infusion of calcium salts or excessive intake of vitamin D, the parathyroid glands decrease in function and show atrophic changes. Instances of primary hyperparathyroidism in humans are a result of parathyroid hyperplasia or an adenoma of one or more of the parathyroid glands. The parathyroids are also stimulated in chronic renal insufficiency where retained phosphate leads to a fall in blood calcium. This is known as secondary hyperparathyroidism.

As noted above, a depression of the blood calcium stimulates the secretion of parathyroid hormone, which causes the calcium to rise. The blood calcium may be kept from overshooting the optimal level by a second blood-calcium-regulating hormone, calcitonin. In mammals this hormone originates from the thyroid gland and is secreted by the parafollicular or C cells which are derived embryologically from the ultimobranchial body (see Chap. 29). Calcitonin counters the action of parathyroid hormone by inhibiting bone resorption and thereby prevents the blood calcium from rising above the optimal level.

The structure of calcitonin has been determined and the hormone synthesized. The molecule consists of a polypeptide of 32 amino acids with a seven-member ring at the N terminus. The sequence of amino acids in caltitonin prepared from different species varies considerably, but the function served by the hormone is the same.

In fish, amphibia, reptiles, and birds, the ultimobranchial gland develops separately from the thyroid gland. In these animals, calcitonin is secreted by the ultimobranchial gland and not by the thyroid gland. Although calcitonin has been found in abundance in the ultimobranchial glands of the elasmobranchs, what function, if any, it may serve in these animals having only a cartilaginous skeleton is unknown. The parathyroids appear to have a large-reserve functional capacity. Little, if any, compensatory hypertrophy occurs following removal of all but one gland, and parathyroid autografts are successful only when all the glands in situ are excised.

On the phyletic scale, the parathyroid glands are not found in the fishes or gill-bearing amphibia but are constantly present in all other vertebrates. They appear to have originated with the disappearance of the branchial apparatus, that is, at the time the ancestors of our modern amphibia made their appearance on land. (For comparative aspects, see the review by Greep, 1963.)

REFERENCES

BAKER, B. L.: A Study of the Parathyroid Glands of the Normal and Hypophysectomized Monkey (*Macaca mulatta*), *Anat. Rec.*, **83:**47 (1942).

BARNICOT, N. A.: The Local Action of the Parathyroid and Other Tissues on Bone in Intracerebral Grafts, *J. Anat.*, **82:**233 (1948).

CHANG, H. Y.: Grafts of Parathyroid and Other Tissues to Bone, *Anat. Rec.*, **111:**23 (1951).

DE ROBERTIS, E.: The Cytology of the Parathyroid Gland of Rats Injected with Parathyroid Extract, *Anat. Rec.*, **78:**473 (1940).

GAILLARD, P. J.: Parathyroid and Bone in Tissue Culture, in R. O. Greep and R. V. Talmage (eds.), ''The Parathyroids,'' Charles C Thomas, Publisher, Springfield, Ill., 1961.

GOLDHABER, P.: Some Chemical Factors Influencing Bone Resorption in Tissue Culture, in R. F. Sognnaes (ed.), "Mechanism of Hard Tissue Destruction," American Association for the Advancement of Science, Washington, D.C., 1963.

GRAY, T. K., C. W. COOPER, and P. L. MUNSON: Parathyroid Hormone, Thyrocalcitonin and the Control of Mineral Metabolism, in S. M. McCann (ed.), "Endocrine Physiology," Butterworth & Co., (Publishers), Ltd., London, 1974.

GREEP, R. O.: Parathyroid Glands, in U.S. Von Euler and H. Heller (eds.), "Comparative Endocrinology," vol. 1, Academic Press, Inc., New York, 1963.

GREEP, R. O.: The Chemistry and Physiology of the Parathyroid Hormone, in G. Pincus and K. V. Thimann (eds.), "The Hormones," vol. 1, Academic Press, Inc., New York, 1948.

HAMILTON, J. W., R. R. MACGREGOR, L. L. H. CHU, and D. V. COHN: Isolation and Partial Purification of a Non-parathyroid Hormone Calcemic Fraction from Bovine Parathyroid Glands, *Endocrinology,* **89:**144 (1971).

KEMPER, B., J. F. HABENER, J. T. POTTS, JR., and A. RICH: Proparathyroid Hormone, Identification of a Biosynthetic Precursor to Parathyroid Hormone, *Proc. Nat. Acad. Sci., (U.S.A.),* **69:**143 (1972).

KEMPER, B., J. F. HABENER, A. RICH, and J. T. POTTS, JR.: Microtubules and the Intracellular Conversion of Proparathyroid Hormone to Parathyroid Hormone, *Endocrinology,* **96:**903 (1975).

LANGE, R.: Zur Histologie und Zytologie der Glandula parathyreoidea des Menschen. Licht und Electronenmikroskopische untersuchungen an Epithelkörperadenomen, *Z. Zellforsch.,* **53:**765 (1961).

LEVER, J. D.: Cytological Appearances in the Normal and Activated Parathyroid of the Rat. A Combined Study by Electron and Light Microscopy with Certain Quantitative Assessments, *J. Endocrinol.,* **17:**210 (1958).

MARSHALL, R. B., D. K. ROBERTS, and R. A. TURNER: Adenomas of the Human Parathyroid, *Cancer,* **20:**512 (1967).

MECCA, C. E., G. P. MARTIN, and P. GOLDHABER: Alterations of Bone Metabolism in Tissue Culture in Response to Parathyroid Extract, *Proc. Soc. Exp. Biol. Med.,* **113:**538 (1963).

MUNGER, B. L. and S. I. ROTH: The Cytology of the Normal Parathyroid Glands of Man and Virginia Deer. A Light and Electron Microscopic Study with Morphologic Evidence of Secretory Activity, *J. Cell Biol.,* **16:**379 (1963).

WONG, E. T. and A. W. LINDALL: Subcellular Location of Human Parathyroid Hormone Immunoreactive Peptides and Preliminary Evidence for a Precursor to Human PTH, *Proc. Soc. Exp. Biol. Med.,* **148:**387 (1975).

The Adrenal Gland

JOHN A. LONG

The adrenal glands constitute one of the major homeostatic organs of the mammalian body. They are composed of two separate endocrine organs which differ in embryologic origin, type of secretion, and function. In mammals, the two organs are arranged as an outer cortex and an inner medulla surrounded by a common capsule (Fig. 31-1). In the other vertebrate classes, the two tissues may be completely unassociated or intermingled to a greater or lesser degree. In these cases, the homologue of the mammalian medulla is referred to as a *chromaffin tissue,* whereas the tissue corresponding to the cortex of mammals is called *interrenal tissue.*

The *cortex,* whose secretory rate is controlled by hormones produced in the adenohypophysis and the kidney, produces steroid hormones that affect carbohydrate and protein metabolism, resistance to physiologic stresses, and electrolyte distribution. The *medulla,* which is under nervous control, secretes catecholamines that affect heart rate and smooth muscle function in blood vessels and other viscera as well as influence various aspects of carbohydrate and lipid metabolism.

It is convenient to describe the two components of the gland separately; it should be kept in mind, however, that there appears to be a phylogenetic trend toward the more intimate structural relationship between the two glandular tissues as seen in mammals. In addition, an interesting functional relationship has been described which will be referred to later.

GROSS ANATOMY

The adrenal glands (called *suprarenal glands* in human beings because of their upright posture) lie retroperitoneally near the anterior poles of the kidneys and embedded in the perirenal adipose tissue. The right and left glands are of somewhat different shape in human beings, with the left gland being somewhat broader. The combined weight of the adrenals from adult human beings dying immediately of accidental causes is about 8 g. It should be borne in mind that both weight and size of the glands may vary considerably with age and physiologic condition of the organism. In gross section, the cortex, which constitutes the largest part of the gland, appears yellow as a result of the presence of lipids. The medulla, which represents approximately 10 percent of the weight of the adrenal, is reddish or brown.

BLOOD SUPPLY

Three main groups of arteries supply the human adrenal gland: (1) superior suprarenal arteries which arise as branches of the inferior phrenic artery and which are the major blood supply, (2) middle suprarenals arising from the aorta, and (3) inferior suprarenals, which arise from the renal artery (Fig. 31-2). The adrenal arteries form a plexus in the capsule from which three types of intraglandular vessels arise. (1) Arteriae capsulae supply the connective tissue capsule of the organ. (2) Arteriae corticis arise from the capsular plexus by repeated branching and then descend into the cortex and break up into the capillary bed supplying the cortical parenchyma. These capillaries anastomose in the inner cortex and empty into the medullary vascular bed via relatively few small channels. (3) Arteriae medullae penetrate the cortex via connective tissue trabeculae and directly supply the medullary tissue (Fig. 31-3). Thus, the medulla has two blood supplies—one via the cortical capillaries and the other from the direct medullary arteries. Several

orders of venules ultimately join to form the large central vein, which in human beings has conspicuous bundles of longitudinally oriented smooth muscle in the intraglandular portions of its wall. The adrenal vein exits at the hilum of the gland and on the left side empties into the left renal vein; the right adrenal vein joins the vena cava directly.

LYMPHATICS

The lymphatic drainage is not well known, but it appears that the capsule possesses a set of lymphatics which pass out along the adrenal arteries; the central vein has a separate set which follows this vein to the exterior of the gland. No small lymphatic vessels have been detected within the parenchyma of the adrenal.

INNERVATION

The main innervation of the adrenal is composed of preganglionic sympathetic fibers arising from T_8 to T_{11} and passing to the gland via the greater and lesser splanchnic nerves. These fibers penetrate to the me-

FIGURE 31-1 Human adrenal gland, Mallory Axan. Note that the central vein is surrounded by a cuff of cortical tissue. ×3.

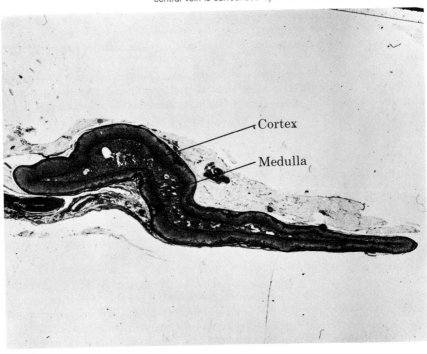

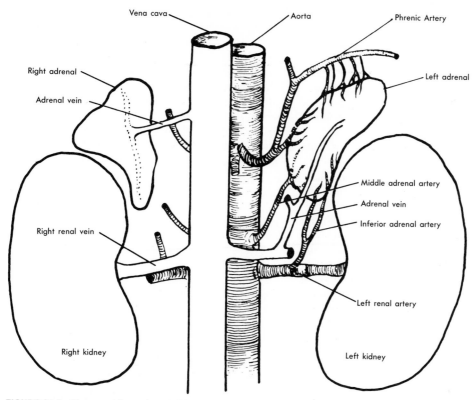

FIGURE 31-2 Diagram of the major arterial supply and venous drainage of the human adrenal gland.

dulla and synapse with the chromaffin cells, which are thus homologous with sympathetic ganglion cells. There is no parasympathetic innervation of medullary parenchymal cells. Recent ultrastructural studies have revealed efferent nerve endings (possibly adrenergic) on the endocrine parenchymal cells of the adrenal cortex in several species including humans. The role of these nerves in the physiology of the adrenal cortex has not been determined.

HISTOLOGY OF THE ADRENAL CORTEX

In all mammals, except monotremes, the adrenal cortex can be divided into three concentric zones, which were named *zona glomerulosa, zona fasciculata,* and *zona reticularis* by Arnold in 1866 (Fig. 31-4). These structural subdivisions of the cortex have functional implications which will be referred to later. In humans, the zona glomerulosa accounts for approximately 15 percent of the total cortical volume, the zona fasciculata about 78 percent, and the zona reticularis about 7 percent. The gland is surrounded by a capsule composed of fibroblasts, collagen, and elastic fibers, as well as a few smooth muscle fibers in some species. Connective tissue trabeculae penetrate the cortex, carrying nerves and blood vessels to the medulla. Reticular fibers which are continuous with the fibers of the capsule form a meshwork around the parenchymal cells of the cortex and medulla.

Lying immediately beneath the capsule, the cells of the zona glomerulosa are ovoid to columnar in shape and are arranged in spherical masses or arcades. These cells are relatively small (12 to 15 μm in diameter), contain a single spherical nucleus, and possess a small amount of homogeneously staining cytoplasm in which are suspended a few small lipid droplets. In the adrenal of humans, the zona glomerulosa may be absent in restricted areas of the cortex; in these regions, cells of the zona fasciculata are found immediately beneath the capsule.

The zona fasciculata is composed of long, radially arranged cords that are generally one or two cells thick and are separated from adjacent cords by capillary vessels which form the blood supply of the cortex. The cells are larger than those of the other zones (approximately 20 μm in diameter) and are packed with numerous large lipid droplets in the living state. After treatment with the organic solvents necessary for the preparation of routine histologic sections, lipids are extracted, leaving spaces which give the cytoplasm a reticulated appearance and a poor affinity for the usual histologic stains. These cells have sometimes been called spongiocytes or clear cells because of this artifact of specimen preparation.

The innermost zone of the adrenal cortex, the zona reticularis, is characterized by the disruption of the regular, parallel alignment of the cords of the zona fasciculata and the formation of an anastomosing network of cellular cords interspersed by capillaries. The component cells are smaller than those of the zona fasciculata and contain relatively few small lipid inclusions. Hence, the cytoplasm is compact and readily stained. Cells of this zone are notable for large accumulations of lipofuscin pigment which is visible with the light microscope as golden-brown deposits.

FIGURE 31-3 Stereogram of a mammalian adrenal gland, showing the medulla (M) with its central vein (CV), and the cortex with its three zones, the zona glomerulosa (ZG), zona fasciculata (ZF), and zona reticularis (ZR) enclosed by the capsule (C). Two arteriae medullae (AM) and an arteria corticis (RAC) are shown. (Reproduced by permission from R. G. Harrison, ''A Textbook of Human Embryology,'' 1st ed., Blackwell Scientific Publications, Ltd., Oxford, 1959.)

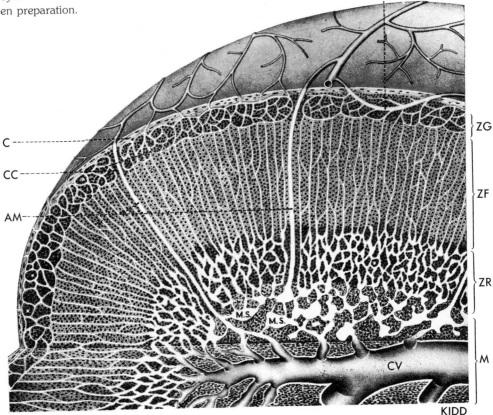

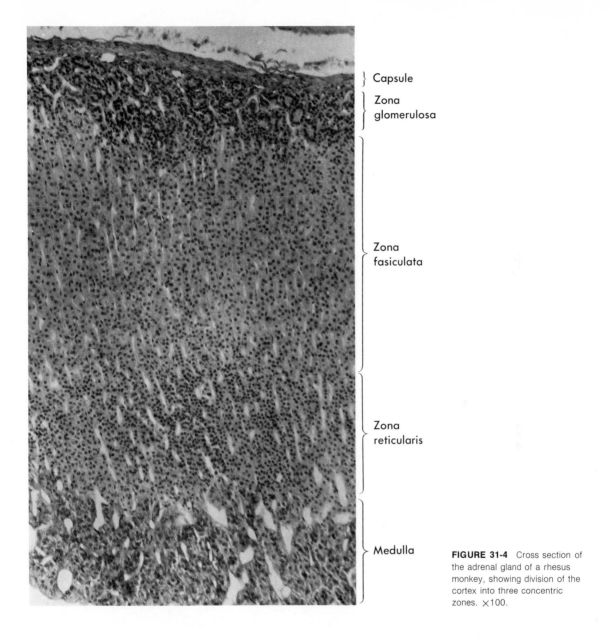

Capsule

Zona glomerulosa

Zona fasiculata

Zona reticularis

Medulla

FIGURE 31-4 Cross section of the adrenal gland of a rhesus monkey, showing division of the cortex into three concentric zones. ×100.

ULTRASTRUCTURE OF THE ADRENAL CORTEX

The ultrastructure of adrenocortical cells is similar in many ways to that of other steroid-secreting cells, including the corpus luteum of the ovary and interstitial cells of the testis. These similarities include an abundant amount of smooth ER, a numerous quantity of lipid inclusions, and a frequent occurrence of mitochondria with tubular or vesicular cristae. Despite these general similarities, cells of each of the zones of the adrenal cortex are sufficiently different to warrant separate description.

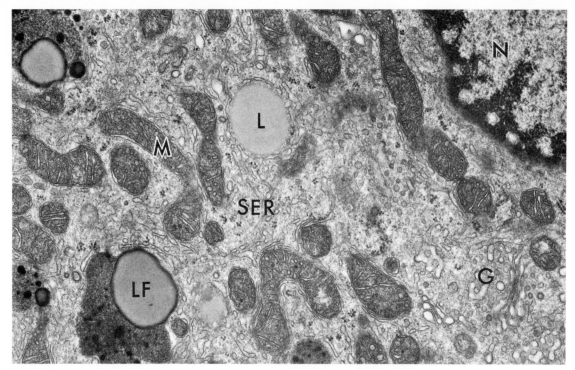

FIGURE 31-5 Electron micrograph of a cell of the zona glomerulosa of the human adrenal cortex. N, nucleus; M, mitochondrion; Ser, smooth-surfaced endoplasmic reticulum; L, lipid droplet; LF, lipofuscin; G, Golgi complex. ×22,500.

FIGURE 31-6 Electron micrograph of a cell of the zona fasciculata from the human adrenal cortex. M, mitochondrion; RER, rough-surfaced endoplasmic reticulum; SER, smooth-surfaced endoplasmic reticulum; L, lipid droplet; LF, lipofuscin pigment. ×19,250.

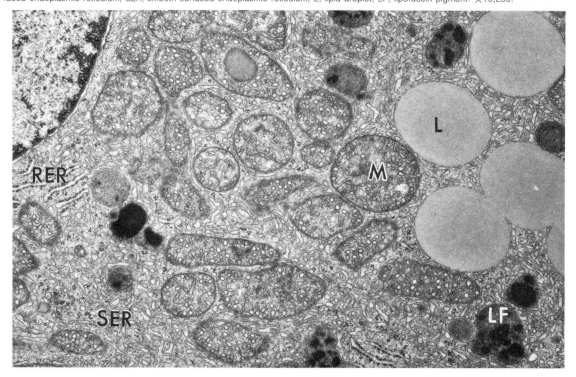

Each cell of the zona glomerulosa possesses a spherical nucleus bounded by a typical nuclear envelope. The cytoplasm is full of smooth ER membranes (Fig. 31-5) which form a tubular, anastomosing network. A few profiles of rough ER are seen; most of the ribosomes are free in the cytoplasm, many being arranged in spirals and rosettes. Stacks of smooth membrane-bounded cisternae associated with numerous small vesicles constitute the Golgi complex, usually seen close to the nucleus. A pair of centrioles is present. The mitochondria are usually elongated and the cristae are broad, flattened extensions of the inner mitochondrial membrane.

Cells of the zona fasciculata differ from those of the zona glomerulosa in several respects. Most prominent is the large number of lipid droplets, which may be so numerous as to almost fill the cell (Fig. 31-6). Mitochondria are distinctive in this zone, usually being more rounded than those of the zona glomerulosa. Their cristae are short, tubular extensions of the inner

mitochondrial membrane. The rough ER is well developed. It is common to find several cisternae aligned parallel to one another forming structures which may be seen, in appropriate light-microscopic preparations, as basophilic bodies. The plasma membrane is thrown into short, irregular microvilli over parts of the cell surface, whereas in other regions the membranes of adjacent cells are parallel and separated by a space of approximately 20 nm. In restricted regions, the membranes of adjacent cells are much closer together and form "gap junctions," which are thought to be sites of high electrical conductivity between cells.

The ultrastructure of the zona reticularis differs only slightly from that of the zona fasciculata. In the reticularis, mitochondria tend to be more elongate and fewer lipid droplets are present (Fig. 31-7). Large numbers of membrane-bounded inclusions with heterogeneous contents are present. These structures correspond to the lipofuscin pigment granules seen by light microscopy. They seem to be accumulations of

FIGURE 31-7 Electron micrograph of a cell from the zona reticularis of the human adrenal cortex. SER, smooth-surfaced endoplasmic reticulum; M, mitochondrion; LF, lipofuscin pigment. ×32,500.

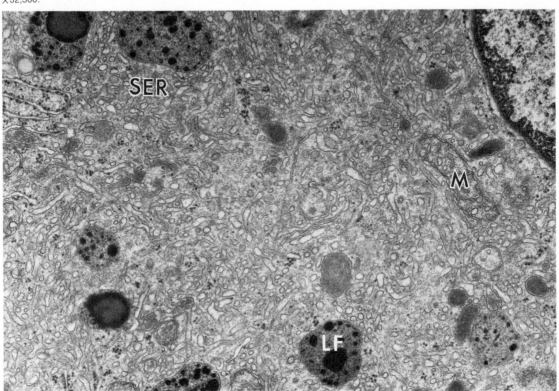

waste materials, some of which are probably oxidized, polymerized products of unsaturated lipids. Acid phosphatase, a typical lysosomal enzyme, has been detected in lipofuscin granules. Their number increases with age.

Certain ultrastructural changes of adrenocortical cells can be observed when the rate of synthesis of adrenocortical steroids is caused to decrease or increase (for example, when the animal is hypophysectomized or injected with adrenocorticotropic hormone). When adrenocortical cells are stimulated, their cytoplasmic volume enlarges and the quantity of smooth ER increases. The fate of the lipid droplets depends upon the degree of stimulation. With a severe stimulus, the droplets may completely disappear, whereas with a more moderate stimulus, they become smaller than usual but very numerous. These responses reflect the fact that stainable lipid is stored precursor material, not the hormone itself. If the cell secretes hormone at the same rate that it manufactures the precursor, no storage of precursor occurs (Fig. 31-8).

When stimulation is withdrawn, as in hypophysectomy, there is an atrophy of the cells of the zonae fasciculata and reticularis and a decrease in the quantity of smooth ER. Lipid droplets at first enlarge and coalesce, reflecting decreased utilization for hormone production. Eventually lipid disappears altogether, as though the cell had utilized this material for its own nutrition.

Close study of adrenocortical cells has not revealed visible evidence for the mechanisms of intracellular transport and release of secretory products, the various steroid hormones. Present evidence indicates that steroid hormones are not stored in large

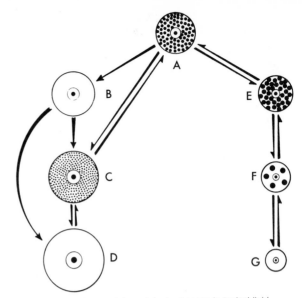

FIGURE 31-8 Some of the cytologic changes in typical lipid-containing adrenocortical cells (A) when their activity is stimulated or inhibited. Left: With stimulation, adrenocortical cells, their nuclei, and the nucleoli enlarge. With acute (B) or prolonged (D) stimulation, there may be a loss of lipid stores; with more moderate but chronic (C) stimulation, the lipid droplets become small and lose detectable cholesterol stores but retain a high titer of unsaturated fatty acids. Right: With removal of stimulus, adrenocortical cells, their nuclei, and their nucleoli shrink (E to G). The lipid droplets apparently coalesce and gradually disappear. Initially there may be an increase in cholesterol concentration. Gradually both the fatty acids and the cholesterol stores decline. Both the severely stimulated and long-term inactive cells lack lipid stores; they are distinguishable only by size. (From Deane, 1962, by permission from Springer-Verlag.)

quantity in adrenocortical cells and that they are released continuously as individual molecules and not discontinuously in packets, as is the case in many protein-secreting cells.

CAPILLARY ENDOTHELIUM

The endothelium of the capillary vessels of the cortex is of the fenestrated or visceral type (Fig. 31-9). The cell is quite thin except near the nucleus where thickenings occur to accommodate the nucleus and most of the other cytoplasmic organelles such as Golgi material and mitochondria. Individual profiles of granular reticulum are sometimes found in the thin cytoplasmic extensions. At intervals, the wall becomes so thin that it appears to be a single layer which does not have the structure of a unit membrane. These regions are termed *fenestrae*. A continuous basal lamina is present beneath the endothelium. A space which may be oc-

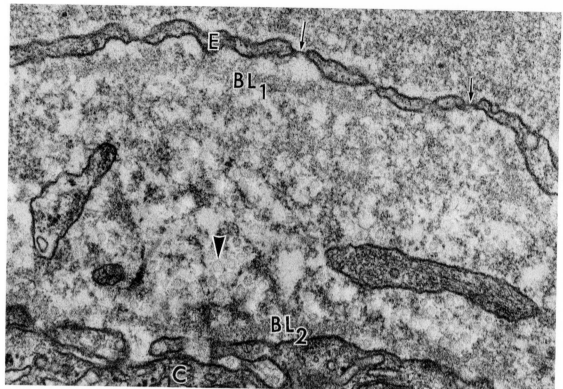

FIGURE 31-9 Electron micrograph of capillary endothelium in the human adrenal cortex. Endothelial cell (E) with fenestrae at arrows; basal lamina beneath endothelium labeled BL_1. Cross sections of reticular fibers are faintly seen at the end of the arrow head. Basal lamina adjacent to cortical parenchymal cell (C) labeled BL_2. ×66,000.

cupied by fibroblasts and macrophages is present between the endothelium and the endocrine parenchyma. Individual fibrils with the characteristic 64-nm repeat of collagen are present in the subendothelial space. They correspond to the elements demonstrated by silver-impregnation methods and are termed reticular fibers by light microscopists. A basal lamina is present on the surfaces of parenchymal cells which abut on the subendothelial space.

HISTOPHYSIOLOGY OF THE ADRENAL CORTEX

A wide variety of steroid hormones are secreted by the adrenal cortex. They are derived from cholesterol stored in the lipid inclusions as fatty acyl esters of cholesterol. However, in human beings, the most important source of substrate for adrenocorticoid biosynthesis is cholesterol taken up from the blood plasma.

Although almost 100 different steroids have been extracted from adrenal glands of humans and experimental animals, only a few are normally released from the gland and are hormonally active. In human beings, the most important adrenal steroid is cortisol, an example of a class of hormones called *glucocorticoids* because of their pronounced effects on carbohydrate metabolism. Another member of this class is corticosterone, which is secreted in small amounts by the human adrenal gland but which is the principal glucocorticoid secreted by the rat. Aldosterone is the most potent *mineralocorticoid,* so called because of the effects of this class of corticosteroids on electrolyte balance. A weak *androgen* (dehydroepiandrosterone and its sulfate) is secreted in large quantities by the human adrenal. The secretion of *estrogens* has not been unequivocally demonstrated and it is probable that the estrogens found in postmenopausal or oophorectomized women originate from the aromatization of precursors, such as dehydroepiandrosterone, in the liver.

The morphologic zonation of the adrenal cortex is paralleled by an important functional zonation. By this is meant the specialization of cells of a given zone for the synthesis and release of certain classes of steroid hormones. Thus, aldosterone is secreted by cells of the zona glomerulosa, whereas cortisol and dehydroepiandrosterone are formed by cells of the zonae fasciculata and reticularis. There are some indications that the zona reticularis may be more active in androgen secretion than the zona fasciculata.

Steroid hormones are formed from cholesterol by removal of a six-carbon fragment of the side chain followed by a dehydrogenation at carbon 3 and a series of hydroxylations at specific sites. A simplified scheme showing the biosynthesis of the principal adrenal steroids is given in Fig. 31-10. In addition, the subcellular localization of the enzymes involved is given. Note that a precursor may move from one compartment to another (for example, mitochondria to microsome) several times before the final product is formed. How this is accomplished in a controlled fashion is not understood at present.

CONTROL OF SECRETION

The adenohypophysis is essential for the maintenance of the structure and function of the adrenal cortex. If the pituitary is removed from an animal, a striking decline in the weight of the adrenal gland ensues and is paralleled by a decline in secretion of most of the adrenal hormones. Upon histologic examination, it is seen that the inner zones of the cortex are atrophied but that the zona glomerulosa is well maintained (Fig. 31-11). The hormone secreted by the adenohypophysis which maintains the adrenal cortex is *adrenocorticotropic hormone,* or ACTH. ACTH is a polypeptide composed of 39 amino acids whose sequence is known for a number of species, including humans. The main effects of ACTH are to stimulate steroid synthesis and release, to promote growth of the adrenal cortex, to increase blood flow through the adrenal, and to cause ascorbic acid depletion in a few species, most notably the rat.

If ACTH is given to a hypophysectomized animal, it will prevent the decline in weight and secretory activity of the adrenal cortex that would ordinarily ensue. If ACTH is given to an animal with an intact pituitary gland, this hormone will cause a hypertrophy of the inner zones of the adrenal cortex and an elevation of the circulating levels of many of the adrenal corticoids. ACTH will not cause a hypertrophy of the zona glomerulosa nor will it increase the secretory rate of aldosterone except when given in large doses and then only transiently. It has been concluded that the inner zones of the adrenal cortex, the zona fasciculata and the zona reticularis, are regulated by ACTH and that the zona glomerulosa is controlled by a different mechanism. This evidence also indicates that aldosterone is formed only by cells of the zona glomerulosa, and careful microchemical investigations have shown that the enzymes necessary for the final steps in aldosterone biosynthesis are found only in these cells. The zona glomerulosa is found to hypertrophy if the animal is maintained on a sodium-deficient diet, but if a potent mineralocorticoid such as aldosterone or deoxycorticosterone is given over a long period, the zona glomerulosa will atrophy and the other zones will remain normal.

If experimental animals or human beings are given large quantities of a glucocorticoid such as cortisol over a long period of time, subsequent histologic examination of the adrenal glands will reveal a pronounced atrophy of the zona fasciculata and zona reticularis. For many years it was thought that the high levels of glucocorticoids directly suppressed the synthesis and release of ACTH by the adenohypophysis which led, in turn, to the observed atrophy. It is now known that an additional link in the feedback loop is present: the hypothalamus. Certain neurons in this region of the brain are believed to produce a substance called *corticotropin-releasing factor* (CRF), which is thought to be a low-molecular-weight peptide. The rate of secretion of CRF is inversely related to the circulating levels of glucocorticoids to which these neurons are exposed. The axons of these hypothalamic neurons end on portal blood vessels in the median eminence which transport CRF to the adeno-

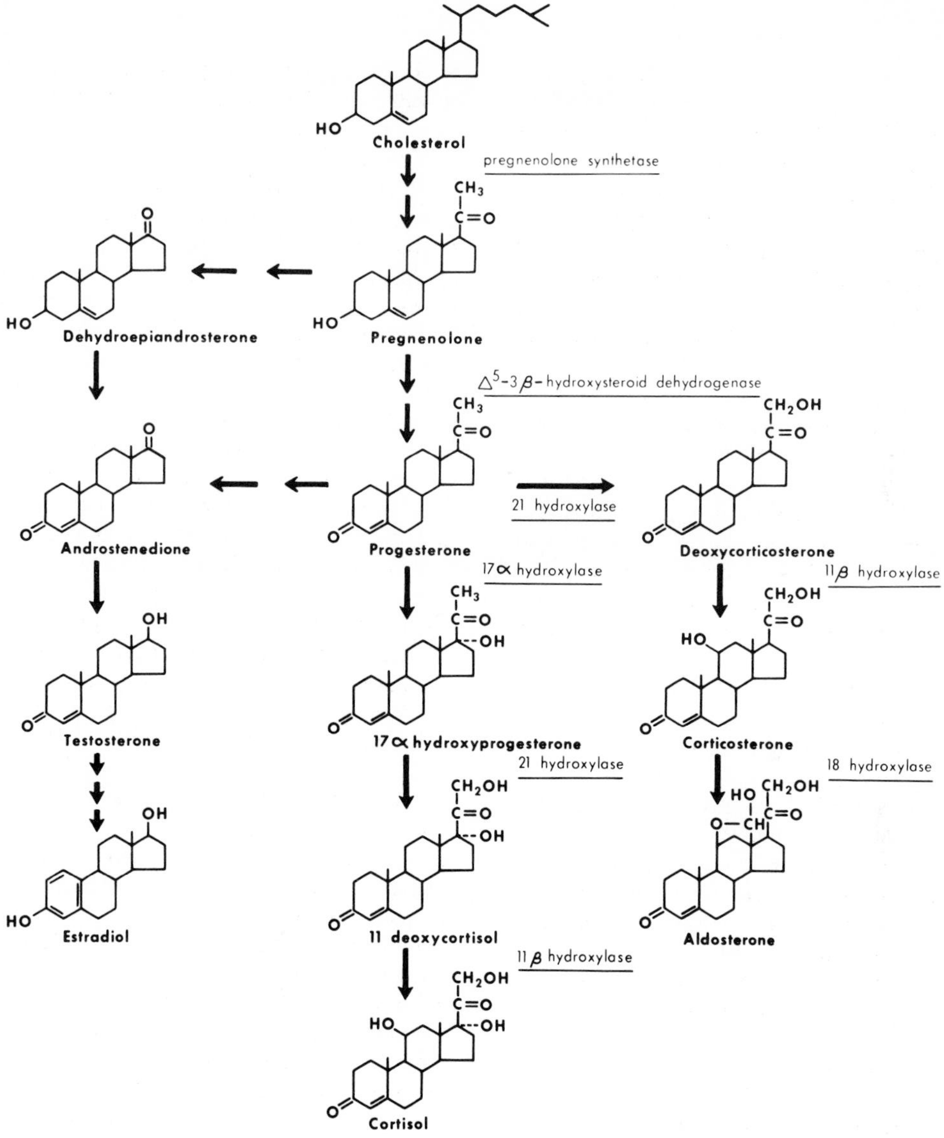

Enzyme	Zonal Localization	Subcellular Localization
Pregnenolone synthetase	All zones	Mitochondria
Δ^5-3β-hydroxy-steroid dehydrogenase	All zones	Microsomes
21 hydroxylase	All zones	Microsomes
11 β hydroxylase	All zones	Mitochondria
17 α hydroxylase	Fasciculata and reticularis	Microsomes
18 hydroxylase	Glomerulosa	Mitochondria

FIGURE 31-10 Diagram showing the pathways taken in the biosynthesis of the principal corticosteroids. The zonal distribution and subcellular distribution of the most important enzymes are given in the table.

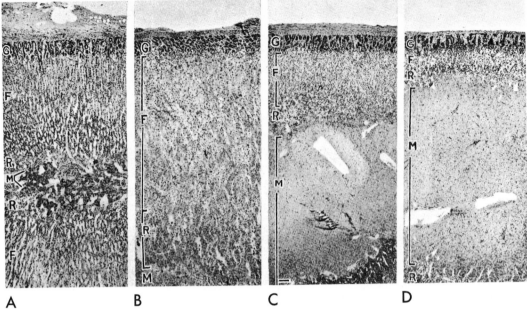

A   B   C   D

FIGURE 31-11 Sections of rhesus monkey adrenal glands.
A. Normal adrenal cortex. B. After treatment with ACTH. Note the increase in width of zonae fasciculata (F) and reticularis (R).
C. After treatment with cortisone. The inner zones are reduced in width. D. Hypophysectomized for 90 days. Extensive atrophy of inner zones. Note that the width of the zona glomerulosa (G) is the same in each instance. M, medulla. ×36. (By permission from Knobil et al., *Acta Endocrinol. (Kobh.)*, **17:**229, 1954.)

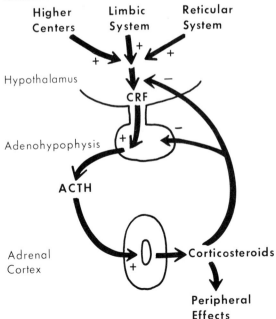

FIGURE 31-12 Diagram illustrating current concepts of the neuroendocrine control of the adrenal cortex.

hypophysis. Here, CRF stimulates the synthesis and release of ACTH. Figure 31-12 diagrams this feedback loop.

The effects of glucocorticoids are numerous and widespread. Most cells possess cytoplasmic receptors for glucocorticoids which bind the steroid. The complex then migrates into the nucleus where it interacts with chromatin and, in some way, modifies the transcription of DNA into messenger RNAs. These RNAs then code for specific proteins which elicit the observed hormonal effects. In general, glucocorticoids are catabolic in the periphery (muscle, lymphoid tissue, skin, adipose tissue) and anabolic in the liver.

Glucocorticoids cause inhibition of protein synthesis in fibroblasts and other cells, but protein catabolism continues normally or is increased. This provides amino acids that can enter the gluconeogenesis pathway in the liver. These hormones decrease peripheral uptake of glucose by cells of muscle, skin, etc., and are necessary for lipolysis to occur under the influence of catecholamines or glucagon. Glucocorticoids enhance amino acid uptake by the liver and

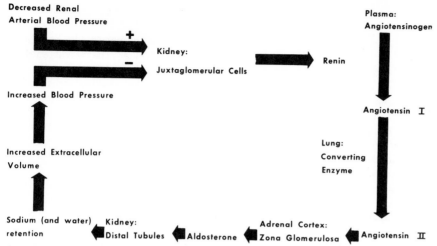

FIGURE 31-13 Diagram illustrating one of the mechanisms controlling secretion of aldosterone by the zona glomerulosa.

appear to induce the formation of certain key enzymes for gluconeogenesis in this organ. The net result is increased glucose concentration in the blood (hyperglycemia), increased urinary nitrogen excretion, and fat loss.

Glucocorticoids also depress the inflammatory response, and wounds heal poorly in the face of high levels of these hormones. In order for the organism to cope with stresses such as burning, cold, or starvation, glucocorticoid hormones are necessary. Finally, glucocorticoids, such as cortisol, have a feedback influence on those hypothalamic neurons which produce the corticotropin-releasing factor.

Aldosterone, the principal secretory product of cells of the zona glomerulosa, is a potent mineralocorticoid first identified in 1953. Aldosterone promotes the resorption of sodium ions in the distal tubule of the nephron, increases potassium excretion by the kidney, and causes a lowering of the sodium concentration in sweat, saliva, and intestinal secretions.

The rate of aldosterone secretion is regulated by the renin-angiotensin system, ACTH, and the plasma concentrations of potassium and sodium. The primary control system is the renin-angiotensin mechanism which is a complex feedback loop involving the kidney (Fig. 31-13). The signal sensed by the juxtaglomerular apparatus is not known with certainty. It may be a decrease in the degree of stretch of the juxtaglomerular cells themselves or it may be a decrease in the sodium load at the macula densa. In either case, this signal causes release of renin from the juxtaglomerular cells. Renin is an enzyme which catalyzes the conversion of angiotensinogen, a circulating α_2 globulin, to angiotensin I. Angiotensin I is then converted to angiotensin II, which acts on the zona glomerulosa of the adrenal to stimulate the secretion of aldosterone. Aldosterone acts on the distal tubules of the nephron to promote sodium retention leading to an increase in intravascular fluid volume and consequent increase in blood pressure. This, in turn, stretches the receptor cells of the juxtaglomerular apparatus, thus closing the feedback loop.

ADRENAL MEDULLA

The adrenal medulla is composed of an endocrine parenchyma (*chromaffin cells*) supported by connective tissue elements and profusely supplied with nerves and blood vessels (Fig. 31-14). Ganglion cells are present but are usually difficult to find in routine sections. Chromaffin cells have been defined by

Coupland (1965) as cells derived from neuroectoderm and innervated by preganglionic sympathetic fibers, which synthesize and release catecholamines (epinephrine and norepinephrine). These cells show a brown coloration when exposed to an aqueous solution of potassium dichromate. This "chromaffin reaction'' is thought to result from the oxidation and polymerization of catecholamines contained within granules in the cells. Catecholamines also form yellow-green fluorescent compounds after reacting with formaldehyde (Fig. 31-15, *see color insert*). This technique has been of great value in recent years in mapping the distribution of catecholamines in organs such as the adrenal medulla and the nervous system.

Chromaffin cells are arranged as epithelioid cords in close association with vascular spaces. The cells are round, polyhedral, or in some species, columnar in shape. In most species, the application of a battery of histochemical methods permits the identification of two types of cells, one of which contains norepinephrine and the other epinephrine. When viewed in the electron microscope, the most prominent feature of these cells is the abundance of membrane-bounded electron-dense granules, 150 to 350 nm in diameter, which are thought to be the site of storage of catecholamines (Fig. 31-16). These granules also contain high

concentrations of ATP, specific proteins called chromogranins, as well as soluble dopamine β-hydroxylase, the enzyme responsible for converting dopamine to norepinephrine. The membranes of these granules are characterized by relatively high concentrations of lysolecithin and the presence of specific membrane proteins, one of which (chromomembrin A) has been found to be membrane-bound dopamine β-hydroxylase. After special preparative methods, it is possible to demonstrate with the electron microscope that two populations of cells exist. Some of the cells, which are thought to be the sites of storage of norepinephrine, possess granules of very high electron density, whereas most of the cells possess granules of lesser electron density and correspond to epinephrine-storing cells (Fig. 31-17).

Typical elongate mitochondria and rough ER are present in both cell types. A Golgi apparatus is situated close to the nucleus, and within the cisternae of this organelle, a dense material may be seen. It is believed that the chromaffin granules are formed in

FIGURE 31-14 Photomicrograph of a section of the human adrenal medulla. A ganglion cell is indicated by the arrow. ×600.

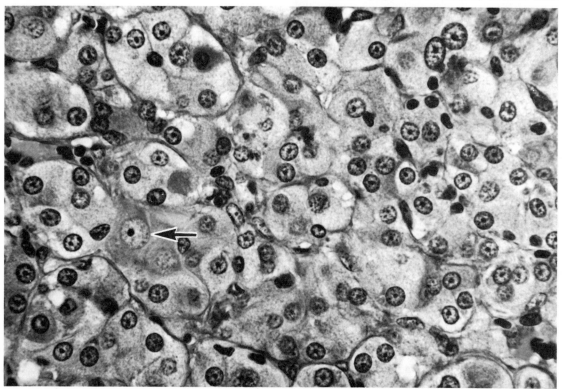

the Golgi complex in a manner similar to that described for zymogen granules in pancreatic acinar cells. A few microvilli may be present at the cell surface, and a single cilium is probably present on each cell. Maculae adhaerantes are frequently seen at the surface of adjacent parenchymal cells. Each chromaffin cell is innervated by a cholinergic preganglionic sympathetic nerve the stimulation of which initiates the release of stored catecholamine from the medullary cell (Fig. 31-18).

Morphologic events accompanying the release of catecholamines are the subject of controversy. Some workers have reported that chromaffin granules retain their integrity and that catecholamine diffuses out of, or is actively transported out of, the granules and the cell. Others have reported that the granule membrane fuses with the plasmalemma and that the entire content of the granule is emptied into the extracellular space and eventually enters the circulation (quantal

release). Physiologic evidence is consistent with the quantal-release mechanism.

As previously noted, the adrenal medulla receives a dual blood supply, one from the arteriae medullae and the other from those formed by vessels which are continuous with the capillaries of the cortex. It has been reported that norepinephrine-storing cells are usually more closely associated with vessels arising from arteriae medullae, whereas epinephrine-storing cells are supplied with blood which has previously perfused the cortex and which thereby contains a higher concentration of corticosteroids. There is evidence that phenylethanolamine-N-methyl transferase, the enzyme which transfers a methyl group from S-adenosyl methionine to norepinephrine, yielding epinephrine, is induced in the presence of glucocorticoids (Fig. 31-19).

In a hypophysectomized animal which does not secrete ACTH and thus does not secrete normal levels of glucocorticoids, the amount of epinephrine which

FIGURE 31-16 Electron micrograph of an epinephrine-storing cell from the rat. C, chromaffin granules; M, mitochondrion; G, Golgi complex. ×14,700.

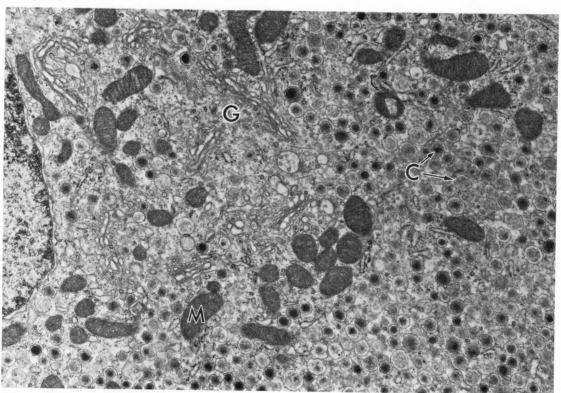

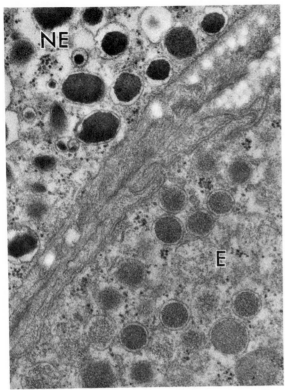

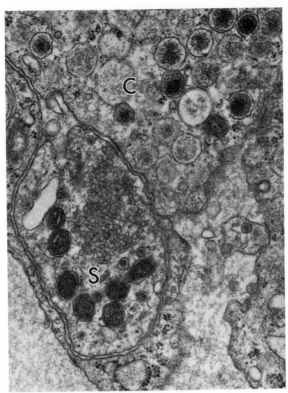

FIGURE 31-17 Electron micrograph to compare the chromaffin granules in a norepinephrine-storing cell (upper left, NE) and an epinephrine-storing cell (lower right, E) in the cat adrenal medulla. ×33,600.

FIGURE 31-18 Electron micrograph showing cholinergic preganglionic fiber (S) ending on a chromaffin cell (C) in the rat adrenal medulla. ×34,700.

can be isolated from the adrenal medulla declines, with a concomitant slight rise in the concentration of norepinephrine. In rat and rabbit fetuses, the accumulation of epinephrine in the adrenal medulla coincides with the initiation of adrenocortical function. If the fetus is deprived of its hypophysis by decapitation in utero, the rise in epinephrine content is not seen, but the levels of norepinephrine are above normal. Injection of ACTH or cortisol into the decapitated fetuses restores the normal ratio of epinephrine to norepinephrine. Comparative histologic and endocrinologic studies provide additional evidence for this interesting interaction between cortex and medulla. In the shark, where interrenal and chromaffin tissues are separate, norepinephrine is the main catecholamine, whereas in mammals, where the cortex (interrenal tissue) surrounds the medulla (chromaffin tissue), the principal catecholamine is epinephrine.

The effects of the hormones of the adrenal medulla are widespread and will be touched upon only briefly here. Epinephrine causes glycogenolysis in the liver and skeletal muscle, with a consequent rise in blood glucose levels. Free fatty acids are mobilized from adipose tissue under the influence of catecholamines. Epinephrine causes an elevation of blood pressure, an acceleration of the heart, a cutaneous vasoconstriction, and a dilation of coronary and skeletal muscle vessels, but vasoconstriction in other organs such as the intestinal tract. Under the influence of catecholamines, the threshold of the reticular-activating system of the brain is lowered and the subject becomes more alert. It can be seen that all these effects have an obvious adaptive value when the organism is confronted with an emergency situation.

Secretion of adrenal medullary hormones is under sympathetic nervous control. During sleep or

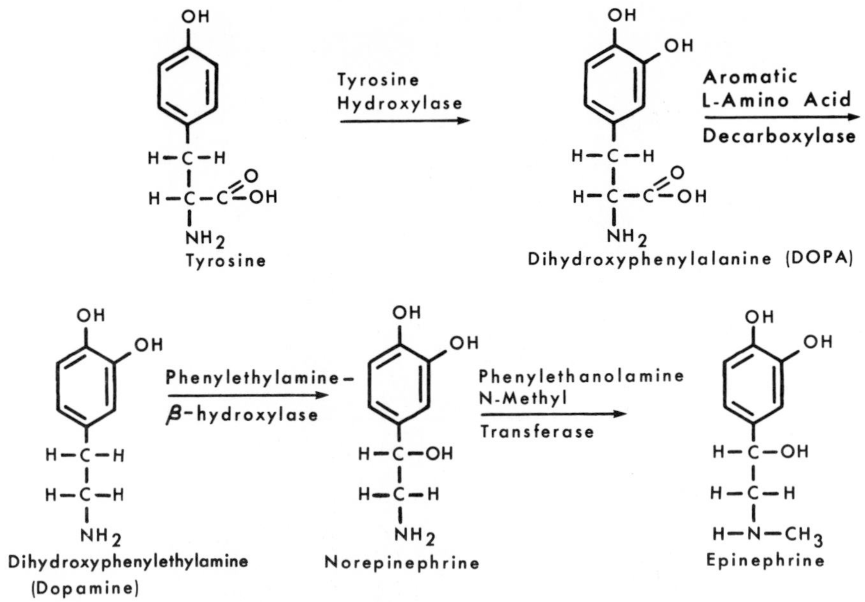

FIGURE 31-19 Biosynthetic pathway of catecholamines in the adrenal medulla.

narcosis, little or no secretion can be detected; but while the organism is carrying on normal activities, low quantities of catecholamines can be detected in the circulation. When the animal is exposed to pain, cold, anoxia, hypoglycemia, emotional excitement, or other stress, the secretion of catecholamines rises sharply and the homeostatic mechanisms mentioned above are brought into play.

DEVELOPMENT

In 4- to 5-week human fetuses, mesothelial cells in the region of the dorsal mesentery and near the cranial pole of the mesonephros begin to proliferate and penetrate into the subjacent, highly vascular mesenchyme. Continued growth of these primordia results in bilaterally placed organs which protrude into the coelomic cavity and become encapsulated. The gland becomes differentiated into two regions: an outer zone composed of small, compact cells, which form the *definitive cortex* of the adult; and an inner zone of larger, eosinophilic cells, which is termed the *fetal zone* (Fig. 31-20). The fetal zone constitutes approximately 80 percent of the cortex at term, but it undergoes rapid degeneration after birth; whereas the definitive cortex enlarges and eventually becomes differentiated into the familiar three zones of the adult gland.

Chromaffin cells from the neural crest begin to migrate into the adrenal anlagen at 6 to 7 weeks of fetal life and subsequently aggregate in the center of the gland to form the adrenal medulla.

Cells of the fetal cortex have the ultrastructural appearance of other steroid-secreting cells (Fig. 31-21). The smooth ER is elaborately developed, lipid droplets are abundant, and the Golgi complex is prominent. The appearance of the mitochondria in cells of the fetal zone is similar to that of mitochondria of the adult zona fasciculata.

The fetal adrenal is under the control of ACTH secreted by the pituitary of the fetus. Anencephalic fetuses possess very small adrenal glands, and the fetal zone is lacking. The physiologic role of the fetal zone of human adrenals in intrauterine life is slowly becoming clearer, but progress in this area is hampered by the fact that none of the commonly used experimental animals has a comparable fetal zone.

The human fetal adrenal gland is a steroidogenic

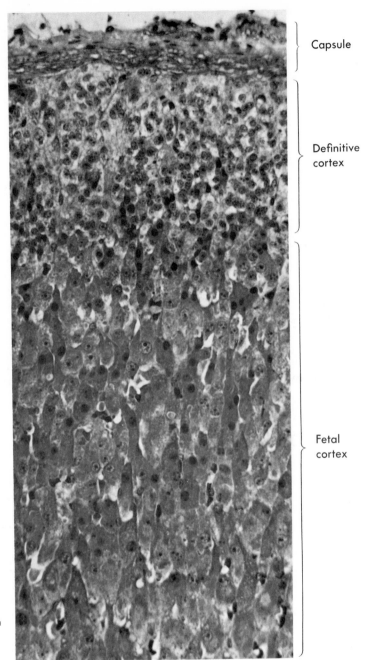

Capsule

Definitive cortex

Fetal cortex

FIGURE 31-20 Section of a human fetal adrenal at 18 weeks of gestation, showing the division into fetal and definitive cortex. ×300.

organ which is part of a "fetal-placental" unit. The fetal adrenal is incapable of carrying out certain steroidogenic reactions; in particular, the Δ^5-3β-hydroxysteroid dehydrogenase system has a very low activity in the gland. This enzyme is present in high quantity in the placenta. The products of this enzymatic reaction are transferred to the fetus where the adrenal gland carries out a series of hydroxylations which result in the production of cortisol, corticosterone, deoxycorticosterone, and aldosterone. A 17-21

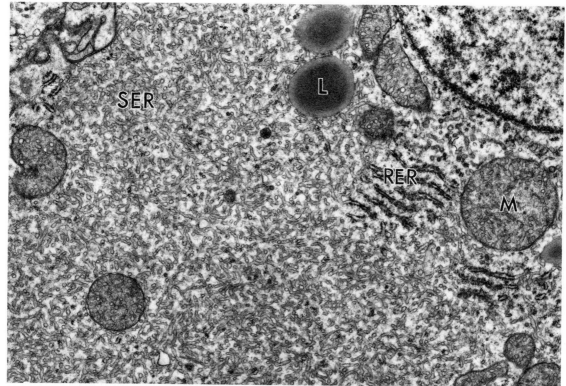

FIGURE 31-21 Electron micrograph of a cell of the human fetal adrenal cortex at 14 weeks of gestation. SER, smooth-surfaced endoplasmic reticulum; RER, rough-surfaced endoplasmic reticulum; M, mitochondrion; L, lipid inclusion. ×13,000. (Courtesy of Dr. N. S. McNutt and Dr. A. L. Jones.)

lyase is present which converts C_{21} steroids to C_{19} products, particularly dehydroepiandrosterone (DHA). This enzyme is not found in the placenta. A sulfokinase is present in the adrenal which converts DHA to DHA sulfate, the principal precursor of placental estrogens.

Although much has been learned about the role of the fetal adrenal in steroidogenesis, the full biological significance of this activity during pregnancy remains to be elucidated.

REFERENCES

BAXTER, J. D., and P. H. FORSHAM: Tissue Effects of Glucocorticoids, *Am. J. Med.,* **53:**573–589 (1972).

BLASCHKO, H., G. SAYERS, and A. D. SMITH (eds.): Adrenal Gland, in "Handbook of Physiology," sec. 7, "Endocrinology," vol. 6, American Physiological Society, Washington, D.C., 1975.

CHRISTY, N. P. (ed.): "The Human Adrenal Cortex." Harper & Row, Publishers, Incorporated, New York, 1971.

COUPLAND, R. E.: "The Natural History of the Chromaffin Cell," Longmans, Green and Co., Ltd., London, 1965.

DEANE, H. W.: The Anatomy, Chemistry and Physiology of Adrenocortical Tissue, in "Handbuch der Experimentellen Pharmakologie," vol. 14, pt. 1, pp. 1–185, Springer-Verlag OHG, Berlin, 1962.

EISENSTEIN, A. B. (ed.): "The Adrenal Cortex," Little, Brown and Company, Boston, 1967.

GRIFFITHS, K., and E. H. D. CAMERON: Steroid Biosynthetic Pathways in the Human Adrenal, *Adv. Steroid Biochem. Pharmacol.,* **2:**223–265 (1970).

IDELMAN, S.: Ultrastructure of the Mammalian Adrenal Cortex, *Int. Rev. Cytol.,* **27:**181–281 (1970).

JOHANNISSON, E.: The Foetal Adrenal Cortex in the Human. Its ultrastructure at different stages of development and in different functional states, *Acta Endocrinol.* (Kbh.), **130** (suppl.) (1968).

JONES, I. CHESTER: "The Adrenal Cortex," Cambridge University Press, New York, 1957.

LANMAN, J. T.: The Fetal Zone of the Adrenal Gland, *Medicine,* **32:**389–430 (1953).

LONG, J. A., and A. L. JONES: Observations on the Fine Structure of the Adrenal Cortex of Man, *Lab. Invest.,* **17:**355–370 (1967).

POHORECKY, L. A., and R. J. WURTMAN: Adrenocortical Control of Epinephrine Synthesis, *Pharmacol. Rev.,* **23:**1–35 (1971).

SYMINGTON, T.: "Functional Pathology of the Human Adrenal Gland," The Williams & Wilkins Company, Baltimore, 1969.

WINKLER, H., F. H. SCHNEIDER, C. RUFENER, P. K. NAKANE, and H. HORTNAGL: Membranes of Adrenal Medulla: Their Role in Exocytosis, In B. Ceccarelli et al. (eds.): "Advances in Cytopharmacology," vol 2, Raven Books, Abeland-Schuman, Limited, New York, pp. 127–139, 1974.

The Eye

TOICHIRO KUWABARA AND DAVID G. COGAN

GENERAL STRUCTURE

The human eye is an approximate sphere, 2.5 cm in diameter. It forms an image of the environment on its photoreceptor layer, the retina, and transmits the information from that image to the optic nerve and thence to the brain. Human eyes have a wide range of motility. They can scan the visual field or track a moving object while maintaining precise coordination with one another. The histologic architecture of the eye serves these optical, photoreceptive, and motility requirements.

The eye is often compared with a camera. The rigid box of the camera is analogous to the corneoscleral coat; the black lining of the camera is the uvea of the eye; and the photosensitive film of the camera is the retina of the eye. The mechanism for focusing differs, however, in that the lens of the camera moves back and forth whereas the lens of the eye changes its accommodation by varying its convexity in situ. The diaphragm of the camera is analogous to the iris of the eye; both control the amount of entering light and the depth of field. With extremes of pupillary size at 2 and 7 mm, the *f* stop of the eye varies from 12.0 to 3.5.

The eyeball is positioned within the bony orbital socket, which contains the adipose tissue, extraocular muscle, blood vessels, and nerve fibers. Eyelids protect the anterior opening of the orbit.

PARTS OF EYE AND ADNEXA

The eye and adnexa lend themselves to the following divisions:

Protective Tissue
These consist of *lids, conjunctiva,* and surface of the *cornea* (Fig. 32-1). To these must be added *lacrimal glands* in the orbit and adnexal sebaceous glands of the lids. The orbital adipose tissue serves as a shock absorbent.

Tissue Giving Form and Relative Rigidity of the Eye
This is chiefly the corneoscleral coat, which together with the intraocular pressure maintains the relatively constant size and shape of the eye.

Nutritional and Light-excluding Tissue

This layer lies just internal to the sclera and is called the *uvea*. Its major anatomic divisions are *choroid, ciliary body,* and *iris.* The uvea is heavily pigmented and vascularized.

Photoreceptive and Neural Tissues

These are located in a membrane called the *retina,* lining much of the interior of the *eye* and connected with the brain by way of the *optic nerve* (Fig. 32-2).

Optical or Refractive Tissues

These consist of the smooth anterior surface of the cornea (where most of the stationary refraction occurs), the *lens* (where the variable refraction occurs), and clear ocular media, consisting of *aqueous humor* in front of the lens and *vitreous humor* behind the lens (Fig. 32-3). Blood vessels are absent in these tissues.

Intraocular Fluid

Most of the fluid turnover in the *eye* occurs by way of the aqueous humor. This is believed to be secreted by the *ciliary epithelium* into the *posterior chamber,* a pyramidal space bounded anteriorly by the iris, posteriorly by the lens and zonular fibers, and laterally by the ciliary body. The aqueous humor drains out of the *eye* at the periphery of the anterior chamber through the *trabecular meshwork* and *Schlemm's canal.*

Ocular Motor System

Each *eye* is provided with three sets of *extraocular muscles* that arise from the apex of the orbit (Fig. 32-4). The lateral and medial recti move the eye in the horizontal plane; the superior and inferior recti move the eye chiefly in the vertical plane but have a small

FIGURE 32-1 Lids and eye. Noteworthy are the conspicuous folds of the upper lid, with the eyelashes coming from the anterior portion of the lid margin: the puncta (arrows) for drainage of tears; the white sclera covered by transparent conjunctiva; the iris with its characteristic radial structure; and the central black pupil. The cornea, being transparent, is not visible, but the central light spot reflected from the surface of the cornea indicates its smooth and convex surface.

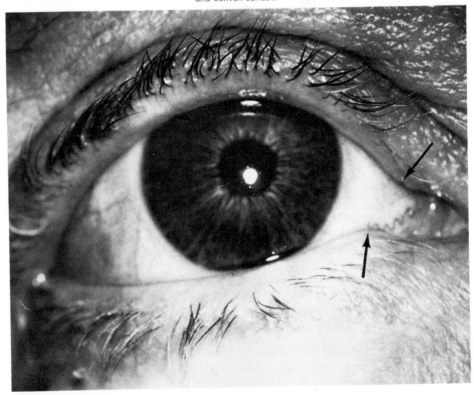

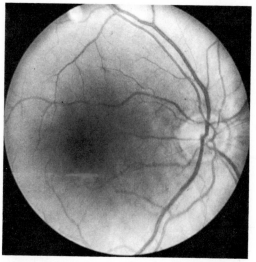

FIGURE 32-2 Ophthalmoscopic view of the interior of the eye. The nerve head, measuring about 1.5 mm in diameter, is the light, circular structure to the right of center. The blood vessels emerge from the center of this nerve. The smaller and lighter vessels are the arteries; the larger and darker vessels are the veins. The central, relatively dark area corresponds to the macula.

ORIGIN

The anlagen of the eyes are recognizable early in the embryo as a pair of lateral outpouching of the diencephalon. As it approaches the surface ectoderm, each pouch invaginates to form an optic cup. The inner layer of this cup is destined to form the retina, and the outer layer is destined to form the pigment epithelium of the choroid.

The surface ectoderm overlying the optic cup thickens, invaginates, and eventually becomes the lens. The embryonic tissue surrounding the optic vesicle and lying in front of the lens then differentiates to form the other structures of the eye.

By reason of this unique outpouching and subsequent invagination, the inner surface of the retina, ciliary body, and iris come to represent the basal surface of the tissue, and the intraocular contents (the vitreous space and anterior chamber) represent a modified tissue space. During the embryonic period, these spaces contain a rich vascular plexus, the hyaloid system, which disappears almost entirely before birth.

The invagination of the surface ectoderm has a similarly unique development, so that the outer surface of the lens consists of the basement membrane.

By the third month of gestation the eye has already attained its definitive shape and structure (Fig. 32-5). Differentiation of the neural elements of the retina occurs at a relatively late stage of gestation.

torsional component; and the superior and inferior obliques have both a torsional component (increasing as the eye is turned outward) and a vertical component (increasing as the eye is turned inward). The two eyes are coordinated to move in remarkable symmetry.

The lids are provided with two sets of muscles. The levator palpebral arise at the apex of the orbit and function to open the eyes. The orbicularis oculi is a sphincterlike muscle within the skin of the lid and functions to close the eyes.

LIDS

The upper and lower lids both protect and lubricate the anterior portions of the eyeballs. The skin surface is covered by stratified squamous epithelium like that of the rest of the face, but the connective tissue stroma is more delicate and contains little fat. The superficial dermis also contains lymph vessels, sweat glands, and sebaceous glands (Fig. 32-6). Superficial muscle fibers, constituting the *orbicularis oculi*, are innervated by the VIIth nerve and serve to close the lids. The orbicularis muscle consists of bundles of fine striated muscle fibers. The transverse tube system is well de-

veloped in this muscle fiber. A small group of bundles of the similar striated muscle at the lid margin is called Riolan's muscle.

The deep stroma of the upper and lower lids contains a plaque of compact connective tissue containing large sebaceous glands that open onto the lid margins. These plaques, called the *tarsal plates,* give a measure of solidity to the lids. The plate consists of compact collagen fibers and abundant elastica. The sebaceous structures within the plates are called *Meibomian glands* (Fig. 32-7); they secrete an oily

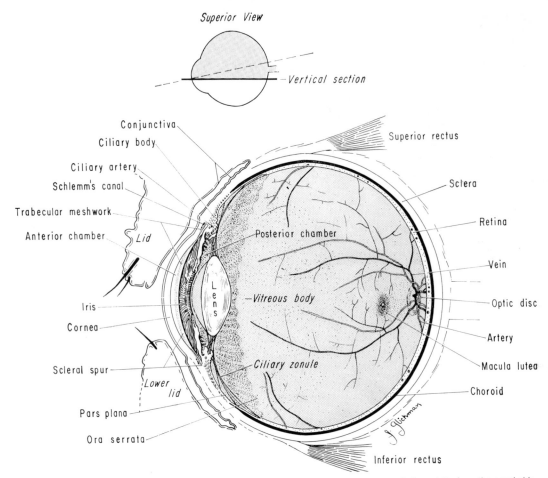

Superior View

Vertical section

Conjunctiva
Ciliary body
Ciliary artery
Schlemm's canal
Trabecular meshwork
Anterior chamber
Lid
Iris
Cornea
Scleral spur
Lower lid
Pars plana
Ora serrata

Posterior chamber
Lens
Vitreous body
Ciliary zonule

Superior rectus
Sclera
Retina
Vein
Optic disc
Artery
Macula lutea
Choroid

Inferior rectus

FIGURE 32-3 Schematic drawing of lids and eye. The interior of the eye has been exposed by removal of a calotte from the nasal side of the globe, as indicated in the insert.

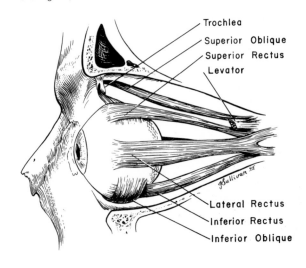

Trochlea
Superior Oblique
Superior Rectus
Levator

Lateral Rectus
Inferior Rectus
Inferior Oblique

material that seals the lid margins when the eyes are closed and prevent overflow of tears when the eyes are open. The glands consists of numerous alveoli which are connected to straight opening ducts and are arranged in a plane parallel to one another. Their orifices are situated slightly posterior to the row of the eyelashes. The gland cells at the margin of the alveoli are stratified epithelium, but the cells deposit abundant lipid droplets toward the center (Fig. 32-7). Cells in the alveoli contain few microorganelles.

The *levator palpebrae muscle* that raises the upper lid inserts into the connective tissue in the subdermal zone and in the superior margin of the

FIGURE 32-4 Origins and insertions of the ocular muscles. (Reprinted with permission of Charles C Thomas, Publisher.)

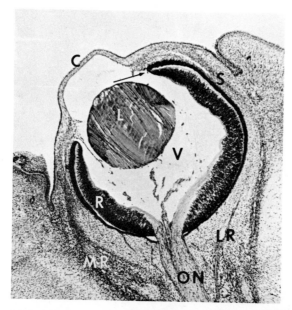

FIGURE 32-5 Horizontal section of the eye and adjacent structures of a 7-week human embryo. MR, medial rectus; LR, lateral rectus; ON, optic nerve; S, sclera; R, retina; V, vitreous; L, lens; C, cornea. Note the hairpin folding of the neuroepithelium at the margin (arrow).

FIGURE 32-6 Vertical section of lids, globe, and orbit of an adult human being. The upper lid has been somewhat displaced forward but otherwise shows an approximately normal relationship of structures. UL, upper lid; LL, lower lid; C, cornea; AC, anterior chamber; I, iris; L, lens (artefactitiously fragmented); CB, ciliary body; R, retina (artefactitiously separated from choroid); V, vitreous body, ON, optic nerve; Lev, levator muscle; MM, Müller's muscle; SR, superior rectus; CN, ciliary nerve; OF, orbital fat. ×4.

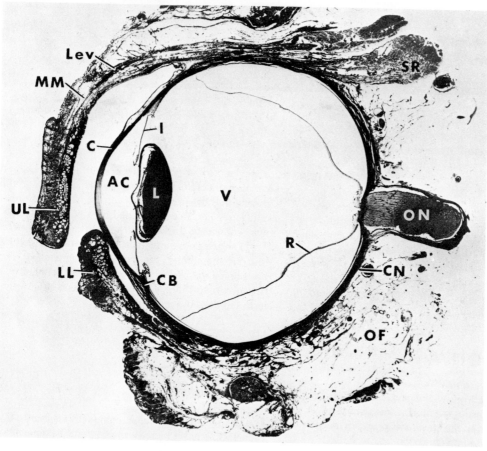

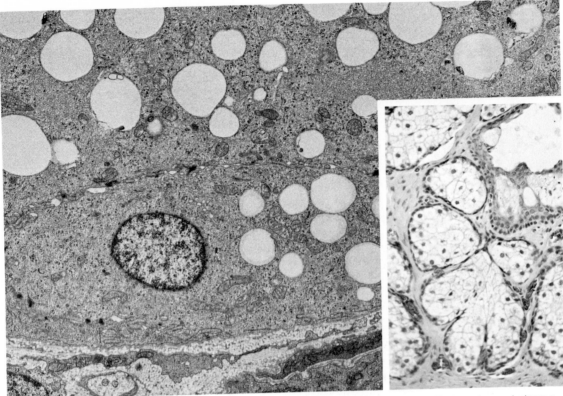

FIGURE 32-7 Meibomian gland. Electron micrograph shows a few cells in the basal portion of the acinus. Cells are joined to each other by desmosomes. Numerous lipid droplets are present. Insert ×7000. H & E stain. ×100.

tarsus. Clusters of smooth muscle, *Muller's lid muscle,* intermingle with the striated muscle fiber at the anterior end of the levator muscle (Fig. 32-8). Similar smooth muscle cells are also present in the lower eyelid.

The lid margins mark the transition between skin and mucous membrane. The stratified squamous ectoderm of the former becomes the mucous epithelium of the latter. But the most noteworthy structures of these lid margins are the *eyelashes,* which emerge from the anterior edge of the lid margin and the 15 to 20 orifices of the Meibomian glands that open into the intermarginal space. The most medial portions of the upper and lower lid margins contain the orifices and canals that conduct the tears into the lacrimal sac and thence into the nose. These canals, called the *upper* and *lower canaliculi,* are lined by a stratified epithelium somewhat thicker than that of the conjunctiva.

The posterior surfaces of the lids are covered by a mucous membrane, the *palpebral conjunctiva.* The transitional zones where the palpebral conjuctiva is reflected onto the eye to become bulbar conjunctiva form cul-de-sacs, or *fornices.*

CONJUNCTIVA

Except for the cornea with which it is continuous, the conjunctiva provides the mucous membrane cover for the eye (*bulbar conjunctiva*) and posterior portion of the lids (*palpebral conjunctiva*).

BULBAR CONJUNCTIVA

The epithelium of the bulbar conjunctiva is four to five cells thick, but this increases to as many as ten cells at

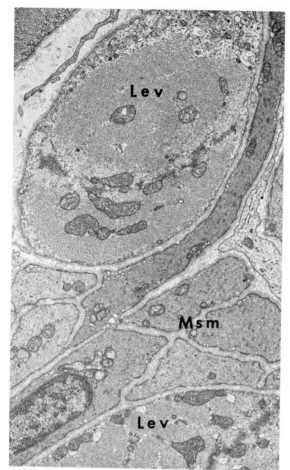

FIGURE 32-8 Anterior end of the levator muscle. Striated muscle fibers (Lev) are intermingled with Müller's smooth muscle cells (Msm). ×12,400.

the junction with the cornea. The epithelium of the conjunctiva is continuous with that of the cornea; the zone of transition is known as the *limbus*. The mucus-forming cells, *goblet cells*, are distributed in the epithelium and are especially abundant in the nasal angle of the bulbar conjunctiva. The folded conjunctiva is modified to form the *caruncle*, a skin tissue which contains hairs and sweat glands.

The epithelial cells are polygonal in shape and are loosely packed with a relatively small number of desmosomes (Fig. 32-9). Cell membranes are sparsely interdigitated and form intercellular spaces. The surface cells are held tightly with zonules occludens.

The cytoplasm of the goblet cell is rich in rough endoplasmic reticulum and Golgi apparatus and the cell contains abundant mucin granules.

PALPEBRAL CONJUNCTIVA

The palpebral conjunctiva has an epithelium only two to three cells thick and a variable abundance of subepithelial lymphoid tissue. The epithelial cells in the fornix are tall and form large intercellular spaces in which wandering cells are commonly present. Goblet cells are abundant in the palpebral conjunctiva (Fig. 32-10).

The subepithelial connective tissue consists of loose collagen fibers, occasional elastica and abundant blood vessels, lymphatic vessels, and nerve fibers. The connective tissue has a great capacity for reversible swelling and congestion.

CORNEA

The clear window constituting the most anterior portion of the eye is the cornea. In the adult it is about 11 mm in diameter and slightly more than 0.5 mm thick. Having a greater curvature than the sclera, the cornea has the gross appearance of a watch crystal (Figs. 32-3 and 32-6).

It is important, although possibly disappointing, to note that the cornea shows meager histologic basis for its transparency. With routine stains, the corneal stroma is much like that of the sclera with no clear-cut demarcation at the limbus corresponding to the sharp optical difference that exists between cornea and sclera. The basis for transparency is physiologic rather than anatomic: the opical homogeneity is maintained by a continual pumping out of the interstitial fluid across the semipermeable surface membranes so that the cornea is kept in a deturgesced state.

The histologic composition of the cornea is notably uniform (Fig. 32-11). The constituent layers listed in an anterior to posterior direction are *epithelium*,

Bowman's membrane, stroma, Descemet's membrane, and *endothelium* (or, as it is called by some authors, "mesenchymal epithelium").

EPITHELIUM

The epithelium, accounting for about one-tenth of the total corneal thickness, is five cells thick, with a uniquely smooth anterior surface (Fig. 32-12). The columnar basal layers have a robust basement membrane, as delineated by the PAS reagent. Except for stratification, the epithelial cells show no differentiation toward either mucous cell formation or other specialization. Mitoses are rarely seen in conventional sections but are readily found in flat whole mounts of the cornea.

By electron microscopy the epithelium is seen to consist of closely packed cells having a fine fibrillary cytoplasm with relatively few microorganelles (Fig. 32-13). The mitochondria are small and sparse. Only a small amount of rough endoplasmic reticulum and Golgi apparatus are present. The matrix contains a large amount of glycogen particles (Fig. 32-13, insert). The cell boundaries show interlacing undulations and an abundance of desmosomes.

The superficial cells are nucleated and have a fine vermiform ridge structure on the surface (Fig. 32-14). This structure may be related to the maintenance of the moisture of the epithelial surface.

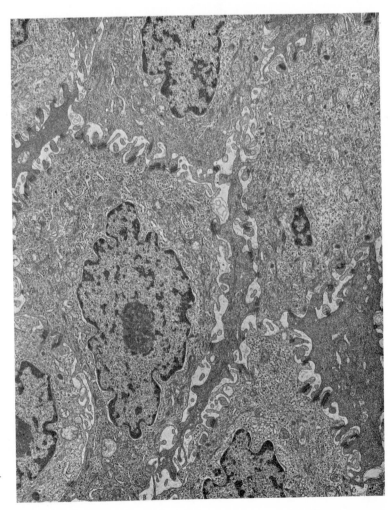

FIGURE 32-9 Bulbar conjunctiva. Polygonal epithelial cells are loosely packed. Cells are joined by a small number of desmosomes. Large intercellular spaces are present. ×13,300.

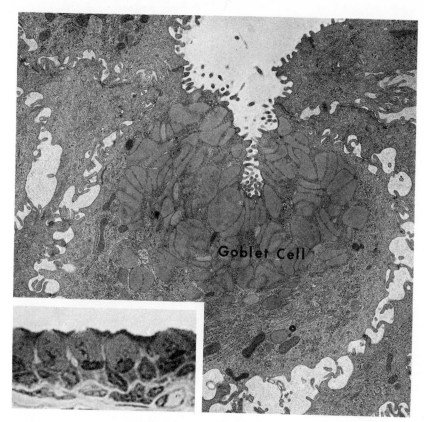

Goblet Cell

FIGURE 32-10 Palpebral conjunctiva. The goblet cell contains numerous mucin granules in the apical cytoplasma. Rough endoplasmic reticulum and Golgi apparatus are abundant in the rest of the cytoplasm. Intercellular spaces are extremely large. ×8400. Insert shows light microscopic view of the palpebral conjunctiva. ×400.

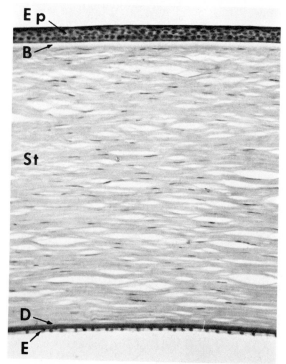

E p

B

St

D

E

FIGURE 32-11 Cross section of the cornea. Ep, epithelium; B, Bowman's membrane; St, stroma; D, Descemet's membrane; E, endothelium. H & E stain. ×155.

FIGURE 32-12 Anterior portion of the cornea. The epithelium shows columnar basal cells, polygonal wing cells, and flat superficial cells. B, acellular Bowman's membrane; St, stroma. ×380.

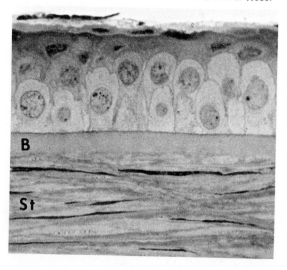

B

St

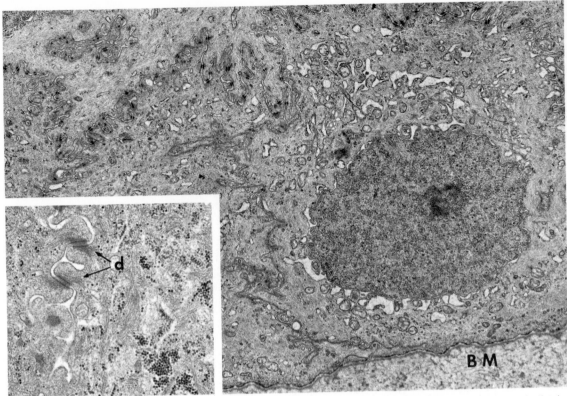

FIGURE 32-13 Basal cells of the corneal epithelium. The lateral cell membranes are markedly interdigitated and joined to each other by numerous desmosomes. The basal surface is flat. BM, Bowman's membrane. ×12,000. Insert shows details of the cytoplasm: abundant keratofibrils; glycogen particles; d, desmosome; membranous microorganelles are sparse. ×30,400.

FIGURE 32-14 A. Superficial epithelial cell of the cornea. The most superficial cell is nucleated. Cells are attached to each other by gap junctions (arrow) and desmosomes. The cytoplasm contains rich glycogen. The surface cells have fine ridges. ×20,000. Scanning electron microscopic view of the corneal surface. The surface is covered with vermiform ridges except at the cell border. ×10,000.

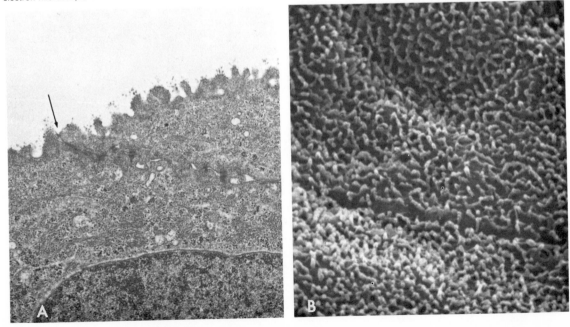

Named in honor of a nineteenth-century ophthalmologist and anatomist, Bowman's membrane is not a distinct membrane in the usual sense but is an acellular layer measuring approximately 30 μm in thickness. This layer stains negatively for mucopolysaccharide, but other physical properties are similar to those of the rest of the corneal stroma (Figs. 32-12 and 32-15). It lies immediately beneath the epithelium throughout the entire extent of the cornea and terminates abruptly at the limbus. It is most highly developed in the human eye. Bowman's membrane maintains the optical smoothness of the anterior corneal layers. This layer consists of short, randomly arranged collagen fibers and fine fibrils. The fibrils seemingly originate from the basement membrane of the basal epithelium (Fig. 32-15).

STROMA

The *stroma* constitutes the bulk of the cornea and accounts for its characteristic shape and resistance. It consists of laminae of collagen fibers parallel to the surface, with *keratocytes* sandwiched between them (Fig. 32-16A). When examined with the polarizing microscope, the corneal fibers show a birefringence that differs from that of most collagenous structures in being unusually fine and regular. Except for occasional wandering cells and inconspicuous nerves in its most anterior layers, the stroma shows no specialized elements. Specifically no blood vessels, lymphatics, or other formed structures are present in the normal cornea. The stroma stains, however, in a characteristically metachromatic fashion with toluidine blue and other thiazine dyes. The metachromatic substances, which have been identified chemically, are chondroitin sulfate and keratosulfate; they probably aid the reversible swelling properties (and transparency) of the cornea. These sulfated polysaccharides are not present in the sclera.

Collagen fibers are small (about 300 Å in diameter) and uniform in size. The 700 Å banding is present but not conspicuous by ordinary electron microscopic staining. Abundant fine fibrils are present among the

FIGURE 32-15 Bowman's membrane consists of fine fibrils and short collagen fibers. ×5000. Higher magnification on the right shows their randomly intermingled arrangement. ×30,000.

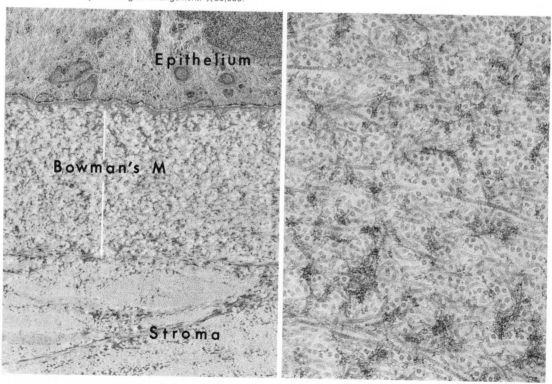

Epithelium

Bowman's M

Stroma

collagen fibers. Collagen fibers form lamellae, approximately 2 μm in thickness, which are arranged parallel to the epithelial surface (Fig. 32-16B). The lamellae in the anterior portion of the stroma are somewhat smaller and not so regular as they are in the central and posterior portion.

The *keratocyte* (stroma cell) is an extremely flat cell which projects stellate processes over a wide area. The cytoplasm consists of an electron-dense matrix in which moderate numbers of membranous micro-organelles are present (Fig. 32-17). The amount of rough endoplasmic reticulum increases markedly in various pathological conditions.

DESCEMET'S MEMBRANE

Descemet's membrane, named for a Parisian ophthalmologist, botanist, and general physician of the eighteenth century, is an acellular layer about 10 μm thick, situated just posterior to the corneal stroma (Fig. 32-18). It stains lightly with eosin (less than the stroma), lightly although definitely with elastic tissue dyes, but heavily with the PAS reagent (like the lens capsule and certain other basement membranes). It does not stain metachromatically. When incised or ruptured, Descemet's membrane coils inward like a watch spring. At the periphery of the cornea it is frequently thickened by a bundle of circular fibers, forming *Schwalbe's line.*

The anterior border of Descemet's membrane is smooth and firmly attached to the deep corneal stroma. Its posterior surface is also smooth and attached to the endothelium, but wartlike excrescenes develop regularly with age toward the periphery of the cornea.

Because of its coiling tendency, Descemet's membrane can take up slack with the reversible swelling of the cornea. Like the elastic lamina of blood vessels, it distributes tension evenly and prevents gross deformation of the tissue.

Descemet's membrane, which appears structureless by light microscopy, also shows little structure by electron microscpy. It is the thick basement membrane of the endothelial cell and is divided into two ill-defined layers (Fig. 32-18). The posterior half is made up chiefly of a uniform, fine basal lamina substance, whereas the anterior half consists of aggregating fibril

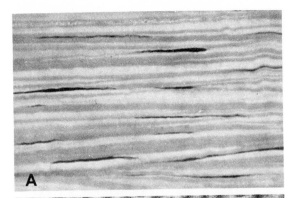

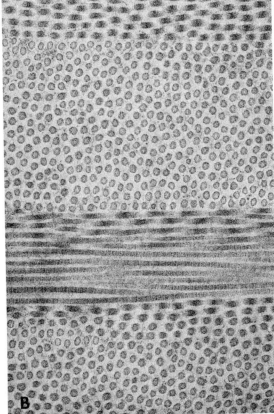

FIGURE 32-16 Lamellar arrangement of the corneal collagen fibers. A. Light microscopy of the central portion of the corneal stroma. Keratocytes distribute between lamellae. ×388. B. Collagen fibers are uniform in size (about 300 Å in diameter) and regularly spaced. Fibers are arranged parallel to the surface of the cornea. ×58,200.

substances arranged somewhat regularly. The anterior portion of Descemet's membrane is considered to be an old form and is absent in the embryonal and infantile corneas. The thickness of Descemet's membrane increases with age. Toward the periphery of the cornea, there are thick collagen fibers with a periodicity of 1000 Å. These are particularly common in senescent corneas and are thought to be a unique form of collagen. Descemet's membrane becomes uneven toward the periphery, permitting processes of endothelial cells to insinuate into fine clefts of Descemet's membrane. A deposit of lipid in the anterior half of Descemet's membrane is common in corneas of adults (arcus lipoides).

ENDOTHELIUM

The *endothelium,* covering the posterior surface of the cornea, is a single layer of cells which are thin and inconspicuous in conventional cross sections (Figs. 32-11 and 32-18) but which appear as a regular mosaic of hexagonal cells in flat preparations (Fig.

32-19). Despite its thinness, the endothelium is an essential structure for the maintenance of normal deturgescence and transparency of the cornea. Mitoses are rarely seen, although the endothelium has the capacity for vigorous proliferation in pathologic states.

At the periphery of the cornea, approximately 1 mm central to the termination of Descemet's membrane, the normally thin endothelium becomes even more tenous and then extends over the pores of the *trabecular meshwork.*

In electron micrographs the endothelium is seen to consist of overlapping cells (Fig. 32-20) with marked interdigitations. However, desmosomes are seldom present. Cells are joined tightly at the apical portion with zonule occludens. In contrast to the epithelium, the endothelial cells are rich in mitochondria, vesicles, and Golgi apparatus but lack the finely filamentous cytoplasm. Metabolically, the endothelium appears to be the more active tissue. Disruption of the endothelium causes sudden and severe edema of the corneal stroma.

FIGURE 32-17 A portion of a stroma cell between collagenous laminae. The paranuclear cytoplasm contains rich mitochondria and rough endoplasmic reticulum. ×18,000.

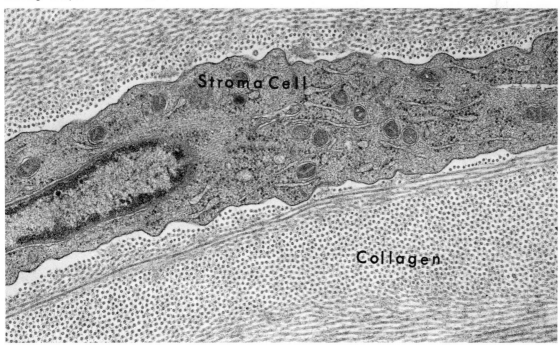

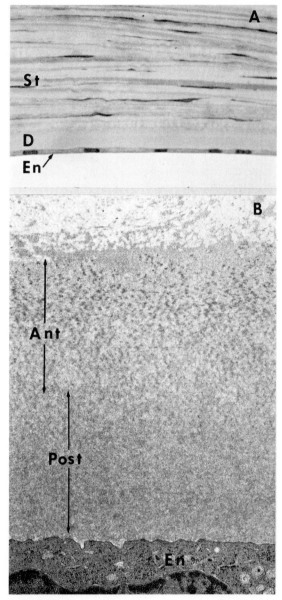

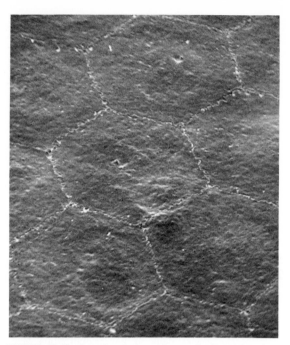

FIGURE 32-19 Scanning electron microscopic view of the surface of the corneal endothelium. Hexagonal shaped endothelial cells have a flat surface. ×4850.

FIGURE 32-18 A. Posterior portion of the cornea. St, stroma; D, Descemet's membrane; En, endothelium. ×380. B. Two layers of Descemet's membrane. Ant, anterior; and Post, posterior portions; En, endothelium. ×15,800.

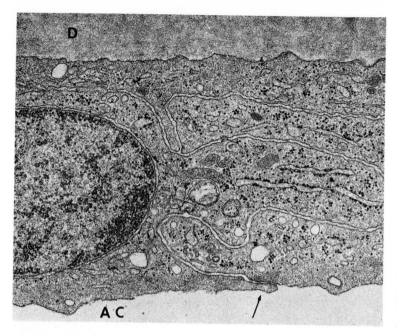

FIGURE 32-20 Endothelial cells have well-interdigitated lateral cell membranes. Apicolateral junction is not always conspicuous (arrow). The cytoplasm contains rich microorganelles. D, Descemet's membrane; AC, anterior chamber. ×28,600.

LIMBUS

An imaginary line connecting the peripheral terminations of Bowman's and Descemet's membranes is the boundary of the cornea with the sclera (Fig. 32-21). The region of this line is called the limbus; it corresponds to the abrupt optical change from the transparent cornea to the opaque *sclera*. Aside from the terminations of Bowman's and Descemet's membranes, it contains the sites of transition of conjunctival epithelium into corneal epithelium, the peripheral boundary of metachromatic staining of the corneal stroma, and the important trabecular meshwork in the angle of the anterior chamber.

The corneal epithelium becomes seven to eight cells thick at the limbus and it gradually transforms into the conjunctival epithelium with the formation of intercellular spaces and basal infoldings. The lamellar arrangement of the corneal collagen fibers become irregular and individual collagen becomes larger as they merge into the sclera. Numerous blood vessels and myelinated nerve fibers are present in this zone.

TRABECULAR MESHWORK AND SCHLEMM'S CANAL

Just peripheral to the end of Descemet's membrane is the *trabeculum*, or *trabecular meshwork*, that marks the site for drainage of aqueous humor (Figs. 32-6 and 32-21). The trabecular strands, which are continuous with Descemet's membranes and endothelium, enclose spaces, called the *spaces of Fontana*, that communicate with the anterior chamber (Fig. 32-22). The central or axial border of the trabeculum coincides with Schwalbe's line and the peripheral border coincides with a prominent ridge, the *scleral spur*, from which the ciliary muscle arises.

Anterior and lateral to the trabecular meshwork are one or more endothelium-lined channels coursing circumferentially about the cornea. These are collectively called *Schlemm's canal* (Figs. 32-21 and 32-22). They collect the aqueous humor which filtered through the spaces of Fontana and which then passes out of the eye and into the episcleral vessels (Fig. 32-23; see color insert). It is obstruction of drainage in these structures at the angle of the anterior chamber that causes a pathologic rise in the intraocular pressure and the eye disease *glaucoma*.

Electron microscopy shows the trabecular meshwork to consist of central cores of collagenous fibers ensheathed by homogeneous ground substance and a lining of endothelial cells (Fig. 32-24). The trabecular connective tissue contains elastica among collagen fibers. The endothelial cells which form bridges con-

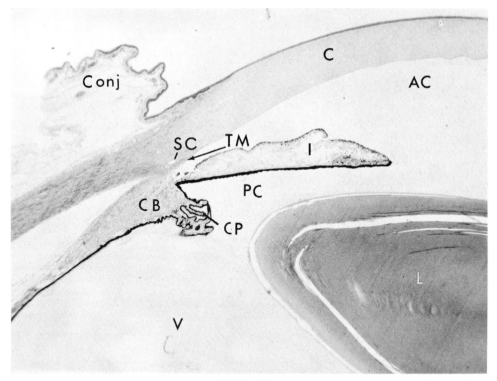

FIGURE 32-21 Portion of the anterior segment of the eye. C, cornea; Conj, conjunctiva; SC, Schlemm's canal; TM, trabecular meshwork; AC, anterior chamber; PC, posterior chamber; CP, ciliary process; CB, ciliary body (artefactitiously separated from the sclera); L, lens; V, vitreous.

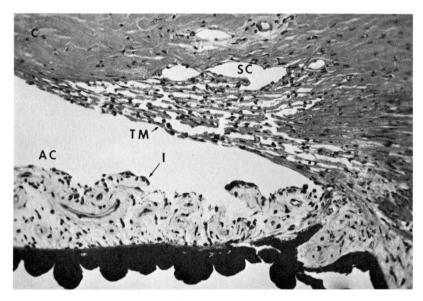

FIGURE 32-22 Angle of the eye. C, cornea; SC, Schlemm's canal; TM, trabecular meshwork; AC, anterior chamber; I, iris. ×180.

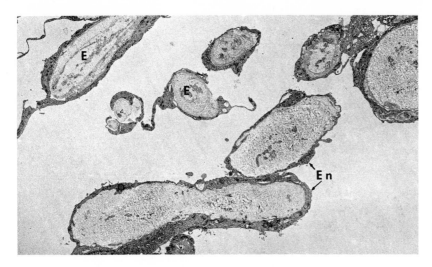

FIGURE 32-24 Trabecular meshwork. The trabecular connective tissue contains elastica (E). En, endothelial covering. ×1800.

necting trabecula in several locations are rich in membranous microorganelles. The covering is often interrupted. The trabecula become less conspicuous toward Schlemm's canal and may disappear altogether, leaving a meshwork of the connective tissue.

The endothelial cells of Schlemm's canal are uninterrupted but they contain large vacuoles measuring 0.5 to 1.5 μm in diameter. It is a moot question whether or not these vacuoles open directly into Schlemm's canal for passage of fluid and particles.

ANTERIOR AND POSTERIOR CHAMBERS

The *anterior chamber* is the area bounded by the cornea anteriorly and by the iris and lens posteriorly (Figs. 32-6 and 32-21). It has a depth of approximately 3 mm at its center, a volume of 0.2 ml, and a fluid turnover rate of 2 mm^3 per min. The *aqueous humor,* which fills the anterior chamber, is a water-clear fluid containing most of the soluble constituents of the blood with an extremely small concentration of proteins (0.02 percent, in contrast to 7 percent in the blood).

The chamber is lined by endothelial cells of the cornea and the trabecular meshwork, but there are no specific lining cells on the anterior surface of the iris. Also, the anterior surface of the lens consists of the basement membrane.

The *posterior chamber* is the pyramidal area bounded by the iris anteriorly, the lens and zonules posteriorly, and the ciliary body laterally (Fig. 32-21). The aqueous humor which fills the posterior chamber is believed to be secreted by the ciliary epithelium and circulates through the pupil into the anterior chamber. The pupillary margin of the iris rests on the lens and thereby provides a ball valve which allows fluid to pass from posterior chamber to anterior chamber but not in the reverse direction.

The posterior chamber is lined by the basement membranes of the iris and ciliary epithelium. The zonules, the posterior boundary of the chamber, form substantial bundles, though they are grossly inconspicuous. Since no apical cell surface bounds the space, the structure of the posterior chamber is not the same as the lumens of other tissues.

SCLERA

The *sclera* is that portion of the outer tunic of the *eye* extending posteriorly to constitute about fourth-fifths of the *eye's* capsule (Fig. 32-3). With an average thickness of 0.5 mm, it varies from a maximal thickness at the posterior pole to a minimal thickness beneath the extraocular muscles. Like the corneal stroma with which it is continuous, the sclera consists chiefly of compact fibrous tissue. Finely branched fibroblastlike cells are present between collagen bundles. In contrast to the cornea, however, the collagenous laminae are less regularly arranged (seen especially well with crossed polaroids); there is more elastic tissue, blood vessels are present (especially at the limbus); the acidic mucoploysaccharides are absent; and there is no tendency to imbibe water.

The sclera shows several regional modifications. Abutting the limbus, the sclera contains a fairly rich plexus of blood vessels in anastomotic connection with Schlemm's canal and with the anterior ciliary vessels. The four rectus muscles insert in the superficial layers of the sclera at 5 to 8 mm from the limbus and the two oblique muscles insert farther posteriorly. However, the most noteworthy modification is at the site of exit of the optic nerve. Here, the sclera is reduced to a fenestrated membrane, the *lamina cribrosa,* through which the nerves pass like filaments through a sieve (Fig. 32-58). This "hole" has a diameter of a little more than 1 mm and is situated about 3 mm nasal to the posterior pole of the eye. It represents a weak spot in the sclera's resistance, and its fibers become bowed outward with abnormal elevations of the intraocular pressure (glaucoma).

Together with the corneal stroma, the sclera maintains the size and form of the eye. That this is of the utmost optical importance is evident from the observation that increasing the axial length of the eye by only 1 mm would cause a person to be severely incapacitated by nearsightedness (*myopia*), whereas a decrease of the length by only 1 mm from the norm would cause the individual to have a refractive deviation (*hyperoria*) of the same magnitude in the opposite direction.

UVEA

The uvea is the pigmented and predominantly vascular coat of the eye. It consists of the *iris,* the *ciliary body,* and the *choroid.*

IRIS

The *iris,* the most anterior portion of the uvea, extends from the angle of the anterior chamber to the pupillary margin (Fig. 32-21). It thus has the form of a disc with a hole in its center (Fig. 32-1). Because of its reaction to light, it is properly considered the diaphragm of the eye.

The iris consists of a spongy *stroma* facing the anterior chamber, constituting the bulk of the iris, and a *pigment epithelial layer* facing the posterior chamber and resting on the lens at the pupillary margin (Fig. 32-25). In addition, the iris contains a substantial *sphincter muscle* near its pupillary margin and a tenuous *dilator muscle* lying just anterior to the pigment epithelium.

The tissue spaces of the iris stroma are continuous with the anterior chamber. There is no endothelium or epithelium at the anterior surface (Fig. 32-26). No junctional apparatus is present between the cells at the anterior margin. Collagen fibers often protrude into the anterior chamber through the wide intercellular spaces. Aside from the fibroblasts, the stroma contains the pigmented cells of two distinctive shapes. First, there are the melanophores with elongated processes and melanin pigment granules in uniform sizes. These are most heavily concentrated along the anterior border layers of the iris. Then there are the round and more heavily pigmented *clump cells,* which are more numerous toward the sphincter regions. These are phagocytes and become numerous in pathological conditions. The relative number of pigment cells varies with the individual's complexion. In dark-skinned persons with brown eyes the pigment cells are abundant; in light-skinned persons with blue eyes the stromal pigment may be absent altogether (Fig. 32-25).

The blood vessels of the iris are noteworthy for having a thick, although not compact, layer about them. This forms a fibrous acellular "wall" that is unique for vessels of the iris. The blood vessel itself consists of a thin endothelial cytoplasm surrounded by a thin basement membrane and thin proesses of the pericyte.

The *sphincter muscle,* which differentiated from the epithelial cells in the embryo, is comprised of a compact bundle of smooth muscle fibers arranged circularly near the pupillary margin (Fig. 32-25). Muscle fibers are completely separated from the epithelial layer. The fine structure of the sphincter muscle cell is

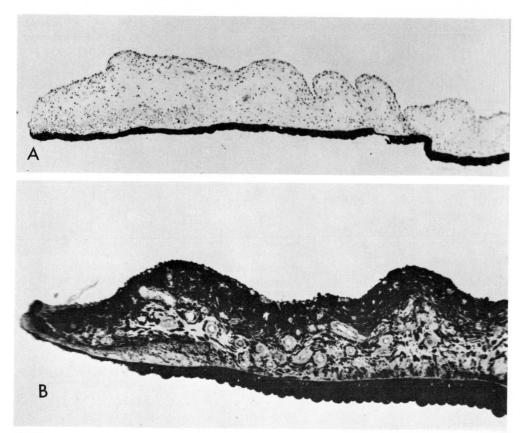

FIGURE 32-25 Contrasting irises of lightly pigmented (blonde) and heavily pigmented (Negro) eyes. The former has a spongy stroma whereas the latter has a relatively compact stroma in which the pigment is concentrated anteriorly. The abundant blood vessels with their characteristically thick walls are seen especially well in the pigmented iris. The sphincter muscle forms a delicate lamina of smooth muscle fibers near the pupillary edge (to the left of center). Both irises contain a heavily pigmented epithelium lining their posterior surfaces.

not different from that of other smooth muscles. It receives innervation for contraction from the parasympathetic ganglion in the orbit by way of the long ciliary nerves within the eye. The *dilator muscle* is formed within the basal portion of the anterior epithelial cell layer (Fig. 32-27). There is no separated cellular layer of the dilator muscle. The apical half of this cell has all the characteristics of the epithelial cell, but the basal half is markedly infolded and the cytoplasm contains smooth muscle elements. The muscle portion of the cell is ramified and covered with basal lamina. Numerous nerve fibers and their endings are present in the muscle tissue. Schwann's cells are often closely

situated at the dilator muscle. Although the layer of the dilator muscle takes PAS staining because of its basement membrane, it is so indistinct that it can scarcely be identified by light microscopy. These dilator muscle fibers are arranged radially to the pupil and run the length of the iris except for the pupillary zone. They receive innervation for positive contraction from the sympathetic nervous system.

The dilator and sphincter muscles function reciprocally and provide an excellent example of the opposite action of the two components of the autonomic nervous system.

The pigment epithelium on the posterior surface of the iris, having developed from the anterior rim of the optic cup of the neuroepithelium, is a double layer of cells attached to each other apically. The surface of the posterior cell is markedly infolded and is covered with the basement membrane, which loosely attach to that of the lens capsule. The anterior layer of cells has the muscular elements in its basal portion (dilator muscle). Cells of both layers are heavily pigmented,

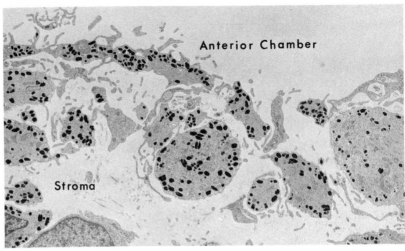

FIGURE 32-26 Anterior surface of the iris. There is no specific cell at the anterior surface. Tissue space of the spongy stroma is continuous to the anterior chamber. ×4100.

FIGURE 32-27 Dilator muscle is developed within the basal infolds of the anterior epithelial cell. Apical portion of the dilator muscle cell is heavily pigmented. BM, basement membrane of the dilator muscle. ×18,000.

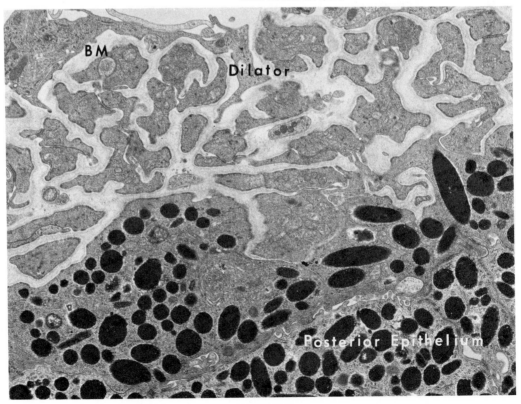

whether the eye is that of a light- or dark-skinned person. The details of the cells are masked by the pigment, but both cells contain relatively rich micro-organelles and glycogen particles. There are numerous intercellular spaces between apexes of the epithelial cells. At the pupillary margin, the cells extend more centrally than does the stroma; hence the pupillary border of the iris normally has a collarette of pigment epithelial cells. The cells of the two layers are continuous in a hairpin fashion at the pupillary margin.

CILIARY BODY

The *ciliary body*, extending from the root of the iris anteriorly to the beginning of the retina at the *ora serrata* posteriorly, is the intermediate portion of the uvea (Fig. 32-21).

The anterior portion of the ciliary body is ar-

FIGURE 32-28 View of the lens and ciliary body from the back of the eye. The most central, white disc corresponds to the pupil: the lozenge-shaped structure is the lens; the radiating ridges constitute the processes of the ciliary body (pars plicata). Peripheral to the white ridges is the flat portion of the ciliary body (pars plana) ending most peripherally in the ora serrata.

ranged in approximately 70 sagittally oriented folds or processes (pars plicata). In the opened eye these form regular ridges, radiating posteriorly (Fig. 32-28). These folds or processes contain a highly vascular stroma and are believed to be the main sites for the formation of the aqueous humor.

The posterior portion of the ciliary body is flat; accordingly, it is called *pars plana*. If the whole eye is cut coronally at its equator, the pars plana may be seen to join abruptly with the retina in a characteristically scalloped manner; this anatomic landmark is called the *ora serrata*.

CILIARY MUSCLE

In cross section the ciliary body has a roughly triangular shape, occupied chiefly with a smooth muscular mass, the *ciliary muscle*, which controls the focal power of the lens. The muscle is subdivided into a circular band situated at the inner anterior angle of the triangle and a radial-meridional portion that extends

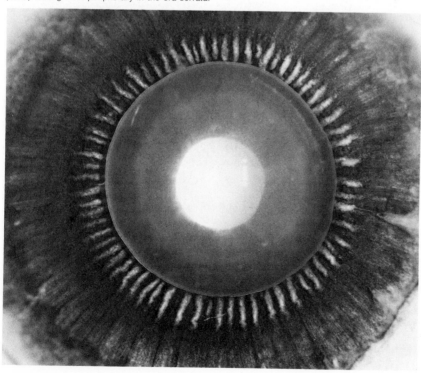

from the scleral insertion just behind the trabecular meshwork to the posterior and inner portions of the ciliary body. The circular fibers, called *Müller's muscle*, relax the tension on the lens and afford the lens the ability to accommodate for near vision; they are innervated by the parasympathetic system through the ciliary ganglion. The radial and meridional fibers (sometimes called *Brücke's muscle*) have no clearly proved function; some evidence suggests that they are innervated by the sympathetic system and allow the lens to focus for distant vision.

The ciliary muscle, which has developed from the mesenchymal tissue, is divided into small compartments with a thick basement membrane (Fig. 32-29). The structure is identical to that of other smooth muscles, but the distribution of the nerve element is more abundant.

The anterior portion of the ciliary body contains a circular artery that provides the main blood supply to the iris and ciliary body. It is in turn connected to the anterior ciliary arteries and the long posterior ciliary arteries.

CILIARY EPITHELIUM

The inner lining of the ciliary body is comprised of two layers of cuboidal cells of neuroectodermal origin and is derived from the marginal zone of the optic cup in the embryo. The inner layer with basement membrane abutting the vitreous is nonpigmented, whereas the outer layer with basement membrane abutting the stroma is pigmented (Fig. 32-30).

Cells of the two epithelial layers are joined to each other by their apical ends with a well-developed junctional complex. Small intercellular spaces are formed between the two cells (Fig. 32-31A and C). The apical

FIGURE 32-29 Ciliary muscle. Smooth muscle cells are divided by thick basement membranes. Cells have rich mitochondria. Marginal patches are apparent (arrow). Muscle is richly innervated. N, nerve endings. ×25,000.

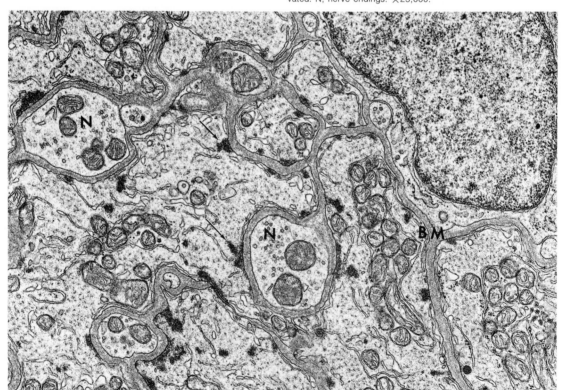

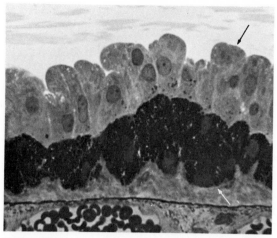

FIGURE 32-30 Ciliary epithelium. The epithelium consists of two layers of cuboidal cells: the nonpigmented inner layer and the pigmented outer layer. Arrows indicate positions of the basement membranes. ×380.

CHOROID

The *choroid* is that portion of the uvea extending posteriorly from the region of the ora serrata (Fig. 32-3). It lies immediately beneath the sclera and is comprised of a heavily vascularized and variably pigmented layer of choroid proper, a hyaline membrane called *Bruch's membrane*, and a pigment epithelial layer.

The choroid proper contains relatively large vessels, mostly veins, in its outer portions and a single layer of small sinuses called the *choriocapillaris* just beneath Bruch's membrane in its inner portions (Fig. 32-33). The endothelial cell, lining the retinal side of the choriocapillaris, is extremely thin and fenestrated (Figs. 32-33B and 32-34). The fenestrae have membranous diaphragms. The cytoplasm of the scleral side of the capillary is thick. Pericytes are present only in the scleral side of the choriocapillaris. This structure indicates an active fluid transport from the choriocapillaris to the *pigment epithelium.*

The blood drains out of the choroid by the four *vortex veins,* one in each posterior quadrant, and, to a lesser extent, by way of the ciliary body into the anterior ciliary vessels. The arterial supply to the choroid comes in part from the short ciliary arteries entering about the optic nerve and in part from anterior ciliary arteries entering the eye from the extraocular muscles. In addition, the choroid contains two large ciliary arteries and two long ciliary nerves passing to the ciliary body in the horizontal meridian.

The *stroma* of the choroid contains pigment cells, the *melanophores,* that vary in abundance according to the complexion of the individual. These cells are also the sites of the common melanotic tumors of the eye. Less common in the choroid are mast cells, seen best with metachromatic stains, and rarely, isolated ganglion cells.

Bruch's membrane is a thin lamina that interdigitates with the choriocapillaris on its outer surface end constitutes the basement membrane of the pigment epithelium on its inner surface (Fig. 32-33B). The basement membrane of the choriocapillaris forms the partial outer limit. The membrane consists of sparse collagen fibers and elastic tissue. Flat sections show that the elastica has a stellate configuration and forms a sievelike lamina at the center of the mem-

junctional complex serves as the blood-aqueous barrier. The basal portion of the inner nonpigmented epithelial cells, which faces the posterior chamber, is markedly infolded (Fig. 32-31B). The cytoplasm of this zone contains numerous mitochondria. The apical portion of the cytoplasm is rich in rough endoplasmic reticulum and Golgi apparatus (Fig. 32-20). These cells have an active phagocytotic activity. The *zonule* fibers are produced mainly by the nonpigmented ciliary epithelium and they insert into the basement membrane of these cells, especially at the valley of the ciliary processes. Although the zonules appear inconspicuous, scanning electron microscopy shows them to be surprisingly abundant (Fig. 32-32).

The pigmented cells in the outer layer also have well-developed basal infoldings. Several nerve fibers are present in the connective tissue between the infoldings. The cytoplasm contains rough endoplasmic reticulum among numerous melanin granules. Lateral cell membranes are closely apposed, but desmosomes are infrequent.

Structure of the nonpigmented epithelium of the *pars plana* is somewhat different from that of the pars plicata. Cells are tall and often their basal ends extend into the vitreous. The basal infoldings are widely open and large intercellular spaces are formed. The cytoplasm contains numerous large mitochondria but only a moderate number of membranous microorganelles.

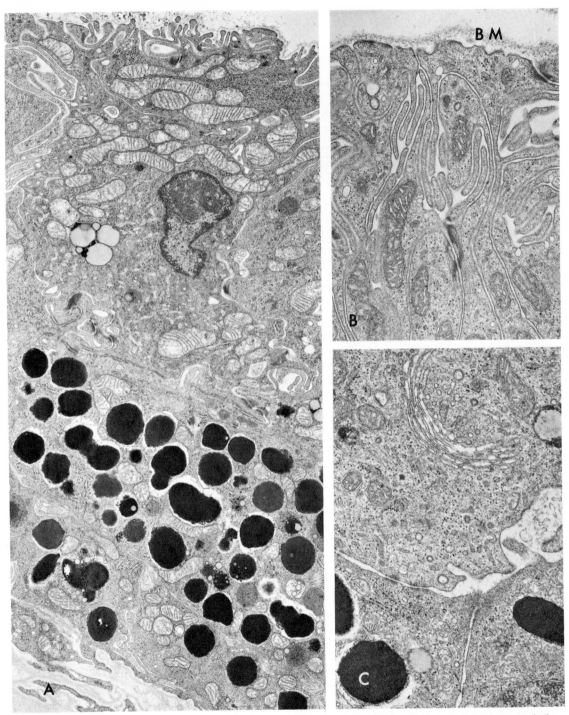

FIGURE 32-31 Electron micrograph of the epithelium of the ciliary body. Two-cell-layer epithelium has basement membranes on both surfaces. A. Outer-layer cells contain abundant melanin pigment. Inner layer is rich in mitochondria. Base of the inner-layer cell forms the posterior chamber surface. B. Inner layer adjacent to posterior chamber showing abundant infolding of the cell wall. C. Intercellular space is formed between the apical ends of the two cell layers.

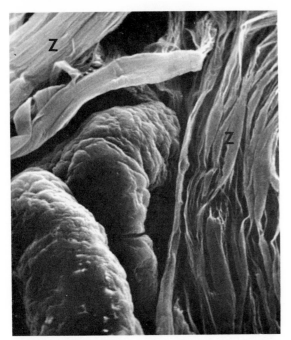

FIGURE 32-32 Scanning electron microscopic view of the ciliary process and the zonule (Z). ×2900.

brane. Bruch's membrane contains deposits of lipid and calcium in old age.

PIGMENT EPITHELIUM

The *pigment epithelium* is a single layer of cuboidal cells situated just internal to Bruch's membrane. This layer is absent at the nerve head and transforms into the pigmented layer of the ciliary epithelium at the ora serrata.

The pigment epithelium is of a neuroepithelial origin and is developed from the outer layer of the optic cup. This layer has a close anatomical and functional relation with the retina and is often called *retinal pigment epithelium*.

The *subretinal space*, containing a mucopolysaccharide rich fluid, is formed between the pigment epithelium and the retina. This space corresponds to the embryonal neuro vesicle. The apical surface of the cell has a multitude of microvilli that extend forward to

FIGURE 32-33 Choroid and the pigment epithelium. PE, pigment epithelium; BM, Bruch's membrane; CC, choriocapillaris; V, vein; A, artery. ×400. Electron micrograph on the right shows the choriocapillaris is fenestrated. E, elastica. ×28,000.

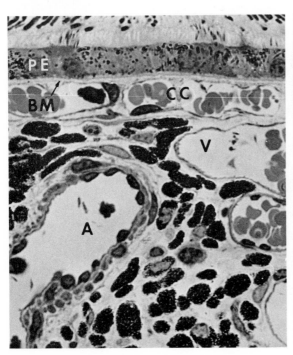

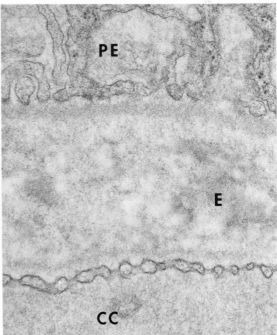

interdigitate with the rods and cones (Fig. 32-34). Thus the rods and cones are not anatomically bound to the outer coats of the eye, and most histologic sections show artifactitious separation of the retina from the choroid. Separation of the retina is also a common clinical abnormality.

The pigment epithelial cell contains smooth endoplasmic reticulum which occupies the major part of the cytoplasm, numerous Golgi apparatus in the parakaryon zone, rough endoplasmic reticulum in the apical zone, and abundant mitochondria in the basal portion. The cell contains a heavy concentration of melanin granules in the apical portion. These granules are round or oval, several times larger than the gran-

ules of melanocytes. Large spindle-shaped melanin granules are present in large microvilli. Primary and secondary lysosomes are abundantly present in the cytoplasm, and the high activity of lysosomal enzymes has been demonstrated. Also, regularly contained with the epithelial cells are myelin bodies with a laminated structure similar to that seen in photoreceptors (Fig. 32-35). The myelin bodies are the phagocytized tips of the outer segment of the photoreceptor element and are called *lamellar phagosomes*. Lamellar phagosomes and their degrading products in various ap-

FIGURE 32-34 Electron micrograph of the junction between choroid and retina. In the lower left corner is a vessel of the choriocapillaris adjacent to Bruch's membrane. The endothelium of the choriocapillaris is fenestrated (arrows). Occupying the center portion of the photograph is the pigment epithelium. The photoreceptor outer segments are interdigitating with microvilli of the pigment epithelium.

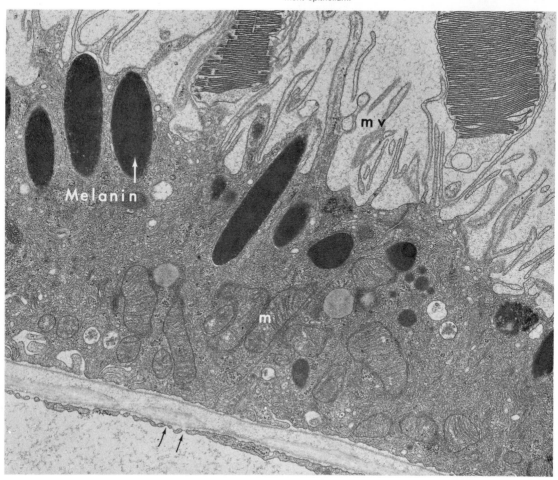

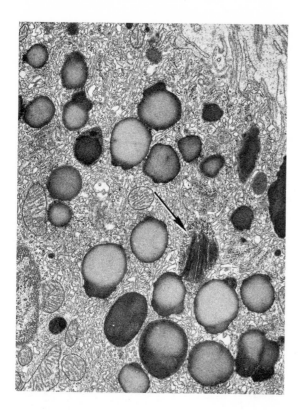

FIGURE 32-35 Pigment epithelial cell of an old human. Melanin granules are sparse whereas lipofuscin particles are abundant. Arrow indicates lamellar phagosome. ×14,500.

pearances are abundant in the cytoplasm, especially in pathological conditions. These substances appear to change into lipofuscin granules. The number of lipofuscin granules increases with age whereas the number of melanin granules decrease in these cells (Fig. 32-35). Microperoxisomes, which contain catalases for digestion of lipidic substances, are rich in this cell.

The pigment epithelium apparently has a secretory function. Pits and vacuoles are abundant in the apical cytoplasm together with rough endoplasmic reticulum and Golgi apparatus. Incorporation of radioactive sulfate has been demonstrated experimentally.

Large oil droplets are present in the pigment epithelial cell of many animals (rabbits, birds, frogs). Certain animals (opposum, fish) have reflectile substances within the cytoplasm. Also, myeloid bodies and regularly packed smooth endoplasmic reticulum are found in the pigment epithelial cells of lower animals.

LENS

The *lens* is a transparent structure situated behind the iris and in front of the vitreous; it is held in place by the *zonular fibers*. In the adult human eye it measures approximately 10 mm in diameter and 5 mm in thickness. The anterior surface of the lens has an approximately spherical convexity, whereas the posterior surface has a paraboloid convexity.

Changes in refraction of the lens occur by the interplay between its inherent tendency to become more spherical and the tension on the zonules which flatten it.

The outer surface of the lens is bounded by a capsule, the basement membrane of the lens cells, which has the same physical and tinctorial properties as Descemet's membrane (Fig. 32-36). The anterior portion of the capsule averages approximately 10 μm in thickness (disregarding minor regional variations), whereas the posterior portion is less than half this.

One of the intriguing features of the lens is its isolation, not only from a blood supply but from an interchange of cells with the rest of the body. The lens epithelium is derived from surface ectoderm and is enclosed in a permanent capsule early in gestation. This capsule is impermeable to cells and permits no ingress of macrophages nor egress of the lens' own cells; the lens carries on its metabolism throughout life in a sort of tissue culture. Moreover, it permits an isolation of antigenic proteins that are foreign to the rest of the body.

Another intriguing feature is the remarkable transparency of the lens despite its densely proteinaceous nature. With age, some of this transparency is lost; opacification of the lens sufficient to disturb vision is called *cataract*.

Beneath the anterior capsule is a layer of cuboidal anterior lens cells (Fig. 32-36) that are remarkable for their uniformity and mode of differentiation. Although these cells are called *lens epithelium*, their structure is different from the conventional covering epithelium. The cell faces inwardly and its apical end attaches to the lens fibers, and the outside is covered with the thick basement membrane. The cytoplasm of the anterior lens cell contains a fine granular substance, a characteristic lens protein and sparse microorganelles. The paucity of mitochondria accords with the relative insignificance of respiratory metabolism in the lens substance. The cells have conspicuous interdigitations, especially toward the equator. Cell membranes form a junctional complex with the lens fiber cells at the apical ends.

At the equator the cells elongate end insinuate beneath the lens epithelium layer anteriorly and beneath the posterior capsule posteriorly (Figs. 32-36 and 32-37). Since each nucleus retains its central location within the cell, the elongation of the cells causes a shifting of the nuclear distribution. Thus the *bow* configuration of the nuclei at the equator is formed. The elongated cells lose their nuclei and basal attachment. These differentiated cells are called *lens fibers*. The lens grows superficially throughout life by continual addition of these fibers. (As in the growth of a tree trunk, the youngest fibers are just beneath the capsule.) Mitoses are practically never seen in conventional sections of the lens, but a few mitoses may be found in the equatorial regions in flat preparations of the epithelium.

The *lens substance* consists of concentrically arranged lens fibers that have undergone varying degrees of condensation (Fig. 32-38). The individual fiber structure is most evident in the superficial layers of the lens substance, called the *cortex;* toward the center, or *nucleus, of the lens,* the fibers become progressively more homogeneous and less readily distinguishable as fibers histologically. The adult lens substance represents one of the most dense concentrations of protein in any tissue of the body. It stains strongly with eosin and other acid dyes. Because of its density, the adult lens substance is poorly infiltrated by ordinary embedding media; hence it is rare, except with embryonic or fetal specimens, to obtain sections of the lens without disturbing artifacts.

By scanning electron microscopy the lens fibers are seen to vary their shape according to their position. Cells in the bow zone have irregular large protrusions which interdigitate with those of adjacent cells. They thus form a regularly spaced knob and socket interlocking in the cortex. Also, lens fibers in the cortex and deeper zones, including the lenticular nu-

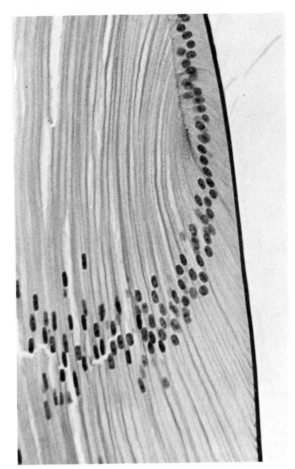

FIGURE 32-36 Equator of the lens of a child. The lens epithelial cells are differentiating into recognizable lens fibers. The nuclei are found at considerable depth in the cortex of the young lens. The capsule is heavily stained with PAS. ×150.

cleus, have fine ridges in a wafflelike pattern (Fig. 32-39).

Sections of the lens show that fibers are closely packed without appreciable interspaces and that cell membranes form several junctions. Gap junctions are common at the knob interlockings. Also, several desmosomes are present. Except for occasional microorganelles in the cells at the bow zone, the lens cells contain only a uniform sprinkling of granules. Cortical cells contain microtubules which run longitudinally in the marginal zone of the lens fiber. Toward the center of the lens, the cytoplasm becomes extremely homogeneous and dense (Fig. 32-38B). No microorganelles are present in these cells.

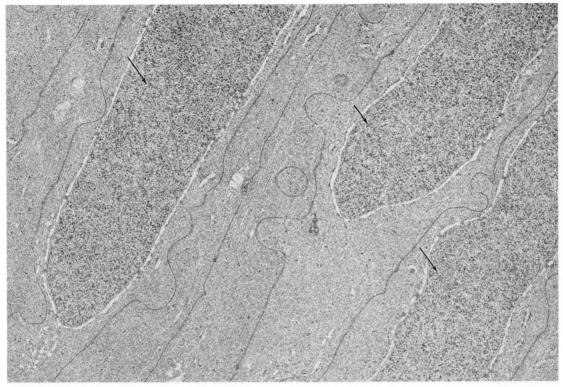

FIGURE 32-37 Bow zone of the lens. Lens cells have nuclei in this area (arrows). Cell membranes are markedly interdigitated. Microtubules are seen frequently. Other microorganelles are sparse.

ZONULES

The *zonules* are hairlike filaments that connect the ciliary body with the lens. They insert into the inner surface of the ciliary body and also into the lens capsule just in front of and just behind the lens equator. They can be seen during life to be the suspensory filaments by which the lens is held in place and through which tension is varied on the lens by contraction of the ciliary muscle. The zonules form the posterior boundary of the posterior chamber and the anterior demarcation of the vitreous space.

The zonules stain poorly with acid dyes but well with the PAS reagent and slightly positive in elastic staining. By electron microscopy the zonules are dense aggregates of filaments similar to those constituting the vitreous structure. Fine filaments often form a tubular arrangement. Although the zonules are grossly and histologically inconspicuous, they are abundant. Scanning electron microscopy reveals the substantial bundles connecting the ciliary epithelium and the lens, and their insertions to the lens are diffusely distributed (Fig. 32-32).

VITREOUS

The large space between the lens, retina, and pars plana of the ciliary body contains a viscid transparent fluid called the *vitreous* (Figs. 32-3 and 32-6). Because of the embryological characteristics of the ocu-

lar tissue, the structure of the ocular cavity is basically different from that of other body cavities: the space is lined by basement membranes of the cells forming the outer wall. Therefore, the vitreous is actually an ex-

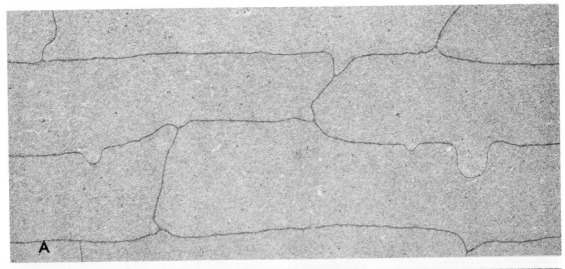

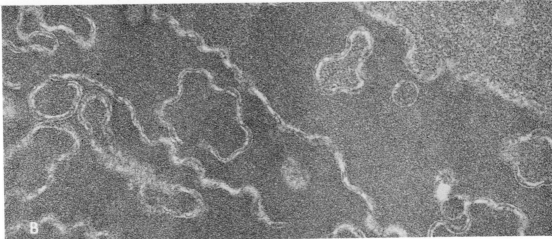

FIGURE 32-38 A. Cross section of lens fibers or cells in the superficial posterior cortex. The cytoplasm consists of fine granular substance. Except for scanty ribosomes, no microorganelles are seen. Cell membranes interdigitate. B. Cross section of the center of the lens. Cell membranes are attenuated. The cytoplasm is extremely compact and homogeneous.

tremely thinned connective tissue but not a cavity content in the ordinary histologic sense.

The intraocular cavity of developing eyes of mammals is rich in blood vessels (*hyaloid vessels*), which disappear upon completion of the differentiation. The thin connective tissue including the basement membranes of the hyaloid blood vessels is called the *primary vitreous.*

The vitreous tissue is made up of minute amounts of filaments and hydrophilic polysaccharides (espe-

cially hyaluronic acid) that stain faintly with the PAS reagent. It is most dense anteriorly in the region of the ciliary body and behind the lens. The vitreous shows considerable shrinkage with most fixatives, however, so that one does not ordinarily find the normal distribution of vitreous in microscopic preparations.

A few cells are present, and PAS staining frequently reveals cells affixed to the outermost portions of the vitreous or between the vitreous and the retina. It has been suggested that these cells are involved with the formation and regeneration of the vitreous. The vitreous cells have histiocytelike processes, and the cytoplasm contains rich Golgi apparatus. Some cells contain membrane-bound inclusion bodies, which may be the PAS-positive granules. The cell has active

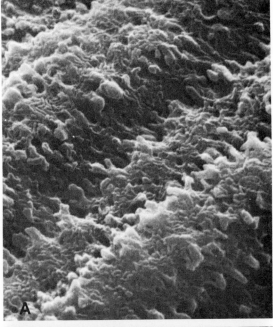

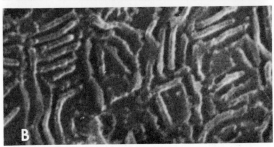

FIGURE 32-39 Scanning electron microscopic view of lens cells in the cortex. The cell has numerous knob and socket junctions. Also the cell membrane is finely reticulated. A. ×3000. B. ×20,000.

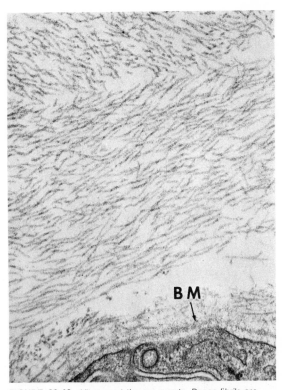

FIGURE 32-40 Vitreous at the ora serrata. Dense fibrils are present in this area. BM, basement membrane of the nonpigmented epithelium at the pars plana. ×34,900.

phagocytic activity. Also, a few wandering cells are present in the vitreous.

Electron microscopy of the vitreous is complicated by artifacts because of high water content (99.9 percent). However, such specimens, having to survive the process of fixation, drying, and staining, show thin fibrils that have a periodicity of 120 Å. The fibrils are apparently of a collagenous nature and attach to the basement membrane of the ciliary epithelium and the retina (Fig. 32-40). The anterior border of the vitreous is comprised of an expecially dense packing of the filaments, thereby constituting the layer known as the *hyaloid membrane*. Also, a condensed layer of the vitreous fibrils are commonly present at the retinal inner limiting membrane. Filaments of the main vitreous body are continuous with those attaching to the basement membrane of the retina.

RETINA

Perhaps the most remarkable tissue of the eye, if not of the body, is the *retina*. In this membrane, which is no more than 0.5 mm thick, a light stimulus is received, converted into a neural impulse, integrated to some extent locally, and transmitted to the optic nerve for relay to the brain. All this is accomplished with an extraordinary degree of adaptability to varying light intensities, discrimination of images, and color perception.

Because of the unique developmental process, the retina is inverted to what one might expect. The inner surface of the retina is covered with the basement membrane and the outer surface is made up of the photoreceptor elements (Figs. 32-41 and 32-42;

FIGURE 32-41 Cross section of the retina. ILM, inner limiting membrane; NFL, nerve fiber layer; GCL, ganglion cell layer; IPL, inner plexiform layer; INL, inner nuclear layer; OPL, outer plexiform layer; ONL, outer nuclear layer; OLM, outer limiting membrane; R & C, rods and cones. PE, pigment epithelium; rods and cones are divided into IS, inner segment and OS, outer segment. ×250.

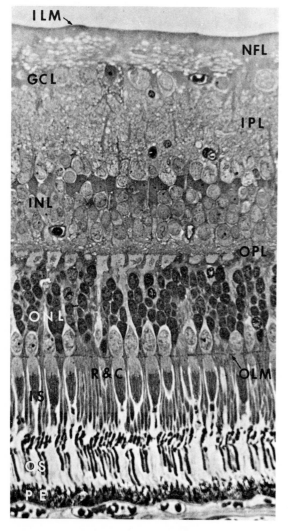

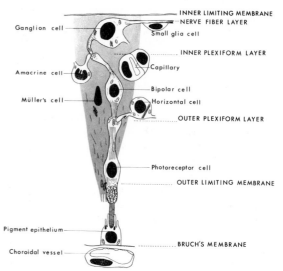

FIGURE 32-43 The major neuronal and glial organization of the retina and pigment epithelium. The Müller cell is shown unrealistically large to emphasize its distribution throughout the whole thickness of the retina.

see color insert). Therefore, light travels through the whole thickness of the retina before reaching the photoreceptors. The photoreceptor cells and the pigment epithelium of the choroid form the *subretinal space*, which corresponds to the embryonal neurovesicular space. The sheetlike retina attaches to the optic nerve head posteriorly and to the ora serrata anteriorly. The rest of the retina has no cytologic attachment to the underlying tissue.

The retina consists of three main categories of neurons: photoreceptor, bipolar, and ganglion cells (Fig. 32-43). These neurons form three clearly defined layers (Figs. 32-41 and 32-42). The photoreceptor cells are often called the *neuroepithelial portion* of the retina. They are analogous to the sensory receptors of the skin or to the first neurons in the efferent arc of other sensory systems. The bipolar cells are analogous to the cells in the dorsal ganglia; the ganglion cells of the retina are analogous to the relay in the spinal cords and brain stem. The optic nerves, the counterparts of the lemnisci in the brainstem, conduct their impulses to the lateral geniculate bodies and thalami. The same number of neuronal relays are thus operative in the retina as in other sensory pathways.

Anterior to the outer nuclear layer is the outer plexiform layer producing synaptic connections between the axons of the rod and cone cells and the dendrites of the next order of cells. The layer between the bipolar cell and ganglion cell is the inner plexiform layer consisting of synaptic organs between these cells.

MACULA

The overall architecture of the retina is modified particularly in two areas. One of these is at the posterior pole of the eye where it forms the *macula* or *fovea*. This is an area about 1.5 mm in diameter at the posterior pole and constitutes the zone of greatest visual acuity (Fig. 32-44). It is the zone of optimal image formation. (The name *macula lutea* refers to the yellow carotenoid pigment in the retina of this region which can be seen in the gross specimen but is not visible by ordinary histologic examination.) At the macula the photoreceptors are modified into long, thin elements called *macula cones*. Morphologically, they resemble rods more closely than cones. The overlying retinal layers are greatly reduced at the center of the macula so that the inner surface of the retina forms a pitlike depression called the *foveola*. The nerve fibers form the regions of the retina which are lateral to the macula arch about it: the ganglion cells, inner plexiform layer, and bipolar cells are displaced away from it; and the inner plexiform layer has a radiating pattern that has been called *Henle's fiber layer*. However, the most distinctive feature of the macula is the abundance of ganglion cells about the foveola.

The thinning of the retina at the macula serves the intensity of visual acuity by reducing to a minimum the

FIGURE 32-44 Cross section through macula. The macula is comprised of a central fossa in which all the layers, except that of the rods and cones, are displaced to the side. ×80.

overlying tissue through which light must pass before reaching the photoreceptors.

MÜLLER'S CELL AND LIMITING MEMBRANES

Certain neuroepithelial cells of the embryonal optic cup keep their basal attachment during development. These cells extend fine cytoplasmic processes and become differentiated retinal glial cells, *Müller's cell*. The basement membrane of these cells is the main part of the *inner limiting membrane* (Fig. 32-45). This membrane forms the inner boundary of the retina and stands out conspicuously with the PAS reagent. Flat preparations of the inner limiting membrane show a gyrate design impressed on it by the arborization of Müller's fibers.

The apical junctions of Müller's cells with photoreceptor cells form a sievelike structure at the outer limit of the outer nuclear layer. This structure is called the *outer limiting membrane* (Fig. 32-46). Fine microvilli of Müller's cells extend beyond the outer limiting membrane into the subretinal space.

Müller's cells have their nuclei in the bipolar cell layer while the cytoplasm is distributed throughout the whole thickness of the retina. Müller's cells are most plentiful in the basal (inner) and apical (outer) layers. The cytoplasm, consisting of rich, smooth endoplasmic reticulum, contains abundant glycogen particles. Also, the cell has considerable glycolytic dehydrogenase activity. This cell serves for the structural as well as

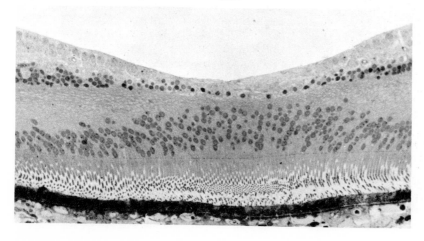

nutritional support system of the retina and is similar to the astrocyte of the central nervous system.

OTHER GLIAL CELLS

A small number of spindle-shaped glial cells are present in the ganglion and nerve-fiber layers. The cytoplasm of these cells contains neurofibrils and usually surrounds bundles of nerve fibers. At the posterior pole, these cells become the main glial element of the retina. The inner limiting membrane in the disc area is mainly made of the basement membrane of these glial cells. Glial cells which extend the cytoplasm to the blood vessel's walls are occasionally present. The number of glial cells in other layers of the retina is extremely small.

FIGURE 32-45 The inner (basal) portion of Müller's cells. The cytoplasm is rich in smooth endoplasmic reticulum and glycogen particles. ILM, inner limiting membrane. ×26,200.

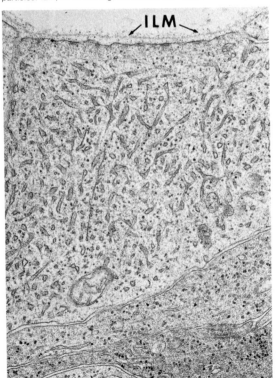

PHOTORECEPTORS

The *photoreceptors* are the *rods* and *cones* situated on the outer surface of the retina (Figs. 32-41, 32-43 and 32-47). These rods and cones consist of an *outer segment* that stains well with eosin and other acid dyes. The outer segment contains the photoreceptive substance (*rhodopsin,* or visual purple in the rods and *iodopsin* in the cones) and is responsible for the absorption of light that triggers off the visual stimulus. As their name implies, the rods have long, thin bodies, whereas the cones have a broad base. The rods have more photoabsorptive pigment, which along with their cumulative neural connections gives them greater sensitivity for low levels of illumination, that is, night vision. The cones, having less summation in the retina, permit greater resolution of images and therefore better visual acuity in daylight. The cones are also responsible for color perception.

The photoreceptor cells have their nuclei in the *outer nuclear layer* and extend their axon processes toward the *outer plexiform layer.* The photoreceptor elements protrude beyond the outer limiting membrane and are divided into two portions: *inner segment* and *outer segment* (Fig. 32-47).

The inner half of the inner segment is called *myoid,* in which abundant Golgi apparatus, smooth endoplasmic reticulum, and microtubules are present. Glycogen particles are rich in this area. A specialized endoplasmic reticulum with abundant glycogen particles is developed in retinas of birds and frogs. The outer half of the inner segment is the *ellipsoid* in which a concentration of mitochondria is present (Fig. 32-48). Wavy filamentous fibrils and scanty microtubules are present among mitochondria. The outer segment is connected to the inner segment by a ciliary connection in which nine pairs of microtubules are present (Fig. 32-49). The central two pairs of the kinocilium are missing.

The *laminated plates* of the rod outer segment have disc shapes measuring about 1 μm in diameter. A stack of these discs is enveloped by the plasma membrane (Fig. 32-50). The disc is formed by two apposing membranes measuring approximately 50 to 60 Å in thickness, and the marginal zone shows a loop configuration in cross sections. These membranes of the rod outer segments are not continuous with the plasma membrane. On the other hand, membranes of the plates of the cone outer segment often connect with the outer plasma membrane (Fig. 32-51). This difference is most striking in the frog retina.

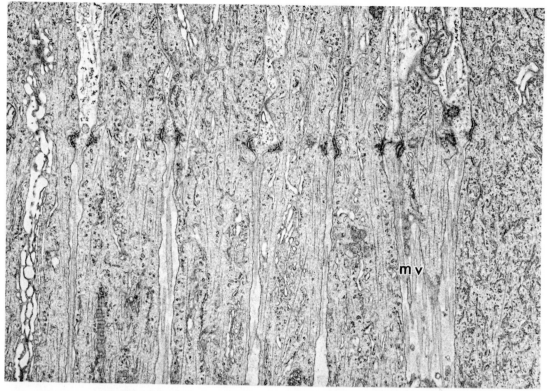

FIGURE 32-46 Outer limiting membrane is a chain of apical junctions of Müller's cells. Microvilli of Müller's cells (mv) extends beyond the limiting membrane. ×20,000.

Lamellated rod membranes are formed at the ciliary connection zone and move centrifugally to be cast off at their outermost tips. They are then phagocytized by the pigment epithelium. In each monkey rod, there are approximately 1,300 plates, each with a life expectancy of about 10 days (Young, 1967).

OUTER NUCLEAR LAYER

The cell bodies and nuclei of the rods and cones constitute the *outer nuclear layer*. The cone nuclei are placed in the outermost portion of this layer. These rod and cone cell bodies are separated from each other by ramifications of the radial glia of the retina, or Müller's cells.

The outermost limit of this layer is the *outer limiting membrane*, a zone of junctional complex be-

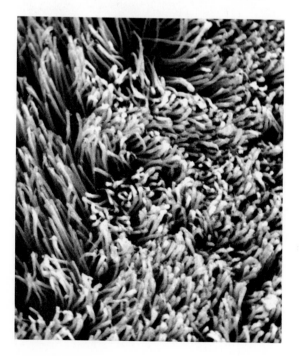

FIGURE 32-47 Scanning electron microscopic view of the photoreceptor outer segments.

tween the photoreceptor cells and apical ends of Müller's cells.

The axonal (inner) and dendritic (outer) portion of the cytoplasm of photoreceptor cells contain regularly arranged microtubules. The parakaryon cytoplasm is scanty.

OUTER PLEXIFORM LAYER

The axonal ends of the photoreceptor cells, dendritic processes of the bipolar cells, and processes of the horizontal cells constitute the *outer plexiform layer* (Fig. 32-41). The cone cell forms a large *synaptic pedicle* in which more than 20 synaptic junctions are present. The rod cell forms a small synaptic spherule which contains a few synaptic junctions (Fig. 32-52).

The synaptic junctions consist of invaginating processes of horizontal cells and superficially located bipolar cell dendrites. The synaptic ends of the photoreceptors contain numerous *synaptic vesicles* which particularly cluster around synaptic bars (Fig. 32-52B). These synaptic ends form rows at the outer half of the layer. The inner half of this plexiform layer is composed of fine processes of bipolar and horizontal cells.

BIPOLAR LAYER

The middle lamina of cells is called the *bipolar cell layer* because it is chiefly made of bipolar neurons that relay impulses from the rod and cone cells to the next

FIGURE 32-48 Photoreceptor elements of the retina. Inner segments of rods and cones contain packs of mitochondria. Outer segments (OS) consist of lamellar membranes. Pigment epithelium (PE) touches lightly at the tips of the outer segments. ×12,000.

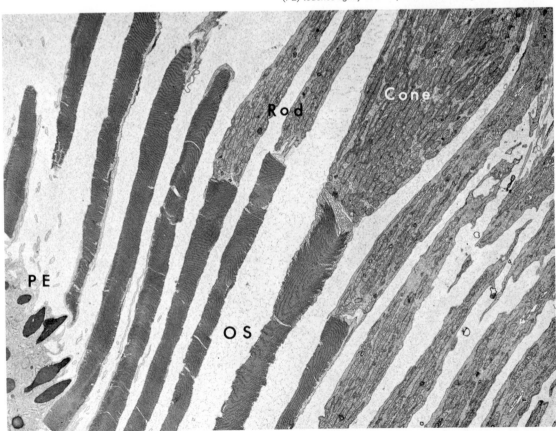

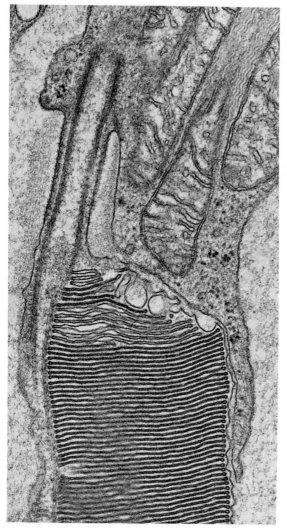

FIGURE 32-49 Electron micrograph through the junctions of the outer and inner segments of the rod. The upper portion of the photograph shows the inner segment containing dense concentrations of mitochondria, whereas the lower portion shows the outer segment, or photoreceptive end organ, containing laminated plates. The two portions are connected by modified cilia. ×32,200.

synaptic junction (Fig. 32-53). The cytoplasm contains rich mitochondria and Golgi apparatus. Microtubules are not conspicuous in the processes, but fine vesicles are present in the tips. Numerous gap junctions are present on the processes of the horizontal cell. The bipolar cells have a relatively small somar cytoplasm but project a large axonal cytoplasm inwardly. The amacrine cells, a monopolar cell, forms a layer in the innermost zone. The amacrine cell has a large cytoplasm which ramifies in the inner plexiform layer. Other nuclei in this layer belong to Müller's glial cells. The parakaryon cytoplasm is usually electron-dense and contains lamellarly arranged rough endoplasmic reticulum. Processes of this cell are chief reservoirs for glycogen and for many enzymes concerned with energy metabolism.

INNER PLEXIFORM LAYER

Anterior to the bipolar cell layer is the *inner plexiform layer* for the synapses of the bipolar layer and the next order of cells. Large bipolar cell axons which contain synaptic vesicles and synaptic bars form a complex of synaptic junctions with amacrine cells and ganglion cell dendrites (Fig. 32-54). Synaptic ends of the amacrine cell contain clusters of vesicles, whereas ganglion cells contain no vesicles. Also, amacrine cell processes form gap junctions with other cell components. This plexiform layer also contains a few glial cells and some blood vessels.

GANGLION CELL LAYER

The ganglion cell layer is the most anterior lamina of cells (Figs. 32-41, 32-42, and 32-43). The ganglion cell layer may be eight to ten cells thick at the posterior pole of the eye (at the macula) but it becomes reduced anteriorly to single scattered cells. Ganglion cells in the posterior retina are small, but the ones in the periphery are extremely large. Several glial cells are present among ganglion cells.

The ganglion cell has a relative abundance of cytoplasm containing rough endoplasmic reticulum organized in masses called *Nissl bodies* (Fig. 32-55). Other microorganelles are rich mitochondria, Golgi apparatus, and lysosomes. The nuclei contain prominent nucleoli. Its dendrites connect with the bipolar

layer of cells inward. It also contains the nuclei of Müller's cells, horizontal cells, and amacrine cells (Figs. 32-41, 32-42 and 32-43). This layer effects some integration of the rods and cones and, in the case of the rods, a summation of impulses.

The outermost zone of the bipolar layer is the horizontal cell which sends fine processes to each

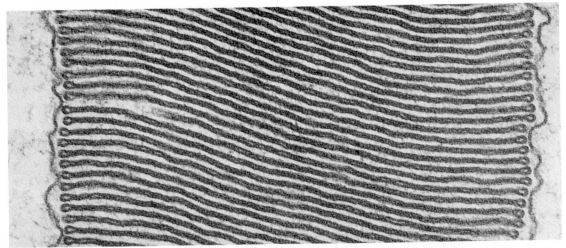

FIGURE 32-50 Higher magnification of the rod outer segment. Saccular discs are separated from each other. ×55,000.

FIGURE 32-51 Cone outer segment. Many membranes of the saccular discs constitute the outer wall of the photoreceptor. Inner side of the disc may communicate with the outside of the cell (arrow). ×50,000.

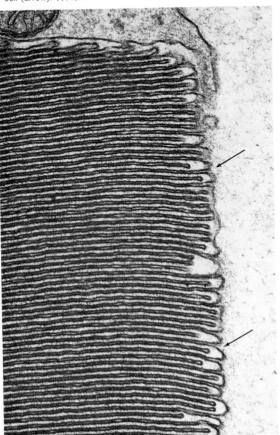

cells in the outer plexiform layer and its axons form the nerve-fiber layer and optic nerve.

NERVE-FIBER LAYER

The *nerve-fiber layer* arises from the ganglion cells and leaves the eye by way of the optic nerve. The layer is, of course, thickest as it approaches the optic nerve. Along with the nerve fibers, this layer also contains blood vessels, miscellaneous glia, and a plexus of Müller's fibers that departmentalize the nerve fibers and fan out toward the innermost surface of the retina.

The axons or nerve fibers contain regularly spaced microtubules and mitochondria. Axons are not myelinated but are often separated by glial cell elements.

NERVE HEAD

The second modification of retinal architecture occurs at the *nerve head,* or *papilla.* This is an area about 1 mm in diameter where the nerve fibers leave the eye to form the optic nerve (Fig. 32-58). The retina is absent in this region, and the visual field shows a corresponding "blind spot." The center of the nerve head is situated about 3 mm nasal to the center of the macula. Only those cross sections of the eye cut near the horizontal meridian will show both macula and optic nerve. Cross sections through the center of the nerve head show a central depression, the physiologic cup, through which the central vessels pass.

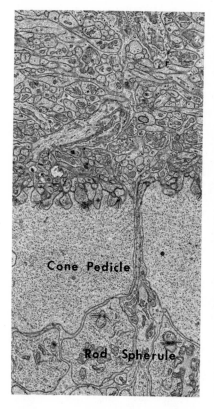

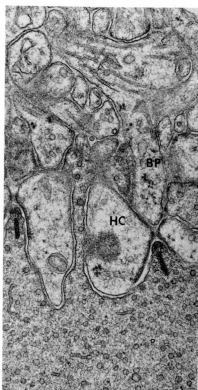

Cone Pedicle

Rod Spherule

BP

HC

FIGURE 32-52 Outer plexiform layer. A. Pedicles of cones and spherules of rods constitute the outer half of the layer. The inner portion of the layer is occupied by processes of bipolar and horizontal cells. Synaptic junctions are seen in the terminal ends of the cones and rods. ×6300. B. Higher magnification of a synaptic end of the cone pedicle. The synapse consists of large horizontal cell processes (HC) and the dendritic end of the bipolar cell (BP). The cone pedicle contains numerous vesicles and synaptic bars. ×37,000.

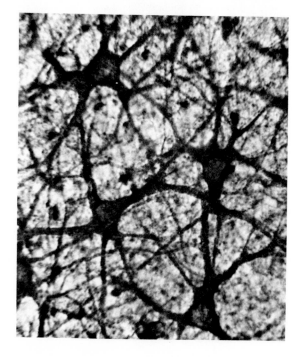

The internal limiting membrane (basement membrane) of this zone is formed mainly by astrocytelike glial cells and is considerably thinner than the rest of the retina. Nerve fibers in this area are not myelinated.

RETINAL VESSELS

The retinal arteries and veins traverse the nerve head but branch immediately once they are within the eye. The larger vessels course horizontally in the nerve fiber and ganglion cell layers but develop elaborate branching and *capillary plexuses* in all the inner layers of the retina (Fig. 32-56).

The retinal vascular tree may either be studied as whole mounts through injection of some material or be digested with the rest of the retina with trypsin. The latter permits subsequent staining of the vessels by ordinary dyes. The capillaries are then seen to contain an unusually thick basement membrane and two types

FIGURE 32-53 Flat section through the outer zone of the bipolar cell layer stained for lactic acid dehydrogenase. Horizontal cells show their stretching processes. ×380.

of cells, one the endothelium lining the capillary lumina and the other enclosed within the basement membrane—hence the name *mural cell,* or intramural pericyte (Fig. 32-57). Cells of the latter type are believed to control the flow through the capillaries.

The endothelial lining is thick and uninterrupted. The cytoplasm of the mural cell contains abundant mitochondria, rough endoplasmic reticulum, Golgi apparatus, and glycogen particles. The cell matrix is filamentous and numerous dense bodies, which are common in smooth muscle cells, are regularly present.

The outer plexiform layer and outer nuclear layers of the retina are vessel-free zones that can derive sufficient nutrition from the choroid to survive when the retinal arteries are obstructed. The fovea is also a capillary-free zone that derives its nutrition from the choriocapillaries.

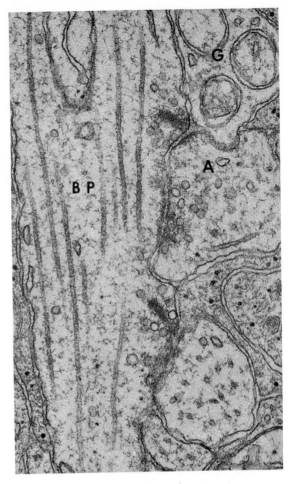

FIGURE 32-54 Synapses in the inner plexiform layer. The axonal end of the bipolar cell (BP) contains synaptic bars and clustering vesicles. Other cell components are ganglion cell (G) and amacrine cells (A). The amacrine cell terminal contains clusters of vesicles. ×48,500.

OPTIC NERVE

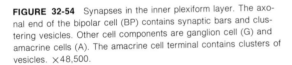

Axons of ganglion cells of the retina converge at the posterior pole and leave the globe (Fig. 32-58). Axon fibers pass through a sievelike connective tissue, *lamina cribrosa* of the sclera where the *optic nerve* begins acquiring myelin. Up to this point myelin is absent. The diameter of the optic nerve increases about twofold beyond this point. With the acquisition of myelin, the optic nerve becomes a tract comparable to white matter of the brain. It is surrounded by meningeal sheaths: a robust dura (continuous with the sclera), a delicate arachnoid, and a thin pia (Fig. 32-59). The subdural and subarachnoid spaces, called collectively the vaginal spaces of the optic nerve, are continuous with those of the intracranial spaces.

The optic nerve contains approximately a million axon fibers, which are strikingly irregular in size and are grouped into small bundles by *astrocytes.* These bundles are then grouped by the connective tissue, *septa,* which contain blood vessels.

Axons consist of electron lucent cytoplasm (axonoplasm) in which regularly spaced microtubules and occasional mitochondria are present. Smooth endoplasmic reticulum is sparsely distributed in the axon.

The cytoplasm of the astrocyte is electron-lucent and contains rich neurofilaments. Other microorganelles are sparse (Fig. 32-60). Fine processes of this cell extend among axon bundles and become the

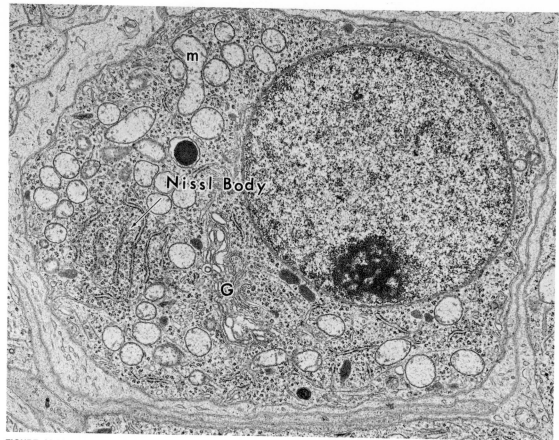

FIGURE 32-55 Ganglion cell in the macula area. The cell contains marked Nissl bodies. The nucleus is located at one edge of the cell and contains a prominent nucleolus. G, Golgi apparatus; m, mitrochondria. ×20,000.

FIGURE 32-56 Flat preparation of the retinal vessels. Fine capillaries form a uniform meshwork. Arrow indicates the avascular zone of the fovea.

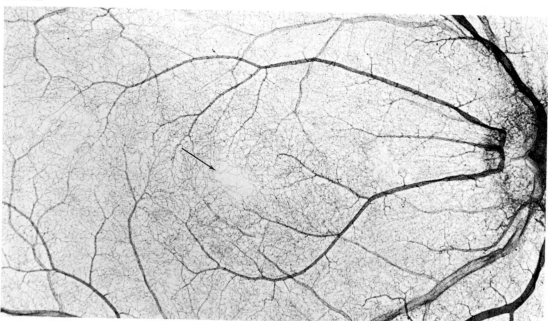

background tissue of the optic nerve. Cell processes are joined to each other by gap junctions and desmosomes in several locations. The astrocytes form thick basement membranes where the cells attach the connective tissue of the lamina cribrosa and septa.

Each axon fiber is surrounded by 5 to 10 layers of the myelin membrane which is believed to be produced by the *oligodendroglia cell.* The *oligondendroglia* cells have electron-dense cytoplasm which contains rich, rough endoplasmic reticulum and Golgi apparatus (Fig. 32-60). Nodes of Ranvier are present regularly.

Glia cells which have very little cytoplasm are infrequently present in the optic nerve. These glia cells are *microglia* and may have a phagocytic function in a certain pathological condition.

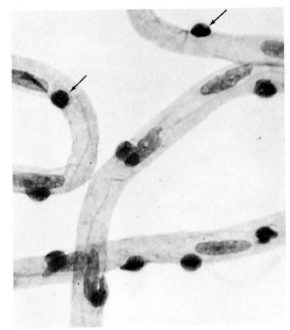

FIGURE 32-57 Capillary wall is made of two types of cells. Endothelial nuclei are ellipsoidal in shape and mural cells (arrow) have dark round nuclei.

FIGURE 32-58 Cross section through the nerve head. ON, myelinated optic nerve; VS, vaginal space; LC, lamina cribrosa; CRV, central retinal vessels; RNF, retinal nerve fibers which are nonmyelinated. ×60.

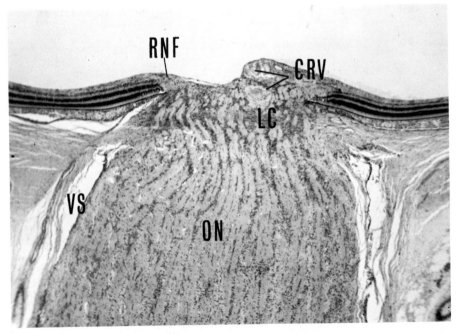

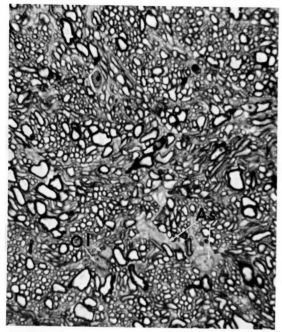

FIGURE 32-59 Cross section of the optic nerve. Myelinated nerve fibers are irregular in size. As, astrocyte; Ol, oligodendroglia cell. ×380.

FIGURE 32-60 Glia cells of the optic nerve. As, astrocyte; Ol, oligodendroglia cell. ×19,300.

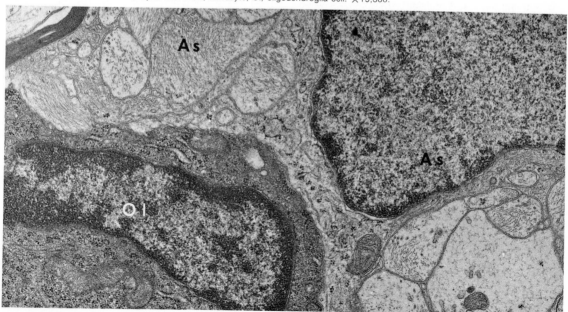

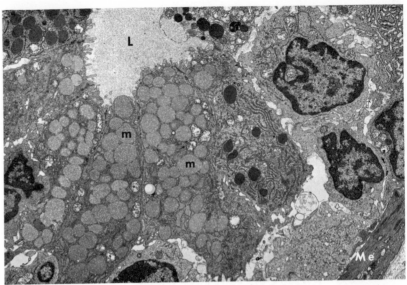

FIGURE 32-61 Cross section of the lacrimal gland. Gland cells are loosely packed. Mucin granules (m) and electron-dense granules are abundantly seen in the cells. L, acinar lumina; Me, myoepithelium. ×3000.

OCULAR ADNEXA AND ORBIT

Surrounding the eye is a sheath of connective tissue called Tenon's capsule. Although this is often looked upon as a socket within which the eye rotates, it has no synovial membrane and no other resemblance to joint structures.

The orbital cavity contains extraocular muscles, optic nerves, blood vessels, and ciliary nerve elements. The rest is filled with adipose and loose connective tissue. The *ciliary ganglion* and plexes of the ciliary nerves are present medial and inferior to the optic nerve.

LACRIMAL GLAND

The *lacrimal gland* is an acinous structure (Fig. 32-61) similar to salivary glands, situated in the upper outer portion of the orbit and opening onto the conjunctiva by 10 to 20 separate ducts. The gland consists of serous glandular cells, surrounded by myoepithelial elements, and ducts containing mucus-forming cells.

The cytoplasm contains mucoid granules and electron-dense secretory substances. Rough endo-plasmic reticulum and Golgi apparatus are abundant. Well-developed myoepithelial cells are present at the basal portion of the gland.

NASOLACRIMAL CANAL

The *nasolacrimal canal* is situated in the bony fossa at the side of the nose. It consists of stratified epithelium, about 10 cells thick, connected with canaliculi from the upper and lower lids and with a nasolacrimal duct that opens into the middle meatus of the nose. The epithelium of the canaliculi consists of columunal ciliated cells. The canaliculi, sac, and duct constitute the effluent channels for tears.

EXTRAOCULAR MUSCLES

The *extraocular muscles* are seven in number; the levator, the four recti (medial, superior lateral, and inferior), and the two obliques (superior and inferior) (Fig. 32-4).

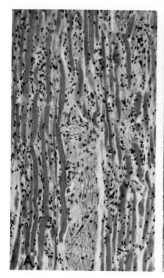
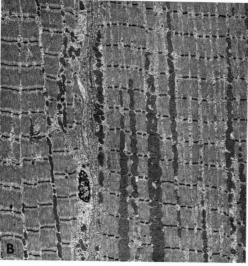

FIGURE 32-62 Rectus muscle. A. The muscle consists of fine muscle fibers, abundant nerves, and considerable connective tissue. ×160. B. Portions of two muscle fibers. Muscle fiber on the left has large myofibrils and sparse mitochondria, whereas the one on the right has fine myofibrils and abundant mitochondria. ×2400.

Fibers of the extraocular muscle are considerably small and irregular in size (10 to 30 μm in diameter). Richly vascularized connective tissue and abundant nerve fibers are present among loosely packed muscle fibers. Two distinct kinds of muscle fibers are intermingled within a muscle bundle; small fibers consisting of well-defined myofibrils and rich mitochondria and large fibers with fused myofibrils and sparse mitochondria (Fig. 32-62). The fine structure of the individual muscle fiber is not different from that of other striated muscles.

REGULAR CHANGES WITH AGE

Certain changes occur with age so regularly that they may be considered normal. These will be mentioned briefly.

1. Sudanophilia of the circumferential portions of Descemet's membrane and, to a lesser extent, of the circumferential stroma of the cornea and of Bowman's membrane. This causes an opacity of the cornea that is known clinically as arcus lipoides.

2. Hyalinization of the stroma in the ciliary processes and between the ciliary muscle and epithelium. Also, the number of the pigmented epithelial cells decreases and the basement membrane of the nonpigmented ciliary epithelium increase in thickness.

3. Condensation of the lens fibers with loss of malleability of the lens substance. This results in a progressive decrease of accommodative power (presbyopia) becoming so marked in middle age that supplementary glasses are needed for near focusing.

4. Occlusion of the capillaries in the peripheral retina with cyst formation in the most anterior portions of the retina. The number of endothelial cells of the retinal capillary decreases considerably.

5. Sudanophilia and basophilia of Bruch's membrane in the posterior portions of the eye.

REFERENCES

DUKE-ELDER, S., and K. C. WYBAR: In S. Duke-Elder (ed), "The Anatomy of the Visual System, System of Ophthalmology," vol. 2, The C. V. Mosby Company, St. Louis, Mo., 1961.

EISLER, P.: Die Anatomie des menschen Auges, in F. Schieck and A. Brückner (eds.), "Kurzes Handbuch der Ophthalmologie," vol. 1, Springer-Verlag OHG, Berlin, 1930.

FINE, B. S., and M. YANOFF: "Ocular Histology," Harper & Row, Publishers, Incorporated, New York, 1972.

HOGAN, M. J., J. A. ALVARADO, and J. E. WEDDELL: "Histology of the Human Eye," W. B. Saunders Company, Philadelphia, 1971.

MANN, I.: "The Development of the Human Eye," 2d ed., Grune & Stratton, Inc., New York, 1950.

POLYAK, S.: "The Retina," The University of Chicago Press, Chicago, 1941.

SMELSER G. K. (ed.): "The Structure of the Eye," Academic Press, Inc., New York, 1961.

WOLFF, E.: "The Anatomy of the Eye and Orbit," 5th ed., McGraw-Hill Book Company, New York, 1961.

YOUNG, R. W.: The Renewal of Photoreceptor Cell Outer Segments, *J. Cell Biol.,* **33:**61 (1967).

The Ear

ÅKE FLOCK

GENERAL STRUCTURE

The ear is composed of three parts, which are illustrated schematically in Fig. 33-1:

1. The external ear, which includes the auricle, or pinna, projecting from the head and the external auditory meatus leading from the surface to the ear drum

2. The middle ear, including the tympanic cavity, the drum, and the chain of three bones extending from the drum to the medial wall of the tympanic cavity, which communicates with the nasopharynx by means of the auditory (eustachian) tube

3. The internal ear, which consists of the membranous labyrinth containing the organs of hearing and equilibrium, the bone surrounding these sense organs, and the acoustic nerve

EXTERNAL EAR

AURICLE

The *auricle* consists of an irregular flap of elastic cartilage. On the lateral surface, the skin adheres tightly to the perichondrium which contains abundant elastic fibers, whereas on the posterior surface a subcutaneous layer is present. Sebaceous glands are often quite large and are associated with small hairs.

EXTERNAL AUDITORY MEATUS

The *external meatus* is lined with skin continuous with the cutaneous layer of the tympanic membrane. In the deep or osseous portion, the skin is very thin and without hairs or glands except along its upper wall. There, and in the outer or cartilaginous part, ceruminous glands

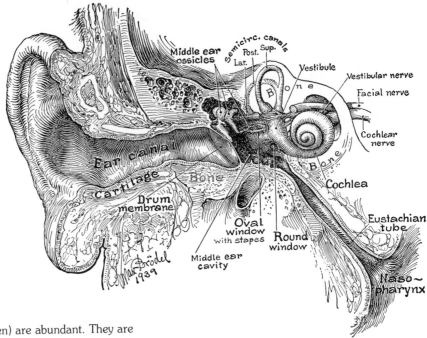

FIGURE 33-1 Schematic drawing of the human ear, illustrating the anatomic relations of the various parts of the ear and the surrounding and connecting structures. (Courtesy of Brödel, three unpublished drawings of the anatomy of the human ear. W. B. Saunders Company, Philadelphia.)

that secrete a wax (cerumen) are abundant. They are branched, tubuloalveolar glands which in many respects resemble large sweat glands. Their ducts are lined with stratified epithelium, and their coils consist of a single layer of secreting cells, generally cuboid, surrounded by smooth muscle fibers and a well-defined basement membrane. They differ from sweat glands in that their coils have a very large lumen, especially in the adult, and their gland cells, often with a distinct cuticular border, contain many pigment granules and lipid droplets. Their narrow ducts end on the surface of the skin or they open together with sebaceous glands into the neck of hair follicles.

MIDDLE EAR

TYMPANIC CAVITY

The air-filled *tympanic cavity*, or *tympanium*, is lined with a mucous membrane closely connected with the surrounding periosteum. It consists of a thin layer of connective tissue covered generally with simple cuboidal epithelium. In places the epithelial cells may be flat or tall, with nuclei in two rows. Cilia are sometimes widely distributed and are usually found on the floor of the cavity. In the anterior part of the tympanic cavity, small alveolar mucous glands occur very sparingly. Capillaries form wide-meshed networks in the connective tissue, and lymphatic vessels are found in the periosteum.

TYMPANIC MEMBRANE

The tympanic cavity is separated from the external auditory canal by the *tympanic membrane* or *ear drum* which consists of the following strata: the outermost cutaneum, the radiatum, the circulare, and the innermost mucosum. The stratum cutaneum is a thin skin without papillae in its corium, except along the handle or manubrium of the malleus. There it is a thicker layer, containing the vessels and nerves which descend along the manubrium and spread from it radially. In addition to the venous plexus which accompanies the artery there, a plexus of veins at the periphery of the membrane receives tributaries from both the stratum cutaneum and the less vascular stratum mucosum. The radiate and circular strata consist of compact bundles of fibrous and elastic tissue which are so arranged as to suggest tendon. The fibers of the radial layer blend with the perichondrium of the hyaline cartilage covering the manubrium. Peripherally the fiber layers form a fibrocartilaginous ring which connects with the surrounding bone. The stratum mucosum is a thin layer of connective tissue covered with a simple, nonciliated, flat epithelium continuous with the lining of the tympanic cavity. Peripherally, in children, its cells may be taller and ciliated. As a whole, the tympanic membrane is divided into tense and flaccid portions. The latter is a relatively small upper part in which the fibrous layers are deficient. The tensor tympani muscle is attached by a tendon to the center of the tympanic membrane.

AUDITORY OSSICLES

The tympanic membrane is connected to the inner ear through a chain of three small bones, the *malleus, incus,* and *stapes* (Fig. 33-1). They articulate against each other by regular joints and are supported in the middle ear cavity by connective tissue strands. The

FIGURE 33-2 Cat stapes with stapedius muscle. The stapes in the oval window. The stapedius muscle is attached to the head of the stapes. Note the sesamoid bone between the head of the stapes and the incus. The facial nerve cut in cross section. TC, tympanic cavity; FN, facial nerve; SB, sesamoid bone; I, incus; HS, head, stapes; FS, footplate, stapes; CS, crura stapes; V, vestibule; SM, stapedius muscle. ×15. (Courtesy of Lurie.)

manubrium of the malleus attaches to the tympanic membrane; the footplate of the stapes is held by an annular fibrous ligament in the *fenestra vestibuli,* or oval window, which opens into the inner ear. The *stapedius muscle* attaches to the head of the stapes (Fig. 33-2).

AUDITORY TUBE

The *auditory,* or *eustachian tube* (Fig. 33-1), includes an osseous part toward the tympanum and a cartiliginous part toward the pharynx. Its mucosa consists of fibrillar connective tissue, with a ciliated columnar epithelium which becomes stratified as it approaches the pharynx. The stroke of the cilia is toward the pharyngeal orifice. In the osseous portion, the mucosa is without glands and very thin; it adheres closely to the surrounding bone. Along its floor there are pockets containing air, the cellulae pneumaticae. In the cartilaginous part the mucosa is thicker; near the pharynx it contains many mixed glands. Lymphocytes are abundant in the surrounding connective tissue, forming nodules near the end of the tube which blend with the pharyngeal tonsil. The cartilage, which only partly surrounds the auditory tube, is hyaline near its junction with the bone of the osseous portion. Here and there are coarse nonelastic fibers. Toward the pharynx the matrix contains thick nets of elastic tissue, so the cartilage there is elastic.

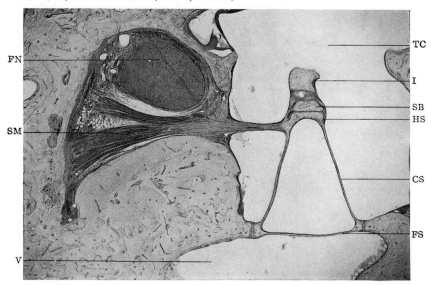

INNER EAR

BONY AND MEMBRANOUS LABYRINTH

The inner ear is located in the pars petrosus of the temporal bone. The bone is pierced by a system of tortuous canals and cavities, the *bony labyrinth,* which is shaped to lodge the *membranous labyrinth.* The bony labyrinth is filled with a fluid, *perilymph,* and communicates with the cerebrospinal space by a narrow canal, the *vestibular aqueduct.*

 The membranous labyrinth (Fig. 33-3) has two subdivisions. The *vestibular labyrinth* contains the organs of equilibrium: the *semicircular canals,* the *utricle,* and the *saccule.* The *cochlea* contains the organ of hearing: the *organ of Corti.* The membranous labyrinth is filled with a fluid called *endolymph.*

VESTIBULAR LABYRINTH

The *utricle* is an elliptical sac which lies in the upper posterior part of the bony vestibule, a cavity on the bony labyrinth. The spherical saccule lies anterior and medial to the utricle and is connected to it by the utriculosaccular duct. From the utriculosaccular duct arises the endolymphatic duct. The three membranous semicircular canals communicate with the utricle. These three canals lie at right angles in the three dimensions of space. Each one has an ampullated end. The ampullae of the anterior (vertical) and lateral (horizontal) canals lie close to each other and open into the superior end of the utricle, whereas the ampulla of the posterior (vertical) canal opens into its inferior end. The common end of the two vertical canals, the *crus commune,* enters the midportion of the utricle, as does also the nonampullated end of the horizontal canal.

 The connective tissue layer of the utricle, saccule, and membranous canals consists of a finely fibrillated intercellular substance and spindle-shaped or stellate fibroblastic cells (Fig. 33-4). From its outer surface, trabeculae run through the perilymphatic spaces to the inner periosteum of the osseous vestibule and the bony semicircular canals. These support the semicircular canals, utricle, and saccule. The spaces and

FIGURE 33-3 Schematic drawing of the membranous labyrinth. Within each sensory area the orientation of the sensory cells is indicated. (Modified from Ebner. Reproduced with permission of W. Engelmann.)

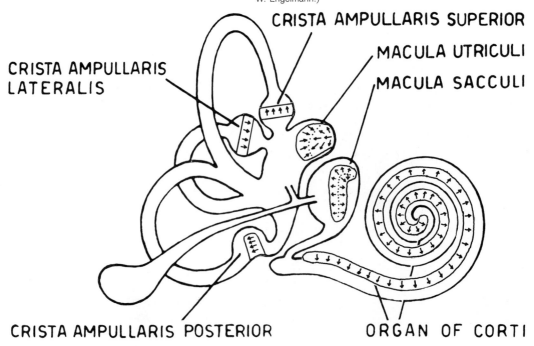

CRISTA AMPULLARIS SUPERIOR

MACULA UTRICULI

MACULA SACCULI

CRISTA AMPULLARIS LATERALIS

CRISTA AMPULLARIS POSTERIOR

ORGAN OF CORTI

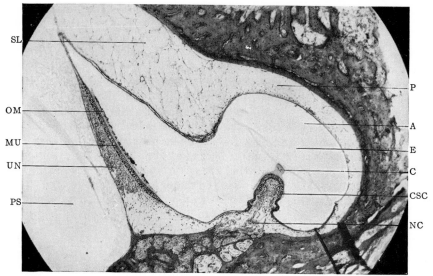

FIGURE 33-4 Macula utriculi and the ampulla of a semicircular canal. Supporting ligaments run from the membranous semicircular canal and utricle to the bony walls of the cavity. The utricle is suspended in the vestibule. PS, perilymphatic space; SL, supporting ligaments; MU, macula utriculi; UN, utricular nerve; OM, otolithic membrane; A, ampulla; CSC, crista, semicircular canal; C, cupula; NC, nerve to crista; E, endolymph; P, perilymph. Guinea pig. ×40. (Courtesy of Lurie.)

FIGURE 33-5 Ampulla of the semicircular canal cut open to expose the sensory epithelium of the crista. The cupula has been removed during dissection. A, ampulla; C, crista; P, planum semilunatum. Scanning microscopy. (Courtesy of Wersäll, Björkroth, Flock, and Lundquist. Reproduced with permission of Springer-Verlag.)

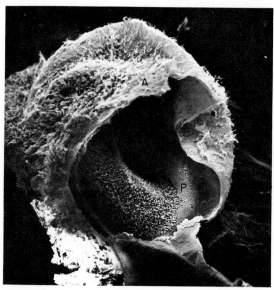

periosteum are lined with a layer of flattened connective tissue cells, which is a mesothelium.

The neuroepithelial areas of the utricle and saccule are called *maculae*. The macula of the utricle, which is about 2 × 2 mm, lies in the superior anterior part of the utricle, approximately in the plane of the base of the skull and also in the plane of the horizontal semicircular canal. The macula of the saccule, which is about 2 × 3 mm, lies in a sagittal plane of the head, so the two maculae are perpendicular to each other.

Semicircular Canals

Each semicircular canal is provided with a sense organ responding to angular acceleration in the plane of the canal. This is the *crista ampullaris* (Figs. 33-5 and 33-6), a ridge of connective tissue which projects into the ampulla of the canal and is covered by a neuro-epithelium consisting of sensory *hair cells* and supporting cells (Fig. 33-7). At both ends, where the crista joins the wall of the ampulla, is a region of tall cylindrical cells called *planum semilunatum*. Each hair cell has a bundle of sensory hairs which project from the luminal surface (Fig. 33-8) and are attached to a gelatinous structure, the *cupula*, which rides on top of the crista and reaches to the roof of the ampulla. The cupula acts as a swinging door to the motion of endolymph and excites the sensory cells by displacing the sensory hairs.

Two types of hair cells are distinguished in vestibular sensory epithelia (Fig. 33-7). *Type I cells* have a constricted neck and a round cell body, most of which is enclosed in a chalicelike afferent nerve terminal. The nerve chalice, in turn, is contacted by endings of efferent nerve fibers which contain abundant vesicles and probably have an inhibitory function. *Type II cells* are cylindrical cells innervated at their base by terminals of afferent and efferent fibers. At the afferent synapse of both types of cells are regions of ultrastructural specialization with a presynaptic dense bar surrounded by vesicles similar to those seen where neurochemical synaptic transmission occurs.

Each sensory hair bundle is composed of 40 to 80 *stereocilia* which progressively increase in length toward one pole of the cell (Fig. 33-7). These sensory hairs are modified microvilli with a core of fibrils, 30 Å in diameter, which continue as a rootlet into a *cuticular plate* in the apical cytoplasm. The cuticular plate is absent near the longest stereocilla, where a single *kinocilium* that has the "9 + 2" pattern of microtubules seen elsewhere is situated, although motility is not expected in this cilium. Each hair cell can thus be given a direction in which the kinocilium is facing. This is functionally important since the sensory nerve fiber connected to that cell increases its firing rate when the sensory hairs are bent in the direction of the kinocilium, whereas opposite displacement causes a

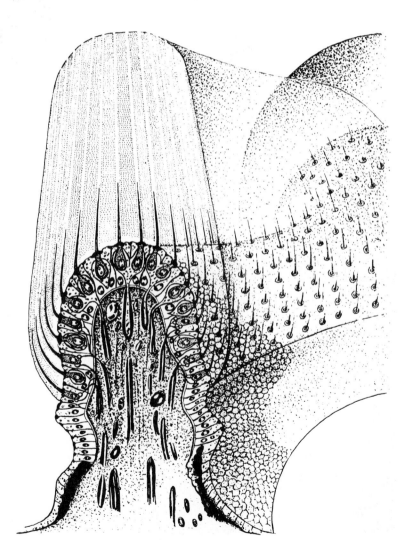

FIGURE 33-6 Sensory epithelium of the crista ampullaris contains hair cells with apical sensory hairs coupled to the cupula. (Courtesy of Wersäll.)

decrease in firing frequency. In each crista all hair cells face the same direction: in the horizontal crista toward the utricle and in the two vertical cristae away from the utricle (Fig. 33-3).

The supporting cells have basal nuclei, an apical cytoplasm containing secretory granules, and a luminal surface provided with microvilli. Their secretory product forms the matrix of the cupula.

Utricle and Saccule

The sensory epithelium of the macula utriculi and macula sacculi has the same structure as that of the crista (Figs. 33-7, 33-9, and 33-10). The surfaces of the maculae are covered with a layer of gelatinous substance, the *otolithic membrane,* into which the

sensory hair bundles penetrate. In the free surface of the otolithic membrane lie many crystals of calcium carbonate, called *otoconia* (Fig. 33-11). Because the otoconia are denser than endolymph, gravitational forces can cause a shear motion of the otolith membrane relative to the sensory epithelium and thus excite or inhibit the sensory cells. Linear acceleration and changes of the position of the head are adequate stimuli. As appears in Fig. 33-3, the pattern of orientation of hair cells is quite complicated in the two maculae. For each direction of motion there is a region of hair cells which will be excited. At the same time, other cells will be inhibited; it is likely that the sensory neurons from different regions project specifically via brainstem nuclei to appropriate muscles which control posture.

FIGURE 33-7 Schematic drawing of vestibular sensory cells. (Modified from Wersäll. Reproduced with permission of Pergamon Press.)

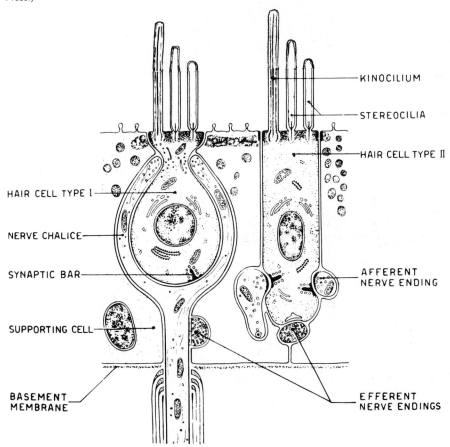

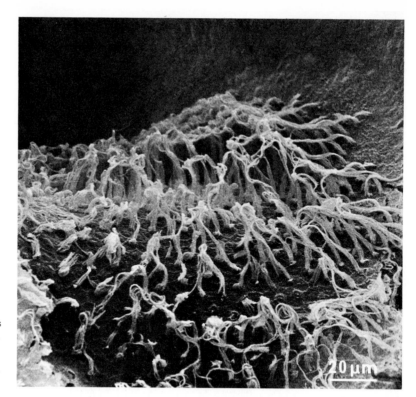

FIGURE 33-8 Scanning picture of the crista toward the planum semilunatum shows sensory hair bundles projecting from the neuroepithelium. The cupula has been removed. (Courtesy of Wersäll, Flock, and Lundquist. Reproduced with permission of Killisch-Horn Verlag.)

20 µm

FIGURE 33-9 Sensory epithelia of the macula utriculi and sacculi have identical structure. (Courtesy of Iurato. Reproduced with permission of Pergamon Press.)

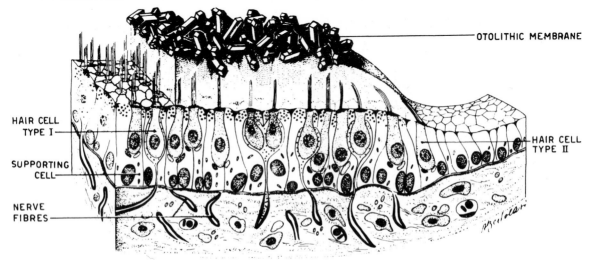

OTOLITHIC MEMBRANE

HAIR CELL TYPE I

HAIR CELL TYPE II

SUPPORTING CELL

NERVE FIBRES

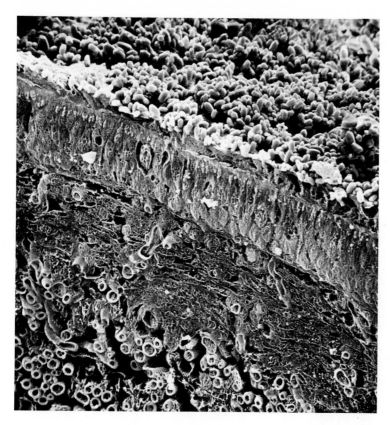

FIGURE 33-10 Freeze fracture through the macula utriculi shows the otolith membrane overlying the sensory epithelium below which myelinated nerve fibers are seen in cross section. Human. (Courtesy of Lundquist, Flock, and Wersäll.)

FIGURE 33-11 Otoconia from the human utricle.

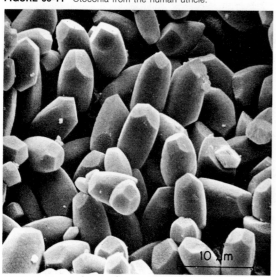

COCHLEA

The bony cochlea provides a rigid protective covering for the membranous cochlea (ductus cochlearis) with its delicate sense organ for hearing. The canal of the bony cochlea makes $2\frac{1}{2}$ turns around its axis, which is a pillar of spongy bone called the *modiolus* (Figs. 33-1 and 33-12). The base of the modiolus (the largest turn) forms the anterior wall of the internal acoustic meatus. The cochlear nerve and blood vessels enter the cochlea through the base of the modiolus. The bony canal is partially divided by a projection of bone from the modiolus, called the *lamina spiralis ossea*. In radial section of the cochlea through the modiolus, this projection looks like the thread of a screw. The lamina spiralis ossea has two lips separated by a sulcus, an upper vestibular lip, or *limbus spiralis,* and a lower tympanic lip (Figs. 33-13 and 33-14).

Attached to the osseous lamina and the outer wall of the canal lies the membranous cochlea, which separates the bony cochlear canal into two partitions: the *scala vestibuli,* which opens into the vestibule; and the scala tympani, which ends basally at the *round window*. The round window faces the middle ear cavity. The lumen of the membranous cochlea is referred to as the *scala media*. It is delimited toward the scala vestibuli by the *Reissner's membrane* and toward the scala tympani by the *basilar membrane*. The membranous cochlea filled with endolymph ends as a blind sac (lagena or cecum cupulare) at the apex of the cochlea.

Just beyond this point the scala vestibuli and scala tympani, which had been separated by the membranous cochlea, join; this is called the *helicotrema*. The aquaeductus cochleae stems from the scala tympani at the base of the cochlea near the round window and passes to the subarachnoid space near the jugular fossa.

The membranous cochlea, which is triangular in shape when seen in cross section, is attached inwardly to the lamina spiralis ossea and outwardly by the *spiral ligament* to the outer wall of the bony canal. The base

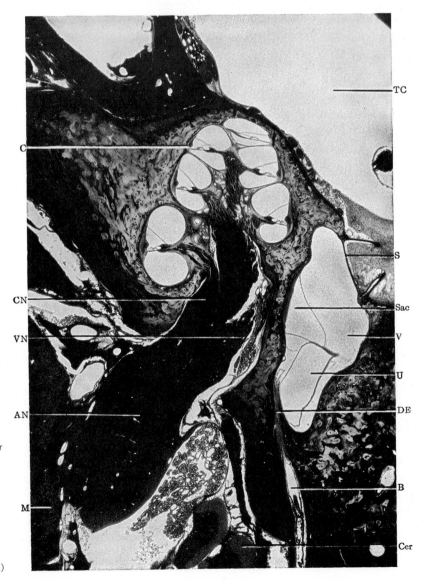

FIGURE 33-12 Cochlea and vestibule of a cat. Horizontal section shows the footplate of the stapes in the oval window, the vestibule showing the relationship of saccule and utricle to the oval window, and the large perilymphatic space around the footplate of the stapes. The ductus endolymphaticus can be followed in the aquaeductus vestibuli. The bulb of the ductus lymphaticus can be seen. The cochlea is cut to show three turns. The cochlear nerve and vesitubular nerve can be seen in their course from the spiral and Scarpa's ganglion into the medulla. TC, tympanic cavity; S, stapes; V, vestibule; Sac, saccule; U, utricle; DE, ductus endolymphaticus; B, bulb (sarcus) of ductus endolymphaticus; C, cochlea; CN, cochlear nerve and spiral ganglia; VN, vestibular nerve. Scarpa's ganglion; AN, auditory nerve; Cer, cerebellum. ×12. (Courtesy of Lurie.)

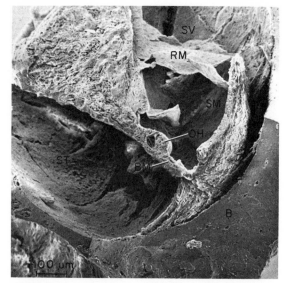

FIGURE 33-13 Freeze fracture through the cochlear portion shows the scala vestibuli (SV), scala media (SM), scale tympani (ST) separated by Reissner's membrane (RM), and the basilar membrane (BM). O, organ of Corti; S, spiral ganglion; B, bone; V, stria vascularis.

FIGURE 33-14 Organ of Corti of a mouse. First turn of the cochlea, showing the relationship of scala vestibuli, scala media, and scala tympani. Reissner's membrane; the stria vascularis; the organ of Corti; techtorial membrane; inner hair cell; pillar cells; outer hair cells; basilar membrane; the spiral ligaments; and the spiral ganglia. SV, scala vestibuli; RM, Reissner's membrane; STV, stria vascularis; SPL, spiral ligament; LSO, lamina spiralis ossea; VL, vestibular lip; TL, tympanic lip; TM, tectorial membrane, ISC, inner sulcus cells; IHC, inner hair cell; EHC, external hair cells; BM, basilar membrane; ST, scala tympani; SpG, spiral ganglia. ×120 (Courtesy of Lurie.)

of the membranous cochlea is made of the tympanic lip of the lamina spiralis ossea and the basilar membrane, which connects the tympanic lip with the spiral ligament. At the attachment of the basilar membrane to the spiral ligament there is a small sulcus called the *external sulcus*. The vestibular lip of the lamina spiralis ossea has attached to it Reissner's membrane and the *tectorial membrane*. The space between the limbus and the tympanic lip is called the *inernal sulcus*.

The basilar membrane is sometimes considered to have two parts, the zona arcuata (inner zone) and the zona pectoralis (outer zone). Its middle layer is formed by fibers which run through both zones. The basilar membrane varies in width from the basal coil at the round window to the apex. It is smallest at the round window, 0.16 mm, and widest at the helicotrema, 0.52 mm. The length of the basilar membrane in man is about 31 mm. On its scala tympani aspect, mesothelial cells and connective tissue line the basilar membrane. There is a small artery running under it, the *vas spirale*. On the upper surface of the basilar membrane in the scala media rests the organ of Corti. Reissner's membrane is attached to the inner superior surface of the vestibular lip of the lamina spiralis ossea and goes to the outer wall of the bony cochlea at the upper end of the spiral ligament. It is two cell layers in thickness and is lined with epithelium on its surface

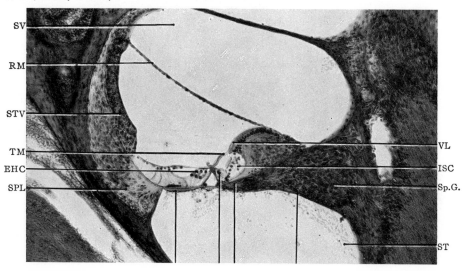

facing the scale media and with mesothelium on its surface facing the scala vestibuli.

The third wall of the scala media is called the *stria vascularis*. It runs from the attachment of Reissner's membrane to the external sulcus. It has a low pseudostratified epithelium in intimate contact with the capillaries. The stria vascularis is believed to secrete the endolymph that fills the membranous cochlea. It runs the whole length of the scala media.

Organ of Corti

On the basilar membrane lies the organ of Corti, which is built up by hair cells and supporting cells arranged in a complicated manner (Figs. 33-15 to 33-22). It runs from the round window to the helicotrema of the cochlea. There are no blood vessels in the organ of Corti. A portion of its rests on the tympanic lip of the lamina spiralis ossea, but most of it lies on the basilar membrane. Between these parts is a free triangular space called the *tunnel*, which is delimited by two rows of supporting cells, the *inner pillar cells* resting on or near the tip of the tympanic lip and the

outer pillar cells on the basilar membrane. The pillar cells have a broad base in which the nucleus lies. The body of the pillar cell contains rigid tonofibrils. The top of the pillar cells is enlarged and covered on its free surface with a cuticular plate. The head of the internal pillar cell is concave so that the rounded head of the external pillar cell can fit into it, like a ball-and-socket joint. There are about 6,000 inner pillar cells and about 4,000 external pillar cells, so that three inner cells articulate with two external cells.

The sensory cells are in two groups: the *inner hair cells*, a single row of about 3,500 cells close to the inner pillar cells, and the *outer hair cells*, about 20,000 cells in three to four rows external to the outer pillar. The outer hair cells are cylindrical with a rounded lower end (Fig. 33-17). They are slanted relative to the surface of the organ of Corti. From the apical end of each outer hair cell a bundle of about 100 stereocilia (Figs. 33-18 and 33-19) project from a cuticular plate in a W pattern (Fig. 33-20), with the row of tallest hairs

FIGURE 13-15 Organ of Corti. TM, tectorial membrane; YH, outer hair cells; ST, phalangeal cells; BM, basilar membrane; P, outer and inner pillars; SP, spiral vessel; N, tunnel of Corti; IH, inner hair cell; MN, myelinated nerve fibers. (Courtesy of Wersäll, Flock, and Lundquist. Reproduced by permission of Cold Spring Harbor Laboratories.)

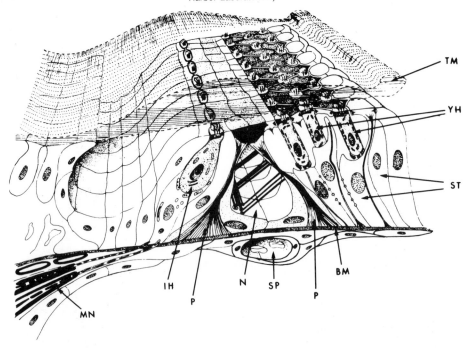

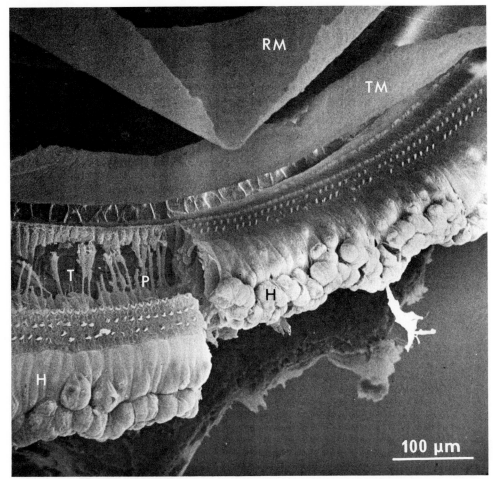

FIGURE 33-16 Scanning micrograph of the organ of Corti. RM, Reissner's membrane; TM, tectorial membrane; H, Hensen cells; P, outer pillar cells; T, tunnel of Corti.

facing away from the modiolus toward the stria vascularis. The cuticular plate is near the stria vascularis. Here is a centriole which sits with its axis perpendicular to the cell membrane and with its upper end close to the membrane (Figs. 33-17 and 33-20). Consequently, the hair cells in the organ of Corti are morphologically polarized like the vestibular hair cells and with similar functional implications. At their base the outer hair cells are innervated by a few afferent nerve endings and several large efferent nerve endings containing abundant vesicles.

The inner hair cells have a roundish cell body (Fig. 33-17), their sensory hairs are lined up in straight rows (Fig. 33-18), and their centriole also faces the stria vascularis. They are innervated by several afferent and a few efferent terminals. The inner hair cells are totally enclosed by supporting cells called *inner phalangeal cells* and the outer hair cells are held by supporting *outer phalangeal cells*. These cells extend as a slender curved process toward the surface of the organ of Corti (Figs. 33-21 and 33-22). At the surface they form a rhomboid plate which interlocks with its neighbors to form the *reticular membrane* that holds the apical ends of the hair cells. Outwardly the phalangeal cells are succeeded by tall *Hensen's cells*. Hensen's cells then pass into a layer of cuboidal *cells of Claudius*, which terminate in the external sulcus just under the spiral prominence.

Lying above the organ of Corti is a gelatinous

tectorial membrane whose lower surface rests on the tips of the tallest row of stereocilia in each hair bundle (Figs. 33-15 and 33-22). It is attached to the limbus spiralis which contains the *interdental cells* that secrete the substance of the membrane.

NERVE SUPPLY

The VIIIth cranial (auditory) nerve supplies the sensory areas of the membranous labyrinth. It divides into a superior posterior part, the *vestibular nerve,* and an inferior anterior part, the *cochlear nerve.*

The vestibular nerve has a superior portion which supplies the macula of the utricle and the cristae of the anterior vertical and the horizontal canals, and an inferior portion which supplies the macula of the saccule and the cristae of the posterior semicircular canals. The ganglion of the vestibular nerve, called the *vestibular ganglion,* or *Scarpa's ganglion,* lies in the internal auditory canal. There is also a small branch from the inferior portion of the vestibular nerve that

joins the cochlear nerve and is called the *nerve of Oort.* Scarpa's ganglion cells are bipolar. The axons of the ganglion cells enter the medulla and end in the vestibular nuclei of the medulla in the region of the fourth ventricle. The vestibular nuclei have connections with the cerebellum and the third, fourth, and sixth eye nuclei, through the posterior longitudinal bundle. They then send nerves down the spinal cord through the vestibular spinal tracts.

The cochlear nerve enters the cochlea through the modiolus, and its ganglion (the *spiral ganglion*) lies in the lamina spiralis ossea. The sensory neurons are bipolar. The nerve fibers go to the hair cell through canals in the lamina spiralis ossea and enter the organ of Corti through small openings called the *foramina*

FIGURE 33-17 Inner (A) and outer (B) hair cells. C, centriole; IP, inner pillar cell; Eff.NE, efferent nerve ending; Aff.NE, afferent nerve ending; H, sensory hairs; M, mitochondria; Nu, nucleus. (Courtesy of Wersäll, Flock, and Lundquist. Reproduced by permission of Cold Spring Harbor Laboratories.)

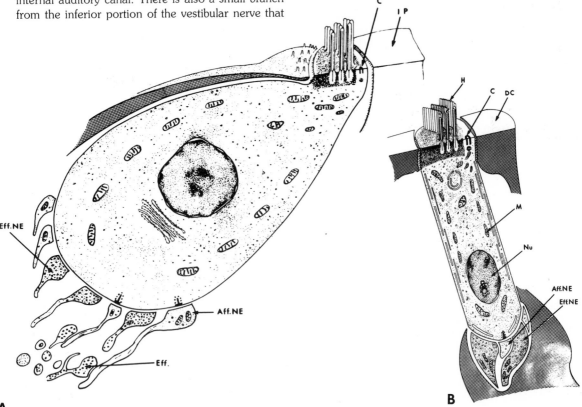

A

B

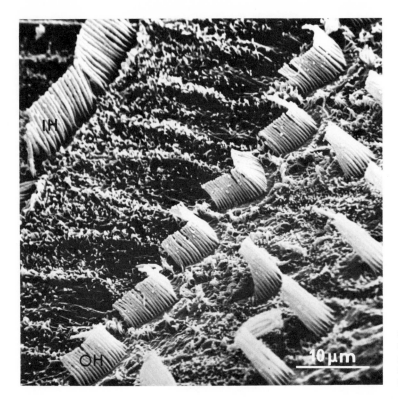

FIGURE 33-18 Sensory hair bundles of inner (IH) and outer (OH) hair cells project from the surface of the organ of Corti. Supporting cells of the reticular lamina have microvilli.

FIGURE 33-19 Sensory hair bundle of an outer hair cell seen from the modiolus side. Human. (Courtesy of Lundquist, Flock, and Wersäll. Reprinted with permission from Urban & Schwarzenberg, Vienna.)

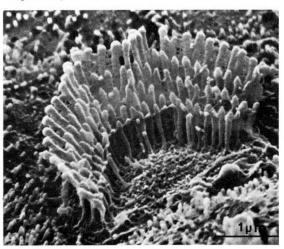

nervosa. When the nerve fibers leave the foramina nervosa, they lose their myelin sheaths.

The pattern of innervation is very complex and is not yet fully understood. It seems that several afferent neurons innervate each inner hair cell, to which they take a direct course (Fig. 33-23). Other fibers cross the tunnel of Corti, turn toward the base of the cochlea, and run as outer spiral fibers to innervate several outer hair cells.

The cochlear nerve enters the medulla and terminates in the cochlear nuclei. From the cochlear nuclei there are connections with other nuclei; the main portion of the cochlear nuclei fibers goes to the medial geniculate of the thalamus and then radiates to the auditory centers of the brain, which lie in the temporal lobe.

The organ of Corti also receives an efferent innervation, as does the vestibular apparatus (Fig. 33-24). These fibers, the olivocochlear bundle, have their cells bodies in the superior olivary nucleus. Fibers from the contralateral side cross the midline of the medulla at the bottom of the fourth ventricle. The efferent fibers leave the medulla with the vestibular nerve and then pass over to the cochlear nerve in

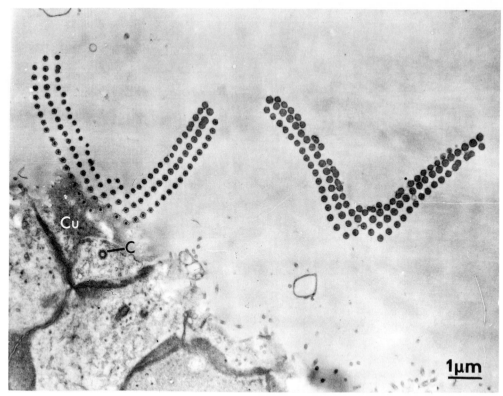

1μm

FIGURE 33-21 Phalangeal cells have slender twisted processes which reach the surface of the organ of Corti where their heads form the reticular lamina. (Courtesy of Wersäll, Flock, and Lundquist. Reproduced with permission from Killisch-Horn Verlag.)

FIGURE 33-20 Section through the sensory hairs of one outer hair cell and through part of the cuticular plate (Cu) and the centriole (C) of its neighbor. (Courtesy of Flock, Kimura, Lundquist, and Wersäll. Reproduced by permission of American Institute of Physics, New York.)

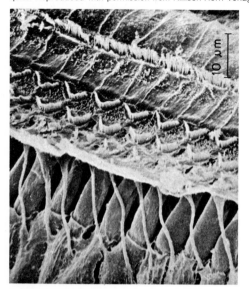

10 μm

Oort's anastomosis. Within the cochlea they travel along a spiral course in the spiral ganglion. Efferent fibers pass the tunnel of Corti to innervate several outer hair cells. Inner hair cells are not as well supplied with efferents.

Sympathetic fibers innervate the blood vessels of the inner ear and also form a plexus of fibers independent of blood vessels. These free fibers have terminals in the vestibular ganglion and in the peripheral vestibular nerve branches. Terminals are seen also in the spiral ganglion and are conspicuous at the point of demyelinization of cochlear nerve fibers in the foramina nervosa of the lamina spiralis ossea. The sympathetic fibers originate in the superior cervical ganglion and reach the inner ear via arteries and via the plexus tympanicus. Their function is as yet unknown.

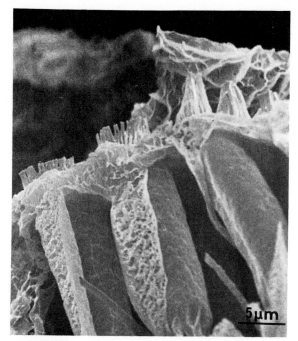

FIGURE 33-22 Tectorial membrane is in contact with the sensory hair bundles. The phalangeal processes are seen. (Courtesy of Wersäll, Flock, and Lundquist. Reproduced with permission from Killisch-Horn Verlag.)

ENDOLYMPHATIC SAC

Utriculus and sacculus are joined by a short duct, the *ductus utriculo saccularis* (Fig. 33-3), from which springs the *ductus endolymphaticus,* which terminates as the endolymphatic sac under the dura. The epithelium outlining the endolymphatic sac is specialized for absorption. The sac often contains cellular debris, and active phagocytosis has been demonstrated.

VESSELS OF THE LABYRINTH

The internal auditory artery is a branch of the basilar artery. It arises along with branches which are distributed to the underside of the cerebellum and the neighboring cerebral nerves, and it passes through the internal acoustic meatus to the ear. It divides into vestibular and cochlear branches. The *vestibular artery* supplies the vestibular nerve and the upper lateral portion of the sacculus, utriculus, and semicircular ducts. The *cochlear artery* sends a vestibulocochlear branch to the lower and medial portion of the sacculus, utriculus, and ducts. This branch also supplies the first third of the first turn of the cochlear. The capillaries formed by the vestibular branches are generally wide-meshed, but near the maculae and cristae the meshes are narrower. The terminal portion of the cochlear artery enters the modiolus and forms three or four spirally ascending branches which divide into about 30 radial branches distributed to three sets of capillaries—to the spiral ganglion, to the lamina spiralis, and to the outer walls of the scalae and the stria vascularis of the cochlear duct.

The veins of the labyrinth form the following three groups.

1. The *vena aquaeductus vestibuli,* which receives blood from the semicircular ducts and a part of the utriculus. It passes toward the brain in a bony canal along with the ductus endolymphaticus and empties into the superior petrosal sinus.

2. The *vena aquaeductus cochleae,* which receives blood from parts of the utriculus, sacculus, and cochlea. It passes through a bony canal to the internal jugular vein. It arises from small vessels, including the vas prominens and the vas spirale. Branches derived from these veins pass toward the modiolus. There are no vessels in Reissner's membrane of the adult, and the vessels in the wall of the scala tympani are arranged so that only veins occur in the part toward the membranous spiral lamina. Thus the latter is not affected by arterial pulsation. Within the modiolus the veins unite in an inferior spiral vein, which receives blood from the basal and a part of a second turn of the cochlea, and a superior spiral vein, which proceeds from the apical portion. These two spiral veins unite with vestibular branches to form the vena aquaeductus cochleae.

3. The *internal auditory vein,* which arises within the modiolus from the veins of the spiral lamina. These anastomose with the spiral veins. It receives branches also from the acoustic nerve and from the bones and empties into the *vena spiralis anterior.*

Lymphatic spaces within the internal ear are represented by the perilymph spaces, which communicate through the aquaeductus cochleae with the arachnoid space. The connecting structure, or *ductus perilymphaticus,* is described as a lymphatic vessel.

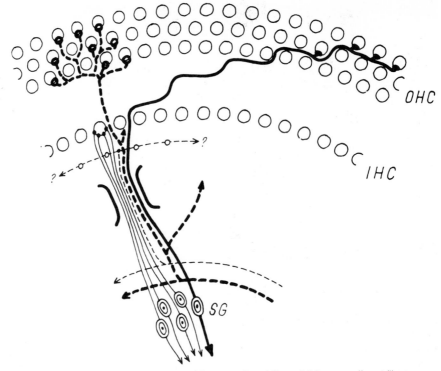

FIGURE 33-23 Innervation pattern of the organ of Corti in the cat. Interrupted lines are afferent fibers; full lines are efferent fibers. OHC, outer hair cells; IHC, inner hair cells; SG, spiral ganglion. (Courtesy of Spoendin. Reproduced with permission from Karger.)

FIGURE 33-24 Efferent nerve supply to the inner ear. (Modified by Iurato from Rossi and Cortesina. Reproduced with permission from Pergamon Press.)

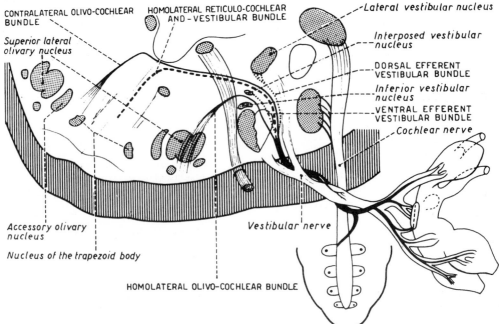

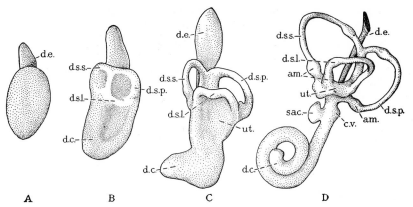

FIGURE 33-25 Lateral or external surfaces of models of the membranous portion of the left internal ear from human embryos. Different enlargements. A. From an embryo of 6.9 mm. B. 10.2 mm. C. 13.5 mm. D. 22 mm. am, ampulla; cv, cecum vestibulare of dc, cochlear duct; de, endolymphatic duct; dsl, dsp, and dss, horizontal, posterior vertical, and anterior vertical semicircular ducts, sac, sacculus; ut, utriculus. (His, Jr.)

EMBRYOLOGIC DEVELOPMENT

The sense organs are derivatives of the ectoderm. The internal ear first appears as a bilateral local thickening of ectoderm opposite that part of the medullary tube which is destined to become the pons. The thickened areas invaginate, as shown in Fig. 33-25, and the pockets thus formed separate from the ectoderm and develop into auditory vesicles (*otocysts*). The point where they become detached from the epidermis is marked by an elevation on the medial side of the vesicle, which elongates and produces the endolymphatic duct.

In two places the medial and lateral walls of the auditory vesicle approach one another and fuse, and the epithelial plates thus formed become thin and are absorbed, leaving two loops, each attached at both ends to the parent vesicle. These are the vertical semicircular canals. Similarly, a third canal forms soon afterward. The lower portion of the otocyst elongates and coils to make $2\frac{1}{2}$ revolutions, forming the ductus cochlearis. A constriction separates the sacculus from the utricle and the cochlea. The surrounding mesenchyme becomes cartilage and then bone.

The middle ear develops from the first pharyngeal pouch and the external ear from the first branchial cleft. At an early stage the ectoderm of the branchial cleft and the entoderm of the pharyngeal pouch meet and fuse to form the tympanic membrane.

REFERENCES

BAST, T. H., and B. J. ANSON: "The Temporal Bone and the Ear," Charles C Thomas, Publisher, Springfield, 1949.

BÉKÉSY, G. VON: "Experiments in Hearing," McGraw-Hill Book Company, New York, 1960.

DE BURLET, H. M.: Vergleichende Anatomie des stato-akustischen Organs, in Bolk et al. (eds.), "Handbüch der Vergleichenden Anatomie der Wirbelthiere," vol. 2, p. 1293, Urban & Schwarzenberg, Vienna, 1934.

DAVIS, H.: A Model for Transducer Action in the Cochlea, *Cold Spring Harbor Symp. Quant. Biol.,* **30:**181 (1965).

ENGSTRÖM, H., H. ADES, and A. ANDERSON: "Structural Pattern of the Organ of Corti," Almqvist and Wiksell, Stockholm, 1966.

FLOCK, Å.: Sensory Transduction in Hair Cells, in W. R. Loewenstein (ed.), "Handbook of Sensory Physiology," vol. 1, "Principles of Receptor Physiology," p. 396, Springer-Verlag OHG, Berlin, 1971.

FLOCK, Å., KIMURA, R., P.-G. LUNDQUIST, and J. WERSÄLL: Morphological Basis of Directional Sensitivity of the Outer Hair Cells in the Organ of Corti, *J. Acoust. Soc. Am.,* **34:**1351 (1962).

HELD, H.: Die Cochlea der Säuger und der Vögel, Entwicklung und ihr Bau, "Handbüch der normale und pathologische Physiologie," vol. 11, p. 467, Julius Springer, Berlin, 1926.

IURATO, S. (ed.): "Submicroscopic Structure of the Inner Ear," Pergamon Press, New York, 1967.

KIMURA, R. S., H. F. SCHUKNECHT, and I. SUNDO: Fine Morphology of the Sensory Cells in the Organ of Corti in Man, *Acta Otolaryngol. (Stockh.),* **58:**390 (1965).

KOLMER, W.: Gehörorgan, in W. von Möllendorff and W. Bargmann (eds.), "Handbüch der mikroskopischen Anatomie des Menschen," vol. 3, p. 250, Springer-Verlag OHG, Berlin, 1927.

LINDEMAN, H.: Studies on the Morphology of the Sensory Regions of the Vestibular Apparatus, *Adv. Anat. Embryol. Cell Biol.,* **42:**1 (1969).

LORENTE DE NÓ, R.: Anatomy of the Eighth Nerve, *Laryngoscope,* **43:**3 (1933).

LUNDQUIST, P-G.: The Endolymphatic Duct and Sac in the Guinea Pig, *Acta Otolaryngol. (Stockh.),* **201** (Suppl.): 1 (1965).

LUNDQUIST, P-G., Å. FLOCK, and J. WERSALL: Rasten-Elektronen-mikroskopie des Menschlichen Labyrinths. Österreich, Monatsschr. HŃO, **105:**285 (1971).

POLYAK, S., G. MCHUGH, and D. K. JUDD, JR.: "The Human Ear in Anatomical Transparencies," T. H. McKenna, Inc., New York, 1946.

RAMÓN Y CAJAL, S.: Histologie du systéme nerveux de l'homme et des vertébrés, 2 vols., A. Maloine, Paris, 1909–1911.

RASMUSSEN, G., and W. F. WINDLE (eds.): "Neural Mechanisms of the Auditory and Vestibular Systems," Charles C Thomas, Publisher, Springfield, Ill., 1961.

SPOENDLIN, H.: The Organization of the Cochlear Receptor, in "Advances in Oto-Rhino-Laryngology," vol. 13, S. Karger, Basel, Switzerland, 1966.

TAKASAKA, T., and C. SMITH: The Structure and Innervation of the Pigeons Basilar Papilla, *J. Ultrastruct. Res.,* **35:**20 (1971).

WERNER, U. F.: "Das Gehörorgan der Wirbeltiere und des Menschen," Thieme Verlag, Leipzig, Georg 1960.

WERSÄLL, J.: Studies on the Structure and Innervation of the Sensory Epithelium of the Cristae Ampullares in the Guinea Pig, *Acta Otolaryngol. (Stockh.),* **126** (Suppl.): (1956).

WERSÄLL, J., Å. FLOCK, and P-G. LUNDQUIST: The Vestibular Sensory Areas and the Organ of Corti. A Scanning Electron Microscopic Study, *Z. Hörgeräte Akustik,* **9:**56 (1970).

WERSÄLL, J., Å. FLOCK, and P-G. LUNDQUIST: Structural Basis for Directional Sensitivity in Cochlear and Vestibular Sensory Receptors, *Cold Spring Harbor Symp. Quant. Biol.,* **30:**133 (1965).

Index